Pediatric ICD-10-CM 2022

A Manual for Provider-Based Coding

7th Edition

American Academy of Pediatrics

Cindy Hughes, CPC, CFPC, Consulting Editor

Becky Dolan, MPH, CPC, CPEDC, Staff Editor

American Academy of Pediatrics

DEDICATED TO THE HEALTH OF ALL CHILDREN®

American Academy of Pediatrics Publishing Staff

Mary Lou White, *Chief Product and Services Officer/SVP, Membership, Marketing, and Publishing*

Mark Grimes, *Vice President, Publishing*

Mary Kelly, *Senior Editor, Professional/Clinical Publishing*

Laura Underhile, *Editor, Professional/Clinical Publishing*

Jason Crase, *Senior Manager, Production and Editorial Services*

Leesa Levin-Doroba, *Production Manager, Practice Management*

Peg Mulcahy, *Manager, Art Direction and Production*

Maryjo Reynolds, *Marketing Manager, Practice Publications*

Published by the American Academy of Pediatrics
345 Park Blvd
Itasca, IL 60143
Telephone: 630/626-6000
Facsimile: 847/434-8000
www.aap.org

The American Academy of Pediatrics is an organization of 67,000 primary care pediatricians, pediatric medical subspecialists, and pediatric surgical specialists dedicated to the health, safety, and well-being of all infants, children, adolescents, and young adults.

While every effort has been made to ensure the accuracy of this publication, the American Academy of Pediatrics (AAP) does not guarantee that it is accurate, complete, or without error.

Any websites, brand names, products, or manufacturers are mentioned for informational and identification purposes only and do not imply an endorsement by the American Academy of Pediatrics (AAP). The AAP is not responsible for the content of external resources. Information was current at the time of publication.

This publication has been developed by the American Academy of Pediatrics. The contributors are expert authorities in the field of pediatrics. No commercial involvement of any kind has been solicited or accepted in development of the content of this publication.

Please visit www.aap.org/coding for an up-to-date list of any applicable errata for this publication.

Special discounts are available for bulk purchases of this publication. Email Special Sales at nationalaccounts@aap.org for more information.

Printed in the United States of America.

11-114F

1 2 3 4 5 6 7 8 9 10

MA1030

ISBN: 978-1-61002-552-2
eBook: 978-1-61002-553-9
ISSN: 2475-9708

Disclaimer

Every effort has been made to include all pediatric-relevant *International Classification of Diseases, 10th Revision, Clinical Modification* (*ICD-10-CM*) codes and their respective guidelines. It is the responsibility of the reader to use this manual as a companion to the official *ICD-10-CM* publication. Do not report new or revised *ICD-10-CM* codes until their published implementation date, at time of publication set for October 1, 2021. Further, it is the reader's responsibility to access the American Academy of Pediatrics (AAP) Coding at the AAP website (www.aap.org/coding) routinely to find any corrections due to errata in the published version.

Equity, Diversity, and Inclusion Statement

The American Academy of Pediatrics is committed to principles of equity, diversity, and inclusion in its publishing program. Editorial boards, author selections, and author transitions (publication succession plans) are designed to include diverse voices that reflect society as a whole. Editor and author teams are encouraged to actively seek out diverse authors and reviewers at all stages of the editorial process. Publishing staff are committed to promoting equity, diversity, and inclusion in all aspects of publication writing, review, and production. Likewise, it is the intent of the authors and publishing team to use visual representations of the diverse range of patients seen in medical settings where children are evaluated and treated.

Contents

Tabular List

Foreword

The American Academy of Pediatrics (AAP) is pleased to publish this seventh edition of *Pediatric ICD-10-CM: A Manual for Provider-Based Coding,* a pediatric version of the *International Classification of Diseases, 10th Revision, Clinical Modification* (*ICD-10-CM*) manual. The AAP believes it is vital to publish an *ICD-10-CM* manual that is more manageable for pediatric providers. The expansive nature of the code set from *International Classification of Diseases, Ninth Revision, Clinical Modification* to *ICD-10-CM* overwhelmed many physicians, providers, and coders, so we condensed the code set by only providing pediatric-relevant diagnoses and their corresponding codes. However, as we move forward, we want members to have access to more codes and those that are less common in pediatrics but still need to be included. We reduced the guidelines so that only those applicable to the physician or provider are included, while those only relevant to facilities are removed. When needed, those codes can be located in the larger *ICD-10-CM* manual. Lastly, guidelines that exist for topic-specific chapters or specific codes can now be found in their respective tabular chapter or right where the specific code is listed. This will aid the user in identifying any chapter- or code-specific guidelines where they are needed most. This should assist in reducing any coding errors caused by reporting services that go against the guidelines that were once solely kept in the front of the manual, away from applicable codes. In addition, tips are included throughout to aid in your coding. These are unique to this manual.

The AAP is committed to the clinical modification of the *ICD* code set and, for the past several years, has sent an AAP liaison to the *ICD* Coordination and Maintenance Committee Meeting. We are especially grateful to Edward A. Liechty, MD, FAAP, and Jeffrey F. Linzer Sr, MD, FAAP, our appointed liaisons. The *ICD* Coordination and Maintenance Meeting is the semiannual meeting where all new *ICD* codes are presented, as well as revisions to the tabular list, index, and guidelines. Having dedicated expert liaisons aids in presenting pediatric and perinatal issues at the meeting. The AAP is also very pleased to continue its work with the *ICD* Editorial Advisory Board for *Coding Clinic for ICD-10-CM and ICD-10-PCS. Coding Clinic* is responsible for publishing *ICD* coding guidance and clarifications to supplement the *ICD-10-CM* manual. Dr Linzer sits on the Editorial Advisory Board, and Dr Liechty is our alternate. They sit on the board to represent pediatric issues, and both are experts on all *ICD-10-CM* matters.

The AAP will continue to support its members on issues regarding coding, and the AAP Health Care Financing Strategy staff at the AAP headquarters stands ready to assist with problem areas not adequately covered in this manual. The AAP Coding Hotline can be accessed at https://form.jotform.com/Subspecialty/aapcodinghotline.

Acknowledgments

Pediatric ICD-10-CM: A Manual for Provider-Based Coding is the product of the efforts of many dedicated individuals. First and foremost, we must thank Cindy Hughes, CPC, CFPC, consulting editor, for her professional input and particularly for her ongoing work to make this manual more user friendly.

We would also like to thank members of the American Academy of Pediatrics (AAP) Committee on Coding and Nomenclature, past and present, and the AAP Coding Publications Editorial Advisory Board. They support all coding efforts here at the AAP. These members contribute extensive time, reviewing and editing various coding content for the AAP.

We would also like to extend a very special thank-you to members of various subspecialty sections of the AAP who contributed their expertise and knowledge to the development of the original manual.

Lastly, we would like to acknowledge the tireless work of Jeffrey F. Linzer Sr, MD, FAAP, and Edward A. Liechty, MD, FAAP. Both Dr Liechty and Dr Linzer are advocates for pediatrics and neonatology and ensure that our issues are heard. They advocate for all pediatric patients in helping get codes established for conditions that need to be tracked for purposes of research and quality. They both keep the AAP and pediatric issues at the forefront of diagnostic coding, and we are very grateful for their time and expertise!

Step 1. Locate the condition in the Alphabetic Index of diagnostic terms (ie, the front section). For example, for a *left ankle fracture of the medial malleolus,* go to **Fracture**
 ↓
 ankle
 ↓
 medial malleolus ──────────────
 The dash at **S82.5-** indicates further characters are needed.
	Fracture (abduction) (adduction) (separation) T14.8
	 ∿∿∿∿∿∿∿∿∿∿∿∿
	 • ankle S82.89-¶
	   – bimalleolar (displaced) S82.84-¶
	     ■ nondisplaced S82.84-¶
	   – lateral malleolus only (displaced) S82.6-¶
	     ■ nondisplaced S82.6-¶
	   – medial malleolus (displaced) S82.5-¶
	     ■ associated with Maisonneuve's fracture—*see* Fracture, Maisonneuve's¶
	     ■ nondisplaced S82.5-¶
	   – talus—*see* Fracture¶
	   – trimalleolar (displaced) S82.85-¶
	     ■ nondisplaced S82.85-¶

Step 2. Next, find the code in the Tabular List (**never code from the index**). Check the Tabular List at the block, chapter, category, and code levels to see if the code has any special considerations. Read any code instructions, if applicable.	**S82** **FRACTURE OF LOWER LEG, INCLUDING ANKLE** Please see full *ICD-10-CM* manual for seventh characters applicable to open fracture types IIIA, IIIB, or IIIC. **Note:** A fracture not indicated as displaced or nondisplaced should be coded to displaced A fracture not indicated as open or closed should be coded to closed The open fracture designations are based on the Gustilo open fracture classification ***Includes:*** fracture of malleolus ***Excludes1:*** traumatic amputation of lower leg (S88.-) ***Excludes2:*** fracture of foot, except ankle (S92.-) periprosthetic fracture around internal prosthetic implant of knee joint (M97.0-)
Step 3. The **5th** indicates that additional code characters are required for this diagnosis. Always code to the highest degree of specificity, including laterality.	**S82.5 Fracture of medial malleolus** ***Excludes1:*** pilon fracture of distal tibia (S82.87-) Salter-Harris type III of lower end of tibia (S89.13-) Salter-Harris type IV of lower end of tibia (S89.14-) **S82.51X Displaced fracture of medial malleolus of right tibia** **S82.52X Displaced fracture of medial malleolus of left tibia** **S82.54X Nondisplaced fracture of medial malleolus of right tibia**
Step 4. If the condition warrants further specificity, an additional character note will be added. For example, an injury code may require a seventh character. Refer to a box on that page or nearby to provide you with that additional information.	7th characters for category S82 except S82.16-, S82.31-, & S81.82 A—initial encounter for closed fracture B—initial encounter for open fracture type I or II C—initial encounter for open fracture NOS D—subsequent encounter for closed fracture with routine healing E—subsequent encounter for open fracture type I or II with routine healing G—subsequent encounter for closed fracture with delayed healing H—subsequent encounter for open fracture type I or II with delayed healing K—subsequent encounter for closed fracture with nonunion M—subsequent encounter for open fracture type I or II with nonunion P—subsequent encounter for closed fracture with malunion Q—subsequent encounter for open fracture type I or II with malunion S—sequela
Step 5. If more than one condition needs to be coded, check all notes, including *Excludes, Code also,* and *Code first.*	

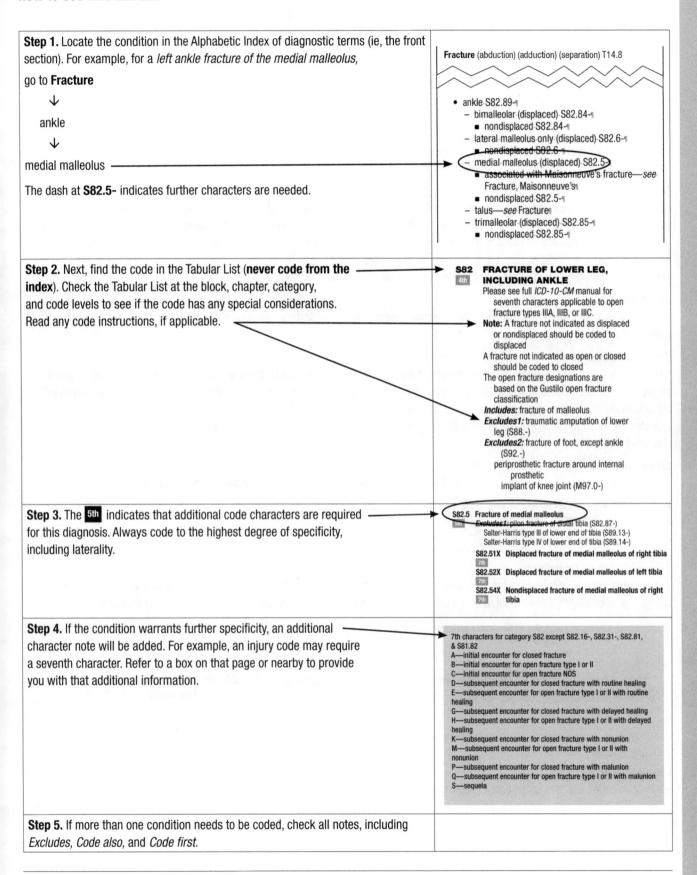

While attempting to stay true to the complete *International Classification of Diseases, 10th Revision, Clinical Modification* (*ICD-10-CM*) manual, *Pediatric ICD-10-CM: A Manual for Provider-Based Coding* is meant specifically for pediatrics and only includes those conditions more commonly seen in pediatrics. We have attempted to remove all adult-only conditions, as well as those conditions not typically found in the United States. Because *ICD* classification is used worldwide, many conditions listed in the official manual are not found in this part of the world.

Some codes are included under *Excludes* notes in the Tabular List for reference purposes only and to be consistent with the coding guidance. However, not every code included under *Excludes* will be found in the Tabular List if the condition is not specific to US pediatric health care. In addition, some codes that can be found in the Alphabetic Index might not also appear in the Tabular List. Again, these conditions are not commonly found in US pediatric health care, and the codes are included in the Alphabetic Index for reference purposes only. These conditions can be found in the larger Tabular List on the National Center for Health Statistics website (https://www.cdc.gov/nchs/icd/icd10cm.htm).

Guidelines

Guidelines relevant to all pediatric codes are still included. Note that some chapter-specific guidelines will appear at the beginning of the related chapter when they are overarching to most of that chapter. However, chapter-specific guidelines that are relevant only at specific category or code levels will be found at those category or code levels. The beginning of each chapter will reference the category(ies) or code(s) where the guidelines can be found. Guidelines that are **bold** have been revised or added for 2022. Guideline updates for the current year in the front matter and chapter-specific guidelines are printed in **bold.**

Abbreviations

We use our own abbreviations throughout that may not appear in *ICD-10-CM;* however, all abbreviations are defined on the inside front cover for easy access as you navigate through the manual.

Unspecified Laterality

While unspecified codes can still be found throughout and in certain instances will be the most appropriate code, we have removed nearly every code that uses unspecified laterality. We feel it is important that laterality is documented in nearly all conditions. You will see a footnote in those chapters where we have specifically left out laterality in nearly all conditions. If you need to report unspecified laterality for a condition and it is not listed in the chapter, refer to the full *ICD-10-CM* manual. Those codes will typically have a final character of 0 (zero) or 9.

Three-Character Codes

Three-character codes still exist in *ICD-10-CM*. Those will be noted specifically throughout the chapters as well.

E15 NONDIABETIC HYPOGLYCEMIC COMA
   Includes: drug-induced insulin coma in nondiabetic
     hyperinsulinism with hypoglycemic coma
     hypoglycemic coma NOS

Abbreviated Code Descriptors

To help keep the size of the manual manageable, some codes are only written out fully at the category or subcategory level. The category or subcategory will be notated with a semicolon (;) and the code will begin with a lowercase letter. For example,

    A37.0 Whooping cough due to Bordetella pertussis;
        A37.00 without pneumonia
        A37.01 with pneumonia

At the subcategory level (**A37.0**) you see the semicolon (;), and at the code levels (**A37.00** and **A37.01**), the codes begin with a lowercase letter. Therefore, code **A37.00** reads, "Whooping cough due to Bordetella pertussis without pneumonia."

Symbols

The following symbols are used throughout the text:

• Identifies new codes

▲ Identifies revised codes

◨ Identifies codes linked to social determinants of health

Reminder: New guidelines have been bolded.

The Centers for Medicare and Medicaid Services (CMS) and the National Center for Health Statistics (NCHS), two departments within the U.S. federal government's Department of Health and Human Services (DHHS), provide the following guidelines for coding and reporting by using the International Classification of Diseases, 10th Revision, Clinical Modification (*ICD-10-CM*). These guidelines should be used as a companion document to the official version of the *ICD-10-CM* as published on the NCHS website. The *ICD-10-CM* is a morbidity classification published by the United States for classifying diagnoses and reason for visits in all health care settings. The *ICD-10-CM* is based on the ICD-10, the statistical classification of disease published by the World Health Organization (WHO).

These guidelines have been approved by the four organizations that make up the Cooperating Parties for the *ICD-10-CM*: the American Hospital Association (AHA), the American Health Information Management Association (AHIMA), CMS, and NCHS.

These guidelines are a set of rules that have been developed to accompany and complement the official conventions and instructions provided within the *ICD-10-CM* itself. The instructions and conventions of the classification take precedence over guidelines. These guidelines are based on the coding and sequencing instructions in the Tabular List and Alphabetic Index of *ICD-10-CM*, but they provide additional instruction. Adherence to these guidelines when assigning *ICD-10-CM* diagnosis codes is required under the Health Insurance Portability and Accountability Act (HIPAA). The diagnosis codes (Tabular List and Alphabetic Index) have been adopted under HIPAA for all healthcare settings. A joint effort between the healthcare provider and the coder is essential to achieve complete and accurate documentation, code assignment, and reporting of diagnoses and procedures. These guidelines have been developed to assist both the healthcare provider and the coder in identifying those diagnoses that are to be reported. The importance of consistent, complete documentation in the medical record cannot be overemphasized. Without such documentation, accurate coding cannot be achieved. The entire record should be reviewed to determine the specific reason for the encounter and the conditions treated.

The term encounter is used for all settings, including hospital admissions. In the context of these guidelines, the term provider is used throughout the guidelines to mean physician or any qualified health care practitioner who is legally accountable for establishing the patient's diagnosis. Only this set of guidelines, approved by the Cooperating Parties, is official.

The guidelines are organized into sections. Section I includes the structure and conventions of the classification and general guidelines that apply to the entire classification and chapter-specific guidelines that correspond to the chapters as they are arranged in the classification. Section II includes guidelines for selection of principal diagnosis for non-outpatient settings. Section III includes guidelines for reporting additional diagnoses in non-outpatient settings. Section IV is for outpatient coding and reporting. It is necessary to review all sections of the guidelines to fully understand all the rules and instructions needed to code properly.

Note: Updates have been bolded.

Section I. Conventions, general coding guidelines, and chapter-specific guidelines

The conventions, general guidelines, and chapter-specific guidelines are applicable to all health care settings unless otherwise indicated. The conventions and instructions of the classification take precedence over guidelines.

A. Conventions for the *ICD-10-CM*

The conventions for the *ICD-10-CM* are the general rules for use of the classification independent of the guidelines. These conventions are incorporated within the Alphabetic Index and Tabular List of the *ICD-10-CM* as instructional notes.

1. The Alphabetic Index and Tabular List

The *ICD-10-CM* is divided into the Alphabetic Index, an alphabetical list of terms and their corresponding code, and the Tabular List, a structured list of codes divided into chapters based on body system or condition. The Alphabetic Index consists of the following parts: the Index of Diseases and Injury, the Index of External Causes of Injury, the Table of Neoplasms, and the Table of Drugs and Chemicals.

> *See Section I.C2. General guidelines*
> *See Section I.C.19. Adverse effects, poisoning, underdosing and toxic effects*

2. Format and Structure

The *ICD-10-CM* Tabular List contains categories, subcategories, and codes. Characters for categories, subcategories, and codes may be either a letter or a number. All categories are 3 characters. A three-character category that has no further subdivision is equivalent to a code. Subcategories are either 4 or 5 characters. Codes may be 3, 4, 5, 6, or 7 characters. That is, each level of subdivision after a category is a subcategory. The final level of subdivision is a code. Codes that have applicable 7th characters are still referred to as codes, not subcategories. A code that has an applicable 7th character is considered invalid without the 7th character.

The *ICD-10-CM* uses an indented format for ease in reference.

3. Use of codes for reporting purposes

For reporting purposes, only codes are permissible, not categories or subcategories, and any applicable 7th character is required.

4. Placeholder character

The *ICD-10-CM* utilizes a placeholder character "X." The "X" is used as a placeholder at certain codes to allow for future expansion. An example of this is at the poisoning, adverse effect, and underdosing codes, categories T36-T50. Where a placeholder exists, the X must be used in order for the code to be considered a valid code.

5. **7th Characters**

Certain *ICD-10-CM* categories have applicable 7th characters. The applicable 7th character is required for all codes within the category, or as the notes in the Tabular List instruct. The 7th character must always be the 7th character in the data field. If a code that requires a 7th character is not 6 characters, a placeholder X must be used to fill in the empty characters.

6. **Abbreviations**

   a. **Alphabetic Index abbreviations**

   NEC "Not elsewhere classifiable"—This abbreviation in the Alphabetic Index represents "other specified." When a specific code is not available for a condition, the Alphabetic Index directs the coder to the "other specified" code in the Tabular List.

   NOS "Not otherwise specified"—This abbreviation is the equivalent of unspecified.

   b. **Tabular List abbreviations**

   NEC "Not elsewhere classifiable"—This abbreviation in the Tabular List represents "other specified." When a specific code is not available for a condition, the Tabular List includes an NEC entry under a code to identify the code as the "other specified" code.

   NOS "Not otherwise specified —This abbreviation is the equivalent of unspecified.

7. **Punctuation**

   [ ] Brackets are used in the Tabular List to enclose synonyms, alternative wording, or explanatory phrases. Brackets are used in the Alphabetic Index to identify manifestation codes.

   ( ) Parentheses are used in both the Alphabetic Index and Tabular List to enclose supplementary words that may be present or absent in the statement of a disease or procedure without affecting the code number to which it is assigned. The terms within the parentheses are referred to as *nonessential modifiers.* The nonessential modifiers in the Alphabetic Index to Diseases apply to subterms following a main term, except when a nonessential modifier and a subentry are mutually exclusive, in which case the subentry takes precedence. For example, in the *ICD-10-CM* Alphabetic Index under the main term *Enteritis,* "acute" is a nonessential modifier and "chronic" is a subentry. In this case, the nonessential modifier "acute" does not apply to the subentry "chronic."

   : Colons are used in the Tabular List after an incomplete term, which needs one or more of the modifiers following the colon to make it assignable to a given category.

8. **Use of "and"**

   Refer to Section I.A.14 (page XV). Use of the term "And"

9. **Other and Unspecified codes**

   a. **"Other" codes**

   Codes titled "other" or "other specified" are for use when the information in the medical record provides detail for which a specific code does not exist. Alphabetic Index entries with NEC in the line designate "other" codes in the Tabular List. These Alphabetic Index entries represent specific disease entities for which no specific code exists so the term is included within an "other" code.

   b. **"Unspecified" codes**

   Codes titled "unspecified" are for use when the information in the medical record is insufficient to assign a more specific code. For those categories for which an unspecified code is not provided, the "other specified" code may represent both other and unspecified.

   See Use of Sign/Symptom/Unspecified Codes, page XVII

10. **Includes Notes**

    This note appears immediately under a three-character code title to further define, or give examples of, the content of the category.

11. **Inclusion terms**

    List of terms is included under some codes. These terms are the conditions for which that code is to be used. The terms may be synonyms of the code title, or, in the case of "other specified" codes, the terms are a list of the various conditions assigned to that code. The inclusion terms are not necessarily exhaustive. Additional terms found only in the Alphabetic Index may also be assigned to a code.

12. **Excludes Notes**

    The *ICD-10-CM* has two types of excludes notes. Each type of note has a different definition for use, but they are all similar in that they indicate that codes excluded from each other are independent of each other.

    a. **Excludes1**

    A type 1 Excludes note is a pure excludes note. It means "NOT CODED HERE!" An Excludes1 note indicates that the code excluded should never be used at the same time as the code above the Excludes1 note. An Excludes1 is used when two conditions cannot occur together, such as a congenital form versus an acquired form of the same condition.

    b. **Excludes2**

    A type 2 Excludes note represents "Not included here." An Excludes2 note indicates that the condition excluded is not part of the condition represented by the code, but a patient may have both conditions at the same time. When an Excludes2 note appears under a code, it is acceptable to use both the code and the excluded code together, when appropriate.

13. **Etiology/manifestation convention ("code first," "use additional code," and "in diseases classified elsewhere" notes)**

Certain conditions have both an underlying etiology and multiple body system manifestations due to the underlying etiology. For such conditions, the *ICD-10-CM* has a coding convention that requires the underlying condition be sequenced first, followed by the manifestation. Wherever such a combination exists, there is a "use additional code" note at the etiology code and a "code first" note at the manifestation code. These instructional notes indicate the proper sequencing order of the codes, etiology followed by manifestation.

In most cases, the manifestation codes will have in the code title, "in diseases classified elsewhere." Codes with this title are a component of the etiology/manifestation convention. The code title indicates that it is a manifestation code. "In diseases classified elsewhere" codes are never permitted to be used as first-listed or principal diagnosis codes. They must be used in conjunction with an underlying condition code, and they must be listed following the underlying condition. See category F02, Dementia in other diseases classified elsewhere, for an example of this convention.

There are manifestation codes that do not have "in diseases classified elsewhere" in the title. For such codes, there is a "use additional code" note at the etiology code and a "code first" note at the manifestation code, and the rules for sequencing apply.

In addition to the notes in the Tabular List, these conditions also have a specific Alphabetic Index entry structure. In the Alphabetic Index, both conditions are listed together with the etiology code first, followed by the manifestation codes in brackets. The code in brackets is always to be sequenced second.

An example of the etiology/manifestation convention is dementia in Parkinson's disease. In the Alphabetic Index, code G20 is listed first, followed by code F02.80 or F02.81 in brackets. Code G20 represents the underlying etiology, Parkinson's disease, and must be sequenced first, whereas codes F02.80 and F02.81 represent the manifestation of dementia in diseases classified elsewhere, with or without behavioral disturbance.

"Code first" and "Use additional code" notes are also used as sequencing rules in the classification for certain codes that are not part of an etiology/manifestation combination.

See Section I.B.7. Multiple coding for a single condition.

14. **"And"**

The word "and" should be interpreted to mean either "and" or "or" when it appears in a title.

For example, cases of "tuberculosis of bones," "tuberculosis of joints," and "tuberculosis of bones and joints" are classified to subcategory A18.0, Tuberculosis of bones and joints.

15. **"With"**

The word "with" or "in" should be interpreted to mean "associated with" or "due to" when it appears in a code title, the Alphabetic Index (either under a main term or subterm), or an instructional note in the Tabular List. The classification presumes a causal relationship between the two conditions linked by these terms in the Alphabetic Index or Tabular List. These conditions should be coded as related even in the absence of provider documentation explicitly linking them, unless the documentation clearly states the conditions are unrelated or when another guideline exists that specifically requires a documented linkage between two conditions (e.g., sepsis guideline for "acute organ dysfunction that is not clearly associated with the sepsis"). For conditions not specifically linked by these relational terms in the classification or when a guideline requires that a linkage between two conditions be explicitly documented, provider documentation must link the conditions in order to code them as related.

The word "with" in the Alphabetic Index is sequenced immediately following the main term or subterm, not in alphabetical order.

16. **"See" and "See Also"**

The "see" instruction following a main term in the Alphabetic Index indicates that another term should be referenced. It is necessary to go to the main term referenced with the "see" note to locate the correct code.

A "see also" instruction following a main term in the Alphabetic Index instructs that there is another main term that may also be referenced that may provide additional Alphabetic Index entries that may be useful. It is not necessary to follow the "see also" note when the original main term provides the necessary code.

17. **"Code also note"**

A "code also" note instructs that two codes may be required to fully describe a condition, but this note does not provide sequencing direction. The sequencing depends on the circumstances of the encounter.

18. **Default codes**

A code listed next to a main term in the *ICD-10-CM* Alphabetic Index is referred to as a default code. The default code represents that condition that is most commonly associated with the main term, or is the unspecified code for the condition. If a condition is documented in a medical record (for example, appendicitis) without any additional information, such as acute or chronic, the default code should be assigned.

B. General Coding Guidelines

1. Locating a code in the *ICD-10-CM*

To select a code in the classification that corresponds to a diagnosis or reason for visit documented in a medical record, first locate the term in the Alphabetic Index, and then verify the code in the Tabular List. Read and be guided by instructional notations that appear in both the Alphabetic Index and the Tabular List.

It is essential to use both the Alphabetic Index and Tabular List when locating and assigning a code. The Alphabetic Index does not always provide the full code. Selection of the full code, including laterality and any applicable 7th character, can only be done in the Tabular List. A dash (-) at the end of an Alphabetic Index entry indicates that additional characters are required. Even if a dash is not included at the Alphabetic Index entry, it is necessary to refer to the Tabular List to verify that no 7th character is required.

2. Level of Detail in Coding

Diagnosis codes are to be used and reported at their highest number of characters available **and to the highest level of specificity documented in the medical record.**

ICD-10-CM diagnosis codes are composed of codes with 3, 4, 5, 6, or 7 characters. Codes with three characters are included in *ICD-10-CM* as the heading of a category of codes that may be further subdivided by the use of fourth and/or fifth characters and/or sixth characters, which provide greater detail.

A three-character code is to be used only if it is not further subdivided. A code is invalid if it has not been coded to the full number of characters required for that code, including the 7th character, if applicable.

3. Code or codes from A00.0 through T88.9, Z00–Z99.8

The appropriate code or codes from A00.0 through T88.9, Z00–Z99.8 **and U00–U85** must be used to identify diagnoses, symptoms, conditions, problems, complaints, or other reason(s) for the encounter/visit.

4. Signs and symptoms

Codes that describe symptoms and signs, as opposed to diagnoses, are acceptable for reporting purposes when a related definitive diagnosis has not been established (confirmed) by the provider. Chapter 18 of *ICD-10-CM*, Symptoms, Signs, and Abnormal Clinical and Laboratory Findings, Not Elsewhere Classified (codes R00.0 – R99), contains many but not all codes for symptoms.

See Use of Sign/Symptom/Unspecified Codes, page XVII

5. Conditions that are an integral part of a disease process

Signs and symptoms that are associated routinely with a disease process should not be assigned as additional codes, unless otherwise instructed by the classification.

6. Conditions that are not an integral part of a disease process

Additional signs and symptoms that may not be associated routinely with a disease process should be coded when present.

7. Multiple coding for a single condition

In addition to the etiology/manifestation convention that requires two codes to fully describe a single condition that affects multiple body systems, there are other single conditions that also require more than one code. "Use additional code" notes are found in the Tabular List at codes that are not part of an etiology/manifestation pair where a secondary code is useful to fully describe a condition. The sequencing rule is the same as the etiology/manifestation pair; "use additional code" indicates that a secondary code should be added, if known.

For example, for bacterial infections that are not included in Chapter 1, a secondary code from category B95, Streptococcus, Staphylococcus, and Enterococcus, as the cause of diseases classified elsewhere, or B96, Other bacterial agents as the cause of diseases classified elsewhere, may be required to identify the bacterial organism causing the infection. A "use additional code" note will normally be found at the infectious disease code, indicating a need for the organism code to be added as a secondary code.

"Code first" notes are also under certain codes that are not specifically manifestation codes but may be due to an underlying cause. When there is a "code first" note and an underlying condition is present, the underlying condition should be sequenced first, if known.

"Code, if applicable, any causal condition first" notes indicate that this code may be assigned as a principal diagnosis when the causal condition is unknown or not applicable. If a causal condition is known, then the code for that condition should be sequenced as the principal or first-listed diagnosis.

Multiple codes may be needed for sequela, complication codes, and obstetric codes to more fully describe a condition. See the specific guidelines for these conditions for further instruction.

8. **Acute and Chronic Conditions**

If the same condition is described as both acute (subacute) and chronic, and separate subentries exist in the Alphabetic Index at the same indentation level, code both and sequence the acute (subacute) code first.

9. **Combination Code**

A combination code is a single code used to classify:

Two diagnoses, or

A diagnosis with an associated secondary process (manifestation)

A diagnosis with an associated complication

Combination codes are identified by referring to subterm entries in the Alphabetic Index and by reading the inclusion and exclusion notes in the Tabular List.

Assign only the combination code when that code fully identifies the diagnostic conditions involved or when the Alphabetic Index so directs. Multiple coding should not be used when the classification provides a combination code that clearly identifies all of the elements documented in the diagnosis. When the combination code lacks necessary specificity in describing the manifestation or complication, an additional code should be used as a secondary code.

10. **Sequela (Late Effects)**

A sequela is the residual effect (condition produced) after the acute phase of an illness or injury has terminated. There is no time limit on when a sequela code can be used. The residual may be apparent early, such as in cerebral infarction, or it may occur months or years later, such as that due to a previous injury. Examples of sequela include: scar formation resulting from a burn, deviated septum due to a nasal fracture, and infertility due to tubal occlusion from old tuberculosis. Coding of sequela generally requires two codes sequenced in the following order: The condition or nature of the sequela is sequenced first. The sequela code is sequenced second.

An exception to the above guidelines are those instances where the code for the sequela is followed by a manifestation code identified in the Tabular List and title, or the sequela code has been expanded (at the fourth, fifth or sixth character levels) to include the manifestation(s). The code for the acute phase of an illness or injury that led to the sequela is never used with a code for the late effect.

Application of 7th characters refer to Chapter 19

11. **Impending or Threatened Condition**

Code any condition described at the time of discharge as "impending" or "threatened" as follows:

If it did occur, code as confirmed diagnosis. If it did not occur, reference the Alphabetic Index to determine if the condition has a subentry term for "impending" or "threatened" and also reference main term entries for "Impending" and for "Threatened." If the subterms are listed, assign the given code. If the subterms are not listed, code the existing underlying condition(s) and not the condition described as impending or threatened.

12. **Reporting Same Diagnosis Code More Than Once**

Each unique *ICD-10-CM* diagnosis code may be reported only once for an encounter. This applies to bilateral conditions when there are no distinct codes identifying laterality or two different conditions classified to the same *ICD-10-CM* diagnosis code.

13. **Laterality**

Some *ICD-10-CM* codes indicate laterality, specifying whether the condition occurs on the left, right or is bilateral. If no bilateral code is provided and the condition is bilateral, assign separate codes for both the left and right side. If the side is not identified in the medical record, assign the code for the unspecified side.

When a patient has a bilateral condition and each side is treated during separate encounters, assign the "bilateral" code (as the condition still exists on both sides), including for the encounter to treat the first side. For the second encounter for treatment after one side has previously been treated and the condition no longer exists on that side, assign the appropriate unilateral code for the side where the condition still exists (e.g., cataract surgery performed on each eye in separate encounters). The bilateral code would not be assigned for the subsequent encounter, as the patient no longer has the condition in the previously-treated site. If the treatment on the first side did not completely resolve the condition, then the bilateral code would still be appropriate.

When laterality is not documented by the patient's provider, code assignment for the affected side may be based on medical record documentation from other clinicians. If there is conflicting medical record documentation regarding the affected side, the patient's attending provider should be queried for clarification. Codes for "unspecified" side should rarely be used, such as when the documentation in the record is insufficient to determine the affected side and it is not possible to obtain clarification.

14. **Documentation by *Clinicians Other Than the Patient's Provider***

Code assignment is based on the documentation by **the** patient's provider (i.e., physician or other qualified healthcare practitioner legally accountable for establishing the patient's diagnosis). There are a few exceptions, **when** code assignment may be based on medical record documentation from clinicians who are not the patient's provider (ie, physician or other qualified healthcare practitioner legally accountable for establishing the patient's diagnosis). **In this context, "clinicians" other than the patient's provider refer to healthcare professionals permitted, based on regulatory or accreditation requirements or internal hospital policies, to document in a patient's official medical record.**

These exceptions include codes for:
- **Body Mass Index (BMI)**
- **Depth of non-pressure chronic ulcers**
- **Pressure ulcer stage**
- **Coma scale**
- **NIH stroke scale (NIHSS)**
- **Social determinants of health (SDOH)**
- **Laterality**
- **Blood alcohol level**

This information is typically, or may be, documented by other clinicians involved in the care of the patient (e.g., a dietitian often documents the BMI, a nurse often documents the pressure ulcer stages, and an emergency medical technician often documents the coma scale). However, the associated diagnosis (such as overweight, obesity, acute stroke, pressure ulcer, or a condition classifiable to category F10, Alcohol related disorders) must be documented by the patient's provider. If there is conflicting medical record documentation, either from the same clinician or different clinicians, the patient's attending provider should be queried for clarification.

The BMI, coma scale, NIHSS, blood alcohol level codes and codes for social determinants of health should only be reported as secondary diagnoses.

See Section I.C.21.c.17 for additional information regarding coding social determinants of health.

15. Syndromes

Follow the Alphabetic Index guidance when coding syndromes. In the absence of Alphabetic Index guidance, assign codes for the documented manifestations of the syndrome. Additional codes for manifestations that are not an integral part of the disease process may also be assigned when the condition does not have a unique code.

16. Documentation of Complications of Care

Code assignment is based on the provider's documentation of the relationship between the condition and the care or procedure. The guideline extends to any complications of care, regardless of the chapter the code is located in. It is important to note that not all conditions that occur during or following medical care or surgery are classified as complications. There must be a cause-and-effect relationship between the care provided and the condition, and an indication in the documentation that it is a complication. Query the provider for clarification, if the complication is not clearly documented.

17. Borderline Diagnosis

If the provider documents a "borderline" diagnosis at the time of discharge, the diagnosis is coded as confirmed, unless the classification provides a specific entry (eg, borderline diabetes). If a borderline condition has a specific index entry in *ICD-10-CM*, it should be coded as such. Since borderline conditions are not uncertain diagnoses, no distinction is made between the care setting (inpatient versus outpatient). Whenever the documentation is unclear regarding a borderline condition, coders are encouraged to query for clarification.

18. Use of Sign/Symptom/Unspecified Codes

Sign/symptom and "unspecified" codes have acceptable, even necessary, uses. While specific diagnosis codes should be reported when they are supported by the available medical record documentation and clinical knowledge of the patient's health condition, there are instances when signs/symptoms or unspecified codes are the best choices for accurately reflecting the healthcare encounter. Each health care encounter should be coded to the level of certainty known for that encounter.

As stated in the introductory section of these official coding guidelines, a joint effort between the healthcare provider and the coder is essential to achieve complete and accurate documentation, code assignment, and reporting of diagnoses and procedures. The importance of consistent, complete documentation in the medical record cannot be overemphasized. Without such documentation accurate coding cannot be achieved. The entire record should be reviewed to determine the specific reason for the encounter and the conditions treated.

If a definitive diagnosis has not been established by the end of the encounter, it is appropriate to report codes for sign(s) and/or symptom(s) in lieu of a definitive diagnosis. When sufficient clinical information isn't known or available about a particular health condition to assign a more specific code, it is acceptable to report the appropriate "unspecified" code (eg, a diagnosis of pneumonia has been determined, but not the specific type). Unspecified codes should be reported when they are the codes that most accurately reflect what is known about the patient's condition at the time of that particular encounter. It would be inappropriate to select a specific code that is not supported by the medical record documentation or conduct medically unnecessary diagnostic testing in order to determine a more specific code.

19. **Coding for Healthcare Encounters in Hurricane Aftermath**
    a. **Use of External Cause of Morbidity Codes**

    An external cause of morbidity code should be assigned to identify the cause of the injury(ies) incurred as a result of the hurricane. The use of external cause of morbidity codes is supplemental to the application of *ICD-10-CM* codes. External cause of morbidity codes are never to be recorded as a principal diagnosis (first-listed in non-inpatient settings). The appropriate injury code should be sequenced before any external cause codes. The external cause of morbidity codes capture how the injury or health condition happened (cause), the intent (unintentional or accidental; or intentional, such as suicide or assault), the place where the event occurred, the activity of the patient at the time of the event, and the person's status (e.g., civilian, military). They should not be assigned for encounters to treat hurricane victims' medical conditions when no injury, adverse effect or poisoning is involved. External cause of morbidity codes should be assigned for each encounter for care and treatment of the injury. External cause of morbidity codes may be assigned in all health care settings. For the purpose of capturing complete and accurate *ICD-10-CM* data in the aftermath of the hurricane, a healthcare setting should be considered as any location where medical care is provided by licensed healthcare professionals.

    b. **Sequencing of External Causes of Morbidity Codes**

    Codes for cataclysmic events, such as a hurricane, take priority over all other external cause codes except child and adult abuse and terrorism and should be sequenced before other external cause of injury codes. Assign as many external cause of morbidity codes as necessary to fully explain each cause. For example, if an injury occurs as a result of a building collapse during the hurricane, external cause codes for both the hurricane and the building collapse should be assigned, with the external causes code for hurricane being sequenced as the first external cause code. For injuries incurred as a direct result of the hurricane, assign the appropriate code(s) for the injuries, followed by the code X37.0-, Hurricane (with the appropriate 7th character), and any other applicable external cause of injury codes. Code X37.0- also should be assigned when an injury is incurred as a result of flooding caused by a levee breaking related to the hurricane. Code X38.-, Flood (with the appropriate 7th character), should be assigned when an injury is from flooding resulting directly from the storm. Code

    X36.0.-, Collapse of dam or man-made structure, should not be assigned when the cause of the collapse is due to the hurricane. Use of code X36.0- is limited to collapses of man-made structures due to earth surface movements, not due to storm surges directly from a hurricane.

    c. **Other External Causes of Morbidity Code Issues**

    For injuries that are not a direct result of the hurricane, such as an evacuee that has incurred an injury as a result of a motor vehicle accident, assign the appropriate external cause of morbidity code(s) to describe the cause of the injury, but do not assign code X37.0-, Hurricane. If it is not clear whether the injury was a direct result of the hurricane, assume the injury is due to the hurricane and assign code X37.0-, Hurricane, as well as any other applicable external cause of morbidity codes. In addition to code X37.0-, Hurricane, other possible applicable external cause of morbidity codes include:

    W54.0-, Bitten by dog
    X30-, Exposure to excessive natural heat
    X31-, Exposure to excessive natural cold
    X38-, Flood

    d. **Use of Z codes**

    Z codes (other reasons for healthcare encounters) may be assigned as appropriate to further explain the reasons for presenting for healthcare services, including transfers between healthcare facilities **or provide additional information relevant to a patient encounter.** The *ICD-10-CM Official Guidelines for Coding and Reporting* identify which codes maybe assigned as principal or first-listed diagnosis only, secondary diagnosis only, or principal/first-listed or secondary (depending on the circumstances). Possible applicable Z codes include:

    Z59.0, Homelessness
    Z59.1, Inadequate housing
    Z59.5, Extreme poverty
    Z75.1, Person awaiting admission to adequate facility elsewhere
    Z75.3, Unavailability and inaccessibility of health-care facilities
    Z75.4, Unavailability and inaccessibility of other helping agencies
    Z76.2, Encounter for health supervision and care of other healthy infant and child
    Z99.12, Encounter for respirator [ventilator] dependence during power failure

    The external cause of morbidity codes and the Z codes listed above are not an all-inclusive list. Other codes may be applicable to the encounter based upon the documentation. Assign as many codes as necessary to fully explain each healthcare encounter. Since patient history information may be very limited, use any available documentation to assign the appropriate external cause of morbidity and Z codes.

C. Chapter-Specific Coding Guidelines

Please refer to each chapter for information on specific guidelines.

Section II. Selection of Principle Diagnosis

Excluded as not relevant to provider-based coding. Refer to the full *ICD-10-CM* manual if needed.

Section III. Reporting Additional Diagnoses

Excluded as not relevant to provider-based coding. Refer to the full *ICD-10-CM* manual if needed.

Section IV. Diagnostic Coding and Reporting Guidelines for Outpatient Services

These coding guidelines for outpatient diagnoses have been approved for use by hospitals/providers in coding and reporting hospital-based outpatient services and provider-based office visits.

Information about the use of certain abbreviations, punctuation, symbols, and other conventions used in the *ICD-10-CM* Tabular List (code numbers and titles), can be found in Section IA of these guidelines, under "Conventions Used in the Tabular List." Section I.B. contains general guidelines that apply to the entire classification. Section I.C. contains chapter-specific guidelines that correspond to the chapters as they are arranged in the classification. Information about the correct sequence to use in finding a code is also described in Section I.

The terms "encounter" and "visit" are often used interchangeably when describing outpatient service contacts and, therefore, appear together in these guidelines without distinguishing one from the other.

Though the conventions and general guidelines apply to all settings, coding guidelines for outpatient and provider reporting of diagnoses will vary in a number of instances from those for inpatient diagnoses, recognizing that:

A. Selection of first-listed condition

In the outpatient setting, the term "first-listed diagnosis" is used in lieu of "principal diagnosis."

In determining the first-listed diagnosis, the coding conventions of *ICD-10-CM*, as well as the general and disease specific guidelines, take precedence over the outpatient guidelines.

Diagnoses are often not established at the time of the initial encounter/visit. It may take two or more visits before the diagnosis is confirmed.

The most critical rule is to begin the search for the correct code assignment through the Alphabetic Index. Never search initially in the Tabular List, as this will lead to coding errors.

1. Outpatient Surgery

When a patient presents for outpatient surgery (same day surgery), code the reason for the surgery as the first-listed diagnosis (reason for the encounter), even if the surgery is not performed due to a contraindication.

2. Observation Stay

When a patient is admitted for observation for a medical condition, assign a code for the medical condition as the first-listed diagnosis.

When a patient presents for outpatient surgery and develops complications requiring admission to observation, code the reason for the surgery as the first reported diagnosis (reason for the encounter), followed by codes for the complications as secondary diagnoses.

B. Codes from A00.0 through T88.9, Z00 – Z99

The appropriate code(s) from A00.0 through T88.9, Z00–Z99 **and U00–U85** must be used to identify diagnoses, symptoms, conditions, problems, complaints, or other reason(s) for the encounter/visit.

C. Accurate reporting of *ICD-10-CM* diagnosis codes

For accurate reporting of *ICD-10-CM* diagnosis codes, the documentation should describe the patient's condition, using terminology which includes specific diagnoses, as well as symptoms, problems, or reasons for the encounter. There are *ICD-10-CM* codes to describe all of these.

D. Codes that describe symptoms and signs

Codes that describe symptoms and signs, as opposed to diagnoses, are acceptable for reporting purposes when a diagnosis has not been established (confirmed) by the provider. Chapter 18 of *ICD-10-CM*, Symptoms, Signs, and Abnormal Clinical and Laboratory Findings Not Elsewhere Classified (codes R00 – R99) contains many, but not all codes for symptoms.

E. Encounters for circumstances other than a disease or injury

ICD-10-CM provides codes to deal with encounters for circumstances other than a disease or injury. The Factors Influencing Health Status and Contact with Health Services codes (Z00 – Z99) are provided to deal with occasions when circumstances other than a disease or injury are recorded as diagnosis or problems.

See Chapter 21, *Factors influencing health status and contact with health services.*

F. Level of Detail in Coding

1. *ICD-10-CM* codes with 3, 4, 5, 6, or 7 characters

ICD-10-CM is composed of codes with 3, 4, 5, 6, or 7 characters. Codes with three characters are included in *ICD-10-CM* as the heading of a category of codes that may be further subdivided by the use of fourth, fifth, sixth, or seventh characters to provide greater specificity.

2. **Use of full number of characters required for a code**
A three-character code is to be used only if it is not further subdivided. A code is invalid if it has not been coded to the full number of characters required for that code, including the 7th character, if applicable.

3. **Highest level of specificity**
Code to the highest level of specificity when supported by the medical record documentation.

G. *ICD-10-CM* **code for the diagnosis, condition, problem, or other reason for encounter/visit**
List first the *ICD-10-CM* code for the diagnosis, condition, problem, or other reason for encounter/visit shown in the medical record to be chiefly responsible for the services provided. List additional codes that describe any coexisting conditions. In some cases, the first-listed diagnosis may be a symptom when a diagnosis has not been established (confirmed) by the **provider.**

H. **Uncertain diagnosis**
<u>Do not code</u> diagnoses documented as "probable," "suspected," "questionable," "rule out," or "working diagnosis" or other similar terms indicating uncertainty. Rather, code the condition(s) to the highest degree of certainty for that encounter/visit, such as symptoms, signs, abnormal test results, or other reason for the visit.

I. **Chronic diseases**
Chronic diseases treated on an ongoing basis may be coded and reported as many times as the patient receives treatment and care for the condition(s)

J. **Code all documented conditions that coexist**
Code all documented conditions that coexist at the time of the encounter/visit, and require or affect patient care treatment or management. Do not code conditions that were previously treated and no longer exist. However, history codes (categories Z80–Z87) may be used as secondary codes if the historical condition or family history has an impact on current care or influences treatment.

K. **Patients receiving diagnostic services only**
For patients receiving diagnostic services only during an encounter/visit, sequence first the diagnosis, condition, problem, or other reason for encounter/visit shown in the medical record to be chiefly responsible for the outpatient services provided during the encounter/visit. Codes for other diagnoses (eg, chronic conditions) may be sequenced as additional diagnoses.

For encounters for routine laboratory/radiology testing in the absence of any signs, symptoms, or associated diagnosis, assign Z01.89, Encounter for other specified special examinations. If routine testing is performed during the same encounter as a test to evaluate a sign, symptom, or diagnosis,

it is appropriate to assign both the Z code and the code describing the reason for the non-routine test.

For outpatient encounters for diagnostic tests that have been interpreted by a physician, and the final report is available at the time of coding, code any confirmed or definitive diagnosis(es) documented in the interpretation. Do not code related signs and symptoms as additional diagnoses.

Please note: This differs from the coding practice in the hospital inpatient setting regarding abnormal findings on test results.

L. **Patients receiving therapeutic services only**
For patients receiving therapeutic services only during an encounter/visit, sequence first the diagnosis, condition, problem, or other reason for encounter/visit shown in the medical record to be chiefly responsible for the outpatient services provided during the encounter/visit. Codes for other diagnoses (eg, chronic conditions) may be sequenced as additional diagnoses.

The only exception to this rule is that when the primary reason for the admission/encounter is chemotherapy or radiation therapy. In this case, the appropriate Z code for the service is listed first, and the diagnosis or problem for which the service is being performed is listed second.

M. **Patients receiving preoperative evaluations only**
For patients receiving preoperative evaluations only, sequence first a code from subcategory Z01.81, Encounter for pre-procedural examinations, to describe the pre-op consultations. Assign a code for the condition to describe the reason for the surgery as an additional diagnosis. Code also any findings related to the pre-op evaluation.

N. **Ambulatory surgery**
For ambulatory surgery, code the diagnosis for which the surgery was performed. If the postoperative diagnosis is known to be different from the preoperative diagnosis at the time the diagnosis is confirmed, select the postoperative diagnosis for coding, since it is the most definitive.

O. **Routine outpatient prenatal visits**
See Chapter 15, *Pregnancy, childbirth and the puerperium.*

P. **Encounters for general medical examinations with abnormal findings**
The subcategories for encounters for general medical examinations, Z00.0-, provide codes for with and without abnormal findings. Should a general medical examination result in an abnormal finding, the code for general medical examination with abnormal finding should be assigned as the first-listed diagnosis. A secondary code for the abnormal finding should also be coded.

Q. **Encounters for routine health screenings**
See Chapter 21, *Factors influencing health status and contact with health services, Screening*

Alphabetic Index

Instructions are listed in *italic font.* The "*see*" instruction indicates it is necessary to reference another term while "*see also*" instruction indicates another main term may provide additional entries. It is not necessary to follow a "*see also*" instruction when the current entry directs to a code for the condition. "*Code*" or "*Code to*" directs to the appropriate reference for a condition.

Punctuation

[ ]—used to identify manifestation codes

( )—enclose nonessential words that do not affect code assignment

:—the colon identifies that a term is incomplete and requires additional modifying terms

- —the hyphen indicates additional characters are found in the tabular list

A

Aarskog's syndrome Q87.19

Abandonment—*see* Maltreatment

Abasia (-astasia) (hysterical) F44.4

Abderhalden-Kaufmann-Lignac syndrome (cystinosis) E72.04

Abdomen, abdominal—*see also* Disease, diseased
- acute R10.0
- angina K55.1
- muscle deficiency syndrome Q79.4

Abdominalgia—*see* Pain(s), abdominal

Abduction contracture, hip or other joint—*see* Contraction, joint

Aberrant (congenital)—*see also* Malposition, congenital
- artery (peripheral) Q27.8
  - eye Q15.8
  - pulmonary Q25.79
  - retina Q14.1
- endocrine gland NEC Q89.2
- hepatic duct Q44.5
- parathyroid gland Q89.2
- pituitary gland Q89.2
- thymus (gland) Q89.2
- thyroid gland Q89.2

Abiotrophy R68.89

Ablepharia, ablepharon Q10.3

Abnormal, abnormality, abnormalities—*see also* Anomaly
- auditory perception H93.29-
- autosomes Q99.9
- basal metabolic rate R94.8
- bleeding time R79.1
- blood amino-acid level R79.83
- blood gas level R79.81
- blood pressure
  - elevated R03.0
- brain scan R94.02
- caloric test R94.138
- chemistry, blood R79.9
  - C-reactive protein R79.82
  - drugs—*see* Findings, abnormal, in blood
  - gas level R79.81
  - pancytopenia D61.818
  - PTT R79.1
- chest sounds (friction) (rales) R09.89
- chromosome, chromosomal Q99.9
  - sex Q99.8
    - female phenotype Q97.9
    - male phenotype Q98.9
- clinical findings NEC R68.89
- coagulation D68.9
  - newborn, transient P61.6
  - profile R79.1
  - time R79.1
- cortisol-binding globulin E27.8
- creatinine clearance R94.4
- development, developmental Q89.9
  - central nervous system Q07.9
- diagnostic imaging
  - abdomen, abdominal region NEC R93.5
  - bladder R93.41
  - coronary circulation R93.1
  - head R93.0

Abnormal, abnormality, abnormalities, *continued*
- heart R93.1
- kidney R93.42-
- lung (field) R91.8
- musculoskeletal system NEC R93.7
- renal pelvis R93.41
- retroperitoneum R93.5
- site specified NEC R93.89
- skull R93.0
- testis R93.81-
- ureter R93.41
- urinary organs, specified R93.49
- echocardiogram R93.1
- electrocardiogram [ECG] [EKG] R94.31
- electroencephalogram [EEG] R94.01
- electrolyte—*see* Imbalance, electrolyte
- electromyogram [EMG] R94.131
- electro-oculogram [EOG] R94.110
- electrophysiological intracardiac studies R94.39
- electroretinogram [ERG] R94.111
- feces (color) (contents) (mucus) R19.5
- function studies
  - auditory R94.120
  - bladder R94.8
  - brain R94.09
  - cardiovascular R94.30
  - ear R94.128
  - endocrine NEC R94.7
  - eye NEC R94.118
  - kidney R94.4
  - liver function test R79.89
  - nervous system
    - central NEC R94.09
    - peripheral NEC R94.138
  - pancreas R94.8
  - placenta R94.8
  - pulmonary R94.2
  - special senses NEC R94.128
  - spleen R94.8
  - thyroid R94.6
  - vestibular R94.121
- gait—*see* Gait abnormality
  - hysterical F44.4
- globulin R77.1
  - cortisol-binding E27.8
- heart
  - rate R00.9
    - specified NEC R00.8
  - shadow R93.1
- hemoglobin (disease) (*see also* Disease, hemoglobin) D58.2
  - trait—*see* Trait, hemoglobin, abnormal
- kidney function test R94.4
- loss of
  - weight R63.4
- Mantoux test R76.11
- movement (disorder)—*see also* Disorder, movement
  - involuntary R25.9
    - spasm R25.2
    - tremor R25.1
- neonatal screening P09.9
  - congenital adrenal hyperplasia P09.2
  - congenital endocrine disease P09.2
  - congenital hematologic disorders P09.3
  - critical congenital heart disease P09.5
  - cystic fibrosis P09.4
  - hemoglobinothies P09.3
  - hypothyroidism P09.2
  - inborn errors of metabolism P09.1
  - neonatal hearing loss P09.6
  - red cell membrane defects P09.3
  - sickle cell P09.3
  - specified NEC P09.8
- oculomotor study R94.113
- palmar creases Q82.8
- partial thromboplastin time (PTT) R79.1
- percussion, chest (tympany) R09.89
- phonocardiogram R94.39
- plasma
  - protein R77.9
    - specified NEC R77.8
  - viscosity R70.1
- posture R29.3

Abnormal, abnormality, abnormalities, *continued*
- prothrombin time (PT) R79.1
- pulmonary
  - artery, congenital Q25.79
  - function, newborn P28.89
  - test results R94.2
- pulsations in neck R00.2
- red blood cell(s) (morphology) (volume) R71.8
- renal function test R94.4
- response to nerve stimulation R94.130
- retinal correspondence H53.31
- retinal function study R94.111
- rhythm, heart—*see also* Arrhythmia
- saliva—*see* Abnormal, specimen
- scan
  - kidney R94.4
  - liver R93.2
  - thyroid R94.6
- serum level (of)
  - acid phosphatase R74.8
  - alkaline phosphatase R74.8
  - amylase R74.8
  - enzymes R74.9
    - specified NEC R74.8
  - lipase R74.8
  - triacylglycerol lipase R74.8
- sinus venosus Q21.1
- specimen
  - specified organ, system and tissue NOS R89.9
- sputum (amount) (color) (odor) R09.3
- stool (color) (contents) (mucus) R19.5
  - bloody K92.1
  - guaiac positive R19.5
- transport protein E88.09
- tumor marker NEC R97.8
- urination NEC R39.198
- urine (constituents) R82.90
  - cytological and histological examination R82.89
  - glucose R81
  - hemoglobin R82.3
  - microbiological examination (positive culture) R82.79
  - pyuria R82.81
  - specified substance NEC R82.998
- vectorcardiogram R94.39
- visually evoked potential (VEP) R94.112
- white blood cells D72.9
  - specified NEC D72.89
- X-ray examination—*see* Abnormal, diagnostic imaging

Abnormity (any organ or part)—*see* Anomaly

Abocclusion M26.29
- hemolytic disease (newborn) P55.1

Abortion (complete) (spontaneous) O03.9
- incomplete (spontaneous) O03.4
- missed O02.1
- spontaneous—*see* Abortion (complete) (spontaneous)
  - threatened O20.0
- threatened (spontaneous) O20.0
- tubal O00.10-
  - with intrauterine pregnancy O00.11

Abramov-Fiedler myocarditis (acute isolated myocarditis) I40.1

Abrasion T14.8
- abdomen, abdominal (wall) S30.811
- alveolar process S00.512
- ankle S90.51-
- antecubital space—*see* Abrasion, elbow
- anus S30.817
- arm (upper) S40.81-
- auditory canal—*see* Abrasion, ear
- auricle—*see* Abrasion, ear
- axilla—*see* Abrasion, arm
- back, lower S30.810
- breast S20.11-
- brow S00.81
- buttock S30.810
- calf—*see* Abrasion, leg
- canthus—*see* Abrasion, eyelid
- cheek S00.81
  - internal S00.512
- chest wall—*see* Abrasion, thorax
- chin S00.81
- clitoris S30.814

Abrasion, *continued*
- cornea S05.0-
- costal region—*see* Abrasion, thorax
- dental K03.1
- digit(s)
  - foot—*see* Abrasion, toe
  - hand—*see* Abrasion, finger
- ear S00.41-
- elbow S50.31-
- epididymis S30.813
- epigastric region S30.811
- epiglottis S10.11
- esophagus (thoracic)
  - cervical S10.11
- eyebrow *S00.21-*
- eyelid S00.21-
- face S00.81
- finger(s) S60.41-
  - index S60.41-
  - little S60.41-
  - middle S60.41-
  - ring S60.41-
- flank S30.811
- foot (except toe(s) alone) S90.81
  - toe—*see* Abrasion, toe
- forearm S50.81-
  - elbow only—*see* Abrasion, elbow
- forehead S00.81
- genital organs, external
  - male S30.815
- groin S30.811
- gum S00.512
- hand S60.51-
- head S00.91
  - ear—*see* Abrasion, ear
  - eyelid—*see* Abrasion, eyelid
  - lip S00.511
  - nose S00.31
  - oral cavity S00.512
  - scalp S00.01
  - specified site NEC S00.81
- heel—*see* Abrasion, foot
- hip S70.21-
- inguinal region S30.811
- interscapular region S20.419
- jaw S00.81
- knee S80.21-
- labium (majus) (minus) S30.814
- larynx S10.11
- leg (lower) S80.81-
  - knee—*see* Abrasion, knee
  - upper—*see* Abrasion, thigh
- lip S00.511
- lower back S30.810
- lumbar region S30.810
- malar region S00.81
- mammary—*see* Abrasion, breast
- mastoid region S00.81
- mouth S00.512
- nail
  - finger—*see* Abrasion, finger
  - toe—*see* Abrasion, toe
- nape S10.81
- nasal S00.31
- neck S10.91
  - specified site NEC S10.81
  - throat S10.11
- nose S00.31
- occipital region S00.01
- oral cavity S00.512
- orbital region—*see* Abrasion, eyelid
- palate S00.512
- palm—*see* Abrasion, hand
- parietal region S00.01
- pelvis S30.810
- penis S30.812
- perineum
  - female S30.814
  - male S30.810
- periocular area—*see* Abrasion, eyelid
- phalanges
  - finger—*see* Abrasion, finger
  - toe—*see* Abrasion, toe

Abrasion, *continued*
- pharynx S10.11
- pinna—*see* Abrasion, ear
- popliteal space—*see* Abrasion, knee
- prepuce S30.812
- pubic region S30.810
- pudendum
  - female S30.816
  - male S30.815
- sacral region S30.810
- scalp S00.01
- scapular region—*see* Abrasion, shoulder
- scrotum S30.813
- shin—*see* Abrasion, leg
- shoulder S40.21
- skin NEC T14.8
- sternal region S20.319
- submaxillary region S00.81
- submental region S00.81
- subungual
  - finger(s)—*see* Abrasion, finger
  - toe(s)—*see* Abrasion, toe
- supraclavicular fossa S10.81
- supraorbital S00.81
- temple S00.81
- temporal region S00.81
- testis S30.813
- thigh S70.31-
- thorax, thoracic (wall) S20.91
  - back S20.41-
  - front S20.31-
- throat S10.11
- thumb S60.31-
- toe(s) (lesser) S90.41-
  - great S90.41-
- tongue S00.512
- tooth, teeth (dentifrice) (habitual) (hard tissues) (occupational) (ritual) (traditional) K03.1
- trachea S10.11
- tunica vaginalis S30.813
- tympanum, tympanic membrane—*see* Abrasion, ear
- uvula S00.512
- vagina S30.814
- vocal cords S10.11
- vulva S30.814
- wrist S60.81-

Abscess (connective tissue) (embolic) (fistulous) (metastatic) (multiple) (pernicious) (pyogenic) (septic) L02.91
- abdomen, abdominal
  - cavity K65.1
  - wall L02.211
- abdominopelvic K65.1
- accessory sinus—*see* Sinusitis
- adrenal (capsule) (gland) E27.8
- alveolar K04.7
- anorectal K61.2
- anus K61.0
- apical (tooth) K04.7
- appendix K35.33
- areola (acute) (chronic) (nonpuerperal) N61.1
- axilla (region) L02.41
  - lymph gland or node L04.2
- back (any part, except buttock) L02.212
- Bartholin's gland N75.1
- brain (any part) (cystic) (otogenic) G06.0
- breast (acute) (chronic) (nonpuerperal) N61.1
  - newborn P39.0
- buccal cavity K12.2
- buttock L02.31
- cecum K35.33
- cerebellum, cerebellar G06.0
  - sequelae G09
- cerebral (embolic) G06.0
  - sequelae G09
- cervical (meaning neck) L02.11
  - lymph gland or node L04.0
- cheek (external) L02.01
  - inner K12.2
- chest J86.9
  - with fistula J86.0
  - wall L02.213
- chin L02.01
- circumtonsillar J36

Abscess, *continued*
- colostomy K94.02
- cranium G06.0
- dental K04.7
- dentoalveolar K04.7
- ear (middle)—*see also* Otitis, media
  - acute—*see* Otitis, media
  - external H60.0-
- epididymis N45.4
- epidural G06.2
  - brain G06.0
  - spinal cord G06.1
- erysipelatous—*see* Erysipelas
- esophagus K20.80
- ethmoid (bone) (chronic) (sinus) J32.2
- extradural G06.2
  - brain G06.0
    - sequelae G09
  - spinal cord G06.1
- eyelid H00.03-
- face (any part, except ear, eye and nose) L02.01
- foot L02.61-
- forehead L02.01
- frontal sinus (chronic) J32.1
- gallbladder K81.0
- gluteal (region) L02.31
- groin L02.214
- hand L02.51-
  - head NEC L02.811 part, except ear, eye and nose) L02.01
- horseshoe K61.31
- heel—*see* Abscess, foot
- ileocecal K35.33
- iliac (region) L02.214
  - fossa K35.33
- inguinal (region) L02.214
  - lymph gland or node L04.1
- intersphincteric K61.4
- intracranial G06.0
- intratonsillar J36
- knee—*see also* Abscess, lower limb
  - joint M00.9
- lateral (alveolar) K04.7
- lingual K14.0
  - tonsil J36
- lip K13.0
- loin (region) L02.211
- lower limb L02.41
- lumbar (tuberculous) A18.01
  - nontuberculous L02.212
- lymph, lymphatic, gland or node (acute)—*see also* Lymphadenitis, acute
  - mesentery I88.0
- marginal, anus K61.0
- maxilla, maxillary M27.2
  - molar (tooth) K04.7
  - premolar K04.7
  - sinus (chronic) J32.0
- mons pubis L02.215
- mouth (floor) K12.2
- myocardium I40.0
- nasal J32.9
- navel L02.216
  - newborn P38.9
    - with mild hemorrhage P38.1
    - without hemorrhage P38.9
- neck (region) L02.11
  - lymph gland or node L04.0
- nipple N61.1
- nose (external) (fossa) (septum) J34.0
  - sinus (chronic)—*see* Sinusitis
- operative wound T81.43
- otogenic G06.0
- palate (soft) K12.2
  - hard M27.2
- parapharyngeal J39.0
- pararectal K61.1
- parietal region (scalp) L02.811
- parotid (duct) (gland) K11.3
  - region K12.2
- pectoral (region) L02.213
- perianal K61.0
- periapical K04.7

Abscess, *continued*

- periappendicular K35.33
- pericardial I30.1
- pericecal K35.33
- perineum, perineal (superficial) L02.215
  – urethra N34.0
- periodontal (parietal)
  – apical K04.7
- peripharyngeal J39.0
- peripleuritic J86.9
  – with fistula J86.0
- perirectal K61.1
- peritoneum, peritoneal (perforated) (ruptured) K65.1
  – with appendicitis K35.33
  – postoperative T81.43
- peritonsillar J36
- perityphlic K35.33
- phagedenic NOS L02.91
  – pituitary (gland) E23.6
- pleura J86.9
  – with fistula J86.0
- pilonidal L05.01
- postcecal K35.33
  – postoperative (any site) T81.43
- postnasal J34.0
- postpharyngeal J39.0
- posttonsillar J36
- presacral K68.19
- rectum K61.1
- retropharyngeal J39.0
- root, tooth K04.7
- rupture (spontaneous) NOS L02.91
- scalp (any part) L02.811
- scrofulous (tuberculous) A18.2
- septal, dental K04.7
- sinus (accessory) (chronic) (nasal)—*see also* Sinusitis
  – intracranial venous (any) G06.0
- specified site NEC L02.818
- sphenoidal (sinus) (chronic) J32.3
- stitch T81.41
- subarachnoid G06.2
  – brain G06.0
  – spinal cord G06.1
- subcecal K35.33
- subcutaneous—*see also* Abscess, by site
- subdural G06.2
  – brain G06.0
    ■ sequelae G09
  – spinal cord G06.1
- subgaleal L02.811
- sublingual K12.2
  – gland K11.3
- submandibular (region) (space) (triangle) K12.2
  – gland K11.3
- submaxillary (region) L02.01
  – gland K11.3
- submental L02.01
  – gland K11.3
- supralevator K61.5
- suprarenal (capsule) (gland) E27.8
- temple L02.01
- temporal region L02.01
- temporosphenoidal G06.0
- testes N45.4
- thorax J86.9
  – with fistula J86.0
- thyroid (gland) E06.0
- tongue (staphylococcal) K14.0
- tonsil(s) (lingual) J36
- tonsillopharyngeal J36
- tooth, teeth (root) K04.7
- trunk L02.219
  – abdominal wall L02.211
  – back L02.212
  – chest wall L02.213
  – groin L02.214
  – perineum L02.215
  – umbilicus L02.216
- umbilicus L02.216
- upper
  – limb L02.41-
- uvula K12.2
- vermiform appendix K35.33

Abscess, *continued*

- vulvovaginal gland N75.1
- wound T81.49

Absence (of) (organ or part) (complete or partial)

- albumin in blood E88.09
- alimentary tract (congenital) Q45.8
  – upper Q40.8
- anus (congenital) Q42.3
  – with fistula Q42.2
- aorta (congenital) Q25.41
- appendix, congenital Q42.8
- artery (congenital) (peripheral) Q27.8
  – pulmonary Q25.79
  – umbilical Q27.0
- atrial septum (congenital) Q21.1
- auditory canal (congenital) (external) Q16.1
- auricle (ear), congenital Q16.0
- bile, biliary duct, congenital Q44.5
- canaliculus lacrimalis, congenital Q10.4
- cervix (with uterus) congenital Q51.5
- cilia (congenital) Q10.3
- corpus callosum Q04.0
- digestive organ(s) or tract, congenital Q45.8
  – acquired NEC Z90.49
  – upper Q40.8
- ear, congenital Q16.9
  – acquired H93.8-
  – auricle Q16.0
  – external Q16.0
  – inner Q16.5
  – lobe, lobule Q17.8
  – middle, except ossicles Q16.4
    ■ ossicles Q16.3
- endocrine gland (congenital) NEC Q89.2
  – acquired E89.89
- eustachian tube (congenital) Q16.2
- eye (acquired)
  – congenital Q11.1
  – muscle (congenital) Q10.3
- eyelid (fold) (congenital) Q10.3
- family member (causing problem in home) NEC (*see also* Disruption, family) Z63.32
- fibrinogen (congenital) D68.2
  – acquired D65
- gallbladder (acquired) Z90.49
  – congenital Q44.0
- gamma globulin in blood D80.1
  – hereditary D80.0
- genital organs
  – acquired (female) (male) Z90.79
  – female, congenital Q52.8
    ■ external Q52.71
    ■ internal NEC Q52.8
  – male, congenital Q55.8
- genitourinary organs, congenital NEC
  – female Q52.8
  – male Q55.8
- ileum (acquired) Z90.49
  – congenital Q41.2
- incus (acquired)
  – congenital Q16.3
- inner ear, congenital Q16.5
- intestine (acquired) (small) Z90.49
  – congenital Q41.9
    ■ specified NEC Q41.8
  – large Z90.49
    ■ congenital Q42.9
      ~ specified NEC Q42.8
- iris, congenital Q13.1
- jejunum (acquired) Z90.49
  – congenital Q41.1
- kidney(s) (acquired) Z90.5
  – congenital
    ■ bilateral Q60.1
    ■ unilateral Q60.0
- labyrinth, membranous Q16.5
- lens (acquired)—*see also* Aphakia
  – congenital Q12.3
- muscle (congenital) (pectoral) Q79.8
  – ocular Q10.3
- organ
  – or site, congenital NEC Q89.8
    ■ acquired NEC Z90.89

Absence, *continued*

- osseous meatus (ear) Q16.4
- parathyroid gland (acquired) E89.2
  – congenital Q89.2
- pituitary gland (congenital) Q89.2
  – acquired E89.3
- punctum lacrimale (congenital) Q10.4
- rectum (congenital) Q42.1
  – with fistula Q42.0
  – acquired Z90.49
- respiratory organ NOS Q34.9
- scrotum, congenital Q55.29
- septum
  – atrial (congenital) Q21.1
- skull bone (congenital) Q75.8
  – with
    ■ anencephaly Q00.0
    ■ encephalocele—*see* Encephalocele
    ■ hydrocephalus Q03.9
      ~ with spina bifida—*see* Spina bifida, by site, with hydrocephalus
    ■ microcephaly Q02
- teeth, tooth (congenital) K00.0
  – acquired (complete) K08.109
    ■ class I K08.101
    ■ class II K08.102
    ■ class III K08.103
    ■ class IV K08.104
    ■ due to
      ~ caries K08.139
        ◊ class I K08.131
        ◊ class II K08.132
        ◊ class III K08.133
        ◊ class IV K08.134
      ~ periodontal disease K08.129
        ◊ class I K08.121
        ◊ class II K08.122
        ◊ class III K08.123
        ◊ class IV K08.124
      ~ specified NEC K08.199
        ◊ class I K08.191
        ◊ class II K08.192
        ◊ class III K08.193
        ◊ class IV K08.194
      ~ trauma K08.119
        ◊ class I K08.111
        ◊ class II K08.112
        ◊ class III K08.113
        ◊ class IV K08.114
    ■ partial K08.409
      ~ class I K08.401
      ~ class II K08.402
      ~ class III K08.403
      ~ class IV K08.404
      ~ due to
        ◊ caries K08.439
          » class I K08.431
          » class II K08.432
          » class III K08.433
          » class IV K08.434
        ◊ periodontal disease K08.429
          » class I K08.421
          » class II K08.422
          » class III K08.423
          » class IV K08.424
        ◊ specified NEC K08.499
          » class I K08.491
          » class II K08.492
          » class III K08.493
          » class IV K08.494
        ◊ trauma K08.419
          » class I K08.411
          » class II K08.412
          » class III K08.413
          » class IV K08.414
- testes (congenital) Q55.0
  – acquired Z90.79
- thymus gland Q89.2
- thyroid (gland) (acquired) E89.0
  – cartilage, congenital Q31.8
  – congenital E03.1
  – tricuspid valve Q22.4
- transverse aortic arch, congenital Q25.49

Absence, *continued*
- umbilical artery, congenital Q27.0
- uterus congenital Q51.0

Absorption
- carbohydrate, disturbance K90.49
- chemical—*see* Table of Drugs and Chemicals
  - through placenta (newborn) P04.9
    - environmental substance P04.6
    - nutritional substance P04.5
    - obstetric anesthetic or analgesic drug P04.0
- drug NEC—*see* Table of Drugs and Chemicals
  - addictive
    - through placenta (newborn) (*see also* newborn, affected by, maternal use of) P04.40
      - ~ cocaine P04.41
      - ~ hallucinogens P04.42
      - ~ specified drug NEC P04.49
  - medicinal
    - through placenta (newborn) P04.19
  - through placenta (newborn) P04.19
    - obstetric anesthetic or analgesic drug P04.0
- fat, disturbance K90.49
  - pancreatic K90.3
- noxious substance—*see* Table of Drugs and Chemicals
- protein, disturbance K90.49
- starch, disturbance K90.49
- toxic substance—*see* Table of Drugs and Chemicals

Abstinence symptoms, syndrome
- alcohol F10.239
- cocaine F14.23
- neonatal P96.1
- nicotine—*see* Dependence, drug, nicotine
- stimulant NEC F15.93
  - with dependence F15.23

Abuse
- alcohol (nondependent) F10.10
  - in remission (early) (sustained) F10.11
  - with
    - intoxication F10.129
      - ~ with delirium F10.121
      - ~ uncomplicated F10.120
    - withdrawal F10.139
      - ~ with
        - ◊ perceptual disturbance F10.132
      - delirium F10.131
      - uncomplicated F10.130
  - counseling and surveillance Z71.41
- amphetamine (or related substance)—*see also* Abuse, drug, stimulant NEC
  - stimulant NEC F15.10
    - with
      - ~ intoxication F15.129
        - ◊ with
          - » delirium F15.121
          - » perceptual disturbance F15.122
- analgesics (non-prescribed) (over the counter) F55.8
- antacids F55.0
- anxiolytic—*see* Abuse, drug, sedative
- barbiturates—*see* Abuse, drug, sedative
- caffeine—*see* Abuse, drug, stimulant NEC
- cannabis, cannabinoids—*see* Abuse, drug, cannabis
- child—*see* Maltreatment, child
- cocaine—*see* Abuse, drug, cocaine
- drug NEC (nondependent) F19.10
  - amphetamine type—*see* Abuse, drug, stimulant NEC
  - anxiolytics—*see* Abuse, drug, sedative
  - barbiturates—*see* Abuse, drug, sedative
  - caffeine—*see* Abuse, drug, stimulant NEC
  - cannabis F12.10
    - in remission (early) (sustained) F12.11
  - cocaine F14.10
    - in remission (early) (sustained) F14.11
    - with
      - ~ intoxication F14.129
        - ◊ uncomplicated F14.120
  - counseling and surveillance Z71.51
  - herbal or folk remedies F55.1
  - hormones F55.3
  - hashish—*see* Abuse, drug, cannabis
  - inhalant F18.10
    - in remission (early) (sustained) F18.11
  - laxatives F55.2

Abuse, *continued*
  - opioid F11.10
    - in remission (early) (sustained) F11.11
  - PCP (phencyclidine) (or related substance)—*see* Abuse, drug, hallucinogen
  - psychoactive NEC F19.10
  - sedative, hypnotic, or anxiolytic F13.10
    - in remission (early) (sustained) F13.11
  - solvent—*see* Abuse, drug, inhalant
  - steroids F55.3
  - stimulant NEC F15.10
    - in remission (early) (sustained) F15.11
    - with
      - ~ intoxication F15.129
        - ◊ uncomplicated F15.120
        - ◊ vitamins F55.4
- hallucinogens F16.1-
- hashish—*see* Abuse, drug, cannabis
- herbal or folk remedies F55.1
- hormones F55.3
- inhalant F18.1-
- laxatives F55.2
- marijuana—*see* Abuse, drug, cannabis
- PCP (phencyclidine) (or related substance) F16.1-
- physical (adult) (child)—*see* Maltreatment
- psychoactive substance F19.1-
- psychological (adult) (child)—*see* Maltreatment
- sexual—*see* Maltreatment
- solvent—*see* Abuse, drug, inhalant

Acalculia R48.8
- developmental F81.2

Acanthamebiasis (with) B60.10
- conjunctiva B60.12
- keratoconjunctivitis B60.13
- meningoencephalitis B60.11
- other specified B60.19

Acanthosis (acquired) (nigricans) L83
- benign Q82.8
- congenital Q82.8
- seborrheic L82.1
  - inflamed L82.0
- tongue K14.3

Acardia, acardius Q89.8

Acardiacus amorphus Q89.8

Acariasis B88.0
- scabies B86

Acarodermatitis (urticarioides) B88.0

Acathisia (drug induced) G25.71

Accelerated atrioventricular conduction I45.6

Accessory (congenital)
- atrioventricular conduction I45.6
- auditory ossicles Q16.3
- biliary duct or passage Q44.5
- carpal bones Q74.0
- cusp
  - pulmonary Q22.3
- cystic duct Q44.5
- endocrine gland NEC Q89.2
- eye muscle Q10.3
- eyelid Q10.3
- face bone(s) Q75.8
- finger(s) Q69.0
- foreskin N47.8
- frontonasal process Q75.8
- gallbladder Q44.1
- genital organ(s)
  - female Q52.8
    - external Q52.79
    - internal NEC Q52.8
  - male Q55.8
- genitourinary organs NEC Q89.8
  - female Q52.8
  - male Q55.8
- hallux Q69.2
- heart Q24.8
  - valve, NEC Q24.8
    - pulmonary Q22.3
- hepatic ducts Q44.5
- lacrimal canal Q10.6

Accessory, *continued*
- liver Q44.7
  - duct Q44.5
- navicular of carpus Q74.0
- nipple Q83.3
- parathyroid gland Q89.2
- pituitary gland Q89.2
- prepuce N47.8
- sesamoid bones Q74.8
  - foot Q74.2
  - hand Q74.0
- skin tags Q82.8
- tarsal bones Q74.2
- thumb Q69.1
- thymus gland Q89.2
- thyroid gland Q89.2
- toes Q69.2
- uterus Q51.28
- valve, heart
  - pulmonary Q22.3

Accident
See also the *ICD-10-CM* External Cause of Injuries Table for codes describing accident details.
- birth—*see* Birth, injury
- cerebrovascular (embolic) (ischemic) (thrombotic) I63.9
  - old (without sequelae) Z86.73

Accretio cordis (nonrheumatic) I31.0

Acculturation difficulty Z60.3

Acephalobrachia monster Q89.8

Acephalochirus monster Q89.8

Acephalogaster Q89.8

Acephalostomus monster Q89.8

Acephalothorax Q89.8

Acetonemia R79.89
- in Type 1 diabetes E10.10
  - with coma E10.11

Achalasia (cardia) (esophagus) K22.0
- congenital Q39.5
- pylorus Q40.0

Achlorhydria, achlorhydric (neurogenic) K31.83
- anemia D50.8
- psychogenic F45.8

Achroma, cutis L80

Achromia parasitica B36.0

Achondrogenesis Q77.0

Achondroplasia (osteosclerosis congenita) Q77.4

Achylia gastrica K31.89
- psychogenic F45.8

Acid
- peptic disease K30
- stomach K30
  - psychogenic F45.8

Acidemia E87.2
- metabolic (newborn) P19.9
  - first noted before onset of labor P19.0
  - first noted during labor P19.1
  - noted at birth P19.2

Acidity, gastric (high) K30
- psychogenic F45.8

Acidocytopenia—*see* Agranulocytosis

Acidocytosis D72.10

Acidosis (lactic) (respiratory) E87.2
- in Type 1 diabetes E10.10
  - with coma E10.11
- metabolic NEC E87.2
  - hyperchlorimic, of newborn P74.421
- mixed metabolic and respiratory, newborn P84
- newborn P84

Aciduria
- 4-hydroxybutyric E72.81
- gamma-hydroxybutyric E72.81
- glutaric (type I)
  - type II E71.313
  - type III E71.5-

Acladiosis (skin) B36.0

Acleistocardia Q21.1

Acne L70.9
- artificialis L70.8
- atrophica L70.2
- cachecticorum (Hebra) L70.8
- conglobata L70.1
- cystic L70.0
- excoriée des jeunes filles L70.5
- frontalis L70.2
- indurata L70.0
- infantile L70.4
- lupoid L70.2
- necrotic, necrotica (miliaris) L70.2
- neonatal L70.4
- nodular L70.0
- occupational L70.8
- picker's L70.5
- pustular L70.0
- rodens L70.2
- specified NEC L70.8
- tropica L70.3
- varioliformis L70.2
- vulgaris L70.0

Acquired—*see also* Disease, diseased
- immunodeficiency syndrome (AIDS) B20

Acroasphyxia, chronic I73.89

Acrocephalopolysyndactyly Q87.0

Acrocephalosyndactyly Q87.0

Acrochondrohyperplasia—*see* Syndrome, Marfan's

Acrocyanosis I73.89
- newborn P28.2
  - meaning transient blue hands and feet—omit code

Acrodermatitis
- infantile papular L44.4

Acromegaly, acromegalia E22.0

Acronyx L60.0

Acroparesthesia (simple) (vasomotor) I73.89

Action, heart
- disorder I49.9
- irregular I49.9
  - psychogenic F45.8

Activation
- mast cell (disorder) (syndrome) D89.40
  - idiopathic D89.42
  - monoclonal D89.41
  - secondary D89.43
  - specified type NEC D89.49

Active—*see* Disease, diseased

Acute—*see also* Disease, diseased
- abdomen R10.0
- gallbladder—*see* Cholecystitis, acute

Acyanotic heart disease (congenital) Q24.9

Adair-Dighton syndrome (brittle bones and blue sclera, deafness) Q78.0

Adamantinoma
- long bones C40.9-
  - lower limb C40.2-
  - upper limb C40.0-
- malignant C41.1
  - jaw (bone) (lower) C41.1
    - upper C41.0
- tibial C40.2-

Adams-Stokes (-Morgagni) disease or syndrome I45.9

Adaption reaction—*see* Disorder, adjustment

Addiction (*see also* Dependence) F19.20
- alcohol, alcoholic (ethyl) (methyl) (wood) (without remission) F10.20
  - with remission F10.21
- drug—*see* Dependence, drug
- ethyl alcohol (without remission) F10.20
  - with remission F10.21
- ethyl alcohol (without remission) F10.20
  - with remission F10.21
- methylated spirit (without remission) F10.20
  - with remission F10.21
- tobacco—*see* Dependence, drug, nicotine

Addisonian crisis E27.2

Addison's
- anemia (pernicious) D51.0
- disease (bronze) or syndrome E27.1

Addison-Schilder complex E71.528

Additional—*see also* Accessory
- chromosome(s) Q99.8
  - sex—*see* Abnormal, chromosome, sex
  - 21—*see* Trisomy, 21

Adduction contracture, hip or other joint—*see* Contraction, joint

Adenitis—*see also* lymphadenitis
- acute, unspecified site L04.9
- axillary I88.9
  - acute L04.2
  - chronic or subacute I88.1
- cervical I88.9
  - acute L04.0
  - chronic or subacute I88.1
- chronic, unspecified site I88.1
- due to Pasteurella multocida (p. septica) A28.0
- gangrenous L04.9
- groin I88.9
  - acute L04.1
  - chronic or subacute I88.1
- inguinal I88.9
  - acute L04.1
  - chronic or subacute I88.1
- lymph gland or node, except mesenteric I88.9
  - acute—*see* Lymphadenitis, acute
  - chronic or subacute I88.1
- mesenteric (acute) (chronic) (nonspecific) (subacute) I88.0
- scrofulous (tuberculous) A18.2
- strumous, tuberculous A18.2
- subacute, unspecified site I88.1

Adenocarcinoma—*see also* Neoplasm, malignant, by site in Table of Neoplasms in the complete *ICD-10-CM* manual
- renal cell C64-

Adenoiditis (chronic) J35.02
- with tonsillitis J35.03
- acute J03.90
  - recurrent J03.91
  - specified organism NEC J03.80
    - recurrent J03.81
  - staphylococcal J03.80
    - recurrent J03.81
  - streptococcal J03.00
    - recurrent J03.01

Adenoma—*see also* Neoplasm, benign, by site in Table of Neoplasms in the complete *ICD-10-CM* manual
- apocrine
  - breast D24-
  - specified site NEC—*see* Neoplasm, skin, benign, by site in Table of Neoplasms in the complete *ICD-10-CM* manual
  - unspecified site D23.9
- ceruminous D23.2-

Adenomatosis
- endocrine (multiple) E31.20
  - single specified site—*see* Neoplasm, uncertain behavior, by site in Table of Neoplasms in the complete *ICD-10-CM* manual
- specified site—*see* Neoplasm, benign, by site in Table of Neoplasms in the complete *ICD-10-CM* manual
- unspecified site D12.6

Adenomatous
- goiter (nontoxic) E04.9
  - with hyperthyroidism—*see* Hyperthyroidism, with, goiter
  - toxic—*see* Hyperthyroidism, with, goiter

Adenopathy (lymph gland) R59.9
- generalized R59.1

Adenosclerosis I88.8

Adenovirus, as cause of disease classified elsewhere B97.0

Adherent—*see also* Adhesions
- labia (minora) N90.89
- pericardium (nonrheumatic) I31.0
  - rheumatic I09.2

Adherent, *continued*
- scar (skin) L90.5
- tendon in scar L90.5

Adhesions, adhesive (postinfective)
- cardiac I31.0
  - rheumatic I09.2
- cervicovaginal N88.1
  - congenital Q52.8
- conjunctiva congenital Q15.8
- joint—*see* Ankylosis
  - temporomandibular M26.61-
- labium (majus) (minus), congenital Q52.5
- meninges (cerebral) (spinal) G96.12
  - congenital Q07.8
  - tuberculous (cerebral) (spinal) A17.0
- nasal (septum) (to turbinates) J34.89
- pericardium (nonrheumatic) I31.0
  - focal I31.8
  - rheumatic I09.2
- preputial, prepuce N47.5
- temporomandibular M26.61-
- vagina (chronic) N89.5

Adiponecrosis neonatorum P83.88

Adiposis—*see also* Obesity
- cerebralis E23.6
- adiposogenital dystrophy E23.6

Admission (for)—*see also* Encounter (for)
- aftercare (*see also* Aftercare) Z51.89
  - radiation therapy (antineoplastic) Z51.0
- attention to artificial opening (of) Z43.9
  - artificial vagina Z43.7
    - colostomy Z43.3
    - cystostomy Z43.5
    - enterostomy Z43.4
    - gastrostomy Z43.1
    - ileostomy Z43.2
    - jejunostomy Z43.4
    - nephrostomy Z43.6
    - specified site NEC Z43.8
      - ~ intestinal tract Z43.4
      - ~ urinary tract Z43.6
    - tracheostomy Z43.0
    - ureterostomy Z43.6
    - urethrostomy Z43.6
- change of
  - dressing (nonsurgical) Z48.00
  - surgical dressing Z48.01
- circumcision, ritual or routine (in absence of diagnosis) Z41.2
- counseling—*see also* Counseling
  - dietary Z71.3
  - HIV Z71.7
  - human immunodeficiency virus Z71.7
  - non-attending third party Z71.0
  - procreative management NEC Z31.69
  - travel Z71.84
- desensitization to allergens Z51.6
- dietary surveillance and counseling Z71.3
- ear piercing Z41.3
- examination at health care facility (adult) (*see also* Examination) Z00.00
  - with abnormal findings Z00.01
  - ear Z01.10
    - with abnormal findings NEC Z01.118
  - eye Z01.00
    - with abnormal findings Z01.01
    - after failed exam Z01.02-
  - hearing Z01.10
    - infant or child (over 28 days old) Z00.129
      - ~ with abnormal findings Z00.121
    - with abnormal findings NEC Z01.118
  - vision Z01.00
    - infant or child (over 28 days old) Z00.129
      - ~ with abnormal findings Z00.121
    - with abnormal findings Z01.01
    - after failed exam Z01.02-
- followup examination Z09
- intrauterine device management Z30.431
  - initial prescription Z30.014
- prophylactic (measure)—*see also* Encounter, prophylactic measure
  - vaccination Z23

Admission (for), *continued*
- radiation therapy (antineoplastic) Z51.0
- removal of
  - dressing (nonsurgical) Z48.00
  - implantable subdermal contraceptive Z30.46
  - intrauterine contraceptive device Z30.432
  - staples Z48.02
  - surgical dressing Z48.01
  - sutures Z48.02
- sensitivity test—*see also* Test, skin
  - allergy NEC Z01.82
  - Mantoux Z11.1
- vision examination Z01.00
  - with abnormal findings Z01.01
  - after failed exam Z01.02-

Adolescent X-linked adrenoleukodystrophy E71.521

Adrenal (gland)—*see* Disease, diseased

Adrenalitis, adrenitis E27.8
- autoimmune E27.1

Adrenogenital syndrome E25.9
- congenital E25.0
- salt loss E25.0

Adrenogenitalism, congenital E25.0

Adrenoleukodystrophy E71.529
- neonatal E71.511
- Xlinked E71.529
  - Addison only phenotype E71.528
  - Addison-Schilder E71.528
  - adolescent E71.521
  - adrenomyeloneuropathy E71.522
  - childhood cerebral E71.520
  - other specified E71.528

Adrenomyeloneuropathy E71.522

Adverse effect—*see* Table of Drugs and Chemicals, categories T36 – T50, with 6th character 5

Aerodermectasia
- subcutaneous (traumatic) T79.7

Aerophagy, aerophagia (psychogenic) F45.8

Afibrinogenemia (*see also* Defect, coagulation) D68.8
- acquired D65
- congenital D68.2

Aftercare (*see also* Care) Z51.89
- following surgery (for) (on)
  - attention to
    - dressings (nonsurgical) Z48.00
      - ~ surgical Z48.01
    - sutures Z48.02
  - circulatory system Z48.812
  - digestive system Z48.815
  - genitourinary system Z48.816
  - nervous system Z48.811
  - oral cavity Z48.814—respiratory system Z48.813
  - sense organs Z48.810
  - skin and subcutaneous tissue Z48.817
  - specified body system
    - circulatory Z48.812
    - digestive Z48.815
    - genitourinary Z48.816
    - nervous Z48.811
    - oral cavity Z48.814
    - respiratory Z48.813
    - sense organs Z48.810
    - skin and subcutaneous tissue Z48.817
    - teeth Z48.814
  - spinal Z47.89
  - teeth Z48.814
- fracture *code to* fracture with seventh character D
- involving
  - removal of
    - dressings (nonsurgical) Z48.00
    - staples Z48.02
    - surgical dressings Z48.01
    - sutures Z48.02

Agammaglobulinemia (acquired) (secondary) (nonfamilial) D80.1
- with
  - immunoglobulin-bearing B-lymphocytes D80.1
  - lymphopenia D81.9
- common variable (CVAgamma) D80.1
- lymphopenic D81.9

Aganglionosis (bowel) (colon) Q43.1

Agenesis
- alimentary tract (complete) (partial) NEC Q45.8
  - upper Q40.8
- anus, anal (canal) Q42.3
  - with fistula Q42.2
- aorta Q25.41
- appendix Q42.8
- artery (peripheral) Q27.9
  - pulmonary Q25.79
  - umbilical Q27.0
- auditory (canal) (external) Q16.1
- auricle (ear) Q16.0
- bile duct or passage Q44.5
- bone Q79.9
- breast (with nipple present) Q83.8
  - with absent nipple Q83.0
- canaliculus lacrimalis Q10.4
- cartilage Q79.9
- cecum Q42.8
- cervix Q51.5
- cilia Q10.3
- clavicle Q74.0
- colon Q42.9
  - specified NEC Q42.8
- corpus callosum Q04.0
- digestive organ(s) or tract (complete) (partial) NEC Q45.8
  - upper Q40.8
- ear Q16.9
  - auricle Q16.0
  - lobe Q17.8
- endocrine (gland) NEC Q89.2
- eustachian tube Q16.2
- eye Q11.1
  - adnexa Q15.8
- eyelid (fold) Q10.3
- face
  - bones NEC Q75.8
- gallbladder Q44.0
- heart Q24.8
  - valve, NEC Q24.8
    - pulmonary Q22.0
- intestine (small) Q41.9
  - large Q42.9
    - specified NEC Q42.8
- iris (dilator fibers) Q13.1
- genitalia, genital (organ(s))
  - female Q52.8
    - external Q52.71
    - internal NEC Q52.8
  - male Q55.8
- incus Q16.3
- labyrinth, membranous Q16.5
- lacrimal apparatus Q10.4
- lens Q12.3
- muscle Q79.8
  - eyelid Q10.3
  - ocular Q15.8
- parathyroid (gland) Q89.2
- pelvic girdle (complete) (partial) Q74.2
- pituitary (gland) Q89.2
- punctum lacrimale Q10.4
- rectum Q42.1
  - with fistula Q42.0
- roof of orbit Q75.8
- round ligament Q52.8
- scapula Q74.0
- scrotum Q55.29
- septum
  - atrial Q21.1
- shoulder girdle (complete) (partial) Q74.0
- skull (bone) Q75.8
  - with
    - anencephaly Q00.0
    - encephalocele—*see* Encephalocele
    - hydrocephalus Q03.9
      - ~ with spina bifida—*see* Spina bifida, by site, with hydrocephalus
    - microcephaly Q02
- spinal cord Q06.0
- testicle Q55.0
- thymus (gland) Q89.2

Agenesis, *continued*
- thyroid (gland) E03.1
  - cartilage Q31.8
  - uterus Q51.0

Aglossia-adactylia syndrome Q87.0

Agnosia (body image) (other senses) (tactile) R48.1
- developmental F88
- verbal R48.1
  - auditory R48.1
    - developmental F80.2
  - developmental F80.2

Agranulocytosis (chronic) (cyclical) (genetic) (infantile) (periodic) (pernicious) (*see also* Neutropenia) D70.9
- congenital D70.0
- cytoreductive cancer chemotherapy sequela D70.1
- drug-induced D70.2
  - due to cytoreductive cancer chemotherapy D70.1
- due to infection D70.3
- secondary D70.4
  - drug-induced D70.2
    - due to cytoreductive cancer chemotherapy D70.1

Agraphia (absolute) R48.8
- with alexia R48.0
- developmental F81.81

Ague (dumb)—*see* Malaria

Ahumada-del Castillo syndrome E23.0

AIDS (related complex) B20

AIPHI (acute idiopathic pulmonary hemorrhage in infants (over 28 days old)) R04.81

Air
- anterior mediastinum J98.2
- hunger, psychogenic F45.8
- sickness T75.3

Airplane sickness T75.3

Akathisia (drug-induced) (treatment-induced) G25.71
- neuroleptic induced (acute) G25.71

Alactasia, congenital E73.0

Albuminuria, albuminuric (acute) (chronic) (subacute) (*see also* Proteinuria) R80.9
- orthostatic R80.2
- postural R80.2
- scarlatinal A38.8

Alcohol, alcoholic, alcohol-induced
- addiction (without remission) F10.20
  - with remission F10.21
- counseling and surveillance Z71.41
  - family member Z71.42
- intoxication (acute) (without dependence) F10.129
  - with
    - delirium F10.121
    - dependence F10.229
      - ~ with delirium F10.221
      - ~ uncomplicated F10.220
    - uncomplicated F10.120

Alcoholism (chronic) (without remission) F10.20
- with
  - psychosis—*see* Psychosis
  - remission F10.21

Alder (-Reilly) anomaly or syndrome (leukocyte granulation) D72.0

Aldrich (-Wiskott) syndrome (eczema-thrombocytopenia) D82.0

Aleukia
- congenital D70.0
- hemorrhagica D61.9
  - congenital D61.09

Alexia R48.0
- developmental F81.0
- secondary to organic lesion R48.0

Alkalosis E87.3
- metabolic E87.3
  - of newborn P74.41

Allergy, allergic (reaction) (to) T78.40
- air-borne substance NEC (rhinitis) J30.89
- anaphylactic reaction or shock T78.2
- angioneurotic edema T78.3
- animal (dander) (epidermal) (hair) (rhinitis) J30.81

Allergy, allergic, *continued*
- bee sting (anaphylactic shock)—*see* Table of Drugs and Chemicals, by animal or substance, poisoning
- biological—*see* Allergy, drug
- colitis K52.29
  - food protein-induced K52.22
- dander (animal) (rhinitis) J30.81
- dandruff (rhinitis) J30.81
- desensitization to allergens, encounter for Z51.6
- drug, medicament & biological (any) (external) (internal) T78.40
  - correct substance properly administered—*see* Table of Drugs and Chemicals, by drug, adverse effect
  - wrong substance given or taken NEC (by accident)— *see* Table of Drugs and Chemicals, by drug, poisoning
- due to pollen J30.1
- dust (house) (stock) (rhinitis) J30.89
  - with asthma—*see* Asthma, allergic extrinsic
- eczema—*see* Dermatitis, contact, allergic
- epidermal (animal) (rhinitis) J30.81
- feathers (rhinitis) J30.89
- food (any) (ingested) NEC T78.1
  - anaphylactic shock—*see* Shock, anaphylactic, due to food
  - dermatitis—*see* Dermatitis, due to, food
  - dietary counseling and surveillance Z71.3
  - in contact with skin L23.6
  - rhinitis J30.5
  - status (without reaction) Z91.018
    - beef Z91.014
    - eggs Z91.012
    - lamb Z91.014
    - mammalian meats Z91.014
    - milk products Z91.011
    - peanuts Z91.010
    - pork Z91.014
    - red meats Z91.014
    - seafood Z91.013
    - specified NEC Z91.018
- gastrointestinal K52.29
  - food protein-induced K52.22
  - meaning colitis or gastroenteritis K52.59
  - meaning other adverse food reaction NEC T78.1
- grain J30.1
- grass (hay fever) (pollen) J30.1
  - asthma—*see* Asthma, allergic extrinsic
- hair (animal) (rhinitis) J30.81
- history (of)—*see* History, family of, allergy
- horse serum—*see* Allergy, serum
- inhalant (rhinitis) J30.89
  - pollen J30.1
- kapok (rhinitis) J30.89
- medicine—*see* Allergy, drug
- milk protein Z91.011
  - anaphylactic reaction T78.07
  - dermatitis L27.2
  - enterocolitis syndrome K52.21
  - enteropathy K52.22
  - gastroenteritis K52.29
  - gastroesophageal reflux (*see also* Reaction, adverse, food) K21.9
    - with esophagitis K21.0-
  - proctocolitis K52.29
  - nasal, seasonal due to pollen J30.1
- pollen (any) (hay fever) J30.1
  - asthma—*see* Asthma, allergic extrinsic
- primrose J30.1
- primula J30.1
- purpura D69.0
- ragweed (hay fever) (pollen) J30.1
  - asthma—*see* Asthma, allergic extrinsic
- rose (pollen) J30.1
- seasonal NEC J30.2
- Senecio jacobae (pollen) J30.1
- serum (*see also* Reaction, serum) T80.69
  - anaphylactic shock T80.59
- shock (anaphylactic) T78.2
  - due to
    - administration of blood and blood products T80.51
    - immunization T80.52
    - serum NEC T80.59
    - vaccination T80.52

Allergy, allergic, *continued*
- specific NEC T78.49
- tree (any) (hay fever) (pollen) J30.1
  - asthma—*see* Asthma, allergic extrinsic
- upper respiratory J30.9
- urticaria L50.0
- vaccine—*see* Allergy, serum
- wheat—*see* Allergy, food

Alopecia (hereditaria) (seborrheica) L65.9
- due to cytotoxic drugs NEC L65.8
- postinfective NEC L65.8
- specified NEC L65.8

Alport syndrome Q87.81

ALTE (apparent life threatening event) **in newborn and infant** R68.13

Alteration (of), Altered
- mental status R41.82
- pattern of family relationships affecting child Z62.898

Alymphocytosis D72.810
- thymic (with immunodeficiency) D82.1

Alymphoplasia, thymic D82.1

Amastia (with nipple present) Q83.8
- with absent nipple Q83.0

Amaurosis (acquired) (congenital)—*see also* Blindness
- hysterical F44.6
- Leber's congenital H35.50

Ambiguous genitalia Q56.4

Amblyopia (congenital) (ex anopsia) (partial) (suppression) H53.00-
- anisometropic—*see* Amblyopia
- hysterical F44.6
- suspect H53.04-

Amebiasis
- acute A06.0
- intestine A06.0

Ameloblastoma—*see also* Cyst
- long bones C40.9-
  - lower limb C40.2-
  - upper limb C40.0-
- malignant C41.1
  - jaw (bone) (lower) C41.1
    - upper C41.0
- tibial C40.2-

Amenorrhea N91.2

Amsterdam dwarfism Q87.19

Amyelia Q06.0

Amygdalitis—*see* Tonsillitis

Amygdalolith J35.8

Amyotonia M62.89
- congenita G70.2

Anacidity, gastric K31.83
- psychogenic F45.8

Anaerosis of newborn P28.89

Analbuminemia E88.09

Anaphylactic
- purpura D69.0
- shock or reaction—*see* Shock, anaphylactic

Anaphylactoid shock or reaction—*see* Shock, anaphylactic

Anaphylaxis—*see* Shock, anaphylactic

Anaplasmosis [*A. phagocytophilum*] (transfusion transmitted) A79.82
- human A77.49

Anarthria R47.1

Anasarca R60.1
- renal N04.9

Anastomosis
- arteriovenous ruptured brain I60.8-
  - intracerebral I61.8
  - intraparenchymal I61.8
  - intraventricular I61.5
  - subarachnoid I60.8-

Android pelvis Q74.2

Anemia (essential) (general) (hemoglobin deficiency) (infantile) (primary) (profound) D64.9
- achlorhydric D50.8
- aplastic D61.9
  - congenital D61.09
  - drug-induced D61.1
  - due to
    - drugs D61.1
    - external agents NEC D61.2
    - infection D61.2
    - radiation D61.2
    - red cell (pure) D60.9
      - chronic D60.0
      - specified type NEC D60.8
      - transient D60.1
  - idiopathic D61.3
  - red cell (pure) D60.9
    - chronic D60.0
    - congenital D61.01
  - specified type NEC D61.89
  - toxic D61.2
- aregenerative
  - congenital D61.09
- atypical D64.9
- Baghdad spring D55.0
- blood loss (chronic) D50.0
  - acute D62
- chlorotic D50.8
- chronic
  - hemolytic D58.9
    - idiopathic D59.9
- chronica congenita aregenerativa D61.09
- congenital P61.4
  - aplastic D61.09
  - Heinz body D58.2
  - spherocytic D58.0
- Cooley's (erythroblastic) D56.1
- deficiency D53.9
  - 2, 3 diphosphoglycurate mutase D55.29
  - 2, 3 PG D55.29
  - enzyme D55.9
    - drug-induced (hemolytic) D59.2
    - glucose-6-phosphate dehydrogenase (G6PD) with anemia D55.0
    - glycolytic D55.29
  - folate D52.9
    - dietary D52.0
    - drug-induced D52.1
  - folic acid D52.9
    - dietary D52.0
    - drug-induced D52.1
  - glucose-6-phosphate dehydrogenase
    - with anemia D55.0
  - glyceraldehyde phosphate dehydrogenase D55.29
  - G6PD with anemia D55.0
  - hexokinase D55.29
  - nutritional D53.9
    - with
      - poor iron absorption D50.8
  - phosphoglycerate kinase D55.29
  - PK D55.21
  - pyruvate kinase D55.21
  - triose-phosphate isomerase D55.29
- Diamond-Blackfan (congenital hypoplastic) D61.01
- due to (in) (with)
  - antineoplastic chemotherapy D64.81
  - blood loss (chronic) D50.0
    - acute D62
  - chemotherapy, antineoplastic D64.81
  - chronic disease classified elsewhere NEC D63.8
  - chronic kidney disease D63.1
  - end stage renal disease D63.1
  - hemorrhage (chronic) D50.0
    - acute D62
  - loss of blood (chronic) D50.0
    - acute D62
  - myxedema E03.9 [D63.8]
  - prematurity P61.2
- Dyke-Young type (secondary) (symptomatic) D59.19
- enzyme-deficiency, drug-induced D59.2

Anemia, *continued*
- erythroblastic
  - familial D56.1
  - newborn (*see also* Disease, hemolytic) P55.9
  - of childhood D56.1
- erythropoietin-resistant anemia (EPO resistant anemia) D63.1
- familial erythroblastic D56.1
- Fanconi's (congenital pancytopenia) D61.09
- favism D55.0
- glucose-6-phosphate dehydrogenase (G6PD) deficiency D55.0
  - with anemia D55.0
  - without anemia D75.A
- Heinz body, congenital D58.2
- hemolytic D58.9
  - acquired D59.9
    - autoimmune NEC D59.19
      - acute D59.9
      - Lederer's D59.19
  - autoimmune D59.10
    - cold D59.12
    - mixed D59.13
    - warm D59.11
  - cold type (primary) (secondary) (symptomatic) D59.12
  - mixed type (primary) (secondary) (symptomatic) D59.13
  - nonspherocytic
    - congenital or hereditary NEC D55.8
      - glucose-6-phosphate dehydrogenase deficiency with anemia D55.0
      - glucose-6-phosphate dehydrogenase deficiency without anemia D75.A
      - pyruvate kinase deficiency D55.21
      - type
        ◊ II D55.29
  - primary
    - autoimmune
      - cold type D59.12
      - mixed type D59.13
      - warm type D59.11
  - secondary D59.4
    - autoimmune D59.1
    - autoimmune
    - cold type D59.12
    - mixed type D59.13
    - warm type D59.11
    - autoimmune
      - cold type D59.12
      - mixed type D59.13
      - warm type D59.11
  - warm type (primary) (secondary) (symptomatic) D59.11
- hemorrhagic (chronic) D50.0
  - acute D62
- Herrick's D57.1
- hookworm B76.9 [D63.8]
- hypochromic (idiopathic) (microcytic) (normoblastic) D50.9
  - due to blood loss (chronic) D50.0
    - acute D62
- hypoplasia, red blood cells D61.9
  - congenital or familial D61.01
- hypoplastic (idiopathic) D61.9
  - congenital or familial (of childhood) D61.01
- hypoproliferative (refractive) D61.9
- idiopathic D64.9
- iron deficiency D50.9
  - secondary to blood loss (chronic) D50.0
    - acute D62
  - specified type NEC D50.8
- Joseph-Diamond-Blackfan (congenital hypoplastic) D61.01
- leukoerythroblastic D61.82
- malarial (*see also* Malaria) B54 [D63.8]
- marsh (*see also* Malaria) B54 [D63.8]
- Mediterranean (with other hemoglobinopathy) D56.9
- microcytic (hypochromic) D50.9
  - due to blood loss (chronic) D50.0
    - acute D62
  - familial D56.8
- microdrepanocytosis D57.40

Anemia, *continued*
- microelliptopoikilocytic (RiettiGreppi Micheli) D56.9
- myelofibrosis D75.81
- myelophthisic D61.82
- myeloproliferative D47.Z9
- newborn P61.4
  - due to
    - ABO (antibodies, isoimmunization, maternal/fetal incompatibility) P55.1
    - Rh (antibodies, isoimmunization, maternal/fetal incompatibility) P55.0
  - following fetal blood loss P61.3
  - posthemorrhagic (fetal) P61.3
- normocytic (infectional) D64.9
  - due to blood loss (chronic) D50.0
    - acute D62
  - myelophthisic D61.82
- nutritional (deficiency) D53.9
  - with
    - poor iron absorption D50.8
- of prematurity P61.2
- paludal (*see also* Malaria) B54 [D63.8]
- posthemorrhagic (chronic) D50.0
  - acute D62
  - newborn P61.3
- postoperative (postprocedural)
  - due to (acute) blood loss D62
    - chronic blood loss D50.0
  - specified NEC D64.9
- progressive D64.9
  - malignant D51.0
  - pernicious D51.0
- pure red cell D60.9
  - congenital D61.01
- pyruvate kinase deficiency D55.21
- Rietti-Greppi-Micheli D56.9
- secondary to
  - blood loss (chronic) D50.0
    - acute D62
  - hemorrhage (chronic) D50.0
    - acute D62
- semiplastic D61.89
- sickle-cell—*see* Disease, sickle-cell
- sideropenic (refractory) D50.9
  - due to blood loss (chronic) D50.0
    - acute D62
- syphilitic (acquired) (late) A52.79 [D63.8]
- thalassemia D56.9
- thrombocytopenic—*see* Thrombocytopenia
- toxic D61.2
- tuberculous A18.89 [D63.8]
- Witts' (achlorhydric anemia) D50.8

Anesthesia, anesthetic R20.0
- dissociative F44.6
- functional (hysterical) F44.6
- hysterical F44.6
- testicular N50.9

Aneurysm (anastomotic) (artery) (cirsoid) (diffuse) (false) (fusiform) (multiple) (saccular)
- aorta, aortic (nonsyphilitic) I71.9
  - congenital Q25.4
  - root Q25.43
  - sinus Q25.43
  - valve (heart) (*see also* Endocarditis, aortic) I35.8
- arteriovenous (congenital)—*see also* Malformation, arteriovenous
  - brain Q28.2
    - ruptured I60.8-
      - intracerebral I61.8
      - intraparenchymal I61.8
      - intraventricular I61.5
      - subarachnoid I60.8-
- berry (congenital) (nonruptured) I67.1
  - ruptured I60.7
- brain I67.1
  - arteriovenous (congenital) (nonruptured) Q28.2
    - acquired I67.1
      - ruptured I60.8-
    - ruptured I60.8-
  - berry (congenital) (nonruptured) I67.1
    - ruptured (*see also* Hemorrhage, intracranial, subarachnoid) I60.7

Aneurysm, *continued*
- congenital Q28.3
  - ruptured I60.7
- meninges I67.1
  - ruptured I60.8-
- miliary (congenital) (nonruptured) I67.1
  - ruptured (*see also* Hemorrhage, intracranial, subarachnoid) I60.7
- mycotic I33.0ruptured into brain I60.0-
- cavernous sinus I67.1
  - arteriovenous (congenital) (nonruptured) Q28.3
    - ruptured I60.8-
- circle of Willis I67.1
  - congenital Q28.3
    - ruptured I60.6
  - ruptured I60.6
- congenital (peripheral) Q27.8
  - brain Q28.3
    - ruptured I60.7
  - pulmonary Q25.79
- ductus arteriosus Q25.0
- endocardial, infective (any valve) I33.0
- infective
  - endocardial (any valve) I33.0
- mycotic
  - endocardial (any valve) I33.0
  - ruptured, brain—*see* Hemorrhage, intracerebral, subarachnoid
- patent ductus arteriosus Q25.0
- pulmonary I28.1
  - arteriovenous Q25.72
- tricuspid (heart) (valve) I07.8

Angelman syndrome Q93.51

Anger R45.4

Angina (attack) (cardiac) (chest) (heart) (pectoris) (syndrome) (vasomotor) I20.9
- aphthous B08.5
- croupous J05.0
- exudative, chronic J37.0
- Ludovici K12.2
- Ludwig's K12.2
- membranous J05.0
- monocytic—*see* Mononucleosis, infectious
- phlegmonous J36
- tonsil J36
- trachealis J05.0

Angioedema (allergic) (any site) (with urticaria) T78.3
- episodic, with eosinophilia D72.118

Angioendothelioma—*see* Neoplasm, uncertain behavior, by site in Table of Neoplasms in the complete *ICD-10-CM* manual
- benign D18.00
  - skin D18.01
  - specified site NEC D18.09
- bone—*see* Neoplasm, bone, malignant in Table of Neoplasms in the complete *ICD-10-CM* manual
- Ewing's—*see* Neoplasm, bone, malignant in Table of Neoplasms in the complete *ICD-10-CM* manual

Angiohemophilia (A) (B) D68.0

Angioma—*see also* Hemangioma, by site
- capillary I78.1
- hemorrhagicum hereditaria I78.0
- malignant—*see* Neoplasm, connective tissue, malignant in Table of Neoplasms in the complete *ICD-10-CM* manual
- plexiform D18.00
  - skin D18.01
  - specified site NEC D18.09
- senile I78.1
- skin D18.01
- specified site NEC D18.09
- spider I78.1
- stellate I78.1

Angiomatosis Q82.8
- encephalotrigeminal Q85.8
- hemorrhagic familial I78.0
- hereditary familial I78.0

Angioneurosis F45.8

Angioneurotic edema (allergic) (any site) (with urticaria) T78.3

Angiopathia, angiopathy I99.9
- peripheral I73.9
  - specified type NEC I73.89

Angiospasm (peripheral) (traumatic) (vessel) I73.9
- cerebral G45.9

Angulation
- femur (acquired)—*see also* Deformity, limb, specified type NEC, thigh
  - congenital Q74.2
- tibia (acquired)—*see also* Deformity, limb, specified type NEC, lower leg
  - congenital Q74.2
- wrist (acquired)—*see also* Deformity, limb, specified type NEC, forearm
  - congenital Q74.0

Angulus infectiosus (lips) K13.0

Anhydration, anhydremia E86.0
- with
  - hypernatremia E87.0
  - hyponatremia E87.1

Anhydremia E86.0
- with
  - hypernatremia E87.0
  - hyponatremia E87.1

Aniridia (congenital) Q13.1

Anisocoria (pupil) H57.02
- congenital Q13.2

Ankyloblepharon (eyelid) (acquired)
- filiforme (adnatum) (congenital) Q10.3
- total Q10.3

Ankyloglossia Q38.1

Ankylosis (fibrous) (osseous) (joint) M24.60
- jaw (temporomandibular) M26.61-
- specified site NEC M24.69
- temporomandibular M26.61-

Anodontia (complete) (partial) (vera) K00.0
- acquired K08.10

Anomaly, anomalous (congenital) (unspecified type) Q89.9
- Alder (-Reilly) (leukocyte granulation) D72.0
- alimentary tract Q45.9
  - upper Q40.9
- ankle (joint) Q74.2
- aorta (arch) NEC Q25.40
  - absence and aplasia Q25.41
  - aneurysm (congenital) Q25.43
  - coarctation (preductal) (postductal) Q25.1
  - dilation (congenital) Q25.44
  - double arch Q25.45
  - hypoplasia Q25.42
  - right aortic arch Q25.47
  - tortuous arch Q25.46
- aqueduct of Sylvius Q03.0
  - with spina bifida—*see* Spina bifida, with hydrocephalus
- arm Q74.0
- artery (peripheral) Q27.9
  - eye Q15.8
  - pulmonary NEC Q25.79
  - retina Q14.1
  - subclavian Q27.8
    - origin Q25.48
  - umbilical Q27.0
- atrial
  - septa Q21.1
- atrioventricular
  - excitation I45.6
  - septum Q21.0
- Axenfeld's Q15.0
- biliary duct or passage Q44.5
- bladder Q64.70
  - absence Q64.5
  - diverticulum Q64.6
  - exstrophy Q64.10
    - cloacal Q64.12
    - extroversion Q64.19
    - specified type NEC Q64.19
    - supravesical fissure Q64.11
  - neck obstruction Q64.31
  - specified type NEC Q64.79
- bone Q79.9
  - arm Q74.0

Anomaly, *continued*
- leg Q74.2
- pelvic girdle Q74.2
- shoulder girdle Q74.0
- skull Q75.9
  - with
    - anencephaly Q00.0
    - encephalocele—*see* Encephalocele
    - hydrocephalus Q03.9
      - with spina bifida—*see* Spina bifida, by site, with hydrocephalus
    - microcephaly Q02
- broad ligament Q50.6
- bursa Q79.9
- canthus Q10.3
- cardiac Q24.9
- carpus Q74.0
- caruncle, lacrimal Q10.6
- cervix Q51.9
- cheek Q18.9
- chin Q18.9
- chromosomes, chromosomal Q99.9
  - D (1)—*see* condition, chromosome 13
  - E (3)—*see* condition, chromosome 18
  - G—*see* condition, chromosome 21
  - sex
    - female phenotype Q97.8
    - gonadal dysgenesis (pure) Q99.1
    - Klinefelter's Q98.4
    - male phenotype Q98.9
    - Turner's Q96.9
  - specified NEC Q99.8
- cilia Q10.3
- clavicle Q74.0
- common duct Q44.5
- communication
  - left ventricle with right atrium Q21.0
- connection
  - pulmonary venous Q26.4
    - partial Q26.3
    - total Q26.2
- cystic duct Q44.5
- dental
  - arch relationship M26.20
    - specified NEC M26.29
- dentofacial M26.9
  - dental arch relationship M26.20
    - specified NEC M26.29
  - jaw size M26.00
    - mandibular
      - hypoplasia M26.04
  - malocclusion M26.4
    - dental arch relationship NEC M26.29
  - specified type NEC M26.89
  - temporomandibular joint M26.60-
    - adhesions M26.61-
    - ankylosis M26.61-
    - arthralgia M26.62-
    - articular disc M26.63-
    - specified type NEC M26.69
- dermatoglyphic Q82.8
- digestive organ(s) or tract Q45.9
  - lower Q43.9
  - upper Q40.9
- ductus
  - arteriosus Q25.0
  - botalli Q25.0
- ear (external) Q17.9
- elbow Q74.0
- endocrine gland NEC Q89.2
- eye Q15.9
  - anterior segment Q13.9
    - specified NEC Q13.89
  - posterior segment Q14.9
    - specified NEC Q14.8
  - ptosis (eyelid) Q10.0
  - specified NEC Q15.8
- eyelid Q10.3
  - ptosis Q10.0
- face Q18.9
- fallopian tube Q50.6
- fascia Q79.9
- femur NEC Q74.2

Anomaly, *continued*
- fibula NEC Q74.2
- finger Q74.0
- flexion (joint) NOS Q74.9
  - hip or thigh Q65.89
- foot NEC Q74.2
  - varus (congenital) Q66.3-
- foramen
  - Botalli Q21.1
  - ovale Q21.1
- forearm Q74.0
- forehead Q75.8
- gastrointestinal tract Q45.9
- gallbladder (position) (shape) (size) Q44.1
- genitalia, genital organ(s) or system
  - female Q52.9
    - external Q52.70
    - internal Q52.9
  - male Q55.9
    - hydrocele P83.5
    - specified NEC Q55.8
- genitourinary NEC
  - female Q52.9
  - male Q55.9
- Gerbode Q21.0
- granulation or granulocyte, genetic (constitutional) (leukocyte) D72.0
- gyri Q07.9
- hand Q74.0
- heart Q24.9
  - patent ductus arteriosus (Botalli) Q25.0
  - septum Q21.9
    - auricular Q21.1
    - interatrial Q21.1
    - interventricular Q21.0
      - with pulmonary stenosis or atresia, dextraposition of aorta and hypertrophy of right ventricle Q21.3
    - specified NEC Q21.8
    - ventricular Q21.0
      - with pulmonary stenosis or atresia, dextraposition of aorta and hypertrophy of right ventricle Q21.3
  - tetralogy of Fallot Q21.3
  - valve NEC Q24.8
    - aortic
      - stenosis Q23.0
    - pulmonary Q22.3
      - stenosis Q22.1
- heel NEC Q74.2
- Hegglin's D72.0
- hepatic duct Q44.5
- hip NEC Q74.2
- humerus Q74.0
- hydatid of Morgagni
  - female Q50.5
  - male (epididymal) Q55.4
    - testicular Q55.29
- hypersegmentation of neutrophils, hereditary D72.0
- hypophyseal Q89.2
- ilium NEC Q74.2
- integument Q84.9
- ischium NEC Q74.2
- joint Q74.9
- Jordan's D72.0
- lens Q12.9
- leukocytes, genetic D72.0
  - granulation (constitutional) D72.0
- ligament Q79.9
  - broad Q50.6
  - round Q52.8
- limb Q74.9
  - lower NEC Q74.2
    - reduction deformity—*see* Defect, reduction, limb, lower
  - upper Q74.0
- liver Q44.7
  - duct Q44.5
- lower limb NEC Q74.2
- May (-Hegglin) D72.0
- meningeal bands or folds Q07.9
  - constriction of Q07.8
  - spinal Q06.9

Anomaly, *continued*
- meninges Q07.9
  - cerebral Q04.8
  - spinal Q06.9
- meningocele Q05.9
- mesentery Q45.9
- metacarpus Q74.0
- metatarsus NEC Q74.2
- multiple NEC Q89.7
- muscle Q79.9
- musculoskeletal system, except limbs Q79.9
- neck (any part) Q18.9
- nerve Q07.9
  - acoustic Q07.8
  - optic Q07.8
- nervous system (central) Q07.9
- omphalomesenteric duct Q43.0
- origin
  - artery
    - pulmonary Q25.79
- ovary Q50.39
- oviduct Q50.6
- parathyroid gland Q89.2
- Pelger-Huët (hereditary hyposegmentation) D72.0
- pelvic girdle NEC Q74.2
- pelvis (bony) NEC Q74.2
- penis (glans) Q55.69
- pigmentation L81.9
  - congenital Q82.8
- pituitary (gland) Q89.2
- prepuce Q55.69
- pulmonary Q33.9
  - artery NEC Q25.79
  - valve Q22.3
    - stenosis Q22.1
  - venous connection Q26.4
    - partial Q26.3
    - total Q26.2
- radius Q74.0
- respiratory system Q34.9
  - specified NEC Q34.8
- rotation
  - hip or thigh Q65.89
- round ligament Q52.8
- sacroiliac (joint) NEC Q74.2
- scapula Q74.0
- sex chromosomes NEC—*see also* Anomaly, chromosomes
  - female phenotype Q97.8
  - male phenotype Q98.9
- shoulder Q74.0
- simian crease Q82.8
- sinus of Valsalva Q25.49
- skull Q75.9
  - with
    - anencephaly Q00.0
    - encephalocele—*see* Encephalocele
    - hydrocephalus Q03.9
      - ~ with spina bifida—*see* Spina bifida, by site, with hydrocephalus
    - microcephaly Q02
- specified organ or site NEC Q89.8
- tarsus NEC Q74.2
- tendon Q79.9
- thigh NEC Q74.2
- thumb Q74.0
- thymus gland Q89.2
- thyroid (gland) Q89.2
  - cartilage Q31.8
- tibia NEC Q74.2
- toe NEC Q74.2
- tooth, teeth K00.9
  - eruption K00.6
- tragus Q17.9
- ulna Q74.0
- umbilical artery Q27.0
- upper limb Q74.0
- ureter Q62.8
  - obstructive NEC Q62.39
    - orthotopic ureterocele Q62.31
- urinary tract Q64.9
- uterus Q51.9
- ventricular

Anomaly, *continued*
- septa Q21.0
- vitelline duct Q43.0
- wrist Q74.0

Anonychia (congenital) Q84.3
- acquired L60.8

Anorchia, anorchism, anorchidism Q55.0

Anorexia R63.0
- nervosa F50.00
  - atypical F50.9
  - binge-eating type with purging F50.02
  - restricting type F50.01

Anosmia R43.0
- hysterical F44.6

Anovulatory cycle N97.0

Anoxemia R09.02
- newborn P84

Anoxia (pathological) R09.02
- cerebral G93.1
  - newborn P84
- due to
  - drowning T75.1
  - high altitude T70.29
- intrauterine P84
- newborn P84

Anteversion
- femur (neck), congenital Q65.89

Anthrax
- with pneumonia A22.1
- cutaneous A22.0
- colitis A22.2
- gastrointestinal A22.2
- inhalation A22.1
- intestinal A22.2
- pulmonary A22.1
- respiratory A22.1

Anthropoid pelvis Q74.2

Antibody
- antiphospholipid R76.0
  - with
    - hemorrhagic disorder D68.312
    - hypercoagulable state D68.61

Anticardiolipin syndrome D68.61

Anticoagulant, circulating (intrinsic)—*see also* Disorder, hemorrhagic D68.318
- drug-induced (extrinsic)—*see also* Disorder, hemorrhagic D68.32
- iatrogenic D68.32

Antidiuretic hormone syndrome E22.2

Antiphospholipid
- antibody
  - with hemorrhagic disorder D68.312
  - syndrome D68.61

Antisocial personality F60.2

Antritis J32.0
- maxilla J32.0
  - acute J01.00
    - recurrent J01.01

Anuria R34
- postrenal N13.8

Anusitis K62.89

Anxiety F41.9
- depression F41.8
- episodic paroxysmal F41.0
- hysteria F41.8
- panic type F41.0
- separation, abnormal (of childhood) F93.0
- social F40.1-
- specified NEC F41.8

Aorta (aortic arch) anomaly Q25.4-

Apepsia K30
- psychogenic F45.8

Apertognathia M26.09

Apert's syndrome Q87.0

Aphagia R13.0
- psychogenic F50.9

Aphakia (acquired) (postoperative) H27.0-
- congenital Q12.3

Aphasia (amnestic) (global) (nominal) (semantic) (syntactic)
- developmental (receptive type) F80.2
  - expressive type F80.1
  - Wernicke's F80.2
- sensory F80.2
- Wernicke's F80.2

Aphonia (organic) R49.1
- hysterical F44.4
- psychogenic F44.4

Aphthae, aphthous—*see also* Disease, diseased
- Bednar's K12.0
- cachectic K14.0
- oral (recurrent) K12.0
- stomatitis (major) (minor) K12.0
- thrush B37.0
- ulcer (oral) (recurrent) K12.0

Aplasia—*see also* Agenesis
- abdominal muscle syndrome Q79.4
- aorta (congenital) Q25.41
- bone marrow (myeloid) D61.9
  - congenital D61.01
- cervix (congenital) Q51.5
- congenital pure red cell D61.01
- corpus callosum Q04.0
- erythrocyte congenital D61.01
- gallbladder, congenital Q44.0
- parathyroid-thymic D82.1
- red cell (with thymoma) D60.9
  - acquired D60.9
    - due to drugs D60.9
  - chronic D60.0
  - congenital D61.01
  - constitutional D61.01
  - due to drugs D60.9
  - hereditary D61.01
  - of infants D61.01
  - primary D61.01
  - pure D61.01
    - due to drugs D60.9
    - transient D60.1
- round ligament Q52.8
- testicle Q55.0
- thymic, with immunodeficiency D82.1
- thyroid (congenital) (with myxedema) E03.1
- uterus Q51.0

Apnea, apneic (of) (spells) R06.81
- newborn NEC P28.4
  - obstructive P28.4
  - sleep (central) (obstructive) (primary) P28.3
- prematurity P28.4
- sleep G47.30
  - central (primary) G47.31
    - idiopathic G47.31
    - in conditions classified elsewhere G47.37
  - obstructive (adult) (pediatric) G47.33
    - hypopnea G47.33
  - primary central G47.31
  - specified NEC G47.39

Apneumatosis, newborn P28.0

Apophysitis (bone)—*see also* Osteochondropathy
- juvenile M92.9

Apoplexia, apoplexy, apoplectic
- heat T67.01

Appendage
- testicular (organ of Morgagni) Q55.29

Appendicitis (pneumococcal) (retrocecal) K37
- with
  - gangrene K35.891
  - perforation NOS K35.32
  - peritoneal abscess K35.33
  - peritonitis NEC K35.33
    - generalized (with perforation or rupture) K35.20
    - with abscess K35.21
    - localized K35.30
      - ~ with
        - ◊ gangrene K35.31
        - ◊ perforation K35.32
          - » and abscess K35.33

Appendicitis, *continued*
- ■ rupture K35.32
- • acute (catarrhal) (fulminating) (gangrenous) (obstructive) (retrocecal) (suppurative) K35.80
  - – with
    - ■ gangrene K35.891
    - ■ peritoneal abscess K35.33
    - ■ peritonitis NEC K35.33
      - ~ generalized (with perforation or rupture) K35.20
        - ◊ with abscess K35.21
      - ~ localized K35.30
        - ◊ with
          - » gangrene K35.31
          - » perforation K35.32
            - ❖ and abscess K35.33
  - – specified NEC K35.890
    - ■ with gangrene K35.891
- • ruptured NOS (with local peritonitis) K35.32

Appendicopathia oxyurica B80

Appendix, appendicular—*see also* Disease, diseased
- • Morgagni
  - – female Q50.5
  - – male (epididymal) Q55.4
    - ■ testicular Q55.29
- • testis Q55.29

Appetite
- • depraved—*see* Pica
- • excessive R63.2
- • lack or loss (*see also* Anorexia) R63.0
  - – nonorganic origin F50.89
  - – psychogenic F50.89
- • perverted (hysterical)—*see* Pica

Apprehensiveness, abnormal F41.9

ARC (AIDS-related complex) B20

Arch
- • aortic Q25.49
- • bovine Q25.49

Arcuate uterus Q51.810

Arcuatus uterus Q51.810

Arnold-Chiari disease, obstruction or syndrome (type II) Q07.00
- • with
  - – hydrocephalus Q07.02
    - ■ with spina bifida Q07.03
  - – spina bifida Q07.01
    - ■ with hydrocephalus Q07.03
- • type III—*see* Encephalocele
- • type IV Q04.8

Arousals, confusional G47.51

Arrest, arrested
- • cardiac I46.9
  - – due to
    - ■ cardiac condition I46.2
    - ■ specified condition NEC I46.8
  - – newborn P29.81
  - – postprocedural I97.12-
- • development or growth
  - – child R62.50
- • epiphyseal
  - – complete
    - ■ femur M89.15-
    - ■ humerus M89.12-
    - ■ tibia M89.16-
    - ■ ulna M89.13-
  - – forearm M89.13-
    - ■ specified NEC M89.13-
    - ■ ulna—*see* Arrest, epiphyseal, by type, ulna
  - – lower leg M89.16-
    - ■ specified NEC M89.168
    - ■ tibia—*see* Arrest, epiphyseal, by type, tibia
  - – partial
    - ■ femur M89.15-
    - ■ humerus M89.12-
    - ■ tibia M89.16-
    - ■ ulna M89.13-
  - – specified NEC M89.18
- • growth plate—*see* Arrest, epiphyseal
- • physeal—*see* Arrest, epiphyseal
- • respiratory R09.2
  - – newborn P28.81

Arrhythmia (auricle) (cardiac) (juvenile) (nodal) (reflex) (supraventricular) (transitory) (ventricle) I49.9
- • block I45.9
- • newborn
  - – bradycardia P29.12
  - – occurring before birth P03.819
    - ■ before onset of labor P03.810
    - ■ during labor P03.811
  - – tachycardia P29.11
- • psychogenic F45.8
- • sinus I49.8
- • vagal R55

Arrillaga-Ayerza syndrome (pulmonary sclerosis with pulmonary hypertension) I27.0

Arsenical pigmentation L81.8
- • from drug or medicament—*see* Table of Drugs and Chemicals

Arteriosclerosis, arteriosclerotic (diffuse) (obliterans) (of) (senile) (with calcification) I70.90
- • pulmonary (idiopathic) I27.0

Arteritis I77.6
- • cerebral I67.7
  - – in
    - ■ systemic lupus erythematosus M32.19
- • coronary (artery) I25.89
  - – rheumatic I01.8
    - ■ chronic I09.89

Artery, arterial—*see also* Disease, diseased
- • single umbilical Q27.0

Arthralgia (allergic)—*see also* Pain, joint
- • temporomandibular M26.62-

Arthritis, arthritic (acute) (chronic) (nonpyogenic) (subacute) M19.9-
- • due to or associated with
  - – acromegaly (*see also* subcategory M14.8-) E22.0
  - – bacterial disease (*see also* subcategory M01) A49.9
  - – erysipelas (*see also* category M01) A46
  - – erythema
    - ■ nodosum L52
  - – hemophilia D66 [M36.2]
  - – Henoch- (Schönlein) purpura D69.0 [M36.4]
  - – human parvovirus (*see also* category M01) B97.6
  - – Lyme disease A69.23
  - – rat bite fever (*see also* M01) A25.1
  - – serum sickness (*see also* Reaction, serum) T80.69
- • in (due to)
  - – acromegaly (*see also* subcategory M14.8-) E22.0
  - – endocrine disorder NEC (*see also* subcategory M14.8-) E34.9
  - – enteritis, infectious NEC (*see also* category M01) A09
  - – erythema
    - ■ multiforme (*see also* subcategory M14.8-) L51.9
    - ■ nodosum (*see also* subcategory M14.8-) L52
  - – hemochromatosis (*see also* subcategory M14.8-) E83.118
  - – hemoglobinopathy NEC D58.2 [M36.3]
  - – hemophilia NEC D66 [M36.2]
  - – Hemophilus influenzae M00.8- [B96.3]
  - – Henoch (-Schönlein)purpura D69.0 [M36.4]
  - – hypogammaglobulinemia (*see also* subcategory M14.8-) D80.1
  - – hypothyroidism NEC (*see also* subcategory M14.8-) E03.9
  - – infection—*see* Arthritis, pyogenic or pyemic
  - – infectious disease NEC—*see* category M01
  - – Lyme disease A69.23
  - – metabolic disorder NEC (*see also* subcategory M14.8-) E88.9
  - – respiratory disorder NEC (*see also* subcategory M14.8-) J98.9
  - – Salmonella (arizonae) (choleraesuis) (typhimurium) A02.23
    - ■ specified organism NEC (*see also* category M01) A08.8
  - – sarcoidosis D86.86
  - – thalassemia NEC D56.9 [M36.3]
- • juvenile M08.90
  - – with systemic onset—*see* Still's disease
  - – ankle M08.97-
  - – elbow M08.92-
  - – foot joint M08.97-

Arthritis, arthritic, *continued*
- – hand joint M08.94-
- – hip M08.95-
- – knee M08.96-
- – multiple site M08.99
- – pauciarticular M08.40
  - ■ ankle M08.47-
  - ■ elbow M08.42-
  - ■ foot joint M08.47-
  - ■ hand joint M08.44-
  - ■ hip M08.45-
  - ■ knee M08.46-
  - ■ shoulder M08.41-
  - ■ specified site NEC M08.4A
  - ■ vertebrae M08.48
  - ■ wrist M08.43-
- – rheumatoid—*see* Arthritis, rheumatoid, juvenile
- – shoulder M08.91-
- – specified site NEC M08.9A
- – vertebra M08.98
- – specified type NEC M08.8-
  - ■ ankle M08.87-
  - ■ elbow M08.82-
  - ■ foot joint M08.87-
  - ■ hand joint M08.84-
  - ■ hip M08.85-
  - ■ knee M08.86-
  - ■ multiple site M08.89
  - ■ shoulder M08.81-
  - ■ specified joint NEC M08.88
  - ■ vertebrae M08.88
  - ■ wrist M08.83-
- – wrist M08.93-
- • pneumococcal M00.10
  - – ankle M00.17-
  - – elbow M00.12-
  - – foot joint M00.17-
  - – hand joint M00.14-
  - – hip M00.15-
  - – knee M00.16-
  - – multiple site M00.19
  - – shoulder M00.11-
  - – vertebra M00.18
  - – wrist M00.13-
- • pyogenic or pyemic (any site except spine) M00.9
  - – bacterial NEC M00.80
    - ■ ankle M00.87-
    - ■ elbow M00.82-
    - ■ foot joint M00.87-
    - ■ hand joint M00.84-
    - ■ hip M00.85-
    - ■ knee M00.86-
    - ■ multiple site M00.89
    - ■ shoulder M00.81-
    - ■ vertebra M00.88
    - ■ wrist M00.83-
  - – pneumococcal—*see* Arthritis, pneumococcal
  - – spine—*see* Spondylopathy, infective
  - – staphylococcal—*see* Arthritis, staphylococcal
  - – streptococcal—*see* Arthritis, streptococcal NEC
    - ■ pneumococcal—*see* Arthritis, pneumococcal
- • rheumatoid M06.9
  - – juvenile (with or without rheumatoid factor) M08.00
    - ■ ankle M08.07-
    - ■ elbow M08.02-
    - ■ foot joint M08.07-
    - ■ hand joint M08.04-
    - ■ hip M08.05-
    - ■ knee M08.06-
    - ■ multiple site M08.09
    - ■ shoulder M08.01-
    - ■ vertebra M08.08
    - ■ wrist M08.03-
- • septic (any site except spine)—*see* Arthritis, pyogenic or pyemic
- • staphylococcal M00.00
  - – ankle M00.07-
  - – elbow M00.02-
  - – foot joint M00.07-
  - – hand joint M00.04-
  - – hip M00.05-
  - – knee M00.06-
  - – multiple site M00.09

Arthritis, arthritic, *continued*
- – shoulder M00.01-
- – vertebra M00.08
- – wrist M00.03-
- • streptococcal NEC M00.20
  - – ankle M00.27-
  - – elbow M00.22-
  - – foot joint M00.07-
  - – hand joint M00.24-
  - – hip M00.25-
  - – knee M00.26-
  - – multiple site M00.29
  - – shoulder M00.21-
  - – vertebra M00.28
  - – wrist M00.23-
- • suppurative—*see* Arthritis, pyogenic or pyemic
- • temporomandibular M26.64-

Arthrodysplasia Q74.9

Arthrogryposis (congenital) Q68.8
- • multiplex congenita Q74.3

Arthropathy (*see also* Arthritis) M12.9
- • hemophilic NEC D66 [M36.2]
- • in (due to)
  - – acromegaly E22.0 [M14.8-]
  - – *blood disorder NOS D75.9 [M36.3]*
  - – endocrine disease NOS E34.9 [M14.8-]
  - – erythema
    - ◾ multiforme L51.9 [M14.8-]
    - ◾ nodosum L52 [M14.8-]
  - – hemochromatosis E83.118 [M14.8-]
  - – hemoglobinopathy NEC D58.2 [M36.3]
  - – hemophilia NEC D66 [M36.2]
  - – Henoch-Schönlein purpura D69.0 [M36.4]
  - – hypothyroidism E03.9 [M14.8-]
  - – infective endocarditis I33.0 [M12.8-]
  - – metabolic disease NOS E88.9 [M14.8-]
  - – neoplastic disease NOS (*see also* Table of Neoplasms in the complete *ICD-10-CM* manual) D49.9 [M36.1]
  - – nutritional deficiency (*see also* subcategory M14.8-) E63.9
  - – sarcoidosis D86.86
  - – thyrotoxicosis (*see also* subcategory M14.8-) E05.90
  - – ulcerative colitis K51.90 [M07.6-]
  - – viral hepatitis (postinfectious) NEC B19.9 [M12.8-]
  - – Whipple's disease (*see also* subcategory M14.8-) K90.81
- • postinfectious NEC B99 [M12.8-]
  - – in (due to)
    - ◾ viral hepatitis NEC B19.9 [M12.8-]
- • temporomandibular joint M26.65-
- • traumatic M12.50
  - – ankle M12.57-
  - – elbow M12.52-
  - – foot joint M12.57-
  - – hand joint M12.54-
  - – hip M12.55-
  - – knee M12.56-
  - – multiple site M12.59
  - – shoulder M12.51-
  - – specified joint NEC M12.58
  - – vertebrae M12.58
  - – wrist M12.53-

Artificial
- • opening status (functioning) (without complication) Z93.9
  - – gastrostomy Z93.1

Ascariasis B77.9
- • with
  - – complications NEC B77.89
  - – intestinal complications B77.0
  - – pneumonia, pneumonitis B77.81

Ascites (abdominal) R18.8
- • cardiac I50.9
- • heart I50.9
- • malignant R18.0
- • pseudochylous R18.8

Asocial personality F60.2

Aspartylglucosaminuria E77.1

Asperger's disease or syndrome F84.5

Asphyxia, asphyxiation (by) R09.01
- • antenatal P84
- • birth P84
- • bunny bag—*see* Asphyxia, due to, mechanical threat to breathing, trapped in bed clothes
- • drowning T75.1
- • gas, fumes, or vapor—*see* Table of Drugs and Chemicals
- • inhalation—*see* Inhalation
- • intrauterine P84
- • newborn P84
- • pathological R09.01
- • postnatal P84
  - – mechanical—*see* Asphyxia, due to, mechanical threat to breathing
- • prenatal P84
- • reticularis R23.1
- • strangulation—*see* Asphyxia, due to, mechanical threat to breathing
- • submersion T75.1
- • traumatic T71.9
  - – due to
    - ◾ foreign body (in)—*see* Foreign body, respiratory tract, causing, asphyxia
    - ◾ low oxygen content of ambient air T71.2-
      - ~ due to
        - ◊ being trapped in
          - » low oxygen environment T71.29
            - ❖ in car trunk T71.221
              - ★ circumstances undetermined T71.224
              - ★ done with intent to harm by
                - ✓ another person T71.223
                - ✓ self T71.222
            - ❖ in refrigerator T71.231
              - ★ circumstances undetermined T71.234
              - ★ done with intent to harm by
                - ✓ another person T71.233
                - ✓ self T71.232
        - ◊ cave-in T71.21
    - ◾ mechanical threat to breathing (accidental) T71.191
      - ~ circumstances undetermined T71.194
      - ~ done with intent to harm by
        - ◊ another person T71.193
        - ◊ self T71.192
      - ~ hanging T71.161
        - ◊ circumstances undetermined T71.164
        - ◊ done with intent to harm by
          - » another person T71.163
          - » self T71.162
      - ~ plastic bag T71.121
        - ◊ circumstances undetermined T71.124
        - ◊ done with intent to harm by
          - » another person T71.123
          - » self T71.122
      - ~ smothering
        - ◊ in furniture T71.151
          - » circumstances undetermined T71.154
          - » done with intent to harm by
            - ❖ another person T71.153
            - ❖ self T71.152
        - ◊ under
          - » another person's body T71.141
            - ❖ circumstances undetermined T71.144
            - ❖ done with intent to harm T71.143
          - » pillow T71.111
            - ❖ circumstances undetermined T71.114
            - ❖ done with intent to harm by
              - ★ another person T71.113
              - ★ self T71.112
      - ~ trapped in bed clothes T71.131
        - ◊ circumstances undetermined T71.134
        - ◊ done with intent to harm by
          - » another person T71.133
          - » self T71.132
- • vomiting, vomitus—*see* Foreign body, respiratory tract, causing, asphyxia

Aspiration
- • amniotic (clear) fluid (newborn) P24.10
  - – with
    - ◾ pneumonia (pneumonitis) P24.11
    - ◾ respiratory symptoms P24.11

Aspiration, *continued*
- • blood
  - – newborn (without respiratory symptoms) P24.20
    - ◾ with
      - ~ pneumonia (pneumonitis) P24.21
      - ~ respiratory symptoms P24.21
  - – specified age NEC—*see* Foreign body, respiratory tract
- • bronchitis J69.0
- • food or foreign body (with asphyxiation)—*see* Asphyxia
- • liquor (amnii) (newborn) P24.10
  - – with
    - ◾ pneumonia (pneumonitis) P24.11
    - ◾ respiratory symptoms P24.11
- • meconium (newborn) (without respiratory symptoms) P24.00
  - – with
    - ◾ pneumonitis (pneumonitis) P24.01
    - ◾ respiratory symptoms P24.01
- • milk (newborn) (without respiratory symptoms) P24.30
  - – with
    - ◾ pneumonia (pneumonitis) P24.31
    - ◾ respiratory symptoms P24.31
  - – specified age NEC—*see* Foreign body, respiratory tract
- • mucus—*see also* Foreign body, by site
  - – newborn P24.10
    - ◾ with
      - ~ pneumonia (pneumonitis) P24.11
      - ~ respiratory symptoms P24.11
- • neonatal P24.9
  - – specific NEC (without respiratory symptoms) P24.80
    - ◾ with
      - ~ pneumonia (pneumonitis) P24.81
      - ~ respiratory symptoms P24.81
- • newborn P24.9
  - – specific NEC (without respiratory symptoms) P24.80
    - ◾ with
      - ~ pneumonia (pneumonitis) P24.81
      - ~ respiratory symptoms P24.81
- • pneumonia J69.0
- • pneumonitis J69.0
- • syndrome of newborn—*see* Aspiration, by substance, with pneumonia
- • vernix caseosa (newborn) P24.80
  - – with
    - ◾ pneumonia (pneumonitis) P24.81
    - ◾ respiratory symptoms P24.81
- • vomitus—*see also* Foreign body, respiratory tract
  - – newborn (without respiratory symptoms) P24.30
    - ◾ with
      - ~ pneumonia (pneumonitis) P24.31
      - ~ respiratory symptoms P24.31

Asplenia (congenital) Q89.01

Astasia (-abasia) (hysterical) F44.4

Asthenia, asthenic R53.1
- • cardiac (*see also* Failure, heart) I50.9
  - – psychogenic F45.8
- • cardiovascular (*see also* Failure, heart) I50.9
  - – psychogenic F45.8
- • heart (*see also* Failure, heart) I50.9
  - – psychogenic F45.8
- • hysterical F44.4
- • myocardial (*see also* Failure, heart) I50.9
  - – psychogenic F45.8
- • nervous F48.8
- • neurocirculatory F45.8

Asthenopia
- • hysterical F44.6
- • psychogenic F44.6

Asthma, asthmatic (bronchial) (catarrh) (spasmodic) J45.909
- • with
  - – exacerbation (acute) J45.901
  - – hay fever—*see* Asthma, allergic extrinsic
  - – rhinitis, allergic—*see* Asthma, allergic extrinsic
  - – status asthmaticus J45.902
- • allergic extrinsic J45.909
  - – with
    - ◾ exacerbation (acute) J45.901
    - ◾ status asthmaticus J45.902
- • atopic—*see* Asthma, allergic extrinsic

Asthma, asthmatic, *continued*
- childhood J45.909
  - with
    - exacerbation (acute) J45.901
    - status asthmaticus J45.902
- cough variant J45.991
- detergent J69.8
- due to
  - detergent J69.8
- extrinsic, allergic—*see* Asthma, allergic extrinsic
- hay—*see* Asthma, allergic extrinsic
- idiosyncratic—*see* Asthma, nonallergic
- intermittent (mild) J45.20
  - with
    - exacerbation (acute) J45.21
    - status asthmaticus J45.22
- intrinsic, nonallergic—*see* Asthma, nonallergic
- late onset J45.909
  - with
    - exacerbation (acute) J45.901
    - status asthmaticus J45.902
- mild intermittent J45.20
  - with
    - exacerbation (acute) J45.21
    - status asthmaticus J45.22
- mild persistent J45.30
  - with
    - exacerbation (acute) J45.31
    - status asthmaticus J45.32
- mixed J45.909
  - with
    - exacerbation (acute) J45.901
    - status asthmaticus J45.902
- moderate persistent J45.40
  - with
    - exacerbation (acute) J45.41
    - status asthmaticus J45.42
- nervous—*see* Asthma, nonallergic
- nonallergic (intrinsic) J45.909
  - with
    - exacerbation (acute) J45.901
    - status asthmaticus J45.902
- persistent
  - mild J45.30
    - with
      - ~ exacerbation (acute) J45.31
      - ~ status asthmaticus J45.32
  - moderate J45.40
    - with
      - ~ exacerbation (acute) J45.41
      - ~ status asthmaticus J45.42
  - severe J45.50
    - with
      - ~ exacerbation (acute) J45.51
      - ~ status asthmaticus J45.52
- predominantly allergic J45.909
- severe persistent J45.50
  - with
    - exacerbation (acute) J45.51
    - status asthmaticus J45.52
- specified NEC J45.998

Astroblastoma
- specified site—*see* Neoplasm, malignant, by site in Table of Neoplasms in the complete *ICD-10-CM* manual
- unspecified site C71.9

Astrocytoma (cystic)
- anaplastic
  - specified site—*see* Neoplasm, malignant, by site in Table of Neoplasms in the complete *ICD-10-CM* manual
  - unspecified site C71.9
- fibrillary
  - specified site—*see* Neoplasm, malignant, by site in Table of Neoplasms in the complete *ICD-10-CM* manual
  - unspecified site C71.9
- fibrous
  - specified site—*see* Neoplasm, malignant, by site in Table of Neoplasms in the complete *ICD-10-CM* manual
  - unspecified site C71.9

Astrocytoma (cystic), *continued*
- gemistocytic
  - specified site—*see* Neoplasm, malignant, by site in Table of Neoplasms in the complete *ICD-10-CM* manual
  - unspecified site C71.9
- juvenile
  - specified site—*see* Neoplasm, malignant, by site in Table of Neoplasms in the complete *ICD-10-CM* manual
  - unspecified site C71.9
- pilocytic
  - specified site—*see* Neoplasm, malignant, by site in Table of Neoplasms in the complete *ICD-10-CM* manual
  - unspecified site C71.9
- piloid
  - specified site—*see* Neoplasm, malignant, by site in Table of Neoplasms in the complete *ICD-10-CM* manual
  - unspecified site C71.9
- protoplasmic
  - specified site—*see* Neoplasm, malignant, by site in Table of Neoplasms in the complete *ICD-10-CM* manual
  - unspecified site C71.9
- unspecified site C71.9

Astroglioma
- specified site—*see* Neoplasm, malignant, by site in Table of Neoplasms in the complete *ICD-10-CM* manual
- unspecified site C71.9

Asymmetrical face Q67.0

At risk
- for
  - dental caries Z91.849
    - high Z91.843
    - low Z91.841
    - moderate Z91.842
  - falling Z91.81

Ataxia, ataxy, ataxic R27.0
- autosomal recessive Friedreich G11.11
- cerebellar (hereditary) G11.9
  - with defective DNA repair G11.3
  - early-onset G11.10
  - in
    - myxedema E03.9 *[G13.2]*
    - neoplastic disease (*see also* Table of Neoplasms in the complete *ICD-10-CM* manual) D49.9 *[G32.81]*
    - specified disease NEC G32.81
  - late-onset (Marie's) G11.2
  - with
    - essential tremor G11.19
    - myoclonus [Hunt's ataxia] G11.19
    - retained tendon reflexes G11.19
- Friedreich's (heredofamilial) (cerebellar) (spinal) G11.11
- gait R26.0
  - hysterical F44.4
- gluten M35.9 *[G32.81]*
  - with celiac disease K90.0 *[G32.81]*
- hereditary G11.9
  - cerebellar—*see* Ataxia, cerebellar
  - spinal (Friedreich's) G11.11
- heredofamilial—*see* Ataxia, hereditary
- Hunt's G11.19
- hysterical F44.4
- Marie's (cerebellar) (heredofamilial) (late- onset) G11.2
- nonorganic origin F44.4
- nonprogressive, congenital G11.0
- psychogenic F44.4
- SangerBrown's (hereditary) G11.2
- spinal
  - hereditary (Friedreich's) G11.11
- spinocerebellar, Xlinked recessive G11.11
- telangiectasia (LouisBar) G11.3

Ataxia-telangiectasia (Louis-Bar) G11.3

Atelectasis (massive) (partial) (pressure) (pulmonary) J98.11
- newborn P28.10
  - due to resorption P28.11
  - partial P28.19
  - primary P28.0
  - secondary P28.19
- primary (newborn) P28.0

Atelocardia Q24.9

Atheroma, atheromatous (*see also* Arteriosclerosis) I70.90
- aorta, aortic I70.0
  - valve (*see also* Endocarditis, aortic) I35.8
- pulmonary valve (heart) (*see also* Endocarditis, pulmonary) I37.8
- tricuspid (heart) (valve) I36.8
- valve, valvular—*see* Endocarditis

Athlete's
- foot B35.3
- heart I51.7

Athyrea (acquired)—*see also* Hypothyroidism
- congenital E03.1

Atonia, atony, atonic
- capillary I78.8
- congenital P94.2
- esophagus K22.89
- intestine K59.89
  - psychogenic F45.8
- stomach K31.89
  - neurotic or psychogenic F45.8
- uterus (during labor)
  - without hemorrhage O75.89

Atransferrinemia, congenital E88.09

Atresia, atretic
- alimentary organ or tract NEC Q45.8
  - upper Q40.8
- ani, anus, anal (canal) Q42.3
  - with fistula Q42.2
- aortic (orifice) (valve) Q23.0
  - congenital with hypoplasia of ascending aorta and defective development of left ventricle (with mitral stenosis) Q23.4
  - in hypoplastic left heart syndrome Q23.4
- aqueduct of Sylvius Q03.0
  - with spina bifida—*see* Spina bifida, with hydrocephalus
- artery NEC Q27.8
  - umbilical Q27.0
- bile duct (common) (congenital) (hepatic) Q44.2
  - acquired—*see* Obstruction, bile duct
- cecum Q42.8
- cervix (acquired) N88.2
  - congenital Q51.828
- choana Q30.0
- colon Q42.9
  - specified NEC Q42.8
- common duct Q44.2
- cystic duct Q44.2
  - acquired K82.8
    - with obstruction K82.0
- digestive organs NEC Q45.8
- esophagus Q39.0
  - with tracheoesophageal fistula Q39.1
- fallopian tube (congenital) Q50.6
  - acquired N97.1
- follicular cyst N83.0-
- foramen of
  - Luschka Q03.1
    - with spina bifida—*see* Spina bifida, with hydrocephalus
  - Magendie Q03.1
    - with spina bifida—*see* Spina bifida, with hydrocephalus
- gallbladder Q44.1
- genital organ
  - external
    - female Q52.79
    - male Q55.8
  - internal
    - female Q52.8
    - male Q55.8
- gullet Q39.0
  - with tracheoesophageal fistula Q39.1
- hymen Q52.3
  - acquired (postinfective) N89.6
- intestine (small) Q41.9
  - large Q42.9
    - specified NEC Q42.8
- iris, filtration angle Q15.0

Atresia, atretic, *continued*
- mitral valve Q23.2
  - in hypoplastic left heart syndrome Q23.4
- nares (anterior) (posterior) Q30.0
- nose, nostril Q30.0
  - acquired J34.89
- organ or site NEC Q89.8
- oviduct (congenital) Q50.6
  - acquired N97.1
- rectum Q42.1
  - with fistula Q42.0
- ureter Q62.10
  - pelvic junction Q62.11
  - vesical orifice Q62.12
- ureteropelvic junction Q62.11
- ureterovesical orifice Q62.12
- uterus Q51.818
  - acquired N85.8
- vagina (congenital) Q52.4
  - acquired (postinfectional) (senile) N89.5
- vein NEC Q27.8
  - pulmonary Q26.4
    - partial Q26.3
    - total Q26.2

Atrophy, atrophic (of)
- adrenal (capsule) (gland) E27.49
  - primary (autoimmune) E27.1
- buccal cavity K13.79
- facioscapulohumeral (Landouzy-Déjérine) G71.02
- hemifacial Q67.4
  - Romberg G51.8
- Landouzy-Déjérine G71.02
- laryngitis, infective J37.0
- lip K13.0
- muscle, muscular (diffuse) (general) (idiopathic) (primary)
  - infantile spinal G12.0
  - progressive (bulbar) G12.21
    - infantile (spinal) G12.0
    - spinal G12
      - infantile G12.0
  - pseudohypertrophic G71.02
  - spinal G12.9
    - infantile, type I (Werdnig-Hoffmann) G12.0
- nail L60.3
- pseudohypertrophic (muscle) G71.0
- rhinitis J31.0
- scar L90.5
- suprarenal (capsule) (gland) E27.49
  - primary E27.1
- systemic affecting central nervous system
  - in
    - myxedema E03.9 *[G13.2]*
    - neoplastic disease (*see also* Table of Neoplasms in the complete *ICD-10-CM* manual) D49.9 *[G13.1]*
    - specified disease NEC G13.8
- testes N50.0
- thyroid (gland) (acquired) E03.4
  - with cretinism E03.1
  - congenital (with myxedema) E03.1
- turbinate J34.89
- WerdnigHoffmann G12.0

Attack, attacks
- AdamsStokes I45.9
- benign shuddering G25.83
- cyanotic, newborn P28.2
- drop NEC R55
- epileptic—*see* Epilepsy
- hysterical F44.9
- panic F41.0
- shuddering, benign G25.83
- StokesAdams I45.9
- syncope R55
- transient ischemic (TIA) G45.9
  - specified NEC G45.8
- unconsciousness R55
  - hysterical F44.89
- vasomotor R55
- vasovagal (paroxysmal) (idiopathic) R55
- without alteration of consciousness—*see* Epilepsy, syndromes, localization-related, symptomatic, with simple partial seizure

Attention (to)
- artificial
  - opening (of) Z43.9
    - digestive tract NEC Z43.4
      - ~ stomach Z43.1
    - specified NEC Z43.8
    - trachea Z43.0
    - urinary tract NEC Z43.6
      - ~ cystostomy Z43.5
      - ~ nephrostomy Z43.6
      - ~ ureterostomy Z43.6
      - ~ urethrostomy Z43.6
- colostomy Z43.3
- cystostomy Z43.5
- deficit disorder or syndrome F98.8
  - with hyperactivity—*see* Disorder, attention-deficit hyperactivity
- gastrostomy Z43.1
- ileostomy Z43.2
- jejunostomy Z43.4
- nephrostomy Z43.6
- surgical dressings Z48.01
- sutures Z48.02
- tracheostomy Z43.0
- ureterostomy Z43.6
- urethrostomy Z43.6

Austin Flint murmur (aortic insufficiency) I35.1

Autism, autistic (childhood) (infantile) F84.0
- atypical F84.9
- spectrum disorder F84.0

Autoerythrocyte sensitization (syndrome) D69.2

Autographism L50.3

Autoimmune
- disease (systemic) M35.9
- lymphoproliferative syndrome *[ALPS]* D89.82
- thyroiditis E06.3

Automatism G93.89
- with temporal sclerosis G93.81
- epileptic—*see* Epilepsy, localization-related, symptomatic, with complex partial seizures
- paroxysmal, idiopathic—*see* Epilepsy, localization-related, symptomatic, with complex partial seizures

Autosensitivity, erythrocyte D69.2

Aversion
- oral R63.39
  - newborn P92.-
  - nonorganic origin F98.2

Avitaminosis (multiple) (*see also* Deficiency, vitamin) E56.9
- D E55.9
  - with rickets E55.0

AVNRT (atrioventricular nodal re-entrant tachycardia) I47.1

AVRT (atrioventricular nodal re-entrant tachycardia) I47.1

Avulsion (traumatic)
- spleen S36.032

Awareness of heart beat R00.2

Axenfeld's
- anomaly or syndrome Q15.0

Ayerza's disease or syndrome (pulmonary artery sclerosis with pulmonary hypertension) I27.0

Azotemia R79.89
- meaning uremia N19

B

Babesiosis B60.00
- due to
  - Babesia
    - divergens B60.03
    - duncani B60.02
    - KO-1 B60.09
    - microti B60.01
    - MO-1 B60.03
    - species
      - ~ unspecified B60.00
    - venatorum B60.09
  - specified NEC B60.09

Babington's disease (familial hemorrhagic telangiectasia) I78.0

Baby
- crying constantly R68.11
- floppy (syndrome) P94.2

Bacilluria R82.71

Bacillus
- coli infection (*see also* Escherichia coli) B96.20
- Shiga's A03.0
- suipestifer infection—*see* Infection, salmonella

Backache (postural) M54.9
- sacroiliac M53.3

Backward reading (dyslexia) F81.0

Bacteremia R78.81
- with sepsis—*see* Sepsis

Bacterium, bacteria, bacterial
- agent NEC, as cause of disease classified elsewhere B96.89
- in blood—*see* Bacteremia
- in urine R82.71

Bacteriuria, bacteruria R82.71
- asymptomatic R82.71
- urinary tract infection N39.0

Baelz's disease (cheilitis glandularis apostematosa) K13.0

Baerensprung's disease (eczema marginatum) B35.6

Balanitis (circinata) (erosiva) (gangrenosa) (phagedenic) (vulgaris) N48.1
- candidal B37.42

Balanoposthitis N47.6

Band(s)
- gallbladder (congenital) Q44.1
- vagina N89.5

Bandemia D72.825

Bankruptcy, anxiety concerning Z59.89

Bannister's disease T78.3

Bartonellosis A44.9
- cutaneous A44.1
- mucocutaneous A44.1
- specified NEC A44.8
- systemic A44.0

Barton's fracture S52.56-

Basophilia D72.824

Basophilism (cortico-adrenal) (Cushing's) (pituitary) E24.0

Bateman's
- disease B08.1
- purpura (senile) D69.2

Bathing cramp T75.1

Battle exhaustion F43.0

Beach ear—*see* Swimmer's, ear

Beat(s)
- atrial, premature I49.1
- premature I49.40
  - atrial I49.1
  - auricular I49.1
  - supraventricular I49.1

Becker's
- disease
  - myotonia congenita, recessive form G71.12
- dystrophy G71.01

Beckwith-Wiedemann syndrome Q87.3

Bedbug bite(s)—*see* Bite(s), by site, superficial, insect

Bedclothes, asphyxiation or suffocation by—*see* Asphyxia, traumatic

Bednar's
- aphthae K12.0

Bedwetting—*see* Enuresis

Bee sting (with allergic or anaphylactic shock)—*see* Table of Drugs and Chemicals, by animal or substance, poisoning

Behavior
- drug seeking Z76.5
- self-damaging (lifestyle) Z72.89

Bell's
- palsy, paralysis G51.0
  - infant or newborn P11.3

Bence Jones albuminuria or proteinuria NEC R80.3

Bennett's fracture (displaced) S62.21-

Bite(s), *continued*
- malar region—*see* Bite, head, specified site NEC
- mammary—*see* Bite, breast
- marine animals (venomous)—*see* Table of Drugs and Chemicals, by animal or substance, poisoning
- mastoid region—*see* Bite, head, specified site NEC
- mouth—*see* Bite, oral cavity
- nail
  - finger—*see* Bite, finger
  - toe—*see* Bite, toe
- nape—*see* Bite, neck, specified site NEC
- nasal (septum) (sinus)—*see* Bite, nose
- nasopharynx—*see* Bite, head, specified site NEC
- neck (code to Bite by specific site for esophagus, larynx, pharynx, or trachea) S11.95
  - involving
  - specified site NEC S11.85
    - superficial NEC S10.87
      - ~ insect S10.86
  - superficial NEC S10.97
    - insect S10.96
  - throat S11.85
    - superficial NEC S10.17
      - ~ insect S10.16
- nose (septum) (sinus) S01.25
  - superficial NEC S00.37
    - insect S00.36
- occipital region—*see* Bite, scalp
- oral cavity S01.552
  - superficial NEC S00.572
    - insect S00.562
- orbital region—*see* Bite, eyelid
- palate—*see* Bite, oral cavity
- palm—*see* Bite, hand
- parietal region—*see* Bite, scalp
- pelvis S31.050
  - superficial NEC S30.870
    - insect S30.860
- penis S31.25
  - superficial NEC S30.872
    - insect S30.862
- perineum
  - female—*see* Bite, vulva
  - male—*see* Bite, pelvis
- periocular area (with or without lacrimal passages)—*see* Bite, eyelid
- phalanges
  - finger—*see* Bite, finger
  - toe—*see* Bite, toe
- pharynx
  - superficial NEC S10.17
    - insect S10.16
- pinna—*see* Bite, ear
- poisonous—*see* Table of Drugs and Chemicals, by animal or substance, poisoning
- popliteal space—*see* Bite, knee
- prepuce—*see* Bite, penis
- pubic region—*see* Bite, abdomen, wall
- rectovaginal septum—*see* Bite, vulva
- red bug B88.0
- reptile NEC—*see* Table of Drugs and Chemicals, by animal or substance, poisoning
  - nonvenomous—*see* Bite, by site
  - snake—*see* Table of Drugs and Chemicals, by animal or substance, poisoning
- sacral region—*see* Bite, back, lower
- sacroiliac region—*see* Bite, back, lower
- salivary gland—*see* Bite, oral cavity
- scalp S01.05
  - superficial NEC S00.07
    - insect S00.06
- scapular region—*see* Bite, shoulder
- scrotum S31.35
  - superficial NEC S30.873
    - insect S30.863
- sea-snake (venomous)—*see* Table of Drugs and Chemicals, by animal or substance, poisoning
- shin—*see* Bite, leg
- shoulder S41.05-
  - superficial NEC S40.27-
    - insect S40.26-

Bite(s), *continued*
- snake—*see* Table of Drugs and Chemicals, by animal or substance, poisoning
  - nonvenomous—*see* Bite, by site
- spermatic cord—*see* Bite, testis
- spider (venomous)—*see* Table of Drugs and Chemicals, by animal or substance, poisoning
  - nonvenomous—*see* Bite, by site, superficial, insect
- sternal region—*see* Bite, thorax, superficial, front
- submaxillary region—*see* Bite, head, specified site NEC
- submental region—*see* Bite, head, specified site NEC
- subungual
  - finger(s)—*see* Bite, finger
  - toe—*see* Bite, toe
- superficial—*see* Bite, by site, superficial
- supraclavicular fossa S11.85
- supraorbital—*see* Bite, head, specified site NEC
- temple, temporal region—*see* Bite, head, specified site NEC
- temporomandibular area—*see* Bite, cheek
- testis S31.35
  - superficial NEC S30.873
    - insect S30.863
- thigh S71.15-
  - superficial NEC S70.37-
    - insect S70.36-
- thorax, thoracic (wall) S21.95
  - breast—*see* Bite, breast
  - superficial NEC S20.97
    - back S20.47-
    - front S20.37-
    - insect S20.96
      - ~ back S20.46-
      - ~ front S20.36-
- throat—*see* Bite, neck, throat
- thumb S61.05-
  - with
    - damage to nail S61.15-
  - superficial NEC S60.37-
    - insect S60.36-
- thyroid
  - superficial NEC S10.87
    - insect S10.86
- toe(s) S91.15-
  - with
    - damage to nail S91.25-
  - great S91.15-
    - with
      - ~ damage to nail S91.25-
  - lesser S91.15-
    - with
      - ~ damage to nail S91.25-
  - superficial NEC S90.47-
    - great S90.47-
    - insect S90.46-
      - ~ great S90.46-
- tongue S01.552
- trachea
  - superficial NEC S10.17
    - insect S10.16
- tunica vaginalis—*see* Bite, testis
- tympanum, tympanic membrane—*see* Bite, ear
- umbilical region S31.155
- uvula—*see* Bite, oral cavity
- vagina—*see* Bite, vulva
- venomous—*see* Table of Drugs and Chemicals, by animal or substance, poisoning
- vulva S31.45
  - superficial NEC S30.874
    - insect S30.864
- wrist S61.55-
  - superficial NEC S60.87-
    - insect S60.86-

Biting, cheek or lip K13.1

Biventricular failure (heart) I50.9

Blackfan-Diamond anemia or syndrome (congenital hypoplastic anemia) D61.01

Blackhead L70.0

Blackout R55

Blastomycosis, blastomycotic B40.9
- cutaneous B40.3
- disseminated B40.7
- generalized B40.7
- North American B40.9
- primary pulmonary B40.0
- pulmonary
  - acute B40.0
  - chronic B40.1
  - skin B40.3
  - specified NEC B40.89

Bleeding—*see also* Hemorrhage
- anal K62.5
- anovulatory N97.0
- gastrointestinal K92.2
- intermenstrual (regular) N92.3
  - irregular N92.1
- irregular N92.6
- nipple N64.59
- nose R04.0
- ovulation N92.3
- pre-pubertal vaginal N93.1
- puberty (excessive, with onset of menstrual periods) N92.2
- rectum, rectal K62.5
  - newborn P54.2
- tendencies—*see* Defect, coagulation
- uterus, uterine NEC N93.9
  - dysfunctional or functional N93.8
- vagina, vaginal (abnormal) N93.9
  - dysfunctional or functional N93.8
  - newborn P54.6
  - pre-pubertal N93.1
- vicarious N94.89

Blennorrhea (acute) (chronic)—*see also* Gonorrhea
- inclusion (neonatal) (newborn) P39.1
- lower genitourinary tract (gonococcal) A54.00
- neonatorum (gonococcal ophthalmia) A54.31

Blepharitis (angularis) (ciliaris) (eyelid) (marginal) (nonulcerative) H01.00-
- left H01.006
  - lower H01.005
  - upper H01.004
  - upper and lower H01.00B
- right H01.003
  - lower H01.002
  - upper H01.001
  - upper and lower H01.00A

Blepharochalasis H02.3-
- congenital Q10.0

Blepharoconjunctivitis H10.50-

Blepharoptosis H02.40-
- congenital Q10.0

Blindness (acquired) (congenital) (both eyes) H54.0X
- emotional (hysterical) F44.6
- hysterical F44.6
- one eye (other eye normal) H54.4-
  - left (normal vision on right) H54.42-
    - low vision on right H54.12-
  - right (normal vision on left) H54.41-
    - low vision on left H54.11-
- sac, fallopian tube (congenital) Q50.6
- word (developmental) F81.0
  - acquired R48.0
  - secondary to organic lesion R48.0

Blister (nonthermal)
- abdominal wall S30.821
- alveolar process S00.522
- ankle S90.52-
- antecubital space—*see* Blister, elbow
- anus S30.827
- arm (upper) S40.82-
- auditory canal—*see* Blister, ear
- auricle—*see* Blister, ear
- axilla—*see* Blister, arm
- back, lower S30.820
- beetle dermatitis L24.89
- breast S20.12-
- brow S00.82
- calf—*see* Blister, leg
- canthus—*see* Blister, eyelid

Blister, *continued*
- cheek S00.82
  - internal S00.522
- chest wall—*see* Blister, thorax
- chin S00.82
- costal region—*see* Blister, thorax
- digit(s)
  - foot—*see* Blister, toe
  - hand—*see* Blister, finger
- due to burn—*see* Burn, by site, second degree
- ear S00.42-
- elbow S50.32-
- epiglottis S10.12
- esophagus, cervical S10.12
- eyebrow—*see* Blister, eyelid
- eyelid S00.22-
- face S00.82
- fever B00.1
- finger(s) S60.42-
  - index S60.42-
  - little S60.42-
  - middle S60.42-
  - ring S60.42-
- foot (except toe(s) alone) S90.82-
  - toe—*see* Blister, toe
- forearm S50.82-
  - elbow only—*see* Blister, elbow
- forehead S00.82
- fracture omit code
- genital organ
  - female S30.826
  - male S30.825
- gum S00.522
- hand S60.52-
- head S00.92
  - ear—*see* Blister, ear
  - eyelid—*see* Blister, eyelid
  - lip S00.521
  - nose S00.32
  - oral cavity S00.522
  - scalp S00.02
  - specified site NEC S00.82
- heel—*see* Blister, foot
- hip S70.22-
- interscapular region S20.429
- jaw S00.82
- knee S80.22-
- larynx S10.12
- leg (lower) S80.82-
  - knee—*see* Blister, knee
  - upper—*see* Blister, thigh
- lip S00.521
- malar region S00.82
- mammary—*see* Blister, breast
- mastoid region S00.82
- mouth S00.522
- multiple, skin, nontraumatic R23.8
- nail
  - finger—*see* Blister, finger
  - toe—*see* Blister, toe
- nasal S00.32
- neck S10.92
  - specified site NEC S10.82
  - throat S10.12
- nose S00.32
- occipital region S00.02
- oral cavity S00.522
- orbital region—*see* Blister, eyelid
- palate S00.522
- palm—*see* Blister, hand
- parietal region S00.02
- pelvis S30.820
- penis S30.822
- periocular area—*see* Blister, eyelid
- phalanges
  - finger—*see* Blister, finger
  - toe—*see* Blister, toe
- pharynx S10.12
- pinna—*see* Blister, ear
- popliteal space—*see* Blister, knee
- scalp S00.02
- scapular region—*see* Blister, shoulder
- scrotum S30.823

Blister, *continued*
- shin—*see* Blister, leg
- shoulder S40.22-
- sternal region S20.32-
- submaxillary region S00.82
- submental region S00.82
- subungual
  - finger(s)—*see* Blister, finger
  - toe(s)—*see* Blister, toe
- supraclavicular fossa S10.82
- supraorbital S00.82
- temple S00.82
- temporal region S00.82
- testis S30.823
- thermal—*see* Burn, second degree, by site
- thigh S70.32-
- thorax, thoracic (wall) S20.92
  - back S20.42-
  - front S20.32-
- throat S10.12
- thumb S60.32-
- toe(s) S90.42-
  - great S90.42-
- tongue S00.522
- trachea S10.12
- tympanum, tympanic membrane—*see* Blister, ear
- upper arm—*see* Blister, arm (upper)
- uvula S00.522
- vagina S30.824
- vocal cords S10.12
- vulva S30.824
- wrist S60.82-

Bloating R14.0

Block, blocked
- arrhythmic I45.9
- atrioventricular (incomplete) (partial) I44.30
  - with atrioventricular dissociation I44.2
  - complete I44.2
    - congenital Q24.6
  - congenital Q24.6
  - first degree I44.0
  - second degree (types I and II) I44.1
  - specified NEC I44.39
  - third degree I44.2
  - types I and II I44.1
- cardiac I45.9
- conduction I45.9
  - complete I44.2
- foramen Magendie (acquired) G91.1
  - congenital Q03.1
    - with spina bifida—*see* Spina bifida, with hydrocephalus
- heart I45.9
  - complete (atrioventricular) I44.2
  - congenital Q24.6
  - first degree (atrioventricular) I44.0
  - second degree (atrioventricular) I44.1
  - third degree (atrioventricular) I44.2
- Mobitz (types I and II) I44.1
- portal (vein) I81
- second degree (types I and II) I44.1
- third degree I44.2
- Wenckebach (types I and II) I44.1

Blocq's disease F44.4

Blood
- constituents, abnormal R78.9
- disease D75.9
- in
  - feces K92.1
    - occult R19.5
  - urine—*see* Hematuria
- occult in feces R19.5
- pressure
  - decreased, due to shock following injury T79.4
  - examination only Z01.30
  - high—*see* Hypertension
    - borderline R03.0
    - incidental reading, without diagnosis of hypertension R03.0

Blood, *continued*
- transfusion
  - reaction or complication—*see* Complications, transfusion
- type Z67-

Blood-forming organs, disease D75.9

Bloom (-Machacek) (-Torre) syndrome Q82.8

Blount disease or osteochondrosis M92.51-

Blue
- baby Q24.9
- dot cataract Q12.0
  - sclera Q13.5

Blurring, visual H53.8

Blushing (abnormal) (excessive) R23.2

BMI—*see* Body, mass index

Boarder, hospital NEC Z76.4
- healthy infant or child Z76.2
  - foundling Z76.1

Blue
- baby Q24.9
- dot cataract Q12.0
- sclera Q13.5
  - with fragility of bone and deafness Q78.0

Boder-Sedgwick syndrome (ataxia-telangiectasia) G11.3

Body, bodies
- mass index (BMI)
  - adult Z68-
  - pediatric
    - 5th percentile to less than 85th percentile for age Z68.52
    - 85th percentile to less than 95th percentile for age Z68.53
    - greater than or equal to ninety-fifth percentile for age Z68.54
    - less than fifth percentile for age Z68.51
- rocking F98.4

Boeck's
- disease or sarcoid—*see* Sarcoidosis
- lupoid (miliary) D86.3

Bonnevie-Ullrich syndrome Q87.19

Borderline
- diabetes mellitus (prediabetes) R73.03
- hypertension R03.0
- personality F60.3

Botalli, ductus (patent) (persistent) Q25.0

Botulism (foodborne intoxication) A05.1
- infant A48.51
- non-foodborne A48.52
- wound A48.52

Bouillaud's disease or syndrome (rheumatic heart disease) I01.9

Bourneville's disease Q85.1

Bowleg(s) (acquired) M21.16-
- congenital Q68.5

Brachycardia R00.1

Bradycardia (sinoatrial) (sinus) (vagal) R00.1
- neonatal P29.12
- tachycardia syndrome I49.5

Bradypnea R06.89

Bradytachycardia I49.5

Brailsford's disease or osteochondrosis—*see* Osteochondrosis, juvenile, radius

Brain—*see also* Disease, diseased
- death G93.82
- syndrome—*see* Syndrome, brain

Brash (water) R12

BRBPR K62.5

Breast—*see also* Disease, diseased
- buds E30.1
  - in newborn P96.89
- nodule N63.0

Breath
- foul R19.6
- holder, child R06.89
- holding spell R06.89
- shortness R06.02

Breathing
- labored—*see* Hyperventilation
- mouth R06.5
- periodic R06.3
  - high altitude G47.32

Breathlessness R06.81

Brennemann's syndrome I88.0

Bright red blood per rectum (BRBPR) K62.5

Briquet's disorder or syndrome F45.0

Brissaud's
- infantilism or dwarfism E23.0
- motor-verbal tic F95.2

Brittle
- bones disease Q78.0
- nails L60.3

Broad—*see also* Disease, diseased
- beta disease E78.2

Broad- or floating-betalipoproteinemia E78.2

Broken
- arm (meaning upper limb)—*see* Fracture, arm
- bone—*see* Fracture
- leg (meaning lower limb)—*see* Fracture, leg
- nose S02.2-
- tooth, teeth—*see* Fracture, tooth

Bromidism, bromism G92.8
- due to
  - correct substance properly administered—*see* Table of Drugs and Chemicals, by drug, adverse effect
  - overdose or wrong substance given or taken—*see* Table of Drugs and Chemicals, by drug, poisoning

Bronchiolitis (acute) (infective) (subacute) J21.9
- with
  - bronchospasm or obstruction J21.9
  - influenza, flu or grippe—*see* Influenza, with, respiratory manifestations NEC
- due to
  - external agent—*see* Bronchitis, acute, due to
  - human metapneumovirus J21.1
  - respiratory syncytial virus (RSV) J21.0
  - specified organism NEC J21.8
- influenzal—*see* Influenza, with, respiratory manifestations NEC

Bronchitis (diffuse) (fibrinous) (hypostatic) (infective) (membranous) J40
- with
  - influenza, flu or grippe—*see* Influenza, with, respiratory manifestations NEC
  - tracheitis (I5 years of age and above) J40
    - acute or subacute J20.9
    - under I5 years of age J20.9
- acute or subacute (with bronchospasm or obstruction) J20.9
  - due to
    - Haemophilus influenzae J20.1
    - Mycoplasma pneumoniae J20.0
    - specified organism NEC J20.8
    - Streptococcus J20.2
    - virus
      - ~ coxsackie J20.3
      - ~ echovirus J20.7
      - ~ parainfluenza J20.4
      - ~ respiratory syncytial (RSV) J20.5
      - ~ rhinovirus J20.6
  - viral NEC J20.8
- allergic (acute) J45.909
  - with
    - exacerbation (acute) J45.901
    - status asthmaticus J45.902
- asthmatic J45.9
- catarrhal (I5 years of age and above) J40
  - acute—*see* Bronchitis, acute
  - under I5 years of age J20.9
- chronic J42
- mucopurulent
  - acute or subacute J20.9
- pneumococcal, acute or subacute J20.2
- viral NEC, acute or subacute (*see also* Bronchitis, acute) J20.8

Bronchoalveolitis J18.0

Bronchocele meaning goiter E04.0

Bronchomycosis NOS B49 *[J99]*
- candidal B37.1

Bronchorrhea J98.09
- acute J20.9

Bronchospasm (acute) J98.01
- with
  - bronchiolitis, acute J21.9
  - bronchitis, acute (conditions in J20)—*see* Bronchitis, acute
- due to external agent—*see* Disease, diseased, respiratory, acute, due to
- exercise induced J45.990

Bronze baby syndrome P83.88

Bruck-de Lange disease Q87.19

BRUE (brief resolved unexplained event) R68.13

Brugsch's syndrome Q82.8

Bruise (skin surface intact)—*see also* Contusion
- with
  - open wound—*see* Wound, open
- internal organ—*see* Injury, by site
- newborn P54.5
- scalp, due to birth injury, newborn P12.3

Bruit (arterial) R09.89
- cardiac R01.1

Bruxism
- psychogenic F45.8

Bubo I88.8
- indolent (nonspecific) I88.8
- inguinal (nonspecific) I88.8
  - infective I88.8
- scrofulous (tuberculous) A18.2
- syphilitic (primary) A51.0

Buds
- breast E30.1
  - in newborn P96.89

Bulimia (nervosa) F50.2
- atypical F50.9
- normal weight F50.9

Bulky
- stools R19.5

Bunion M21.61-
- tailor's M21.62-

Bunionette M21.62-

Buphthalmia, buphthalmos (congenital) Q15.0

Buried
- penis (congenital) Q55.64

Burkitt
- cell leukemia C91.0-
- lymphoma (malignant) C83.7-
  - small noncleaved, diffuse C83.7-
  - spleen C83.77
  - undifferentiated C83.7-
- tumor C83.7-
- type
  - acute lymphoblastic leukemia C91.0-
  - undifferentiated C83.7-

Burn (electricity) (flame) (hot gas, liquid or hot object) (radiation) (steam) (thermal) T30.0
- abdomen, abdominal (muscle) (wall) T21.02
  - first degree T21.12
  - second degree T21.22
  - third degree T21.32
- above elbow T22.03-
  - first degree T22.13-
  - left T22.032
    - first degree T22.132
    - second degree T22.232
    - third degree T22.332
  - right T22.031
    - first degree T22.131
    - second degree T22.231
    - third degree T22.331
  - second degree T22.23-
  - third degree T22.33-
- acid (caustic) (external) (internal)—*see* Corrosion, by site

Burn, *continued*
- alimentary tract
  - esophagus T28.1
  - mouth T28.0
  - pharynx T28.0
- alkaline (caustic) (external) (internal)—*see* Corrosion, by site
- ankle T25.01-
  - first degree T25.11-
  - left T25.012
    - first degree T25.112
    - second degree T25.212
    - third degree T25.312
  - multiple with foot—*see* Burn, lower, limb, multiple sites, ankle and foot
  - right T25.011
    - first degree T25.111
    - second degree T25.211
    - third degree T25.311
  - second degree T25.21-
  - third degree T25.31-
- anus—*see* Burn, buttock
- arm (lower) (upper)—*see* Burn, upper limb
- axilla T22.04-
  - first degree T22.14-
  - left T22.042
    - first degree T22.142
    - second degree T22.242
    - third degree T22.342
  - right T22.041
    - first degree T22.141
    - second degree T22.241
    - third degree T22.341
  - second degree T22.24-
  - third degree T22.34-
- back (lower) T21.04
  - first degree T21.14
  - second degree T21.24
  - third degree T21.34
  - upper T21.03
    - first degree T21.13
    - second degree T21.23
    - third degree T21.33
- blisters *code as* Burn, second degree, by site
- breast(s)—*see* Burn, chest wall
- buttock(s) T21.05
  - first degree T21.15
  - second degree T21.25
  - third degree T21.35
- calf T24.03-
  - first degree T24.13-
  - left T24.032
    - first degree T24.132
    - second degree T24.232
    - third degree T24.332
  - right T24.031
    - first degree T24.131
    - second degree T24.231
    - third degree T24.331
  - second degree T24.23-
  - third degree T24.33-
- canthus (eye)—*see* Burn, eyelid
- caustic acid or alkaline—*see* Corrosion, by site
- cheek T20.06
  - first degree T20.16
  - second degree T20.26
  - third degree T20.36
- chemical (acids) (alkalines) (caustics) (external) (internal)—*see* Corrosion, by site
- chest wall T21.01
  - first degree T21.11
  - second degree T21.21
  - third degree T21.31
- chin T20.03
  - first degree T20.13
  - second degree T20.23
  - third degree T20.33
- conjunctiva (and cornea)—*see* Burn, cornea
- cornea (and conjunctiva) T26.1- (see complete *ICD-10-CM* Manual)
- corrosion (external) (internal)—*see* Corrosion, by site
- deep necrosis of underlying tissue *code as* Burn, third degree, by site

Burn, *continued*
- dorsum of hand T23.069
  - first degree T23.16-
  - left T23.062
    - first degree T23.162
    - second degree T23.262
    - third degree T23.362
  - right T23.061
    - first degree T23.161
    - second degree T23.261
    - third degree T23.361
  - second degree T23.26-
  - third degree T23.36-
- due to ingested chemical agent—*see* Corrosion, by site
- ear (auricle) (external) (canal) T20.01
  - first degree T20.11
  - second degree T20.21
  - third degree T20.31
- elbow T22.02-
  - first degree T22.12-
  - left T22.022
    - first degree T22.122
    - second degree T22.222
    - third degree T22.322
  - right T22.021
    - first degree T22.121
    - second degree T22.221
    - third degree T22.321
  - second degree T22.22-
  - third degree T22.32-
- epidermal loss *code as* Burn, second degree, by site
- erythema, erythematous *code as* Burn, first degree, by site
- esophagus T28.1
- extent (percentage of body surface)
  - less than 10 percent T31.0
  - 10 –19 percent T31.10
    - with 0 – 9 percent third degree burns T31.10
    - with 10 –19 percent third degree burns T31.11
- extremity—*see* Burn, limb
- eye(s) and adnexa T26.4- (see complete *ICD-10-CM* Manual)
- eyelid(s) T26.0- (See complete *ICD-10-CM* Manual for codes)
- face—*see* Burn, head
- finger T23.029
  - first degree T23.12-
  - left T23.022
    - first degree T23.122
    - second degree T23.222
    - third degree T23.322
  - multiple sites (without thumb) T23.03-
    - with thumb T23.04-
      - ~ first degree T23.14-
      - ~ left T23.042
        - ◊ first degree T23.142
        - ◊ second degree T23.242
        - ◊ third degree T23.342
      - ~ right T23.041
        - ◊ first degree T23.141
        - ◊ second degree T23.241
        - ◊ third degree T23.341
      - ~ second degree T23.24-
      - ~ third degree T23.34-
    - first degree T23.13-
    - left T23.032
      - ~ first degree T23.132
      - ~ second degree T23.232
      - ~ third degree T23.332
    - right T23.031
      - ~ first degree T23.131
      - ~ second degree T23.231
      - ~ third degree T23.331
    - second degree T23.23-
    - third degree T23.33-
  - right T23.021
    - first degree T23.121
    - second degree T23.221
    - third degree T23.321
  - second degree T23.22-
  - third degree T23.32-
- flank—*see* Burn, abdomen, abdominal (muscle) (wall)

Burn, *continued*
- foot T25.02-
  - first degree T25.12-
  - left T25.022
    - first degree T25.122
    - second degree T25.222
    - third degree T25.322
  - multiple with ankle—*see* Burn, lower, limb, multiple sites
  - right T25.021
    - first degree T25.121
    - second degree T25.221
    - third degree T25.321
  - second degree T25.22-
  - third degree T25.32-
- forearm T22.01-
  - first degree T22.11-
  - left T22.012
    - first degree T22.112
    - second degree T22.212
    - third degree T22.312
  - right T22.011
    - first degree T22.111
    - second degree T22.211
    - third degree T22.311
  - second degree T22.219
  - third degree T22.319
- forehead T20.06
  - first degree T20.16
  - second degree T20.26
  - third degree T20.36
- fourth degree *code as* Burn, third degree, by site
- friction—*see* Burn, by site
- from swallowing caustic or corrosive substance NEC—*see* Corrosion, by site
- full thickness skin loss *code as* Burn, third degree, by site
- genital organs
  - external
    - female T21.07
      - ~ first degree T21.17
      - ~ second degree T21.27
      - ~ third degree T21.37
    - male T21.06
      - ~ first degree T21.16
      - ~ second degree T21.26
      - ~ third degree T21.36
- groin—*see* Burn, abdomen, abdominal (muscle) (wall)
- hand(s) T23.009
  - back—*see* Burn, dorsum of hand
  - finger—*see* Burn, finger
  - first degree T23.10-
  - left T23.002
    - first degree T23.102
    - second degree T23.202
    - third degree T23.302
  - multiple sites with wrist T23.09-
    - first degree T23.19-
    - left T23.092
      - ~ first degree T23.192
      - ~ second degree T23.292
      - ~ third degree T23.392
    - right T23.091
      - ~ first degree T23.191
      - ~ second degree T23.291
      - ~ third degree T23.391
    - second degree T23.29-
    - third degree T23.39-
  - palm—*see* Burn, palm
  - right T23.001
    - first degree T23.101
    - second degree T23.201
    - third degree T23.301
  - second degree T23.20-
  - third degree T23.30-
  - thumb—*see* Burn, thumb
- head (and face) (and neck) (*Code by* Burn to specific site for cheek, chin, ear, eye, forehead, lip, neck, nose, or scalp) T20.00
  - first degree T20.10
  - multiple sites T20.09
    - first degree T20.19
    - second degree T20.29

Burn, *continued*
    - third degree T20.39
  - second degree T20.20
  - third degree T20.30
- hip(s)—*see* Burn, thigh
- inhalation—*see* Burn, respiratory tract
  - caustic or corrosive substance (fumes)—*see* Corrosion
- internal organ(s)
  - esophagus T28.1
  - from caustic or corrosive substance (swallowing) NEC—*see* Corrosion, by site
  - mouth T28.0
  - pharynx T28.0
- interscapular region—*see* Burn, back, upper
- knee T24.02-
  - first degree T24.12-
  - left T24.022
    - first degree T24.122
    - second degree T24.222
    - third degree T24.322
  - right T24.021
    - first degree T24.121
    - second degree T24.221
    - third degree T24.321
  - second degree T24.22-
  - third degree T24.32-
- labium (majus) (minus)—*see* Burn, genital organs, external, female
- lacrimal apparatus, duct, gland or sac—*see* Burn, eye, specified site NEC
- larynx T27.0- (See complete *ICD-10-CM* Manual for codes)
  - with lung T27.1-
- leg(s) (lower) (upper)—*see* Burn, lower, limb
- lightning—*see* Burn, by site
- limb(s)
  - lower (except ankle or foot alone)—*see* Burn, lower, limb
  - upper—*see* Burn, upper limb
- lip(s) T20.02
  - first degree T20.12
  - second degree T20.22
  - third degree T20.32
- lower
  - back—*see* Burn, back
  - limb T24.00- (*Code to* Burn *by specific site for ankle, calf, foot, thigh, knee*)
    - first degree T24.109
    - left T24.002
      - ~ first degree T24.102
      - ~ second degree T24.202
      - ~ third degree T24.302
    - multiple sites, except ankle and foot T24.099
      - ~ ankle and foot T25.09-
        - ◊ first degree T25.19-
        - ◊ left T25.092
          - » first degree T25.192
          - » second degree T25.292
          - » third degree T25.392
        - ◊ right T25.091
          - » first degree T25.191
          - » second degree T25.291
          - » third degree T25.391
        - ◊ second degree T25.29-
        - ◊ third degree T25.39-
      - ~ first degree T24.19-
      - ~ left T24.092
        - ◊ first degree T24.192
        - ◊ second degree T24.292
        - ◊ third degree T24.392
      - ~ right T24.091
        - ◊ first degree T24.191
        - ◊ second degree T24.291
        - ◊ third degree T24.391
      - ~ second degree T24.29-
      - ~ third degree T24.39-
    - right T24.001
      - ~ first degree T24.101
      - ~ second degree T24.201
      - ~ third degree T24.301
    - second degree T24.20-
    - thigh—*see* Burn, thigh

Burn, *continued*
- ■ third degree T24.30-
- ■ toe—*see* Burn, toe
- • mouth T28.0
- • neck T20.07
  - – first degree T20.17
  - – second degree T20.27
  - – third degree T20.37
- • nose (septum) T20.04
  - – first degree T20.14
  - – second degree T20.24
  - – third degree T20.34
- • ocular adnexa—*see* Burn, eye
- • orbit region—*see* Burn, eyelid
- • palm T23.059
  - – first degree T23.15-
  - – left T23.052
    - ■ first degree T23.152
    - ■ second degree T23.252
    - ■ third degree T23.352
  - – right T23.051
    - ■ first degree T23.151
    - ■ second degree T23.251
    - ■ third degree T23.351
  - – second degree T23.25-
  - – third degree T23.35-
- • partial thickness *code as* Burn, unspecified degree, by site
- • pelvis—*see* Burn, trunk
- • penis—*see* Burn, genital organs, external, male
- • perineum
  - – female—*see* Burn, genital organs, external, female
  - – male—*see* Burn, genital organs, external, male
- • periocular area—*see* Burn, eyelid
- • pharynx T28.0
- • respiratory tract T27.- (See complete *ICD-10-CM* Manual for codes)
- • scalp T20.05
  - – first degree T20.15
  - – second degree T20.25
  - – third degree T20.35
- • scapular region T22.06-
  - – first degree T22.16-
  - – left T22.062
    - ■ first degree T22.162
    - ■ second degree T22.262
    - ■ third degree T22.362
  - – right T22.061
    - ■ first degree T22.161
    - ■ second degree T22.261
    - ■ third degree T22.361
  - – second degree T22.26-
  - – third degree T22.36-
- • scrotum—*see* Burn, genital organs, external, male
- • shoulder T22.05-
  - – first degree T22.15-
  - – left T22.052
    - ■ first degree T22.152
    - ■ second degree T22.252
    - ■ third degree T22.352
  - – right T22.051
    - ■ first degree T22.151
    - ■ second degree T22.251
    - ■ third degree T22.351
  - – second degree T22.25-
  - – third degree T22.35-
- • temple—*see* Burn, head
- • testis—*see* Burn, genital organs, external, male
- • thigh T24.01-
  - – first degree T24.11-
  - – left T24.012
    - ■ first degree T24.112
    - ■ second degree T24.212
    - ■ third degree T24.312
  - – right T24.011
    - ■ first degree T24.111
    - ■ second degree T24.211
    - ■ third degree T24.311
  - – second degree T24.21-
  - – third degree T24.31-
- • thorax (external)—*see* Burn, trunk
- • throat (meaning pharynx) T28.0

Burn, *continued*
- • thumb(s) T23.01-
  - – first degree T23.11-
  - – left T23.012
    - ■ first degree T23.112
    - ■ second degree T23.212
    - ■ third degree T23.312
  - – multiple sites with fingers T23.04-
    - ■ first degree T23.14-
    - ■ left T23.042
      - ~ first degree T23.142
      - ~ second degree T23.242
      - ~ third degree T23.342
    - ■ right T23.041
      - ~ first degree T23.141
      - ~ second degree T23.241
      - ~ third degree T23.341
    - ■ second degree T23.24-
    - ■ third degree T23.34-
  - – right T23.011
    - ■ first degree T23.111
    - ■ second degree T23.211
    - ■ third degree T23.311
  - – second degree T23.21-
  - – third degree T23.31-
- • toe T25.039
  - – first degree T25.139
  - – left T25.032
    - ■ first degree T25.132
    - ■ second degree T25.232
    - ■ third degree T25.332
  - – right T25.031
    - ■ first degree T25.131
    - ■ second degree T25.231
    - ■ third degree T25.331
  - – second degree T25.23-
  - – third degree T25.33-
- • tongue T28.0
- • tonsil(s) T28.0
- • trachea T27.- (See complete *ICD-10-CM* Manual for codes)
- • trunk T21.00 *(Code to Burn by specific site for abdominal wall, buttock, upper limb, back, chest wall, genital organs, or scapular region)*
  - – first degree T21.10
  - – second degree T21.20
  - – specified site NEC T21.09
    - ■ first degree T21.19
    - ■ second degree T21.29
    - ■ third degree T21.39
  - – third degree T21.30
- • unspecified site with extent of body surface involved specified
  - – less than 10 percent T31.0
  - – 10 –19 percent (0 – 9 percent third degree) T31.10
    - ■ with 10 –19 percent third degree T31.11
- • upper limb *(Code to Burn by specific site for above elbow, axilla, elbow, forearm, hand, scapular region, shoulder, upper back, or wrist)* T22.00
  - – first degree T22.10
  - – multiple sites T22.09-
    - ■ first degree T22.19-
    - ■ left T22.092
      - ~ first degree T22.192
      - ~ second degree T22.292
      - ~ third degree T22.392
    - ■ right T22.091
      - ~ first degree T22.191
      - ~ second degree T22.291
      - ~ third degree T22.391
    - ■ second degree T22.29-
    - ■ third degree T22.39-
  - – second degree T22.20
  - – third degree T22.3-
- • vulva—*see* Burn, genital organs, external, female
- • wrist T23.07-
  - – first degree T23.17-
  - – left T23.072
    - ■ first degree T23.172
    - ■ second degree T23.272
    - ■ third degree T23.372

Burn, *continued*
- – multiple sites with hand T23.09-
  - ■ first degree T23.19-
  - ■ left T23.092
    - ~ first degree T23.192
    - ~ second degree T23.292
    - ~ third degree T23.392
  - ■ right T23.091
    - ~ first degree T23.191
    - ~ second degree T23.291
    - ~ third degree T23.391
  - ■ second degree T23.29-
  - ■ third degree T23.39-
- – right T23.071
  - ■ first degree T23.171
  - ■ second degree T23.271
  - ■ third degree T23.371
- – second degree T23.27-
- – third degree T23.37-

Burnett's syndrome E83.52

Bursitis M71.9
- • hip NEC M70.7-
  - – trochanteric M70.6-
- • radiohumeral M70.3-
- • specified NEC M71.50
  - – ankle M71.57-
  - – due to use, overuse or pressure—*see* Disorder
  - – elbow M71.52-
  - – foot M71.57-
  - – hand M71.54-
  - – hip M71.55-
  - – knee M71.56-
  - – specified site NEC M71.58
  - – tibial collateral M76.4-
  - – wrist M71.53-

C

Cachexia R64
- • dehydration E86.0
  - – with
    - ■ hypernatremia E87.0
    - ■ hyponatremia E87.1
    - ■ hypophyseal E23.0
    - ■ hypopituitary E23.0
    - ■ pituitary E23.0
    - ■ Simmonds' E23.0
- • pulmonary R64

CADASIL (cerebral autosomal dominate arteriopathy with subcortical infarcts and leukocephalopathy) I67.850

Café au lait spots L81.3

Caked breast (puerperal, postpartum) O92.79

Calciferol (vitamin D) deficiency E55.9
- • with rickets E55.0

Calcification
- • adrenal (capsule) (gland) E27.49
- • cerebral (cortex) G93.89
- • choroid plexus G93.89
- • kidney N28.89
  - – tuberculous B90.9
- • lymph gland or node (postinfectional) I89.8
  - – tuberculous B90.8
- • pericardium (*see also* Pericarditis) I31.1
- • pleura
  - – tuberculous NEC B90.9
- • subcutaneous L94.2
- • suprarenal (capsule) (gland) E27.49

Calcinosis (interstitial) (tumoral) (universalis) E83.59
- • circumscripta (skin) L94.2
- • cutis L94.2

Calciuria 82.994

Calculus, calculi, calculous
- • biliary—*see also* Calculus, gallbladder
  - – specified NEC K80.80
    - ■ with obstruction K80.81
- • bilirubin, multiple—*see* Calculus, gallbladder
- • bladder (encysted) (impacted) (urinary) (diverticulum) N21.0

Calculus, calculi, calculous, *continued*
- gallbladder K80.20
  - with
    - bile duct calculus—*see* Calculus, gallbladder, with, bile duct calculus
    - cholecystitis K80.10
      - ~ with obstruction K80.11
      - ~ acute K80.00
        - ◊ with
          - » chronic cholecystitis K80.12
            - ❖ with obstruction K80.13
          - » obstruction K80.01
      - ~ chronic K80.10
        - ◊ with
          - » acute cholecystitis K80.12
            - ❖ with obstruction K80.13
          - » obstruction K80.11
      - ~ specified NEC K80.18
        - ◊ with obstruction K80.19
    - obstruction K80.21
- intestinal (impaction) (obstruction) K56.49
- kidney (impacted) (multiple) (pelvis) (recurrent) (staghorn) N20.0
  - with calculus, ureter N20.2
  - congenital Q63.8
- nose J34.89
- pyelitis (impacted) (recurrent) N20.0
  - with hydronephrosis N13.6
- pyelonephritis (impacted) (recurrent)—*see* category N20
  - with hydronephrosis N13.2
- tonsil J35.8
- ureter (impacted) (recurrent) N20.1
  - with calculus, kidney N20.2
    - with hydronephrosis N13.6
      - ~ with infection N13.6
      - ~ ureteropelvic junction N20.1
- urethra (impacted) N21.1
- urinary (duct) (impacted) (passage) (tract) N20.9
  - with hydronephrosis N13.2
    - with infection N13.6
- vagina N89.8
- xanthine E79.8 [N22]

California
- encephalitis A83.5

Callositas, callosity (infected) L84

Callus (infected) L84

CALME (Childhood asymmetric labium majus enlargement) N90.61

Calorie deficiency or malnutrition (*see also* Malnutrition) E46

Calvé-Perthes disease M91.1-

Camptocormia (hysterical) F44.4

Canal—*see also* Disease, diseased
- atrioventricular common Q21.2

Candidiasis, candidal B37.9
- balanitis B37.42
- bronchitis B37.1
- cheilitis B37.83
- congenital P37.5
- cystitis B37.41
- disseminated B37.7
- endocarditis B37.6
- enteritis B37.82
- esophagitis B37.81
- intertrigo B37.2
- lung B37.1
- meningitis B37.5
- mouth B37.0
- nails B37.2
- neonatal P37.5
- onychia B37.2
- oral B37.0
- osteomyelitis B37.89
- otitis externa B37.84
- paronychia B37.2
- perionyxis B37.2
- pneumonia B37.1
- proctitis B37.82
- pulmonary B37.1
- pyelonephritis B37.49

Candidiasis, candidal, *continued*
- sepsis B37.7
- skin B37.2
- specified site NEC B37.89
- stomatitis B37.0
- systemic B37.7
- urethritis B37.41
- urogenital site NEC B37.49
- vagina B37.3
- vulva B37.3
- vulvovaginitis B37.3

Canker (mouth) (sore) K12.0
- rash A38.9

Caput
- crepitus Q75.8

Carbuncle L02.93
- abdominal wall L02.231
- anus K61.0
- axilla L02.43-
- back (any part) L02.232
- breast N61.1
- buttock L02.33
- cheek (external) L02.03
- chest wall L02.233
- chin L02.03
- face NEC L02.03
- finger L02.53-
- flank L02.231
- foot L02.63-
- forehead L02.03
- gluteal (region) L02.33
- groin L02.234
- hand L02.53-
- head NEC L02.831
- heel L02.63-
- hip L02.43-
- knee L02.43-
- lower limb L02.43-
- navel L02.236
- neck L02.13
- nose (external) (septum) J34.0
- partes posteriores L02.33
- pectoral region L02.233
- perineum L02.235
- pinna—*see* Abscess, ear, external
- scalp L02.831
- specified site NEC L02.838
- temple (region) L02.03
- thumb L02.53-
- toe L02.63-
- trunk L02.239
  - abdominal wall L02.231
  - back L02.232
  - chest wall L02.233
  - groin L02.234
  - perineum L02.235
  - umbilicus L02.236
- umbilicus L02.236
- upper limb L02.43-
- urethra N34.0
- vulva N76.4

Carcinoma (malignant)—*see also* Neoplasm, by site, malignant in the Table of Neoplasms in the complete *ICD-10-CM* manual.
- Merkel cell C4A.-
- renal cell C64-

Cardiac—*see also* Disease, diseased
- death, sudden—*see* Arrest, cardiac
- pacemaker
  - in situ Z95.0
  - management or adjustment Z45.018
- tamponade I31.4

Cardiochalasia K21.9

Cardiomegaly—*see also* Hypertrophy, cardiac
- congenital Q24.8
- idiopathic I51.7

Cardiomyopathy (familial) (idiopathic) I42.9
- constrictive NOS I42.5
- due to
  - Friedreich's ataxia G11.11
  - progressive muscular dystrophy G71.0

Cardiomyopathy, *continued*
- hypertrophic (nonobstructive) I42.2
  - obstructive I42.1
    - congenital Q24.8
- in
  - sarcoidosis D86.85
- metabolic E88.9 [I43]
  - thyrotoxic E05.90 [I43]
    - with thyroid storm E05.91 [I43]
- nutritional E63.9 [I43]
- restrictive NEC I42.5
- secondary I42.9
- specified NEC I42.8
- thyrotoxic E05.90 [I43]
  - with thyroid storm E05.91 [I43]

Cardiopathia nigra I27.0

Cardiopathy
- idiopathic I42.9
- mucopolysaccharidosis E76.3 [I52]

Cardiosymphysis I31.0

Care (of) (for) (following)
- family member (handicapped) (sick)
  - unavailable, due to
    - absence (person rendering care) (sufferer) Z74.2
    - inability (any reason) of person rendering care Z74.2
- foundling Z76.1
- palliative Z51.5
- unavailable, due to
  - absence of person rendering care Z74.2
  - inability (any reason) of person rendering care Z74.2
- well baby Z76.2

Caries
- dental K02.9

Carnitine insufficiency E71.40

Carpenter's syndrome Q87.0

Carrier (suspected) **of**
- bacterial disease NEC Z22.39
  - diphtheria Z22.2
  - intestinal infectious NEC Z22.1
    - typhoid Z22.0
  - meningococcal Z22.31
  - sexually transmitted Z22.4
  - specified NEC Z22.39
  - staphylococcal (Methicillin susceptible) Z22.321
    - Methicillin resistant Z22.322
  - streptococcal Z22.338
    - group B Z22.330
- genetic Z14.8
  - cystic fibrosis Z14.1
  - hemophilia A (asymptomatic) Z14.01
    - symptomatic Z14.02
- gonorrhea Z22.4
- HAA (hepatitis Australian-antigen) Z22.5
- HB (c)(s)-AG Z22.5
- hepatitis (viral) Z22.5
  - Australia-antigen (HAA) Z22.5
  - B surface antigen (HBsAg) Z22.5
  - C Z22.5
  - specified NEC Z22.5
- infectious organism Z22.9
  - specified NEC Z22.8
- meningococci Z22.31
- serum hepatitis—*see* Carrier, hepatitis
- staphylococci (Methicillin susceptible) Z22.321
  - Methicillin resistant Z22.322
- streptococci Z22.338
  - group B Z22.330
- syphilis Z22.4
- venereal disease Z22.4

Car sickness T75.3

Caruncle (inflamed)
- myrtiform N89.8

Caseation lymphatic gland (tuberculous) A18.2

Casts in urine R82.998

Cat
- cry syndrome Q93.4

Cataract (cortical) (immature) (incipient) H26.9
- anterior
  - and posterior axial embryonal Q12.0
  - pyramidal Q12.0
- blue Q12.0
- central Q12.0
- cerulean Q12.0
- congenital Q12.0
- coraliform Q12.0
- coronary Q12.0
- crystalline Q12.0
- in
  - hypoparathyroidism E20.9 [H28]
  - nutritional disease E63.9 [H28]
- infantile—*see* Cataract, presenile
- juvenile—*see* Cataract, presenile
- nuclear
  - embryonal Q12.0
- presenile H26.00-
- zonular (perinuclear) Q12.0

Cataracta—*see also* Cataract
- centralis pulverulenta Q12.0
- cerulea Q12.0
- congenita Q12.0
- coralliformis Q12.0
- coronaria Q12.0
- membranacea
  - congenita Q12.0

Catarrh, catarrhal (acute) (febrile) (infectious) (inflammation) (*see also* Disease, diseased) J00
- chronic J31.0
- gingivitis K05.00
  - plaque induced K05.00
- larynx, chronic J37.0
- liver B15.9
- middle ear, chronic H65.2-
- mouth K12.1
- nasal (chronic)—*see* Rhinitis
- nasopharyngeal (chronic) J31.1
  - acute J00
- pulmonary—*see* Bronchitis
- spring (eye) (vernal)—*see* Conjunctivitis, acute, atopic
- summer (hay)—*see* Fever, hay
- throat J31.2
- tubotympanal—*see also* Otitis, media, acute, subacute, nonsuppurative NEC
  - chronic H65.2-

Catatonic
- stupor R40.1

Cat-scratch disease or fever A28.1

Cavovarus foot, congenital Q66.1-

Cavus foot (congenital) Q66.7-

CDKL5 (Cyclin-Dependent Kinase-Like 5 Deficiency Disorder) G40.42

Cecitis K52.9
- with perforation, peritonitis, or rupture K65.8

Cecoureterocele Q62.32

Celiac
- disease (with steatorrhea) K90.0
- infantilism K90.0

Cells (see Disease, diseased)
- in urine R82.998

Cellulitis (diffuse) (phlegmonous) (septic) (suppurative) L03.90
- abdominal wall L03.311
- ankle L03.11-
- anus K61.0
- axilla L03.11-
- back (any part) L03.312
- breast (acute) (nonpuerperal) N61.0
  - nipple N61.0
- buttock L03.317
- cervical (meaning neck) L03.221
- cheek (external) L03.211
  - internal K12.2
- chest wall L03.313
- chronic L03.90
- drainage site (following operation) T81.49
- ear (external) H60.1-
- erysipelatous—*see* Erysipelas

Cellulitis, *continued*
- face NEC L03.211
- finger (intrathecal) (periosteal) (subcutaneous) (subcuticular) L03.01-
- foot L03.11-
- gangrenous—*see* Gangrene
- gluteal (region) L03.317
- groin L03.314
- head NEC L03.811
  - face (any part, except ear, eye and nose) L03.211
- jaw (region) L03.211
- knee L03.11-
- lip K13.0
- lower limb L03.11-
  - toe—*see* Cellulitis, toe
- mouth (floor) K12.2
- multiple sites, so stated L03.90
- navel L03.316
  - newborn P38.9
    - with mild hemorrhage P38.1
    - without hemorrhage P38.9
- neck (region) L03.221
- nose (septum) (external) J34.0
- orbit, orbital H05.01-
  - periorbital L03.213
- palate (soft) K12.2
- pectoral (region) L03.313
- pelvis, pelvic (chronic)
  - female (*see also* Disease, pelvis, inflammatory) N73.2
    - acute N73.0
  - male K65.0
- perineal, perineum L03.315
- periorbital L03.213
- perirectal K61.1peritonsillar J36
- preseptal L03.213
- rectum K61.1
- scalp (any part) L03.811
- specified site NEC L03.818
- submandibular (region) (space) (triangle) K12.2
  - gland K11.3
- submaxillary (region) K12.2
  - gland K11.3
- toe (intrathecal) (periosteal) (subcutaneous) (subcuticular) L03.03
- tonsil J36
- trunk L03.319
  - abdominal wall L03.311
  - back (any part) L03.312
  - buttock L03.317
  - chest wall L03.313
  - groin L03.314
  - perineal, perineum L03.315
  - umbilicus L03.316
- umbilicus L03.316
- upper limb L03.11-
  - axilla L03.11-
  - finger L03.01-
  - thumb L03.01-
- vaccinal T88.0

Central auditory processing disorder H93.25

Cephalematoma, cephalhematoma (calcified)
- newborn (birth injury) P12.0

Cephalgia, cephalalgia—*see also* Headache
- histamine G44.009
  - intractable G44.001
  - not intractable G44.009

Cerumen (accumulation) (impacted) H61.2-

Cervicalgia M54.2

Cervicitis (acute) (chronic) (nonvenereal) (senile (atrophic)) (subacute) (with ulceration) N72
- chlamydial A56.09
- gonococcal A54.03
- trichomonal A59.09

Cervicocolpitis (emphysematosa) (*see also* Cervicitis) N72

Cestode infestation B71.9
- specified type NEC B71.8

Cestodiasis B71.9

Chafing L30.4

Chalasia (cardiac sphincter) K21.9

Chalazion H00.10
- left H00.16
  - lower H00.15
  - upper H00.14
- right H00.13
  - lower H00.12
  - upper H00.11

Chancre (any genital site) (hard) (hunterian) (mixed) (primary) (seronegative) (seropositive) (syphilitic) A51.0
- conjunctiva NEC A51.2
- extragenital A51.2
- eyelid A51.2
- lip A51.2
- nipple A51.2
- palate, soft A51.2
- soft
  - palate A51.2
- urethra A51.0

Change(s) (in) (of)—*see also* Removal
- circulatory I99.9
- contraceptive device Z30.433
- dressing (nonsurgical) Z48.00
  - surgical Z48.01
- hypertrophic
  - nasal sinus J34.89
  - turbinate, nasal J34.3
  - upper respiratory tract J39.8
- mental status R41.82
- sacroiliac joint M53.3
- skin R23.9
  - acute, due to ultraviolet radiation L56.9
    - specified NEC L56.8
  - cyanosis R23.0
  - flushing R23.2
  - pallor R23.1
  - petechiae R23.3
  - specified change NEC R23.8
  - swelling—*see* Mass, localized
- vascular I99.9
- voice R49.9
  - psychogenic F44.4

CHARGE association Q89.8

Charley-horse (quadriceps) M62.831
- traumatic (quadriceps) S76.11-

Checking (of)
- implantable subdermal contraceptive Z30.46
- intrauterine contraceptive device Z30.431

Cheese itch B88.0

Cheilitis (acute) (angular) (catarrhal) (chronic) (exfoliative) (gangrenous) (glandular) (infectional) (suppurative) (ulcerative) (vesicular) K13.0
- actinic (due to sun) L56.8
  - other than from sun L56.9
- candidal B37.83

Cheilodynia K13.0

Cheiloschisis—*see* Cleft, lip

Cheilosis (angular) K13.0

Cheiropompholyx L30.1

Chemotherapy (session) (for)
- cancer Z51.11
- neoplasm Z51.11

Cheyne-Stokes breathing (respiration) R06.3

Chickenpox—*see* Varicella

Chigger (infestation) B88.0

Child
- custody dispute Z65.3

Childhood
- cerebral X-linked adrenoleukodystrophy E71.520
- period of rapid growth Z00.2

Chill(s) R68.83
- with fever R50.9
- congestive in malarial regions B54
- without fever R68.83

Chinese dysentery A03.9

Chlamydia, chlamydial A74.9
- cervicitis A56.09
- conjunctivitis A74.0
- cystitis A56.01

Chlamydia, chlamydial, *continued*
- endometritis A56.11
- epididymitis A56.19
- female
  - pelvic inflammatory disease A56.11
    - pelviperitonitis A56.11
- orchitis A56.19
- peritonitis A74.81
- pharyngitis A56.4
- proctitis A56.3
- salpingitis A56.11
- sexually-transmitted infection NEC A56.8
- specified NEC A74.89
- urethritis A56.01
- vulvovaginitis A56.02

Chlamydiosis—*see* Chlamydia

Chlorotic anemia D50.8

Cholecystitis K81.9
- with
  - gangrene of gallbladder K82.A1
  - perforation of gallbladder K82.A2
- acute (emphysematous) (gangrenous) (suppurative) K81.0
  - with
    - calculus, stones in
      - cystic duct—*see* Calculus, gallbladder, with, cholecystitis, acute
      - gallbladder—*see* Calculus, gallbladder, with, cholecystitis, acute
    - choledocholithiasis—*see* Calculus, gallbladder, with, cholecystitis, acute
    - cholelithiasis—*see* Calculus, gallbladder, with, cholecystitis, acute
    - chronic cholecystitis K81.2
      - with gallbladder calculus K80.12
        ◊ with obstruction K80.13
- chronic K81.1
  - with acute cholecystitis K81.2
    - with gallbladder calculus K80.12
      - with obstruction K80.13
- emphysematous (acute)—*see* Cholecystitis, acute
- gangrenous—*see* Cholecystitis, acute
- suppurative—*see* Cholecystitis, acute

Choking sensation R09.89

Cholesteremia E78.0

Cholesterol
- elevated (high) E78.00
  - with elevated (high) triglycerides E78.2
  - screening for Z13.220

Cholesterolemia (essential) (pure) E78.00
- familial E78.01
- hereditary E78.01

Chondritis M94.8X-
- costal (Tietze's) M94.0
- patella, posttraumatic M22.4-

Chondrodysplasia Q78.9
- with hemangioma Q78.4
- calcificans congenita Q77.3
- fetalis Q77.4
- metaphyseal (Jansen's) (McKusick's) (Schmid's) Q78.8
- punctata Q77.3

Chondrodystrophy, chondrodystrophia (familial) (fetalis) (hypoplastic) Q78.9
- calcificans congenita Q77.3
- myotonic (congenital) G71.13
- punctata Q77.3

Chondroectodermal dysplasia Q77.6

Chondrogenesis imperfecta Q77.4

Chondromalacia (systemic) M94.2-
- knee M94.26-
  - patella M22.4-

Chondro-osteodysplasia (Morquio-Brailsford type) E76.219

Chondro-osteodystrophy E76.29

Chondropathia tuberosa M94.0

Chordee (nonvenereal) N48.89
- congenital Q54.4

Chorea (chronic) (gravis) (posthemiplegic) (senile) (spasmodic) G25.5
- drug-induced G25.4
- hysterical F44.4
- progressive G25.5
- with
  - heart involvement I02.0
    - active or acute (conditions in I01-) I02.0
    - rheumatic I02.9
      ~ with valvular disorder I02.0
  - rheumatic heart disease (chronic) (inactive) (quiescent)—*code to* rheumatic heart condition involved

Choreoathetosis (paroxysmal) G25.5

Chorioretinitis
- in (due to)
  - toxoplasmosis (acquired) B58.01
    - congenital (active) P37.1 *[H32]*

Chromophytosis B36.0

Chylopericardium I31.3
- acute I30.9

Cicatricial (deformity)—*see* Cicatrix

Cicatrix (adherent) (contracted) (painful) (vicious) (*see also* Scar) L90.5
- adenoid (and tonsil) J35.8
- anus K62.89
- brain G93.89
- mouth K13.79
- muscle M62.89
  - with contracture—*see* Contraction, muscle NEC
- palate (soft) K13.79
- rectum K62.89
- skin L90.5
  - postinfective L90.5
  - specified site NEC L90.5
  - tuberculous B90.8
- tonsil (and adenoid) J35.8
- tuberculous NEC B90.9
- vagina N89.8
  - postoperative N99.2
- wrist, constricting (annular) L90.5

CINCA (chronic infantile neurological, cutaneous and articular syndrome) M04.2

Circulation
- failure (peripheral) R57.9
  - newborn P29.89
- fetal, persistent P29.38

Circumcision (in absence of medical indication) (ritual) (routine) Z41.2

Cirrhosis, cirrhotic (hepatic) (liver) K74.60
- due to
  - xanthomatosis E78.2
- fatty K76.0
- liver K74.60
  - congenital P78.81
- pigmentary E83.110
- xanthomatous (biliary) K74.5
  - due to xanthomatosis (familial) (metabolic) (primary) E78.2

Clam digger's itch B65.3

Clammy skin R23.1

Clark's paralysis G80.9

Claudication, intermittent I73.9
- cerebral (artery) G45.9

Clavus (infected) L84

Clawfoot (congenital) Q66.89
- acquired M21.53-

Clawtoe (congenital) Q66.89
- acquired M20.5X-

Cleft (congenital)—*see also* Imperfect, closure
- foot Q72.7
- hand Q71.6
- lip (unilateral) Q36.9
  - with cleft palate Q37.9
    - hard Q37.1
      ~ with soft Q37.5
    - soft Q37.3
      ~ with hard Q37.5

Cleft, *continued*
  - bilateral Q36.0
    - with cleft palate Q37.8
      ~ hard Q37.0
        ◊ with soft Q37.4
      ~ soft Q37.2
        ◊ with hard Q37.4
  - median Q36.1
- palate Q35.9
  - with cleft lip (unilateral) Q37.9
    - bilateral Q37.8
  - hard Q35.1
    - with
      ~ cleft lip (unilateral) Q37.1
        ◊ bilateral Q37.0
      ~ soft Q35.5
        ◊ with cleft lip (unilateral) Q37.5
          » bilateral Q37.4
  - medial Q35.5
  - soft Q35.3
    - with
      ~ cleft lip (unilateral) Q37.3
        ◊ bilateral Q37.2
      ~ hard Q35.5
        ◊ with cleft lip (unilateral) Q37.5
          » bilateral Q37.4
- penis Q55.69
- scrotum Q55.29
- uvula Q35.7

Cleidocranial dysostosis Q74.0

Clicking hip (newborn) R29.4

Closed bite M26.29

Closure
- congenital, nose Q30.0
- foramen ovale, imperfect Q21.1
- hymen N89.6
- interauricular septum, defective Q21.1
- interventricular septum, defective Q21.0
- lacrimal duct—*see also* Stenosis, lacrimal, duct
  - congenital Q10.5
- nose (congenital) Q30.0
  - acquired M95.0
- vagina N89.5

Clot (blood)—*see also* Embolism
- artery (obstruction) (occlusion)—*see* Embolism
- circulation I74.9

Clouded state R40.1
- epileptic—*see* Epilepsy, specified NEC
- paroxysmal—*see* Epilepsy, specified NEC

Cloudy antrum, antra J32.0

Clubfoot (congenital) Q66.89
- acquired M21.54-
- equinovarus Q66.0-
- paralytic M21.54-

Clubhand (congenital) (radial) Q71.4-
- acquired M21.51-

Clumsiness, clumsy child syndrome F82

Cluttering F80.81

Coagulopathy—*see also* Defect, coagulation
- consumption D65
- intravascular D65
  - newborn P60

Coalition
- calcaneo-scaphoid Q66.89
- tarsal Q66.89

Coarctation
- aorta (preductal) (postductal) Q25.1
- pulmonary artery Q25.71

Coccydynia, coccygodynia M53.3

Cockayne's syndrome Q87.19

Cock's peculiar tumor L72.3

Cold J00
- with influenza, flu, or grippe—*see* Influenza, with, respiratory manifestations NEC
- agglutinin disease or hemoglobinuria (chronic) D59.12
- bronchial—*see* Bronchitis
- chest—*see* Bronchitis
- common (head) J00

Cold, *continued*
- head J00
- on lung—*see* Bronchitis
- rose J30.1
- virus J00
- sensitivity, auto-immune D59.12
- symptoms J00

Colibacillosis A49.8
- as the cause of other disease (*see also* Escherichia coli) B96.20
- generalized A41.50

Colic (bilious) (infantile) (intestinal) (recurrent) (spasmodic) R10.83
- abdomen R10.83
  - psychogenic F45.8
- hysterical F45.8
- kidney N23
- mucous K58.9
  - with constipation K58.1
  - with diarrhea K58.0
  - mixed K58.2
  - other K58.8
  - psychogenic F54
- nephritic N23
- psychogenic F45.8
- renal N23
- ureter N23
- uterus NEC N94.89
  - menstrual—*see* Dysmenorrhea

Colitis (acute) (catarrhal) (chronic) (noninfective) (hemorrhagic) (*see also* Enteritis) K52.9
- allergic K52.29
  - with
    - food protein-induced enterocolitis syndrome K52.21
    - proctocolitis K52.29
- amebic (acute) (*see also* Amebiasis) A06.0
- anthrax A22.2
- C. difficile
  - not specified as recurrent A04.72
  - recurrent A04.71
- collagenous K52.831
- cystica superficialis K52.89
- dietary counseling and surveillance (for) Z71.3
- dietetic K52.29
- eosinophilic K52.82
- food hypersensitivity K52.29
- giardial A07.1
- granulomatous—*see* Enteritis, regional, large intestine
- infectious—*see* Enteritis, infectious
- indeterminate, so stated K52.3
- left sided K51.50
  - with
    - abscess K51.514
    - complication K51.519
      - ~ specified NEC K51.518
    - fistula K51.513
    - obstruction K51.512
    - rectal bleeding K51.511
- lymphocytic K52.832
- microscopic, other K52.838
  - unspecified K52.839
- noninfective K52.9
  - specified NEC K52.89
- septic—*see* Enteritis, infectious
- spastic K58.9
  - with constipation K58.1
  - with diarrhea K58.0
  - mixed K58.2
  - other K58.8
  - psychogenic F54
- staphylococcal A04.8
  - foodborne A05.0
- ulcerative (chronic) K51.90
  - with
    - complication K51.919
      - ~ abscess K51.914
      - ~ fistula K51.913
      - ~ obstruction K51.912
      - ~ rectal bleeding K51.911
      - ~ specified complication NEC K51.918
  - enterocolitis—*see* Pancolitis, ulcerative

Colitis, *continued*
- ileocolitis—*see* Ileocolitis, ulcerative
- mucosal proctocolitis—*see* Rectosigmoiditis, ulcerative
- proctitis—*see* Proctitis, ulcerative
- pseudopolyposis—*see* Polyp, colon, inflammatory
- psychogenic F54
- rectosigmoiditis—*see* Rectosigmoiditis, ulcerative
- specified type NEC K51.80
  - with
    - ~ complication K51.819
      - ◊ abscess K51.814
      - ◊ fistula K51.813
      - ◊ obstruction K51.812
      - ◊ rectal bleeding K51.811
      - ◊ specified complication NEC K51.818

Collagenosis, collagen disease (nonvascular) (vascular) M35.9
- specified NEC M35.8

Collapse R55
- adrenal E27.2
- cardiorespiratory R57.0
- cardiovascular R57.0
  - newborn P29.89
- circulatory (peripheral) R57.9
- during or
  - resulting from a procedure, not elsewhere classified T81.10
- general R55
- neurocirculatory F45.8
- postoperative T81.10
- valvular—*see* Endocarditis
- vascular (peripheral) R57.9
  - newborn P29.89

Colles' fracture S52.53-

Collet (-Sicard) syndrome G52.7

Collodion baby Q80.2

Coloboma (iris) Q13.0
- eyelid Q10.3
- fundus Q14.8
- lens Q12.2
- optic disc (congenital) Q14.2

Colonization
- MRSA (Methicillin resistant Staphylococcus aureus) Z22.322
- MSSA (Methicillin susceptible Staphylococcus aureus) Z22.321
- status—*see* Carrier (suspected) of

Colostomy
- attention to Z43.3
- fitting or adjustment Z46.89
- malfunctioning K94.03
- status Z93.3

Coma R40.20
- with
  - motor response (none) R40.231
    - abnormal R40.233
    - extension R40.232
    - flexion withdrawal R40.234
    - localizes pain R40.235
    - obeys commands R40.236
    - score of
      - ~ 1 R40.231
      - ~ 2 R40.232
      - ~ 3 R40.233
      - ~ 4 R40.234
      - ~ 5 R40.235
      - ~ 6 R40.236
  - opening of eyes (never) R40.211
    - in response to
      - ~ pain R40.212
      - ~ sound R40.213
    - score of
      - ~ 1 R40.211
      - ~ 2 R40.212
      - ~ 3 R40.213
      - ~ 4 R40.214
    - spontaneous R40.214
  - verbal response (none) R40.221
    - confused conversation R40.224
    - inappropriate words R40.223

Coma, *continued*
- incomprehensible words R40.222
- oriented R40.225
- score of
  - ~ 1 R40.221
  - ~ 2 R40.222
  - ~ 3 R40.223
  - ~ 4 R40.224
  - ~ 5 R40.225
- hyperosmolar (diabetic)—*see* Diabetes
- hypoglycemic (diabetic)—*see* Diabetes
  - nondiabetic E15
- in diabetes—*see* Diabetes
- insulin-induced—*see* Diabetes, coma
- newborn P91.5
- persistent vegetative state R40.3
- specified NEC, without documented Glasgow coma scale score, or with partial Glasgow coma scale score reported R40.244

Comatose—*see* Coma

Comedo, comedones (giant) L70.0

Common
- arterial trunk Q20.0
- atrioventricular canal Q21.2
- atrium Q21.1
- cold (head) J00
- truncus (arteriosus) Q20.0

Communication
- between
  - pulmonary artery and pulmonary vein, congenital Q25.72
- congenital between uterus and digestive or urinary tract Q51.7
- disorder
  - social pragmatic F80.82

Complaint—*see also* Disease
- bowel, functional K59.9
  - psychogenic F45.8
- intestine, functional K59.9
  - psychogenic F45.8
- kidney—*see* Disease, renal

Complex
- Addison-Schilder E71.528
- Costen's M26.69
- Eisenmenger's (ventricular septal defect) I27.83
- Schilder-Addison E71.528

Complication(s) (from) (of)
- arteriovenous
  - fistula, surgically created T82.9
    - infection or inflammation T82.7
  - shunt, surgically created T82.9
    - infection or inflammation T82.7
  - vascular (counterpulsation) T82.9
    - infection or inflammation T82.7
- cardiac—*see also* Disease, heart
  - device, implant or graft T82.9
    - infection or inflammation T82.7
- cardiovascular device, graft or implant T82.9
  - infection or inflammation T82.7
- catheter (device) NEC—*see also* Complications, prosthetic device or implant
  - cystostomy T83.9
    - infection and inflammation T83.510
    - mechanical
      - ~ obstruction T83.090
      - ~ perforation T83.090
      - ~ protrusion T83.090
      - ~ specified NEC T83.090
  - dialysis (vascular) T82.9
    - infection and inflammation T82.7
  - intravenous infusion T82.9
    - infection or inflammation T82.7
  - urethral T83.9
    - indwelling
      - ~ infection and inflammation T83.511
      - ~ specified complication NEC T83.091
    - infection and inflammation T83.511
    - obstruction (mechanical)
    - perforation T83.091
    - protrusion T83.091
    - specified type NEC T83.091

Complication(s), *continued*
- – urinary NEC
  - ■ infection and inflammation T83.518
  - ■ specified complication NEC T83.098
- chimeric antigen receptor (CAR-T) cell therapy T80.82
- circulatory system I99.8
  - – postprocedural I97.89
    - ■ following cardiac surgery I97.19-
      - ~ postcardiotomy syndrome I97.0
    - ■ postcardiotomy syndrome I97.0
- delivery (*see also* Complications, obstetric) O75.9
  - – specified NEC O75.89
- extracorporeal circulation T80.90
- gastrointestinal K92.9
  - – postoperative
    - ■ malabsorption NEC K91.2
- gastrostomy (stoma) K94.20
  - – hemorrhage K94.21
  - – infection K94.22
  - – malfunction K94.23
  - – mechanical K94.23
  - – specified complication NEC K94.29
- genitourinary
  - – device or implant T83.9
    - ■ urinary system T83.9
      - ~ infection or inflammation T83.598
        - ◊ indwelling urethral catheter T83.511
- graft (bypass) (patch)—*see also* Complications, prosthetic device or implant
  - – urinary organ
    - ■ infection and inflammation T83.598
      - ~ indwelling urethral catheter T83.511
- IEC (immune effector cellular) therapy T80.82
- immune effector cellular (IEC) therapy T80.82
- infusion (procedure) T80.90
  - – infection T80.29
  - – sepsis T80.29
  - – serum reaction (*see also* Reaction, serum) T80.69
    - ■ anaphylactic shock (*see also* Shock, anaphylactic) T80.59
- injection (procedure) T80.90
  - – drug reaction—*see* Reaction, drug
  - – infection T80.29
  - – sepsis T80.29
- labor O75.9
  - – specified NEC O75.89
- metabolic E88.9
  - – postoperative E89.89
    - ■ specified NEC E89.89
- obstetric O75.9
  - – specified NEC O75.89
- perfusion NEC T80.90
- postprocedural—*see also* Complications, surgical procedure
  - – cardiac arrest
    - ■ following cardiac surgery I97.120
    - ■ following other surgery I97.121
  - – cardiac functional disturbance NEC
    - ■ following cardiac surgery I97.190
    - ■ following other surgery I97.191
  - – cardiac insufficiency
    - ■ following cardiac surgery I97.110
    - ■ following other surgery I97.111
  - – heart failure
    - ■ following cardiac surgery I97.130
    - ■ following other surgery I97.131
  - – hemorrhage (hematoma) (of)
    - ■ genitourinary organ or structure
      - ~ following procedure on genitourinary organ or structure N99.820
  - – specified NEC
    - ■ respiratory system J95.89
- prosthetic device or implant T85
  - – mechanical NEC T85.698
    - ■ ventricular shunt
      - ~ breakdown T85.01
      - ~ displacement T85.02
      - ~ leakage T85.03
      - ~ malposition T85.02
      - ~ obstruction T85.09
      - ~ perforation T85.09
      - ~ protrusion T85.09
      - ~ specified NEC T85.09

Complication(s), *continued*
- respiratory system J98.9
  - – postoperative J95.89
    - ■ air leak J95.812
    - ■ specified NEC J95.89
- surgical procedure (on) T81.9
  - – malabsorption (postsurgical) NEC K91.2
  - – postcardiotomy syndrome I97.0
  - – postcommissurotomy syndrome I97.0
  - – postvalvulotomy syndrome I97.0
  - – shock (hypovolemic) T81.19
  - – stitch abscess T81.41
  - – wound infection T81.49
  - – transfusion (blood) (lymphocytes) (plasma) T80.92
- transfusion (blood) (lymphocytes) (plasma) T80.92
  - – circulatory overload E87.71
  - – febrile nonhemolytic transfusion reaction R50.84
  - – hemochromatosis E83.111
  - – hemolytic reaction (antigen unspecified) T80.919
  - – incompatibility reaction (antigen unspecified) T80.919
    - ■ acute (antigen unspecified) T80.910
    - ■ delayed (antigen unspecified) T80.911
    - ■ delayed serologic (DSTR) T80.89
  - – infection T80.29
    - ■ acute T80.22
  - – reaction NEC T80.89
  - – sepsis T80.29
  - – shock T80.89
- transplant T86.90
  - – bone marrow T86.00
    - ■ failure T86.02
    - ■ rejection T86.01
  - – failure T86.-
  - – heart T86.2-
    - ■ with lung T86.30
    - ■ cardiac allograft vasculopathy T86.290
      - ~ failure T86.32
      - ~ rejection T86.31
    - ■ failure T86.22
    - ■ rejection T86.21
  - – infection T86.-
  - – kidney T86.10
    - ■ failure T86.12
    - ■ rejection T86.11
  - – liver T86.4-
    - ■ failure T86.42
    - ■ rejection T86.41
  - – lung T86.81-
    - ■ with heart T86.30
      - ~ failure T86.32
      - ~ rejection T86.31
    - ■ failure T86.811
    - ■ rejection T86.810
  - – malignant neoplasm C80.2
  - – peripheral blood stem cells T86.5
  - – post-transplant lymphoproliferative disorder (PTLD) D47.Z1
  - – rejection T86.-
  - – specified
    - ■ type NEC T86.-
  - – stem cell (from peripheral blood) (from umbilical cord) T86.5
  - – umbilical cord stem cells T86.5
- vaccination T88.1-
  - – anaphylaxis NEC T80.52-
  - – cellulitis T88.0-
  - – encephalitis or encephalomyelitis G04.02
  - – infection (general) (local) NEC T88.0-
    - ■ meningitis G03.8
  - – myelitis G04.89
  - – protein sickness T80.62-
  - – rash T88.1-
  - – reaction (allergic) T88.1-
    - ■ serum T80.62-
  - – sepsis T88.0-
  - – serum intoxication, sickness, rash, or other serum reaction NEC T80.62-
    - ■ anaphylactic shock T80.52-
  - – shock (allergic) (anaphylactic) T80.52-
  - – vaccinia (generalized) (localized) T88.1-
- vascular I99.9
  - – device or implant T82.9
    - ■ infection or inflammation T82.7

Complication(s), *continued*
- ventricular (communicating) shunt (device) T85-
  - – mechanical
    - ■ breakdown T85.01
    - ■ displacement T85.02
    - ■ leakage T85.03
    - ■ malposition T85.02
    - ■ obstruction T85.09
    - ■ perforation T85.09
    - ■ protrusion T85.09
    - ■ specified NEC T85.09

Compression
- brain (stem) G93.5
  - – due to
    - ■ contusion (diffuse) (see also Injury, intracranial, diffuse) S06.A0
      - ~ with herniation S06.A1
    - ■ focal (see also Injury, intracranial, focal) S06.A0
      - ~ with herniation S06.A1
    - ■ injury NEC (see also Injury, intracranial, diffuse) S06.A0
      - ~ nontraumatic G93.5
    - ■ traumatic (see also Injury, intracranial, diffuse) S06.A0
      - ~ with herniation S06.A1
- facies Q67.1
- with injury *code by* Nature of injury
- laryngeal nerve, recurrent G52.2
  - – with paralysis of vocal cords and larynx J38.00
    - ■ bilateral J38.02
    - ■ unilateral J38.01
- nerve (*see also* Disorder, nerve) G58.9
  - – root or plexus NOS (in) G54.9
    - ■ neoplastic disease (*see also* Table of Neoplasms in the complete *ICD-10-CM* manual) D49.9 [G55]

Compulsion, compulsive
- neurosis F42.8
- personality F60.5
- states F42.9
- swearing F42.8
  - – in Gilles de la Tourette's syndrome F95.2
- tics and spasms F95.9

Concato's disease (pericardial polyserositis) A19.9
- nontubercular I31.1
- pleural—*see* Pleurisy, with, effusion

Concealed penis Q55.64

Concretio cordis I31.1
- rheumatic I09.2

Concretion—*see also* Calculus
- prepuce (male) N47.8
- tonsil J35.8

Concussion (brain) (cerebral) (current) S06.0X-
- syndrome F07.81
- with
  - – loss of consciousness of 30 minutes or less S06.0X1
  - – loss of consciousness of unspecified duration S06.0X9
- without loss of consciousness S06.0X0

Condition—*see also* Disease
- post COVID-19 U09.9

Conditions arising in the perinatal period—*see* Newborn, affected by

Conduct disorder—*see* Disorder, conduct

Condyloma A63.0
- acuminatum A63.0
- gonorrheal A54.09
- latum A51.31
- syphilitic A51.31
  - – congenital A50.07
- venereal, syphilitic A51.31

Conflagration—*see also* Burn
- asphyxia (by inhalation of gases, fumes or vapors) *see* Table of Drugs and Chemicals

Conflict (with)—*see also* Discord
- family Z73.9
- marital Z63.0
  - – involving divorce or estrangement Z63.5
- parent-child Z62.820
  - – parent-adopted child Z62.821

Conflict, *continued*
- – parent-biological child Z62.820
- – parent-foster child Z62.822

Confusional arousals G47.51

Congestion, congestive
- • brain G93.89
- • breast N64.59
- • catarrhal J31.0
- • chest R09.89
- • glottis J37.0
- • larynx J37.0
- • lung R09.89
  - – active or acute—*see* Pneumonia

Conjunctivitis (staphylococcal) (streptococcal) NOS H10.9
- • acute H10.3-
  - – atopic H10.1-
  - – chemical H10.21-
  - – mucopurulent H10.02-
    - ▪ viral—*see* Conjunctivitis, viral
  - – toxic H10.21-
- • blennorrhagic (gonococcal) (neonatorum) A54.31
- • chemical (acute) H10.21-
- • chlamydial A74.0
  - – neonatal P39.1
- • epidemic (viral) B30.9
- • gonococcal (neonatorum) A54.31
- • in (due to)
  - – Chlamydia A74.0
  - – gonococci A54.31
  - – rosacea H10.82-
- • inclusion A74.0
- • infantile P39.1
  - – gonococcal A54.31
- • neonatal P39.1
  - – gonococcal A54.31
- • viral B30.9

Conradi (-Hunermann) disease Q77.3

Conscious simulation (of illness) Z76.5

Consecutive—*see* Disease, diseased

Consolidation lung (base)—*see* Pneumonia, lobar

Constipation (atonic) (neurogenic) (simple) (spastic) K59.00
- • chronic K59.09
  - – idiopathic K59.04
- • drug-induced K59.03
- • functional K59.04
- • outlet dysfunction K59.02
- • psychogenic F45.8
- • slow transit K59.01
- • specified NEC K59.09

Constriction—*see also* Stricture
- • external
  - – abdomen, abdominal (wall) S30.841
  - – alveolar process S00.542
  - – ankle S90.54-
  - – antecubital space S50.84-
  - – arm (upper) S40.84-
  - – auricle S00.44-
  - – axilla S40.84-
  - – back, lower S30.840
  - – breast S20.14-
  - – brow S00.84
  - – buttock S30.840
  - – calf S80.84-
  - – canthus S00.24-
  - – cheek S00.84
    - ▪ internal S00.542
  - – chest wall—*see* Constriction, external, thorax
  - – chin S00.84
  - – clitoris S30.844
  - – costal region—*see* Constriction, external, thorax
  - – digit(s)
    - ▪ foot—*see* Constriction, external, toe
    - ▪ hand—*see* Constriction, external, finger
  - – ear S00.44-
  - – elbow S50.34-
  - – epididymis S30.843
  - – epigastric region S30.841
  - – esophagus, cervical S10.14
  - – eyebrow S00.24-
  - – eyelid S00.24-
  - – face S00.84

Constriction, *continued*
- – finger(s) S60.44-
  - ▪ index S60.44-
  - ▪ little S60.44-
  - ▪ middle S60.44-
  - ▪ ring S60.44-
- – flank S30.841
- – foot (except toe(s) alone) S90.84-
  - ▪ toe—*see* Constriction, external, toe
- – forearm S50.84-
  - ▪ elbow only S50.34-
- – forehead S00.84
- – genital organs, external
  - ▪ female S30.846
  - ▪ male S30.845
- – groin S30.841
- – gum S00.542
- – hand S60.54-
- – head S00.94
  - ▪ ear S00.44-
  - ▪ eyelid S00.24-
  - ▪ lip S00.541
  - ▪ nose S00.34
  - ▪ oral cavity S00.542
  - ▪ scalp S00.04
  - ▪ specified site NEC S00.84
- – heel S90.84-
- – hip S70.24-
- – inguinal region S30.841
- – interscapular region S20.449
- – jaw S00.84
- – knee S80.24-
- – labium (majus) (minus) S30.844
- – larynx S10.14
- – leg (lower) S80.84-
  - ▪ knee S80.24-
  - ▪ upper S70.34-
- – lip S00.541
- – lower back S30.840
- – lumbar region S30.840
- – malar region S00.84
- – mammary S20.14-
- – mastoid region S00.84
- – mouth S00.542
- – nail
  - ▪ finger—*see* Constriction, external, finger
  - ▪ toe—*see* Constriction, external, toe
- – nasal S00.34
- – neck S10.94
  - ▪ specified site NEC S10.84
  - ▪ throat S10.14
- – nose S00.34
- – occipital region S00.04
- – oral cavity S00.542
- – orbital region S00.24-
- – palate S00.542
- – palm S60.54-
- – parietal region S00.04
- – pelvis S30.840
- – penis S30.842
- – perineum
  - ▪ female S30.844
  - ▪ male S30.840
- – periocular area S00.24-
- – phalanges
  - ▪ finger—*see* Constriction, external, finger
  - ▪ toe—*see* Constriction, external, toe
- – pharynx S10.14
- – pinna S00.44-
- – popliteal space S80.24-
- – prepuce S30.842
- – pubic region S30.840
- – pudendum
  - ▪ female S30.846
  - ▪ male S30.845
- – sacral region S30.840
- – scalp S00.04
- – scapular region S40.24-
- – scrotum S30.843
- – shin S80.84-
- – shoulder S40.24-
- – sternal region S20.349
- – submaxillary region S00.84

Constriction, *continued*
- – submental region S00.84
- – subungual
  - ▪ finger(s)—*see* Constriction, external, finger
  - ▪ toe(s)—*see* Constriction, external, toe
- – supraclavicular fossa S10.84
- – supraorbital S00.84
- – temple S00.84
- – temporal region S00.84
- – testis S30.843
- – thigh S70.34-
- – thorax, thoracic (wall) S20.94
  - ▪ back S20.44-
  - ▪ front S20.34-
- – throat S10.14
- – thumb S60.34-
- – toe(s) (lesser) S90.44-
  - ▪ great S90.44-
- – tongue S00.542
- – trachea S10.14
- – tunica vaginalis S30.843
- – uvula S00.542
- – vagina S30.844
- – vulva S30.844
- – wrist S60.84-
- • prepuce (acquired) (congenital) N47.1
- • pylorus (adult hypertrophic) K31.1
  - – congenital or infantile Q40.0
  - – newborn Q40.0

Constrictive—*see* Disease, diseased

Consultation
- • medical—*see* Counseling
- • specified reason NEC Z71.89
- • without complaint or sickness Z71.9
  - – specified reason NEC Z71.89

Consumption—*see* Tuberculosis

Contact (with)—*see also* Exposure (to)
- • AIDS virus Z20.6
- • anthrax Z20.810
- • aromatic amines Z77.020
- • arsenic Z77.010
- • asbestos Z77.090
- • bacterial disease NEC Z20.818
- • body fluids (potentially hazardous) Z77.21
- • benzene Z77.021
- • chemicals (chiefly nonmedicinal) (hazardous) NEC Z77.098
- • chromium compounds Z77.018
- • communicable disease Z20.9
  - – bacterial NEC Z20.818
  - – specified NEC Z20.89
  - – viral NEC Z20.828
  - – Zika virus Z20.821
- • coronavirus (disease) (novel) 2019 Z20.822
- • dyes Z77.098
- • Escherichia coli (E. coli) Z20.01
- • German measles Z20.4
- • gonorrhea Z20.2
- • hazardous metals NEC Z77.018
- • hazardous substances NEC Z77.29
- • hazards in the physical environment NEC Z77.128
- • hazards to health NEC Z77.9
- • HIV Z20.6
- • HTLV-III/LAV Z20.6
- • human immunodeficiency virus Z20.6
- • infection Z20.9
  - – specified NEC Z20.89
- • intestinal infectious disease NEC Z20.09
  - – Escherichia Coli (E. coli) Z20.01
- • lead Z77.011
- • meningococcus Z20.811
- • mold (toxic) Z77.120
- • nickel dust Z77.018
- • poliomyelitis Z20.89
- • positive maternal group B streptococcus P00.82
- • rabies Z20.3
- • rubella Z20.4
- • sexually-transmitted disease Z20.2
- • smallpox (laboratory) Z20.89
- • syphilis Z20.2
- • tuberculosis Z20.1
- • varicella Z20.820

Contact, *continued*
- venereal disease Z20.2
- viral disease NEC Z20.828
- viral hepatitis Z20.5
- Zika virus Z20.821

Contamination, food—*see* Intoxication, foodborne

Contraception, contraceptive
- advice Z30.09
- counseling Z30.09
- device (intrauterine) (in situ) Z97.5
  - checking Z30.431
  - in place Z97.5
  - initial prescription Z30.014
    - barrier Z30.018
    - diaphragm Z30.018
    - subdermal implantable Z30.017
    - transdermal patch hormonal Z30.016
    - vaginal ring hormonal Z30.015
  - maintenance Z30.40
    - barrier Z30.49
    - diaphragm Z30.49
    - subdermal implantable Z30.46
    - transdermal patch hormonal Z30.45
    - vaginal ring hormonal Z30.44
  - reinsertion Z30.433
  - removal Z30.432
  - replacement Z30.433
- emergency (postcoital) Z30.012
- initial prescription Z30.019
  - injectable Z30.013
  - intrauterine device Z30.014
  - pills Z30.011
  - postcoital (emergency) Z30.012
  - specified type NEC Z30.018
  - subdermal implantable Z30.019
- maintenance Z30.40
  - examination Z30.8
  - injectable Z30.42
  - intrauterine device Z30.431
  - pills Z30.41
  - specified type NEC Z30.49
  - subdermal implantable Z30.46
  - transdermal patch Z30.45
  - vaginal ring Z30.44
- management Z30.9
  - specified NEC Z30.8
- postcoital (emergency) Z30.012
- prescription Z30.019
  - repeat Z30.40
- surveillance (drug)—*see* Contraception, maintenance

Contraction(s), contracture, contracted
- Achilles tendon—*see also* Short, tendon, Achilles
  - congenital Q66.89
- bladder N32.89
  - neck or sphincter N32.0
- congenital Q65.89
  - hysterical F44.4
  - knee M24.56-
  - shoulder M24.51-
  - wrist M24.53-
- hip Q65.89
  - elbow M24.52-
  - foot joint M24.57-
  - hand joint M24.54-
  - hip M24.55-
- hourglass
  - bladder N32.89
    - congenital Q64.79
  - gallbladder K82.0
    - congenital Q44.1
  - stomach K31.89
    - congenital Q40.2
    - psychogenic F45.8
- hysterical F44.4
- joint (abduction) (acquired) (adduction) (flexion) (rotation) M24.5-
  - ankle M24.57-
  - congenital NEC Q68.8
- muscle (postinfective) (postural) NEC M62.40
  - with contracture of joint—*see* Contraction, joint
  - congenital Q79.8
    - sternocleidomastoid Q68.0

Contraction(s), contracture, contracted, *continued*
- hysterical F44.4
- posttraumatic—*see* Strabismus, paralytic
- psychogenic F45.8
  - conversion reaction F44.4
- psychogenic F45.8
  - conversion reaction F44.4
- premature
  - atrium I49.1
  - supraventricular I49.1
- pylorus NEC—*see also* Pylorospasm
  - psychogenic F45.8
- sternocleidomastoid (muscle), congenital Q68.0
- stomach K31.89
  - hourglass K31.89
    - congenital Q40.2
    - psychogenic F45.8
  - psychogenic F45.8
- tendon (sheath) M62.40
  - ankle M62.47-
  - foot M62.47-
  - forearm M62.43-
  - hand M62.44-
  - lower leg M62.46-
  - multiple sites M62.49
  - neck M62.48
  - pelvic region M62.45-
  - shoulder region M62.41-
  - specified site NEC M62.48
  - thigh M62.45-
  - thorax M62.48
  - trunk M62.48
  - upper arm M62.42-
- urethra—*see also* Stricture, urethra
  - orifice N32.0
- vagina (outlet) N89.5
- vesical N32.89
  - neck or urethral orifice N32.0

Contusion (skin surface intact) T14.8
- abdomen, abdominal (muscle) (wall) S30.1
- adnexa, eye NEC S05.8X-
- alveolar process S00.532
- ankle S90.0-
- antecubital space S50.1-
- anus S30.3
- arm (upper) S40.02-
  - lower (with elbow) S50.1-
- auditory canal S00.43-
- auricle S00.43-
- axilla S40.02-
- back S20.22-
  - lower S30.0
- bone NEC T14.8
- brainstem S06.38-
- breast S20.0-
- brow S00.83
- buttock S30.0
- canthus, eye S00.1-
- cauda equina S34.3
- cerebellar, traumatic S06.37-
- cheek S00.83
  - internal S00.532
- chest (wall)—*see* Contusion, thorax
- chin S00.83
- clitoris S30.23
- conus medullaris (spine) S34.139
- corpus cavernosum S30.21
- costal region—*see* Contusion, thorax
- ear S00.43-
- elbow S50.0-
  - with forearm S50.1-
- epididymis S30.22
- epigastric region S30.1
- epiglottis S10.0
- esophagus (thoracic)
  - cervical S10.0
- eyebrow S00.1-
- eyelid (and periocular area) S00.1-
- face NEC S00.83
- femoral triangle S30.1
- finger(s) S60.00
  - with damage to nail (matrix) S60.1-

Contusion, *continued*
- index S60.02-
  - with damage to nail S60.12-
- little S60.05-
  - with damage to nail S60.15-
- middle S60.03-
  - with damage to nail S60.13-
- ring S60.04-
  - with damage to nail S60.14-
- thumb—*see* Contusion, thumb
- flank S30.1
- foot (except toe(s) alone) S90.3-
  - toe—*see* Contusion, toe
- forearm S50.1-
  - elbow only S50.0-
- forehead S00.83
- genital organs, external
  - female S30.202
  - male S30.201
- groin S30.1
- gum S00.532
- hand S60.22-
  - finger(s)—*see* Contusion, finger
  - wrist S60.21-
- head S00.93
  - ear S00.43-
  - eyelid S00.1-
  - lip S00.531
  - nose S00.33
  - oral cavity S00.532
  - scalp S00.03
  - specified part NEC S00.83
- heel S90.3-
- hip S70.0-
- iliac region S30.1
- inguinal region S30.1
- interscapular region S20.229
- intra-abdominal organ S36.92
  - refer to specific organ under contusion
- jaw S00.83
- kidney S37.01-
  - major (greater than 2 cm) S37.02-
  - minor (less than 2 cm) S37.01-
- knee S80.0-
- labium (majus) (minus) S30.23
- lacrimal apparatus, gland or sac S05.8X-
- larynx S10.0
- leg (lower) S80.1-
  - knee S80.0-
- lip S00.531
- lower back S30.0
- lumbar region S30.0
- lung S27.329
  - bilateral S27.322
  - unilateral S27.321
- malar region S00.83
- mastoid region S00.83
- mouth S00.532
- muscle—*see* Contusion, by site
- nail
  - finger—*see* Contusion, finger, with damage to nail
  - toe—*see* Contusion, toe, with damage to nail
- nasal S00.33
- neck S10.93
  - specified site NEC S10.83
  - throat S10.0
- nerve—*see* Injury, nerve
- newborn P54.5
- nose S00.33
- occipital
  - region (scalp) S00.03
- palate S00.532
- parietal
  - region (scalp) S00.03
  - kidney—*see* Contusion, kidney
- pelvis S30.0
- penis S30.21
- perineum
  - female S30.23
  - male S30.23
- periocular area S00.1-
- pharynx S10.0
- pinna S00.43-

Contusion, *continued*
- popliteal space S80.0-
- prepuce S30.21
- pubic region S30.1
- pudendum
  - female S30.202
  - male S30.201
- quadriceps femoris S70.1-
- rectum S36.62
- sacral region S30.0
- scalp S00.03
  - due to birth injury P12.3
- scapular region S40.01-
- scrotum S30.22
- shoulder S40.01-
- skin NEC T14.8
- spermatic cord S30.22
- spinal cord—*see* Injury, spinal cord, by region
  - cauda equina S34.3
  - conus medullaris S34.139
- spleen S36.02-
  - major S36.021
  - minor S36.020
- sternal region S20.219
- stomach S36.32
- subcutaneous NEC T14.8
- submaxillary region S00.83
- submental region S00.83
- subperiosteal NEC T14.8
- subungual
  - finger—*see* Contusion, finger, with damage to nail
  - toe—*see* Contusion, toe, with damage to nail
- supraclavicular fossa S10.83
- supraorbital S00.83
- temple (region) S00.83
- testis S30.22
- thigh S70.1-
- thorax (wall) S20.20
  - back S20.22-
  - front S20.21-
- throat S10.0
- thumb S60.01-
  - with damage to nail S60.11-
- toe(s) (lesser) S90.12-
  - with damage to nail S90.22-
  - great S90.11-
    - with damage to nail S90.21-
    - specified type NEC S90.221
- tongue S00.532
- trachea (cervical) S10.0
- tunica vaginalis S30.22
- tympanum, tympanic membrane S00.43-
- uvula S00.532
- vagina S30.23
- vocal cord(s) S10.0
- vulva S30.23
- wrist S60.21-

Conversion hysteria, neurosis or reaction F44.9

Converter, tuberculosis (test reaction) R76.11

Convulsions (idiopathic) (*see also* Seizure(s)) R56.9
- febrile R56.00
  - with status epilepticus G40.901
  - complex R56.01
    - with status epilepticus G40.901
  - simple R56.00
- infantile P90
  - epilepsy—*see* Epilepsy
- myoclonic G25.3
- neonatal, benign (familial)—*see* Epilepsy, generalized, idiopathic
- newborn P90
- post traumatic R56.1
- recurrent R56.9
- scarlatinal A38.8

Convulsive—*see also* Convulsions

Cooley's anemia D56.1

Copra itch B88.0

Coprophagy F50.89

Cor
- pulmonale (chronic) I27.81
- triloculare Q20.8
  - biventriculare Q21.1

Corbus' disease (gangrenous balanitis) N48.1

Corn (infected) L84

Cornelia de Lange syndrome Q87.19

Cornual gestation or pregnancy O00.8-

Coronavirus (Infection)
- as cause of diseases classified elsewhere B97.29
- coronavirus-19 U07.1
- COVID-19 U07.1
- SARS-associated B97.21

Corrosion (injury) (acid) (caustic) (chemical) (lime) (external) (internal) T30.4
- extent (percentage of body surface)
  - less than 10 percent T32.0

Coryza (acute) J00
- with grippe or influenza—*see* Influenza, with, respiratory manifestations NEC

Costen's syndrome or complex M26.69

Costochondritis M94.0

Cot death R99

Cough (affected) (chronic) (epidemic) (nervous) R05.9
- with hemorrhage—*see* Hemoptysis
- acute R05.1
- bronchial R05
  - with grippe or influenza—*see* Influenza, with, respiratory manifestations NEC
- chronic R05.3
- functional F45.8
- hysterical F45.8
- laryngeal, spasmodic R05
- paroxysmal, due to Bordetella pertussis (without pneumonia) A37.00
  - with pneumonia A37.01
- persistent R05.3
- psychogenic F45.8
- refractory R05.3
- specified NEC R05.8
- subacute R05.2
- syncope R05.4
- unexplained R05.3

Counseling (for) Z71.9
- abuse NEC
  - perpetrator Z69.82
  - victim Z69.81
- alcohol abuser Z71.41
  - family Z71.42
- child abuse
  - non-parental
    - perpetrator Z69.021
    - victim Z69.020
  - parental
    - perpetrator Z69.011
    - victim Z69.010
- contraceptive Z30.09
- dietary Z71.3
- drug abuser Z71.51
  - family member Z71.52
- exercise Z71.82
- family Z71.89
- for non-attending third party Z71.0
  - related to sexual behavior or orientation Z70.2
- genetic
  - nonprocreative Z71.83
  - procreative NEC Z31.5
- health (advice) (education) (instruction)—*see* Counseling
- human immunodeficiency virus (HIV) Z71.7
- immunization safety Z71.85
- insulin pump use Z46.81
- medical (for) Z71.9
  - human immunodeficiency virus (HIV) Z71.7
  - on behalf of another Z71.0
  - specified reason NEC Z71.89
- natural family planning
  - to avoid pregnancy Z30.02
- perpetrator (of)
  - abuse NEC Z69.82
  - child abuse

Counseling, *continued*
- non-parental Z69.021
- parental Z69.011
  - rape NEC Z69.82
  - spousal abuse Z69.12
- procreative NEC Z31.69
- rape victim Z69.81
- safety for (international) travel Z71.84
- specified reason NEC Z71.89
- spousal abuse (perpetrator) Z69.12
  - victim Z69.11
- substance abuse Z71.89
  - alcohol Z71.41
  - drug Z71.51
  - tobacco Z71.6
- tobacco use Z71.6
- travel (international) Z71.84
- use (of)
  - insulin pump Z46.81
- vaccine product safety Z71.85
- victim (of)
  - abuse Z69.81
  - child abuse
    - by parent Z69.010
    - non-parental Z69.020
  - rape NEC Z69.81

COVID-19 U07.1
- condition post U09.9
- contact (with) Z20.822
- exposure (to) Z20.822
- history of (personal) Z86.16
- long (haul) U09.9
  - sequelae (post acute) U09.9

Coxsackie (virus) (infection) B34.1
- as cause of disease classified elsewhere B97.11
- enteritis A08.3
- meningitis (aseptic) A87.0
- pharyngitis B08.5

Crabs, meaning pubic lice B85.3

Crack baby P04.41

Cracked tooth K03.81

Cradle cap L21.0

Cramp(s) R25.2
- abdominal—*see* Pain, abdominal
- bathing T75.1
- colic R10.83
  - psychogenic F45.8
- due to immersion T75.1
- fireman T67.2
- heat T67.2
- immersion T75.1
- intestinal—*see* Pain, abdominal
  - psychogenic F45.8
- limb (lower) (upper) NEC R25.2
  - sleep related G47.62
- muscle (limb) (general) R25.2
  - due to immersion T75.1
  - psychogenic F45.8
- salt-depletion E87.1
- stoker's T67.2
- swimmer's T75.1

Craniocleidodysostosis Q74.0

Craniofenestria (skull) Q75.8

Craniolacunia (skull) Q75.8

Cranioschisis Q75.8

Crepitus
- caput Q75.8
- joint—*see* Derangement, joint, specified type NEC

Crib death R99

Cribriform hymen Q52.3

Cri-du-chat syndrome Q93.4

Crigler-Najjar disease or syndrome E80.5

Crisis
- abdomen R10.0
- acute reaction F43.0
- addisonian E27.2
- adrenal (cortical) E27.2
- celiac K90.0
- Dietl's N13.8

Crisis, *continued*
- emotional—*see also* Disorder, adjustment
  - acute reaction to stress F43.0
  - specific to childhood and adolescence F93.8
- oculogyric H51.8
  - psychogenic F45.8
- psychosexual identity F64.2
- sickle-cell D57.00
  - with
    - acute chest syndrome D57.01
    - cerebral vascular involvement D57.03
    - crisis (painful) D57.00
      - with complication specified NEC D57.09
    - splenic sequestration D57.02
    - vasoocclusive pain D57.00
- state (acute reaction) F43.0

Crocq's disease (acrocyanosis) I73.89

Crohn's disease—*see* Enteritis, regional

Crooked septum, nasal J34.2

Croup, croupous (catarrhal) (infectious) (inflammatory) (nondiphtheritic) J05.0
- bronchial J20.9

Crush, crushed, crushing T14.8
- ankle S97.0-
- arm (upper) (and shoulder) S47.- (See complete *ICD-10-CM* Manual for codes)
- finger(s) S67.1-
  - with hand (and wrist) S67.2-
  - index S67.19-
  - little S67.19-
  - middle S67.19-
  - ring S67.19-
  - thumb—*see* Crush, thumb
- foot S97.8-
  - toe—*see* Crush, toe
- hand (except fingers alone) S67.2-
  - with wrist S67.4-
- thumb S67.0-
  - with hand (and wrist) S00.44-
- toe(s) S97.10-
  - great S97.11-
  - lesser S97.12-
- wrist S67.3-
  - with hand S67.4-

Crusta lactea L21.0

Crying (constant) (continuous) (excessive)
- child, adolescent, or adult R45.83
- infant (baby) (newborn) R68.11

Cryptitis (anal) (rectal) K62.89

Cryptopapillitis (anus) K62.89

Cryptophthalmos Q11.2
- syndrome Q87.0

Cryptorchid, cryptorchism, cryptorchidism Q53.9
- bilateral Q53.20
  - abdominal Q53.211
  - perineal Q53.22
- unilateral Q53.10
  - abdominal Q53.111
  - perineal Q53.12

Cryptosporidiosis A07.2
- hepatobiliary B88.8
- respiratory B88.8

Crystalluria R82.998

Cubitus
- congenital Q68.8
- valgus (acquired) M21.0-
  - congenital Q68.8
- varus (acquired) M21.1-
  - congenital Q68.8

Cultural deprivation or shock Z60.3

Curvature
- organ or site, congenital NEC—*see* Distortion
- penis (lateral) Q55.61
- Pott's (spinal) A18.01
- radius, idiopathic, progressive (congenital) Q74.0
- spine (acquired) (angular) (idiopathic) (incorrect) (postural)
  - congenital Q67.5
  - due to or associated with

Curvature, *continued*
- osteitis
  - deformans M88.88
  - tuberculosis (Pott's curvature) A18.01
- tuberculous A18.01

Cushingoid due to steroid therapy E24.2
- correct substance properly administered—*see* Table of Drugs and Chemicals, by drug, adverse effect
- overdose or wrong substance given or taken—*see* Table of Drugs and Chemicals, by drug, poisoning

Cushing's
- syndrome or disease E24.9
  - drug-induced E24.2
  - iatrogenic E24.2
  - pituitary-dependent E24.0
  - specified NEC E24.8
- ulcer—*see* Ulcer, peptic, acute

Cutaneous—*see also* Disease, diseased
- hemorrhage R23.3

Cutis—*see also* Disease, diseased
- hyperelastica Q82.8
- osteosis L94.2
- verticis gyrata Q82.8
  - acquired L91.8

Cyanosis R23.0
- due to
  - patent foramen botalli Q21.1
  - persistent foramen ovale Q21.1
- enterogenous D74.8

Cyanotic heart disease I24.9
- congenital Q24.9

Cycle
- anovulatory N97.0
- menstrual, irregular N92.6

Cyclical vomiting, in migraine (*see also* Vomiting, cyclical) G43.A0
- psychogenic F50.89

Cyclical vomiting syndrome unrelated to migraine R11.15

Cycloid personality F34.0

Cyclopia, cyclops Q87.0

Cyclopism Q87.0

Cyclothymia F34.0

Cyclothymic personality F34.0

Cylindruria R82.998

Cynanche
- tonsillaris J36

Cyst (colloid) (mucous) (simple) (retention)
- adenoid (infected) J35.8
- antrum J34.1
- anus K62.89
- arachnoid, brain (acquired) G93.0
  - congenital Q04.6
- Baker's M71.2-
  - choroid plexus Q04.6
- Bartholin's gland N75.0
- bone (local) NEC M85.60
  - specified type NEC M85.60
    - ankle M85.67-
    - foot M85.67-
    - forearm M85.63-
    - hand M85.64-
    - jaw M27.40
      - developmental (nonodontogenic) K09.1
        - odontogenic K09.0
    - lower leg M85.66-
    - multiple site M85.69
    - neck M85.68
    - rib M85.68
    - shoulder M85.61-
    - skull M85.68
    - specified site NEC M85.68
    - thigh M85.65-
    - toe M85.67-
    - upper arm M85.62-
    - vertebra M85.68
- brain (acquired) G93.0
  - congenital Q04.6
  - third ventricle (colloid), congenital Q04.6

Cyst, *continued*
- breast (benign) (blue dome) (pedunculated) (solitary) N60.0-
- canal of Nuck (female) N94.89
  - congenital Q52.4
- choledochus, congenital Q44.4
- common (bile) duct
  - congenital NEC Q89.8
  - fallopian tube Q50.4
  - kidney Q61.00
    - more than one (multiple) Q61.02
    - specified as polycystic Q61.3
      - infantile type NEC Q61.19
  - ovary Q50.1
  - oviduct Q50.4
- congenital NEC Q89.8
  - kidney Q61.00
    - more than one (multiple) Q61.02
      - specified as polycystic Q61.3
        - infantile type NEC Q61.19
          - collecting duct dilation Q61.11
    - solitary Q61.01
  - prepuce Q55.69
  - thymus (gland) Q89.2
- corpus
  - albicans N83.29-
  - luteum (hemorrhagic) (ruptured) N83.1-
- craniobuccal pouch E23.6
- craniopharyngeal pouch E23.6
- Dandy-Walker Q03.1
  - with spina bifida—*see* Spina bifida
- dental (root) K04.8
  - developmental K09.0
  - eruption K09.0
  - primordial K09.0
- dentigerous (mandible) (maxilla) K09.0
- dermoid—*see* Neoplasm, benign, by site in Table of Neoplasms in the complete *ICD-10-CM* manual
  - implantation
    - vagina N89.8
- developmental K09.1
  - odontogenic K09.0
- dura (cerebral) G93.0
  - spinal G96.198
- epoophoron Q50.5
- eruption K09.0
- esophagus K22.89
- ethmoid sinus J34.1
- eye NEC H57.89
- eyelid (sebaceous) H02.82-
  - infected—*see* Hordeolum
  - left H02.826
    - lower H02.825
    - upper H02.824
  - right H02.823
    - lower H02.822
    - upper H02.821
- fallopian tube N83.8
  - congenital Q50.4
- follicle (graafian) (hemorrhagic) N83.0-
- follicular (atretic) (hemorrhagic) (ovarian) N83.0-
  - dentigerous K09.0
  - odontogenic K09.0
  - skin L72.9
    - specified NEC L72.8
- frontal sinus J34.1
- gingiva K09.0
- graafian follicle (hemorrhagic) N83.0-
- granulosal lutein (hemorrhagic) N83.1-
- hemangiomatous D18.00
  - skin D18.01
  - specified site NEC D18.09
- hydatid (*see also* Echinococcus)
  - Morgagni
    - male (epididymal) Q55.4
    - testicular Q55.29
- hymen N89.8
  - embryonic Q52.4
- hypophysis, hypophyseal (duct) (recurrent) E23.6
  - cerebri E23.6
- implantation (dermoid)
  - vagina N89.8

Cyst, *continued*
- intrasellar E23.6
- jaw (bone) M27.40
  - developmental (odontogenic) K09.0
- kidney (acquired) N28.1
  - congenital Q61.00
  - more than one (multiple) Q61.02
    - specified as polycystic Q61.3
      - ~ infantile type (autosomal recessive) NEC Q61.19
        - ◊ collecting duct dilation Q61.11
  - simple N28.1
  - solitary (single) Q61.01
    - acquired N28.1
- lateral periodontal K09.0
- lens H27.8
  - congenital Q12.8
- lip (gland) K13.0
- lutein N83.1-
- mandible M27.40
  - dentigerous K09.0
- maxilla M27.40
  - dentigerous K09.0
- meninges (cerebral) G93.0
  - spinal G96.19-
- Morgagni (hydatid)
  - male (epididymal) Q55.4
    - testicular Q55.29
- Müllerian duct Q50.4
  - appendix testis Q55.29
  - cervix Q51.6
  - fallopian tube Q50.4
  - female Q50.4
  - male Q55.29
- nerve root
  - cervical G96.191
  - lumbar G96.191
  - sacral G96.191
  - thoracic G96.191
- nervous system NEC G96.89
- nose (turbinates) J34.1
  - sinus J34.1
- odontogenic, developmental K09.0
- omentum (lesser) congenital Q45.8
- ovary, ovarian (twisted) N83.20-
  - adherent N83.20-
  - corpus
    - albicans N83.29-
    - luteum (hemorrhagic) N83.1-
  - developmental Q50.1
  - due to failure of involution NEC N83.20-
  - follicular (graafian) (hemorrhagic) N83.0-
  - hemorrhagic N83.20-
  - retention N83.29-
  - serous N83.20-
  - specified NEC N83.29-
  - theca lutein (hemorrhagic) N83.1-
- paramesonephric duct Q50.4
  - female Q50.4
  - male Q55.29
- paranephric N28.1
- paraphysis, cerebri, congenital Q04.6
- paroophoron Q50.5
- parovarian Q50.5
- pericardial (congenital) Q24.8
  - acquired (secondary) I31.8
- pericoronal K09.0
- periodontal K04.8
  - lateral K09.0
- perineural G96.191
- peripelvic (lymphatic) N28.1
- periventricular, acquired, newborn P91.1
- pilar L72.11
- pilonidal (infected) (rectum) L05.91
  - with abscess L05.01
- pituitary (duct) (gland) E23.6
- porencephalic Q04.6
  - acquired G93.0
- prepuce N47.4
  - congenital Q55.69
- primordial (jaw) K09.0
- Rathke's pouch E23.6
- rectum (epithelium) (mucous) K62.89
- renal—*see* Cyst, kidney

Cyst, *continued*
- retention (ovary) N83.29-
- sebaceous (duct) (gland) L72.3
  - eyelid—*see* Cyst, eyelid
  - genital organ NEC
    - female N94.89
    - male N50.89
  - scrotum L72.3
- serous (ovary) N83.20-
- sinus (accessory) (nasal) J34.1
- skin L72.9
  - sebaceous L72.3
- solitary
  - bone—*see* Cyst, bone
  - jaw M27.40
  - kidney N28.1
- sphenoid sinus J34.1
- spinal meninges G96.198
- subdural (cerebral) G93.0
  - spinal cord G96.198
- Tarlov G96.191
- testis N44.2
  - tunica albuginea N44.1
- theca lutein (ovary) N83.1-
- thyroglossal duct (infected) (persistent) Q89.2
- thyrolingual duct (infected) (persistent) Q89.2
- tonsil J35.8
- trichilemmal (proliferating) L72.12
- trichodermal L72.12
- turbinate (nose) J34.1
- vagina, vaginal (implantation) (inclusion) (squamous cell) (wall) N89.8
  - embryonic Q52.4
- wolffian
  - female Q50.5
  - male Q55.4

Cystic—*see also* Disease, diseased
- corpora lutea (hemorrhagic) N83.1-
- kidney (congenital) Q61.9
  - infantile type NEC Q61.19
    - collecting duct dilatation Q61.11
  - medullary Q61.5
- ovary N83.20-

Cysticerosis, cysticerciasis B69.9
- with
  - epileptiform fits B69.0
- brain B69.0
- central nervous system B69.0
- cerebral B69.0
- specified NEC B69.89

Cystinosis (malignant) E72.04

Cystitis (exudative) (hemorrhagic) (septic) (suppurative) N30.90
- acute N30.00
  - with hematuria N30.01
  - of trigone N30.00
    - with hematuria N30.31
- blennorrhagic (gonococcal) A54.01
- chlamydial A56.01
- gonococcal A54.01
- trichomonal A59.03

Cystoma—*see also* Neoplasm, benign, by site in Table of Neoplasms in the complete *ICD-10-CM* manual
- simple (ovary) N83.29-

Cytomegalic inclusion disease
- congenital P35.1

Cytomegalovirus infection B25.9

Cytopenia D75.9

D

Da Costa's syndrome F45.8

Dacryocystitis
- neonatal P39.1

Dacryostenosis—*see also* Stenosis, lacrimal
- **congenital** Q10.5

Dactylitis
- bone—*see* Osteomyelitis
- sickle-cell D57.00
  - Hb C D57.219

Dactylitis, *continued*
- Hb SS D57.00
- specified NEC D57.819
- skin L08.9
- tuberculous A18.03

Dactylosymphysis Q70.9
- fingers—*see* Syndactylism, complex, fingers
- toes—*see* Syndactylism, complex, toes

Damage
- brain (nontraumatic) G93.9
  - anoxic, hypoxic G93.1
  - child NEC G80.9
  - due to birth injury P11.2
- cerebral NEC—*see* Damage, brain
- eye, birth injury P15.3
- lung
  - dabbing (related) U07.0
  - electronic cigarette (related) U07.0
  - vaping (associated) (device) (product) (use) U07.0
- organ
  - dabbing (related) U07.0
  - electronic cigarette (related) U07.0
  - vaping (device) (product) (use) (associated) U07.0
- vascular I99.9

Dandruff L21.0

Dandy-Walker syndrome Q03.1
- with spina bifida—*see* Spina bifida

Danlos' syndrome Q79.60
- classical Ehlers-Danlos syndrome Q79.61
- hypermobile Ehlers-Danlos syndrome Q79.62
- other Ehlers-Danlos syndromes Q79.69
- vascular Ehlers-Danlos syndrome Q79.63

Darier (-White) disease (congenital) Q82.8
- meaning erythema annulare centrifugum L53.1

Darier-Roussy sarcoid D86.3

De la Tourette's syndrome F95.2

De Lange's syndrome Q87.19

De Morgan's spots (senile angiomas) I78.1

De Toni-Fanconi (-Debré) syndrome E72.09
- with cystinosis E72.04

Dead
- fetus, retained (mother) O36.4
  - early pregnancy O02.1

Deaf-mutism (acquired) (congenital) NEC H91.3
- hysterical F44.6

Deafness (acquired) (complete) (hereditary) (partial) H91.9-
- with blue sclera and fragility of bone Q78.0
- central—*see* Deafness, sensorineural
- conductive H90.2
  - and sensorineural, mixed H90.8
    - bilateral H90.6
  - bilateral H90.0
  - unilateral H90.1-
    - with restrictive hearing on contralateral side H90.A-
- congenital H90.5
  - with blue sclera and fragility of bone Q78.0
- emotional (hysterical) F44.6
- functional (hysterical) F44.6
- high frequency H91.9-
- hysterical F44.6
- low frequency H91.9-
- mixed conductive and sensorineural H90.8
  - bilateral H90.6
  - unilateral H90.7-
- nerve—*see* Deafness, sensorineural
- neural—*see* Deafness, sensorineural
- noise-induced—*see also* subcategory H83.3
- psychogenic (hysterical) F44.6
- sensorineural H90.5
  - and conductive, mixed H90.8
    - bilateral H90.6
  - bilateral H90.3
  - unilateral H90.4-
- sensory—*see* Deafness, sensorineural
- word (developmental) H93.25

Death (cause unknown) (of) (unexplained) (unspecified cause) R99
- brain G93.82
- cardiac (sudden) (with successful resuscitation)—*code to* underlying disease
  - family history of Z82.41
  - personal history of Z86.74
- family member (assumed) Z63.4

Debility (chronic) (general) (nervous) R53.81
- congenital or neonatal NOS P96.9
- nervous R53.81

Débove's disease (splenomegaly) R16.1

Decalcification
- teeth K03.89

Decrease(d)
- absolute neutrophil count—*see* Neutropenia
- blood
  - platelets—*see* Thrombocytopenia
  - pressure R03.1
    - due to shock following
      - ~ injury T79.4
      - ~ operation T81.19
- function
  - ovary in hypopituitarism E23.0
  - pituitary (gland) (anterior) (lobe) E23.0
    - posterior (lobe) E23.0
- hematocrit R71.0
- hemoglobin R71.0
- leukocytes D72.819
  - specified NEC D72.818
- lymphocytes D72.810
- respiration, due to shock following injury T79.4
- tolerance
  - fat K90.49
  - glucose R73.09
  - salt and water E87.8
- vision NEC H54.7
- white blood cell count D72.819
  - specified NEC D72.818

Defect, defective Q89.9
- 3-beta-hydroxysterioid dehydrogenase E25.0
- 11-hydroxylase E25.0
- 21-hydroxylase E25.0
- atrial septal (ostium secundum type) Q21.1
  - ostium primum type Q21.2
- atrioventricular
  - canal Q21.2
  - septum Q21.2
- auricular septal Q21.1
- bilirubin excretion NEC E80.6
- bulbar septum Q21.0
- cell membrane receptor complex (CR3) D71
- circulation I99.9
  - congenital Q28.9
  - newborn Q28.9
- coagulation (factor) (*see also* Deficiency) D68.9
  - newborn, transient P61.6
- conduction (heart) I45.9
  - bone—*see* Deafness, conductive
- coronary sinus Q21.1
- cushion, endocardial Q21.2
- degradation, glycoprotein E77.1
- diaphragm
  - with elevation, eventration or hernia—*see* Hernia, diaphragm
  - congenital Q79.1
    - with hernia Q79.0
    - gross (with hernia) Q79.0
- extensor retinaculum M62.89
- filling
  - bladder R93.41
  - kidney R93.42-
  - renal pelvis R93.41
  - ureter R93.41
  - urinary organs, specified NEC R93.49
- GABA (gamma aminobutyric acid) metabolic E72.81
- Gerbode Q21.0
- glucose transport, blood-brain barrier E74.810
- glycoprotein degradation E77.1
- interatrial septal Q21.1
- interauricular septal Q21.1

Defect, defective, *continued*
- interventricular septal Q21.0
  - with dextroposition of aorta, pulmonary stenosis and hypertrophy of right ventricle Q21.3
  - in tetralogy of Fallot Q21.3
- learning (specific)—*see* Disorder, learning
- lymphocyte function antigen-1 (LFA-1) D84.0
- lysosomal enzyme, post-translational modification E77.0
- modification, lysosomal enzymes, post-translational E77.0
- obstructive, congenital
  - ureter Q62.39
    - orthotopic ureterocele Q62.31
- osteochondral NEC—*see also* Deformity M95.8
- ostium
  - primum Q21.2
  - secundum Q21.1
- platelets, qualitative D69.1
  - constitutional D68.0
- reduction
  - limb
    - lower Q72.9-
      - ~ longitudinal
        - ◊ femur Q72.4-
        - ◊ fibula Q72.6-
        - ◊ tibia Q72.5-
      - ~ specified type NEC Q72.89-
    - upper Q71.9-
      - ~ longitudinal
        - ◊ radius Q71.4-
        - ◊ ulna Q71.5-
      - ~ specified type NEC Q71.89-
- respiratory system, congenital Q34.9
- septal (heart) NOS Q21.9
  - atrial Q21.1
  - ventricular (*see also* Defect, ventricular septal) Q21.0
- sinus venosus Q21.1
- speech R47.9
  - developmental F80.9
  - specified NEC R47.89
- vascular (local) I99.9
  - congenital Q27.9
- ventricular septal Q21.0
  - in tetralogy of Fallot Q21.3
- vision NEC H54.7

Defibrination (syndrome) D65
- newborn P60

Deficiency, deficient
- 3-beta-hydroxysterioid dehydrogenase E25.0
- 11-hydroxylase E25.0
- 21-hydroxylase E25.0
- AADC (aromatic L-amino acid decarboxylase) E70.81
- abdominal muscle syndrome Q79.4
- acid sphingomyelinase (ASMD) E75.249
  - type
    - A E75.240
    - A/B E75.244
    - B E75.241
- adenosine deaminase (ADA) D81.30
  - deaminase 2 D81.32
  - other adenosine deaminase D81.39
  - severe combined immunodeficiency due to adenosine deaminase deficiency D81.31
    - type 1 (without SCID) (without severe combined immunodeficiency) D81.39
    - type 2 D81.32
- anti-hemophilic
  - factor (A) D66
    - B D67
    - C D68.1
  - globulin (AHG) NEC D66
- antidiuretic hormone E23.2
- aromatic L-amino acid decarboxylase (AADC) E70.81
- attention (disorder) (syndrome) F98.8
  - with hyperactivity—*see* Disorder, attention-deficit hyperactivity
- beta-glucuronidase E76.29
- calcium (dietary) E58
- carnitine E71.40
  - due to
    - hemodialysis E71.43
    - inborn errors of metabolism E71.42

Deficiency, deficient, *continued*
- Valproic acid therapy E71.43
- iatrogenic E71.43
- muscle palmityltransferase E71.314
- primary E71.41
- secondary E71.448
- cell membrane receptor complex (CR3) D71
- central nervous system G96.89
- clotting (blood) (*see also* Deficiency) D68.9
- coagulation NOS D68.9
- combined glucocorticoid and mineralocorticoid E27.49
- corticoadrenal E27.40
  - primary E27.1
- dehydrogenase
  - long chain/very long chain acyl CoA E71.310
  - medium chain acyl CoA E71.311
  - short chain acyl CoA E71.312
- diet E63.9
- disaccharidase E73.9
- enzymes, circulating NEC E88.09
- essential fatty acid (EFA) E63.0
- factor—*see also* Deficiency
  - IX (congenital) (functional) (hereditary) (with functional defect) D67
  - VIII (congenital) (functional) (hereditary) (with functional defect) D66
    - with vascular defect D68.0
  - XI (congenital) (hereditary) D68.1
- fibrinogen (congenital) (hereditary) D68.2
  - acquired D65
- GABA (gamma aminobutyric acid) metabolic E72.81
- GABA-T (gamma aminobutyric acid) metabolic E72.81
- gammaglobulin in blood D80.1
  - hereditary D80.0
- glucocorticoid E27.49
  - mineralocorticoid E27.49
- glucose-6-phosphate dehydrogenase (G6PD) with anemia D55.0
- glucose-6-phosphate dehydrogenase (G6PD) without anemia D75.A
- glucose transporter protein type 1 E74.810
- glucuronyl transferase E80.5
- Glut1 E74.810
- gonadotropin (isolated) E23.0
- growth hormone (idiopathic) (isolated) E23.0
- hearing—*see* Deafness
- high grade F70
- hemoglobin D64.9
- hormone
  - anterior pituitary (partial) NEC E23.0
    - growth E23.0
  - growth (isolated) E23.0
  - pituitary E23.0
- hypoxanthine- (guanine)-phosphoribosyltransferase (HG-PRT) (total H-PRT) E79.1
- immunity D84.9
  - cell-mediated D84.89
    - with thrombocytopenia and eczema D82.0
  - combined D81.9
- infantile neurovisceral acid sphingomyelinase E75.240
- kappa-light chain D80.8
- lacrimal fluid (acquired)—*see also* Syndrome
  - congenital Q10.6
- lactase
  - congenital E73.0
  - secondary E73.1
- menadione (vitamin K) E56.1
  - newborn P53
- mineralocorticoid E27.49
  - with glucocorticoid E27.49
- moral F60.2
- multiple sulfatase (MSD) E75.26
  - *Add-* succinic semialdehyde dehydrogenase E72.81
  - *Revise from-* sulfatase E75.29
  - *Revise to-* sulfatase E75.26
- muscle
  - carnitine (palmityltransferase) E71.314
- NADH diaphorase or reductase (congenital) D74.0
- NADH-methemoglobin reductase (congenital) D74.0
- natrium E87.1
- parathyroid (gland) E20.9
- phosphoenolpyruvate carboxykinase E74.4
- phosphomannomutuse E74.818

Deficiency, deficient, *continued*
- phosphomannose isomerase E74.818
- phosphomannosyl mutase E74.818
- pituitary hormone (isolated) E23.0
- plasma thromboplastin
  - antecedent (PTA) D68.1
  - component (PTC) D67
- plasminogen (type 1) (type 2) E88.02
- platelet NEC D69.1
  - constitutional D68.0
- protein (*see also* Malnutrition) E46
- pseudocholinesterase E88.09
- PTA (plasma thromboplastin antecedent) D68.1
- pyruvate
  - carboxylase E74.4
  - dehydrogenase E74.4
- salt E87.1
- secretion
  - urine R34
- short stature homeobox gene (SHOX)
  - with
    - dyschondrosteosis Q78.8
    - short stature (idiopathic) E34.3
    - Turner's syndrome Q96.9
- sodium (Na) E87.1
- thrombokinase D68.2
  - newborn P53
- vascular I99.9
- vasopressin E23.2
- vitamin (multiple) NOS E56.9
  - K E56.1
    - of newborn P53

Deficit—*see also* Deficiency
- attention and concentration R41.840
  - disorder—*see* Attention, deficit
- concentration R41.840
- oxygen R09.02

Deflection
- radius M21.83-
- septum (acquired) (nasal) (nose) J34.2
- spine—*see* Curvature, spine
- turbinate (nose) J34.2

Defluvium
- capillorum—*see* Alopecia
- unguium L60.8

Deformity Q89.9
- abdominal wall
  - acquired M95.8
  - congenital Q79.59
- alimentary tract, congenital Q45.9
  - upper Q40.9
- anus (acquired) K62.89
  - congenital Q43.9
- aorta (arch) (congenital) Q25.40
- aortic
  - cusp or valve (congenital) Q23.8
    - acquired (*see also* Endocarditis, aortic) I35.8
- artery (congenital) (peripheral) NOS Q27.9
  - umbilical Q27.0
- atrial septal Q21.1
- bile duct (common) (congenital) (hepatic) Q44.5
  - acquired K83.8
- biliary duct or passage (congenital) Q44.5
  - acquired K83.8
- bladder (neck) (trigone) (sphincter) (acquired) N32.89
  - congenital Q64.79
- bone (acquired) NOS M95.9
  - congenital Q79.9
- brain (congenital) Q04.9
  - acquired G93.89
- bursa, congenital Q79.9
- cerebral, acquired G93.89
  - congenital Q04.9
- cheek (acquired) M95.2
  - congenital Q18.9
- chin (acquired) M95.2
  - congenital Q18.9
- choroid (congenital) Q14.3
  - plexus Q07.8
    - acquired G96.198
- clavicle (acquired) M95.8
  - congenital Q68.8

Deformity, *continued*
- cystic duct (congenital) Q44.5
  - acquired K82.8
- Dandy-Walker Q03.1
  - with spina bifida—*see* Spina bifida
- diaphragm (congenital) Q79.1
  - acquired J98.6
- digestive organ NOS Q45.9
- ductus arteriosus Q25.0
- ear (acquired) H61.1-
  - congenital (external) Q17.9
- ectodermal (congenital) NEC Q84.9
- endocrine gland NEC Q89.2
- eye, congenital Q15.9
- face (acquired) M95.2
  - congenital Q18.9
- flexion (joint) (acquired) (*see also* Deformity, limb, flexion) M21.20
  - congenital NOS Q74.9
    - hip Q65.89
- foot (acquired)—*see also* Deformity, limb, lower leg
  - cavovarus (congenital) Q66.1-
  - congenital NOS Q66.9-
    - specified type NEC Q66.89
  - specified type NEC M21.6X-
  - valgus (congenital) Q66.6
    - acquired M21.07-
  - varus (congenital) NEC Q66.3-
    - acquired M21.17-
- forehead (acquired) M95.2
  - congenital Q75.8
- frontal bone (acquired) M95.2
  - congenital Q75.8
- gallbladder (congenital) Q44.1
  - acquired K82.8
- gastrointestinal tract (congenital) NOS Q45.9
  - acquired K63.89
- genitalia, genital organ(s) or system NEC
  - female (congenital) Q52.9
    - acquired N94.89
    - external Q52.70
  - male (congenital) Q55.9
    - acquired N50.89
- head (acquired) M95.2
  - congenital Q75.8
- heart (congenital) Q24.9
  - septum Q21.9
    - auricular Q21.1
    - ventricular Q21.0
- hepatic duct (congenital) Q44.5
  - acquired K83.8
- humerus (acquired) M21.82-
  - congenital Q74.0
- hypophyseal (congenital) Q89.2
- ilium (acquired) M95.5
  - congenital Q74.2
- integument (congenital) Q84.9
- ischium (acquired) M95.5
  - congenital Q74.2
- ligament (acquired)—*see* Disorder
  - congenital Q79.9
- limb (acquired) M21.90
  - congenital Q38.0
  - congenital, except reduction deformity Q74.9
  - flat foot M21.4-
  - flexion M21.20
    - ankle M21.27-
    - elbow M21.22-
    - finger M21.24-
    - hip M21.25-
    - knee M21.26-
    - shoulder M21.21-
    - toe M21.27-
    - wrist M21.23-
  - foot
    - drop M21.37-
    - flat—*see* Deformity, limb, flat foot
    - specified NEC M21.6X-
  - forearm M21.93-
  - hand M21.94-
  - lower leg M21.96-
  - specified type NEC M21.80
    - forearm M21.83-

Deformity, *continued*
    - lower leg M21.86-
    - thigh M21.85-
      - ~ unequal length M21.70
    - thigh M21.95-
    - upper arm M21.82-
- lip (acquired) NEC K13.0
- liver (congenital) Q44.7
  - acquired K76.89
- Madelung's (radius) Q74.0
- meninges or membrane (congenital) Q07.9
  - cerebral Q04.8
    - acquired G96.198
  - spinal cord (congenital) Q06.-
    - acquired G96.198
- metacarpus (acquired)—*see* Deformity, limb, forearm
  - congenital Q74.0
- mitral (leaflets) (valve) I05.8
  - parachute Q23.2
  - stenosis, congenital Q23.2
- mouth (acquired) K13.79
  - congenital Q38.6
- multiple, congenital NEC Q89.7
- muscle (acquired) M62.89
  - congenital Q79.9
    - sternocleidomastoid Q68.0
- musculoskeletal system (acquired) M95.9
  - congenital Q79.9
  - specified NEC M95.8
- nail (acquired) L60.8
  - congenital Q84.6
- nasal—*see* Deformity, nose
- neck (acquired) M95.3
  - congenital Q18.9
    - sternocleidomastoid Q68.0
- nervous system (congenital) Q07.9
- nose (acquired) (cartilage) M95.0
  - bone (turbinate) M95.0
  - congenital Q30.9
    - bent or squashed Q67.4
  - septum (acquired) J34.2
  - congenital Q30.8
- ovary (congenital) Q50.39
- parathyroid (gland) Q89.2
- pelvis, pelvic (acquired) (bony) M95.5
  - congenital Q74.2
- penis (glans) (congenital) Q55.69
  - acquired N48.89
- pinna, acquired H61.1-
  - congenital Q17.9
- pituitary (congenital) Q89.2
  - posture—*see* Dorsopathy
- prepuce (congenital) Q55.69
  - acquired N47.8
- rectum (congenital) Q43.9
  - acquired K62.89
- respiratory system (congenital) Q34.9
- rotation (joint) (acquired)—*see* Deformity, limb, specified site NEC
  - congenital Q74.9
  - hip M21.85-
    - congenital Q65.89
- sacroiliac joint (congenital) Q74.2
- septum, nasal (acquired) J34.2
- scapula (acquired) M95.8
  - congenital Q68.8
- shoulder (joint) (acquired) M21.92-
  - congenital Q74.0
- skull (acquired) M95.2
  - congenital Q75.8
    - with
      - ~ anencephaly Q00.0
      - ~ encephalocele—*see* Encephalocele
      - ~ hydrocephalus Q03.9
        - ◊ with spina bifida—*see* Spina bifida, by site, with hydrocephalus
      - ~ microcephaly Q02
- spinal
  - nerve root (congenital) Q07.9
- Sprengel's (congenital) Q74.0
- sternocleidomastoid (muscle), congenital Q68.0
- thymus (tissue) (congenital) Q89.2
- thyroid (gland) (congenital) Q89.2

Deformity, *continued*
- toe (acquired) M20.6-
  - congenital Q66.9-
  - hallux valgus M20.1-
- tricuspid (leaflets) (valve) I07.8
  - atresia or stenosis Q22.4
  - Ebstein's Q22.5
- trunk (acquired) M95.8
  - congenital Q89.9
- urachus (congenital) Q64.4
- urinary tract (congenital) Q64.9
  - urachus Q64.4
- vagina (acquired) N89.8
  - congenital Q52.4
- valgus NEC M21.00
  - knee M21.06-
- varus NEC M21.10
  - knee M21.16-
- vesicourethral orifice (acquired) N32.89
  - congenital NEC Q64.79
  - wrist drop M21.33-

Degeneration, degenerative
- brain (cortical) (progressive) G31.9
  - childhood G31.9
    - specified NEC G31.89
  - cystic G31.89
    - congenital Q04.6
  - in
    - congenital hydrocephalus Q03.9
      ~ with spina bifida—*see also* Spina bifida
    - Hunter's syndrome E76.1
- cerebrovascular I67.9
  - due to hypertension I67.4
- cortical (cerebellar) (parenchymatous) G31.89
- cutis L98.8
- extrapyramidal G25.9
- fatty
  - liver NEC K76.0
- intervertebral disc NOS
  - sacrococcygeal region M53.3
- kidney N28.89
  - cystic, congenital Q61.9
  - fatty N28.89
  - polycystic Q61.3
    - infantile type (autosomal recessive) NEC Q61.19
      ~ collecting duct dilatation Q61.11
- muscle (fatty) (fibrous) (hyaline) (progressive) M62.89
  - heart—*see* Degeneration, myocardial
- myocardial, myocardium (fatty) (hyaline) (senile) I51.5
  - with rheumatic fever (conditions in I00) I09.0
    - active, acute or subacute I01.2
      ~ with chorea I02.0
    - inactive or quiescent (with chorea) I09.0
- nasal sinus (mucosa) J32.9
  - frontal J32.1
  - maxillary J32.0
- nervous system G31.9
  - fatty G31.89
  - specified NEC G31.89
- ovary N83.8
  - cystic N83.20-
  - microcystic N83.20-
- pituitary (gland) E23.6
- pulmonary valve (heart) I37.8
- sinus (cystic)—*see also* Sinusitis
- skin L98.8
  - colloid L98.8
- spinal (cord) G31.89
  - familial NEC G31.89
  - fatty G31.89
- tricuspid (heart) (valve) I07.9
- turbinate J34.89

Deglutition
- paralysis R13.0
  - hysterical F44.4
- pneumonia J69.0

Dehiscence (of)
- closure
  - laceration (internal) (external) T81.33
  - traumatic laceration (external) (internal) T81.33
- traumatic injury wound repair T81.33

Dehiscence, *continued*
- wound T81.30
  - traumatic repair T81.33

Dehydration E86.0
- hypertonic E87.0
- hypotonic E87.1
- newborn P74.1

Delay, delayed
- closure, ductus arteriosus (Botalli) P29.38
- conduction (cardiac) (ventricular) I45.9
- development R62.50
  - intellectual (specific) F81.9
  - language F80.9
    - due to hearing loss F80.4
  - learning F81.9
  - pervasive F84.9
  - physiological R62.50
    - specified stage NEC R62.0
  - reading F81.0
  - sexual E30.0
  - speech F80.9
    - due to hearing loss F80.4
  - spelling F81.81
- gastric emptying K30
- menarche E30.0
- milestone R62.0
- passage of meconium (newborn) P76.0
- primary respiration P28.9
- puberty (constitutional) E30.0
- separation of umbilical cord P96.82
- sexual maturation, female E30.0
- sleep phase syndrome G47.21
- vaccination Z28.9

Deletion(s)
- autosome Q93.9
  - identified by fluorescence in situ hybridization (FISH) Q93.89
  - identified by in situ hybridization (ISH) Q93.89
- chromosome
  - seen only at prometaphase Q93.89
  - part of NEC Q93.59
  - short arm
    - 5p Q93.4
    - 22q11.2 Q93.81
  - specified NEC Q93.89
- microdeletions NEC Q93.88

Delinquency (juvenile) (neurotic) F91.8
- group Z72.810

Delinquent immunization status Z28.3

Delirium, delirious (acute or subacute) (not alcohol- or drug-induced) (with dementia) R41.0
- exhaustion F43.0

Delivery (childbirth) (labor)
- cesarean (for)
  - fetal-maternal hemorrhage O43.01-
  - placental insufficiency O36.51-
  - placental transfusion syndromes
    - fetomaternal O43.01-
    - fetus to fetus O43.02-
    - maternofetal O43.01-
  - pre-eclampsia O14.9-
    - mild O14.0-
    - moderate O14.0-
    - severe
      ~ with hemolysis, elevated liver enzymes and low platelet count (HELLP) O14.2-
- complicated O75.9
  - by
    - premature rupture, membranes (*see also* Pregnancy, complicated by, premature rupture of membranes) O42.90
- missed (at or near term) O36.4

Dementia (degenerative (primary)) (old age) (persisting)
- in (due to)
  - hypercalcemia E83.52 [*F02.80*]
    - with behavioral disturbance E83.52 [*F02.81*]
  - hypothyroidism, acquired E03.9 [*F02.80*]
    - with behavioral disturbance E03.9 [*F02.81*]
    - due to iodine deficiency E01.8 [*F02.80*]
      ~ with behavioral disturbance E01.8 [*F02.81*]

Demodex folliculorum (infestation) B88.0

Demyelination, demyelinization
- central nervous system G37.9
  - specified NEC G37.8
- corpus callosum (central) G37.1
- disseminated, acute G36.9
  - specified NEC G36.8
- global G35
- in optic neuritis G36.0

Dentia praecox K00.6

Dentigerous cyst K09.0

Dentin
- sensitive K03.89

Dentition (syndrome) K00.7
- delayed K00.6
- difficult K00.7
- precocious K00.6
- premature K00.6
- retarded K00.6

Dependence (on) (syndrome) F19.20
- with remission F19.21
- alcohol (ethyl) (methyl) (without remission) F10.20
  - with
    - anxiety disorder F10.280
    - intoxication F10.229
      ~ with delirium F10.221
      ~ uncomplicated F10.220
  - counseling and surveillance Z71.41
  - in remission F10.21
- amphetamine(s) (type)—*see* Dependence, drug, stimulant NEC
- benzedrine—*see* Dependence, drug, stimulant NEC
- bhang—*see* Dependence, drug, cannabis
- caffeine—*see* Dependence, drug, stimulant NEC
- cannabis (sativa) (indica) (resin) (derivatives) (type) F12.20
  - withdrawal F12.23
- coca (leaf) (derivatives)—*see* Dependence, drug, cocaine
- cocaine—*see* Dependence, drug, cocaine
- combinations of drugs F19.20
- dagga—*see* Dependence, drug, cannabis
- dexamphetamine—*see* Dependence, drug, stimulant NEC
- dexedrine—*see* Dependence, drug, stimulant NEC
- dextro-nor-pseudo-ephedrine—*see* Dependence, drug, stimulant NEC
- diazepam—*see* Dependence, drug
- drug NEC F19.20
  - cannabis F12.20
    - with
      ~ intoxication F12.229
        ◊ uncomplicated F12.220
    - in remission F12.21
  - cocaine F14.20
    - with
      ~ intoxication F14.229
        ◊ uncomplicated F14.220
      ~ withdrawal F14.23
    - in remission F14.21
    - withdrawal symptoms in newborn P96.1
  - counseling and surveillance Z71.51
  - inhalant F18.20
    - with
      ~ intoxication F18.229
        ◊ uncomplicated F18.220
    - in remission F18.21
  - nicotine F17.200
    - with disorder F17.209
      ~ in remission F17.201
      ~ specified disorder NEC F17.208
      ~ withdrawal F17.203
    - chewing tobacco F17.220
      ~ with disorder F17.229
        ◊ in remission F17.221
        ◊ specified disorder NEC F17.228
        ◊ withdrawal F17.223
    - cigarettes F17.210
      ~ with disorder F17.219
        ◊ in remission F17.211
        ◊ specified disorder NEC F17.218
    - specified product NEC F17.290
      ~ with disorder F17.299

Dependence, *continued*
- ◊ in remission F17.291
- ◊ specified disorder NEC F17.298
- ◊ withdrawal F17.293
- – psychoactive NEC F19.20
- – sedative, anxiolytic or hypnotic F13.-
- – stimulant NEC F15.20
  - ■ with
    - ~ intoxication F15.229
      - ◊ uncomplicated F15.220
    - ~ withdrawal F15.23
  - ■ in remission F15.21
- ethyl
  - – alcohol (without remission) F10.20
    - ■ with remission F10.21
- ganja—*see* Dependence, drug, cannabis
- glue (airplane) (sniffing)—*see* Dependence, drug, inhalant
- hashish—*see* Dependence, drug, cannabis
- hemp—*see* Dependence, drug, cannabis
- Indian hemp—*see* Dependence, drug, cannabis
- inhalants—*see* Dependence, drug, inhalant
- maconha—*see* Dependence, drug, cannabis
- marijuana—*see* Dependence, drug, cannabis
- methyl
  - – alcohol (without remission) F10.20
    - ■ with remission F10.21
- nicotine—*see* Dependence, drug, nicotine
- on
  - – assistance with personal care Z74.1
  - – care provider (because of) Z74.9
    - ■ no other household member able to render care Z74.2
  - – machine Z99.89
    - ■ enabling NEC Z99.89
    - ■ specified type NEC Z99.89
  - – renal dialysis (hemodialysis) (peritoneal) Z99.2
  - – respirator Z99.11
  - – ventilator Z99.11
  - – wheelchair Z99.3
- oxygen (long-term) (supplemental) Z99.81
- PCP (phencyclidine) (*see also* Abuse, drug) F16.20
- phencyclidine (PCP) (and related substances) (*see also* Abuse, drug) F16.20
- phenmetrazine—*see* Dependence, drug, stimulant NEC
- polysubstance F19.20
- psychostimulant NEC—*see* Dependence, drug, stimulant NEC
- sedative, anxiolytic or hypnotic F13.-
- specified drug NEC—*see* Dependence, drug
- stimulant NEC—*see* Dependence, drug, stimulant NEC
- substance NEC—*see* Dependence, drug
- supplemental oxygen Z99.81
- tobacco—*see* Dependence, drug, nicotine
  - – counseling and surveillance Z71.6
- volatile solvents—*see* Dependence, drug, inhalant

Depletion
- extracellular fluid E86.9
- plasma E86.1
- salt or sodium E87.1
  - – causing heat exhaustion or prostration T67.4
  - – nephropathy N28.9
- volume NOS E86.9

Depolarization, premature I49.40
- atrial I49.1
- specified NEC I49.49

Deposit
- bone in Boeck's sarcoid D86.89

Depression (acute) (mental) F32.A
- anaclitic—*see* Disorder, adjustment
- anxiety F41.8
  - – persistent F34.1
- atypical (single episode) F32.89
- basal metabolic rate R94.8
- bone marrow D75.89
- central nervous system R09.2
- cerebral R29.818
  - – newborn P91.4
- major F32.9
- medullary G93.89
- nervous F34.1
- neurotic F34.1

Depression, *continued*
- psychogenic (reactive) (single episode) F32.9
- psychoneurotic F34.1
- reactive (psychogenic) (single episode) F32.9
  - – psychotic (single episode) F32.3
- recurrent—*see* Disorder, depressive, recurrent
- respiratory center G93.89
- situational F43.21
- skull Q67.4
- specified NEC (single episode) F32.89

Deprivation
- cultural Z60.3
- emotional NEC Z65.8
  - – affecting infant or child—*see* Maltreatment, child, psychological
- social Z60.4
  - – affecting infant or child—*see* Maltreatment, child, psychological abuse

De Quervain's
- syndrome E34.51
- thyroiditis (subacute granulomatous thyroiditis) E06.1

Derangement
- joint (internal) M24.9
  - – ankylosis—*see* Ankylosis
  - – specified type NEC M24.8-
    - ■ ankle M24.87-
    - ■ elbow M24.82-
    - ■ foot joint M24.87-
    - ■ hand joint M24.84-
    - ■ hip M24.85-
    - ■ shoulder M24.81-
  - – temporomandibular M26.69

Dermatitis (eczematous) L30.9
- acarine B88.0
- ammonia L22
- arsenical (ingested) L27.8
- artefacta L98.1
  - – psychogenic F54
- atopic L20.9
  - – psychogenic F54
  - – specified NEC L20.89
- cercarial B65.3
- contact (occupational) L25.9
  - – allergic L23.9
    - ■ due to
      - ~ adhesives L23.1
      - ~ cement L24.5
      - ~ chemical products NEC L23.5
      - ~ chromium L23.0
      - ~ cosmetics L23.2
      - ~ dander (cat) (dog) L23.81
      - ~ drugs in contact with skin L23.3
      - ~ dyes L23.4
      - ~ food in contact with skin L23.6
      - ~ hair (cat) (dog) L23.81
      - ~ insecticide L23.5
      - ~ metals L23.0
      - ~ nickel L23.0
      - ~ plants, non-food L23.7
      - ~ plastic L23.5
      - ~ rubber L23.5
      - ~ specified agent NEC L23.89
  - – due to
    - ■ dander (cat) (dog) L23.81
    - ■ hair (cat) (dog) L23.81
  - – irritant L24.9
    - ■ due to
      - ~ body fluids L24.A0
      - ~ digestive L24.B1
      - ~ fecal or urinary L24.B3
      - ~ incontinence (dual) (fecal) (urinary) L24.A2
      - ~ saliva L24.A1
      - ~ specified NEC L24.A9
    - ■ related to
      - ~ colostomy L24.B3
      - ~ endotracheal tube L24.A9
      - ~ enterocutaneous fistula L24.B3
      - ~ gastrostomy L24.B1
      - ~ ileostomy L24.B3
      - ~ jejunostomy L24.B1
      - ~ respiratory L24.B2
      - ~ saliva or spit fistula L24.B1

Dermatitis, *continued*
- ~ stoma or fistula L24.B0
- ~ tracheostomy L24.B2
- contusiformis L52
- desquamative L30.8
- diabetic—*see* E08-E13 with .620
- diaper L22
- due to
  - – adhesive(s) (allergic) (contact) (plaster) L23.1
  - – alcohol (irritant) (skin contact) L24.2
    - ■ taken internally L27.8
  - – alkalis (contact) (irritant) L24.5
  - – arsenic (ingested) L27.8
  - – cereal (ingested) L27.2
  - – chemical(s) NEC L25.3
    - ■ taken internally L27.8
  - – coffee (ingested) L27.2
  - – cosmetics (contact) L25.0
    - ■ allergic L23.2
  - – dander (cat) (dog) L23.81
  - – Demodex species B88.0
  - – Dermanyssus gallinae B88.0
  - – drugs and medicaments (generalized) (internal use) L27.0
    - ■ in contact with skin L25.1
      - ~ allergic L23.3
    - ■ localized skin eruption L27.1
    - ■ specified substance—*see* Table of Drugs and Chemicals
  - – dyes (contact) L25.2
    - ■ allergic L23.4
  - – fish (ingested) L27.2
  - – flour (ingested) L27.2
  - – food (ingested) L27.2
    - ■ in contact with skin L25.4
  - – fruit (ingested) L27.2
  - – furs (allergic) (contact) L23.81
  - – hair (cat) (dog) L23.81
  - – infrared rays
  - – ingestion, ingested substance L27.9
    - ■ chemical NEC L27.8
    - ■ drugs and medicaments—*see* Dermatitis, due to, drugs and medicaments
    - ■ food L27.2
    - ■ specified NEC L27.8
  - – insecticide in contact with skin L24.5
  - – internal agent L27.9
    - ■ drugs and medicaments (generalized)—*see* Dermatitis, due to, drugs and medicaments
    - ■ food L27.2
  - – irradiation—*see* Dermatitis, due to, radiation
  - – lacquer tree (allergic) (contact) L23.7
  - – light (sun) NEC
    - ■ acute L56.8
  - – Lyponyssoides sanguineus B88.0
  - – milk (ingested) L27.2
  - – petroleum products (contact) (irritant) (substances in T52.0) L24.2
  - – plants NEC (contact) L25.5
    - ■ allergic L23.7
  - – plasters (adhesive) (any) (allergic) (contact) L23.1
  - – primrose (allergic) (contact) L23.7
  - – primula (allergic) (contact) L23.7
  - – radiation
    - ■ nonionizing (chronic exposure)
    - ■ sun NEC
      - ~ acute L56.8
  - – ragweed (allergic) (contact) L23.7
  - – Rhus (allergic) (contact) (diversiloba) (radicans) (toxicodendron) (venenata) (verniciflua) L23.7
  - – Senecio jacobaea (allergic) (contact) L23.7
  - – solvents (contact) (irritant) (substances in categories T52) L24.2
  - – specified agent NEC (contact) L25.8
    - ■ allergic L23.89
  - – sunshine NEC
    - ■ acute L56.8
  - – ultraviolet rays (sun NEC) (chronic exposure)
    - ■ acute L56.8
  - – vaccine or vaccination L27.0
    - ■ specified substance—*see* Table of Drugs and Chemicals
- dyshydrotic L30.1

Dermatitis, *continued*
- dysmenorrheica N94.6
- exfoliative, exfoliativa (generalized) L26
  - neonatorum L00
- eyelid H01.9
  - allergic H01.11-
    - left H01.116
      - ~ lower H01.115
      - ~ upper H01.114
    - right H01.113
      - ~ lower H01.112
      - ~ upper H01.111
  - due to
    - Demodex species B88.0
- facta, factitia, factitial L98.1
  - psychogenic F54
- flexural NEC L20.82
- friction L30.4
- gangrenosa, gangrenous infantum L08.0
- harvest mite B88.0
- infectious eczematoid L30.3
- infective L30.3
- irritant—*see* Dermatitis, contact
- Jacquet's (diaper dermatitis) L22
- Leptus B88.0
- mite B88.0
- napkin L22
- purulent L08.0
- pyococcal L08.0
- pyogenica L08.0
- Ritter's (exfoliativa) L00
- schistosome B65.3
- seborrheic L21.9
  - infantile L21.1
  - specified NEC L21.8
- sensitization NOS L23.9
- septic L08.0
- suppurative L08.0
- traumatic NEC L30.4
- ultraviolet (sun) (chronic exposure)
  - acute L56.8

Dermatographia L50.3

Dermatolysis (exfoliativa) (congenital) Q82.8

Dermatomegaly NEC Q82.8

Dermatomycosis B36.9
- furfuracea B36.0
- specified type NEC B36.8

Dermatomyositis (acute) (chronic)—*see also* Dermatopolymyositis
- in (due to) neoplastic disease (*see also* Table of Neoplasms in the complete *ICD-10-CM* manual) D49.9 [M36.0]
- juvenile M33.00
  - with
    - myopathy M33.02
    - respiratory involvement M33.01
    - specified organ involvement NEC M33.09
  - without myopathy M33.03
- specified NEC M33.10
  - with
    - myopathy M33.12
    - respiratory involvement M33.11
    - specified organ involvement NEC M33.19
  - without myopathy M33.13

Dermatoneuritis of children—*see* Poisoning

Dermatophytosis (epidermophyton) (infection) (Microsporum) (tinea) (Trichophyton) B35.9
- beard B35.0
- body B35.4
- capitis B35.0
- corporis B35.4
- deep-seated B35.8
- disseminated B35.8
- foot B35.3
- granulomatous B35.8
- groin B35.6
- hand B35.2
- nail B35.1
- perianal (area) B35.6
- scalp B35.0
- specified NEC B35.8

Dermatophytosis M33.90
- with
  - myopathy M33.92
  - respiratory involvement M33.91
  - specified organ involvement NEC M33.99
- juvenile M33.00
  - with
    - myopathy M33.02
    - respiratory involvement M33.01
    - specified organ involvement NEC M33.09
- without myopathy M33.93

Dermatopolyneuritis—*see* Poisoning

Dermatorrhexis (Ehlers-Danos) Q79.60

Dermatosis L98.9
- eyelid (noninfectious) H01.9
- factitial L98.1
- menstrual NEC L98.8

Dermophytosis—*see* Dermatophytosis

Despondency F32.A

Destruction, destructive—*see also* Damage
- joint—*see also* Derangement, joint, specified type NEC
  - sacroiliac M53.3
- rectal sphincter K62.89
- septum (nasal) J34.89

Detergent asthma J69.8

Deterioration
- general physical R53.81

Development
- abnormal, bone Q79.9
- arrested R62.50
  - bone—*see* Arrest, development or growth, bone
  - child R62.50
  - due to malnutrition E45
- defective, congenital—*see also* Anomaly, by site
  - left ventricle Q24.8
    - in hypoplastic left heart syndrome Q23.4
- delayed (*see also* Delay, development) R62.50
  - arithmetical skills F81.2
  - language (skills) (expressive) F80.1
  - learning skill F81.9
  - mixed skills F88
  - motor coordination F82
  - reading F81.0
  - specified learning skill NEC F81.89
  - speech F80.9
  - spelling F81.81
  - written expression F81.81
- imperfect, congenital—*see also* Anomaly, by site
  - heart Q24.9
  - lungs Q33.6
- incomplete
  - bronchial tree Q32.4
  - organ or site not listed—*see* Hypoplasia, by site
  - respiratory system Q34.9
- sexual, precocious NEC E30.1
- tardy, mental (*see also* Disability, intellectual) F79

Developmental—*see* Disease, diseased
- testing, infant or child—*see* Examination, child

Deviation (in)
- midline (jaw) (teeth) (dental arch) M26.29
  - specified site NEC—*see* Malposition
- nasal septum J34.2
  - congenital Q67.4
- septum (nasal) (acquired) J34.2
  - congenital Q67.4
- sexual transvestism F64.1
- teeth, midline M26.29

Device
- cerebral ventricle (communicating) in situ Z98.2
- drainage, cerebrospinal fluid, in situ Z98.2

Devil's
- pinches (purpura simplex) D69.2

Dextraposition, aorta Q20.3
- in tetralogy of Fallot Q21.3

Dextrocardia (true) Q24.0
- with
  - complete transposition of viscera Q89.3
  - situs inversus Q89.3

Dextrotransposition, aorta Q20.3

Dhobi itch B35.6

Di George's syndrome D82.1

Diabetes, diabetic (mellitus) (sugar) E11.9
- with
  - coma due to
    - hyperosmolarity E11.01
    - hypoglycemia E11.641
    - ketoacidosis E11.11
- bronzed E83.110
- dietary counseling and surveillance Z71.3
- due to drug or chemical E09.9
  - with
    - amyotrophy E09.44
    - arthropathy NEC E09.618
    - autonomic (poly)neuropathy E09.43
    - cataract E09.36
    - Charcot's joints E09.610
    - chronic kidney disease E09.22
    - circulatory complication NEC E09.59
    - complication E09.8
      - ~ specified NEC E09.69
    - dermatitis E09.620
    - foot ulcer E09.621
    - gangrene E09.52
    - gastroparesis E09.43
    - glomerulonephrosis, intracapillary E09.21
    - glomerulosclerosis, intercapillary E09.21
    - hyperglycemia E09.65
    - hyperosmolarity E09.00
      - ~ with coma E09.01
    - hypoglycemia E09.649
      - ~ with coma E09.641
    - ketoacidosis E09.10
      - ~ with coma E09.11
    - kidney complications NEC E09.29
    - Kimmelstiel-Wilson disease E09.21
    - mononeuropathy E09.41
    - myasthenia E09.44
    - necrobiosis lipoidica E09.620
    - nephropathy E09.21
    - neuralgia E09.42
    - neurologic complication NEC E09.49
    - neuropathic arthropathy E09.610
    - neuropathy E09.40
    - ophthalmic complication NEC E09.39
    - oral complication NEC E09.638
    - periodontal disease E09.630
    - peripheral angiopathy E09.51
      - ~ with gangrene E09.52
    - polyneuropathy E09.42
    - renal complication NEC E09.29
    - renal tubular degeneration E09.29
    - retinopathy E09.319
      - ~ with macular edema E09.311
      - ~ nonproliferative E09.329
        - ◊ with macular edema E09.321
        - ◊ mild E09.329
          - » with macular edema E09.321
        - ◊ moderate E09.339
          - » with macular edema E09.331
        - ◊ severe E09.349
          - » with macular edema E09.341
      - ~ proliferative E09.359
        - ◊ with macular edema E09.351
    - skin complication NEC E09.628
    - skin ulcer NEC E09.622
- due to underlying condition E08.9
  - with
    - amyotrophy E08.44
    - arthropathy NEC E08.618
    - autonomic (poly)neuropathy E08.43
    - cataract E08.36
    - Charcot's joints E08.610
    - chronic kidney disease E08.22
    - circulatory complication NEC E08.59
    - complication E08.8
      - ~ specified NEC E08.69
    - dermatitis E08.620
    - foot ulcer E08.621
    - gangrene E08.52
    - gastroparesis E08.43
    - glomerulonephrosis, intracapillary E08.21
    - glomerulosclerosis, intercapillary E08.21

Diabetes, diabetic (mellitus) (sugar), *continued*
- hyperglycemia E08.65
- hyperosmolarity E08.00
  - ~ with coma E08.01
- hypoglycemia E08.649
  - ~ with coma E08.641
- ketoacidosis E08.10
  - ~ with coma E08.11
- kidney complications NEC E08.29
- Kimmelstiel-Wilson disease E08.21
- mononeuropathy E08.41
- myasthenia E08.44
- necrobiosis lipoidica E08.620
- nephropathy E08.21
- neuralgia E08.42
- neurologic complication NEC E08.49
- neuropathic arthropathy E08.610
- neuropathy E08.40
- ophthalmic complication NEC E08.39
- oral complication NEC E08.638
- periodontal disease E08.630
- peripheral angiopathy E08.51
  - ~ with gangrene E08.52
- polyneuropathy E08.42
- renal complication NEC E08.29
- renal tubular degeneration E08.29
- retinopathy E08.319
  - ~ with macular edema E08.311
  - ~ nonproliferative E08.329
    - ◊ with macular edema E08.321
    - ◊ mild E08.329
      - » with macular edema E08.321
    - ◊ moderate E08.339
      - » with macular edema E08.331
    - ◊ severe E08.349
      - » with macular edema E08.341
  - ~ proliferative E08.359
    - ◊ with macular edema E08.351
- skin complication NEC E08.628
- skin ulcer NEC E08.622
- gestational (in pregnancy)
  - affecting newborn P70.0
  - diet controlled O24.410
  - insulin (and diet) controlled O24.414
  - oral hypoglycemic drug controlled O24.415
- inadequately controlled—*code to* Diabetes, by type, with hyperglycemia
- insipidus E23.2
  - nephrogenic N25.1
  - pituitary E23.2
- insulin dependent—*code to* type of diabetes
- juvenile-onset—*see* Diabetes, type 1
- ketosis-prone—*see* Diabetes, type 1
- latent R73.09
- neonatal (transient) P70.2
- non-insulin dependent—*code to* type of diabetes
- out of control—*code to* Diabetes, by type, with hyperglycemia
- poorly controlled—*code to* Diabetes, by type, with hyperglycemia
- postpancreatectomy—*see* Diabetes
- postprocedural—*see* Diabetes
- prediabetes R73.03
- secondary diabetes mellitus NEC—*see* Diabetes
- steroid-induced—*see* Diabetes, due to drug or chemical
- type 1 E10.9
  - with
    - amyotrophy E10.44
    - arthropathy NEC E10.618
    - autonomic (poly)neuropathy E10.43
    - cataract E10.36
    - Charcot's joints E10.610
    - chronic kidney disease E10.22
    - circulatory complication NEC E10.59
    - complication E10.8
      - ~ specified NEC E10.69
    - dermatitis E10.620
    - foot ulcer E10.621
    - gangrene E10.52
    - gastroparesis E10.43
    - glomerulonephrosis, intracapillary E10.21
    - glomerulosclerosis, intercapillary E10.21
    - hyperglycemia E10.65

Diabetes, diabetic (mellitus) (sugar), *continued*
- hypoglycemia E10.649
  - ~ with coma E10.641
- ketoacidosis E10.10
  - ~ with coma E10.11
- kidney complications NEC E10.29
- Kimmelstiel-Wilson disease E10.21
- mononeuropathy E10.41
- myasthenia E10.44
- necrobiosis lipoidica E10.620
- nephropathy E10.21
- neuralgia E10.42
- neurologic complication NEC E10.49
- neuropathic arthropathy E10.610
- neuropathy E10.40
- ophthalmic complication NEC E10.39
- oral complication NEC E10.638
- periodontal disease E10.630
- peripheral angiopathy E10.51
  - ~ with gangrene E10.52
- polyneuropathy E10.42
- renal complication NEC E10.29
- renal tubular degeneration E10.29
- retinopathy E10.319
  - ~ with macular edema E10.311
  - ~ nonproliferative E10.329
    - ◊ with macular edema E10.321
    - ◊ mild E10.329
      - » with macular edema E10.321
    - ◊ moderate E10.339
      - » with macular edema E10.331
    - ◊ severe E10.349
      - » with macular edema E10.341
  - ~ proliferative E10.359
    - ◊ with macular edema E10.351
- skin complication NEC E10.628
- skin ulcer NEC E10.622
- type 2 E11.9
  - with
    - amyotrophy E11.44
    - arthropathy NEC E11.618
    - autonomic (poly)neuropathy E11.43
    - cataract E11.36
    - Charcot's joints E11.610
    - chronic kidney disease E11.22
    - circulatory complication NEC E11.59
    - complication E11.8
      - ~ specified NEC E11.69
    - dermatitis E11.620
    - foot ulcer E11.621
    - gangrene E11.52
    - gastroparesis E11.43
    - glomerulonephrosis, intracapillary E11.21
    - glomerulosclerosis, intercapillary E11.21
    - hyperglycemia E11.65
    - hyperosmolarity E11.00
      - ~ with coma E11.01
    - hypoglycemia E11.649
      - ~ with coma E11.641
    - ketoacidosis E11.10
      - ~ with coma E11.11
    - kidney complications NEC E11.29
    - Kimmelstiel-Wilson disease E11.21
    - mononeuropathy E11.41
    - myasthenia E11.44
    - necrobiosis lipoidica E11.620
    - nephropathy E11.21
    - neuralgia E11.42
    - neurologic complication NEC E11.49
    - neuropathic arthropathy E11.610
    - neuropathy E11.40
    - ophthalmic complication NEC E11.39
    - oral complication NEC E11.638
    - periodontal disease E11.630
    - peripheral angiopathy E11.51
      - ~ with gangrene E11.52
    - polyneuropathy E11.42
    - renal complication NEC E11.29
    - renal tubular degeneration E11.29
    - retinopathy E11.319
      - ~ with macular edema E11.311
      - ~ nonproliferative E11.329
        - ◊ with macular edema E11.321

Diabetes, diabetic (mellitus) (sugar), *continued*
- ◊ mild E11.329
  - » with macular edema E11.321
- ◊ moderate E11.339
  - » with macular edema E11.331
- ◊ severe E11.349
  - » with macular edema E11.341
- ~ proliferative E11.359
  - ◊ with macular edema E11.351
- skin complication NEC E11.628
- skin ulcer NEC E11.622

Diagnosis deferred R69

Dialysis (intermittent) (treatment)
- noncompliance (with) Z91.15
- renal (hemodialysis) (peritoneal), status Z99.2

Diamond-Blackfan anemia (congenital hypoplastic) D61.01

Diamond-Gardener syndrome (autoerythrocyte sensitization) D69.2

Diaper rash L22

Diaphoresis (excessive) R61

Diaphragmatitis, diaphragmitis J98.6

Diarrhea, diarrheal (disease) (infantile) (inflammatory) R19.7
- allergic K52.29
- amebic (*see also* Amebiasis) A06.0
  - acute A06.0
- cachectic NEC K52.89
- chronic (noninfectious) K52.9
- dietetic K52.29
- due to
  - Campylobacter A04.5
  - C. difficile A04.7-
  - Escherichia coli A04.4
    - enteroaggregative A04.4
    - enterohemorrhagic A04.3
    - enteropathogenic A04.0
    - enterotoxigenic A04.1
    - specified NEC A04.4
  - food hypersensitivity K52.29
  - specified organism NEC A08.8
    - bacterial A04.8
    - viral A08.39
- dysenteric A09
- endemic A09
- epidemic A09
- functional K59.1
  - following gastrointestinal surgery K91.89
  - psychogenic F45.8
- Giardia lamblia A07.1
- giardial A07.1
- infectious A09
- mite B88.0
- neonatal (noninfectious) P78.3
- nervous F45.8
- noninfectious K52.9
- psychogenic F45.8
- specified
  - bacterial A04.8
  - virus NEC A08.39

Diastasis
- cranial bones M84.88
  - congenital NEC Q75.8
- joint (traumatic)—*see* Dislocation

Diathesis
- hemorrhagic (familial) D69.9
  - newborn NEC P53

Didymytis N45.1
- with orchitis N45.3

Dietary
- surveillance and counseling Z71.3

Dietl's crisis N13.8

Difficult, difficulty (in)
- acculturation Z60.3
- feeding R63.30
  - newborn P92.9
    - breast P92.5
    - specified NEC P92.8
  - nonorganic (infant or child) F98.29
- reading (developmental) F81.0
  - secondary to emotional disorders F93.9

Difficult, difficulty (in), *continued*
- spelling (specific) F81.81
  - with reading disorder F81.89
  - due to inadequate teaching Z55.8
- swallowing—*see* Dysphagia
- walking R26.2

DiGeorge's syndrome (thymic hypoplasia) D82.1

Dilatation
- aorta (congenital) Q25.44
- bladder (sphincter) N32.89
  - congenital Q64.79
- colon K59.39
  - congenital Q43.1
  - psychogenic F45.8
  - toxic K59.31
- common duct (acquired) K83.8
  - congenital Q44.5
- cystic duct (acquired) K82.8
  - congenital Q44.5
- ileum K59.89
  - psychogenic F45.8
- jejunum K59.89
  - psychogenic F45.8
- Meckel's diverticulum (congenital) Q43.0
- rectum K59.39
- sphincter ani K62.89
- stomach K31.89
  - acute K31.0
  - psychogenic F45.8
- vesical orifice N32.89

Dilated, dilation—*see* Dilatation

Diminished, diminution
- hearing (acuity)—*see* Deafness
- sense or sensation (cold) (heat) (tactile) (vibratory) R20.8
- vision NEC H54.7

Dimitri-Sturge-Weber disease Q85.8

Dimple
- congenital, sacral Q82.6
  - parasacral Q82.6
- parasacral, pilonidal or postanal—*see* Cyst, pilonidal

Diphallus Q55.69

Diphtheria, diphtheritic (gangrenous) (hemorrhagic) A36.9
- carrier Z22.2

Diplegia (upper limbs) G83.0
- lower limbs G82.20

Dipsomania F10.20
- with
  - remission F10.21

Dirt-eating child F98.3

Disability, disabilities
- intellectual F79
  - with
    - autistic features F84.9
    - pathogenic CHAMP1 (genetic) (variant) F78.A9
    - pathogenic HNRNPH2 (genetic) (variant) F78.A9
    - pathogenic SATB2 (genetic) (variant) F78.A9
    - pathogenic SETBP1 (genetic) (variant) F78.A9
    - pathogenic STXBP1 (genetic) (variant) F78.A9
    - pathogenic SYNGAP1 (genetic) (variant) F78.A1
      - autosomal dominant F78.A9
      - autosomal recessive F78.A9
      - genetic related F78.A9
    - with
      - pathogenic CHAMP1 (variant) F78.A9
      - pathogenic HNRNPH2 (variant) F78.A9
      - pathogenic SATB2 (variant) F78.A9
      - pathogenic SETBP1 (variant) F78.A9
      - pathogenic STXBP1 (variant) F78.A9
      - pathogenic SYNGAP1 (variant) F78.A1
    - specified NEC F78.A9
    - SYNGAP1-related F78.A1
      - in
        ◊ autosomal dominant mental retardation F78.A9
        ◊ autosomal recessive mental retardation F78.A9
        ◊ SATB2-associated syndrome F78.A9
        ◊ SETBP1 disorder F78.A9

Disability, disabilities, *continued*
        ◊ STXBP1 encephalopathy with epilepsy (*see also* Encephalopathy; and see also Epilepsy) F78.A9
        ◊ X-linked mental retardation (syndromic) (Bain type) F78.A9
  - mild (I.Q.50 – 69) F70
  - moderate (I.Q.35 – 49) F71
  - profound (I.Q. under 20) F73
  - severe (I.Q.20 – 34) F72
  - specified level NEC F78
- knowledge acquisition F81.9
- learning F81.9
- limiting activities Z73.6
- spelling, specific F81.81

Disappearance of family member Z63.4

Discharge (from)
- abnormal finding in—*see* Abnormal, specimen
- breast (female) (male) N64.52
- diencephalic autonomic idiopathic—*see* Epilepsy, specified NEC
- ear—*see also* Otorrhea
- excessive urine R35.89
- nipple N64.52
- penile R36.9
- postnasal R09.82
- urethral R36.9
  - without blood R36.0
- vaginal N89.8

Discoloration
- nails L60.8

Discord (with)
- family Z63.8

Discordant connection
- ventriculoarterial Q20.3

Discrepancy
- leg length (acquired)—*see* Deformity, limb, unequal length
  - congenital—*see* Defect, reduction, limb, lower

Disease, diseased—*see also* Syndrome
- acid-peptic K30
- Adams-Stokes (-Morgagni) (syncope with heart block) I45.9
- adenoids (and tonsils) J35.9
- airway
  - reactive—*see* Asthma
- alligator-skin Q80.9
- angiospastic I73.9
  - cerebral G45.9
- anus K62.9
  - specified NEC K62.89
- aortic (heart) (valve) I35.9
  - rheumatic I06.9
- autoimmune (systemic) NOS M35.9
  - hemolytic D59.1
    - cold type (primary) (secondary) (symptomatic) D59.12
    - drug-induced D59.0
    - mixed type (primary) (secondary) (symptomatic) D59.13
    - warm type (primary) (secondary) (symptomatic) D59.11
  - thyroid E06.3
- autoinflammatory M04.9
  - NOD2-associated M04.8
- Ayerza's (pulmonary artery sclerosis with pulmonary hypertension) I27.0
- Babington's (familial hemorrhagic telangiectasia) I78.0
- Baelz's (cheilitis glandularis apostematosa) K13.0
- Bannister's T78.3
- basal ganglia G25.9
  - specified NEC G25.89
- Bateman's B08.1
- Becker
  - myotonia congenita G71.12
- bladder N32.9
  - specified NEC N32.89
- bleeder's D66
- blood D75.9
  - vessel I99.9
- Blount M92.51-

Disease, diseased, *continued*
- Bouillaud's (rheumatic heart disease) I01.9
- Bourneville (-Brissaud) (tuberous sclerosis) Q85.1
- bowel K63.9
  - functional K59.9
    - psychogenic F45.8
- brain G93.9
  - parasitic NEC B71.9 *[G94]*
  - specified NEC G93.89
- broad
  - beta E78.2
- bronze Addison's E27.1
- cardiopulmonary, chronic I27.9
- cardiovascular (atherosclerotic) I25.10
- celiac (adult) (infantile) K90.0
- cerebrovascular I67.9
  - acute I67.89
  - hereditary NEC I67.858
  - specified NEC I67.89
- chigo, chigoe B88.1
- childhood granulomatous D71
- chlamydial A74.9
  - specified NEC A74.89
- cold
  - agglutinin or hemoglobinuria D59.12
  - hemagglutinin (chronic) D59.12
- collagen NOS (nonvascular) (vascular) M35.9
  - specified NEC M35.8
- colon K63.9
  - functional K59.9
    - congenital Q43.2
- Concato's (pericardial polyserositis) A19.9
  - nontubercular I31.1
  - pleural—*see* Pleurisy, with, effusion
- congenital Q07.9
  - nonautoimmune hemolytic D59.4
- conjunctiva H11.9
  - chlamydial A74.0
  - viral B30.9
- connective tissue, systemic (diffuse) M35.9
  - in (due to)
    - hypogammaglobulinemia D80.1 *[M36.8]*
  - specified NEC M35.8
  - COVID-19 U07.1
- Crocq's (acrocyanosis) I73.89
- cystic
  - kidney, congenital Q61.9
- cytomegalic inclusion (generalized) B25.9
  - congenital P35.1
- cytomegaloviral B25.9
- Débove's (splenomegaly) R16.1
- de Quervain's (tendon sheath) M65.4
  - thyroid (subacute granulomatous thyroiditis) E06.1
- diaphorase deficiency D74.0
- diaphragm J98.6
- diarrheal, infectious NEC A09
- disruptive F91.9
  - mood dysregulation F34.81
  - specified NEC F91.8
- disruptive behavior F91.9
- Duchenne-Griesinger G71.01
- Duchenne's
  - muscular dystrophy G71.01
  - pseudohypertrophy, muscles G71.01
- Dupré's (meningism) R29.1
- dysmorphic body F45.22
- Eddowes' (brittle bones and blue sclera) Q78.0
- Edsall's T67.2
- Eichstedt's (pityriasis versicolor) B36.0
- Eisenmenger's (irreversible) I27.83
- Ellis-van Creveld (chondroectodermal dysplasia) Q77.6
- end stage renal (ESRD) N18.6
- English (rickets) E55.0
- Erb (-Landouzy) G71.02
- esophagus K22.9
  - functional K22.4
  - psychogenic F45.8
- eustachian tube—*see* Disorder, eustachian tube
- facial nerve (seventh) G51.9
  - newborn (birth injury) P11.3
- Fanconi's (congenital pancytopenia) D61.09

Disease, diseased, *continued*

- fascia NEC—*see also* Disorder, muscle
  - inflammatory—*see* Myositis
  - specified NEC M62.89
- Fede's K14.0
- female pelvic inflammatory (*see also* Disease, pelvis, inflammatory) N73.9
- fifth B08.3
- Fothergill's
  - scarlatina anginosa A38.9
- Friedreich's
  - combined systemic or ataxia G11.11
  - myoclonia G25.3
- frontal sinus—*see* Sinusitis, frontal
- fungus NEC B49
- Gaisböck's (polycythemia hypertonica) D75.1
- gastroesophageal reflux (GERD) K21.9
  - with esophagitis K21.0-
- gastrointestinal (tract) K92.9
  - functional K59.9
    - psychogenic F45.8
  - specified NEC K92.89
- Gee (-Herter) (-Heubner) (-Thaysen) (nontropical sprue) K90.0
- genital organs
  - female N94.9
  - male N50.9
- Gibert's (pityriasis rosea) L42
- Gilles de la Tourette's (motor-verbal tic) F95.2
- Goldstein's (familial hemorrhagic telangiectasia) I78.0
- graft-versus-host (GVH) D89.813
  - acute D89.810
  - acute on chronic D89.812
  - chronic D89.811
- granulomatous (childhood) (chronic) D71
- Grisel's M43.6
- Gruby's (tinea tonsurans) B35.0
- Guinon's (motor-verbal tic) F95.2
  - follicles L73.9
    - specified NEC L73.8
- Hamman's (spontaneous mediastinal emphysema) J98.2
- hand, foot, and mouth B08.4
- heart (organic) I51.9
  - with
    - pulmonary edema (acute) (*see also* Failure, ventricular, left) I50.1
    - rheumatic fever (conditions in I00)
      - ~ active I01.9
        - ◊ with chorea I02.0
        - ◊ specified NEC I01.8
      - ~ inactive or quiescent (with chorea) I09.9
        - ◊ specified NEC I09.89
  - aortic (valve) I35.9
  - black I27.0
  - congenital Q24.9
    - cyanotic Q24.9
    - specified NEC Q24.8
  - fibroid—*see* Myocarditis
  - functional I51.89
    - psychogenic F45.8
  - hyperthyroid (*see also* Hyperthyroidism) E05.90 [I43]
    - with thyroid storm E05.91 [I43]
  - kyphoscoliotic I27.1
  - mitral I05.9
    - specified NEC I0
  - psychogenic (functional) F45.8
  - pulmonary (chronic) I27.9
    - in schistosomiasis B65.9 [I52]
    - specified NEC I27.89
  - rheumatic (chronic) (inactive) (old) (quiescent) (with chorea) I09.9
    - active or acute I01.9
      - ~ with chorea (acute) (rheumatic) (Sydenham's) I02.0
  - thyrotoxic (*see also* Thyrotoxicosis) E05.90 [I43]
    - with thyroid storm E05.91 [I43]
- Hebra's
  - pityriasis
    - maculata et circinata L42
- hemoglobin or Hb
  - abnormal (mixed) NEC D58.2
    - with thalassemia D56.9
  - AS genotype D57.3

Disease, diseased, *continued*

- Bart's D56.0
- C (Hb-C) D58.2
  - with other abnormal hemoglobin NEC D58.2
  - elliptocytosis D58.1
  - Hb-S D57.2-
  - sickle-cell D57.2-
  - thalassemia D56.8
- Constant Spring D58.2
- D (Hb-D) D58.2
- E (Hb-E) D58.2
- E-beta thalassemia D56.5
- elliptocytosis D58.1
- H (Hb-H) (thalassemia) D56.0
  - with other abnormal hemoglobin NEC D56.9
  - Constant Spring D56.0
- I thalassemia D56.9
- M D74.0
- S or SS D57.1
  - with
    - ~ acute chest syndrome D57.01
    - ~ cerebral vascular involvement D57.03
    - ~ crisis (painful) D57.00
      - ◊ with complication specified NEC D57.09
    - ~ splenic sequestration D57.02
    - ~ vasoocclusive pain D57.00
  - beta plus D57.44
    - with
      - ◊ acute chest syndrome D57.451
      - ◊ cerebral vascular involvement D57.453
      - ◊ crisis D57.459
        - » with specified complication NEC D57.458
      - ◊ splenic sequestration D57.452
        - » vasoocclusive pain D57.459
    - ~ without crisis D57.44
  - beta zero D57.42
    - with
      - ◊ acute chest syndrome D57.431
      - ◊ cerebral vascular involvement D57.433
      - ◊ crisis D57.439
        - » with specified complication NEC D57.438
      - ◊ splenic sequestration D57.432
      - ◊ vasoocclusive pain D57.439
    - ~ without crisis D57.42
- SC D57.2-
- SD D57.8-
- SE D57.8-
- spherocytosis D58.0
- unstable, hemolytic D58.2
- hemolytic (newborn) P55.9
  - autoimmune D59.10
    - cold type (primary) (secondary) (symptomatic) D59.12
    - mixed type (primary) (secondary) (symptomatic) D59.13
    - warm type (primary) (secondary) (symptomatic) D59.11
    - drug-induced D59.0
  - due to or with
    - incompatibility
      - ~ ABO (blood group) P55.1
      - ~ blood (group) (Duffy) (K) (Kell) (Kidd) (Lewis) (M) (S) NEC P55.8
- hemorrhagic D69.9
  - newborn P53
- Henoch (-Schönlein) (purpura nervosa) D69.0
- hepatic—*see* Disease, liver
- Herter (-Gee) (-Heubner) (nontropical sprue) K90.0
- Heubner-Herter (nontropical sprue) K90.0
- high fetal gene or hemoglobin thalassemia D56.9
- hip (joint) M25.9
  - congenital Q65.89
  - suppurative M00.9
- host-versus-graft D89.813
  - acute D89.810
  - acute on chronic D89.812
  - chronic D89.811
- human immunodeficiency virus (HIV) B20
- hyaline (diffuse) (generalized)
  - membrane (lung) (newborn) P22.0
- hypophysis E23.7
- I-cell E77.0
- immune D89.9

Disease, diseased, *continued*

- inclusion B25.9
  - salivary gland B25.9
- infectious, infective B99.9
  - congenital P37.9
    - specified NEC P37.8
    - viral P35.9
      - ~ specified type NEC P35.8
  - specified NEC B99.8
- inflammatory
  - prepuce
    - balanoposthitis N47.6
- intestine K63.9
  - functional K59.9
    - psychogenic F45.8
    - specified NEC K59.89
- jigger B88.1
- joint—*see also* Disorder, joint
  - sacroiliac M53.3
- Jourdain's (acute gingivitis) K05.00
  - plaque induced K05.00
- kidney (functional) (pelvis) N28.9
  - chronic N18.9
    - hypertensive—*see* Hypertension, kidney
    - stage 1 N18.1
    - stage 2 (mild) N18.2
    - stage 3 (moderate) N18.30
    - stage 3a N18.31
    - stage 3b N18.32
    - stage 4 (severe) N18.4
    - stage 5 N18.5
  - cystic (congenital) Q61.9
  - in (due to)
  - multicystic Q61.4
  - polycystic Q61.3
    - childhood type NEC Q61.19
      - ~ collecting duct dilatation Q61.11
- Kimmelstiel (-Wilson) (intercapillary polycystic (congenital) glomerulosclerosis)—*see* E08-E13 with .21
- kissing—*see* Mononucleosis, infectious
- Kok Q89.8
- Kostmann's (infantile genetic agranulocytosis) D70.0
- Lenegre's I44.2
- Lev's (acquired complete heart block) I44.2
- lip K13.0
- liver (chronic) (organic) K76.9
  - fatty, nonalcoholic (NAFLD) K76.0
    - gestational alloimmune (GALD) P78.84
- Lobstein's (brittle bones and blue sclera) Q78.0
- Ludwig's (submaxillary cellulitis) K12.2
- lung J98.4
  - dabbing (related) U07.0
  - electronic cigarette (related) U07.0
  - in
    - sarcoidosis D86.0
    - systemic
      - ~ lupus erythematosus M32.13
  - interstitial J84.9
    - of childhood, specified NEC J84.848
    - specified NEC J84.89
  - vaping (device) (product) (use) (associated) U07.0
- Lutembacher's (atrial septal defect with mitral stenosis) Q21.1
- Lyme A69.20
- lymphoproliferative D47.9
  - specified NEC D47.Z9
  - T-gamma D47.Z9
  - X-linked D82.3
- maple-syrup-urine E71.0
- Marion's (bladder neck obstruction) N32.0
- medullary center (idiopathic) (respiratory) G93.89
- metabolic, metabolism E88.9
  - bilirubin E80.7
  - glycoprotein E77.9
    - specified NEC E77.8
- minicore G71.29
- Minot's (hemorrhagic disease, newborn) P53
- Minot-von Willebrand-Jürgens (angiohemophilia) D68.0
- mitral (valve) I05.9
- Morgagni-Adams-Stokes (syncope with heart block) I45.9
- Morvan's G60.8
- multicore G71.29

Disease, diseased, *continued*
- muscle M62.9
  - specified type NEC M62.89
  - tone, newborn P94.9
    - specified NEC P94.8
- myocardium, myocardial (*see also* Degeneration, myocardial) I51.5
  - primary (idiopathic) I42.9
- myoneural G70.9
- nails L60.9
  - specified NEC L60.8
- nasal J34.9
- nemaline body G71.21
- neuromuscular system G70.9
- neutropenic D70.9
- nerve—*see* Disorder, nerve
  - nervous system G98.8 central G96.9
    - specified NEC G96.89
- nose J34.9
- organ
  - dabbing (related) U07.0
  - electronic cigarette (related) U07.0
  - vaping (device) (product) (use) (associated) U07.0
- Osler-Rendu (familial hemorrhagic telangiectasia) I78.0
- ovary (noninflammatory) N83.9
  - cystic N83.20-
  - inflammatory—*see* Salpingo-oophoritis
  - polycystic E28.2
  - specified NEC N83.8
- pancreas K86.9
  - cystic K86.2
  - fibrocystic E84.9
  - specified NEC K86.89
- parasitic B89
  - cerebral NEC B71.9 *[G94]*
  - intestinal NOS B82.9
  - mouth B37.0
  - skin NOS B88.9
  - *specified type—see* Infestation
  - tongue B37.0
- pelvis, pelvic
  - gonococcal (acute) (chronic) A54.24
  - inflammatory (female) N73.9
    - acute N73.0
    - chronic N73.1
    - specified NEC N73.8
- Pick's I31.1
- pinworm B80
- pituitary (gland) E23.7
- Pollitzer's (hidradenitis suppurativa) L73.2
- polycystic
  - kidney or renal Q61.3
    - childhood type NEC Q61.19
      - collecting duct dilatation Q61.11
  - ovary, ovaries E28.2
- prepuce N47.8
  - inflammatory N47.7
    - balanoposthitis N47.6
- Pringle's (tuberous sclerosis) Q85.1
- Puente's (simple glandular cheilitis) K13.0
- pulmonary—*see also* Disease, lung
  - heart I27.9
    - specified NEC I27.89
  - hypertensive (vascular) I27.20
    - primary (idiopathic) I27.0
  - valve I37.9
    - rheumatic I09.89
- rag picker's or rag sorter's A22.1
- rectum K62.9
  - specified NEC K62.89
- renal (functional) (pelvis) (*see also* Disease, kidney) N28.9
  - with
    - edema—*see* Nephrosis
    - glomerular lesion—*see* Glomerulonephritis
      - with edema—*see* Nephrosis
    - interstitial nephritis N12
  - acute N28.9
  - chronic (*see also* Disease, kidney, chronic) N18.9
  - cystic, congenital Q61.9
  - diabetic—*see* E08-E13 with .22
  - end-stage (failure) N18.6
  - fibrocystic (congenital) Q61.8

Disease, diseased, *continued*
- lupus M32.14
- polycystic (congenital) Q61.3
  - childhood type NEC Q61.19
    - collecting duct dilatation Q61.11
- Rendu-Osler-Weber (familial hemorrhagic telangiectasia) I78.0
- respiratory (tract) J98.9
  - acute or subacute NOS J06.9
    - due to
      - smoke inhalation J70.5
  - newborn P28.9
    - specified type NEC P28.89
  - upper J39.9
    - acute or subacute J06.9
    - streptococcal J06.9
- rickettsial NOS A79.9
  - specified type NEC A79.89
- Riga (-Fede) (cachectic aphthae) K14.0
- Ritter's L00
- Roger's (congenital interventricular septal defect) Q21.0
- Rosenthal's (factor XI deficiency) D68.1
- Rossbach's (hyperchlorhydria) K30
- sacroiliac NEC M53.3
- salivary gland or duct K11.9
  - inclusion B25.9
  - *specified NEC K11.8*
  - virus B25.9
- Schönlein (-Henoch) (purpura rheumatica) D69.0
- scrofulous (tuberculous) A18.2
- scrotum N50.9
- serum NEC (*see also* Reaction, serum) T80.69
- sexually transmitted A64
  - anogenital
    - herpesviral infection—*see* Herpes, anogenital
    - warts A63.0
  - chlamydial infection—*see* Chlamydia
  - gonorrhea—*see* Gonorrhea
  - specified organism NEC A63.8
  - syphilis—*see* Syphilis
  - trichomoniasis—*see* Trichomoniasis
- sickle-cell D57.1
  - with crisis (vasoocclusive pain) D57.00
  - with
    - acute chest syndrome D57.01
    - cerebral vascular involvement D57.03
    - crisis (painful) D57.00
      - with complication specified NEC D57.09
    - splenic sequestration D57.02
    - vasoocclusive pain D57.00
  - Hb-C D57.20
    - with
      - acute chest syndrome D57.211
      - cerebral vascular involvement D57.213
      - crisis D57.219
        - with specified complication NEC D57.218
      - splenic sequestration D57.212
      - vasoocclusive pain D57.219
  - Hb-SD D57.80
    - with
      - acute chest syndrome D57.811
      - cerebral vascular involvement D57.813
      - crisis D57.819
        - with complication specified NEC D57.818
      - splenic sequestration D57.812
      - vasoocclusive pain D57.819
    - without crisis D57.80
  - Hb-SE D57.80
    - with crisis D57.819
    - with
      - acute chest syndrome D57.811
      - cerebral vascular involvement D57.813
      - crisis D57.819
        - with complication specified NEC D57.818
      - splenic sequestration D57.812
      - vasoocclusive pain D57.819
    - without crisis D57.80
  - specified NEC D57.80
    - with
      - acute chest syndrome D57.811
      - cerebral vascular involvement D57.813
      - crisis D57.819
        - with complication specified NEC D57.818

Disease, diseased, *continued*
- splenic sequestration D57.812
- vasoocclusive pain D57.819
  - without crisis D57.80
- spherocytosis D57.80
  - with
    - acute chest syndrome D57.811
    - cerebral vascular involvement D57.813
    - crisis D57.819
      - with complication specified NEC D57.818
    - splenic sequestration D57.812
    - vasoocclusive pain D57.819
  - without crisis D57.80
- thalassemia D57.40
  - with
    - acute chest syndrome D57.411
    - cerebral vascular involvement D57.413
    - crisis (painful) D57.419
      - with specified complication NEC D57.418
    - splenic sequestration D57.412
    - vasoocclusive pain D57.419
  - beta plus D57.44
    - with
      - acute chest syndrome D57.451
      - cerebral vascular involvement D57.453
      - crisis D57.459
        - with specified complication NEC D57.458
      - splenic sequestration D57.452
      - vasoocclusive pain D57.459
    - without crisis D57.44
  - beta zero D57.42
    - with
      - acute chest syndrome D57.431
      - cerebral vascular involvement D57.433
      - crisis D57.439
        - with specified complication NEC D57.438
      - splenic sequestration D57.432
      - vasoocclusive pain D57.439
    - without crisis D57.42
  - elliptocytosis D57.8-
- sixth B08.20
  - due to human herpesvirus 6 B08.21
  - due to human herpesvirus 7 B08.22
- skin L98.9
  - due to metabolic disorder NEC E88.9 [L99]
  - specified NEC L98.8
- slim (HIV) B20
- South African creeping B88.0
- Startle Q89.8
- Sticker's (erythema infectiosum) B08.3
- Stokes-Adams (syncope with heart block) I45.9
- stomach K31.9
  - functional, psychogenic F45.8
  - specified NEC K31.89
- striatopallidal system NEC G25.89
- testes N50.9
- thalassemia Hb-S—*see* Disease, sickle-cell, thalassemia
- Thaysen-Gee (nontropical sprue) K90.0
- Thomsen G71.12
- throat J39.2
  - septic J02.0
- thyroid (gland) E07.9
  - heart (*see also* Hyperthyroidism) E05.90 [I43]
    - with thyroid storm E05.91 [I43]
  - specified NEC E07.89
- Tietze's M94.0
- tonsils, tonsillar (and adenoids) J35.9
- tooth, teeth K08.9
  - hard tissues K03.9
    - specified NEC K03.89
- Tourette's F95.2
- tricuspid I07.9
  - nonrheumatic I36.9
- Underwood's (sclerema neonatorum) P83.0
- urinary (tract) N39.9
  - bladder N32.9
    - specified NEC N32.89
  - specified NEC N39.8
- vagabond's B85.1
- vagina, vaginal (noninflammatory) N89.9
  - inflammatory NEC N76.89
  - specified NEC N89.8

Disease, diseased, *continued*
- vascular I99.9
- venereal (*see also* Disease, sexually transmitted) A64
  – chlamydial NEC A56.8
    ∎ anus A56.3
    ∎ genitourinary NOS A56.2
    ∎ pharynx A56.4
    ∎ rectum A56.3
- viral, virus (*see also* Disease, by type of virus) B34.9
  – human immunodeficiency (HIV) B20
  – Powassan A84.81
- von Willebrand (-Jürgens) (angiohemophilia) D68.0
- Vrolik's (osteogenesis imperfecta) Q78.0
- Werdnig-Hoffmann G12.0
- Werner-Schultz (neutropenic splenomegaly) D73.81
- white blood cells D72.9
  – specified NEC D72.89
- wool sorter's A22.1

Disfigurement (due to scar) L90.5

Dislocation (articular)
- finger S63.2-
  – index S63.2-
  – interphalangeal S63.27-
    ∎ distal S63.29-
      ~ index S63.29-
      ~ little S63.29-
      ~ middle S63.29-
      ~ ring S63.29-
    ∎ index S63.2-
    ∎ little S63.2-
    ∎ middle S63.2-
    ∎ proximal S63.28-
      ~ index S63.28-
      ~ little S63.28-
      ~ middle S63.28-
      ~ ring S63.28-
    ∎ ring S63.2-
  – little S63.2-
  – metacarpophalangeal S63.26-
    ∎ index S63.26-
    ∎ little S63.26-
    ∎ middle S63.26-
    ∎ ring S63.26-
  – middle S63.2-
  – ring S63.2-
  – thumb—*see* Dislocation
- hip S73.0-
  – congenital (total) Q65.2
    ∎ bilateral Q65.1
    ∎ partial Q65.5
      ~ bilateral Q65.4
      ~ unilateral Q65.3-
    ∎ unilateral Q65.0-
- interphalangeal (joint(s))
  – finger S63.2-
    ∎ distal S63.29-
      ~ index S63.29-
      ~ little S63.29-
      ~ middle S63.29-
      ~ ring S63.29-
    ∎ index S63.2-
    ∎ little S63.2-
    ∎ middle S63.2-
    ∎ proximal S63.28-
      ~ index S63.28-
      ~ little S63.28-
      ~ middle S63.28-
      ~ ring S63.28-
    ∎ ring S63.2-
    – thumb S63.12-
- jaw (cartilage) (meniscus) S03.0-
- knee S83.10-
  – cap—*see* Dislocation, patella
  – congenital Q68.2
  – old M23.8X-
  – patella—*see* Dislocation, patella
  – proximal tibia
    ∎ anteriorly S83.11-
    ∎ laterally S83.14-
    ∎ medially S83.13-
    ∎ posteriorly S83.12-
  – specified type NEC S83.19-

Dislocation, *continued*
- lens (complete) H27.10
  – anterior H27.12-
  – congenital Q12.1
  – partial H27.11-
  – posterior H27.13-
  – traumatic S05.8X-
- mandible S03.0-
- metacarpophalangeal (joint)
  – finger S63.26-
    ∎ index S63.26-
    ∎ little S63.26-
    ∎ middle S63.26-
    ∎ ring S63.26-
  – thumb S63.11-
- partial—*see* Subluxation, by site
- patella S83.00-
  – congenital Q74.1
  – lateral S83.01-
  – recurrent (nontraumatic) M22.0-
    ∎ incomplete M22.1-
  – specified type NEC S83.09-
- sacroiliac (joint) (ligament) S33.2
  – congenital Q74.2
- septum (nasal) (old) J34.2
- temporomandibular S03.0-
- thumb S63.10-

Disorder (of)—*see also* Disease
- acute
  – psychotic—*see* Psychosis, acute
  – stress F43.0
- adjustment (grief) F43.20
  – with
    ∎ anxiety F43.22
      ~ with depressed mood F43.23
    ∎ conduct disturbance F43.24
      ~ with emotional disturbance F43.25
    ∎ depressed mood F43.21
      ~ with anxiety F43.23
    ∎ other specified symptom F43.29
- adrenogenital E25.9
- aggressive, unsocialized F91.1
- alcohol-related
  – with
    ∎ intoxication F10.929
      ~ uncomplicated F10.920
- allergic—*see* Allergy
- alveolar NEC J84.09
- amino-acid
  – metabolism—*see* Disturbance, metabolism, amino-acid
    ∎ specified NEC E72.89
  – neonatal, transitory P74.8
- anaerobic glycolysis with anemia D55.29
- anxiety F41.9
  – illness F45.21
  – mixed
    ∎ with depression (mild) F41.8
  – phobic F40.9
    ∎ of childhood F40.8
  – social F40.1-
  – specified NEC F41.8
- aromatic amino-acid metabolism E70.9
  – specified NEC E70.89
- attention-deficit hyperactivity (adolescent) (adult) (child) F90.9
  – combined type F90.2
  – hyperactive type F90.1
  – inattentive type F90.0
  – specified type NEC F90.8
- attention-deficit without hyperactivity (adolescent) (adult) (child) F90.0
- auditory processing (central) H93.25
- autistic F84.0
- autoimmune D89.89
- avoidant
  – restrictive food intake F50.82
- balance
  – acid-base E87.8
    ∎ mixed E87.4
  – electrolyte E87.8
  – fluid NEC E87.8

Disorder, *continued*
- beta-amino-acid metabolism E72.89
- bilirubin excretion E80.6
- binge-eating F50.81
- bipolar (I) (type1) F31.9
  – current (or most recent) episode
    ∎ depressed F31.9
      ~ without psychotic features F31.30
        ◊ mild F31.31
        ◊ moderate F31.32
        ◊ severe (without psychotic features) F31.4
    ∎ hypomanic F31.0
    ∎ manic F31.9
      ~ without psychotic features F31.10
        ◊ mild F31.11
        ◊ moderate F31.12
        ◊ severe (without psychotic features) F31.13
    ∎ mixed F31.60
      ~ mild F31.61
      ~ moderate F31.62
- bladder N32.9
  – specified NEC N32.89
- bleeding D68.9
- body dysmorphic F45.22
- breast
  – associated with
    ∎ cracked nipple O92.1-
    ∎ galactorrhea O92.6
    ∎ hypogalactia O92.4
    ∎ lactation O92.70
      – specified NEC O92.79
    ∎ lactation disorder NEC O92.79
    ∎ pregnancy O92.20
      – specified NEC O92.29
    ∎ puerperium O92.20
      – specified NEC O92.29
- Briquet's F45.0
- cannabis use
  – due to drug abuse—*see* Abuse, drug, cannabis
  – due to drug dependence—*see* Dependence, drug, cannabis
- carbohydrate
  – metabolism (congenital) E74.9
    ∎ specified NEC E74.89
- carnitine metabolism E71.40
- central auditory processing H93.25
- character NOS F60.9
- coagulation (factor) (*see also* Defect, coagulation) D68.9
  – newborn, transient P61.6
- coccyx NEC M53.3
- conduct (childhood) F91.9
  – adjustment reaction—*see* Disorder, adjustment
  – adolescent onset type F91.2
  – childhood onset type F91.1
  – depressive F91.8
  – group type F91.2
  – hyperkinetic—*see* Disorder, attention-deficit hyperactivity
  – oppositional defiance F91.3
  – socialized F91.2
  – solitary aggressive type F91.1
  – specified NEC F91.8
  – unsocialized (aggressive) F91.1
- conduction, heart I45.9
- congenital glycosylation (CDG) E74.89
- cornea H18.9
  – due to contact lens H18.82-
  – Cyclin-Dependent Kinase-Like 5 Deficiency (CDKL5) G40.42
- cyclothymic F34.0
- defiant oppositional F91.3
- depressive F32.A
  – major F32.9
    ∎ with psychotic symptoms F32.3
    ∎ in remission (full) F32.5
      – partial F32.4
    ∎ recurrent F33.9
    ∎ single episode F32.9
      ~ mild F32.0
      ~ moderate F32.1
      ~ severe (without psychotic symptoms) F32.2
        ◊ with psychotic symptoms F32.3

Disorder, *continued*
- developmental F89
  - arithmetical skills F81.2
  - coordination (motor) F82
  - expressive writing F81.81
  - language F80.9
    - expressive F80.1
    - mixed receptive and expressive F80.2
    - receptive type F80.2
    - specified NEC F80.89
  - learning F81.9
    - arithmetical F81.2
    - reading F81.0
  - mixed F88
  - motor coordination or function F82
  - pervasive F84.9
    - specified NEC F84.8
  - phonological F80.0
  - reading F81.0
  - scholastic skills—*see also* Disorder, learning
    - mixed F81.89
  - specified NEC F88
  - speech F80.9
    - articulation F80.0
    - specified NEC F80.89
  - written expression F81.81
- diaphragm J98.6
- digestive (system) K92.9
  - newborn P78.9
    - specified NEC P78.89
  - postprocedural—*see* Complication, gastrointestinal
  - psychogenic F45.8
- disc (intervertebral)
  - with
    - myelopathy
      ~ sacroiliac region M53.3
      ~ sacrococcygeal region M53.3
    - specified NEC
      - sacrococcygeal region M53.3
- disruptive F91.9
  - mood dysregulation F34.81
  - specified NEC F91.8
- dissocial personality F60.2
- dissociative F44.9
  - affecting
    - motor function F44.4
      ~ and sensation F44.7
    - sensation F44.6
      ~ and motor function F44.7
  - brief reactive F43.0
  - drug induced hemorrhagic D68.32
- drug related
  - abuse—*see* Abuse, drug
  - dependence—*see* Dependence, drug
- dysthymic F34.1
- eating (adult) (psychogenic) F50.9
  - anorexia—*see* Anorexia
  - binge F50.81
  - bulimia F50.2
  - child F98.29
    - pica F98.3
    - rumination disorder F98.21
  - other F50.89
  - pica F50.89
    - childhood F98.3
- electrolyte (balance) NEC E87.8
  - acidosis (metabolic) (respiratory) E87.2
  - alkalosis (metabolic) (respiratory) E87.3
- emotional (persistent) F34.9
  - of childhood F93.9
    - specified NEC F93.8
- esophagus K22.9
  - functional K22.4
  - psychogenic F45.8
- eustachian tube H69.9-
  - specified NEC H69.8-
- factor, coagulation—*see* Defect, coagulation
- fatty acid
  - metabolism E71.30
    - specified NEC E71.39
  - oxidation
    - LCAD E71.310
    - MCAD E71.311

Disorder, *continued*
  - SCAD E71.312
  - specified deficiency NEC E71.318
- feeding (infant or child) (*see also* Disorder, eating) R63.30
  - or eating disorder F50.9
  - pediatric
    - acute R63.31
    - chronic R63.32
  - specified NEC F50.9
- feigned (with obvious motivation) Z76.5
- fibroblastic M72.9
- fluency
  - childhood onset F80.81
  - in conditions classified elsewhere R47.82
- fluid balance E87.8
- follicular (skin) L73.9
  - specified NEC L73.8
- functional polymorphonuclear neutrophils D71
- gamma-glutamyl cycle E72.89
- gastric (functional) K31.9
  - motility K30
  - psychogenic F45.8
  - secretion K30
- gastrointestinal (functional) NOS K92.9
  - newborn P78.9
  - psychogenic F45.8
- gender-identity or -role F64.9
  - childhood F64.2
  - effect on relationship F66
  - of adolescence or adulthood (nontranssexual) F64.0
  - specified NEC F64.8
  - uncertainty F66
- genitourinary system
  - female N94.9
  - male N50.9
  - psychogenic F45.8
- glomerular (in) N05.9
  - disseminated intravascular coagulation D65 [N08]
  - hemolytic-uremic syndrome D59.3
  - Henoch (-Schönlein) purpura D69.0 [N08]
  - sepsis NEC A41. - [N08]
  - subacute bacterial endocarditis I33.0 [N08]
  - systemic lupus erythematosus M32.14
- gluconeogenesis E74.4
- glucose transport E74.819
  - specified NEC E74.818
- glycine metabolism E72.50
  - hyperoxaluria R82.992
    - primary E72.53
- glycoprotein E77.9
  - specified NEC E77.8
- habit (and impulse) F63.9
  - specified NEC F63.89
- heart action I49.9
- hemorrhagic NEC D69.9
  - drug-induced D68.32
  - due to
    - extrinsic circulating anticoagulants D68.32
    - increase in
      ~ anti-IIa D68.32
      ~ anti-Xa D68.32
- hoarding F42.3
- hypochondriacal F45.20
  - body dysmorphic F45.22
- identity
  - dissociative F44.81
  - of childhood F93.8
- immune mechanism (immunity) D89.9
  - specified type NEC D89.89
- integument, newborn P83.9
  - specified NEC P83.88
- intestine, intestinal
  - carbohydrate absorption NEC E74.39
    - postoperative K91.2
  - functional NEC K59.9
  - psychogenic F45.8
- joint M25.9
  - psychogenic F45.8
- lacrimal system H04.9
- lactation NEC O92.79
- language (developmental) F80.9
  - expressive F80.1

Disorder, *continued*
  - mixed receptive and expressive F80.2
  - receptive F80.2
- learning (specific) F81.9
  - acalculia R48.8
  - alexia R48.0
  - mathematics F81.2
  - reading F81.0
  - specified NEC F81.89
    - with impairment in
      ~ mathematics F81.2
      ~ reading F81.0
      ~ written expression F81.81
  - spelling F81.81
  - written expression F81.81
- liver K76.9
  - malarial B54 [K77]
- lung, interstitial, drug-induced J70.4
  - dabbing (related) U07.0
  - e-cigarette (related) U07.0
  - electronic cigarette (related) U07.0
  - vaping (device) (product) (use) (associated) (related) U07.0
- lymphoproliferative, post-transplant (PTLD) D47.Z1
- meninges, specified type NEC G96.198
- menstrual N92.6
  - psychogenic F45.8
  - specified NEC N92.5
- mental (or behavioral) (nonpsychotic) F99
  - following organic brain damage F07.9
    - postconcussional syndrome F07.81
    - specified NEC F07.89
  - infancy, childhood or adolescence F98.9
  - neurotic—*see* Neurosis
- metabolic, amino acid, transitory, newborn P74.8
- metabolism NOS E88.9
  - amino-acid E72.9
    - aromatic
      ~ hyperphenylalaninemia E70.1
      ◊ classical phenylketonuria E70.0
      ~ other specified E70.89
    - branched chain E71.2
      ~ maple syrup urine disease E71.0
    - glycine E72.50
      ~ hyperoxaluria R82.992
      ◊ primary E72.53
    - other specified E72.8
      ~ beta-amino acid E72.8
      ~ gamma-glutamyl cycle E72.8
    - straight-chain E72.8
  - bilirubin E80.7
    - specified NEC E80.6
  - calcium E83.50
    - hypercalcemia E83.52
    - hypocalcemia E83.51
    - other specified E83.59
  - carbohydrate E74.9
    - specified NEC E74.89
  - congenital E88.9
  - glutamine E72.89
  - glycoprotein E77.9
    - specified NEC E77.8
  - mitochondrial E88.40
    - MELAS syndrome E88.41
    - MERRF syndrome (myoclonic epilepsy associated with ragged-red fibers) E88.42
    - other specified E88.49
      ~ beta-amino acid E72.89
      ~ gamma-glutamyl cycle E72.89
  - plasma protein NEC E88.09
  - purine E79.9
  - pyrimidine E79.9
  - pyruvate E74.4
  - serine E72.8
  - sodium E87.8
  - straight chain E72.89
  - threonine E72.89
- micturition NEC R39.198
  - feeling of incomplete emptying R39.14
  - hesitancy R39.11
  - need to immediately re-void R39.191
  - poor stream R39.12
  - position dependent R39.192

Disorder, *continued*
- – psychogenic F45.8
- – split stream R39.13
- – straining R39.16
- – urgency R39.15
- • mitochondrial metabolism E88.40
- • mixed
  - – anxiety and depressive F41.8
  - – of scholastic skills (developmental) F81.89
  - – receptive expressive language F80.2
- • mood (affective), unspecified F39
- • movement G25.9
  - – drug-induced G25.70
    - ■ akathisia G25.71
    - ■ specified NEC G25.79
  - – treatment-induced G25.9
  - – hysterical F44.4
  - – stereotyped F98.4
- • muscle M62.9
  - – psychogenic F45.8
  - – specified type NEC M62.89
  - – tone, newborn P94.9
    - ■ specified NEC P94.8
- • musculoskeletal system, soft tissue
  - – psychogenic F45.8
- • myoneural G70.9
  - – due to lead G70.1
  - – specified NEC G70.89
  - – toxic G70.1
- • nerve G58.9
  - – cranial G52.9
    - ■ multiple G52.7
    - ■ seventh NEC G51.8
    - ■ sixth NEC—*see* Strabismus, paralytic, sixth nerve
  - – facial G51.9
    - ■ specified NEC G51.8
- • neurodevelopmental F89
  - – specified NEC F88
- • neurohypophysis NEC E23.3
- • neuromuscular G70.9
  - – hereditary NEC G71.9
  - – specified NEC G70.89
  - – toxic G70.1
- • neurotic F48.9
  - – specified NEC F48.8
- • neutrophil, polymorphonuclear D71
- • non-rapid eye movement sleep arousal
  - – sleep terror type F51.4
  - – sleepwalking type F51.3
- • nose J34.9
  - – specified NEC J34.89
- • obsessive-compulsive F42.9
  - – excoriation (skin picking) disorder F42.4
  - – hoarding disorder F42.3
  - – mixed obsessional thoughts and acts F42.2
  - – other F42.8
- • oppositional defiant F91.3
- • overanxious F41.1
  - – of childhood F93.8
- • pain
  - – with related psychological factors F45.42
  - – exclusively related to psychological factors F45.41
- • panic F41.0
- • parietoalveolar NEC J84.09
- • paroxysmal, mixed R56.9
- • peroxisomal E71.50
  - – biogenesis
    - ■ neonatal adrenoleukodystrophy E71.511
    - ■ specified disorder NEC E71.518
    - ■ Zellweger syndrome E71.510
  - – rhizomelic chondrodysplasia punctata E71.540
  - – specified form NEC E71.548
    - ■ group 1 E71.518
    - ■ group 2 E71.53
    - ■ group 3 E71.542
  - – X-linked adrenoleukodystrophy E71.529
    - ■ adolescent E71.521
    - ■ adrenomyeloneuropathy E71.522
    - ■ childhood E71.520
    - ■ specified form NEC E71.528
  - – Zellweger-like syndrome E71.54

Disorder, *continued*
- • persistent
  - – (somatoform) pain F45.41
  - – affective (mood) F34.9
- • personality (*see also* Personality) F60.9
  - – affective F34.0
  - – aggressive F60.3
  - – amoral F60.2
  - – anankastic F60.5
  - – antisocial F60.2
  - – anxious F60.6
  - – asocial F60.2
  - – avoidant F60.6
  - – borderline F60.3
  - – compulsive F60.5
  - – cyclothymic F34.0
  - – dissocial F60.2
  - – emotional instability F60.3
  - – expansive paranoid F60.0
  - – explosive F60.3
  - – histrionic F60.4
  - – hysterical F60.4
  - – labile F60.3
  - – moral deficiency F60.2
  - – obsessional F60.5
  - – obsessive (-compulsive) F60.5
  - – paranoid F60.0
  - – pseudosocial F60.2
  - – psychopathic F60.2
  - – schizoid F60.1
  - – type A F60.5
  - – unstable (emotional) F60.3
- • pervasive, developmental F84.9
- • pigmentation L81.9
  - – choroid, congenital Q14.3
  - – diminished melanin formation L81.6
  - – iron L81.8
  - – specified NEC L81.8
- • pituitary gland E23.7
  - – specified NEC E23.6
- • polymorphonuclear neutrophils D71
- • postconcussional F07.81
- • postprocedural (postoperative)—*see* Complications, postprocedural
- • post-traumatic stress (PTSD) F43.10
  - – acute F43.11
  - – chronic F43.12
- • premenstrual dysphoric (PMDD) F32.81
- • prepuce N47.8
- • psychogenic NOS (*see also* Disease, diseased) F45.9
  - – anxiety F41.8
  - – appetite F50.9
  - – asthenic F48.8
  - – cardiovascular (system) F45.8
  - – compulsive F42.8
  - – cutaneous F54
  - – depressive F32.9
  - – digestive (system) F45.8
  - – dysmenorrheic F45.8
  - – dyspneic F45.8
  - – endocrine (system) F54
  - – eye NEC F45.8
  - – feeding—*see* Disorder, eating
  - – functional NEC F45.8
  - – gastric F45.8
  - – gastrointestinal (system) F45.8
  - – genitourinary (system) F45.8
  - – heart (function) (rhythm) F45.8
  - – hyperventilatory F45.8
  - – hypochondriacal—*see* Disorder, hypochondriacal
  - – intestinal F45.8
  - – joint F45.8
  - – learning F81.9
  - – limb F45.8
  - – lymphatic (system) F45.8
  - – menstrual F45.8
  - – micturition F45.8
  - – monoplegic NEC F44.4
  - – motor F44.4
  - – muscle F45.8
  - – musculoskeletal F45.8
  - – neurocirculatory F45.8
  - – obsessive F42.8

Disorder, *continued*
- – organ or part of body NEC F45.8
- – paralytic NEC F44.4
- – phobic F40.9
- – physical NEC F45.8
- – rectal F45.8
- – respiratory (system) F45.8
- – rheumatic F45.8
- – specified part of body NEC F45.8
- – stomach F45.8
- • psychomotor NEC F44.4
  - – hysterical F44.4
- • psychoneurotic—*see also* Neurosis
  - – mixed NEC F48.8
- • psychophysiologic—*see* Disorder, somatoform
- • psychosexual development F66
  - – identity of childhood F64.2
- • psychosomatic NOS—*see* Disorder, somatoform
  - – multiple F45.0
  - – undifferentiated F45.1
- • psychotic—*see* Psychosis
  - – puberty E30.9
  - – specified NEC E30.8
- • pulmonary (valve)—*see* Endocarditis, pulmonary
- • pyruvate metabolism E74.4
- • reading R48.0
  - – developmental (specific) F81.0
- • REM sleep behavior G47.52
- • receptive language F80.2
- • refraction H52.7
- • respiratory function, impaired—*see also* Failure, respiration
  - – postprocedural—*see* Complication
  - – psychogenic F45.8
- • sacrum, sacrococcygeal NEC M53.3
- • schizoid of childhood F84.5
- • seizure (*see also* Epilepsy) G40.909
- • semantic pragmatic F80.89
  - – with autism F84.0
- • sense of smell R43.1
  - – psychogenic F45.8
- • separation anxiety, of childhood F93.0
- • shyness, of childhood and adolescence F40.10
- • sibling rivalry F93.8
- • sickle-cell (sickling) (homozygous)—*see* Disease, sickle-cell
  - – heterozygous D57.3
  - – specified type NEC D57.8-
  - – trait D57.3
- • sinus (nasal) J34.9
  - – specified NEC J34.89
- • skin L98.9
  - – hypertrophic L91.9
    - ■ specified NEC L91.8
  - – newborn P83.9
    - ■ specified NEC P83.88
  - – picking F42.4
- • sleep G47.9
  - – circadian rhythm G47.20
    - ■ advanced sleep phase type G47.22
    - ■ delayed sleep phase type G47.21
    - ■ free running type G47.24
    - ■ in conditions classified elsewhere G47.27
    - ■ irregular sleep wake type G47.23
    - ■ jet lag type G47.25
    - ■ non-24 hour sleep-wake type G47.24
    - ■ specified NEC G47.29
  - – terrors F51.4
  - – walking F51.3
- • sleep-wake pattern or schedule—*see* Disorder, sleep, circadian rhythm G47.9
- • social
  - – anxiety (of childhood) F40.10
    - ■ generalized F40.11
  - – functioning in childhood F94.9
    - ■ specified NEC F94.8
  - – pragmatic F80.82
- • somatization F45.0
- • somatoform F45.9
  - – pain (persistent) F45.41
  - – somatization (multiple) (long-lasting) F45.0
  - – specified NEC F45.8
  - – undifferentiated F45.1

Disorder, *continued*
- specific
  - arithmetical F81.2
  - developmental, of motor F82
  - reading F81.0
  - speech and language F80.9
  - spelling F81.81
  - written expression F81.81
- speech R47.9
  - articulation (functional) (specific) F80.0
  - developmental F80.9
  - specified NEC R47.89
- spelling (specific) F81.81
- stereotyped, habit or movement F98.4
- stomach (functional)—*see* Disorder, gastric
- stress F43.9
  - acute F43.0
  - post-traumatic F43.10
    - acute F43.11
    - chronic F43.12
- temperature regulation, newborn P81.9
- thyroid (gland) E07.9
  - function NEC, neonatal, transitory P72.2
  - iodine-deficiency related E01.8
  - specified NEC E07.89
- tic—*see* Tic
- tobacco use
  - mild F17.200
  - moderate or severe F17.200
- tooth K08.9
  - eruption K00.6
- Tourette's F95.2
- trauma and stressor related F43.9
- tubulo-interstitial (in)
  - lymphoma NEC C85.9- [N16]
  - Salmonella infection A02.25
  - sarcoidosis D86.84
  - sepsis A41.9 [N16]
    - streptococcal A40.9 [N16]
  - systemic lupus erythematosus M32.15
  - toxoplasmosis B58.83
  - transplant rejection T86.-- [N16]
- unsocialized aggressive F91.1
- vision, binocular H53.30
  - abnormal retinal correspondence H53.31
  - diplopia H53.2
- white blood cells D72.9
  - specified NEC D72.89

Disorientation R41.0

Displacement, displaced
- acquired traumatic of bone, cartilage, joint, tendon NEC—*see* Dislocation
- bladder (acquired) N32.89
  - congenital Q64.19
- canaliculus (lacrimalis), congenital Q10.6
- fallopian tube (acquired) N83.4-
  - congenital Q50.6
  - opening (congenital) Q50.6
- gallbladder (congenital) Q44.1
- intervertebral disc NEC
  - sacrococcygeal region M53.3
- lachrymal, lacrimal apparatus or duct (congenital) Q10.6
- lens, congenital Q12.1
- macula (congenital) Q14.1
- Meckel's diverticulum Q43.0
- nail (congenital) Q84.6
  - acquired L60.8
- ovary (acquired) N83.4-
  - congenital Q50.39
- oviduct (acquired) N83.4-
  - congenital Q50.6
- sacro-iliac (joint) (congenital) Q74.2
  - current injury S33.2
- uterine opening of oviducts or fallopian tubes Q50.6
- ventricular septum Q21.0

Disproportion
- fiber-type G71.20
  - congenital G71.29

Disruption (of)
- closure of
  - laceration (external) (internal) T81.33
  - traumatic laceration (external) (internal) T81.33

Disruption, *continued*
- family Z63.8
  - due to
    - absence of family member due to military deployment Z63.31
    - absence of family member NEC Z63.32
    - alcoholism and drug addiction in family Z63.72
    - bereavement Z63.4
    - death (assumed) or disappearance of family member Z63.4
    - divorce or separation Z63.5
    - drug addiction in family Z63.72
    - stressful life events NEC Z63.79
- wound T81.30
  - traumatic injury repair T81.33
- traumatic injury wound repair T81.33

Dissociation
- auriculoventricular or atrioventricular (AV) (any degree) (isorhythmic) I45.89
  - with heart block I44.2

Dissociative reaction, state F44.9

Distension, distention
- abdomen R14.0
- bladder N32.89
- stomach K31.89
  - acute K31.0
  - psychogenic F45.8

Distortion(s) (congenital)
- bile duct or passage Q44.5
- cervix (uteri) Q51.9
- clavicle Q74.0
- common duct Q44.5
- cystic duct Q44.5
- ear (auricle) (external) Q17.3
  - inner Q16.5
  - middle Q16.4
  - ossicles Q16.3
- endocrine NEC Q89.2
- eustachian tube Q17.8
- eye (adnexa) Q15.8
- face bone(s) NEC Q75.8
- fallopian tube Q50.6
- foot Q66.9-
- genitalia, genital organ(s)
  - female Q52.8
    - external Q52.79
    - internal NEC Q52.8
- hepatic duct Q44.5
- intrafamilial communications Z63.8
- lens Q12.8
- oviduct Q50.6
- parathyroid (gland) Q89.2
- pituitary (gland) Q89.2
- sacroiliac joint Q74.2
- scapula Q74.0
- shoulder girdle Q74.0
- skull bone(s) NEC Q75.8
  - with
    - anencephalus Q00.0
    - encephalocele—*see* Encephalocele
    - hydrocephalus Q03.9
      - with spina bifida—*see* Spina bifida, with hydrocephalus
    - microcephaly Q02
- thymus (gland) Q89.2
- thyroid (gland) Q89.2
- toe(s) Q66.9-

Distress
- abdomen—*see* Pain, abdominal
- acute respiratory R06.03
  - syndrome (adult) (child) J80
- epigastric R10.13
- fetal P84
- gastrointestinal (functional) K30
  - psychogenic F45.8
- intestinal (functional) NOS K59.9
  - psychogenic F45.8
- relationship, with spouse or intimate partner Z63.0
- respiratory R06.03
  - distress syndrome, child J80
  - newborn P22.9

Distress, *continued*
  - specified NEC P22.8
  - orthopnea R06.01
  - psychogenic F45.8
  - shortness of breath R06.02

Disturbance(s)—*see also* Disease
- absorption K90.9
  - calcium E58
  - carbohydrate K90.49
  - fat K90.49
    - pancreatic K90.3
  - protein K90.49
  - starch K90.49
  - vitamin—*see* Deficiency
- acid-base equilibrium E87.8
  - mixed E87.4
- activity and attention (with hyperkinesis)—*see* Disorder, attention-deficit hyperactivity
- assimilation, food K90.9
- blood clotting (mechanism) (*see also* Defect, coagulation) D68.9
- cerebral
  - status, newborn P91.9
    - specified NEC P91.88
- circulatory I99.9
- conduct (*see also* Disorder, conduct) F91.9
  - adjustment reaction—*see* Disorder, adjustment
  - disruptive F91.9
  - hyperkinetic—*see* Disorder, attention-deficit hyperactivity
  - socialized F91.2
  - specified NEC F91.8
  - unsocialized F91.1
- digestive K30
  - psychogenic F45.8
- electrolyte—*see also* Imbalance, electrolyte
  - newborn, transitory P74.49
    - hyperchloremia P74.421
    - hyperchloremic metabolic acidosis P74.421
    - hypochloremia P74.422
    - potassium balance
      - hyperkalemia P74.31
      - hypokalemia P74.32
    - sodium balance
      - hypernatremia P74.21
      - hyponatremia P74.22
    - specified type NEC P74.49
- emotions specific to childhood and adolescence F93.9
  - endocrine (gland)
  - involving relationship problems F93.8
  - mixed F93.8
  - neonatal, transitory specified P72.8
  - specified NEC F93.8
  - with
    - anxiety and fearfulness NEC F93.8
    - oppositional disorder F91.3
    - sensitivity (withdrawal) F40.10
    - shyness F40.10
    - social withdrawal F40.10
- equilibrium R42
- gait—*see* Gait abnormality
  - hysterical F44.4
  - psychogenic F44.4
- gastrointestinal (functional) K30
  - psychogenic F45.8
- heart, functional (conditions in I44-I50)
  - due to presence of (cardiac) prosthesis I97.19-
  - postoperative I97.89
    - cardiac surgery I97.19-
- keratinization NEC
  - lip K13.0
- metabolism E88.9
  - amino-acid E72.9
    - straight-chain E72.89
  - general E88.9
  - glutamine E72.89
  - neonatal, transitory P74.9
    - calcium and magnesium P71.9
      - specified type NEC P71.8
    - carbohydrate metabolism P70.9
      - specified type NEC P70.8
    - specified NEC P74.8
  - threonine E72.8

Disturbance(s), *continued*
- nervous, functional R45.0
- nutritional E63.9
  - nail L60.3
- ocular motion H51.9
  - psychogenic F45.8
- oculogyric H51.8
  - psychogenic F45.8
- oculomotor H51.9
  - psychogenic F45.8
- personality (pattern) (trait) (*see also* Disorder, personality) F60.9
- potassium balance, newborn
  - hyperkalemia P74.31
  - hypokalemia P74.32
- psychomotor F44.4
- rhythm, heart I49.9
- sensation (cold) (heat) (localization) (tactile discrimination) (texture) (vibratory) NEC R20.9
  - hysterical F44.6
- sensory—*see* Disturbance
- situational (transient)—*see also* Disorder, adjustment
  - acute F43.0
- sleep G47.9
  - nonorganic origin F51.9
- smell R43.9
  - and taste (mixed) R43.8
  - anosmia R43.0
  - parosmia R43.1
  - specified NEC R43.8
- sodium balance, newborn
  - hypernatremia P74.21
  - hyponatremia P74.22
- speech R47.9
  - developmental F80.9
  - specified NEC R47.89
- taste R43.9
  - and smell (mixed) R43.8
  - parageusia R43.2
  - specified NEC R43.8
- temperature
  - regulation, newborn P81.9
    - specified NEC P81.8
  - sense R20.8
    - hysterical F44.6
- tooth
  - eruption K00.6
- vascular I99.9
- vision, visual H53.9
  - specified NEC H53.8
- voice R49.9
  - psychogenic F44.4
  - specified NEC R49.8

Diuresis R35.89

Diverticulum, diverticula (multiple)
- Meckel's (displaced) (hypertrophic) Q43.0
- pericardium (congenital) (cyst) Q24.8
  - acquired I31.8

Division
- glans penis Q55.69

Divorce, causing family disruption Z63.5

Dizziness R42
- hysterical F44.89
- psychogenic F45.8

DNR (do not resuscitate) Z66

Dohle body panmyelopathic syndrome D72.0

Dorsalgia M54.9
- psychogenic F45.41

Dorsopathy M53.9

Double
- albumin E88.09
- aortic arch Q25.45
- uterus Q51.2-

Doubled up Z59.01

Down syndrome Q90.9

Drinking (alcohol)
- excessive, to excess NEC (without dependence) F10.10
  - habitual (continual) (without remission) F10.20
    - with remission F10.21

Drip, postnasal (chronic) R09.82
- due to
  - allergic rhinitis—*see* Rhinitis, allergic
  - common cold J00
  - nasopharyngitis—*see* Nasopharyngitis
  - other know condition—*code to* condition
  - sinusitis—*see* Sinusitis

Drop (in)
- attack NEC R55
- hematocrit (precipitous) R71.0
- hemoglobin R71.0

Dropped heart beats I45.9

Dropsy, dropsical—*see also* Hydrops
- abdomen R18.8
- brain—*see* Hydrocephalus
- newborn due to isoimmunization P56.0

Drowned, drowning (near) T75.1

Drowsiness R40.0

Drug
- abuse counseling and surveillance Z71.51
- addiction—*see* Dependence
- dependence—*see* Dependence
- habit—*see* Dependence
- harmful use—*see* Abuse, drug
- induced fever R50.2
- overdose—*see* Table of Drugs and Chemicals, by drug, poisoning
- poisoning—*see* Table of Drugs and Chemicals, by drug, poisoning
- resistant organism infection (*see also* Resistant, organism, to, drug) Z16.30
- therapy
  - long term (current) (prophylactic)—*see* Therapy, drug long-term (current) (prophylactic)
  - short term—omit code
- wrong substance given or taken in error—*see* Table of Drugs and Chemicals, by drug, poisoning

Drunkenness (without dependence) F10.129
- acute in alcoholism F10.229
- chronic (without remission) F10.20
  - with remission F10.21
- pathological (without dependence) F10.129
  - with dependence F10.229

Dry, dryness—*see also* Disease, diseased
- mouth R68.2
  - due to dehydration E86.0
- nose J34.89

Dubin-Johnson disease or syndrome E80.6

Dubowitz' syndrome Q87.19

Duchenne-Griesinger disease G71.01

Duchenne's
- disease or syndrome
  - muscular dystrophy G71.01
- paralysis
  - birth injury P14.0
  - due to or associated with
    - muscular dystrophy G71.01

Duodenitis (nonspecific) (peptic) K29.80
- with bleeding K29.81

Duplication, duplex—*see also* Accessory
- alimentary tract Q45.8
- biliary duct (any) Q44.5
- cystic duct Q44.5
- digestive organs Q45.8
- frontonasal process Q75.8

Dupré's disease (meningism) R29.1

Dwarfism E34.3
- achondroplastic Q77.4
- congenital E34.3
- constitutional E34.3
- hypochondroplastic Q77.4
- hypophyseal E23.0
- infantile E34.3
- Laron-type E34.3
- Lorain (-Levi) type E23.0
- metatropic Q77.8
- nephrotic-glycosuric (with hypophosphatemic rickets) E72.09
- nutritional E45

Dwarfism, *continued*
- penis Q55.69
- pituitary E23.0
- renal N25.0
- thanatophoric Q77.1

Dysarthria R47.1

Dysbasia R26.2
- hysterical F44.4
- nonorganic origin F44.4
- psychogenic F44.4

Dysbetalipoproteinemia (familial) E78.2

Dyscalculia R48.8
- developmental F81.2

Dyschezia K59.00

Dyscranio-pygo-phalangy Q87.0
- stomach K31.89
  - psychogenic F45.8

Dysentery, dysenteric (catarrhal) (diarrhea) (epidemic) (hemorrhagic) (infectious) (sporadic) (tropical) A09
- amebic (*see also* Amebiasis) A06.0
  - acute A06.0
- arthritis (*see also* category M01) A09
  - bacillary (*see also* category M01) A03.9
- bacillary A03.9
  - arthritis (*see also* category M01)
  - Shigella A03.9
    - boydii A03.2
    - dysenteriae A03.0
    - flexneri A03.1
    - group A A03.0
    - group B A03.1
    - group C A03.2
    - group D A03.3
    - sonnei A03.3
    - specified type NEC A03.8
- candidal B37.82
- Chinese A03.9
- Giardia lamblia A07.1
- Lamblia A07.1
- monilial B37.82
- Salmonella A02.0
- viral (*see also* Enteritis, viral) A08.4

Dysequilibrium R42

Dysesthesia R20.8
- hysterical F44.6

Dysfunction
- autonomic
  - somatoform F45.8
- bladder N31.9
  - neuromuscular NOS N31.9
- bleeding, uterus N93.8
- cerebral G93.89
- colon K59.9
  - psychogenic F45.8
- feeding, pediatric
  - acute R63.31
  - chronic R63.32
- hypophysis E23.7
- hypothalamic NEC E23.3
- meibomian gland, of eyelid H02.88-
  - left H02.886
    - lower H02.885
    - upper H02.884
    - upper and lower eyelids H02.88B
  - right H02.883
    - lower H02.882
    - upper H02.881
    - upper and lower eyelids H02.88A
- physiological NEC R68.89
  - psychogenic F59
- pituitary (gland) E23.3
- rectum K59.9
  - psychogenic F45.8
- sexual (due to) R37
- sinoatrial node I49.5
- somatoform autonomic F45.8
- temporomandibular (joint) M26.69
  - joint-pain syndrome M26.62-
- ventricular I51.9
  - with congestive heart failure I50.9

Dysgenesis
- gonadal (due to chromosomal anomaly) Q96.9
- renal
  - bilateral Q60.4
  - unilateral Q60.3
- reticular D72.0
- tidal platelet D69.3

Dyshidrosis, dysidrosis L30.1

Dyskeratosis L85.8
- congenital Q82.8

Dyskinesia G24.9
- hysterical F44.4
- nonorganic origin F44.4
- psychogenic F44.4

Dyslalia (developmental) F80.0

Dyslexia R48.0
- developmental F81.0

Dyslipidemia E78.5

Dysmenorrhea (essential) (exfoliative) N94.6
- congestive (syndrome) N94.6
- primary N94.4
- psychogenic F45.8
- secondary N94.5

Dysmetabolic syndrome X E88.81

Dysmorphism (due to)
- alcohol Q86.0

Dysmorphophobia (non-delusional) F45.22

Dysorexia R63.0
- psychogenic F50.89

Dysostosis
- cleidocranial, cleidocranialis Q74.0
- multiplex E76.01

Dyspareunia N94.10
- deep N94.12
- other specified N94.19
- superficial (introital) N94.11

Dyspepsia R10.13
- atonic K30
- functional (allergic) (congenital) (gastrointestinal) (occupational) (reflex) K30
- nervous F45.8
- neurotic F45.8
- psychogenic F45.8

Dysphagia R13.10
- cervical R13.19
- functional (hysterical) F45.8
- hysterical F45.8
- nervous (hysterical) F45.8
- neurogenic R13.19
- oral phase R13.11
- oropharyngeal phase R13.12
- pharyngeal phase R13.13
- pharyngoesophageal phase R13.14
- psychogenic F45.8
- specified NEC R13.19

Dysphagocytosis, congenital D71

Dysphasia
- developmental
  - expressive type F80.1
  - receptive type F80.2

Dysphonia R49.0
- functional F44.4
- hysterical F44.4
- psychogenic F44.4

Dyspituitarism E23.3

Dysplasia—see also Anomaly
- acetabular, congenital Q65.89
- alveolar capillary, with vein misalignment J84.843
- anus (histologically confirmed) (mild) (moderate) K62.82
- asphyxiating thoracic (congenital) Q77.2
- brain Q07.9
- bronchopulmonary, perinatal P27.1
- chondroectodermal Q77.6
- colon D12.6
- dystrophic Q77.5
- ectodermal (anhidrotic) (congenital) (hereditary) Q82.4
  - hydrotic Q82.8
- high grade, focal D12.6

Dysplasia, continued
- hip, congenital Q65.89
- joint, congenital Q74.8
- kidney Q61.4
  - multicystic Q61.4
- leg Q74.2
- lung, congenital (not associated with short gestation) Q33.6
- oculodentodigital Q87.0
- renal Q61.4
  - multicystic Q61.4
- skin L98.8
- spondyloepiphyseal Q77.7
- thymic, with immunodeficiency D82.1

Dysplasminogenemia E88.02

Dyspnea (nocturnal) (paroxysmal) R06.00
- asthmatic (bronchial) J45.909
  - with
    - exacerbation (acute) J45.901
    - bronchitis J45.909
      - with
        - ◊ exacerbation (acute) J45.901
        - ◊ status asthmaticus J45.902
    - status asthmaticus J45.902
- functional F45.8
- hyperventilation R06.4
- hysterical F45.8
- newborn P28.89
- orthopnea R06.01
- psychogenic F45.8
- shortness of breath R06.02

Dyspraxia R27.8
- developmental (syndrome) F82

Dysproteinemia E88.09

Dysrhythmia
- cardiac I49.9
  - newborn
    - bradycardia P29.12
    - occurring before birth P03.819
      - before onset of labor P03.810
      - during labor P03.811
    - tachycardia P29.11
  - postoperative I97.89
- cerebral or cortical—see Epilepsy

Dyssomnia—see Disorder, sleep

Dyssynergia
- cerebellaris myoclonica (Hunt's ataxia) G11.19

Dystocia
- affecting newborn P03.1

Dystonia G24.9
- cervical G24.3
- deformans progressiva G24.1
- drug induced NEC G24.09
  - acute G24.02
  - specified NEC G24.09
- familial G24.1
- idiopathic G24.1
  - familial G24.1
  - nonfamilial G24.2
  - orofacial G24.4
- lenticularis G24.8
- musculorum deformans G24.1
- neuroleptic induced (acute) G24.02
- orofacial (idiopathic) G24.4
- oromandibular G24.4
  - due to drug G24.01
- specified NEC G24.8
- torsion (familial) (idiopathic) G24.1
  - acquired G24.8
  - genetic G24.1
  - symptomatic (nonfamilial) G24.2

Dystonic movements R25.8

Dystrophy, dystrophia
- adiposogenital E23.6
- autosomal recessive, childhood type, muscular dystrophy resembling Duchenne or Becker G71.01
- Becker's type G71.01
- cornea (hereditary) H18.50-
  - endothelial H18.51-
  - epithelial H18.52-

Dystrophy, dystrophia, continued
- granular H18.53-
- lattice H18.54-
- macular H18.55-
- specified type NEC H18.59-
- Duchenne's type G71.01
- Erb's G71.02
- Fuchs' H18.51-
- Gower's muscular G71.01
- infantile neuraxonal G31.89
- Landouzy-Déjérine G71.02
- Leyden-Möbius G71.09
- muscular G71.00
  - autosomal recessive, childhood type, muscular dystrophy resembling Duchenne or Becker G71.01
  - benign (Becker type) G71.01
    - capuloperoneal with early contractures [Emery-Dreifuss] G71.09
  - congenital (hereditary) (progressive) (with specific morphological abnormalities of the muscle fiber) G71.09
  - distal G71.09
  - Duchenne type G71.01
  - Emery-Dreifuss G71.09
  - Erb type G71.02
  - facioscapulohumeral G71.02
  - Gower's G71.01
  - hereditary (progressive) G71.09
  - Landouzy-Déjérine type G71.02
  - limb-girdle G71.09
  - progressive (hereditary) G71.09
  - pseudohypertrophic (infantile) G71.01
  - scapulohumeral G71.02
  - scapuloperoneal G71.09
  - severe (Duchenne type) G71.01
  - specified type NEC G71.09
- nail L60.3
- ocular G71.09
- oculocerebrorenal E72.03
- oculopharyngeal G71.09
- retinal (hereditary) H35.50
  - involving
    - sensory area H35.53
- scapuloperoneal G71.09
- skin NEC L98.8
- thoracic, asphyxiating Q77.2
- unguium L60.3

Dysuria R30.0
- psychogenic F45.8

E

Ear—see also Disease, diseased
- piercing Z41.3
- wax (impacted) H61.2-

Earache—see subcategory H92.0

Ebola virus disease A98.4

Eccentro-osteochondrodysplasia E76.29

Ecchymosis R58
- newborn P54.5
- spontaneous R23.3
- traumatic—see Contusion

Echovirus, as cause of disease classified elsewhere B97.12

Ectasia, ectasis
- annuloaortic I35.8

Ecthyma L08.0
- gangrenosum L08.0

Ectodermosis erosiva pluriorificialis L51.1

Ectopic, ectopia (congenital)
- abdominal viscera Q45.8
  - due to defect in anterior abdominal wall Q79.59
- atrial beats I49.1
- beats I49.49
  - atrial I49.1
- bladder Q64.10
- lens, lentis Q12.1
- testis Q53.00
  - bilateral Q53.02
  - unilateral Q53.01

Ectopic, ectopia, *continued*
- thyroid Q89.2
- vesicae Q64.10

Ectropion H02.10-
- cervix N86
  - with cervicitis N72
- congenital Q10.1
- lip (acquired) K13.0
  - congenital Q38.0

Eczema (acute) (chronic) (erythematous) (fissum) (rubrum) (squamous) (*see also* Dermatitis) L30.9
- contact—*see* Dermatitis, contact
- dyshydrotic L30.1
- flexural L20.82
- infantile L20.83
  - intertriginous L21.1
  - seborrheic L21.1
- intertriginous NEC L30.4
  - infantile L21.1
- intrinsic (allergic) L20.84
- marginatum (hebrae) B35.6
- pustular L30.3
- vaccination, vaccinatum T88.1

Eddowes (-Spurway) syndrome Q78.0

Edema, edematous (infectious) (pitting) (toxic) R60.9
- with nephritis—*see* Nephrosis
- allergic T78.3
- angioneurotic (allergic) (any site) (with urticaria) T78.3
- brain (cytotoxic) (vasogenic) G93.6
  - due to birth injury P11.0
  - newborn (anoxia or hypoxia) P52.4
    - birth injury P11.0
- circumscribed, acute T78.3
- conjunctiva H11.42-
- due to
  - salt retention E87.0
- epiglottis—*see* Edema, glottis
- essential, acute T78.3
- eyelid NEC H02.84-
  - left H02.846
    - lower H02.845
    - upper H02.844
  - right H02.843
    - lower H02.842
    - upper H02.841
- generalized R60.1
- glottis, glottic, glottidis (obstructive) (passive) J38.4
  - allergic T78.3
- intracranial G93.6
- legs R60.0
- localized R60.0
- lower limbs R60.0
- lung J81.1
  - acute J81.0
  - due to
    - high altitude T70.29
    - near drowning T75.1
- newborn P83.30
  - hydrops fetalis—*see* Hydrops, fetalis
  - specified NEC P83.39
- penis N48.89
- periodic T78.3
- Quincke's T78.3
- salt E87.0

Edentulism—*see* Absence, teeth, acquired

Edsall's disease T67.2

Educational handicap Z55.9
- less than a high school diploma or GED Z55.5
- specified NEC Z55.8

Edward's syndrome—*see* Trisomy, 18

Effect, adverse
- abuse—*see* Maltreatment
- altitude (high)—*see* Effect, adverse, high altitude
- biological, correct substance properly administered—*see* Effect, adverse, drugs and medicaments
- blood (derivatives) (serum) (transfusion)—*see* Complications, transfusion
- chemical substance—*see* Table of Drugs and Chemicals
- cold (temperature) (weather)
  - frostbite—*see* Frostbite
- drugs and medicaments T88.7

Effect, adverse, *continued*
- specified drug—*see* Table of Drugs and Chemicals, by drug, adverse effect
- specified effect—*code to* condition
- electric current, electricity (shock) T75.4
  - burn—*see* Burn
- exposure—*see* Exposure
- external cause NEC T75.89
- foodstuffs T78.1
  - allergic reaction—*see* Allergy, food
    - causing anaphylaxis—*see* Shock, anaphylactic, due to food
  - noxious—*see* Poisoning, food, noxious
- gases, fumes, or vapors
  - specified agent—*see* Table of Drugs and Chemicals
- glue (airplane) sniffing
  - due to drug abuse—*see* Abuse, drug, inhalant
  - due to drug dependence—*see* Dependence, drug, inhalant
- heat—*see* Heat
- high altitude NEC T70.29
  - anoxia T70.29
  - on
    - ears T70.0
    - sinuses T70.1
  - polycythemia D75.1
- hot weather—*see* Heat
- hunger T73.0
- immersion, foot—*see* Immersion
- immunization—*see* Complications, vaccination
- immunological agents—*see* Complications, vaccination
- infusion—*see* Complications, infusion
- lack of care of infants—*see* Maltreatment, child
- medical care T88.9
  - specified NEC T88.8
- medicinal substance, correct, properly administered—*see* Effect, adverse, drugs and medicaments
- motion T75.3
- serum NEC (*see also* Reaction, serum) T80.69
- specified NEC T78.8
- strangulation—*see* Asphyxia, traumatic
- submersion T75.1
- toxic—*see* Table of Drugs and Chemicals, by animal or substance, poisoning
- transfusion—*see* Complications, transfusion
- ultraviolet (radiation) (rays) NOS
  - burn—*see* Burn
  - dermatitis or eczema—*see* Dermatitis, due to, ultraviolet rays
    - acute L56.8
- vaccine (any)—*see* Complications, vaccination
- whole blood—*see* Complications, transfusion

Effect(s) (of) (from)—*see* Effect, adverse

Effects, late—*see* Sequelae

Effort syndrome (psychogenic) F45.8

Effusion
- brain (serous) G93.6
- bronchial—*see* Bronchitis
- cerebral G93.6
- cerebrospinal—*see also* Meningitis
  - vessel G93.6
- chest—*see* Effusion, pleura
- intracranial G93.6
- joint M25.40
  - ankle M25.47-
  - elbow M25.42-
  - foot joint M25.47-
  - hand joint M25.44-
  - hip M25.45-
  - knee M25.46-
  - shoulder M25.41-
  - specified joint NEC M25.48
  - wrist M25.43-
- malignant pleural J91.0
- pericardium, pericardial (noninflammatory) I31.3
  - acute—*see* Pericarditis, acute
- peritoneal (chronic) R18.8
- pleura, pleurisy, pleuritic, pleuropericardial J90
  - due to systemic lupus erythematosus M32.13
  - in conditions classified elsewhere J91.8
  - malignant J91.0
  - newborn P28.89

Effusion, *continued*
- spinal—*see* Meningitis
- thorax, thoracic—*see* Effusion, pleura

Ehlers-Danlos syndrome Q79.60
- classical Ehlers-Danlos syndrome Q79.61
- hypermobile Ehlers-Danlos syndrome Q79.62
- other Ehlers-Danlos syndromes Q79.69
- vascular Ehlers-Danlos syndrome Q79.63

Ehrlichiosis A77.4-

Eichstedt's disease B36.0

Eisenmenger's
- complex or syndrome I27.83
- defect Q21.8

Ekbom's syndrome (restless legs) G25.81

Ekman's syndrome (brittle bones and blue sclera) Q78.0

Elastic skin Q82.8

Elastoma (juvenile) Q82.8

Electric current, electricity, effects (concussion) (fatal) (nonfatal) (shock) T75.4
- burn—*see* Burn

Electrocution T75.4
- from electroshock gun (taser) T75.4

Electrolyte imbalance E87.8

Elevated, elevation
- alanine transaminase (ALT) R74.01
- ALT (alanine transaminase) R74.01
- aspartate transaminase (AST) R74.01
- AST (aspartate transaminase) R74.01
- basal metabolic rate R94.8
- blood pressure—*see also* Hypertension
  - reading (incidental) (isolated) (nonspecific), no diagnosis of hypertension R03.0
- blood sugar R73.9
- body temperature (of unknown origin) R50.9
- C-reactive protein (CRP) R79.82
- cancer antigen 125 [CA 125] R97.1
- carcinoembryonic antigen [CEA] R97.0
- cholesterol E78.00
  - with high triglycerides E78.2
- erythrocyte sedimentation rate R70.0
- fasting glucose R73.01
- finding on laboratory examination—*see* Findings, abnormal, inconclusive, without diagnosis
- glucose tolerance (oral) R73.02
- lactic acid dehydrogenase (LDH) level R74.02
- leukocytes D72.829
- lipoprotein a (Lp(a)) level E78.41
- liver function
  - study R94.5
  - test R79.89
    - alkaline phosphatase R74.8
    - aminotransferase R74.01
    - bilirubin R17
    - hepatic enzyme R74.8
    - lactate dehydrogenase R74.02
- lymphocytes D72.820
- scapula, congenital Q74.0
- sedimentation rate R70.0
- SGOT R74.0
- SGPT R74.0
- transaminase level R74.0
- triglycerides E78.1
  - with high cholesterol E78.2
- troponin R77.8
- tumor associated antigens [TAA] NEC R97.8
- tumor specific antigens [TSA] NEC R97.8
- white blood cell count D72.829
  - specified NEC D72.828

Elliptocytosis (congenital) (hereditary) D58.1
- Hb C (disease) D58.1
- hemoglobin disease D58.1
- sickle-cell (disease) D57.8-
  - trait D57.3

Elongated, elongation (congenital)—*see also* Distortion
- bone Q79.9
- cystic duct Q44.5
- frenulum, penis Q55.69
- labia minora (acquired) N90.69

Embolism (multiple) (paradoxical) I74.9
- artery I74.9
- pituitary E23.6
- portal (vein) I81
- pulmonary (acute) (artery) (vein)
  - chronic I27.82
- pyemic (multiple) I76
  - following
    - Hemophilus influenzae A41.3
    - pneumococcal A40.3
      - with pneumonia J13
    - specified organism NEC A41.89
    - staphylococcal A41.2
    - streptococcal A40.9
- renal (artery) N28.0
  - vein I82.3
- vein (acute) I82.90
  - renal I82.3

Embryoma—see also Neoplasm, uncertain behavior, by site in Table of Neoplasms in the complete ICD-10-CM manual
- kidney C64.-
- malignant—see also Neoplasm, malignant, by site in Table of Neoplasms in the complete ICD-10-CM manual
  - kidney C64.-

Emesis—see Vomiting

Emotional lability R45.86

Emotionality, pathological F60.3

Emphysema
- cellular tissue (traumatic) T79.7
- connective tissue (traumatic) T79.7
- eyelid(s) H02.89
  - traumatic T79.7
- interstitial J98.2
  - congenital P25.0
  - perinatal period P25.0
- laminated tissue T79.7
- mediastinal J98.2
  - newborn P25.2
- subcutaneous (traumatic) T79.7
  - nontraumatic J98.2
- traumatic T79.7

Empyema (acute) (chest) (double) (pleura) (supradiaphragmatic) (thorax) J86.9
- with fistula J86.0
- gallbladder K81.0

Enanthema, viral B09

Encephalitis (chronic) (hemorrhagic) (idiopathic) (nonepidemic) (spurious) (subacute) G04.90
- acute A86
  - disseminated G04.00
    - infectious G04.01
    - noninfectious G04.81
    - postimmunization (postvaccination) G04.02
    - postinfectious G04.01
  - inclusion body A85.8
  - necrotizing hemorrhagic G04.30
    - postimmunization G04.32
    - postinfectious G04.31
    - specified NEC G04.39
    - toxic NEC G92.8

Encephalomyelitis (see also Encephalitis) G04.90
- acute disseminated G04.00
  - infectious G04.01
  - noninfectious G04.81
  - postimmunization G04.02
  - postinfectious G04.01
- acute necrotizing hemorrhagic G04.30
  - postimmunization G04.32
  - postinfectious G04.31
  - specified NEC G04.39
- equine A83.9
  - Eastern A83.2
- in diseases classified elsewhere G05.3
- postchickenpox B01.11
- postinfectious NEC G04.01
- postmeasles B05.0
- postvaccinal G04.02
- postvaricella B01.11

Encephalopathy (acute) G93.40
- acute necrotizing hemorrhagic G04.30
  - postimmunization G04.32
  - postinfectious G04.31
  - specified NEC G04.39
- congenital Q07.9
- due to
  - drugs (see also Table of Drugs and Chemicals) G92.-
- hyperbilirubinemic, newborn P57.9
  - due to isoimmunization (conditions in P55) P57.0
- hypertensive I67.4
- hypoglycemic E16.2
- hypoxic—see Damage, brain, anoxic
- hypoxic ischemic P91.60
  - mild P91.61
  - moderate P91.62
  - severe P91.63
- in (due to) (with)
  - birth injury P11.1
  - hyperinsulinism E16.1 [G94]
  - influenza—see Influenza, with, encephalopathy
  - lack of vitamin (see also Deficiency, vitamin) E56.9 [G32.89]
  - neoplastic disease (see also Neoplasm) D49.9 [G13.1]
  - serum (see also Reaction, serum) T80.69
  - trauma (postconcussional) F07.81
    - current injury—see Injury, intracranial
  - vaccination G04.02
- lead—see Poisoning, lead
- metabolic G93.41
  - drug induced G92.8
  - toxic G92.9
- neonatal P91.819
  - in diseases classified elsewhere P91.811
- postcontusional F07.81
  - current injury—see Injury, intracranial, diffuse
- postradiation G93.89
- toxic G92.9
  - metabolic G92.8
- traumatic (postconcussional) F07.81
  - current injury—see Injury, intracranial

Encephalocele Q01.9
- frontal Q01.0
- nasofrontal Q01.1
- occipital Q01.2
- specified NEC Q01.8

Encephalomalacia (brain) (cerebellar) (cerebral)—see Softening, brain

Encephalomyelitis (see also Encephalitis) G04.90
- acute disseminated G04.00
  - infectious G04.01
  - noninfectious G04.81
  - postimmunization G04.02
  - postinfectious G04.01
- acute necrotizing hemorrhagic G04.30
  - postimmunization G04.32
  - postinfectious G04.31
  - specified NEC G04.39
- congenital Q07.9
- due to
  - drugs (see also Table of Drugs and Chemicals) G92
- equine A83.9
  - Eastern A83.2
- hyperbilirubinemic, newborn P57.9
  - due to isoimmunization (conditions in P55) P57.0
- hypertensive I67.4
- hypoglycemic E16.2
- hypoxic—see Damage, brain, anoxic
- hypoxic ischemic P91.60
  - mild P91.61
  - moderate P91.62
  - severe P91.63
- in diseases classified elsewhere G05.3
- in (due to) (with)
  - birth injury P11.1
  - hyperinsulinism E16.1 [G94]
  - influenza—see Influenza, with, encephalopathy
  - lack of vitamin (see also Deficiency, vitamin) E56.9 [G32.89]
  - neoplastic disease (see also Table of Neoplasms in the complete ICD-10-CM manual) D49.9 [G13.1]

Encephalomyelitis, continued
  - serum (see also Reaction, serum) T80.69
  - trauma (postconcussional) F07.81
    - current injury—see Injury, intracranial
  - vaccination G04.02
- lead—see Poisoning, lead
- metabolic G93.41
  - drug induced G92.8
  - toxic G92.9
- neonatal P91.819
  - in diseases classified elsewhere P91.811
- postchickenpox B01.11
- postcontusional F07.81
  - current injury—see Injury, intracranial, diffuse
- postinfectious NEC G04.01
- postmeasles B05.0
- postradiation G93.89
- postvaccinal G04.02
- postvaricella B01.11
  - specified NEC G04.39
- toxic G92.9
  - metabolic G92.8
- traumatic (postconcussional) F07.81
  - current injury—see Injury, intracranial

Encephalorrhagia—see Hemorrhage, intracranial, intracerebral

Encephalosis, posttraumatic F07.81

Encopresis R15.9
- functional F98.1
- nonorganic origin F98.1
- psychogenic F98.1

Encounter (with health service) (for) Z76.89
- administrative purpose only Z02.9
  - examination for
    - adoption Z02.82
    - armed forces Z02.3
    - disability determination Z02.71
    - driving license Z02.4
    - employment Z02.1
    - insurance Z02.6
    - medical certificate NEC Z02.79
    - residential institution admission Z02.2
    - school admission Z02.0
    - sports Z02.5
  - specified reason NEC Z02.89
- aftercare—see Aftercare
- check-up—see Examination
- chemotherapy for neoplasm Z51.11
- counseling—see Counseling
- desensitization to allergens Z51.6
- ear piercing Z41.3
- examination—see Examination
- expectant parent(s) (adoptive) pre-birth pediatrician visit Z76.81
- fluoride varnish application Z29.3
- genetic
  - nonprocreative Z71.83
  - procreative counseling Z31.5
  - testing—see Test
- hearing conservation and treatment Z01.12
- instruction (in)
  - child care (postpartal) (prenatal) Z32.3
  - natural family planning
    - to avoid pregnancy Z30.02
- laboratory (as part of a general medical examination) Z00.00
  - with abnormal findings Z00.01
- mental health services (for)
  - abuse NEC
    - perpetrator Z69.82
    - victim Z69.81
  - child abuse/neglect (psychological) (sexual)
    - non-parental
      ~ perpetrator Z69.021
      ~ victim Z69.020
    - parental
      ~ perpetrator Z69.011
      ~ victim Z69.010
  - spousal or partner abuse (psychological)
    - perpetrator Z69.12
    - victim Z69.11
- observation (for) (ruled out)

Encounter, *continued*
- – exposure to (suspected)
  - ■ anthrax Z03.810
  - ■ biological agent NEC Z03.818
- • pediatrician visit, by expectant parent(s) (adoptive) Z76.81
- • pregnancy
  - – supervision of—*see* Pregnancy, supervision of
  - – test Z32.00
    - ■ result negative Z32.02
    - ■ result positive Z32.01
- • prophylactic measures
  - – antivenin Z29.12
  - – ear piercing Z41.3
  - – fluoride administration Z29.3
  - – other specified Z29.8
  - – rabies immune globulin Z29.14
  - – respiratory syncytial virus (RSV) immune globulin Z29.11
  - – Rho(D) immune globulin Z29.13
  - – unspecified Z29.9
- • radiation therapy (antineoplastic) Z51.0
- • radiological (as part of a general medical examination) Z00.00
  - – with abnormal findings Z00.01
- • repeat cervical smear to confirm findings of recent normal smear following initial abnormal smear Z01.42
- • respiratory syncytial (RSV) virus immune globulin administration Z29.11
- • suspected condition, ruled out
  - – fetal anomaly Z03.73
  - – fetal growth Z03.74
- • suspected exposure (to), ruled out
  - – anthrax Z03.810
  - – biological agents NEC Z03.818
- • therapeutic drug level monitoring Z51.81
- • to determine fetal viability of pregnancy O36.80
- • training
  - – insulin pump Z46.81
- • X-ray of chest (as part of a general medical examination) Z00.00
  - – with abnormal findings Z00.01

Endocarditis (chronic) (marantic) (nonbacterial) (thrombotic) (valvular) I38
- • with rheumatic fever (conditions in I00)
  - – active—*see* Endocarditis, acute, rheumatic
  - – inactive or quiescent (with chorea) I09.1
- • acute or subacute I33.9
  - – infective I33.0
  - – rheumatic (aortic) (mitral) (pulmonary) (tricuspid) I01.1
    - ■ with chorea (acute) (rheumatic) (Sydenham's) I02.0
- • aortic (heart) (nonrheumatic) (valve) I35.8
  - – with
    - ■ mitral disease I08.0
      - ~ with tricuspid (valve) disease I08.3
      - ~ active or acute I01.1
        - ◊ with chorea (acute) (rheumatic) (Sydenham's) I02.0
    - ■ rheumatic fever (conditions in I00)
      - ~ active—*see* Endocarditis, acute, rheumatic
      - ~ inactive or quiescent (with chorea) I06.9
    - ■ tricuspid (valve) disease I08.2
      - ~ with mitral (valve) disease I08.3
  - – acute or subacute I33.9
  - – arteriosclerotic I35.8
  - – rheumatic I06.9
    - ■ with mitral disease I08.0
      - ~ with tricuspid (valve) disease I08.3
      - ~ active or acute I01.1
        - ◊ with chorea (acute) (rheumatic) (Sydenham's) I02.0
    - ■ active or acute I01.1
      - ~ with chorea (acute) (rheumatic) (Sydenham's) I02.0
    - ■ specified NEC I06.8
  - – specified cause NEC I35.8
- • atypical verrucous (Libman-Sacks) M32.11
- • bacterial (acute) (any valve) (subacute) I33.0
- • candidal B37.6
- • constrictive I33.0

Endocarditis, *continued*
- • due to
  - – Serratia marcescens I33.0
- • infectious or infective (acute) (any valve) (subacute) I33.0
- • lenta (acute) (any valve) (subacute) I33.0
- • Libman-Sacks M32.11
- • malignant (acute) (any valve) (subacute) I33.0
- • mitral (chronic) (double) (fibroid) (heart) (inactive) (valve) (with chorea) I05.9
  - – with
    - ■ aortic (valve) disease I08.0
      - ~ with tricuspid (valve) disease I08.3
      - ~ active or acute I01.1
        - ◊ with chorea (acute) (rheumatic) (Sydenham's) I02.0
    - ■ rheumatic fever (conditions in I00)
      - ~ active—*see* Endocarditis, acute, rheumatic
      - ~ inactive or quiescent (with chorea) I05.9
  - – active or acute I01.1
    - ■ with chorea (acute) (rheumatic) (Sydenham's) I02.0
    - ■ bacterial I33.0
  - – nonrheumatic I34.8
    - ■ acute or subacute I33.9
  - – specified NEC I05.8
- • monilial B37.6
- • mycotic (acute) (any valve) (subacute) I33.0
- • pneumococcal (acute) (any valve) (subacute) I33.0
- • pulmonary (chronic) (heart) (valve) I37.8
  - – with rheumatic fever (conditions in I00)
    - ■ active—*see* Endocarditis, acute, rheumatic
    - ■ inactive or quiescent (with chorea) I09.89
      - ~ with aortic, mitral or tricuspid disease I08.8
  - – acute or subacute I33.9
    - ■ rheumatic I01.1
      - ~ with chorea (acute) (rheumatic) (Sydenham's) I02.0
  - – arteriosclerotic I37.8
  - – congenital Q22.2
- • purulent (acute) (any valve) (subacute) I33.0
- • rheumatic (chronic) (inactive) (with chorea) I09.1
  - – active or acute (aortic) (mitral) (pulmonary) (tricuspid) I01.1
    - ■ with chorea (acute) (rheumatic) (Sydenham's) I02.0
- • septic (acute) (any valve) (subacute) I33.0
- • streptococcal (acute) (any valve) (subacute) I33.0
- • subacute—*see* Endocarditis, acute
- • suppurative (acute) (any valve) (subacute) I33.0
- • toxic I33.9
- • tricuspid (chronic) (heart) (inactive) (rheumatic) (valve) (with chorea) I07.9
  - – with
    - ■ aortic (valve) disease I08.2
      - ~ mitral (valve) disease I08.3
    - ■ mitral (valve) disease I08.1
      - ~ aortic (valve) disease I08.3
    - ■ rheumatic fever (conditions in I00)
      - ~ active—*see* Endocarditis, acute, rheumatic
      - ~ inactive or quiescent (with chorea) I07.8
  - – active or acute I01.1
    - ■ with chorea (acute) (rheumatic) (Sydenham's) I02.0
  - – arteriosclerotic I36.8
  - – nonrheumatic I36.8
    - ■ acute or subacute I33.9
  - – specified cause, except rheumatic I36.8
- • ulcerative (acute) (any valve) (subacute) I33.0
- • vegetative (acute) (any valve) (subacute) I33.0
- • verrucous (atypical) (nonbacterial) (nonrheumatic) M32.11

Endocardium, endocardial—*see also* Disease, diseased
- • cushion defect Q21.2

Endocervicitis—*see also* Cervicitis
- • hyperplastic N72

Endometritis (decidual) (nonspecific) (purulent) (senile) (atrophic) (suppurative) N71.9
- • acute N71.0
- • blennorrhagic (gonococcal) (acute) (chronic) A54.24
- • cervix, cervical (with erosion or ectropion)—*see also* Cervicitis

Endometritis, *continued*
- – hyperplastic N72
- • chlamydial A56.11
- • gonococcal, gonorrheal (acute) (chronic) A54.24
- • hyperplastic N85.00-
  - – cervix N72

Engman's disease L30.3

Engorgement
- • breast N64.59
  - – newborn P83.4
  - – puerperal, postpartum O92.79

Enlargement, enlarged—*see also* Hypertrophy
- • adenoids J35.2
  - – with tonsils J35.3
- • gingival K06.1
- • labium majus (childhood asymmetric) CALME N90.61
- • lymph gland or node R59.9
  - – generalized R59.1
  - – localized R59.0
- • tonsils J35.1
  - – with adenoids J35.3
- • vestibular aqueduct Q16.5

Enteritis (acute) (diarrheal) (hemorrhagic) (noninfective) K52.9
- • aertrycke infection A02.0
- • allergic K52.29
  - – with
    - ■ eosinophilic gastritis or gastroenteritis K52.81
    - ■ food protein-induced enterocolitis syndrome (FPIES) K52.21
    - ■ food protein-induced enteropathy K52.22
- • amebic (acute) A06.0
- • bacillary NOS A03.9
- • candidal B37.82
- • chronic (noninfectious) K52.9
  - – ulcerative—*see* Colitis, ulcerative
- • Clostridium
  - – botulinum (food poisoning) A05.1
  - – difficile
    - ■ not specified as recurrent A04.72
    - ■ recurrent A04.71
- • coxsackie virus A08.39
- • dietetic K52.29
- • due to
  - – Clostridium difficile A04.7-
  - – coxsackie virus A08.39
  - – echovirus A08.39
  - – enterovirus NEC A08.39
  - – food hypersensitivity K52.29
  - – torovirus A08.39
- • echovirus A08.39
- • enterovirus NEC A08.39
- • eosinophilic K52.81
- • epidemic (infectious) A09
- • fulminant (*see also* Ischemia, intestine) K55.019
  - – ischemic K55.9
    - ■ acute (*see also* Ischemia, intestine) K55.019
- • giardial A07.1
- • infectious NOS A09
  - – due to
    - ■ Arizona (bacillus) A02.0
    - ■ Campylobacter A04.5
    - ■ Escherichia coli A04.4
      - ~ enteroaggregative A04.4
      - ~ enterohemorrhagic A04.3
      - ~ enteropathogenic A04.0
      - ~ enterotoxigenic A04.1
      - ~ specified NEC A04.4
    - ■ enterovirus A08.39
    - ■ specified
      - ~ bacteria NEC A04.8
      - ~ virus NEC A08.39
    - ■ virus NEC A08.4
      - ~ specified type NEC A08.39
- • necroticans A05.2
- • noninfectious K52.9
- • parasitic NEC B82.9
- • regional (of) K50.90
  - – with
    - ■ complication K50.919
      - ~ abscess K50.914
      - ~ fistula K50.913

Enteritis, *continued*
- ~ intestinal obstruction K50.912
- ~ rectal bleeding K50.911
- ~ specified complication NEC K50.918
- – large intestine (colon) (rectum) K50.10
  - ■ with
    - ~ complication K50.119
      - ◊ abscess K50.114
      - ◊ fistula K50.113
      - ◊ intestinal obstruction K50.112
      - ◊ rectal bleeding K50.111
      - ◊ small intestine (duodenum) (ileum) (jejunum) involvement K50.80
        - » with
          - ❖ complication K50.819
            - ★ abscess K50.814
            - ★ fistula K50.813
            - ★ intestinal obstruction K50.812
            - ★ rectal bleeding K50.811
            - ★ specified complication NEC K50.818
      - ◊ specified complication NEC K50.118
- – rectum—*see* Enteritis, regional, large intestine
- – small intestine (duodenum) (ileum) (jejunum) K50.00
  - ■ with
    - ~ complication K50.019
      - ◊ abscess K50.014
      - ◊ fistula K50.013
      - ◊ intestinal obstruction K50.012
      - ◊ large intestine (colon) (rectum) involvement K50.80
        - » with
          - ❖ complication K50.819
            - ★ abscess K50.814
            - ★ fistula K50.813
            - ★ intestinal obstruction K50.812
            - ★ rectal bleeding K50.811
            - ★ specified complication NEC K50.818
      - ◊ rectal bleeding K50.011
      - ◊ specified complication NEC K50.018
- rotaviral A08.0
- Salmonella, salmonellosis (arizonae) (choleraesuis) (enteritidis) (typhimurium) A02.0
- septic A09
- staphylococcal A04.8
  - – due to food A05.0
- torovirus A08.39
- viral A08.4
  - – enterovirus A08.39
  - – Rotavirus A08.0
  - – specified NEC A08.39
  - – virus specified NEC A08.39

Enterobiasis B80

Enterobius vermicularis (infection) (infestation) B80

Enterocolitis (*see also* Enteritis) K52.9
- due to Clostridium difficile A04.7-
- fulminant ischemic (*see also* Ischemia, intestine) K55.059
- hemorrhagic (acute) (*see also* Ischemia, intestine) K55.059
- infectious NEC A09
- necrotizing
  - – due to Clostridium difficile A04.7-
  - – in newborn P77.9
    - ■ stage 1 (without pneumatosis, without perforation) P77.1
    - ■ stage 2 (with pneumatosis, without perforation) P77.2
    - ■ stage 3 (with pneumatosis, with perforation) P77.3
  - – stage 1 (excluding newborns) K55.31
  - – stage 2 (excluding newborns) K55.32
  - – stage 3 (excluding newborns) K55.33
  - – unspecified K55.30
- noninfectious K52.9
  - – newborn—*see* Enterocolitis, necrotizing
- protein-induced syndrome K52.21
- pseudomembranous (newborn) A04.7-

Enteropathy K63.9
- food protein-induced enterocolitis K52.22
- gluten-sensitive
  - – celiac K90.0
  - – non-celiac K90.41
- protein-losing K90.49

Enterorrhagia K92.2

Enterospasm—*see also* Syndrome, irritable, bowel
- psychogenic F45.8

Enterovirus, as cause of disease classified elsewhere B97.10
- coxsackievirus B97.11
- echovirus B97.12
- other specified B97.19

Enthesopathy (peripheral) M77.9
- ankle and tarsus M77.5
  - – specified type NEC—*see* Enthesopathy, foot, specified type NEC
- elbow region M77.8
  - – lateral epicondylitis—*see* Epicondylitis, lateral
  - – medial epicondylitis—*see* Epicondylitis, medial
- foot NEC M77.9
  - – specified type NEC M77.5-
- forearm M77.9
- hand M77.9
- hip —*see* Enthesopathy, lower limb, specified type NEC
- iliac crest spur—*see* Spur, bone, iliac crest
- lateral epicondylitis—*see* Epicondylitis, lateral
- lower limb (excluding foot) M76.9
  - – Achilles tendinitis—*see* Tendinitis, Achilles
  - – anterior tibial syndrome M76.81-
  - – iliac crest spur—*see* Spur, bone, iliac crest
  - – iliotibial band syndrome—*see* Syndrome, iliotibial band
  - – pelvic region—*see* Enthesopathy, lower limb, specified type NEC
  - – posterior tibial syndrome M76.82-
  - – specified type NEC M76.89-
  - – tibial collateral bursitis—*see* Bursitis, tibial collateral
- medial epicondylitis—*see* Epicondylitis, medial
- metatarsalgia—*see* Metatarsalgia
- multiple sites M77.9
- pelvis M77.9
- posterior tibial syndrome M76.82-
- psoas tendinitis—*see* Tendinitis
- shoulder M77.9
- specified site NEC M77.9
- specified type NEC M77.8
- upper arm M77.9
- wrist and carpus NEC M77.8

Entropion (eyelid) (paralytic)
- congenital Q10.2

Enuresis R32
- functional F98.0
- habit disturbance F98.0
- nocturnal N39.44
  - – psychogenic F98.0
- nonorganic origin F98.0
- psychogenic F98.0

Eosinophilia (allergic) (hereditary) (idiopathic) (secondary) D72.10
- familial D72.19
- hereditary D72.19
- in disease classified elsewhere D72.18
- with
  - – angiolymphoid hyperplasia (ALHE) D18.01

Eosinophilia-myalgia syndrome M35.8

Ependymoblastoma
- specified site—*see* Neoplasm, malignant, by site in Table of Neoplasms in the complete *ICD-10-CM* manual
- unspecified site C71.9

Ependymoma (epithelial) (malignant)
- anaplastic
  - – specified site—*see* Neoplasm, malignant, by site in Table of Neoplasms in the complete *ICD-10-CM* manual
  - – unspecified site C71.9
- benign specified site—*see* Neoplasm, benign, by site in Table of Neoplasms in the complete *ICD-10-CM* manual
- specified site—*see* Neoplasm, malignant, by site in Table of Neoplasms in the complete *ICD-10-CM* manual
- unspecified site C71.9

Ependymopathy G93.89

Epiblepharon (congenital) Q10.3

Epicanthus, epicanthic fold (eyelid) (congenital) Q10.3

Epicondylitis (elbow)
- lateral M77.1-
- medial M77.0-

Epidermodysplasia verruciformis B07.8

Epidermolysis
- bullosa (congenital) Q81.9
  - – dystrophica Q81.2
  - – letalis Q81.1
  - – simplex Q81.0
  - – specified NEC Q81.8
- necroticans combustiformis L51.2
  - – due to drug—*see* Table of Drugs and Chemicals, by drug

Epididymitis (acute) (nonvenereal) (recurrent) (residual) N45.1
- with orchitis N45.3
- blennorrhagic (gonococcal) A54.23
- chlamydial A56.19
- gonococcal A54.23
- syphilitic A52.76

Epididymo-orchitis (*see also* Epididymitis) N45.3

Epiglottitis, epiglottiditis (acute) J05.10
- with obstruction J05.11
- chronic J37.0

Epilepsia partialis continua (*see also* Kozhevnikof's epilepsy) G40.1-

Epilepsy, epileptic, epilepsia (attack) (cerebral) (convulsion) (fit) (seizure) G40.909
- *Note:* the following terms are to be considered equivalent to intractable: pharmacoresistant (pharmacologically resistant), treatment resistant, refractory (medically) and poorly controlled
- benign childhood with centrotemporal EEG spikes—*see* Epilepsy, localization-related, idiopathic
- benign myoclonic in infancy G40.80-
- childhood
  - – with occipital EEG paroxysms—*see* Epilepsy, localization-related, idiopathic
- generalized
  - – specified NEC G40.409
    - ■ intractable G40.419
      - ~ with status epilepticus G40.411
      - ~ without status epilepticus G40.419
    - ■ not intractable G40.409
      - ~ with status epilepticus G40.401
      - ~ without status epilepticus G40.409
- impulsive petit mal—*see* Epilepsy, juvenile myoclonic
- localization-related (focal) (partial)
- not intractable G40.909
  - – with status epilepticus G40.901
  - – without status epilepticus G40.909
- on awakening—*see* Epilepsy, generalized, specified NEC
- parasitic NOS B71.9 *[G94]*
- spasms G40.822
  - – intractable G40.824
    - ■ with status epilepticus G40.823
    - ■ without status epilepticus G40.824
  - – not intractable G40.822
    - ■ with status epilepticus G40.821
    - ■ without status epilepticus G40.822
- specified NEC G40.802
  - – intractable G40.804
    - ■ with status epilepticus G40.803
    - ■ without status epilepticus G40.804
  - – not intractable G40.802
    - ■ with status epilepticus G40.801
    - ■ without status epilepticus G40.802
- syndromes
  - – generalized
  - – localization-related (focal) (partial)
    - ■ idiopathic
      - ~ with seizures of localized onset
        - ◊ intractable G40.019
          - » without status epilepticus G40.019
  - – specified NEC G40.802
    - ■ intractable G40.804
      - ~ with status epilepticus G40.803
      - ~ without status epilepticus G40.804
    - ■ not intractable G40.802
      - ~ with status epilepticus G40.801
      - ~ without status epilepticus G40.802
- tonic (-clonic)—*see* Epilepsy, generalized, specified NEC

Epiloia Q85.1

Epimenorrhea N92.0

Epipharyngitis—*see* Nasopharyngitis

Epiphysitis—*see also* Osteochondropathy
- juvenile M92.9

Episode
- depressive F32.A
  - major F32.9
    - mild F32.0
    - moderate F32.1
    - severe (without psychotic symptoms) F32.2
      ~ with psychotic symptoms F32.3
  - recurrent F33.9
    - brief F33.8
  - specified NEC F32.89

Epispadias (female) (male) Q64.0

Epistaxis (multiple) R04.0
- hereditary I78.0

Equinovarus (congenital) (talipes) Q66.0-

Equivalent
- convulsive (abdominal)—*see* Epilepsy, specified NEC
- epileptic (psychic)—*see* Epilepsy, localization-related, symptomatic, with complex partial seizures

Erb (-Duchenne) paralysis (birth injury) (newborn) P14.0

Erb-Goldflam disease or syndrome G70.00
- with exacerbation (acute) G70.01
- in crisis G70.01

Erb's
- disease G71.02
- palsy, paralysis (brachial) (birth) (newborn) P14.0
- pseudohypertrophic muscular dystrophy G71.02

Erdheim's syndrome (acromegalic macrospondylitis) E22.0

Erosio interdigitalis blastomycetica B37.2

Erosion
- cervix (uteri) (acquired) (chronic) (congenital) N86
  - with cervicitis N72

Eructation R14.2
- nervous or psychogenic F45.8

Eruption
- drug (generalized) (taken internally) L27.0
  - fixed L27.1
  - in contact with skin—*see* Dermatitis, due to drugs and medicaments
  - localized L27.1
- napkin L22
- skin (nonspecific) R21
  - due to inoculation/vaccination (generalized) (*see also* Dermatitis, due to, vaccine) L27.0
    - localized L27.1
  - feigned L98.1
- tooth, teeth, abnormal (incomplete) (late) (premature) (sequence) K00.6

Erysipelas (gangrenous) (infantile) (newborn) (phlegmonous) (suppurative) A46
- external ear A46 [H62.4-]

Erythema, erythematous (infectional) (inflammation) L53.9
- arthriticum epidemicum A25.1
- chronicum migrans (Borrelia burgdorferi) A69.20
- diaper L22
- gluteal L22
- ichthyosiforme congenitum bullous Q80.3
- induratum (nontuberculous) L52
- infectiosum B08.3
- intertrigo L30.4
- marginatum L53.2
  - in (due to) acute rheumatic fever I00
- migrans A26.0
  - chronicum A69.20
  - tongue K14.1
- multiforme (major) (minor) L51.9
  - bullous, bullosum L51.1
  - conjunctiva L51.1
  - specified NEC L51.8
- napkin L22
- neonatorum P83.88
  - toxic P83.1
- nodosum L52
- rash, newborn P83.88

Erythema, erythematous, *continued*
- solare L55.0
- toxic, toxicum NEC L53.0
  - newborn P83.1

Erythremia (acute) C94.0-
- secondary D75.1

Erythroblastopenia (*see also* Aplasia, red cell) D60.9
- congenital D61.01

Erythroblastophthisis D61.09

Erythroblastosis (fetalis) (newborn) P55.9
- due to
  - ABO (antibodies) (incompatibility) (isoimmunization) P55.1

Erythrocyanosis (crurum) I73.89

Erythrocytosis (megalosplenic) (secondary) D75.1
- familial D75.0
- oval, hereditary—*see* Elliptocytosis
- secondary D75.1
- stress D75.1

Erythroderma (secondary) (*see also* Erythema) L53.9
- bullous ichthyosiform, congenital Q80.3
- desquamativum L21.1
- ichthyosiform, congenital (bullous) Q80.3
- neonatorum P83.88
- psoriaticum L40.8

Erythrodysesthesia, palmar plantar (PPE) L27.1

Erythrogenesis imperfecta D61.09

Erythrophagocytosis D75.89

Escherichia coli (E. coli), as cause of disease classified elsewhere B96.20
- non-0157 Shiga toxin-producing (with known O group) B96.22
- non-Shiga toxin-producing B96.29
- 0157 with confirmation of Shiga toxin when H antigen is unknown, or is not H7 B96.21
- 0157:H- (nonmotile)with confirmation of Shiga toxin B96.21
- 0157:H7 with or without confirmation of Shiga toxin-production B96.21
- Shiga toxin-producing (with unspecified O group) (STEC) B96.23
- 0157 B96.21
- 0157:H7 with or without confirmation of Shiga toxin-production B96.21
  - specified NEC B96.22
- specified NEC B96.29

Esophagitis (acute) (alkaline) (chemical) (chronic) (infectional) (necrotic) (peptic) (postoperative) K20.9-
- candidal B37.81
- due to gastrointestinal reflux disease K21.0-
- eosinophilic K20.0
- reflux K21.0-
- specified NEC K20.80

Estrangement (marital) Z63.5
- parent-child NEC Z62.890

Ethmoiditis (chronic) (nonpurulent) (purulent)—*see also* Sinusitis, ethmoidal
- influenzal—*see* Influenza manifestations NEC

Evaluation (for) (of)
- development state
  - adolescent Z00.3
  - period of
    - delayed growth in childhood Z00.70
      ~ with abnormal findings Z00.71
    - rapid growth in childhood Z00.2
  - puberty Z00.3
- growth and developmental state (period of rapid growth) Z00.2
- period of
  - delayed growth in childhood Z00.70
    - with abnormal findings Z00.71
  - rapid growth in childhood Z00.2
- suspected condition—*see* Observation

Evans syndrome D69.41

Event
- apparent life threatening in newborn and infant (ALTE) R68.13
- brief resolved unexplained event (BRUE) R68.13

Eversion
- cervix (uteri) N86
  - with cervicitis N72

Evisceration
- birth injury P15.8

Examination (for) (following) (general) (of) (routine) Z00.00
- with abnormal findings Z00.01
- abuse, physical (alleged), ruled out
  - child Z04.72
- adolescent (development state) Z00.3
- alleged rape or sexual assault (victim), ruled out
  - child Z04.42
- annual (adult) (periodic) (physical) Z00.00
  - with abnormal findings Z00.01
  - gynecological Z01.419
    - with abnormal findings Z01.411
- blood—*see* Examination, laboratory
- blood pressure Z01.30
  - with abnormal findings Z01.31
- cervical Papanicolaou smear Z12.4
  - as part of routine gynecological examination Z01.419
    - with abnormal findings Z01.411
- child (over 28 days old) Z00.129
  - with abnormal findings Z00.121
  - under 28 days old—*see* Newborn, examination
- contraceptive (drug) maintenance (routine) Z30.8
  - device (intrauterine) Z30.431
- developmental—*see* Examination, child
- ear Z01.10
  - with abnormal findings NEC Z01.118
- eye Z01.00
  - with abnormal findings Z01.01
  - after failed exam Z01.02
- following
  - accident NEC Z04.3
    - transport Z04.1
    - work Z04.2
  - assault, alleged, ruled out
    - child Z04.72
  - motor vehicle accident Z04.1
  - treatment (for) Z09
    - combined NEC Z09
      ~ fracture Z09
      ~ malignant neoplasm Z08
    - malignant neoplasm Z08
    - mental disorder Z09
    - specified condition NEC Z09
- follow-up (routine) (following) Z09
  - chemotherapy NEC Z09
    - malignant neoplasm Z08
  - fracture Z09
  - malignant neoplasm Z08
  - radiotherapy NEC Z09
    - malignant neoplasm Z08
  - surgery NEC Z09
    - malignant neoplasm Z08
- forced labor exploitation Z04.82
- forced sexual exploitation Z04.81
- gynecological Z01.419
  - with abnormal findings Z01.411
  - for contraceptive maintenance Z30.8
- health—*see* Examination, medical
- hearing Z01.10
  - with abnormal findings NEC Z01.118
  - following failed hearing screening Z01.110
  - infant or child (28 days and older) Z00.129
    - with abnormal findings Z00.121
- immunity status testing Z01.84
- laboratory (as part of a general medical examination) Z00.00
  - with abnormal findings Z00.01
  - preprocedural Z01.812
- lactating mother Z39.1
- medical (adult) (for) (of) Z00.00
  - with abnormal findings Z00.01
  - administrative purpose only Z02.9
    - specified NEC Z02.89
  - admission to
    - school Z02.0
      ~ following illness or medical treatment Z02.0
    - summer camp Z02.89
  - adoption Z02.82

Examination, *continued*
- blood alcohol or drug level Z02.83
- camp (summer) Z02.89
- general (adult) Z00.00
  - with abnormal findings Z00.01
- medicolegal reasons NEC Z04.89
- participation in sport Z02.5
- pre-operative—*see* Examination, pre-procedural
- pre-procedural
  - cardiovascular Z01.810
  - respiratory Z01.811
  - specified NEC Z01.818
- preschool children
  - for admission to school Z02.0
- sport competition Z02.5
- medicolegal reason NEC Z04.89
  - following
    - forced labor exploitation Z04.82
    - forced sexual exploitation Z04.81
- newborn—*see* Newborn, examination
- pelvic (annual) (periodic) Z01.419
  - with abnormal findings Z01.411
- period of rapid growth in childhood Z00.2
- periodic (adult) (annual) (routine) Z00.00
  - with abnormal findings Z00.01
- physical (adult)—*see also* Examination, medical Z00.00
  - sports Z02.5
- pre-chemotherapy (antineoplastic) Z01.818
- pre-procedural (pre-operative)
  - cardiovascular Z01.810
  - laboratory Z01.812
  - respiratory Z01.811
  - specified NEC Z01.818
- prior to chemotherapy (antineoplastic) Z01.818
- radiological (as part of a general medical examination) Z00.00
  - with abnormal findings Z00.01
- repeat cervical smear to confirm findings of recent normal smear following initial abnormal smear Z01.42
- skin (hypersensitivity) Z01.82
- special (*see also* Examination) Z01.89
  - specified type NEC Z01.89
- specified type or reason NEC Z04.89
- urine—*see* Examination, laboratory
- vision Z01.00
  - following failed vision screening Z01.020
    - with abnormal findings Z01.021
  - infant or child (over 28 days old) Z00.129
    - with abnormal findings Z00.121
  - with abnormal findings Z01.01

Exanthem, exanthema—*see also* Rash
- with enteroviral vesicular stomatitis B08.4
- subitum B08.20
  - due to human herpesvirus 6 B08.21
  - due to human herpesvirus 7 B08.22
- viral, virus B09
  - specified type NEC B08.8

Excess, excessive, excessively
- alcohol level in blood R78.0
- crying
  - in child, adolescent, or adult R45.83
  - in infant R68.11
- development, breast N62
- drinking (alcohol) NEC (without dependence) F10.10
  - habitual (continual) (without remission) F10.20
- eating R63.2
- foreskin N47.8
- gas R14.0
- large
  - colon K59.39
    - congenital Q43.8
    - toxic K59.31
  - infant P08.0
  - organ or site, congenital NEC—*see* Anomaly, by site
- long
  - organ or site, congenital NEC—*see* Anomaly, by site
- menstruation (with regular cycle) N92.0
  - with irregular cycle N92.1
- napping Z72.821
- natrium E87.0
- secretion—*see also* Hypersecretion
  - sweat R61

Excess, excessive, excessively, *continued*
- skin and subcutaneous tissue L98.7
  - eyelid (acquired)—*see* Blepharochalasis
    - congenital Q10.3
- sodium (Na) E87.0
- sweating R61
- thirst R63.1
  - due to deprivation of water T73.1
- weight
  - gain R63.5
  - loss R63.4

Excitability, abnormal, under minor stress (personality disorder) F60.3

Excitation
- anomalous atrioventricular I45.6

Excoriation (traumatic)—*see also* Abrasion
- neurotic L98.1
- skin picking disorder F42.4

Exhaustion, exhaustive (physical NEC) R53.83
- battle F43.0
- cardiac—*see* Failure, heart
- delirium F43.0
- heat (*see also* Heat, exhaustion) T67.5
  - due to
    - salt depletion T67.4
    - water depletion T67.3
- psychosis F43.0

Exomphalos Q79.2
- meaning hernia—*see* Hernia, umbilicus

Exotropia—*see* Strabismus, divergent concomitant

Explanation of
- investigation finding Z71.2
- medication Z71.89

Exploitation
- labor
  - confirmed
    - adult forced T74.61
    - child forced T74.62
  - suspected
    - adult forced T76.61
    - child forced T76.62
- sexual
  - confirmed
    - adult forced T74.51
    - child T74.52
  - suspected
    - adult forced T76.51
    - child T76.52

Exposure (to) (*see also* Contact) T75.89
- AIDS virus Z20.6
- anthrax Z20.810
- aromatic amines Z77.020
- aromatic (hazardous) compounds NEC Z77.028
- aromatic dyes NOS Z77.028
- arsenic Z77.010
- asbestos Z77.090
- bacterial disease NEC Z20.818
- benzene Z77.021
- body fluids (potentially hazardous) Z77.21
- chemicals (chiefly nonmedicinal) (hazardous) NEC Z77.098
- chromium compounds Z77.018
- communicable disease Z20.9
  - bacterial NEC Z20.818
  - specified NEC Z20.89
  - viral NEC Z20.828
- coronavirus (disease) (novel) 2019 Z20.822
- dyes Z77.098
- environmental tobacco smoke (acute) (chronic) Z77.22
- Escherichia coli (E. coli) Z20.01
- German measles Z20.4
- gonorrhea Z20.2
- hazardous metals NEC Z77.018
- hazardous substances NEC Z77.29
- hazards in the physical environment NEC Z77.128
- hazards to health NEC Z77.9
- human immunodeficiency virus (HIV) Z20.6
- human T-lymphotropic virus type-1 (HTLV-1) Z20.89
- infestation (parasitic) NEC Z20.7
- intestinal infectious disease NEC Z20.09
  - Escherichia coli (E. coli) Z20.01

Exposure, *continued*
- lead Z77.011
- meningococcus Z20.811
- mold (toxic) Z77.120
- nickel dust Z77.018
- poliomyelitis Z20.89
- polycyclic aromatic hydrocarbons Z77.028
- prenatal (drugs) (toxic chemicals)—*see* Newborn, noxious substances transmitted via placenta or breast milk
- rabies Z20.3
- rubella Z20.4
- second hand tobacco smoke (acute) (chronic) Z77.22
  - in the perinatal period P96.81
- sexually-transmitted disease Z20.2
- smallpox (laboratory) Z20.89
- syphilis Z20.2
- tuberculosis Z20.1
- varicella Z20.820
- venereal disease Z20.2
- viral disease NEC Z20.828
- Zika virus Z20.821

Exstrophy
- abdominal contents Q45.8
- bladder Q64.10
  - cloacal Q64.12
  - specified type NEC Q64.19
  - supravesical fissure Q64.11

Extrasystoles (supraventricular) I49.49
- atrial I49.1
- auricular I49.1

Extravasation
- pelvicalyceal N13.8
- pyelosinus N13.8
- vesicant agent
  - antineoplastic chemotherapy T80.810
  - other agent NEC T80.818

F

Failure, failed
- aortic (valve) I35.8
  - rheumatic I06.8
- biventricular I50.82
- cardiorenal (chronic) I50.9
- cardiorespiratory (*see also* Failure, heart) R09.2
- circulation, circulatory (peripheral) R57.9
  - newborn P29.89
- compensation—*see* Disease, heart
- compliance with medical treatment or regimen—*see* Noncompliance
- expansion terminal respiratory units (newborn) (primary) P28.0
- gain weight (child over 28 days old) R62.51
  - newborn P92.6
- heart (acute) (senile) (sudden) I50.9
  - biventricular I50.82
  - combined left-right sided I50.82
  - compensated I50.9
  - congestive (compensated) (decompensated) I50.9
    - with rheumatic fever (conditions in I00)
      - ~ active I01.8
      - ~ inactive or quiescent (with chorea) I09.81
    - newborn P29.0
    - rheumatic (chronic) (inactive) (with chorea) I09.81
      - ~ active or acute I01.8
        - ◊ with chorea I02.0
  - decompensated I50.9
    - newborn P29.0
  - diastolic (congestive) (left ventricular) I50.3-
    - combined with systolic (congestive) I50.40
      - ~ acute (congestive) I50.41
        - ◊ and (on) chronic (congestive) I50.43
      - ~ chronic (congestive) I50.42
        - ◊ and (on) acute (congestive) I50.43
  - due to presence of cardiac prosthesis I97.13-
  - following cardiac surgery I97.13-
  - high output NOS I50.83
  - low output (syndrome) NOS I50.9
  - postprocedural I97.13-
  - specified NEC I50.89

Failure, failed, *continued*
- – Note: heart failure stages A, B, C, and D are based on the American College of Cardiology and American Heart Association stages of heart failure, which complement and should not be confused with the New York Heart Association Classification of Heart Failure, into Class I, Class II, Class III, and Class IV
- – stage A Z91.89
- – stage B—*see also* Failure, heart, by type as diastolic or systolic I50.9
- – stage C—*see also* Failure, heart, by type as diastolic or systolic I50.9
- – stage D—*see also* Failure, heart, by type as diastolic or systolic, chronic I50.84
- – systolic (congestive) (left ventricular) I50.2-
  - ■ combined with diastolic (congestive) I50.40
    - ~ acute (congestive) I50.41
    - ~ chronic (congestive) I50.42
    - ◊ and (on) acute (congestive) I50.43
- • kidney (*see also* Disease, kidney, chronic) N19
  - – acute (*see also* Failure, renal, acute) N17.9-
  - – diabetic—*see* E08-E13 with .22
- • lactation (complete) O92.3
  - – partial O92.4
- • mitral I05.8
- • myocardial, myocardium (*see also* Failure, heart) I50.9
  - – chronic (*see also* Failure, heart, congestive) I50.9
  - – congestive (*see also* Failure, heart, congestive) I50.9
- • newborn screening P09.-
- • ovulation causing infertility N97.0
- • renal N19
  - – with
    - ■ tubular necrosis (acute) N17.0
  - – acute N17.9
    - ■ with
      - ~ cortical necrosis N17.1
      - ~ medullary necrosis N17.2
      - ~ tubular necrosis N17.0
    - ■ specified NEC N17.8
  - – chronic N18.9
  - – congenital P96.0
  - – end stage N18.6
    - ■ due to hypertension I12.0
- • respiration, respiratory J96.90
  - – with
    - ■ hypercapnia J96.92
    - ■ hypercarbia J96.92
    - ■ hypoxia J96.91
  - – acute J96.00
    - ■ with
      - ~ hypercapnia J96.02
      - ~ hypercarbia J96.02
      - ~ hypoxia J96.01
  - – center G93.89
  - – chronic J96.10
    - ■ with
      - ~ hypercapnia J96.12
      - ~ hypercarbia J96.12
      - ~ hypoxia J96.11
  - – newborn P28.5
  - – postprocedural (acute) J95.821
    - ■ acute and chronic J95.822
- • to thrive (child over 28 days old) R62.51
  - – newborn P92.6
- • transplant T86.-
  - – bone
    - ■ marrow T86.02
  - – heart T86.22
    - ■ with lung(s) T86.32
  - – kidney T86.12
  - – liver T86.42
  - – lung(s) T86.811
    - ■ with heart T86.32
  - – stem cell (peripheral blood) (umbilical cord) T86.5
- • ventricular (*see also* Failure, heart) I50.9
  - – left I50.1
    - ■ with rheumatic fever (conditions in I00)
      - ~ active I01.8
        - ◊ with chorea I02.0
      - ~ inactive or quiescent (with chorea) I09.81
    - ■ rheumatic (chronic) (inactive) (with chorea) I09.81
      - ~ active or acute I01.8
        - ◊ with chorea I02.0

Failure, failed, *continued*
- – right (*see also* Failure, heart, congestive) I50.9
- • vital centers, newborn P91.88

Fainting (fit) R55

Fallot's
- • tetrad or tetralogy Q21.3

Family, familial—*see also* Disease, diseased
- • disruption Z63.8
  - – involving divorce or separation Z63.5
- • planning advice Z30.09
- • problem Z63.9
  - – specified NEC Z63.8
- • retinoblastoma C69.2-

Fanconi's anemia (congenital pancytopenia) D61.09

Fasciitis M72.9
- • infective M72.8
  - – necrotizing M72.6
- • necrotizing M72.6

Fascioscapulohumeral myopathy G71.02

Fast pulse R00.0

Fat
- • in stool R19.5

Fatigue R53.83
- • auditory deafness—*see* Deafness
- • chronic R53.82
- • combat F43.0
- • general R53.83
- • muscle M62.89

Fatty—*see also* Disease, diseased
- • liver NEC K76.0
  - – nonalcoholic K76.0

Faucitis J02.9

Favism (anemia) D55.0

Favus—*see* Dermatophytosis

Fear complex or reaction F40.9

Fear of—*see* Phobia

Febris, febrile—*see also* Fever
- • rubra A38.9

Fecal
- • incontinence R15.9
- • smearing R15.1
- • soiling R15.1
- • urgency R15.2

Fecalith (impaction) K56.41

Fede's disease K14.0

Feeble rapid pulse due to shock following injury T79.4

Feeble-minded F70

Feeding
- • difficulties R63.30
- • problem R63.39
  - – newborn P92.9
    - ■ specified NEC P92.8
  - – nonorganic (adult)—*see* Disorder, eating

Feeling (of)
- • foreign body in throat R09.89

Feet—*see* Disease, diseased

Feigned illness Z76.5

Fetid
- • breath R19.6

Fetus, fetal—*see also* Disease, diseased
- • alcohol syndrome (dysmorphic) Q86.0
- • lung tissue P28.0

Fever (inanition) (of unknown origin) (persistent) (with chills) (with rigor) R50.9
- • African tick bite A77.8
- • American
  - – mountain (tick) A93.2
  - – spotted A77.0
- • Bullis A77.0
- • catarrhal (acute) J00
  - – chronic J31.0
- • cerebrospinal meningococcal A39.0
- • Colorado tick (virus) A93.2
- • due to
  - – conditions classified elsewhere R50.81
  - – heat T67.0-

Fever, *continued*
- • ephemeral (of unknown origin) R50.9
- • epidemic hemorrhagic A98.5
- • erysipelatous—*see* Erysipelas
- • glandular—*see* Mononucleosis, infectious
- • Haverhill A25.1
- • hay (allergic) J30.1
  - – with asthma (bronchial) J45.909
    - ■ with
      - ~ exacerbation (acute) J45.901
      - ~ status asthmaticus J45.902
  - – due to
    - ■ allergen other than pollen J30.89
    - ■ pollen, any plant or tree J30.1
- • heat (effects) T67.0-
- • hemorrhagic (arthropod-borne) NOS A94
  - – arenaviral A96.9
- • intermittent (bilious)—*see also* Malaria
  - – of unknown origin R50.9
- • Lone Star A77.0
- • mountain
  - – meaning Rocky Mountain spotted fever A77.0
  - – tick (American) (Colorado) (viral) A93.2
- • newborn P81.9
  - – environmental P81.0
- • non-exanthematous tick A93.2
- • persistent (of unknown origin) R50.9
- • petechial A39.0
- • postimmunization R50.83
- • postoperative R50.82
  - – due to infection T81.40
- • posttransfusion R50.84
- • postvaccination R50.83
- • presenting with conditions classified elsewhere R50.81
- • rat-bite A25.9
  - – due to
    - ■ Spirillum A25.0
      - ~ Streptobacillus moniliformis A25.1
- • relapsing (Borrelia) A68.9
  - – louse borne A68.0
  - – Novy's
    - ■ louse-borne A68.0
    - ■ tick-bourne A68.1
  - – tick borne A68.1
- • rheumatic (active) (acute) (chronic) (subacute) I00
  - – with central nervous system involvement I02.9
  - – active with heart involvement (*see* category) I01
  - – inactive or quiescent with
    - ■ cardiac hypertrophy I09.89
    - ■ carditis I09.9
    - ■ endocarditis I09.1
      - ~ aortic (valve) I06.9
        - ◊ with mitral (valve) disease I08.0
      - ~ mitral (valve) I05.9
        - ◊ with aortic (valve) disease I08.0
      - ~ pulmonary (valve) I09.89
      - ~ tricuspid (valve) I07.8
    - ■ heart disease NEC I09.89
    - ■ heart failure (congestive) (conditions in I50) I09.81
    - ■ left ventricular failure (conditions in I50.1–I50.4-) I09.81
    - ■ myocarditis, myocardial degeneration (conditions in I51.4) I09.0
    - ■ pancarditis I09.9
    - ■ pericarditis I09.2
- • Rocky Mountain spotted A77.0
- • rose J30.1
- • Sao Paulo A77.0
- • scarlet A38.9
- • specified NEC A96.8
  - – viral A99
    - ■ specified NEC A98.8
- • spirillary A25.0
- • spotted A77.9
  - – American A77.0
  - – Brazilian A77.0
  - – cerebrospinal meningitis A39.0
  - – Columbian A77.0
  - – due to Rickettsia
    - ■ rickettsii A77.0
  - – Ehrlichiosis A77.40
  - – Rocky Mountain spotted A77.0
- • streptobacillary A25.1

Fever, *continued*
- swine A02.8
- thermic T67.0-
- unknown origin R50.9
- uveoparotid D86.69
- West Nile (viral) A92.30
  - with
    - complications NEC A92.39
    - cranial nerve disorders A92.32
    - encephalitis A92.31
    - encephalomyelitis A92.31
    - neurologic manifestation NEC A92.32
    - optic neuritis A92.32
    - polyradiculitis A92.32
- yellow A95.9
  - jungle A95.0
  - sylvatic A95.0
  - urban A95.1
- Zika virus A92.5

Fibrillation
- atrial or auricular (established) I48.91
  - cardiac I49.8
  - chronic I48.20
    - persistent I48.19
  - paroxysmal I48.0
  - permanent I48.21
  - persistent (chronic) (NOS) (other) I48.19
    - longstanding I48.11
- heart I49.8
  - muscular M62.89
  - ventricular I49.01

Fibrinogenopenia D68.8
- acquired D65
- congenital D68.2

Fibrinolysis (hemorrhagic) (acquired) D65
- newborn, transient P60

Fibrocystic
- disease—*see also* Fibrosis, cystic
  - pancreas E84.9

Fibromatosis M72.9
- gingival K06.1

Fibromyxolipoma D17.9

Fibroplasia, retrolental H35.17-

Fibrosis, fibrotic
- anal papillae K62.89
- cystic (of pancreas) E84.9
  - with
    - distal intestinal obstruction syndrome E84.19
    - fecal impaction E84.19
    - intestinal manifestations NEC E84.19
    - pulmonary manifestations E84.0
    - specified manifestations NEC E84.8
- meninges G96.198
- pericardium I31.0
- rectal sphincter K62.89
- skin L90.5

Fiedler's
- myocarditis (acute) I40.1

Fifth disease B08.3

Filatov's disease—*see* Mononucleosis, infectious

Fimbrial cyst Q50.4

Financial problem affecting care NOS Z59.-

Findings, abnormal, inconclusive, without diagnosis—*see also* Abnormal
- alcohol in blood R78.0
- antenatal screening of mother O28.9
  - biochemical O28.1
  - chromosomal O28.5
  - cytological O28.2
  - genetic O28.5
  - hematological O28.0
  - radiological O28.4
  - specified NEC O28.8
  - ultrasonic O28.3
- bacteriuria R82.71
- bicarbonate E87.8
- blood sugar R73.09
  - high R73.9
  - low (transient) E16.2

Findings, abnormal, inconclusive, without diagnosis, *continued*
- casts or cells, urine R82.998
- chloride E87.8
- cholesterol E78.9
  - high E78.00
    - with high triglycerides E78.2
- creatinine clearance R94.4
- crystals, urine R82.998
- culture
  - blood R78.81
  - positive—*see* Positive, culture
- echocardiogram R93.1
- electrolyte level, urinary R82.998
- function study NEC R94.8
  - bladder R94.8
  - endocrine NEC R94.7
    - kidney R94.4
    - liver R94.5
    - pancreas R94.8
    - placenta R94.8
    - pulmonary R94.2
    - spleen R94.8
    - thyroid R94.6
- glycosuria R81
- heart
  - shadow R93.1
  - sounds R01.2
- hematinuria R82.3
- hemoglobinuria R82.3
- in blood (of substance not normally found in blood) R78.9
  - alcohol (excessive level) R78.0
  - lead R78.71
- lactic acid dehydrogenase (LDH) R74.02
- liver function test (see also Elevated, liver function, test) R79.89
- neonatal screening/newborn state mandated P09.-
- PPD R76.11
- radiologic (X-ray) R93.89
  - abdomen R93.5
  - intrathoracic organs NEC R93.1
  - musculoskeletal
    - limbs R93.6
    - other than limb R93.7
  - retroperitoneum R93.5
  - testis R93.81-
- scan NEC R94.8
  - bladder R94.8
  - bone R94.8
  - kidney R94.4
  - liver R93.2
  - lung R94.2
  - pancreas R94.8
  - placental R94.8
  - spleen R94.8
  - thyroid R94.6
- sedimentation rate, elevated R70.0
- SGOT R74.01
- SGPT R74.01
- sodium (deficiency) E87.1
  - excess E87.0
- stress test R94.39
- thyroid (function) (metabolic rate) (scan) (uptake) R94.6
- transaminase (level) R74.01
- triglycerides E78.9
  - high E78.1
    - with high cholesterol E78.2
- tuberculin skin test (without active tuberculosis) R76.11
- urine
  - bacteriuria R82.71
  - casts or cells R82.998
  - culture positive R82.79
  - glucose R81
  - hemoglobin R82.3
  - sugar R81
- vectorcardiogram (VCG) R94.39

Fire, Saint Anthony's—*see* Erysipelas

Fissure, fissured
- anus, anal K60.2
  - acute K60.0
  - chronic K60.1

Fissure, fissured, *continued*
  - congenital Q43.8
- lip K13.0
  - congenital—*see* Cleft, lip
- nipple N64.0
  - associated with
    - lactation O92.13
    - puerperium O92.12

Fistula (cutaneous) L98.8
- abdominothoracic J86.0
- accessory sinuses—*see* Sinusitis
- anus, anal (recurrent) (infectional) K60.3
  - congenital Q43.6
    - with absence, atresia and stenosis Q42.2
- arteriovenous (acquired) (nonruptured) I77.0
  - brain I67.1
    - congenital Q28.2
      - ~ ruptured—*see* Fistula, arteriovenous, brain, ruptured
    - ruptured I60.8-
      - ~ intracerebral I61.8
      - ~ intraparenchymal I61.8
      - ~ intraventricular I61.5
      - ~ subarachnoid I60.8-
  - cerebral—*see* Fistula, arteriovenous, brain
  - congenital (peripheral)—*see also* Malformation, arteriovenous
    - brain Q28.2
      - ~ ruptured I60.8-
    - pulmonary Q25.72
  - pulmonary I28.0
    - congenital Q25.72
  - surgically created (for dialysis) Z99.2
- brain G93.89
- breast N61.0
- bronchial J86.0
- bronchocutaneous, bronchomediastinal, bronchopleural, bronchopleuro-mediastinal (infective) J86.0
- bronchoesophageal J86.0
  - congenital Q39.2
    - with atresia of esophagus Q39.1
- bronchovisceral J86.0
- buccal cavity (infective) K12.2
- cerebrospinal (fluid) G96.08
- chest (wall) J86.0
- colovesical N32.1
- costal region J86.0
- cystic duct
  - congenital Q44.5
- diaphragm J86.0
- esophagobronchial J86.0
  - congenital Q39.2
    - with atresia of esophagus Q39.1
- esophagocutaneous K22.89
- esophagopleural-cutaneous J86.0
- esophagotracheal J86.0
  - congenital Q39.2
  - with atresia of esophagus Q39.1
- esophagus K22.89
  - congenital Q39.2
    - with atresia of esophagus Q39.1
- ethmoid—*see* Sinusitis, ethmoidal
- hepatopleural J86.0
- hepatopulmonary J86.0
- ischiorectal (fossa) K61.39
- lip K13.0
  - congenital Q38.0
- lung J86.0
- mammary (gland) N61.0
- maxillary J32.0
- mediastinal J86.0
- mediastinobronchial J86.0
- mediastinocutaneous J86.0
- mouth K12.2
- nasal J34.89
  - sinus—*see* Sinusitis
- nose J34.89
- oral (cutaneous) K12.2
  - maxillary J32.0
- oroantral J32.0
- parotid (gland) K11.4
  - region K12.2
- pleura, pleural, pleurocutaneous, pleuroperitoneal J86.0

Fistula, *continued*
- pleuropericardial I31.8
- pulmonary J86.0
  - arteriovenous I28.0
    - congenital Q25.72
- pulmonoperitoneal J86.0
- rectum (to skin) K60.4
  - congenital Q43.6
    - with absence, atresia and stenosis Q42.0
- skin L98.8
- submaxillary (gland) K11.4
  - region K12.2
- thoracic J86.0
- thoracoabdominal J86.0
- thoracogastric J86.0
- thoracointestinal J86.0
- thorax J86.0
- thyroglossal duct Q89.2
- tracheoesophageal J86.0
  - congenital Q39.2
    - with atresia of esophagus Q39.1

Fit R56.9
- epileptic—*see* Epilepsy
- fainting R55
- newborn P90

Flail
- chest S22.5
  - newborn (birth injury) P13.8
- joint (paralytic) M25.2-
  - ankle M25.27-
  - elbow M25.22-
  - foot joint M25.27-
  - hand joint M25.24-
  - hip M25.25-
  - knee M25.26-
  - shoulder M25.21-
  - specified joint NEC M25.28
  - wrist M25.23-

Flat
- foot (acquired) (fixed type) (painful) (postural)—*see also* Deformity, limb, flat foot
  - congenital (rigid) (spastic) (everted) Q66.5-
- pelvis M95.5
  - congenital Q74.2

Flattening
- nose (congenital) Q67.4
  - acquired M95.0

Flatulence R14.3
- psychogenic F45.8

Flexion
- deformity, joint (*see also* Deformity, limb, flexion) M21.20
  - hip, congenital Q65.89

Flint murmur (aortic insufficiency) I35.1

Floating
- gallbladder, congenital Q44.1

Flooding N92.0

Floppy
- baby syndrome (nonspecific) P94.2

Flu—*see also* Influenza
- avian (*see also* Influenza, due to, identified novel influenza A virus) J09.X2
- bird (*see also* Influenza, due to, identified novel influenza A virus) J09.X2
- intestinal NEC A08.4
- swine (viruses that normally cause infections in pigs) (*see also* Influenza, due to, identified novel influenza A virus) J09.X2

Fluid
- abdomen R18.8
- loss (acute) E86.9
- peritoneal cavity R18.8
- retention R60.9

Fluoride varnish application Z29.3

Fluorosis
- dental K00.3

Flutter
- atrial or auricular I48.92
  - atypical I48.4
  - type I I48.3
  - type II I48.4
  - typical I48.3
- heart I49.8
  - atrial or auricular I48.92
  - atypical I48.4
  - type I I48.3
  - type II I48.4
  - typical I48.3
  - ventricular I49.02
- ventricular I49.02

FNHTR (febrile nonhemolytic transfusion reaction) R50.84

Follicle
- graafian, ruptured, with hemorrhage N83.0-

Folliculitis (superficial) L73.9
- cyst N83.0-
- gonococcal (acute) (chronic) A54.01

Folling's disease E70.0

Follow-up—*see* Examination, follow-up

Food
- allergy L27.2
- asphyxia (from aspiration or inhalation)—*see* Foreign body, by site
- choked on—*see* Foreign body, by site
- cyst N83.0-
- deprivation T73.0
  - specified kind of food NEC E63.8
- insecurity Z59.5
- intoxication—*see* Poisoning, food
- lack of T73.0
- poisoning—*see* Poisoning, food
- rejection NEC—*see* Disorder, eating
- strangulation or suffocation—*see* Foreign body, by site
- toxemia—*see* Poisoning, food

Foramen ovale (nonclosure) (patent) (persistent) Q21.1

Foreign body
- alimentary tract T18.9
  - esophagus—*see* Foreign body, esophagus
  - mouth T18.0
  - multiple sites T18.8
  - specified site NEC T18.8
- auditory canal—*see* Foreign body, entering through orifice, ear
- bronchus T17.50 (See complete *ICD-10-CM* Manual for codes)
- canthus—*see* Foreign body, conjunctival sac
- conjunctival sac T15.1-
- cornea T15.0-
- entering through orifice
  - accessory sinus T17.0
  - alimentary canal T18.9
    - multiple parts T18.8
    - specified part NEC T18.8
  - alveolar process T18.0
  - antrum (Highmore's) T17.0
  - anus T18.5
  - appendix T18.4
  - auditory canal T16.-
  - auricle T16.-
  - bronchioles—*see* Foreign body, respiratory tract
  - bronchus (main)—*see* Foreign body, bronchus
  - buccal cavity T18.0
  - canthus (inner) T15.1-
  - conjunctival sac T15.1-
  - digestive organ or tract NOS T18.9
    - multiple parts T18.8
    - specified part NEC T18.8
  - ear (external) T16.-
  - esophagus—*see* Foreign body, esophagus
  - eye (external) NOS T15.-
    - conjunctival sac T15.1-
    - cornea T15.0-
    - specified part NEC T15. -
  - eyeball T15. -
  - eyelid T15.1-
    - with
      - laceration—*see* Laceration, eyelid, with foreign body

Foreign body, *continued*
  - puncture—*see* Puncture, eyelid, with foreign body
  - superficial injury—*see* Foreign body, superficial, eyelid
- gastrointestinal tract T18.9
  - multiple parts T18.8
  - specified part NEC T18.8
- genitourinary tract T19.9
  - multiple parts T19.8
  - specified part NEC T19.8
- Highmore's antrum T17.0
- hypopharynx—*see* Foreign body, pharynx
- lacrimal apparatus (punctum) T15.-
- larynx—*see* Foreign body, larynx
- lung—*see* Foreign body, respiratory tract
- maxillary sinus T17.0
- mouth T18.0
- nasal sinus T17.0
- nasopharynx—*see* Foreign body, pharynx
- nose (passage) T17.1
- nostril T17.1
- pharynx—*see* Foreign body, pharynx
- piriform sinus—*see* Foreign body, pharynx
- respiratory tract—*see* Foreign body, respiratory tract
- sinus (accessory) (frontal) (maxillary) (nasal) T17.0
  - piriform—*see* Foreign body, pharynx
- suffocation by—*see* Foreign body, by site
- tear ducts or glands—*see* Foreign body, entering through orifice, eye, specified part NEC
- throat—*see* Foreign body, pharynx
- tongue T18.0
- tonsil, tonsillar (fossa)—*see* Foreign body, pharynx
- trachea—*see* Foreign body, trachea
- vagina T19.2
- vulva T19.2
- esophagus T18.108
  - causing
    - injury NEC T18.108
      - food (bone) (seed) T18.128
      - gastric contents (vomitus) T18.118
      - specified type NEC T18.19-
    - tracheal compression T18.100
      - food (bone) (seed) T18.120
      - gastric contents (vomitus) T18.110
      - specified type NEC T18.190
- feeling of, in throat R09.89
- fragment—*see* Retained, foreign body fragments (type of)
- genitourinary tract T19.9
  - vagina T19.2
  - vulva T19.2
- granuloma (old) (soft tissue)—*see also* Granuloma, foreign body
  - skin L92.3
- in
  - laceration—*see* Laceration, by site, with foreign body
  - puncture wound—*see* Puncture, by site, with foreign body
  - soft tissue (residual) M79.5
- ingestion, ingested NOS T18.9
- inhalation or inspiration—*see* Foreign body, by site
- larynx T17.308
  - causing
    - asphyxiation T17.300
      - food (bone) (seed) T17.320
      - gastric contents (vomitus) T17.310
      - specified type NEC T17.390
    - injury NEC T17.308
      - food (bone) (seed) T17.328
      - gastric contents (vomitus) T17.318
      - specified type NEC T17.398
- old or residual
  - soft tissue (residual) M79.5
- pharynx T17.208
  - causing
    - asphyxiation T17.200
      - food (bone) (seed) T17.220
      - gastric contents (vomitus) T17.210
      - specified type NEC T17.290
    - injury NEC T17.208
      - food (bone) (seed) T17.228

Fracture, *continued*
- bone NEC T14.8
  - birth injury P13.9
  - following insertion of orthopedic implant, joint prosthesis or bone plate—*see* Fracture
- burst—*see* Fracture, traumatic, by site
- calcaneus—*see* Fracture, tarsal, calcaneus
- carpal bone(s) S62.10-
  - capitate (displaced) S62.13-
    - nondisplaced S62.13-
  - cuneiform—*see* Fracture, carpal bone, triquetrum
  - hamate (body) (displaced) S62.14-
    - hook process (displaced) S62.15-
      - nondisplaced S62.15-
    - nondisplaced S62.14-
  - larger multangular—*see* Fracture, carpal bones, trapezium
  - lunate (displaced) S62.12-
    - nondisplaced S62.12-
  - navicular S62.00-
    - distal pole (displaced) S62.01-
      - nondisplaced S62.01-
    - middle third (displaced) S62.02-
      - nondisplaced S62.02-
    - proximal third (displaced) S62.03-
      - nondisplaced S62.03-
    - volar tuberosity—*see* Fracture, carpal bones, navicular, distal pole
  - os magnum—*see* Fracture, carpal bones, capitate
  - pisiform (displaced) S62.16-
    - nondisplaced S62.16-
  - semilunar—*see* Fracture, carpal bones, lunate
  - smaller multangular—*see* Fracture, carpal bones, trapezoid
  - trapezium (displaced) S62.17-
    - nondisplaced S62.17-
  - trapezoid (displaced) S62.18-
    - nondisplaced S62.18-
  - triquetrum (displaced) S62.11-
    - nondisplaced S62.11-
  - unciform—*see* Fracture, carpal bones, hamate
- clavicle S42.00-
  - acromial end (displaced) S42.03-
    - nondisplaced S42.03-
  - birth injury P13.4
  - lateral end—*see* Fracture, clavicle, acromial end
  - shaft (displaced) S42.02-
    - nondisplaced S42.02-
  - sternal end (anterior) (displaced) S42.01-
    - nondisplaced S42.01-
    - posterior S42.01-
- coccyx S32.2
- collar bone—*see* Fracture, clavicle
- Colles'—*see* Colles' fracture
- coronoid process—*see* Fracture, ulna, upper end, coronoid process
- costochondral, costosternal junction—*see* Fracture, rib
- cranium—*see* Fracture, skull
- cricoid cartilage S12.8
- cuboid (ankle)—*see* Fracture, tarsal, cuboid
- cuneiform
  - foot—*see* Fracture, tarsal, cuneiform
  - wrist—*see* Fracture, carpal, triquetrum
- delayed union—*see* Delay
- due to
  - birth injury—*see* Birth, injury, fracture
- Dupuytren's—*see* Fracture, ankle, lateral malleolus only
- elbow S42.40-
- ethmoid (bone) (sinus)—*see* Fracture, skull, base
- face bone S02.92-
- fatigue—*see also* Fracture, stress
- femur, femoral S72.9-
  - basicervical (basal) S72.0
  - birth injury P13.2
  - capital epiphyseal S79.01-
  - condyles, epicondyles—*see* Fracture, femur, lower end
  - distal end—*see* Fracture, femur, lower end
  - epiphysis
    - head—*see* Fracture, femur, upper end, epiphysis
    - lower—*see* Fracture, femur, lower end, epiphysis
    - upper—*see* Fracture, femur, upper end, epiphysis
  - head—*see* Fracture, femur, upper end, head

Fracture, *continued*
- intertrochanteric—*see* Fracture, femur
- intratrochanteric—*see* Fracture, femur
- lower end S72.40-
  - condyle (displaced) S72.41-
    - lateral (displaced) S72.42-
      - nondisplaced S72.42-
    - medial (displaced) S72.43-
      - nondisplaced S72.43-
    - nondisplaced S72.41-
  - epiphysis (displaced) S72.44-
    - nondisplaced S72.44-
  - physeal S79.10-
    - Salter-Harris
      - Type I S79.11-
      - Type II S79.12-
      - Type III S79.13-
      - Type IV S79.14-
    - specified NEC S79.19-
  - specified NEC S72.49-
  - supracondylar (displaced) S72.45-
    - with intracondylar extension (displaced) S72.46-
      - nondisplaced S72.46-
    - nondisplaced S72.45-
  - torus S72.47-
- neck—*see* Fracture, femur, upper end, neck
- pertrochanteric—*see* Fracture, femur
- shaft (lower third) (middle third) (upper third) S72.30-
  - comminuted (displaced) S72.35-
    - nondisplaced S72.35-
  - oblique (displaced) S72.33-
    - nondisplaced S72.33-
  - segmental (displaced) S72.36-
    - nondisplaced S72.36-
  - specified NEC S72.39-
  - spiral (displaced) S72.34-
    - nondisplaced S72.34-
  - transverse (displaced) S72.32-
    - nondisplaced S72.32-
- specified site NEC—*see* subcategory S72.8
- transcervical—*see* Fracture, femur, upper end, neck
- transtrochanteric—*see* Fracture, femur, trochanteric
- upper end S72.00-
  - cervicotrochanteric—*see* Fracture, femur, upper end, neck, base
  - epiphysis (displaced) S72.02-
    - nondisplaced S72.02-
  - midcervical (displaced) S72.03-
    - nondisplaced S72.03-
  - neck S72.00-
    - base (displaced) S72.04-
      - nondisplaced S72.04-
  - pertrochanteric—*see* Fracture, femur, upper end
  - physeal S79.00-
    - Salter-Harris type I S79.01-
    - specified NEC S79.09-
  - transcervical—*see* Fracture, femur, upper end, midcervical
- fibula (shaft) (styloid) S82.40-
  - comminuted (displaced or nondisplaced) S82.45- (See complete *ICD-10-CM* Manual for codes)
    - involving ankle or malleolus—*see* Fracture, fibula
  - lateral malleolus (displaced) S82.6-
    - nondisplaced S82.6-
  - lower end
    - physeal S89.30-
      - Salter-Harris
        - Type I S89.31-
        - Type II S89.32-
      - specified NEC S89.39-
    - specified NEC S82.83-
    - torus S82.82-
  - oblique (displaced or nondisplaced) S82.43- (See complete *ICD-10-CM* Manual for codes)
  - segmental (displacedor nondisplaced) S82.46- (See complete *ICD-10-CM* Manual for codes)
  - spiral (displaced or nondisplaced) S82.44- (See complete *ICD-10-CM* Manual for codes)
  - transverse (displaced or nondisplaced) S82.42- (See complete *ICD-10-CM* Manual for codes)
  - upper end
    - physeal S89.20-

Fracture, *continued*
      - Salter-Harris
        - Type I S89.21-
        - Type II S89.22-
      - specified NEC S89.29-
    - specified NEC S82.83-
    - torus S82.81-
- finger (except thumb) S62.6-
  - distal phalanx (displaced) S62.63-
    - nondisplaced S62.66-
  - index S62.6-
    - distal phalanx (displaced) S62.63-
      - nondisplaced S62.66-
    - medial phalanx (displaced) S62.62-
      - nondisplaced S62.65-
    - proximal phalanx (displaced) S62.61-
      - nondisplaced S62.64-
  - little S62.6-
    - distal phalanx (displaced) S62.63-
      - nondisplaced S62.66-
    - medial phalanx (displaced) S62.62-
      - nondisplaced S62.65-
    - proximal phalanx (displaced) S62.61-
      - nondisplaced S62.64-
  - medial phalanx (displaced) S62.62-
    - nondisplaced S62.65-
  - middle S62.6-
    - distal phalanx (displaced) S62.63-
      - nondisplaced S62.66-
    - medial phalanx (displaced) S62.62-
      - nondisplaced S62.65-
    - proximal phalanx (displaced) S62.61-
      - nondisplaced S62.64-
  - proximal phalanx (displaced) S62.61-
    - nondisplaced S62.64-
  - ring S62.6-
    - distal phalanx (displaced) S62.63-
      - nondisplaced S62.66-
    - medial phalanx (displaced) S62.62-
      - nondisplaced S62.65-
    - proximal phalanx (displaced) S62.61-
      - nondisplaced S62.64-
  - thumb—*see* Fracture, thumb
- foot S92.90-
  - astragalus—*see* Fracture, tarsal, talus
  - calcaneus—*see* Fracture, tarsal, calcaneus
  - cuboid—*see* Fracture, tarsal, cuboid
  - cuneiform—*see* Fracture, tarsal, cuneiform
  - metatarsal—*see* Fracture, metatarsal bone
  - navicular—*see* Fracture, tarsal, navicular
  - sesamoid S92.81-
  - talus—*see* Fracture, tarsal, talus
  - tarsal—*see* Fracture, tarsal
  - toe—*see* Fracture, toe
- forearm S52.9-
  - radius—*see* Fracture, radius
  - ulna—*see* Fracture, ulna
- fossa (anterior) (middle) (posterior) S02.19-
- frontal (bone) (skull) S02.0-
  - sinus S02.19-
- greenstick—*see* Fracture, by site
- hallux—*see* Fracture, toe, great
- hand
  - carpal—*see* Fracture, carpal bone
  - finger (except thumb)—*see* Fracture, finger
  - metacarpal—*see* Fracture, metacarpal
  - navicular (scaphoid) (hand)—*see* Fracture, carpal bone, navicular
  - thumb—*see* Fracture, thumb
- healed or old
  - with complications—*code by* Nature of the complication
- heel bone—*see* Fracture, tarsal, calcaneus
- Hill-Sachs S42.29-
- hip—*see* Fracture, femur, neck
- humerus S42.30-
  - anatomical neck—*see* Fracture, humerus, upper end
  - articular process—*see* Fracture, humerus, lower end
  - capitellum—*see* Fracture, humerus, lower end, condyle, lateral
  - distal end—*see* Fracture, humerus, lower end
  - epiphysis
    - lower—*see* Fracture, humerus, lower end, physeal

Fracture, *continued*

- upper—*see* Fracture, humerus, upper end, physeal
- external condyle—*see* Fracture, humerus, lower end, condyle, lateral
- great tuberosity—*see* Fracture, humerus, upper end, greater tuberosity
- intercondylar—*see* Fracture, humerus, lower end
- internal epicondyle—*see* Fracture, humerus, lower end, epicondyle, medial
- lesser tuberosity—*see* Fracture, humerus, upper end, lesser tuberosity
- lower end S42.40-
  - condyle
    - lateral (displaced) S42.45-
      - nondisplaced S42.45-
    - medial (displaced) S42.46-
      - nondisplaced S42.46-
  - epicondyle
    - lateral (displaced) S42.43-
      - nondisplaced S42.43-
    - medial (displaced) S42.44-
      - incarcerated S42.44-
      - nondisplaced S42.44-
  - physeal S49.10-
    - Salter-Harris
      - Type I S49.11-
      - Type II S49.12-
      - Type III S49.13-
      - Type IV S49.14-
    - specified NEC S49.19-
  - specified NEC (displaced) S42.49-
    - nondisplaced S42.49-
  - supracondylar (simple) (displaced) S42.41-
    - comminuted (displaced) S42.42-
      - nondisplaced S42.42-
    - nondisplaced S42.41-
  - torus S42.48-
  - transcondylar (displaced) S42.47-
    - nondisplaced S42.47-
- proximal end—*see* Fracture, humerus, upper end
- shaft S42.30-
  - comminuted (displaced) S42.35-
    - nondisplaced S42.35-
  - greenstick S42.31-
  - oblique (displaced) S42.33
    - nondisplaced S42.33-
  - segmental (displaced) S42.36-
    - nondisplaced S42.36-
  - specified NEC S42.39-
  - spiral (displaced) S42.34-
    - nondisplaced S42.34-
  - transverse (displaced) S42.32-
    - nondisplaced S42.32-
- supracondylar—*see* Fracture, humerus, lower end
- surgical neck—*see* Fracture, humerus, upper end, surgical neck
- trochlea—*see* Fracture, humerus, lower end, condyle, medial
- tuberosity—*see* Fracture, humerus, upper end
- upper end S42.20-
  - anatomical neck—*see* Fracture, humerus, upper end, specified NEC
  - articular head—*see* Fracture, humerus, upper end, specified NEC
  - epiphysis—*see* Fracture, humerus, upper end, physeal
  - greater tuberosity (displaced) S42.25-
    - nondisplaced S42.25-
  - lesser tuberosity (displaced) S42.26-
    - nondisplaced S42.26-
  - physeal S49.00-
    - Salter-Harris
      - Type I S49.01-
      - Type II S49.02-
      - Type III S49.03-
      - Type IV S49.04-
    - specified NEC S49.09-
  - specified NEC (displaced) S42.29-
    - nondisplaced S42.29-
  - surgical neck (displaced) S42.21-
    - four-part S42.24-
    - nondisplaced S42.21-

Fracture, *continued*

- three-part S42.23-
- two-part (displaced) S42.22-
  - nondisplaced S42.22-
- torus S42.27-
- transepiphyseal—*see* Fracture, humerus, upper end, physeal
- hyoid bone S12.8
- ilium S32.30-
  - avulsion (displaced) S32.31-
    - nondisplaced S32.31-
  - specified NEC S32.39-
- impaction, impacted—*code as* Fracture, by site
- innominate bone—*see* Fracture, ilium
- instep—*see* Fracture, foot
- ischium S32.60-
  - avulsion (displaced) S32.61-
    - nondisplaced S32.61-
  - specified NEC S32.69-
- jaw (bone) (lower)—*see* Fracture, mandible
- knee cap—*see* Fracture, patella
- larynx S12.8
- late effects—*see* Sequelae
- leg (lower)
  - ankle—*see* Fracture, ankle
  - femur—*see* Fracture, femur
  - fibula—*see* Fracture, fibula
  - malleolus—*see* Fracture, ankle
  - patella—*see* Fracture, patella
  - specified site NEC S82.89-
  - tibia—*see* Fracture, tibia
- lumbosacral spine S32.9
- Maisonneuve's (displaced) S82.86-
  - nondisplaced S82.86-
- malar bone (*see also* Fracture) S02.40-
- malleolus—*see* Fracture, ankle
- malunion—*see* Fracture, by site
- mandible (lower jaw (bone)) S02.609-
  - alveolus S02.67-
  - angle (of jaw) S02.65-
  - body, unspecified S02.60-
  - condylar process S02.61-
  - coronoid process S02.63-
  - ramus, unspecified S02.64-
  - specified site NEC S02.69-
  - subcondylar process S02.62-
  - symphysis S02.66-
- march—*see* Fracture
- metacarpal S62.30-
  - base (displaced) S62.31-
    - nondisplaced S62.34-
  - fifth S62.30-
    - base (displaced) S62.31-
      - nondisplaced S62.34-
    - neck (displaced) S62.33-
      - nondisplaced S62.36-
    - shaft (displaced) S62.32-
      - nondisplaced S62.35-
    - specified NEC S62.39-
  - first S62.20-
    - base NEC (displaced) S62.23-
      - nondisplaced S62.23-
    - Bennett's—*see* Bennett's fracture
    - neck (displaced) S62.25-
      - nondisplaced S62.25-
    - shaft (displaced) S62.24-
      - nondisplaced S62.24-
    - specified NEC S62.29-
  - fourth S62.30-
    - base (displaced) S62.31-
      - nondisplaced S62.34-
    - neck (displaced) S62.33-
      - nondisplaced S62.36-
    - shaft (displaced) S62.32-
      - nondisplaced S62.35-
    - specified NEC S62.39-
  - neck (displaced) S62.33-
    - nondisplaced S62.36-
  - Rolando's—*see* Rolando's fracture
  - second S62.30-
    - base (displaced) S62.31-
      - nondisplaced S62.34-

Fracture, *continued*

- neck (displaced) S62.33-
  - nondisplaced S62.36-
- shaft (displaced) S62.32-
  - nondisplaced S62.35-
- specified NEC S62.39-
- shaft (displaced) S62.32-
  - nondisplaced S62.35-
- third S62.30-
  - base (displaced) S62.31-
    - nondisplaced S62.34-
  - neck (displaced) S62.33-
    - nondisplaced S62.36-
  - shaft (displaced) S62.32-
    - nondisplaced S62.35-
  - specified NEC S62.39-
- specified NEC S62.39-
- metatarsal bone S92.30-
  - fifth (displaced) S92.35-
    - nondisplaced S92.35-
  - first (displaced) S92.31-
    - nondisplaced S92.31-
  - fourth (displaced) S92.34-
    - nondisplaced S92.34-
  - physeal S99.10-
    - Salter-Harris
      - Type I S99.11-
      - Type II S99.12-
      - Type III S99.13-
      - Type IV S99.14-
  - second (displaced) S92.32-
    - nondisplaced S92.32-
  - third (displaced) S92.33-
    - nondisplaced S92.33-
    - specified NEC S99.19-
- Monteggia's—*see* Monteggia's fracture
- multiple
  - hand (and wrist) NEC—*see* Fracture, by site
  - ribs—*see* Fracture, rib, multiple
- nasal (bone(s)) S02.2-
- navicular (scaphoid) (foot)—*see also* Fracture, tarsal bone(s), navicular
  - hand—*see* Fracture, carpal bone(s), navicular
- neck S12.9
  - cervical vertebra S12.9
    - fifth (displaced) S12.400
      - nondisplaced S12.401
    - first (displaced) S12.000
      - burst (stable) S12.0-
        - unstable S12.0-
      - nondisplaced S12.001
      - posterior arch (displaced) S12.030
        - nondisplaced S12.031
    - fourth (displaced) S12.300
      - nondisplaced S12.301
    - second (displaced) S12.100
      - nondisplaced S12.101
    - seventh (displaced) S12.600
      - nondisplaced S12.601~
    - sixth (displaced) S12.500
      - nondisplaced S12.501
    - third (displaced) S12.200
      - nondisplaced S12.201
  - hyoid bone S12.8
  - larynx S12.8
  - specified site NEC S12.8
  - thyroid cartilage S12.8
  - trachea S12.8
- newborn—*see* Birth, injury, fracture
- nonunion—*see* Nonunion, fracture
- nose, nasal (bone) (septum) S02.2-
- occiput—*see* Fracture, skull, base, occiput
- olecranon (process) (ulna)—*see* Fracture, ulna, upper end, olecranon process
- orbit, orbital (bone) (region) S02.85
  - calcis—*see* Fracture, tarsal bone(s), calcaneus
  - floor (blow-out) S02.3-
  - magnum—*see* Fracture, carpal bone(s), capitate
  - pubis—*see* Fracture, pubis
  - roof S02.12-
  - wall
    - lateral S02.83-
    - medial S02.84-

FRACTURE-FRACTURE

Fracture, *continued*
- palate S02.8-
- parietal bone (skull) S02.0-
- patella S82.00-
  - comminuted (displaced or nondisplaced) S82.04- (See complete *ICD-10-CM* Manual for codes)
  - longitudinal (displaced or nondisplaced) S82.02- (See complete *ICD-10-CM* Manual for codes)
  - osteochondral (displaced or nondisplaced) S82.01- (See complete *ICD-10-CM* Manual)
  - transverse (displaced or nondisplaced) S82.03- (See complete *ICD-10-CM* Manual for codes)
- pedicle (of vertebral arch)—*see* Fracture, vertebra
- pelvis, pelvic (bone) S32.9
  - acetabulum—*see* Fracture, acetabulum
  - ilium—*see* Fracture, ilium
  - ischium—*see* Fracture, ischium
  - multiple
    - without disruption of pelvic ring (circle) S32.82
  - pubis—*see* Fracture, pubis
  - specified site NEC S32.89
  - sacrum—*see* Fracture, sacrum
- phalanx
  - foot—*see* Fracture, toe
  - hand—*see* Fracture, finger
- pisiform—*see* Fracture, carpal bone(s), pisiform
- pond—*see* Fracture, skull
- prosthetic device, internal—*see* Complications, prosthetic device, by site, mechanical
- pubis S32.50-
  - with disruption of pelvic ring—*see* Disruption
  - specified site NEC S32.59-
  - superior rim S32.51-
- radius S52.9-
  - distal end—*see* Fracture, radius, lower end
  - head—*see* Fracture, radius, upper end, head
  - lower end S52.50-
    - Barton's—*see* Barton's fracture
    - Colles'—*see* Colles' fracture
    - extraarticular NEC S52.55-
    - intraarticular NEC S52.57-
    - physeal S59.20-
      - Salter-Harris
        - ◊ Type I S59.21-
        - ◊ Type II S59.22-
        - ◊ Type III S59.23-
        - ◊ Type IV S59.24-
      - ~ specified NEC S59.29-
    - Smith's—*see* Smith's fracture
    - specified NEC S52.59-
    - styloid process (displaced) S52.51-
      - ~ nondisplaced S52.51-
    - torus S52.52-
  - neck—*see* Fracture, radius, upper end
  - proximal end—*see* Fracture, radius, upper end
  - shaft S52.30-
    - bent bone S52.38-
    - comminuted (displaced) S52.35-
      - ~ nondisplaced S52.35-
    - Galeazzi's—*see* Galeazzi's fracture
    - greenstick S52.31-
    - oblique (displaced) S52.33-
      - ~ nondisplaced S52.33-
    - segmental (displaced) S52.36-
      - ~ nondisplaced S52.36-
    - specified NEC S52.39-
    - spiral (displaced) S52.34-
      - ~ nondisplaced S52.34-
    - transverse (displaced) S52.32-
      - ~ nondisplaced S52.32-
  - upper end S52.10-
    - head (displaced) S52.12-
      - ~ nondisplaced S52.12-
    - neck (displaced) S52.13-
      - ~ nondisplaced S52.13-
    - specified NEC S52.18-
    - physeal S59.10-
      - Salter-Harris
        - ◊ Type I S59.11-
        - ◊ Type II S59.12-
        - ◊ Type III S59.13-
        - ◊ Type IV S59.14-
      - ~ specified NEC S59.19-

Fracture, *continued*
- torus S52.11-
- ramus
  - inferior or superior, pubis—*see* Fracture, pubis
  - mandible—*see* Fracture, mandible
- rib S22.3-
  - with flail chest—*see* Flail, chest
  - multiple S22.4-
    - with flail chest—*see* Flail, chest
- root, tooth—*see* Fracture, tooth
- sacrum S32.10
  - specified NEC S32.19
  - Type
    - 1 S32.14
    - 2 S32.15
    - 3 S32.16
    - 4 S32.17
  - Zone
    - I S32.119
      - ~ displaced (minimally) S32.111
        - ◊ severely S32.112
      - ~ nondisplaced S32.110
    - II S32.129
      - ~ displaced (minimally) S32.121
        - ◊ severely S32.122
      - ~ nondisplaced S32.120
    - III S32.139
      - ~ displaced (minimally) S32.131
        - ◊ severely S32.132
      - ~ nondisplaced S32.130
- scaphoid (hand)—*see also* Fracture, carpal bone(s), navicular
  - foot—*see* Fracture, tarsal, navicular
- semilunar bone, wrist—*see* Fracture, carpal, lunate
- sequelae—*see* Sequelae
- sesamoid bone
  - foot S92.81-
  - hand—*see* Fracture, carpal bone(s)
  - other—*code by* site under Fracture
- shepherd's—*see* Fracture, tarsal bone(s), talus
- shoulder (girdle) S42.9-
- sinus (ethmoid) (frontal) S02.19-
- skull S02.91-
  - base S02.10-
    - occiput S02.119
      - ~ condyle S02.11-
        - ◊ type I S02.11-
        - ◊ type II S02.11-
        - ◊ type III S02.11
      - ~ specified NEC S02.118-
    - specified NEC S02.19-
  - birth injury P13.0
  - frontal bone S02.0-
  - parietal bone S02.0-
  - specified site NEC S02.8-
  - temporal bone S02.19-
  - vault S02.0-
- Smith's—*see* Smith's fracture
- sphenoid (bone) (sinus) S02.19-
- stave (of thumb)—*see* Fracture, metacarpal, first
- sternum S22.20
  - with flail chest—*see* Flail, chest
  - body S22.22
  - manubrium S22.21
  - xiphoid (process) S22.24
- stress M84.30-
  - ankle M84.37-
  - carpus M84.34-
  - clavicle M84.31-
  - femoral neck M84.359
  - femur M84.35-
  - fibula M84.36-
  - finger M84.34-
  - hip M84.359
  - humerus M84.32-
  - ilium M84.350
  - ischium M84.350
  - metacarpus M84.34-
  - metatarsus M84.37-
  - pelvis M84.350
  - radius M84.33-
  - rib M84.38
  - scapula M84.31-

Fracture, *continued*
- skull M84.38
- tarsus M84.37-
- tibia M84.36-
- toe M84.37-
- ulna M84.33-
- supracondylar, elbow—*see* Fracture, humerus, lower end, supracondylar
- symphysis pubis—*see* Fracture, pubis
- talus (ankle bone)—*see* Fracture, tarsal bone(s), talus
- tarsal bone(s) S92.20-
  - astragalus—*see* Fracture, tarsal bone(s), talus
  - calcaneus S92.00-
    - anterior process (displaced) S92.02-
      - ~ nondisplaced S92.02-
    - body (displaced) S92.01-
      - ~ nondisplaced S92.01-
    - extraarticular NEC (displaced) S92.05-
      - ~ nondisplaced S92.05-
    - intraarticular (displaced) S92.06-
      - ~ nondisplaced S92.06-
    - physeal S99.00-
      - Salter-Harris
        - ◊ Type I S99.01-
        - ◊ Type II S99.02-
        - ◊ Type III S99.03-
        - ◊ Type IV S99.04-
      - ~ specified NEC S99.09-
    - tuberosity (displaced) S92.04-
      - ~ avulsion (displaced) S92.03-
        - ◊ nondisplaced S92.03-
      - ~ nondisplaced S92.04-
  - cuboid (displaced) S92.21-
    - nondisplaced S92.21-
  - cuneiform
    - intermediate (displaced) S92.23-
      - ~ nondisplaced S92.23-
    - lateral (displaced) S92.22-
      - ~ nondisplaced S92.22-
    - medial (displaced) S92.24-
      - ~ nondisplaced S92.24-
  - navicular (displaced) S92.25-
    - nondisplaced S92.25-
  - scaphoid—*see* Fracture, tarsal bone(s), navicular
  - talus S92.10-
    - avulsion (displaced) S92.15-
      - ~ nondisplaced S92.15-
    - body (displaced) S92.12-
      - ~ nondisplaced S92.12-
    - dome (displaced) S92.14-
      - ~ nondisplaced S92.14-
    - head (displaced) S92.12-
      - ~ nondisplaced S92.12-
    - lateral process (displaced) S92.14-
      - ~ nondisplaced S92.14-
    - neck (displaced) S92.11-
      - ~ nondisplaced S92.11-
    - posterior process (displaced) S92.13-
      - ~ nondisplaced S92.13-
    - specified NEC S92.19-
- temporal bone (styloid) S02.19-
- thorax (bony) S22.9
  - with flail chest—*see* Flail, chest
  - rib S22.3-
    - multiple S22.4-
      - ~ with flail chest—*see* Flail, chest
- thumb S62.50-
  - distal phalanx (displaced) S62.52-
    - nondisplaced S62.52-
  - proximal phalanx (displaced) S62.51-
    - nondisplaced S62.51-
- thyroid cartilage S12.8
- tibia (shaft) S82.20-
  - comminuted (displaced or nondisplaced) S82.25- (See complete *ICD-10-CM* Manual)
  - condyles—*see* Fracture, tibia
  - distal end—*see* Fracture, tibia
  - epiphysis
    - lower—*see* Fracture, tibia
    - upper—*see* Fracture, tibia
  - head (involving knee joint)—*see* Fracture, tibia
  - intercondyloid eminence—*see* Fracture, tibia

Fracture, *continued*
- – involving ankle or malleolus—*see* Fracture, ankle, medial malleolus
- – lower end S82.30-
  - ■ physeal S89.10-
    - ~ Salter-Harris
      - ◊ Type I S89.11-
      - ◊ Type II S89.12-
      - ◊ Type III S89.13-
      - ◊ Type IV S89.14-
    - ~ specified NEC S89.19-
  - ■ pilon (displaced) S82.87-
    - ~ nondisplaced S82.87-
  - ■ specified NEC S82.39-
  - ■ torus S82.31-
- – malleolus—*see* Fracture, ankle, medial malleolus
- – oblique (displaced or nondisplaced) S82.23- - (See complete *ICD-10-CM* Manual)
- – pilon—*see* Fracture, tibia
- – proximal end—*see* Fracture, tibia
- – segmental (displaced or nondisplaced) S82.26- - (See complete *ICD-10-CM* Manual)
- – spiral (displaced) S82.24-
  - ■ nondisplaced S82.24-
- – transverse (displaced or nondisplaced) S82.22- - (See complete *ICD-10-CM* Manual)
- – tuberosity—*see* Fracture, tibia
- – upper end S82.10-
  - ■ bicondylar (displaced) or nondisplaced) S82.14— (See complete *ICD-10-CM* Manual)
  - ■ lateral condyle (displaced) or nondisplaced) S82.12—(See complete *ICD-10-CM* Manual)
  - ■ medial condyle (displaced) or nondisplaced) S82.13—(See complete *ICD-10-CM* Manual)
  - ■ physeal S89.00-
    - ~ Salter-Harris
      - ◊ Type I S89.01-
      - ◊ Type II S89.02-
      - ◊ Type III S89.03-
      - ◊ Type IV S89.04-
    - ~ specified NEC S89.09-
  - ■ plateau—*see* Fracture, tibial
  - ■ spine (displaced or nondisplaced) S82.11- (See complete *ICD-10-CM* Manual)
  - ■ torus S82.16-
  - ■ specified NEC S82.19-
  - ■ tuberosity (displacedor nondisplaced) S82.15- (See complete *ICD-10-CM* Manual)
- • toe S92.91-
  - – great (displaced) S92.4-
    - ■ distal phalanx (displaced) S92.42-
      - ~ nondisplaced S92.42-
    - ■ nondisplaced S92.4-
    - ■ proximal phalanx (displaced) S92.41-
      - ~ nondisplaced S92.41-
    - ■ specified NEC S92.49-
  - – lesser (displaced) S92.5-
    - ■ distal phalanx (displaced) S92.53-
      - ~ nondisplaced S92.53-
    - ■ middle phalanx (displaced) S92.52-
      - ~ nondisplaced S92.52-
    - ■ nondisplaced S92.5-
    - ■ proximal phalanx (displaced) S92.51-
      - ~ nondisplaced S92.51-
    - ■ specified NEC S92.59-
- • tooth (root) S02.5-
- • trachea (cartilage) S12.8
- • trapezium or trapezoid bone—*see* Fracture, carpal bone(s)
- • trimalleolar—*see* Fracture, ankle, trimalleolar
- • triquetrum (cuneiform of carpus)—*see* Fracture, carpal bone(s), triquetrum
- • trochanter—*see* Fracture, femur
- • tuberosity (external)—*code by* site under Fracture
- • ulna (shaft) S52.20-
  - – bent bone S52.28-
  - – coronoid process—*see* Fracture, ulna, upper end, coronoid process
  - – distal end—*see* Fracture, ulna, lower end
  - – head S52.60-
  - – lower end S52.60-
    - ■ physeal S59.00-
      - ~ Salter-Harris

Fracture, *continued*
- ◊ Type I S59.01-
- ◊ Type II S59.02-
- ◊ Type III S59.03-
- ◊ Type IV S59.04-
- ~ specified NEC S59.09-
  - ■ specified NEC S52.69-
  - ■ styloid process (displaced) S52.61-
    - ~ nondisplaced S52.61-
  - ■ torus S52.62-
- – proximal end—*see* Fracture, ulna, upper end
- – shaft S52.20-
  - ■ comminuted (displaced) S52.25-
    - ~ nondisplaced S52.25-
  - ■ greenstick S52.21-
  - ■ Monteggia's—*see* Monteggia's fracture
  - ■ oblique (displaced) S52.23-
    - ~ nondisplaced S52.23-
  - ■ segmental (displaced) S52.26-
    - ~ nondisplaced S52.26-
  - ■ specified NEC S52.29-
  - ■ spiral (displaced) S52.24-
    - ~ nondisplaced S52.24-
  - ■ transverse (displaced) S52.22-
    - ~ nondisplaced S52.22-
- – upper end S52.00-
  - ■ coronoid process (displaced) S52.04-
    - ~ nondisplaced S52.04-
  - ■ olecranon process (displaced) S52.02-
    - ~ with intraarticular extension S52.03-
    - ~ nondisplaced S52.02-
      - ◊ with intraarticular extension S52.03-
  - ■ specified NEC S52.09-
  - ■ torus S52.01-
- • unciform—*see* Fracture, carpal bone(s), hamate
- • vault of skull S02.0-
- • vertebra, vertebral (arch) (body) (column) (neural arch) (pedicle) (spinous process) (transverse process)
  - – atlas—*see* Fracture, neck, cervical vertebra, first
  - – axis—*see* Fracture, neck, cervical vertebra, second
  - – cervical (teardrop) S12.9
    - ■ axis—*see* Fracture, neck, cervical vertebra, second
    - ■ first (atlas)—*see* Fracture, neck, cervical vertebra, first
    - ■ second (axis)—*see* Fracture, neck, cervical vertebra, second
- • vertex S02.0-
- • vomer (bone) S02.2-
- • wrist S62.10-
  - – carpal—*see* Fracture, carpal bone
  - – navicular (scaphoid) (hand)—*see* Fracture, carpal bone(s), navicular
- • zygoma S02.402
  - – left side S02.40F
  - – right side S02.40E

Fragile, fragility
- • bone, congenital (with blue sclera) Q78.0
- • X chromosome Q99.2

Fragilitas
- • ossium (with blue sclerae) (hereditary) Q78.0

Frank's essential thrombocytopenia D69.3

Fraser's syndrome Q87.0

Freckle(s) L81.2

Frederickson's hyperlipoproteinemia, type
- • IIA E78.0
- • IIB and III E78.2

Freeman Sheldon syndrome Q87.0

Frenum, frenulum
- • tongue (shortening) (congenital) Q38.1

Frequency micturition (nocturnal) R35.0
- • psychogenic F45.8

Friction
- • burn—*see* Burn, by site
- • sounds, chest R09.89

Friedreich's
- • ataxia G11.11
- • combined systemic disease G11.11
- • facial hemihypertrophy Q67.4
- • sclerosis (cerebellum) (spinal cord) G11.11

Fröhlich's syndrome E23.6

Fucosidosis E77.1

Fugue R68.89
- • reaction to exceptional stress (transient) F43.0

Fulminant, fulminating—*see* Disease, diseased

Functional—*see also* Disease, diseased
- • bleeding (uterus) N93.8

Fungus, fungous
- • cerebral G93.89
- • disease NOS B49
- • infection—*see* Infection, fungus

Funnel
- • breast (acquired) M95.4
  - – congenital Q67.6
- • chest (acquired) M95.4
  - – congenital Q67.6
- • pelvis (acquired) M95.5
  - – congenital Q74.2

FUO (fever of unknown origin) R50.9

Furfur L21.0
- • microsporon B36.0

Furuncle L02.92
- • abdominal wall L02.221
- • ankle L02.42-
- • anus K61.0
- • axilla (region) L02.42-
- • back (any part) L02.222
- • breast N61.1
- • buttock L02.32
- • cheek (external) L02.02
- • chest wall L02.223
- • chin L02.02
- • face L02.02
- • flank L02.221
- • foot L02.62-
- • forehead L02.02
- • gluteal (region) L02.32
- • groin L02.224
- • hand L02.52-
- • head L02.821
  - – face L02.02
- • hip L02.42-
- • knee L02.42-
- • leg (any part) L02.42-
- • lower limb L02.42-
- • malignant A22.0
- • mouth K12.2
- • navel L02.226
- • neck L02.12
- • nose J34.0
- • partes posteriores L02.32
- • pectoral region L02.223
- • perineum L02.225
- • scalp L02.821
- • specified site NEC L02.828
- • submandibular K12.2
- • temple (region) L02.02
- • thumb L02.52-
- • toe L02.62-
- • trunk L02.229
  - – abdominal wall L02.221
  - – back L02.222
  - – chest wall L02.223
  - – groin L02.224
  - – perineum L02.225
  - – umbilicus L02.226
- • umbilicus L02.226
- • upper limb L02.42-
- • vulva N76.4

Fusion, fused (congenital)
- • astragaloscaphoid Q74.2
- • atria Q21.1
- • auricles, heart Q21.1
- • choanal Q30.0
- • cusps, heart valve NEC Q24.8
  - – pulmonary Q22.1
- • fingers Q70.0-
- • hymen Q52.3
- • limb, congenital Q74.8
  - – lower Q74.2
  - – upper Q74.0
- • nares, nose, nasal, nostril(s) Q30.0

Fusion, fused, *continued*
- ossicles Q79.9
  - auditory Q16.3
- pulmonic cusps Q22.1
- sacroiliac (joint) (acquired) M43.28
  - congenital Q74.2
- toes Q70.2
- ventricles, heart Q21.0

Fussy baby R68.12

G

Gain in weight (abnormal) (excessive)—*see also* Weight, gain

Gaisböck's disease (polycythemia hypertonica) D75.1

Gait abnormality R26.9
- ataxic R26.0
- hysterical (ataxic) (staggering) F44.4
- paralytic R26.1
- spastic R26.1
- specified type NEC R26.89
- staggering R26.0
- unsteadiness R26.81
- walking difficulty NEC R26.2

Galactocele (breast)
- puerperal, postpartum O92.79

Galactophoritis N61.0

Galactorrhea O92.6
- not associated with childbirth N64.3

GALD (gestational alloimmune liver disease) P78.84

Galeazzi's fracture S52.37-

Gallbladder—*see also* Disease, diseased
- acute K81.0

Gambling Z72.6

Ganglion (compound) (diffuse) (joint) (tendon (sheath)) M67.40
- ankle M67.47-
- foot M67.47-
- forearm M67.43-
- hand M67.44-
- lower leg M67.46-
- multiple sites M67.49
- pelvic region M67.45-
- shoulder region M67.41-
- specified site NEC M67.48
- thigh region M67.45-
- upper arm M67.42-
- wrist M67.43-

Ganglionitis
- newborn (birth injury) P11.3

Gangliosidosis E75.10
- GM2 E75.00
  - Sandhoff disease E75.01
  - Tay-Sachs disease E75.02

Gangrene, gangrenous (connective tissue) (dropsical) (dry) (moist) (skin) (ulcer) (*see also* Necrosis)
- appendix K35.80
  - with
    - peritonitis, localized (*see also* Appendicitis) K35.31
- epididymis (infectional) N45.1
- erysipelas—*see* Erysipelas
- glossitis K14.0
- laryngitis J04.0
- pancreas
  - idiopathic
    - infected K85.02
    - uninfected K85.01
  - infected K85.82
  - uninfected K85.81
- quinsy J36
- testis (infectional) N45.2
  - noninfective N44.8
- uvulitis K12.2

Gardner-Diamond syndrome (autoerythrocyte sensitization) D69.2

Gargoylism E76.01

Gartner's duct
- cyst Q52.4
- persistent Q50.6

Gas R14.3
- excessive R14.0
- on stomach R14.0
- pains R14.1

Gastrectasis K31.0
- psychogenic F45.8

Gastric—*see* Disease, diseased

Gastritis (simple) K29.70
- with bleeding K29.71
- acute (erosive) K29.00
  - with bleeding K29.01
- dietary counseling and surveillance Z71.3
- eosinophilic K52.81
- viral NEC A08.4

Gastroduodenitis K29.90
- with bleeding K29.91
- virus, viral A08.4
  - specified type NEC A08.39

Gastroenteritis (acute) (chronic) (noninfectious) (*see also* Enteritis) K52.9
- allergic K52.29
  - with
    - eosinophilic gastritis or gastroenteritis K52.81
    - food protein-induced enterocolitis syndrome K52.21
    - food protein-induced enteropathy K52.22
- dietetic K52.29
- eosinophilic K52.81
- epidemic (infectious) A09
- food hypersensitivity K52.29
- infectious—*see* Enteritis, infectious
- noninfectious K52.9
  - specified NEC K52.89
- rotaviral A08.0
- Salmonella A02.0
- viral NEC A08.4
  - acute infectious A08.39
  - infantile (acute) A08.39
  - rotaviral A08.0
  - severe of infants A08.39
  - specified type NEC A08.39

Gastroenteropathy (*see also* Gastroenteritis) K52.9
- infectious A09

Gastrojejunitis (*see also* Enteritis) K52.9

Gastropathy K31.9
- erythematous K29.70
- exudative K90.89

Gastrorrhagia K92.2
- psychogenic F45.8

Gastroschisis (congenital) Q79.3

Gastrospasm (neurogenic) (reflex) K31.89
- neurotic F45.8
- psychogenic F45.8

Gastrostomy
- attention to Z43.1
- status Z93.1

Gee (-Herter) (-Thaysen) disease (nontropical sprue) K90.0

Gemistocytoma
- specified site—*see* Neoplasm, malignant, by site in Table of Neoplasms in the complete *ICD-10-CM* manual
- unspecified site C71.9

General, generalized—*see* Disease, diseased

Genetic
- carrier (status)
  - cystic fibrosis Z14.1
  - hemophilia A (asymptomatic) Z14.01
    - symptomatic Z14.02
  - specified NEC Z14.8

Genu
- congenital Q74.1
- extrorsum (acquired) M21.16-
  - congenital Q74.1
- introrsum (acquired) M21.06-
  - congenital Q74.1
- recurvatum (acquired) M21.86-
  - congenital Q68.2
- valgum (acquired) (knock-knee) M21.06-
  - congenital Q74.1
- varum (acquired) (bowleg) M21.16-
  - congenital Q74.1

Geographic tongue K14.1

Geophagia—*see* Pica

Gerbode defect Q21.0

GERD (gastroesophageal reflux disease) K21.9

Gerhardt's
- syndrome (vocal cord paralysis) J38.00
  - bilateral J38.02
  - unilateral J38.01

German measles—*see also* Rubella
- exposure to Z20.4

Germinoblastoma (diffuse) C85.9-

Gerstmann's syndrome R48.8
- developmental F81.2

Gianotti-Crosti disease L44.4

Giant
- urticaria T78.3

Giardiasis A07.1

Gibert's disease or pityriasis L42

Giddiness R42
- hysterical F44.89
- psychogenic F45.8

Gigantism (cerebral) (hypophyseal) (pituitary) E22.0
- constitutional E34.4

Gilbert's disease or syndrome E80.4

Gilles de la Tourette's disease or syndrome (motor-verbal tic) F95.2

Gingivitis
- acute (catarrhal) K05.00
  - plaque induced K05.00

Gingivoglossitis K14.0

Gingivostomatitis
- herpesviral B00.2

Glaucoma
- childhood Q15.0
- congenital Q15.0
- in (due to)
  - endocrine disease NOS E34.9 *[H42]*
  - Lowe's syndrome E72.03 *[H42]*
  - metabolic disease NOS E88.9 *[H42]*
- infantile Q15.0
- newborn Q15.0
- secondary (to)
  - trauma H40.3-
- traumatic—*see also* Glaucoma, secondary, trauma
  - newborn (birth injury) P15.3

Gleet (gonococcal) A54.01

Glioblastoma (multiforme)
- with sarcomatous component
  - specified site—*see* Neoplasm, malignant, by site in Table of Neoplasms in the complete *ICD-10-CM* manual
  - unspecified site C71.9
- giant cell
  - specified site—*see* Neoplasm, malignant, by site in Table of Neoplasms in the complete *ICD-10-CM* manual
  - unspecified site C71.9
- specified site—*see* Neoplasm, malignant, by site in Table of Neoplasms in the complete *ICD-10-CM* manual
- unspecified site C71.9

Glioma (malignant)
- astrocytic
  - specified site—*see* Neoplasm, malignant, by site in Table of Neoplasms in the complete *ICD-10-CM* manual
  - unspecified site C71.9
- mixed
  - specified site—*see* Neoplasm, malignant, by site in Table of Neoplasms in the complete *ICD-10-CM* manual
  - unspecified site C71.9
- nose Q30.8
- specified site NEC—*see* Neoplasm, malignant, by site in Table of Neoplasms in the complete *ICD-10-CM* manual
  - specified site—*see* Neoplasm, uncertain behavior, by site in Table of Neoplasms in the complete *ICD-10-CM* manual

Glioma, *continued*
- unspecified site C71.9

Gliosarcoma
- specified site—*see* Neoplasm, malignant, by site in Table of Neoplasms in the complete *ICD-10-CM* manual
- unspecified site C71.9

Gliosis (cerebral) G93.89

Globinuria R82.3

Globus (hystericus) F45.8

Glomangioma D18.00
- skin D18.01
- specified site NEC D18.09

Glomangiomyoma D18.00
- intra-abdominal D18.03
- intracranial D18.02
- skin D18.01
- specified site NEC D18.09

Glomerulonephritis (*see also* Nephritis) N05.9
- with
  - C3
    - glomerulonephritis N05.A
    - glomerulopathy N05.A
      - ~ with dense deposit disease N05.6
  - edema—*see* Nephrosis
  - minimal change N05.0
  - minor glomerular abnormality N05.0
- acute N00.9
- chronic N03.9
- in (due to)
  - defibrination syndrome D65 [N08]
  - disseminated intravascular coagulation D65 [N08]
  - *hemolytic-uremic syndrome D59.3*
  - Henoch (-Schönlein) purpura D69.0 [N08]
  - sepsis A41.9 [N08]
    - streptococcal A40- [N08]
  - subacute bacterial endocarditis I33.0 [N08]
  - systemic lupus erythematosus M32.14
- poststreptococcal NEC N05.9
  - acute N00.9
  - chronic N03.9
- proliferative NEC (*see also* N00-N07 with fourth character .8) N05.8
  - diffuse (lupus) M32.14

Glossitis (chronic superficial) (gangrenous) (Moeller's) K14.0
- areata exfoliativa K14.1
- benign migratory K14.1
- cortical superficial, sclerotic K14.0
- interstitial, sclerous K14.0
- superficial, chronic K14.0

Glottitis (*see also* Laryngitis) J04.0

Glue
- ear H65.3-
- sniffing (airplane)—*see* Abuse, drug
  - dependence—*see* Dependence, drug
- GLUT1 deficiency syndrome 1, infantile onset E74.810
- GLUT1 deficiency syndrome 2, childhood onset E74.810

Glycogenosis (diffuse) (generalized)
- pulmonary interstitial J84.842

Glycopenia E16.2

Glycosuria R81
- renal E74.818

Goiter (plunging) (substernal) E04.9
- with
  - hyperthyroidism (recurrent)—*see* Hyperthyroidism, with, goiter
  - thyrotoxicosis—*see* Hyperthyroidism, with, goiter
- adenomatous—*see* Goiter, nodular
- congenital
  - transitory, with normal functioning P72.0
- due to
  - iodine-deficiency (endemic) E01.2
- endemic (iodine-deficiency) E01.2
  - diffuse E01.0
  - multinodular E01.1
- iodine-deficiency (endemic) E01.2
  - diffuse E01.0
  - multinodular E01.1
  - nodular E01.1
- lingual Q89.2

Goiter, *continued*
- lymphadenoid E06.3
- neonatal NEC P72.0
- nodular (nontoxic) (due to) E04.9
  - endemic E01.1
  - iodine-deficiency E01.1
  - sporadic E04.9
- nontoxic E04.9
  - diffuse (colloid) E04.0
  - multinodular E04.2
  - simple E04.0
  - specified NEC E04.8
  - uninodular E04.1
- simple E04.0

Goldberg syndrome Q89.8

Goldberg-Maxwell syndrome E34.51

Goldenhar (-Gorlin) syndrome Q87.0

Goldflam-Erb disease or syndrome G70.00
- with exacerbation (acute) G70.01
- in crisis G70.01

Goldscheider's disease Q81.8

Goldstein's disease (familial hemorrhagic telangiectasia) I78.0

Gonococcus, gonococcal (disease) (infection) (*see also* Disease, diseased) A54.9
- conjunctiva, conjunctivitis (neonatorum) A54.31
- eye A54.30
  - conjunctivitis A54.31
  - newborn A54.31
- fallopian tubes (acute) (chronic) A54.24
- genitourinary (organ) (system) (tract) (acute)
  - lower A54.00
- pelviperitonitis A54.24
- pelvis (acute) (chronic) A54.24
- pyosalpinx (acute) (chronic) A54.24
- urethra (acute) (chronic) A54.01
  - with abscess (accessory gland) (periurethral) A54.1
- vulva (acute) (chronic) A54.02

Gonorrhea (acute) (chronic) A54.9
- Bartholin's gland (acute) (chronic) (purulent) A54.02
  - with abscess (accessory gland) (periurethral) A54.1
- bladder A54.01
- cervix A54.03
- conjunctiva, conjunctivitis (neonatorum) A54.31
- contact Z20.2
- exposure to Z20.2
- fallopian tube A54.24
- lower genitourinary tract A54.00
- ovary (acute) (chronic) A54.24
- pelvis (acute) (chronic) A54.24
  - female pelvic inflammatory disease A54.24
- urethra A54.01
- vagina A54.02
- vulva A54.02

Gorlin-Chaudry-Moss syndrome Q87.0

Gougerot-Carteaud disease or syndrome (confluent reticulate papillomatosis) L83

Gouley's syndrome (constrictive pericarditis) I31.1

Gout, gouty (acute) (attack) (flare)—*see also* Gout M10.9
- idiopathic M10.0-
  - ankle M10.07-
  - elbow M10.02-
  - foot joint M10.07-
  - hand joint M10.04-
  - hip M10.05-
  - knee M10.06-
  - multiple site M10.09
  - shoulder M10.01-
  - vertebrae M10.08

Gower's
- muscular dystrophy G71.01
- syndrome (vasovagal attack) R55

Graft-versus-host disease D89.813
- acute D89.810
- acute on chronic D89.812
- chronic D89.811

Grain mite (itch) B88.0

Granular—*see also* Disease, diseased
- inflammation, pharynx J31.2

Granuloma L92.9
- abdomen
  - from residual foreign body L92.3
  - pyogenicum L98.0
- annulare (perforating) L92.0
- beryllium (skin) L92.3
- brain (any site) G06.0
- candidal (cutaneous) B37.2
- cerebral (any site) G06.0
- foreign body (in soft tissue) NEC M60.2-
  - ankle M60.27-
  - foot M60.27-
  - forearm M60.23-
  - hand M60.24-
  - lower leg M60.26-
  - pelvic region M60.25-
  - shoulder region M60.21-
  - skin L92.3
  - specified site NEC M60.28
  - subcutaneous tissue L92.3
  - thigh M60.25-
  - upper arm M60.22-
- gland (lymph) I88.8
- hepatic NEC K75.3
  - in (due to)
    - sarcoidosis D86.89
- Hodgkin C81.9-
- intracranial (any site) G06.0
- monilial (cutaneous) B37.2
- operation wound T81.89
  - foreign body—*see* Foreign body
  - stitch T81.89
- orbit, orbital H05.11-
- pyogenic, pyogenicum (of) (skin) L98.0
- rectum K62.89
- reticulohistiocytic D76.3
- septic (skin) L98.0
- silica (skin) L92.3
- skin L92.9
  - from residual foreign body L92.3
  - pyogenicum L98.0
- stitch (postoperative) T81.89
- suppurative (skin) L98.0
- telangiectaticum (skin) L98.0
- umbilical (umbilicus) P83.81

Granulomatosis L92.9
- with polyangiitis M31.3
- eosinophilic, with polyangiitis [EGPA] M30.1
- progressive septic D71

Grawitz tumor C64.-

Green sickness D50.8

Grief F43.21
- prolonged F43.29
- reaction (*see also* Disorder, adjustment) F43.20

Grinding, teeth
- psychogenic F45.8
- sleep related G47.63

Grisel's disease M43.6

Growing pains, children R29.898

Growth (fungoid) (neoplastic) (new)—*see also* Table of Neoplasms in the complete *ICD-10-CM* manual
- adenoid (vegetative) J35.8
- benign—*see* Neoplasm, benign, by site in Table of Neoplasms in the complete *ICD-10-CM* manual
- malignant—*see* Neoplasm, malignant, by site in Table of Neoplasms in the complete *ICD-10-CM* manual
- rapid, childhood Z00.2
- secondary—*see* Neoplasm, secondary, by site in Table of Neoplasms in the complete *ICD-10-CM* manual

Gruby's disease B35.0

Guerin-Stern syndrome Q74.3

Guinon's disease (motor-verbal tic) F95.2

Gumboil K04.7

Gynecological examination (periodic) (routine) Z01.419
- with abnormal findings Z01.411

Gynecomastia N62

Gyrate scalp Q82.8

H

Haemophilus (H.) influenzae, as cause of disease classified elsewhere B96.3

Hailey-Hailey disease Q82.8

Hair—*see also* Disease, diseased
- plucking F63.3
  - in stereotyped movement disorder F98.4
- tourniquet syndrome—*see also* Constriction, external, by site
  - finger S60.44-
  - penis S30.842
  - thumb S60.34-
  - toe S90.44-

Hairball in stomach T18.2

Hair-pulling, pathological (compulsive) F63.3

Halitosis R19.6

Hallerman-Streiff syndrome Q87.0

Hallucination R44.3
- auditory R44.0
- gustatory R44.2
- olfactory R44.2
- specified NEC R44.2
- tactile R44.2
- visual R44.1

Hallux
- deformity (acquired) NEC M20.5X-
- limitus M20.5X-
- rigidus congenital Q74.2
- valgus (acquired) M20.1-
  - congenital Q66.6
- varus congenital Q66.3-

Hamartoma, hamartoblastoma Q85.9

Hamartosis Q85.9

Hammer toe (acquired) NEC—*see also* Deformity, toe, hammer toe
- congenital Q66.89

Hand-foot syndrome L27.1

Handicap, handicapped
- educational Z55.9
  - specified NEC Z55.8

Hangover (alcohol) F10.129

Hanhart's syndrome Q87.0

Hardening
- brain G93.89

Harelip (complete) (incomplete)—*see* Cleft, lip

Harlequin (newborn) Q80.4

Harmful use (of)
- alcohol F10.10
- cannabinoids—*see* Abuse, drug, cannabis
- cocaine—*see* Abuse, drug, cocaine
- drug—*see* Abuse, drug
- hallucinogens—*see* Abuse, drug
- PCP (phencyclidine)—*see* Abuse, drug

Hashimoto's (struma lymphomatosa) E06.3

Hashitoxicosis (transient) E06.3

Haverhill fever A25.1

Hay fever (*see also* Fever, hay) J30.1

Hb (abnormal)
- Bart's disease D56.0
- disease—*see* Disease, hemoglobin
- trait—*see* Trait

Head—*see* Disease, diseased

Headache R51.9
- with
  - orthostatic component NEC R51.0
  - positional component NEC R51.0
- cervicogenic G44.86
- chronic daily R51.9
- cluster G44.009
  - intractable G44.001
  - not intractable G44.009
- daily chronic R51.9
- histamine G44.009
  - intractable G44.001
  - not intractable G44.009
- migraine (type)—*see also* Migraine G43.909

Headache, *continued*
- nasal septum R51.9
- periodic syndromes in adults and children G43.C0
  - with refractory migraine G43.C1
  - intractable G43.C1
  - not intractable G43.C0
  - without refractory migraine G43.C0
- tension (-type) G44.209
  - chronic G44.229
    - intractable G44.221
    - not intractable G44.229
  - episodic G44.219
    - intractable G44.211
    - not intractable G44.219
  - intractable G44.201
  - not intractable G44.209

Hearing examination Z01.10
- abnormal findings NEC Z01.118
- following failed hearing screening Z01.110
- for hearing conservation and treatment Z01.12
- infant or child (over 28 days old) Z00.12-

Heart—*see* condition

Heart beat
- abnormality R00.9
  - specified NEC R00.8
- awareness R00.2
- rapid R00.0
- slow R00.1

Heartburn R12
- psychogenic F45.8

Heat (effects) T67.9
- apoplexy T67.01
- burn (*see also* Burn) L55.9
- cramps T67.2
- exertional T67.02
- exhaustion T67.5
  - anhydrotic T67.3
  - due to
    - salt (and water) depletion T67.4
    - water depletion T67.3
      - ~ with salt depletion T67.4
- fatigue (transient) T67.6
- fever T67.01
- hyperpyrexia T67.01
- prickly L74.0
- pyrexia T67.01
- rash L74.0
- stroke T67.01
  - exertional T67.02
  - specified NEC T67.09
- syncope T67.1

Heavy-for-dates NEC (infant) (4000g to 4499g) P08.1
- exceptionally (4500g or more) P08.0

Heerfordt's disease D86.89

Hegglin's anomaly or syndrome D72.0

Heinz body anemia, congenital D58.2

Heloma L84

Hemangioendothelioma—*see also* Neoplasm, uncertain behavior, by site in Table of Neoplasms in the complete *ICD-10-CM* manual
- benign D18.00
  - skin D18.01
  - specified site NEC D18.09
- bone (diffuse)—*see* Neoplasm, bone, malignant in Table of Neoplasms in the complete *ICD-10-CM* manual
- epithelioid—*see also* Neoplasm, uncertain behavior, by site in Table of Neoplasms in the complete *ICD-10-CM* manual
  - malignant—*see* Neoplasm, malignant, by site in Table of Neoplasms in the complete *ICD-10-CM* manual
- malignant—*see* Neoplasm, connective tissue, malignant in Table of Neoplasms in the complete *ICD-10-CM* manual

Hemangiofibroma—*see* Neoplasm, benign, by site in Table of Neoplasms in the complete *ICD-10-CM* manual

Hemangiolipoma—*see* Lipoma

Hemangioma D18.00
- arteriovenous D18.00

Hemangioma, *continued*
- skin D18.01
- specified site NEC D18.09
- capillary I78.1
  - skin D18.01
  - specified site NEC D18.09
- cavernous D18.00
  - skin D18.01
  - specified site NEC D18.09
- epithelioid D18.00
  - skin D18.01
  - specified site NEC D18.09
- histiocytoid D18.00
  - skin D18.01
  - specified site NEC D18.09
- infantile D18.00
  - skin D18.01
  - specified site NEC D18.09
- intramuscular D18.00
  - skin D18.01
  - specified site NEC D18.09
- juvenile D18.00
- malignant—*see* Neoplasm, connective tissue, malignant in Table of Neoplasms in the complete *ICD-10-CM* manual
- plexiform D18.00
  - skin D18.01
  - specified site NEC D18.09
- racemose D18.00
  - skin D18.01
  - specified site NEC D18.09
- sclerosing—*see* Neoplasm, skin, benign in Table of Neoplasms in the complete *ICD-10-CM* manual
- simplex D18.00
  - skin D18.01
  - specified site NEC D18.09
- skin D18.01
- specified site NEC D18.09
- venous D18.00
  - skin D18.01
  - specified site NEC D18.09
- verrucous keratotic D18.00
  - skin D18.01
  - specified site NEC D18.09

Hemangiomatosis (systemic) I78.8
- involving single site—*see* Hemangioma

Hemarthrosis (nontraumatic) M25.00
- ankle M25.07-
- elbow M25.02-
- foot joint M25.07-
- hand joint M25.04-
- hip M25.05-
- in hemophilic arthropathy—*see* Arthropathy, hemophilic
- knee M25.06-
- shoulder M25.01-
- specified joint NEC M25.08
- traumatic—*see* Sprain, by site
- vertebrae M25.08
- wrist M25.03

Hematemesis K92.0
- with ulcer—*code by* site under Ulcer, with hemorrhage K27.4
- newborn, neonatal P54.0
  - due to swallowed maternal blood P78.2

Hematocele
- female NEC N94.89
  - with ectopic pregnancy O00.90
    - with uterine pregnancy O00.91

Hematochezia (*see also* Melena) K92.1

Hematoma (traumatic) (skin surface intact)—*see also* Contusion
- with
  - injury of internal organs—*see* Injury, by site
  - open wound—*see* Wound, open
- auricle—*see* Contusion, ear
  - nontraumatic—*see* Disorder
- birth injury NEC P15.8
- brain (traumatic)
  - with
    - cerebral laceration or contusion (diffuse)—*see* Injury, intracranial, diffuse

Hematoma, *continued*
- cerebellar, traumatic S06.37-
- newborn NEC P52.4
  - birth injury P10.1
- intracerebral, traumatic—*see* Injury, intracranial, intracerebral hemorrhage
- nontraumatic—*see* Hemorrhage, intracranial
- subarachnoid, arachnoid, traumatic—*see* Injury, intracranial, subarachnoid hemorrhage
- subdural, traumatic—*see* Injury, intracranial, subdural hemorrhage
- breast (nontraumatic) N64.89
- cerebral—*see* Hematoma, brain
- cerebrum
  - left S06.35-
  - right S06.34-
- face, birth injury P15.4
- genital organ NEC (nontraumatic)
  - female (nonobstetric) N94.89
    - traumatic S30.202
- internal organs—*see* Injury, by site
- intracerebral, traumatic—*see* Injury, intracranial, intracerebral hemorrhage
- intraoperative—*see* Complications
- labia (nontraumatic) (nonobstetric) N90.89
- pelvis (female) (nontraumatic) (nonobstetric) N94.89
  - traumatic—*see* Injury, by site
- perianal (nontraumatic) K64.5
- pinna H61.12-
- superficial, newborn P54.5
- vagina (ruptured) (nontraumatic) N89.8

Hematomyelitis G04.90

Hematopneumothorax (*See* Hemothorax)

Hematopoiesis, cyclic D70.4

Hematuria R31.9
- benign (familial) (of childhood)
  - essential microscopic R31.1
- gross R31.0
- microscopic NEC (with symptoms) R31.29
  - asymptomatic R31.21
  - benign essential R31.1

Hemiatrophy R68.89
- face, facial, progressive (Romberg) G51.8

Hemichorea G25.5

Hemiplegia G81.9-
- ascending NEC G81.9-
  - spinal G95.89
- flaccid G81.0-
- hysterical F44.4
- newborn NEC P91.88
  - birth injury P11.9
- spastic G81.1-
  - congenital G80.2

Hemispasm (facial) R25.2

Hemitremor R25.1

Hemochromatosis E83.119
- due to repeated red blood cell transfusion E83.111
- hereditary (primary) E83.110
- neonatal P78.84
- primary E83.110
- specified NEC E83.118

Hemoglobin—*see also* Disease, diseased
- abnormal (disease)—*see* Disease, hemoglobin
- AS genotype D57.3
- Constant Spring D58.2
- E-beta thalassemia D56.5
- fetal, hereditary persistence (HPFH) D56.4
- H Constant Spring D56.0
- low NOS D64.9
- S (Hb S), heterozygous D57.3

Hemoglobinemia D59.9
- paroxysmal D59.6
  - nocturnal D59.5

Hemoglobinopathy (mixed) D58.2
- with thalassemia D56.8
- sickle-cell D57.1
  - with thalassemia D57.40
    - with
      ~ acute chest syndrome D57.411
      ~ cerebral vascular involvement D57.413

Hemoglobinopathy, *continued*
- ~ crisis (painful) D57.419
- ~ with specified complication NEC D57.418
  ◊ splenic sequestration D57.412
  ◊ vasoocclusive pain D57.419
  - without crisis D57.40

Hemoglobinuria R82.3
- with anemia, hemolytic, acquired (chronic) NEC D59.6
- cold (paroxysmal) (with Raynaud's syndrome) D59.6
  - agglutinin D59.12
- due to exertion or hemolysis NEC D59.6
- intermittent D59.6
- march D59.6
- nocturnal (paroxysmal) D59.5
- paroxysmal (cold) D59.6
  - nocturnal D59.5

Hemopericardium I31.2
- newborn P54.8

Hemophilia (classical) (familial) (hereditary) D66
- A D66
- B D67
- C D68.1
- acquired D68.311
- autoimmune D68.311
- secondary D68.311
- vascular D68.0

Hemoptysis R04.2
- newborn P26.9

Hemorrhage, hemorrhagic (concealed) R58
- acute idiopathic pulmonary, in infants R04.81
- adenoid J35.8
- adrenal (capsule) (gland) E27.49
  - medulla E27.8
  - newborn P54.4
- alveolar
  - lung, newborn P26.8
- anemia (chronic) D50.0
  - acute D62
- antepartum (with)
  - before 20 weeks gestation O20.9
    - specified type NEC O20.8
    - threatened abortion O20.0
- anus K62.5
- basilar (ganglion) I61.0
- bowel K92.2
  - newborn P54.3
- brain (miliary) (nontraumatic)—*see* Hemorrhage, intracranial, intracerebral
  - due to
    - birth injury P10.1
  - newborn P52.4
    - birth injury P10.1
- brainstem (nontraumatic) I61.3
  - traumatic S06.38-
- breast N64.59
- bulbar I61.5
- cecum K92.2
- cerebellar, cerebellum (nontraumatic) I61.4
  - newborn P52.6
  - traumatic S06.37-
- cerebral, cerebrum—*see also* Hemorrhage, intracranial, intracerebral
  - newborn (anoxic) P52.4
    - birth injury P10.1
  - lobe I61.1
- cerebromeningeal I61.8
- cerebrospinal—*see* Hemorrhage, intracranial, intracerebral
- colon K92.2
- conjunctiva H11.3-
  - newborn P54.8
- corpus luteum (ruptured) cyst N83.1-
- cortical (brain) I61.1
- cranial—*see* Hemorrhage, intracranial
- cutaneous R23.3
  - due to autosensitivity, erythrocyte D69.2
  - newborn P54.5
- disease D69.9
  - newborn P53
- duodenum, duodenal K92.2
  - ulcer—*see* Ulcer, duodenum, with, hemorrhage
- epicranial subaponeurotic (massive), birth injury P12.2

Hemorrhage, hemorrhagic, *continued*
- epidural (traumatic)—*see also* Injury, intracranial
  - nontraumatic I62.1
- esophagus K22.89
  - varix I85.01
- extradural (traumatic)—*see* Injury, intracranial, epidural hemorrhage
  - birth injury P10.8
  - newborn (anoxic) (nontraumatic) P52.8
  - nontraumatic I62.1
- gastric—*see* Hemorrhage, stomach
- gastroenteric K92.2
  - newborn P54.3
- gastrointestinal (tract) K92.2
  - newborn P54.3
- genitourinary (tract) NOS R31.9
- graafian follicle cyst (ruptured) N83.0-
- intermenstrual (regular) N92.3
  - irregular N92.1
- internal (organs) EC R58
  - capsule I61.0
  - newborn P54.8
- intestine K92.2
  - newborn P54.3
- intra-alveolar (lung), newborn P26.8
- intracerebral (nontraumatic)—*see* Hemorrhage, intracranial, intracerebral
- intracranial (nontraumatic) I62.9
  - birth injury P10.9
  - epidural, nontraumatic I62.1
  - extradural, nontraumatic I62.1
  - intracerebral (nontraumatic) (in) I61.9
    - brain stem I61.3
    - cerebellum I61.4
    - hemisphere I61.2
      ~ cortical (superficial) I61.1
      ~ subcortical (deep) I61.0
    - intraventricular I61.5
    - multiple localized I61.6
    - newborn P52.4
      ~ birth injury P10.1
    - specified NEC I61.8
    - superficial I61.1
  - subarachnoid (nontraumatic) (from) I60.9
    - intracranial (cerebral) artery I60.7
      ~ anterior communicating I60.2-
      ~ basilar I60.4
      ~ carotid siphon and bifurcation I60.0-
      ~ communicating I60.7
        ◊ anterior I60.2-
        ◊ posterior I60.3-
      ~ middle cerebral I60.1-
      ~ posterior communicating I60.3-
      ~ specified artery NEC I60.6
      ~ vertebral I60.5-
    - newborn P52.5
      ~ birth injury P10.3
    - specified NEC I60.8-
    - traumatic S06.6X-
  - subdural (nontraumatic) I62.00
    - acute I62.01
    - birth injury P10.0
    - chronic I62.03
    - newborn (anoxic) (hypoxic) P52.8
      ~ birth injury P10.0
    - spinal G95.19
    - subacute I62.02
    - traumatic—*see* Injury, intracranial, subdural hemorrhage
- intrapontine I61.3
- intraventricular I61.5
  - newborn (nontraumatic) (*see also* Newborn, affected by, hemorrhage) P52.3
    - due to birth injury P10.2
    - grade
      ~ 1 P52.0
      ~ 2 P52.1
      ~ 3 P52.21
      ~ 4 P52.22
- lenticular striate artery I61.0
- lung R04.89
  - newborn P26.9
    - massive P26.1

Hemorrhage, hemorrhagic, *continued*
- ▪ specified NEC P26.8
- medulla I61.3
- membrane (brain) I60.8-
- meninges, meningeal (brain) (middle) I60.8-
- mouth K13.79
- mucous membrane NEC R58
  - newborn P54.8
- nail (subungual) L60.8
- nasal turbinate R04.0
  - newborn P54.8
- newborn P54.9
  - specified NEC P54.8
- nipple N64.59
- nose R04.0
  - newborn P54.8
- ovary NEC N83.8
- pericardium, pericarditis I31.2
- peritonsillar tissue J35.8
  - due to infection J36
- pituitary (gland) E23.6
- petechial R23.3
  - due to autosensitivity, erythrocyte D69.2
- pons, pontine I61.3
- posterior fossa (nontraumatic) I61.8
  - newborn P52.6
- postnasal R04.0
- pulmonary R04.89
  - newborn P26.9
    - ▪ massive P26.1
    - ▪ specified NEC P26.8
- purpura (primary) D69.3
- rectum (sphincter) K62.5
  - newborn P54.2
- skin R23.3
  - newborn P54.5
- slipped umbilical ligature P51.8
- stomach K92.2
  - newborn P54.3
  - ulcer—*see* Ulcer, stomach, with, hemorrhage
- subconjunctival—*see also* Hemorrhage, conjunctiva
  - birth injury P15.3
- subcortical (brain) I61.0
- subcutaneous R23.3
- subependymal
  - newborn P52.0
    - ▪ with intraventricular extension P52.1
      - ~ and intracerebral extension P52.22
- subungual L60.8
- suprarenal (capsule) (gland) E27.49
  - newborn P54.4
- tonsil J35.8
- ulcer—*code by* site under Ulcer, with hemorrhage K27.4
- umbilicus, umbilical
  - cord
    - ▪ after birth, newborn P51.9
  - newborn P51.9
    - ▪ massive P51.0
    - ▪ slipped ligature P51.8
  - stump P51.9
- uterus, uterine (abnormal) N93.9
  - dysfunctional or functional N93.8
  - intermenstrual (regular) N92.3
    - ▪ irregular N92.1
  - pubertal N92.2
- vagina (abnormal) N93.9
  - newborn P54.6
- ventricular I61.5
- viscera NEC R58
  - newborn P54.8

Hemorrhoids (bleeding) (without mention of degree) K64.9
- 1st degree (grade/stage I) (without prolapse outside of anal canal) K64.0
- 2nd degree (grade/stage II) (that prolapse with straining but retract spontaneously) K64.1
- 3rd degree (grade/stage III) (that prolapse with straining and require manual replacement back inside anal canal) K64.2
- 4th degree (grade/stage IV) (with prolapsed tissue that cannot be manually replaced) K64.3
- external K64.4
  - with
    - ▪ thrombosis K64.5

Hemorrhoids, *continued*
- internal (without mention of degree) K64.8
- prolapsed K64.8
- skin tags
  - anus K64.4
  - residual K64.4
- specified NEC K64.8
- strangulated (*see also* Hemorrhoids, by degree) K64.8
- thrombosed (*see also* Hemorrhoids, by degree) K64.5
- ulcerated (*see also* Hemorrhoids, by degree) K64.8

Hemothorax
- newborn P54.8

Henoch (-Schönlein) disease or syndrome (purpura) D69.0

Hepatitis K75.9
- acute (infectious) (viral) B17.9
- B B19.10
  - acute B16.9
- C (viral) B19.20
  - acute B17.10
  - chronic B18.2
- catarrhal (acute) B15.9
- chronic K73.9
  - active NEC K73.2
- epidemic B15.9
- fulminant NEC K75.3
  - neonatal giant cell P59.29
- history of
  - B Z86.19
  - C Z86.19
- homologous serum—*see* Hepatitis, viral, type B
- in (due to)
  - congenital (active) P37.1 [K77]
- infectious, infective (acute) (chronic) (subacute) B15.9
- neonatal (idiopathic) (toxic) P59.29
- newborn P59.29
- viral, virus B19.9
  - acute B17.9
    - ▪ C B18.2
  - in remission, any type—*code to* Hepatitis, chronic, by type
  - type
    - ▪ A B15.9
    - ▪ B 19.10
      - ~ acute B16.9
    - ▪ C B19.20
      - ~ acute B17.10
      - ~ chronic B18.2

Hepatomegaly—*see also* Hypertrophy, liver
- in mononucleosis
  - gammaherpesviral B27.09
  - infectious specified NEC B27.89

Hereditary alpha tryptasemia (syndrome) D89.44

Herlitz' syndrome Q81.1

Hernia, hernial (acquired) (recurrent) K46.9
- with
  - gangrene—*see* Hernia, by site, with, gangrene
  - incarceration—*see* Hernia, by site, with, obstruction
  - irreducible—*see* Hernia, by site, with, obstruction
  - obstruction—*see* Hernia, by site, with, obstruction
  - strangulation—*see* Hernia, by site, with, obstruction
- abdomen, abdominal K46.-
- bladder (mucosa) (sphincter)
  - congenital (female) (male) Q79.51
- diaphragm, diaphragmatic K44.9
  - with
    - ▪ gangrene (and obstruction) K44.1
    - ▪ obstruction K44.0
  - congenital Q79.0
- direct (inguinal)—*see* Hernia, inguinal
- diverticulum, intestine—*see* Hernia
- double (inguinal)—*see* Hernia, inguinal, bilateral
- epigastric (*see also* Hernia, ventral) K43.9
- esophageal hiatus—*see* Hernia, hiatal
- external (inguinal)—*see* Hernia, inguinal
- foramen magnum G93.5
  - congenital Q01.8
- hiatal (esophageal) (sliding) K44.9
  - with
    - ▪ gangrene (and obstruction) K44.1
    - ▪ obstruction K44.0
  - congenital Q40.1

Hernia, hernial, *continued*
- indirect (inguinal)—*see* Hernia, inguinal
- incisional K43.2
  - with
    - ▪ gangrene (and obstruction) K43.1
    - ▪ obstruction K43.0
- inguinal (direct) (external) (funicular) (indirect) (internal) (oblique) (scrotal) (sliding) K40.90
  - with
    - ▪ gangrene (and obstruction) K40.40
      - ~ not specified as recurrent K40.40
      - ~ recurrent K40.41
    - ▪ obstruction K40.30
      - ~ not specified as recurrent K40.30
      - ~ recurrent K40.31
  - bilateral K40.20
    - ▪ with
      - ~ gangrene (and obstruction) K40.10
        - ◊ not specified as recurrent K40.10
        - ◊ recurrent K40.11
      - ~ obstruction K40.00
        - ◊ not specified as recurrent K40.00
        - ◊ recurrent K40.01
    - ▪ not specified as recurrent K40.20
    - ▪ recurrent K40.21
  - not specified as recurrent K40.90
  - recurrent K40.91
  - unilateral K40.90
    - ▪ with
      - ~ gangrene (and obstruction) K40.40
        - ◊ not specified as recurrent K40.40
        - ◊ recurrent K40.41
      - ~ obstruction K40.30
        - ◊ not specified as recurrent K40.30
        - ◊ recurrent K40.31
    - ▪ not specified as recurrent K40.90
    - ▪ recurrent K40.91
- irreducible—*see also* Hernia, by site, with obstruction
  - with gangrene—*see* Hernia, by site, with gangrene
- linea (alba) (semilunaris)—*see* Hernia, ventral
- midline—*see* Hernia, ventral
- oblique (inguinal)—*see* Hernia, inguinal
- obstructive—*see also* Hernia, by site, with obstruction
  - with gangrene—*see* Hernia, by site, with gangrene
- scrotum, scrotal—*see* Hernia, inguinal
- sliding (inguinal)—*see also* Hernia, inguinal
  - hiatus—*see* Hernia, hiatal
- spigelian—*see* Hernia, ventral
- spinal—*see* Spina bifida
- strangulated—*see also* Hernia, by site, with obstruction
  - with gangrene—*see* Hernia, by site, with gangrene
- subxiphoid—*see* Hernia, ventral
- supra-umbilicus—*see* Hernia, ventral
- tunica vaginalis Q55.29
- umbilicus, umbilical K42.9
  - with
    - ▪ gangrene (and obstruction) K42.1
    - ▪ obstruction K42.0
- ventral K43.9
  - recurrent—*see* Hernia, incisional
  - incisional K43.2
    - ▪ with
      - ~ gangrene (and obstruction) K43.1
      - ~ obstruction K43.0
  - specified NEC K43.9

Herniation—*see also* Hernia
- brain (stem) G93.5
  - nontraumatic G93.5
  - traumatic S06.A1
- cerebral G93.5
  - nontraumatic G93.5
  - traumatic S06.A1

Herpangina B08.5

Herpes, herpesvirus, herpetic B00.9
- anogenital A60.9
  - urogenital tract A60.00
    - ▪ cervix A60.03
    - ▪ male genital organ NEC A60.02
    - ▪ penis A60.01
    - ▪ specified site NEC A60.09
    - ▪ vagina A60.04
    - ▪ vulva A60.04

Herpes, herpesvirus, herpetic, *continued*
- circinatus B35.4
- encephalitis B00.4
  - due to herpesvirus 7 B10.09
  - specified NEC B10.09
- genital, genitalis A60.00
  - female A60.09
  - male A60.02
- gingivostomatitis B00.2
- human B00.9
  - 1—*see* Herpes, simplex
  - 2—*see* Herpes, simplex
  - 4—*see* Mononucleosis, Epstein-Barr (virus)
  - 7
    - encephalitis B10.09
- meningitis (simplex) B00.3
- pharyngitis, pharyngotonsillitis B00.2
- simplex B00.9
  - complicated NEC B00.89
  - congenital P35.2
  - specified complication NEC B00.89
  - visceral B00.89
- stomatitis B00.2
- tonsurans B35.0 visceral B00.89
- whitlow B00.89

Herter-Gee Syndrome K90.0

Hesitancy
- of micturition R39.11
- urinary R39.11

Heubner-Herter disease K90.0

Hiccup, hiccough R06.6
- psychogenic F45.8

Hidden penis (congenital) Q55.64

Hidradenitis (axillaris) (suppurative) L73.2

High
- altitude effects T70.20
  - anoxia T70.29
  - on
    - ears T70.0
    - sinuses T70.1
  - polycythemia D75.1
- arch
  - foot Q66.7-
  - palate, congenital Q38.5
- basal metabolic rate R94.8
- blood pressure—*see also* Hypertension
  - borderline R03.0
  - reading (incidental) (isolated) (nonspecific), without diagnosis of hypertension R03.0
- cholesterol E78.00
  - with high triglycerides E78.2
- expressed emotional level within family Z63.8
- palate, congenital Q38.5
- risk
  - infant NEC Z76.2
  - sexual behavior (heterosexual) Z72.51
    - bisexual Z72.53
    - homosexual Z72.52
- scrotal testis, testes
  - bilateral Q53.23
  - unilateral Q53.13
- temperature (of unknown origin) R50.9
- triglycerides E78.1
  - with high cholesterol E78.2

Hippel's disease Q85.8

Hirschsprung's disease or megacolon Q43.1

Hirsutism, hirsuties L68.0

Hirudiniasis
- external B88.3

Histiocytosis D76.3
- lipid, lipoid D76.3
- mononuclear phagocytes NEC D76.1
- non-Langerhans cell D76.3
- polyostotic sclerosing D76.3
- sinus, with massive lymphadenopathy D76.3
- syndrome NEC D76.3

Histoplasmosis B39.9
- with pneumonia NEC B39.2
  - capsulati B39.4

Histoplasmosis, *continued*
- disseminated B39.3
- generalized B39.3
- pulmonary B39.2
  - acute B39.0
  - chronic B39.1

History
- family (of)—*see also* History, personal (of)
  - alcohol abuse Z81.1
  - allergy NEC Z84.89
  - anemia Z83.2
  - arthritis Z82.61
  - asthma Z82.5
  - blindness Z82.1
  - cardiac death (sudden) Z82.41
  - carrier of genetic disease Z84.81
  - chromosomal anomaly Z82.79
  - chronic
    - disabling disease NEC Z82.8
    - lower respiratory disease Z82.5
  - colonic polyps Z83.71
  - congenital malformations and deformations Z82.79
    - polycystic kidney Z82.71
  - consanguinity Z84.3
  - deafness Z82.2
  - diabetes mellitus Z83.3
  - disability NEC Z82.8
  - disease or disorder (of)
    - allergic NEC Z84.89
    - behavioral NEC Z81.8
    - blood and blood-forming organs Z83.2
    - cardiovascular NEC Z82.49
    - chronic disabling NEC Z82.8
    - digestive Z83.79
    - ear NEC Z83.52
    - elevated lipoprotein(a) (Lp(a)) Z83.430
    - endocrine NEC Z83.49
    - eye NEC Z83.518
      - glaucoma Z83.511
    - familial hypercholesterolemia Z83.42
    - genitourinary NEC Z84.2
    - glaucoma Z83.511
    - hematological Z83.2
    - immune mechanism Z83.2
    - infectious NEC Z83.1
    - ischemic heart Z82.49
    - kidney Z84.1
    - lipoprotein metabolism Z83.438
    - mental NEC Z81.8
    - metabolic Z83.49
    - musculoskeletal NEC Z82.69
    - neurological NEC Z82.0
    - nutritional Z83.49
    - parasitic NEC Z83.1
    - psychiatric NEC Z81.8
    - respiratory NEC Z83.6
    - skin and subcutaneous tissue NEC Z84.0
    - specified NEC Z84.89
  - drug abuse NEC Z81.3
  - elevated lipoprotein (a) (LP(a)) Z83.430
  - epilepsy Z82.0
  - familial hypercholesterolemia Z83.42
  - genetic disease carrier Z84.81
  - glaucoma Z83.511
  - hearing loss Z82.2
  - human immunodeficiency virus (HIV) infection Z83.0
  - Huntington's chorea Z82.0
  - hypercholesterolemia (familial) Z83.42
  - hyperlipidemia, familial combined Z83.438
  - intellectual disability Z81.0
  - leukemia Z80.6
  - lipidemia NEC Z83.438
  - malignant neoplasm (of) NOS Z80.9
    - bladder Z80.52
    - breast Z80.3
    - bronchus Z80.1
    - digestive organ Z80.0
    - gastrointestinal tract Z80.0
    - genital organ Z80.49
      - ovary Z80.41
      - prostate Z80.42
      - specified organ NEC Z80.49
      - testis Z80.43

History, *continued*
  - hematopoietic NEC Z80.7
  - intrathoracic organ NEC Z80.2
  - kidney Z80.51
  - lung Z80.1
  - lymphatic NEC Z80.7
  - ovary Z80.41
  - prostate Z80.42
  - respiratory organ NEC Z80.2
  - specified site NEC Z80.8
  - testis Z80.43
  - trachea Z80.1
  - urinary organ or tract Z80.59
    - bladder Z80.52
    - kidney Z80.51
  - mental
    - disorder NEC Z81.8
  - multiple endocrine neoplasia (MEN) syndrome Z83.41
  - osteoporosis Z82.62
  - polycystic kidney Z82.71
  - polyps (colon) Z83.71
  - psychiatric disorder Z81.8
  - psychoactive substance abuse NEC Z81.3
  - respiratory condition NEC Z83.6
    - asthma and other lower respiratory conditions Z82.5
  - self-harmful behavior Z81.8
  - SIDS (sudden infant death syndrome) Z84.82
  - skin condition Z84.0
  - specified condition NEC Z84.89
  - stroke (cerebrovascular) Z82.3
  - substance abuse NEC Z81.4
    - alcohol Z81.1
    - drug NEC Z81.3
    - psychoactive NEC Z81.3
    - tobacco Z81.2
  - sudden cardiac death Z82.41
  - sudden infant death syndrome Z84.82
  - tobacco abuse Z81.2
  - violence, violent behavior Z81.8
  - visual loss Z82.1
- personal (of)—*see also* History, family (of)
  - abuse
    - childhood Z62.819
      - forced labor or sexual exploitation in childhood Z62.813
      - physical Z62.810
      - psychological Z62.811
      - sexual Z62.810
  - alcohol dependence F10.21
  - allergy (to) Z88.9
    - antibiotic agent NEC Z88.1
    - drugs, medicaments and biological substances Z88.9
      - specified NEC Z88.8
    - food Z91.018
      - additives Z91.02
      - beef Z91.014
      - eggs Z91.012
      - lamb Z91.014
      - mammalian meats Z91.014
      - milk products Z91.011
      - peanuts Z91.010
      - pork Z91.014
      - red meats Z91.014
      - seafood Z91.013
      - specified food NEC Z91.018
    - insect Z91.038
      - bee Z91.030
    - latex Z91.040
    - medicinal agents Z88.9
      - specified NEC Z88.8
    - narcotic agent Z88.5
    - nonmedicinal agents Z91.048
    - penicillin Z88.0
    - serum Z88.7
    - sulfonamides Z88.2
    - vaccine Z88.7
  - anaphylactic shock Z87.892
  - anaphylaxis Z87.892
  - behavioral disorders Z86.59
  - brain injury (traumatic) Z87.820

History, *continued*
- cancer—*see* History, personal (of), malignant neoplasm (of)
- cardiac arrest (death), successfully resuscitated Z86.74
- CAR-T (Chimeric Antigen Receptor T-cell) therapy Z92.850
- cellular therapy Z92.859
  - specified NEC Z92.858
- cerebral infarction without residual deficit Z86.73
- chemotherapy for neoplastic condition Z92.21
- Chimeric Antigen Receptor T-cell (CAR-T) therapy Z92.850
- cleft lip (corrected) Z87.730
- cleft palate (corrected) Z87.730
- congenital malformation (corrected) Z87.798
  - circulatory system (corrected) Z87.74
  - digestive system (corrected) NEC Z87.738
  - ear (corrected) Z87.721
  - eye (corrected) Z87.720
  - face and neck (corrected) Z87.790
  - genitourinary system (corrected) NEC Z87.718
  - heart (corrected) Z87.74
  - integument (corrected) Z87.76
  - limb(s) (corrected) Z87.76
  - musculoskeletal system (corrected) Z87.76
  - neck (corrected) Z87.790
  - nervous system (corrected) NEC Z87.728
  - respiratory system (corrected) Z87.75
  - sense organs (corrected) NEC Z87.728
  - specified NEC Z87.798
- coronavirus (disease) (novel) 2019 Z86.16
- disease or disorder (of) Z87.898
  - blood and blood-forming organs Z86.2
  - connective tissue NEC Z87.39
  - ear Z86.69
  - endocrine Z86.39
    - ~ specified type NEC Z86.39
  - eye Z86.69
  - hematological Z86.2
  - Hodgkin Z85.71
  - immune mechanism Z86.2
  - infectious Z86.19
    - ~ Methicillin resistant Staphylococcus aureus (MRSA) Z86.14
    - ~ tuberculosis Z86.11
  - mental NEC Z86.59
  - metabolic Z86.39
    - ~ specified type NEC Z86.39
  - musculoskeletal NEC Z87.39
  - nervous system Z86.69
  - nutritional Z86.39
  - respiratory system NEC Z87.09
  - sense organs Z86.69
  - specified site or type NEC Z87.898
  - urinary system NEC Z87.448
- drug therapy
  - antineoplastic chemotherapy Z92.21
  - immunosupression Z92.25
  - inhaled steroids Z92.240
  - monoclonal drug Z92.22
  - specified NEC Z92.29
  - steroid Z92.241
  - systemic steroids Z92.241
- encephalitis Z86.61
- extracorporeal membrane oxygenation (ECMO) Z92.81
- fall, falling Z91.81
- forced labor or sexual exploitation in childhood Z62.813
- gene therapy Z92.86
- hepatitis
  - B Z86.19
  - C Z86.19
- Hodgkin disease Z85.71
- hypospadias (corrected) Z87.710
- immunosupression therapy Z92.25
- infection NEC Z86.19
  - central nervous system Z86.61
  - latent tuberculosis Z86.15
  - Methicillin resistant Staphylococcus aureus (MRSA) Z86.14

History, *continued*
- in situ neoplasm
  - breast Z86.000
  - cervix uteri Z86.001
  - digestive organs, specified NEC Z86.004
  - esophagus Z86.003
  - genital organs, specified NEC Z86.002
  - melanoma Z86.006
  - middle ear Z86.005
  - oral cavity Z86.003
  - respiratory system Z86.005
  - skin Z86.007
  - specified NEC Z86.008
  - stomach Z86.003
- in utero procedure while a fetus Z98.871
- latent tuberculosis Z86.15
- leukemia Z85.6
- lymphoma (non-Hodgkin) Z85.72
- malignant melanoma (skin) Z85.820
- malignant neoplasm (of) Z85.9
  - bone Z85.830
  - brain Z85.841
  - carcinoid—*see* History, personal (of), malignant neoplasm, by site, carcinoid
  - endocrine gland NEC Z85.858
  - eye Z85.840
  - hematopoietic NEC Z85.79
  - kidney NEC Z85.528
    - ~ carcinoid Z85.520
- maltreatment Z91.89
- melanoma Z85.820
- meningitis Z86.61
- mental disorder Z86.59
- Methicillin resistant Staphylococcus aureus (MRSA) Z86.14
- neglect (in)
  - childhood Z62.812
- neoplasm
  - in situ—*see* Table of Neoplasms in the complete *ICD-10-CM* manual
  - malignant—*see* Table of Neoplasms in the complete *ICD-10-CM* manual
  - uncertain behavior Z86.03
- nephrotic syndrome Z87.441
- nicotine dependence Z87.891
- noncompliance with medical treatment or regimen—*see* Noncompliance
- nutritional deficiency Z86.39
- parasuicide (attempt) Z91.51
- physical trauma NEC Z87.828
  - self-harm or suicide attempt Z91.51
- pneumonia (recurrent) Z87.01
- poisoning NEC Z91.89
  - self-harm or suicide attempt Z91.51
- procedure while a fetus Z98.871
- prolonged reversible ischemic neurologic deficit (PRIND) Z86.73
- psychological
  - abuse
    - ~ child Z62.811
  - trauma, specified NEC Z91.49
- respiratory condition NEC Z87.09
- retained foreign body fully removed Z87.821
- risk factors NEC Z91.89
- self-harm
  - nonsuicidal Z91.52
  - suicidal Z91.51
- self-inflicted injury without suicidal intent Z91.52
  - self-injury Z91.52
  - nonsuicidal Z91.52
- self-mutilation Z91.52
- self-poisoning attempt Z91.51
- specified NEC Z87.898
- steroid therapy (systemic) Z92.241
  - inhaled Z92.240
- stroke without residual deficits Z86.73
- substance abuse NEC F10-F19
- sudden cardiac arrest Z86.74
- sudden cardiac death successfully resuscitated Z86.74
- suicidal behavior Z91.51
- suicide attempt Z91.51
- surgery NEC Z98.890

History, *continued*
- tobacco dependence Z87.891
- transient ischemic attack (TIA) without residual deficits Z86.73
- trauma (physical) NEC Z87.828
  - psychological NEC Z91.49
  - self-harm Z91.51
- traumatic brain injury Z87.820

HIV (*see also* Human, immunodeficiency virus) B20
- laboratory evidence (nonconclusive) R75
- positive, seropositive Z21
- nonconclusive test (in infants) R75

Hives (bold)—*see* Urticaria

Hoarseness R49.0

Hoffmann's syndrome E03.9 *[G73.7]*

Homelessness Z59.00
- sheltered Z59.01
- unsheltered Z59.02

Homocysteinemia R79.83

Hooded
- clitoris Q52.6
- penis Q55.69

Hordeolum (eyelid) (externum) (recurrent) H00.01-
- internum H00.02-
  - left H00.026
    - lower H00.025
    - upper H00.024
  - right H00.023
    - lower H00.022
    - upper H00.021
- left H00.016
  - lower H00.015
  - upper H00.014
- right H00.013
  - lower H00.012
  - upper H00.011

Horseshoe kidney (congenital) Q63.1

Hospitalism in children—*see* Disorder, adjustment

Household, housing circumstance affecting care Z59.9
- specified NEC Z59.89

HSCT-TMA (hematopoietic stem cell transplantation-associated thrombotic microangiopathy) M31.11

Human
- bite (open wound)—*see also* Bite
  - intact skin surface—*see* Bite
- herpesvirus—*see* Herpes
- immunodeficiency virus (HIV) disease (infection) B20
  - asymptomatic status Z21
  - contact Z20.6
  - counseling Z71.7
  - exposure to Z20.6
  - laboratory evidence R75
- papillomavirus (HPV)
  - screening for Z11.51

Hunger T73.0
- air, psychogenic F45.8

Hunter's
- syndrome E76.1

Hunt's
- dyssynergia cerebellaris myoclonica G11.19

Hutchinson's
- disease, meaning
  - pompholyx (cheiropompholyx) L30.1

Hyaline membrane (disease) (lung) (pulmonary) (newborn) P22.0

Hydatid
- Morgagni
  - female Q50.5
  - male (epididymal) Q55.4
    - testicular Q55.29

Hydradenitis (axillaris) (suppurative) L73.2

Hydramnios O40.-

Hydrarthrosis—*see also* Effusion, joint
- intermittent M12.4-
  - ankle M12.47-
  - elbow M12.42-
  - foot joint M12.47-

Hydrarthrosis, *continued*
- – hand joint M12.44-
- – hip M12.45-
- – knee M12.46-
- – multiple site M12.49
- – shoulder M12.41-
- – specified joint NEC M12.48
- – wrist M12.43-

Hydroadenitis (axillaris) (suppurative) L73.2

Hydrocele (spermatic cord) (testis) (tunica vaginalis) N43.3
- • communicating N43.2
  - – congenital P83.5
- • congenital P83.5
- • encysted N43.0
- • female NEC N94.89
- • infected N43.1
- • newborn P83.5
- • round ligament N94.89
- • specified NEC N43.2
- • spinalis—*see* Spina bifida
- • vulva N90.89

Hydrocephalus (acquired) (external) (internal) (malignant) (recurrent) G91.9
- • aqueduct Sylvius stricture Q03.0
- • communicating G91.0
- • congenital (external) (internal) Q03.9
  - – with spina bifida Q05.4
    - ■ cervical Q05.0
    - ■ dorsal Q05.1
    - ■ lumbar Q05.2
    - ■ lumbosacral Q05.2
    - ■ sacral Q05.3
    - ■ thoracic Q05.1
    - ■ thoracolumbar Q05.1
  - – specified NEC Q03.8
- • due to toxoplasmosis (congenital) P37.1
- • foramen Magendie block (acquired) G91.1
  - – congenital (*see also* Hydrocephalus, congenital) Q03.1
- • in (due to)
  - – infectious disease NEC B89 [G91.4]
  - – neoplastic disease NEC (*see also* Table of Neoplasms in the complete *ICD-10-CM* manual) G91.4
  - – parasitic disease B89 [G91.4]
- • newborn Q03.9
  - – with spina bifida—*see* Spina bifida, with hydrocephalus
- • noncommunicating G91.1
- • normal pressure G91.2
  - – secondary G91.0
- • obstructive G91.1
- • otitic G93.2
- • post-traumatic NEC G91.3
- • secondary G91.4
  - – post-traumatic G91.3
- • specified NEC G91.8

Hydromicrocephaly Q02

Hydromphalos (since birth) Q45.8

Hydronephrosis (atrophic) (early) (functionless) (intermittent) (primary) (secondary) NEC N13.30
- • with
  - – obstruction (by) (of)
    - ■ renal calculus N13.2
    - ■ ureteral NEC N13.1
      - ~ calculus N13.2
    - ■ ureteropelvic junction N13.0
      - ~ congenital Q62.11
      - ~ with infection N13.6
  - – ureteral stricture NEC N13.1
- • congenital Q62.0
- • specified type NEC N13.39

Hydroperitoneum R18.8

Hydrophthalmos Q15.0

Hydrops R60.9
- • abdominis R18.8
- • endolymphatic H81.0-
- • fetalis P83.2
  - – due to
    - ■ ABO isoimmunization P56.0
    - ■ alpha thalassemia D56.0
    - ■ hemolytic disease P56.90
      - ~ specified NEC P56.99

Hydrops, *continued*
- - ■ isoimmunization (ABO) (Rh) P56.0
  - ■ other specified nonhemolytic disease NEC P83.2
  - ■ Rh incompatibility P56.0
- • newborn (idiopathic) P83.2
  - – due to
    - ■ ABO isoimmunization P56.0
    - ■ alpha thalassemia D56.0
    - ■ hemolytic disease P56.90
      - ~ specified NEC P56.99
    - ■ isoimmunization (ABO) (Rh) P56.0
    - ■ Rh incompatibility P56.0
- • pericardium—*see* Pericarditis
- • spermatic cord—*see* Hydrocele

Hydropyonephrosis N13.6

Hydrorrhea (nasal) J34.89

Hydrosadenitis (axillaris) (suppurative) L73.2

Hydroxykynureninuria E70.89

Hyperacidity (gastric) K31.89
- • psychogenic F45.8

Hyperactive, hyperactivity F90.9
- • bowel sounds R19.12
- • child F90.9
  - – attention deficit—*see* Disorder, attention-deficit hyperactivity
- • detrusor muscle N32.81
- • gastrointestinal K31.89
  - – psychogenic F45.8
- • nasal mucous membrane J34.3

Hyperadrenocorticism E24.9
- • congenital E25.0
- • iatrogenic E24.2
  - – correct substance properly administered—*see* Table of Drugs and Chemicals, by drug, adverse effect
  - – overdose or wrong substance given or taken—*see* Table of Drugs and Chemicals, by drug, poisoning
- • not associated with Cushing's syndrome E27.0
- • pituitary-dependent E24.0

Hyperalimentation R63.2

Hyperbetalipoproteinemia (familial) E78.0
- • with prebetalipoproteinemia E78.2

Hyperbicarbonatemia P74.41

Hyperbilirubinemia
- • constitutional E80.6
- • familial conjugated E80.6
- • neonatal (transient)—*see* Jaundice, newborn

Hypercalcemia, hypocalciuric, familial E83.52

Hypercalciuria, idiopathic R82.994

Hypercapnia R06.89
- • newborn P84

Hyperchloremia E87.8

Hyperchlorhydria K31.89
- • neurotic F45.8
- • psychogenic F45.8

Hypercholesterolemia (essential) (primary) (pure) E78.00
- • with hyperglyceridemia, endogenous E78.2
- • dietary counseling and surveillance Z71.3
- • familial E78.01
- • family history of Z83.42
- • hereditary E78.01

Hyperchylia gastrica, psychogenic F45.8

Hypercorticalism, pituitary-dependent E24.0

Hypercorticosolism—*see* Cushing's, syndrome

Hypercorticosteronism E24.2
- • correct substance properly administered—*see* Table of Drugs and Chemicals, by drug, adverse effect
- • overdose or wrong substance given or taken—*see* Table of Drugs and Chemicals, by drug, poisoning

Hypercortisonism E24.2
- • correct substance properly administered—*see* Table of Drugs and Chemicals, by drug, adverse effect
- • overdose or wrong substance given or taken—*see* Table of Drugs and Chemicals, by drug, poisoning

Hyperekplexia Q89.8

Hyperelectrolytemia E87.8

Hyperemesis R11.10
- • with nausea R11.2
- • projectile R11.12
- • psychogenic F45.8

Hyperemia (acute) (passive) R68.89
- • anal mucosa K62.89
- • ear internal, acute—*see* subcategory H83.0
- • labyrinth—*see* subcategory H83.0

Hyperexplexia Q89.8

Hyperfunction
- • adrenal cortex, not associated with Cushing's syndrome E27.0
  - – virilism E25.9
    - ■ congenital E25.0

Hyperglycemia, hyperglycemic (transient) R73.9
- • coma—*see* Diabetes, by type, with coma
- • postpancreatectomy E89.1

Hyperheparinemia D68.32

Hyperhidrosis, hyperidrosis R61
- • generalized R61
- • psychogenic F45.8
- • secondary R61
  - – focal L74.52

Hyperinsulinism (functional) E16.1
- • therapeutic misadventure (from administration of insulin)—*see* subcategory T38.3

Hyperkeratosis (*see also* Keratosis) L85.9
- • follicularis Q82.8
- • universalis congenita Q80.8

Hyperlipemia, hyperlipidemia E78.5
- • combined E78.2
  - – familial E78.49
- • group
  - – A E78.00
  - – C E78.2
- • mixed E78.2
  - – specified NEC E78.49

Hyperlipoproteinemia E78.5
- • Fredrickson's type
  - – IIa E78.00
  - – IIb E78.2
  - – III E78.2
- • low-density-lipoprotein-type (LDL) E78.00
- • very-low-density-lipoprotein-type (VLDL) E78.1

Hypermagnesemia E83.41
- • neonatal P71.8

Hypermenorrhea N92.0

Hypermetropia (congenital) H52.0-

Hypermobility, hypermotility
- • colon—*see* Syndrome, irritable bowel
  - – psychogenic F45.8
- • intestine (*see also* Syndrome, irritable bowel) K58.9
  - – psychogenic F45.8
- • stomach K31.89
  - – psychogenic F45.8
- • syndrome M35.7

Hypernatremia E87.0

Hypernephroma C64.-

Hyperopia—*see* Hypermetropia

Hyperorexia nervosa F50.2

Hyperosmolality E87.0

Hyperostosis (monomelic)—*see also* Disorder
- • skull M85.2
  - – congenital Q75.8

Hyperperistalsis R19.2
- • psychogenic F45.8

Hyperpigmentation—*see also* Pigmentation
- • melanin NEC L81.4

Hyperplasia, hyperplastic
- • adenoids J35.2
- • adrenal (capsule) (cortex) (gland) E27.8
  - – with
    - ■ sexual precocity (male) E25.9
      - ~ congenital E25.0
    - ■ virilism, adrenal E25.9
      - ~ congenital E25.0

Hyperplasia, hyperplastic, *continued*
- virilization (female) E25.9
  - ~ congenital E25.0
  - congenital E25.0
    - salt-losing E25.0
- angiolymphoid, eosinophilia (ALHE) D18.01
- bone NOS Q79.9
  - face Q75.8
  - skull—*see* Hypoplasia, skull
- cervix (uteri) (basal cell) (endometrium) (polypoid)
  - congenital Q51.828
- endocervicitis N72
- epithelial L85.9
  - nipple N62
  - skin L85.9
- face Q18.8
  - bone(s) Q75.8
- genital
  - female NEC N94.89
  - male N50.89
- gingiva K06.1
- gum K06.1
- nose
  - lymphoid J34.89
  - polypoid J33.9
- tonsils (faucial) (infective) (lingual) (lymphoid) J35.1
  - with adenoids J35.3

Hyperpnea—*see* Hyperventilation

Hyperproteinemia E88.09

Hyperpyrexia R50.9
- heat (effects) T67.01
- rheumatic—*see* Fever, rheumatic
- unknown origin R50.9

Hypersecretion
- ACTH (not associated with Cushing's syndrome) E27.0
  - pituitary E24.0
- corticoadrenal E24.9
- cortisol E24.9
- gastric K31.89
  - psychogenic F45.8
- hormone(s)
  - ACTH (not associated with Cushing's syndrome) E27.0
    - pituitary E24.0
  - antidiuretic E22.2
  - growth E22.0

Hypersegmentation, leukocytic, hereditary D72.0

Hypersensitive, hypersensitiveness, hypersensitivity—*see also* Allergy
- gastrointestinal K52.29
  - psychogenic F45.8
- reaction T78.40

Hypertension, hypertensive (accelerated) (benign) (essential) (idiopathic) (malignant) (systemic) I10
- benign, intracranial G93.2
- borderline R03.0
- complicating
  - pregnancy
    - gestational (pregnancy induced) (transient) (without proteinuria)
      - ~ with proteinuria O14.9
        - ◊ mild pre-eclampsia O14.0-
        - ◊ moderate pre-eclampsia O14.0-
        - ◊ severe pre-eclampsia O14.1-
          - » with hemolysis, elevated liver enzymes and low platelet count (HELLP) O14.2-
    - pre-existing
      - ~ with
        - ◊ pre-eclampsia O11.-
      - ~ essential O10.01-
      - ~ secondary O10.41-
- crisis I16.9
- emergency I16.1
- encephalopathy I67.4
- kidney I12.9
  - with
    - stage 5 chronic kidney disease (CKD) or end stage renal disease (ESRD) I12.0
- lesser circulation I27.0
- newborn P29.2
  - pulmonary (persistent) P29.30

Hypertension, hypertensive, *continued*
- psychogenic F45.8
- pulmonary I27.20
  - with
    - cor pulmonale (chronic) I27.29
      - ~ right heart ventricular strain/failure I27.29
  - due to
    - hematologic disorders I27.29
    - left heart disease I27.22
    - lung diseases and hypoxia I27.23
    - metabolic disorders I27.29
    - specified systemic disorders NEC I27.29
  - group 1 (associated) (drug-induced) (toxin-induced) I27.21
  - group 2 I27.22
  - group 3 I27.23
  - group 4 I27.24
  - group 5 I27.29
  - of newborn (persistent) P29.3
  - primary (idiopathic) I27.0
    - secondary
      - ~ arterial I27.21
      - ~ specified NEC I27.29
- urgency I16.0

Hyperthermia (of unknown origin)—*see also* Hyperpyrexia
- newborn P81.9
  - environmental P81.0

Hyperthyroidism (latent) (pre-adult) (recurrent) E05.90
- with
  - goiter (diffuse) E05.00
    - with thyroid storm E05.01
  - storm E05.91
- intracranial (benign) G93.2
- neonatal, transitory P72.1

Hypertony, hypertonia, hypertonicity
- stomach K31.89
  - psychogenic F45.8

Hypertrophy, hypertrophic
- adenoids (infective) J35.2
  - with tonsils J35.3
- anal papillae K62.89
- bladder (sphincter) (trigone) N32.89
- brain G93.89
- breast N62
  - newborn P83.4
  - pubertal, massive N62
- cardiac (chronic) (idiopathic) I51.7
  - with rheumatic fever (conditions in I00)
    - active I01.8
    - inactive or quiescent (with chorea) I09.89
  - congenital NEC Q24.8
  - rheumatic (with chorea) I09.89
    - active or acute I01.8
    - ~ with chorea I02.0
- foot (congenital) Q74.2
- frenulum, frenum (tongue) K14.8
  - lip K13.0
- gland, glandular R59.9
  - generalized R59.1
  - localized R59.0
- gum (mucous membrane) K06.1
- hemifacial 67.4
- lingual tonsil (infective) J35.1
  - with adenoids J35.3
- lip K13.0
  - congenital Q18.6
- liver R16.0
- lymph, lymphatic gland R59.9
  - generalized R59.1
  - localized R59.0
- Meckel's diverticulum (congenital) Q43.0
- mucous membrane
  - gum K06.1
  - nose (turbinate) J34.3
- myocardium—*see also* Hypertrophy, cardiac
  - idiopathic I42.2
- nasal J34.89
  - alae J34.89
  - bone J34.89
  - cartilage J34.89
  - mucous membrane (septum) J34.3
  - sinus J34.89

Hypertrophy, hypertrophic, *continued*
- turbinate J34.3
- nasopharynx, lymphoid (infectional) (tissue) (wall) J35.2
- nipple N62
- palate (hard) M27.8
  - soft K13.79
- pharyngeal tonsil J35.2
- pharynx J39.2
  - lymphoid (infectional) (tissue) (wall) J35.2
- pituitary (anterior) (fossa) (gland) E23.6
- prepuce (congenital) N47.8
  - female N90.89
- pseudomuscular G71.09
- pylorus (adult) (muscle) (sphincter) K31.1
  - congenital or infantile Q40.0
- rectal, rectum (sphincter) K62.89
- rhinitis (turbinate) J31.0
- scar L91.0
  - specified NEC L91.8
- skin L91.9
- testis N44.8
  - congenital Q55.29
- toe (congenital) Q74.2
  - acquired—*see also* Deformity, toe
- tonsils (faucial) (infective) (lingual) (lymphoid) J35.1
  - with adenoids J35.3
- uvula K13.79
- ventricle, ventricular (heart)—*see also* Hypertrophy, cardiac
  - congenital Q24.8
  - in tetralogy of Fallot Q21.3
- vulva N90.60
  - childhood asymmetric labium majus enlargement (CALME) N90.61
  - other specified N90.69

Hyperuricemia (asymptomatic) E79.0

Hyperuricosuria R82.993

Hyperventilation (tetany) R06.4
- hysterical F45.8
- psychogenic F45.8
- syndrome F45.8

Hypoacidity, gastric K31.89
- psychogenic F45.8

Hypoadrenalism, hypoadrenia E27.40
- primary E27.1

Hypoadrenocorticism E27.40
- pituitary E23.0
- primary E27.1

Hypoalbuminemia E88.09

Hypoaldosteronism E27.40

Hypocalcemia E83.51
- dietary E58
- neonatal P71.1
  - due to cow's milk P71.0
- phosphate-loading (newborn) P71.1

Hypochloremia E87.8

Hypochlorhydria K31.89
- neurotic F45.8
- psychogenic F45.8

Hypochondria, hypochondriac, hypochondriasis (reaction) F45.21
- sleep F51.03

Hypochondrogenesis Q77.0

Hypochondroplasia Q77.4

Hypochromasia, blood cells D50.8

Hypocitraturia R82.991

Hypoeosinophilia D72.89

Hypofibrinogenemia D68.8
- acquired D65
- congenital (hereditary) D68.2

Hypofunction
- adrenocortical E27.40
  - primary E27.1
- corticoadrenal NEC E27.40
- pituitary (gland) (anterior) E23.0

Hypogalactia O92.4

Hypogammaglobulinemia (*see also* Agammaglobulinemia) D80.1
- hereditary D80.0
- nonfamilial D80.1
- transient, of infancy D80.7

Hypoglycemia (spontaneous) E16.2
- coma E15
  - diabetic—*see* Diabetes
- diabetic—*see* Diabetes
- dietary counseling and surveillance Z71.3
- due to insulin E16.0
  - therapeutic misadventure—*see* subcategory T38.3
- neonatal (transitory) P70.4
- transitory neonatal P70.4

Hypogonadism
- female E28.39
- hypogonadotropic E23.0
- ovarian (primary) E28.39
- pituitary E23.0

Hypometabolism R63.8

Hypomotility
- gastrointestinal (tract) K31.89
  - psychogenic F45.8
- intestine K59.89
  - psychogenic F45.8
- stomach K31.89
  - psychogenic F45.8

Hyponatremia E87.1

Hypo-osmolality E87.1

Hypoparathyroidism E20.9
- familial E20.8
- idiopathic E20.0
- neonatal, transitory P71.4
- postprocedural E89.2
- specified NEC E20.8

Hypoperfusion (in)
- newborn P96.89

Hypophyseal, hypophysis—*see also* Disease, diseased
- gigantism E22.0

Hypopituitarism (juvenile) E23.0
- drug-induced E23.1
- iatrogenic NEC E23.1

Hypoplasia, hypoplastic
- alimentary tract, congenital Q45.8
  - upper Q40.8
- anus, anal (canal) Q42.3
  - with fistula Q42.2
- aorta, aortic Q25.42
  - ascending, in hypoplastic left heart syndrome Q23.4
  - valve Q23.1
    - in hypoplastic left heart syndrome Q23.4
- artery (peripheral) Q27.8
  - pulmonary Q25.79
  - umbilical Q27.0
- biliary duct or passage Q44.5
- bone NOS Q79.9
  - marrow D61.9
    - megakaryocytic D69.49
  - skull—*see* Hypoplasia, skull
- brain Q02
- cecum Q42.8
- cephalic Q02
- clavicle (congenital) Q74.0
- colon Q42.9
  - specified NEC Q42.8
- corpus callosum Q04.0
- digestive organ(s) or tract NEC Q45.8
  - upper (congenital) Q40.8
- ear (auricle) (lobe) Q17.2
  - middle Q16.4
- endocrine (gland) NEC Q89.2
- erythroid, congenital D61.01
- eye Q11.2
- eyelid (congenital) Q10.3
- focal dermal Q82.8
- gallbladder Q44.0
- genitalia, genital organ(s)
  - female, congenital Q52.8
    - external Q52.79
    - internal NEC Q52.8

Hypoplasia, hypoplastic, *continued*
- in adiposogenital dystrophy E23.6
- intestine (small) Q41.9
  - large Q42.9
    - specified NEC Q42.8
- jaw M26.09
  - lower M26.04
- kidney(s)
  - bilateral Q60.4
  - unilateral Q60.3
- left heart syndrome Q23.4
- lung (lobe) (not associated with short gestation) Q33.6
  - associated with immaturity, low birth weight, prematurity, or short gestation P28.0
- mandible, mandibular M26.04
- medullary D61.9
- megakaryocytic D69.49
- metacarpus—*see* Defect, reduction, limb, upper, specified type NEC
- metatarsus—*see* Defect, reduction, limb, lower, specified type NEC
- optic nerve H47.03-
- ovary, congenital Q50.39
- parathyroid (gland) Q89.2
- pelvis, pelvic girdle Q74.2
- penis (congenital) Q55.62
- pituitary (gland) (congenital) Q89.2
- pulmonary (not associated with short gestation) Q33.6
  - associated with short gestation P28.0
- rectum Q42.1
  - with fistula Q42.0
- scapula Q74.0
- shoulder girdle Q74.0
- skin Q82.8
- skull (bone) Q75.8
  - with
    - anencephaly Q00.0
    - encephalocele—*see* Encephalocele
    - hydrocephalus Q03.9
      ~ with spina bifida—*see* Spina bifida, by site, with hydrocephalus
    - microcephaly Q02
- thymic, with immunodeficiency D82.1
- thymus (gland) Q89.2
  - with immunodeficiency D82.1
- thyroid (gland) E03.1
  - cartilage Q31.2
- umbilical artery Q27.0
- zonule (ciliary) Q12.8

Hypoplasminogenemia E88.02

Hypopnea, obstructive sleep apnea G47.33

Hypoproteinemia E77.8

Hypopyrexia R68.0

Hyposecretion
- ACTH E23.0
- antidiuretic hormone E23.2
- ovary E28.39
- vasopressin E23.2

Hyposegmentation, leukocytic, hereditary D72.0

Hypospadias Q54.9
- balanic Q54.0
- coronal Q54.0
- glandular Q54.0
- penile Q54.1
- penoscrotal Q54.2
- perineal Q54.3
- specified NEC Q54.8

Hypotension (arterial) (constitutional) I95.9
- intracranial G96.810
  - following
    - lumbar cerebrospinal fluid shunting G97.83
    - specified procedure NEC G97.84
    - ventricular shunting (ventriculostomy) G97.2
  - specified NEC G96.819
  - spontaneous G96.811
- orthostatic (chronic) I95.1
- postural I95.1

Hypothermia (accidental) T68
- low environmental temperature T68
- neonatal P80.9

Hypothermia, *continued*
- environmental (mild) NEC P80.8
- mild P80.8
- severe (chronic) (cold injury syndrome) P80.0
- specified NEC P80.8
- not associated with low environmental temperature R68.0

Hypothyroidism (acquired) E03.9
- congenital (without goiter) E03.1
  - with goiter (diffuse) E03.0
- due to
  - iodine-deficiency, acquired E01.8
    - subclinical E02
- iodine-deficiency (acquired) E01.8
  - congenital—*see* Syndrome
  - subclinical E02
- neonatal, transitory P72.2
- specified NEC E03.8

Hypotonia, hypotonicity, hypotony
- congenital (benign) P94.2

Hypoventilation R06.89

Hypovolemia E86.1
- surgical shock T81.19
- traumatic (shock) T79.4

Hypoxemia R09.02
- newborn P84

Hypoxia (*see also* Anoxia) R09.02
- intrauterine P84
- newborn P84

Hysteria, hysterical (conversion) (dissociative state) F44.9
- anxiety F41.8
- psychosis, acute F44.9

I

Ichthyoparasitism due to Vandellia cirrhosa B88.8

Ichthyosis (congenital) Q80.9
- fetalis Q80.4
- hystrix Q80.8
- lamellar Q80.2
- palmaris and plantaris Q82.8
- simplex Q80.0
- vera Q80.8
- vulgaris Q80.0
- X-linked Q80.1

Icterus—*see also* Jaundice
- conjunctiva R17
  - newborn P59.9
- hemorrhagic (acute) (leptospiral) (spirochetal) A27.0
  - newborn P53
- infectious B15.9

Ictus solaris, solis T67.01

Ideation
- homicidal R45.850
- suicidal R45.851

Identity disorder (child) F64.9
- gender role F64.2
- psychosexual F64.2

Idioglossia F80.0

Idiopathic—*see* Disease, diseased

Idiot, idiocy (congenital) F73
- microcephalic Q02

IgE asthma J45.909

IIAC (idiopathic infantile arterial calcification) Q28.8

Ileitis (chronic) (noninfectious) (*see also* Enteritis) K52.9
- infectious A09
- regional (ulcerative)—*see* Enteritis, regional, small intestine
- segmental—*see* Enteritis, regional
- terminal (ulcerative)—*see* Enteritis, regional, small intestine

Ileocolitis (*see also* Enteritis) K52.9
- regional—*see* Enteritis, regional
- infectious A09
- ulcerative K51.0-

Ileus (bowel) (colon) (inhibitory) (intestine) K56.7
- adynamic K56.0
- meconium P76.0

Ileus, *continued*
- in cystic fibrosis E84.11
- meaning meconium plug (without cystic fibrosis) P76.0
- neurogenic K56.0
  - Hirschsprung's disease or megacolon Q43.1
- newborn
  - due to meconium P76.0
    - in cystic fibrosis E84.11
    - meaning meconium plug (without cystic fibrosis) P76.0
  - transitory P76.1
- obstructive K56.69
- paralytic K56.0

Illness (*see also* Disease) R69

Imbalance R26.89
- constituents of food intake E63.1
- electrolyte E87.8
  - neonatal, transitory NEC P74.49
    - potassium
      - ~ hyperkalemia P74.31
      - ~ hypokalemia P74.32
    - sodium
      - ~ hypernatremia P74.21
      - ~ hyponatremia P74.22
- endocrine E34.9
- eye muscle NOS H50.9
- hysterical F44.4
- posture R29.3
- protein-energy—*see* Malnutrition

Immaturity (less than 37 completed weeks)—*see also* Preterm, newborn
- extreme of newborn (less than 28 completed weeks of gestation) (less than 196 completed days of gestation) (unspecified weeks of gestation) P07.20
  - gestational age
    - 23 completed weeks (23 weeks, 0 days through 23 weeks, 6 days) P07.22
    - 24 completed weeks (24 weeks, 0 days through 24 weeks, 6 days) P07.23
    - 25 completed weeks (25 weeks, 0 days through 25 weeks, 6 days) P07.24
    - 26 completed weeks (26 weeks, 0 days through 26 weeks, 6 days) P07.25
    - 27 completed weeks (27 weeks, 0 days through 27 weeks, 6 days) P07.26
    - less than 23 completed weeks P07.21
- fetus or infant light-for-dates—*see* Light-for-dates
- lung, newborn P28.0
- organ or site NEC—*see* Hypoplasia
- pulmonary, newborn P28.0
- sexual (female) (male), after puberty E30.0

Immersion T75.1

Immunization—*see also* Vaccination
- ABO—*see* Incompatibility, ABO
  - in newborn P55.1
- complication—*see* Complications, vaccination
- encounter for Z23
- not done (not carried out) Z28.9
  - because (of)
    - acute illness of patient Z28.01
    - allergy to vaccine (or component) Z28.04
    - caregiver refusal Z28.82
    - chronic illness of patient Z28.02
    - contraindication NEC Z28.09
    - delay in delivery of vaccine Z28.83
    - group pressure Z28.1
    - guardian refusal Z28.82
    - immune compromised state of patient Z28.03
    - lack of availability of vaccine Z28.83
    - manufacturer delay of vaccine Z28.83
    - parent refusal Z28.82
    - patient's belief Z28.1
    - patient had disease being vaccinated against Z28.81
    - patient refusal Z28.21
    - religious beliefs of patient Z28.1
    - specified reason NEC Z28.89
      - ~ of patient Z28.29
    - unavailability of vaccine Z28.83
    - unspecified patient reason Z28.20

Immunization, *continued*
- Rh factor
  - affecting management of pregnancy NEC O36.09-
    - anti-D antibody O36.01-

Immunocompromised NOS D84.9

Immunodeficiency D84.9
- with
  - adenosine-deaminase deficiency D81.30
    - adenosine deaminase 2 D81.32
    - other adenosine deaminase D81.39
    - severe combined immunodeficiency due to adenosine deaminase deficiency D81.31
  - antibody defects D80.9
    - specified type NEC D80.8
  - thrombocytopenia and eczema D82.0
- common variable D83.9
  - with
    - abnormalities of B-cell numbers and function D83.0
    - autoantibodies to B- or T-cells D83.2
    - immunoregulatory T-cell disorders D83.1
    - specified type NEC D83.8
- due to
  - conditions classified elsewhere D84.81
  - drugs D84.821
  - external causes D84.822
  - medication (current or past) D84.821
- combined D81.9
  - severe D81.9
    - due to adenosine deaminase deficiency D81.31
- following hereditary defective response to Epstein-Barr virus (EBV) D82.3
- severe combined (SCID) D81.9
  - due to adenosine deaminase deficiency D81.31
- specified type NEC D84.89

Immunodeficient NOS D84.9

Immunosuppressed NOS D84.9

Impaction, impacted
- bowel, colon, rectum (*see also* Impaction, fecal) K56.49
- cerumen (ear) (external) H61.2-
- fecal, feces K56.41
- intestine (calculous) NEC (*see also* Impaction, fecal) K56.49
- turbinate J34.89

Impaired, impairment (function)
- auditory discrimination—*see* Abnormal, auditory perception
- dual sensory Z73.82
- fasting glucose R73.01
- glucose tolerance (oral) R73.02
- hearing—*see* Deafness
- heart—*see* Disease, heart
- rectal sphincter R19.8
- vision NEC H54.7
  - both eyes H54.3

Impediment, speech R47.9
- psychogenic (childhood) F98.8
- slurring R47.81
- specified NEC R47.89

Imperception auditory (acquired)—*see also* Deafness
- congenital H93.25

Imperfect
- aeration, lung (newborn) NEC—*see* Atelectasis
- closure (congenital)
  - alimentary tract NEC Q45.8
    - lower Q43.8
    - upper Q40.8
  - atrioventricular ostium Q21.2
  - atrium (secundum) Q21.1
  - branchial cleft NOS Q18.2
    - cyst Q18.0
    - fistula Q18.0
    - sinus Q18.0
  - choroid Q14.3
  - ductus
    - arteriosus Q25.0
    - Botalli Q25.0
  - ear drum (causing impairment of hearing) Q16.4
  - esophagus with communication to bronchus or trachea Q39.1
  - eyelid Q10.3

Imperfect, *continued*
- foramen
  - botalli Q21.1
  - ovale Q21.1
- genitalia, genital organ(s)or system
  - female Q52.8
    - ~ external Q52.79
    - ~ internal NEC Q52.8
  - male Q55.8
- interatrial ostium or septum Q21.1
- interauricular ostium or septum Q21.1
- interventricular ostium or septum Q21.0
- omphalomesenteric duct Q43.0
- ostium
  - interatrial Q21.1
  - interauricular Q21.1
  - interventricular Q21.0
- roof of orbit Q75.8
- septum
  - atrial (secundum) Q21.1
  - interatrial (secundum) Q21.1
  - interauricular (secundum) Q21.1
  - interventricular Q21.0
    - ~ in tetralogy of Fallot Q21.3
  - ventricular Q21.0
    - ~ with pulmonary stenosis or atresia, dextraposition of aorta, and hypertrophy of right ventricle Q21.3
    - ~ in tetralogy of Fallot Q21.3
- skull Q75.0
  - with
    - ~ anencephaly Q00.0
    - ~ encephalocele—*see* Encephalocele
    - ~ hydrocephalus Q03.9
      - ◊ with spina bifida—*see* Spina bifida, by site, with hydrocephalus
    - ~ microcephaly Q02
- spine (with meningocele)—*see* Spina bifida
- vitelline duct Q43.0
- posture R29.3
- rotation, intestine Q43.3
- septum, ventricular Q21.0

Imperfectly descended testis—*see* Cryptorchid

Imperforate (congenital)—*see also* Atresia
- anus Q42.3
  - with fistula Q42.2
- esophagus Q39.0
  - with tracheoesophageal fistula Q39.1
- hymen Q52.3
- jejunum Q41.1
- rectum Q42.1
  - with fistula Q42.0

Impervious (congenital)—*see also* Atresia
- anus Q42.3
  - with fistula Q42.2
- bile duct Q44.2
- esophagus Q39.0
  - with tracheoesophageal fistula Q39.1
- intestine (small) Q41.9
  - large Q42.9
    - specified NEC Q42.8
- rectum Q42.1
  - with fistula Q42.0

Impetigo (any organism) (any site) (circinate) (contagiosa) (simplex) (vulgaris) L01.00
- external ear L01.00 [H62.4-]
- furfuracea L30.5

Implantation
- cyst
  - vagina N89.8

Impression, basilar Q75.8

Improper care (child) (newborn)—*see* Maltreatment

Improperly tied umbilical cord (causing hemorrhage) P51.8

Impulsiveness (impulsive) R45.87

Inability to swallow—*see* Aphagia

Inadequate, inadequacy
- development
  - child R62.50
  - genitalia
    - after puberty NEC E30.0

Inadequate, inadequacy, *continued*
- congenital
  - ~ female Q52.8
    - ◊ external Q52.79
    - ◊ internal Q52.8
  - ~ male Q55.8
  - lungs Q33.6
    - associated with short gestation P28.0
  - organ or site not listed—*see* Anomaly, by site
- drinking-water supply Z58.6
- eating habits Z72.4
- environment, household Z59.1
- family support Z63.8
- food (supply) NEC Z59.48
  - hunger effects T73.0
- household care, due to
  - family member
    - handicapped or ill Z74.2
    - temporarily away from home Z74.2
- housing (heating) (space) Z59.1
- intrafamilial communication Z63.8
- mental—*see* Disability, intellectual
- pulmonary
  - function R06.89
    - newborn P28.5
  - ventilation, newborn P28.5
- social
  - insurance Z59.7
  - skills NEC Z73.4

Inanition R64
- fever R50.9

Inappropriate
- diet or eating habits Z72.4
- secretion
  - antidiuretic hormone (ADH) (excessive) E22.2
  - pituitary (posterior) E22.2

Inattention at or after birth—*see* Neglect

Incarceration, incarcerated
- exomphalos K42.0
  - gangrenous K42.1
- hernia—*see also* Hernia, by site, with obstruction
  - with gangrene—*see* Hernia, by site, with gangrene
- omphalocele K42.0
- rupture—*see* Hernia, by site
- sarcoepiplomphalocele K42.0
  - with gangrene K42.1

Incision, incisional
- hernia K43.2
  - with
    - gangrene (and obstruction) K43.1
    - obstruction K43.0

Inclusion
- azurophilic leukocytic D72.0
- blennorrhea (neonatal) (newborn) P39.1
- gallbladder in liver (congenital) Q44.1

Incompatibility
- ABO
  - affecting management of pregnancy O36.11-
    - anti-A sensitization O36.11-
    - anti-B sensitization O36.19-
    - specified NEC O36.19-
  - infusion or transfusion reaction T80.30-
  - newborn P55.1
- blood (group) (Duffy) (K(ell)) (Kidd) (Lewis) (M) (S) NEC
  - affecting management of pregnancy O36.11-
    - anti-A sensitization O36.11-
    - anti-B sensitization O36.19-
  - infusion or transfusion reaction T80.89
  - newborn P55.8
- Rh (blood group) (factor)
  - affecting management of pregnancy NEC O36.09-
    - anti-D antibody O36.01-
  - infusion or transfusion reaction—*see* Complication(s), transfusion, incompatibility reaction, Rh (factor)
  - newborn P55.0
- rhesus—*see* Incompatibility, Rh

Incompetency, incompetent, incompetence
- annular
  - aortic (valve)—*see* Insufficiency, aortic
  - mitral (valve) I34.0

Incompetency, incompetent, incompetence, *continued*
- pulmonary valve (heart) I37.1
- aortic (valve)—*see* Insufficiency, aortic
- cardiac valve—*see* Endocarditis
- pulmonary valve (heart) I37.1
  - congenital Q22.3

Incomplete—*see also* Disease, diseased
- bladder, emptying R33.9
- defecation R15.0
- expansion lungs (newborn) NEC—*see* Atelectasis
- rotation, intestine Q43.3

Incontinence R32
- anal sphincter R15.9
- feces R15.9
  - nonorganic origin F98.1
- psychogenic F45.8
- rectal R15.9
- urethral sphincter R32
- urine (urinary) R32
  - nocturnal N39.44
  - nonorganic origin F98.0

Increase, increased
- abnormal, in development R63.8
- function
  - adrenal
    - cortex—*see* Cushing's, syndrome
    - pituitary (gland) (anterior) (lobe) E22.9
    - posterior E22.2
- intracranial pressure (benign) G93.2
- pressure, intracranial G93.2
- sphericity, lens Q12.4

Indeterminate sex Q56.4

India rubber skin Q82.8

Indigestion (acid) (bilious) (functional) K30
- due to decomposed food NOS A05.9
- nervous F45.8
- psychogenic F45.8

Induration
- brain G93.89
- breast (fibrous) N64.51
- chancre
  - congenital A50.07
  - extragenital NEC A51.2

Inertia
- stomach K31.89
  - psychogenic F45.8

Infancy, infantile, infantilism—*see also* Disease, diseased
- celiac K90.0
- genitalia, genitals (after puberty) E30.0
- Herter's (nontropical sprue) K90.0
- intestinal K90.0
- Lorain E23.0
- pituitary E23.0
- uterus—*see* Infantile, genitalia

Infant(s)—*see also* Infancy
- excessive crying R68.11
- irritable child R68.12
- lack of care—*see* Neglect
- liveborn (singleton) Z38.2
  - born in hospital Z38.00
    - by cesarean Z38.01
  - born outside hospital Z38.1
  - multiple NEC Z38.8
    - born in hospital Z38.68
      - ~ by cesarean Z38.69
    - born outside hospital Z38.7
  - quadruplet Z38.8
    - born in hospital Z38.63
      - ~ by cesarean Z38.64
    - born outside hospital Z38.7
  - quintuplet Z38.8
    - born in hospital Z38.65
      - ~ by cesarean Z38.66
    - born outside hospital Z38.7
  - triplet Z38.8
    - born in hospital Z38.61
      - ~ by cesarean Z38.62
    - born outside hospital Z38.7
  - twin Z38.5
    - born in hospital Z38.30

Infant(s), *continued*
- ~ by cesarean Z38.31
- born outside hospital Z38.4
- of diabetic mother (syndrome of) P70.1
  - gestational diabetes P70.0

Infantile—*see also* Disease, diseased
- genitalia, genitals E30.0
- os, uterine E30.0
- penis E30.0
- uterus E30.0

Infantilism—*see* Infancy

Infarct, infarction
- adrenal (capsule) (gland) E27.49
- cerebral (acute) (chronic) (*see also* Occlusion, artery) I63.9-
  - neonatal P91.82-
  - perinatal (arterial ischemic) P91.82-
- hypophysis (anterior lobe) E23.6
  - diffuse acute K55.062
  - focal (segmental) K55.061
  - intestine, part unspecified
  - unspecified extent K55.069
- large intestine
  - diffuse acute K55.042
  - focal (segmental) K55.041
  - unspecified extent K55.049
- myocardium, myocardial (acute) (with stated duration of 4 weeks or less)
  - postprocedural
    - following cardiac surgery I97.190
    - following other surgery I97.191
- pituitary (gland) E23.6
- small intestine
  - diffuse acute K55.022
  - focal (segmental) K55.021
  - unspecified extent K55.029
- suprarenal (capsule) (gland) E27.49

Infection
- with
  - drug resistant organism—*see* Resistance, organism(s), to, drug—*see also* specific organism
  - organ dysfunction (acute) R65.20
    - with septic shock R65.21
- acromioclavicular M00.9
- adenoid (and tonsil) J03.90
  - chronic J35.02
- adenovirus NEC
  - as cause of disease classified elsewhere B97.0
  - unspecified nature or site B34.0
- alveolus, alveolar (process) K04.7
- antrum (chronic)—*see* Sinusitis, acute, maxillary
- anus, anal (papillae) (sphincter) K62.89
- axillary gland (lymph) L04.2
- bacterial NOS A49.9
  - as cause of disease classified elsewhere B96.89
    - Enterococcus B95.2
    - Escherichia coli [E. coli] (*see also* Escherichia coli) B96.20
    - Helicobacter pylori [H. pylori] B96.81
    - Hemophilus influenzae [H. influenzae] B96.3
    - Mycoplasma pneumoniae [M. pneumoniae] B96.0
    - Proteus (mirabilis) (morganii) B96.4
    - Pseudomonas (aeruginosa) (mallei) (pseudomallei) B96.5
    - Staphylococcus B95.8
      - ~ aureus (methicillin susceptible) (MSSA) B95.61
        - ◊ methicillin resistant (MRSA) B95.62
      - ~ specified NEC B95.7
    - Streptococcus B95.5
      - ~ group A B95.0
      - ~ group B B95.1
      - ~ pneumoniae B95.3
      - ~ specified NEC B95.4
  - specified NEC A48.8
- Blastomyces, blastomycotic—*see also* Blastomycosis
  - North American B40.9
- Borrelia burgdorferi A69.20
- brain (*see also* Encephalitis) G04.90
  - membranes—*see* Meningitis
  - septic G06.0
    - meninges—*see* Meningitis, bacterial
- buttocks (skin) L08.9

Infection, *continued*

- Campylobacter, intestinal A04.5
  - as cause of disease classified elsewhere B96.81
- Candida (albicans) (tropicalis)—*see* Candidiasis
- candiru B88.8
- central line-associated T80.219
  - bloodstream (CLABSI) T80.211
  - specified NEC T80.218
- cervical gland (lymph) L04.0
- Chlamydia, chlamydial A74.9
  - anus A56.3
  - genitourinary tract A56.2
    - lower A56.00
    - specified NEC A56.19
  - pharynx A56.4
  - rectum A56.3
  - sexually transmitted NEC A56.8
- Clostridium NEC
  - botulinum (food poisoning) A05.1
    - infant A48.51
    - wound A48.52
  - difficile
    - foodborne (disease) A04.7-
    - necrotizing enterocolitis A04.7-
    - sepsis A41.4
  - perfringens
    - due to food A05.2
    - foodborne (disease) A05.2
    - necrotizing enterocolitis A05.2
    - sepsis A41.4
  - welchii
    - foodborne (disease) A05.2
    - sepsis A41.4
- congenital P39.9
  - Candida (albicans) P37.5
  - cytomegalovirus P35.1
  - herpes simplex P35.2
  - infectious or parasitic disease P37.9
    - specified NEC P37.8
  - listeriosis (disseminated) P37.2
  - rubella P35.0
  - toxoplasmosis (acute) (subacute) (chronic) P37.1
  - urinary (tract) P39.3
- coronavirus-2019 U07.1
- coronavirus NEC B34.2
  - as cause of disease classified elsewhere B97.29
  - severe acute respiratory syndrome (SARS associated) B97.21
- COVID-19 U07.1
- cytomegalovirus, cytomegaloviral B25.9
  - congenital P35.1
  - maternal, maternal care for (suspected) damage to fetus O35.3
  - mononucleosis B27.10
    - with
      ~ complication NEC B27.19
      ~ meningitis B27.12
      ~ polyneuropathy B27.11
- dental (pulpal origin) K04.7
- due to or resulting from
  - central venous catheter T80.219
    - bloodstream T80.211
    - exit or insertion site T80.212
    - localized T80.212
    - port or reservoir T80.212
    - specified NEC T80.218
    - tunnel T80.212
  - device, implant or graft (*see also* Complications, by site and type, infection or inflammation) T85.79
    - arterial graft NEC T82.7
    - catheter NEC T85.79
      ~ dialysis (renal) T82.7
      ~ infusion NEC T82.7
      ~ urinary T83.518
        ◊ cystostomy T83.510
        ◊ Hopkins T83.518
        ◊ ileostomy T83.518
        ◊ nephrostomy T83.512
        ◊ specified NEC T83.518
        ◊ urethral indwelling T83.511
        ◊ urostomy T83.518
  - Hickman catheter T80.219
    - bloodstream T80.211

Infection, *continued*

- localized T80.212
- specified NEC T80.218
  - immunization or vaccination T88.0
  - infusion, injection or transfusion NEC T80.29
    - acute T80.22
  - peripherally inserted central catheter (PICC) T80.219
    - bloodstream T80.211
    - localized T80.212
    - specified NEC T80.218
  - portacath (port-a-cath) T80.219
    - bloodstream T80.211
    - localized T80.212
    - specified NEC T80.218
  - postoperative (postprocedural) T81.4
    - sepsis T81.49
    - specified surgical site NEC T81.4-
    - superficial incisional surgical site T81.41
  - surgery T81.40
  - triple lumen catheter T80.219
    - bloodstream T80.211
    - localized T80.212
    - specified NEC T80.218
  - umbilical venous catheter T80.219
    - bloodstream T80.211
    - localized T80.212
    - specified NEC T80.218
- ear (middle)—*see also* Otitis, media
  - external—*see* Otitis, externa, infective
  - inner—*see* subcategory H83.0
- echovirus
  - as cause of disease classified elsewhere B97.12
  - unspecified nature or site B34.1
- endocardium I33.0
- Enterobius vermicularis B80
- enterovirus B34.1
  - as cause of disease classified elsewhere B97.10
    - coxsackievirus B97.11
    - echovirus B97.12
    - specified NEC B97.19
- erythema infectiosum B08.3
- Escherichia (E.) coli NEC A49.8
  - as cause of disease classified elsewhere (*see also* Escherichia coli) B96.20
  - congenital P39.8
    - sepsis P36.4
  - generalized A41.51
  - intestinal—*see* Enteritis, infectious, due to, Escherichia coli
- eyelid H01.-
  - abscess—*see* Abscess, eyelid
  - blepharitis—*see* Blepharitis
  - chalazion—*see* Chalazion
  - dermatosis (noninfectious)—*see* Dermatitis, eyelid
  - hordeolum—*see* Hordeolum
  - specified NEC H01.8
- finger (skin) L08.9
  - nail L03.01-
    - fungus B35.1
- focal
  - teeth (pulpal origin) K04.7
  - tonsils J35.01
- foot (skin) L08.9
  - dermatophytic fungus B35.3
- fungus NOS B49
  - beard B35.0
  - dermatophytic—*see* Dermatophytosis
  - foot B35.3
  - groin B35.6
  - hand B35.2
  - nail B35.1
  - perianal (area) B35.6
  - scalp B35.0
  - skin B36.9
    - foot B35.3
    - hand B35.2
    - toenails B35.1
- Giardia lamblia A07.1
- gingiva (chronic)
  - acute K05.00
    - plaque induced K05.00
- gram-negative bacilli NOS A49.9
- gum (chronic)

Infection, *continued*

- acute K05.00
  - plaque induced K05.00
- Helicobacter pylori A04.8
  - as the cause of disease classified elsewhere B96.81
- Hemophilus
  - influenzae NEC A49.2
    - as cause of disease classified elsewhere B96.3
  - generalized A41.3
- herpes (simplex)—*see also* Herpes
  - congenital P35.2
  - disseminated B00.7
  - herpesvirus, herpesviral—*see* Herpes
- hip (joint) NEC M00.9
  - skin NEC L08.9
- human
  - papilloma virus A63.0
- hydrocele N43.0
- inguinal (lymph) glands L04.1
- joint NEC M00.9
- knee (joint) NEC M00.9
  - joint M00.9
  - skin L08.9
- leg (skin) NOS L08.9
- listeria monocytogenes—*see also* Listeriosis
  - congenital P37.2
- local, skin (staphylococcal) (streptococcal) L08.9
  - abscess—*code by* site under Abscess
  - cellulitis—*code by* site under Cellulitis
  - ulcer—*see* Ulcer
- lung (*see also* Pneumonia) J18.9
  - virus—*see* Pneumonia, viral
- lymph gland—*see also* Lymphadenitis, acute
  - mesenteric I88.0
- lymphoid tissue, base of tongue or posterior pharynx, NEC (chronic) J35.03
- Malassezia furfur B36.0
- mammary gland N61.0
- meningococcal (*see also* Disease, diseased) A39.9
  - cerebrospinal A39.0
  - meninges A39.0
  - meningococcemia A39.4
    - acute A39.2
    - chronic A39.3
- mesenteric lymph nodes or glands NEC I88.0
- metatarsophalangeal M00.9
- mouth, parasitic B37.0
- Mycoplasma NEC A49.3
  - pneumoniae, as cause of disease classified elsewhere B96.0
- myocardium NEC I40.0
- nail (chronic)
  - with lymphangitis—*see* Lymphangitis, acute
  - finger L03.01-
    - fungus B35.1
  - ingrowing L60.0
  - toe L03.03-
    - fungus B35.1
- newborn P39.9
  - intra-amniotic NEC P39.2
  - skin P39.4
  - specified type NEC P39.8
- nipple N61.0
- Oidium albicans B37.9
- operative wound T81.49
- Oxyuris vermicularis B80
- pancreas (acute) K85.92
  - abscess—*see* Pancreatitis, acute
  - specified NEC K85.82
- parameningococcus A39.9
- paraurethral ducts N34.2
- parvovirus NEC B34.3
  - as the cause of disease classified elsewhere B97.6
- Pasteurella NEC A28.0
  - multocida A28.0
  - pseudotuberculosis A28.0
  - septica (cat bite) (dog bite) A28.0
- perinatal period P39.9
  - specified type NEC P39.8
- perirectal K62.89
- perirenal—*see* Infection, kidney
- peritoneal—*see* Peritonitis

Infection, *continued*
- pharynx—*see also* Pharyngitis
  - coxsackievirus B08.5
  - posterior, lymphoid (chronic) J35.03
- pinworm B80
- pityrosporum furfur B36.0
- pleuro-pneumonia-like organism (PPLO) NEC A49.3
  - as cause of disease classified elsewhere B96.0
- pneumococcus, pneumococcal NEC A49.1
  - as cause of disease classified elsewhere B95.3
  - generalized (purulent) A40.3
    - with pneumonia J13
- port or reservoir T80.212
- postoperative T81.40
  - surgical site
    - deep incisional T81.42
    - organ and space T81.43
    - specified NEC T81.49
    - superficial incisional T81.41
- postprocedural T81.40
- prepuce NEC N47.7
  - with penile inflammation N47.6
- Proteus (mirabilis) (morganii) (vulgaris) NEC A49.8
  - as cause of disease classified elsewhere B96.4
- Pseudomonas NEC A49.8
  - as cause of disease classified elsewhere B96.5
  - pneumonia J15.1
- rectum (sphincter) K62.89
- renal
  - pelvis and ureter (cystic) N28.85
- respiratory (tract) NEC J98.8
  - acute J22
  - chronic J98.8
  - influenzal (upper) (acute)—*see* Influenza, with, respiratory manifestations NEC
  - lower (acute) J22
    - chronic—*see* Bronchitis
  - rhinovirus J00
  - syncytial virus (RSV) J06.9 [B97.4]
  - upper (acute) NOS J06.9
    - streptococcal J06.9
    - viral NOS J06.9
- rhinovirus
  - as cause of disease classified elsewhere B97.89
  - unspecified nature or site B34.8
- rickettsial NOS A79.9
- roundworm (large) NEC B82.0
  - Ascariasis (*see also* Ascariasis) B77.9
- Salmonella (aertrycke) (arizonae) (callinarum) (choleraesuis) (enteritidis) (suipestifer) (typhimurium)
  - with
    - (gastro) enteritis A02.0
    - specified manifestation NEC A02.8
  - due to food (poisoning) A02.9
- scabies B86
- Shigella A03.9
  - boydii A03.2
  - dysenteriae A03.0
  - flexneri A03.1
  - group
    - A A03.0
    - B A03.1
    - C A03.2
    - D A03.3
- shoulder (joint) NEC M00.9
  - skin NEC L08.9
- skin (local) (staphylococcal) (streptococcal) L08.9
  - abscess—*code by* site under Abscess
  - cellulitis—*code by* site under Cellulitis
- spinal cord NOS (*see also* Myelitis) G04.91
  - abscess G06.1
  - meninges—*see* Meningitis
  - streptococcal G04.89
- staphylococcal, unspecified site
  - aureus (methicillin susceptible) (MSSA) A49.01
    - methicillin resistant (MRSA) A49.02
  - as cause of disease classified elsewhere B95.8
    - aureus (methicillin susceptible) (MSSA) B95.61
      ~ methicillin resistant (MRSA) B95.62
    - specified NEC B95.7
  - food poisoning A05.0
  - generalized (purulent) A41.2
  - pneumonia—*see* Pneumonia, staphylococcal

Infection, *continued*
- streptobacillus moniliformis A25.1
- streptococcal NEC A49.1
  - as the cause of disease classified elsewhere B95.5
  - congenital
    - sepsis P36.10
      ~ group B P36.0
      ~ specified NEC P36.19
  - generalized (purulent) A40.9
- subcutaneous tissue, local L08.9
- threadworm B80
- toe (skin) L08.9
  - cellulitis L03.03-
    - fungus B35.1
  - nail L03.03-
    - fungus B35.1
- tongue NEC K14.0
  - parasitic B37.0
- tooth, teeth K04.7
  - periapical K04.7
- TORCH—*see* Infection, congenital
  - without active infection P00.2
- Trichomonas A59.9
  - cervix A59.09
  - specified site NEC A59.8
  - urethra A59.03
  - urogenitalis A59.00
  - vagina A59.01
  - vulva A59.01
- Trombicula (irritans) B88.0
- tuberculous
  - latent (LTBI) Z22.7
  - NEC—*see* Tuberculosis
- tunnel T80.212
- urinary (tract) N39.0
  - bladder—*see* Cystitis
  - newborn P39.3
  - urethra—*see* Urethritis
- varicella B01.9
- Vibrio
  - parahaemolyticus (food poisoning) A05.3
  - vulnificus
    - foodborne intoxication A05.5
- virus, viral NOS B34.9
  - adenovirus
    - as the cause of disease classified elsewhere B97.0
    - unspecified nature or site B34.0
  - as the cause of disease classified elsewhere B97.89
    - adenovirus B97.0
    - coxsackievirus B97.11
    - echovirus B97.12
    - enterovirus B97.10
      ~ coxsackievirus B97.11
      ~ echovirus B97.12
      ~ specified NEC B97.19
    - parvovirus B97.6
    - specified NEC B97.89
  - central nervous system A89
    - enterovirus NEC A88.8
      ~ meningitis A87.0
  - coxsackie B34.1
    - as cause of disease classified elsewhere B97.11
  - ECHO
    - as cause of disease classified elsewhere B97.12
    - unspecified nature or site B34.1
  - enterovirus, as cause of disease classified elsewhere B97.10
    - coxsackievirus B97.11
    - echovirus B97.12
    - specified NEC B97.19
  - exanthem NOS B09
  - respiratory syncytial (RSV)
    - as cause of disease classified elsewhere B97.4
    - bronchiolitis J21.0
    - bronchitis J20.5
    - bronchopneumonia J12.1
    - otitis media H65.- [B97.4]
    - pneumonia J12.1
    - upper respiratory infection J06.9 [B97.4]
  - rhinovirus
    - as the cause of disease specified elsewhere B97.89

Infection, *continued*
- specified type NEC B33.8
  - as the cause of disease specified elsewhere B97.89
- yeast (*see also* Candidiasis) B37.9
- Zika virus A92.5
  - congenital P35.4

Infertility
- female N97.9
  - associated with
    - anovulation N97.0
    - Stein-Leventhal syndrome E28.2
  - due to
    - Stein-Leventhal syndrome E28.2

Infestation B88.9
- Acariasis B88.0
  - demodex folliculorum B88.0
  - sarcoptes scabiei B86
  - trombiculae B88.0
- arthropod NEC B88.2
- Ascaris lumbricoides—*see* Ascariasis
- candiru B88.8
- cestodes B71.9
- chigger B88.0
- chigo, chigoe B88.1
- crab-lice B85.3
- Demodex (folliculorum) B88.0
- Dermanyssus gallinae B88.0
- Enterobius vermicularis B80
- eyelid
  - in (due to)
    - phthiriasis B85.3
- fluke B66.9
  - specified type NEC B66.8
- Giardia lamblia A07.1
- helminth
  - intestinal B82.0
    - enterobiasis B80
- intestinal NEC B82.9
- Linguatula B88.8
- Lyponyssoides sanguineus B88.0
- mites B88.9
  - scabic B86
- Monilia (albicans)—*see* Candidiasis
- mouth B37.0
- nematode NEC (intestinal) B82.0
  - Enterobius vermicularis B80
  - physaloptera B80
- Oxyuris vermicularis B80
- parasite, parasitic B89
  - eyelid B89
  - intestinal NOS B82.9
  - mouth B37.0
  - skin B88.9
  - tongue B37.0
- Pediculus B85.2
  - body B85.1
  - capitis (humanus) (any site) B85.0
  - corporis (humanus) (any site) B85.1
  - mixed (classifiable to more than one of the titles B85.0–B85.3) B85.4
  - pubis (any site) B85.3
- Pentastoma B88.8
- Phthirus (pubis) (any site) B85.3
  - with any infestation classifiable to B85.0-B85.2 B85.4
- pinworm B80
- pubic louse B85.3
- red bug B88.0
- sand flea B88.1
- Sarcoptes scabiei B86
- scabies B86
- Schistosoma B65.9
  - cercariae B65.3
- skin NOS B88.9
- specified type NEC B88.8
- tapeworm B71.9
- Tetranychus molestissimus B88.0
- threadworm B80
- tongue B37.0
- Trombicula (irritans) B88.0
- Tunga penetrans B88.1
- Vandella cirrhosa B88.8

Infiltrate, infiltration
- leukemic—*see* Leukemia
- lung R91.8
- lymphatic (*see also* Leukemia) C91.9-
  - gland I88.9
- on chest x-ray R91.8
- pulmonary R91.8
- vesicant agent
  - antineoplastic chemotherapy T80.810
  - other agent NEC T80.818

Inflammation, inflamed, inflammatory (with exudation)
- anal canal, anus K62.89
- areola N61.0
- areolar tissue NOS L08.9
- breast N61.0
- bronchi—*see* Bronchitis
- catarrhal J00
- cerebrospinal
  - meningococcal A39.0
- due to device, implant or graft—*see also* Complications, by site and type, infection or inflammation
  - arterial graft T82.7
  - catheter T85.79
    - cardiac T82.7
    - dialysis (renal) T82.7
    - infusion T82.7
    - urinary T83.518
      - ~ cystostomy T83.510
      - ~ Hopkins T83.518
      - ~ ileostomy T83.518
      - ~ nephrostomy T83.512
      - ~ specified NEC T83.518
      - ~ urethral indwelling T83.511
      - ~ urostomy T83.518
  - electronic (electrode) (pulse generator) (stimulator) T82.7
  - vascular NEC T82.7
- duodenum K29.80
  - with bleeding K29.81
- esophagus K20.9-
- follicular, pharynx J31.2
- gland (lymph)—*see* Lymphadenitis
- glottis—*see* Laryngitis
- granular, pharynx J31.2
- leg NOS L08.9
- lip K13.0
- mouth K12.1
- nipple N61.0
- orbit (chronic) H05.10-
  - acute H05.00
    - abscess—*see* Abscess
  - granuloma—*see* Granuloma, orbit
- parotid region L08.9
- perianal K62.89
- pericardium—*see* Pericarditis
- perineum (female) (male) L08.9
- perirectal K62.89
- peritoneum—*see* Peritonitis
- polyp, colon (*see also* Polyp, colon, inflammatory) K51.40
- rectum (*see also* Proctitis) K62.89
- respiratory, upper (*see also* Infection, respiratory, upper) J06.9
- skin L08.9
- subcutaneous tissue L08.9
- tongue K14.0
- tonsil—*see* Tonsillitis
- vein—*see also* Phlebitis
  - intracranial or intraspinal (septic) G08
  - thrombotic I80.9
    - leg—*see* Phlebitis, leg
    - lower extremity—*see* Phlebitis, leg

Influenza (bronchial) (epidemic) (respiratory) (upper) (unidentified influenza virus) J11.1
- with
  - digestive manifestations J11.2
  - encephalopathy J11.81
  - enteritis J11.2
  - gastroenteritis J11.2
  - gastrointestinal manifestations J11.2
  - laryngitis J11.1
  - myocarditis J11.82
  - otitis media J11.83

Influenza, *continued*
- pharyngitis J11.1
- pneumonia J11.00
  - specified type J11.08
- respiratory manifestations NEC J11.1
- specified manifestation NEC J11.89
- A (non-novel) J10-
- A/H5N1 (*see also* Influenza, due to, identified novel influenza A virus) J09.X2
- avian (*see also* Influenza, due to, identified novel influenza A virus) J09.X2
- B J10-
- bird (*see also* Influenza, due to, identified novel influenza A virus) J09.X2
- C J10-
- novel (2009) H1N1 influenza (*see also* Influenza, due to, identified influenza virus NEC) J10.1
- novel influenza A/H1N1 (*see also* Influenza, due to, identified influenza virus NEC) J10.1
- due to
  - avian (*see also* Influenza, due to, identified novel influenza A virus) J09.X2
  - identified influenza virus NEC J10.1
    - with
      - ~ digestive manifestations J10.2
      - ~ encephalopathy J10.81
      - ~ enteritis J10.2
      - ~ gastroenteritis J10.2
      - ~ gastrointestinal manifestations J10.2
      - ~ laryngitis J10.1
      - ~ myocarditis J10.82
      - ~ otitis media J10.83
      - ~ pharyngitis J10.1
      - ~ pneumonia (unspecified type) J10.00
        - ◊ with same identified influenza virus J10.01
        - ◊ specified type NEC J10.08
      - ~ respiratory manifestations NEC J10.1
      - ~ specified manifestation NEC J10.89
  - identified novel influenza A virus J09.X2
    - with
      - ~ digestive manifestations J09.X3
      - ~ encephalopathy J09.X9
      - ~ enteritis J09.X3
      - ~ gastroenteritis J09.X3
      - ~ gastrointestinal manifestations J09.X3
      - ~ laryngitis J09.X2
      - ~ myocarditis J09.X9
      - ~ otitis media J09.X9
      - ~ pharyngitis J09.X2
      - ~ pneumonia J09.X1
      - ~ respiratory manifestations NEC J09.X2
      - ~ specified manifestation NEC J09.X9
      - ~ upper respiratory symptoms J09.X2
- of other animal origin, not bird or swine (*see also* Influenza, due to, identified novel influenza A virus) J09.X2
- swine (viruses that normally cause infections in pigs) (*see also* Influenza, due to, identified novel influenza A virus) J09.X2

Influenza-like disease—*see* Influenza

Influenzal—*see* Influenza

Ingestion
- chemical—*see* Table of Drugs and Chemicals, by substance, poisoning
- drug or medicament
  - correct substance properly administered—*see* Table of Drugs and Chemicals, by drug, adverse effect
  - overdose or wrong substance given or taken—*see* Table of Drugs and Chemicals, by drug, poisoning
- foreign body—*see* Foreign body, alimentary tract

Ingrowing
- hair (beard) L73.1
- nail (finger) (toe) L60.0

Inguinal—*see also* Disease, diseased
- testicle Q53.9
  - bilateral Q53.212
  - unilateral Q53.112

Inhalation
- anthrax A22.1
- gases, fumes, or vapors
  - specified agent—*see* Table of Drugs and Chemicals, by substance T59.89-
- liquid or vomitus—*see* Asphyxia
- meconium (newborn) P24.00
  - with
    - pneumonia (pneumonitis) P24.01
    - with respiratory symptoms P24.01
- mucus—*see* Asphyxia
- oil or gasoline (causing suffocation)—*see* Foreign body, by site
- smoke T59.81-
  - with respiratory conditions J70.5

Injury (*see also* specified type of injury) T14.90
See also the *ICD-10-CM* External Cause of Injuries Table for codes describing accident details.
- ankle S99.91-
  - specified type NEC S99.81-
- blood vessel NEC T14.8
  - hand (level) S65.9-
    - laceration S65.91-
    - specified
      - ~ type NEC S65.99-
  - neck S15.9
    - specified site NEC S15.8
  - palmar arch (superficial) S65.2-
    - deep S65.30-
      - ~ laceration S65.31-
      - ~ specified type NEC S65.39-
    - laceration S65.21-
    - specified type NEC S65.29-
- brachial plexus S14.3
  - newborn P14.3
- cord
  - spermatic (pelvic region)
    - scrotal region S39.848
- eye S05.9-
  - conjunctiva S05.0-
  - cornea
    - abrasion S05.0-
- foot S99.92-
  - specified type NEC S99.82-
- genital organ(s)
  - external S39.94
    - specified NEC S39.848
- head S09.90
  - with loss of consciousness S06.9-
  - specified NEC S09.8
- heart (traumatic)
  - non-traumatic (acute) (chronic) (non-ischemic) I5A
- internal T14.8
  - pelvis, pelvic (organ) S39.9-
  - specified NEC S39.83
- intra-abdominal S36.90
- intracranial (traumatic) (*see also*, if applicable, Compression, brain, traumatic) S06.9-
  - intracerebral hemorrhage, traumatic
    - intracranial (trauma)
      - ~ epidural, hemorrhage (traumatic) S06.4X
    - left side S06.35-
    - right side S06.34-
  - subarachnoid hemorrhage, traumatic S06.6X-
  - subdural hemorrhage, traumatic S06.5X-
- intrathoracic
  - lung S27.30-
    - aspiration J69.0
    - bilateral S27.302
    - contusion S27.329
      - ~ bilateral S27.322
      - ~ unilateral S27.321
    - unilateral S27.301
  - pneumothorax S27.0-
- kidney S37.0-
  - acute (nontraumatic) N17.9
  - contusion—*see* Contusion, kidney
- lung—*see also* Injury, intrathoracic, lung
  - aspiration J69.0
  - dabbing (related) U07.0
  - electronic cigarette (related) U07.0
  - EVALI- [e-cigarette, or vaping, product use associated] U07.0

Injury, *continued*
- – transfusion-related (TRALI) J95.84
- – vaping (device) (product) (use) (associated) U07.0
- • multiple NOS T07
- • muscle
  - – finger
    - ▪ extensor S56.4-
      - ~ hand level S66.3-
        - ◊ strain S66.31-
      - ~ laceration S56.42-
      - ~ strain S56.41-
    - ▪ flexor (forearm level) S56.1-
      - ~ hand level S66.1-
        - ◊ laceration S66.12- (See complete *ICD-10-CM* Manual)
        - ◊ strain S66.11-
      - ~ laceration S56.12-
      - ~ strain S56.11-
    - ▪ intrinsic S66.5-
      - ~ strain S66.51-
  - – foot S96.9-
    - ▪ intrinsic S96.2-
      - ~ laceration S96.22-
      - ~ strain S96.21-
    - ▪ laceration S96.92-
    - ▪ specified
      - ~ site NEC S96.8-
        - ◊ strain S96.81-
    - ▪ strain S96.91-
  - – forearm (level) S56.90-
    - ▪ extensor S56.5-
      - ~ laceration S56.52-
      - ~ strain S56.51-
    - ▪ flexor
      - ~ laceration S56.22-
      - ~ strain S56.21-
    - ▪ laceration S56.92-
    - ▪ specified
      - ~ site NEC S56.8-
        - ◊ laceration S56.82-
        - ◊ strain S56.81-
    - ▪ strain S56.91-
  - – hand (level) S66.9-
    - ▪ strain S66.91-
  - – thumb
    - ▪ abductor (forearm level) S56.3-
      - ~ laceration S56.32-
      - ~ strain S56.31-
    - ▪ extensor (forearm level) S56.3-
      - ~ hand level S66.2-
        - ◊ strain S66.21-
      - ~ laceration S56.32-
      - ~ specified type NEC S56.39-
      - ~ strain S56.31-
    - ▪ flexor (forearm level) S56.0 -
      - ~ hand level S66.0-
        - ◊ laceration S66.02-
        - ◊ strain S66.01-
      - ~ laceration S56.02-
      - ~ strain S56.01-
    - ▪ intrinsic S66.4-
      - ~ strain S66.41-
  - – toe—*see also* Injury, muscle, foot
    - ▪ extensor, long S96.1-
      - ~ laceration S96.12-
      - ~ strain S96.11-
    - ▪ flexor, long S96.0-
      - ~ laceration S96.02-
      - ~ strain S96.01-
  - – neck (level) S16.9
    - ▪ laceration S16.2
    - ▪ specified type NEC S16.8
    - ▪ strain S16.1
- • nerve NEC T14.8
  - – facial S04.5-
    - ▪ newborn P11.3
  - – lumbar spinal
    - ▪ peripheral S34.6
    - ▪ root S34.21
    - ▪ sympathetic S34.5
    - ▪ sacral spinal peripheral S34.6

Injury, *continued*
- ▪ root S34.22
- ▪ sympathetic S34.5
- • pelvis, pelvic (floor) S39.93
  - – specified NEC S39.83
- • postcardiac surgery (syndrome) I97.0
- • rectovaginal septum NEC S39.83
- • scalp S09.90
  - – newborn (birth injury) P12.9
    - ▪ due to monitoring (electrode) (sampling incision) P12.4
    - ▪ specified NEC P12.89
      - ~ caput succedaneum P12.81
- • self-inflicted, without suicidal intent R45.88
- • spermatic cord (pelvic region)
  - – scrotal region S39.848
- • spinal (cord)
  - – cervical (neck) S14.109
    - ▪ C1 level S14.101
    - ▪ C2 level S14.102
    - ▪ C3 level S14.103
    - ▪ C4 level S14.104
    - ▪ C5 level S14.105
    - ▪ C6 level S14.106
    - ▪ C7 level S14.107
    - ▪ C8 level S14.108
  - – lumbar S34.109
    - ▪ complete lesion S34.11- (See complete *ICD-10-CM* Manual)
    - ▪ incomplete lesion S34.129
      - ~ L1 level S34.121
      - ~ L2 level S34.122
      - ~ L3 level S34.123
      - ~ L4 level S34.124
      - ~ L5 level S34.125
    - ▪ L1 level S34.101
    - ▪ L2 level S34.102
    - ▪ L3 level S34.103
    - ▪ L4 level S34.104
    - ▪ L5 level S34.105
  - – sacral S34.139
    - ▪ complete lesion S34.131
    - ▪ incomplete lesion S34.132
  - – thoracic S24.109
    - ▪ T1 level S24.101
    - ▪ T2–T6 level S24.102
    - ▪ T7–T10 level S24.103
    - ▪ T11–T12 level S24.104
- • spleen S36.0-
  - – laceration S36.03-
    - ▪ superficial (capsular) (minor) S36.030
- • toe S99.92-
  - – specified type NEC S99.82-
- • transfusion-related acute lung (TRALI) J95.84
- • vagina S39.93
  - – abrasion S30.814
  - – bite S31.45
    - ▪ insect S30.864
    - ▪ superficial NEC S30.874
  - – contusion S30.23
  - – external constriction S30.844
  - – insect bite S30.864
  - – laceration S31.41
    - ▪ with foreign body S31.42
  - – open wound S31.4-
  - – puncture S31.43
    - ▪ with foreign body S31.44
  - – superficial S30.95
    - ▪ foreign body S30.854
- • vulva S39.94
  - – abrasion S30.814
  - – bite S31.45
    - ▪ insect S30.864
    - ▪ superficial NEC S30.874
  - – contusion S30.23
  - – external constriction S30.844
  - – insect bite S30.864
  - – laceration S31.41
    - ▪ with foreign body S31.42
  - – open wound S31.4-
  - – puncture S31.43
    - ▪ with foreign body S31.44

Injury, *continued*
- – superficial S30.95
  - ▪ foreign body S30.854
- – whiplash (cervical spine) S13.4

Insecurity, food Z59.41

Insensitivity
- • adrenocorticotropin hormone (ACTH) E27.49
- • androgen E34.50
  - – complete E34.51
  - – partial E34.52

Insolation (sunstroke) T67.01

Insomnia (organic) G47.00
- • adjustment F51.02
  - – adjustment disorder F51.02
- • behavioral, of childhood Z73.819
  - – combined type Z73.812
  - – limit setting type Z73.811
  - – sleep-onset association type Z73.810
- • childhood Z73.819
- • chronic F51.04
  - – somatized tension F51.04
- • conditioned F51.04
- • due to
  - – anxiety disorder F51.05
  - – depression F51.05
  - – medical condition G47.01
  - – mental disorder NEC F51.05
- • idiopathic F51.01
- • learned F51.3
- • nonorganic origin F51.01
- • not due to a substance or known physiological condition F51.01
  - – specified NEC F51.09
- • paradoxical F51.03
- • primary F51.01
- • psychiatric F51.05
- • psychophysiologic F51.04
- • related to psychopathology F51.05
- • short-term F51.02
- • specified NEC G47.09
- • stress-related F51.02
- • transient F51.02
- • without objective findings F51.02

Inspissated bile syndrome (newborn) P59.1

Instability
- • emotional (excessive) F60.3
- • housing
  - – housed Z59.819
    - ▪ with risk of homelessness Z59.811
    - ▪ homelessness in past 12 months Z59.812
- • joint (post-traumatic) M25.30
  - – specified site NEC M25.39
- • personality (emotional) F60.3
- • vasomotor R55

Insufficiency, insufficient
- • adrenal (gland) E27.40
  - – primary E27.1
- • adrenocortical E27.40
  - – primary E27.1
- • anus K62.89
- • aortic (valve) I35.1
  - – with
    - ▪ mitral (valve) disease I08.0
      - ~ with tricuspid (valve) disease I08.3
    - ▪ stenosis I35.2
    - ▪ tricuspid (valve) disease I08.2
      - ~ with mitral (valve) disease I08.3
  - – congenital Q23.1
  - – rheumatic I06.1
    - ▪ with
      - ~ mitral (valve) disease I08.0
        - ◊ with tricuspid (valve) disease I08.3
      - ~ stenosis I06.2
        - ◊ with mitral (valve) disease I08.0
          - » with tricuspid (valve) disease I08.3
      - ~ tricuspid (valve) disease I08.2
        - ◊ with mitral (valve) disease I08.3
  - – specified cause NEC I35.1
- • cardiac—*see also* Insufficiency, myocardial
  - – due to presence of (cardiac) prosthesis I97.11-
  - – postprocedural I97.11-

Insufficiency, insufficient, *continued*
- corticoadrenal E27.40
  - primary E27.1
- kidney N28.9
  - acute N28.9
  - chronic N18.9
- mitral (valve) I34.0
  - with
    - aortic valve disease I08.0
      - ~ with tricuspid (valve) disease I08.3
    - obstruction or stenosis I05.2
      - ~ with aortic valve disease I08.0
    - tricuspid (valve) disease I08.1
      - ~ with aortic (valve) disease I08.3
  - congenital Q23.3
  - rheumatic I05.1
    - with
      - ~ aortic valve disease I08.0
        - ◊ with tricuspid (valve) disease I08.3
      - ~ obstruction or stenosis I05.2
        - ◊ with aortic valve disease I08.0
          - » with tricuspid (valve) disease I08.3
      - ~ tricuspid (valve) disease I08.1
        - ◊ with aortic (valve) disease I08.3
    - active or acute I01.1
      - ~ with chorea, rheumatic (Sydenham's) I02.0
  - specified cause, except rheumatic I34.0
- muscle—*see also* Disease, muscle
  - heart—*see* Insufficiency, myocardium, myocardial
  - ocular NEC H50.9
- myocardial, myocardium (with arteriosclerosis) I50.9
  - with
    - rheumatic fever (conditions in I00) I09.0
      - ~ active, acute or subacute I01.2
        - ◊ with chorea I02.0
      - ~ inactive or quiescent (with chorea) I09.0
  - congenital Q24.8
  - newborn P29.0
  - rheumatic I09.0
    - active, acute, or subacute I01.2
- placental (mother) O36.51
- pulmonary J98.4
  - newborn P28.89
  - valve I37.1
    - with stenosis I37.2
    - congenital Q22.2
    - rheumatic I09.89
      - ~ with aortic, mitral or tricuspid (valve) disease I08.8
- renal (acute) N28.9
  - chronic N18.9
- respiratory R06.89
  - newborn P28.5
- rotation—*see* Malrotation
- suprarenal E27.40
  - primary E27.1
- tarso-orbital fascia, congenital Q10.3
- thyroid (gland) (acquired) E03.9
  - congenital E03.1
- tricuspid (valve) (rheumatic) I07.1
  - with
    - aortic (valve) disease I08.2
      - ~ with mitral (valve) disease I08.3
    - mitral (valve) disease I08.1
      - ~ with aortic (valve) disease I08.3
    - obstruction or stenosis I07.2
      - ~ with aortic (valve) disease I08.2
        - ◊ with mitral (valve) disease I08.3
  - congenital Q22.8
  - nonrheumatic I36.1
    - with stenosis I36.2
- urethral sphincter R32
- velopharyngeal
  - acquired K13.79
  - congenital Q38.8

Intertrigo L30.4
- labialis K13.0

Intolerance
- carbohydrate K90.49
- disaccharide, hereditary E73.0
- fat NEC K90.49
  - pancreatic K90.3

Intolerance, *continued*
- food K90.49
  - dietary counseling and surveillance Z71.3
- gluten
  - celiac K90.0
  - non-celiac K90.41
- lactose E73.9
  - specified NEC E73.8
- milk NEC K90.49
  - lactose E73.9
- protein K90.49
- starch NEC K90.49

Intoxication
- drug
  - acute (without dependence)—*see* Abuse, drug, by type, with intoxication
    - with dependence—*see* Dependence, drug, by type with intoxication
  - addictive
    - via placenta or breast milk—*see* Absorption, drug
  - newborn P93.8
    - gray baby syndrome P93.0
  - overdose or wrong substance given or taken—*see* Table of Drugs and Chemicals, by drug, poisoning
- foodborne A05.9
  - bacterial A05.9
  - classical (Clostridium botulinum) A05.1
  - due to
    - Bacillus cereus A05.4
    - bacterium A05.9
      - ~ specified NEC A05.8
    - Clostridium
      - ~ botulinum A05.1
      - ~ perfringens A05.2
      - ~ welchii A05.2
    - Salmonella A02.9
      - ~ with
        - ◊ (gastro) enteritis A02.0
        - ◊ specified manifestation NEC A02.8
    - Staphylococcus A05.0
    - Vibrio
      - ~ parahaemolyticus A05.3
      - ~ vulnificus A05.5
  - enterotoxin, staphylococcal A05.0
  - noxious—*see* Poisoning, food, noxious
- meaning
  - inebriation—*see* category F10
  - poisoning—*see* Table of Drugs and Chemicals
- serum (*see also* Reaction, serum) T80.69

Intraabdominal testis, testes
- bilateral Q53.211
- unilateral Q53.111

Intrahepatic gallbladder Q44.1

Intrauterine contraceptive device
- checking Z30.431
- insertion Z30.430
  - immediately following removal Z30.433
- in situ Z97.5
- management Z30.431
- reinsertion Z30.433
- removal Z30.432
- replacement Z30.433

Intussusception (bowel) (colon) (enteric) (ileocecal) (ileocolic) (intestine) (rectum) K56.1

Invagination (bowel, colon, intestine or rectum) K56.1

Inversion
- albumin-globulin (A-G) ratio E88.09
- nipple N64.59
- testis (congenital) Q55.29

Investigation (*see also* Examination) Z04.9

I. Q.
- under 20 F73
- 20–34 F72
- 35–49 F71
- 50–69 F70

IRDS (type I) P22.0
- type II P22.1

Iritis
- diabetic—*see* E08 –E13 with .39

Irradiated enamel (tooth, teeth) K03.89

Irradiation effects, adverse T66

Irregular, irregularity
- action, heart I49.9
- bleeding N92.6
- breathing R06.89
- menstruation (cause unknown) N92.6
- periods N92.6
- respiratory R06.89
- septum (nasal) J34.2
- sleep-wake pattern (rhythm) G47.23

Irritable, irritability R45.4
- bladder N32.89
- bowel (syndrome) K58.9
  - with constipation K58.1
  - with diarrhea K58.0
  - mixed K58.2
  - other K58.8
  - psychogenic F45.8
- cerebral, in newborn P91.3
- colon K58.9
  - with constipation K58.1
  - with diarrhea K58.0
  - mixed K58.2
  - other K58.8
  - psychogenic F45.8
- heart (psychogenic) F45.8
- infant R68.12stomach K31.89
  - psychogenic F45.8

Irritation
- anus K62.89
- bladder N32.89
- gastric K31.89
  - psychogenic F45.8
- nervous R45.0
- perineum NEC L29.3
- stomach K31.89
  - psychogenic F45.8
- vaginal N89.8

Ischemia, ischemic I99.8
- brain—*see* Ischemia, cerebral
- cerebral (chronic) (generalized) I67.82
  - intermittent G45.9
  - newborn P91.0
  - recurrent focal G45.8
  - transient G45.9
- intestine, unspecified part
  - diffuse acute (reversible) K55.052
  - focal (segmental) acute (reversible) K55.051
  - unspecified extent K55.059
- large intestine
  - diffuse acute (reversible) K55.032
  - focal (segmental) acute (reversible) K55.031
  - unspecified extent K55.039
- small intestine
  - diffuse acute (reversible) K55.012
  - focal (segmental) acute (reversible) K55.011
  - unspecified extent K55.019

Ischuria R34

Isoimmunization NEC—*see also* Incompatibility
- affecting management of pregnancy (ABO) (with hydrops fetalis) O36.11-
  - anti-A sensitization O36.11-
  - anti-B sensitization O36.19-
  - anti-c sensitization O36.09-
  - anti-C sensitization O36.09-
  - anti-e sensitization O36.09-
  - anti-E sensitization O36.09-
  - Rh NEC O36.09-
    - anti-D antibody O36.01-
  - specified NEC O36.19-
- newborn P55.9
  - with
    - hydrops fetalis P56.0
    - kernicterus P57.0
  - ABO (blood groups) P55.1
  - Rhesus (Rh) factor P55.0
  - specified type NEC P55.8

Isolation, isolated
- dwelling Z59.89
- family Z63.79

Issue of
- medical certificate Z02.79
  - for disability determination Z02.71
- repeat prescription (appliance) (glasses) (medicinal substance, medicament, medicine) Z76.0
  - contraception—*see* Contraception

Itch, itching—*see also* Pruritus
- baker's L23.6
- barber's B35.0
- cheese B88.0
- clam digger's B65.3
- copra B88.0
- dhobi B35.6
- grain B88.0
- grocer's B88.0
- harvest B88.0
- jock B35.6
- Malabar B35.5
  - beard B35.0
  - foot B35.3
  - scalp B35.0
- meaning scabies B86
- Norwegian B86
- perianal L29.0
- poultrymen's B88.0
- sarcoptic B86
- scabies B86
- scrub B88.0
- straw B88.0
- swimmer's B65.3
- winter L29.8

Ixodiasis NEC B88.8

J

Jacquet's dermatitis (diaper dermatitis) L22
Jamaican
- neuropathy G92.8
- paraplegic tropical ataxic-spastic syndrome G92.8

Jaundice (yellow) R17
- breast-milk (inhibitor) P59.3
- catarrhal (acute) B15.9
- cholestatic (benign) R17
- due to or associated with
  - delayed conjugation P59.8
    - associated with (due to) preterm delivery P59.0
  - preterm delivery P59.0
- epidemic (catarrhal) B15.9
- familial nonhemolytic (congenital) (Gilbert) E80.4
  - Crigler-Najjar E80.5
- febrile (acute) B15.9
- infectious (acute) (subacute) B15.9
- neonatal—*see* Jaundice, newborn
- newborn P59.9
  - due to or associated with
    - ABO
      - ~ antibodies P55.1
      - ~ incompatibility, maternal/fetal P55.1
      - ~ isoimmunization P55.1
    - breast milk inhibitors to conjugation P59.3
      - ~ associated with preterm delivery P59.0
    - Crigler-Najjar syndrome E80.5
    - delayed conjugation P59.8
      - ~ associated with preterm delivery P59.0
    - Gilbert syndrome E80.4
    - hemolytic disease P55.9
      - ~ ABO isoimmunization P55.1
    - hepatocellular damage P59.20
      - ~ specified NEC P59.29
    - hypothyroidism, congenital E03.1
    - inspissated bile syndrome P59.1
    - mucoviscidosis E84.9
    - preterm delivery P59.0
  - spherocytosis (congenital) D58.0
- nonhemolytic congenital familial (Gilbert) E80.4
- symptomatic R17
  - newborn P59.9

Jealousy
- childhood F93.8
- sibling F93.8

Jejunitis—*see* Enteritis

Jejunostomy status Z93.4
Jejunum, jejunal—*see* Disease, diseased
Jerks, myoclonic G25.3
Jervell-Lange-Nielsen syndrome I45.81
Jeune's disease Q77.2
Jigger disease B88.1
Job's syndrome (chronic granulomatous disease) D71
Joseph-Diamond-Blackfan anemia (congenital hypoplastic) D61.01

K

Kallmann's syndrome E23.0
Kaposi's
- vaccinia T88.1
Kartagener's syndrome or triad (sinusitis, bronchiectasis, situs inversus) Q89.3
Karyotype
- 46,XX Q98.3
  - with streak gonads Q50.32
  - hermaphrodite (true) Q99.1
  - male Q98.3
- 47,XXX Q97.0
- 47,XYY Q98.5
Kawasaki's syndrome M30.3
Kaznelson's syndrome (congenital hypoplastic anemia) D61.01
Kelis L91.0
Keloid, cheloid L91.0
- Hawkin's L91.0
- scar L91.0
Keloma L91.0
Keratitis (nodular) (nonulcerative) (simple) (zonular) H16.9
- dendritic (a) (herpes simplex) B00.52
- disciform (is) (herpes simplex) B00.52
  - varicella B01.81
- gonococcal (congenital or prenatal) A54.33
- herpes, herpetic (simplex) B00.52
- in (due to)
  - exanthema (*see also* Exanthem) B09
  - herpes (simplex) virus B00.52
  - measles B05.81
- postmeasles B05.81
Keratoconjunctivitis H16.20-
- herpes, herpetic (simplex) B00.52
- in exanthema (*see also* Exanthem) B09
- postmeasles B05.81
Keratoderma, keratodermia (congenital) (palmaris et plantaris) (symmetrical) Q82.8
Keratoglobus H18.79
- congenital Q15.8
  - with glaucoma Q15.0
Keratoma
- palmaris and plantaris hereditarium Q82.8
Keratosis
- congenital, specified NEC Q80.8
- female genital NEC N94.89
- follicularis Q82.8
  - congenita Q82.8
  - spinulosa (decalvans) Q82.8
- gonococcal A54.89
- nigricans L83
- palmaris et plantaris (inherited) (symmetrical) Q82.8
  - acquired L85.1
- tonsillaris J35.8
- vegetans Q82.8
Kerion (celsi) B35.0
Kink, kinking
- ureter (pelvic junction) N13.5
  - with
    - hydronephrosis N13.1
Klinefelter's syndrome Q98.4
Klumpke (-Déjerine) palsy, paralysis (birth) (newborn) P14.1
Knee—*see* Disease, diseased
Knock knee (acquired) M21.06-
- congenital Q74.1

Knot(s)
- intestinal, syndrome (volvulus) K56.2
Knotting (of)
- intestine K56.2
Köebner's syndrome Q81.8
Koplik's spots B05.9
Kraft-Weber-Dimitri disease Q85.8
Kraurosis
- ani K62.89
Kreotoxism A05.9
Kwashiokor E40
Kyphoscoliosis, kyphoscoliotic (acquired) (*see also* Scoliosis) M41.9
- congenital Q67.5
- heart (disease) I27.1
Kyphosis, kyphotic (acquired) M40.209
- Morquio-Brailsford type (spinal) E76.219

L

Labile
- blood pressure R09.89
Labium leporinum—*see* Cleft, lip
Labyrinthitis (circumscribed) (destructive) (diffuse) (inner ear) (latent) (purulent) (suppurative) H83.0
Laceration
- abdomen, abdominal
  - wall S31.119
    - with
      - ~ foreign body S31.129
    - epigastric region S31.112
      - ~ with
        - ◊ foreign body S31.122
    - left
      - ~ lower quadrant S31.114
        - ◊ with
          - » foreign body S31.124
      - ~ upper quadrant S31.111
        - ◊ with
          - » foreign body S31.121
    - periumbilic region S31.115
      - ~ with
        - ◊ foreign body S31.125
    - right
      - ~ lower quadrant S31.113
        - ◊ with
          - » foreign body S31.123
      - ~ upper quadrant S31.110
        - ◊ with
          - » foreign body S31.120
- Achilles tendon S86.02-
- ankle S91.01-
  - with
    - foreign body S91.02-
- antecubital space—*see* Laceration
- anus (sphincter) S31.831
  - with
    - foreign body S31.832
  - nontraumatic, nonpuerperal—*see* Fissure, anus
- arm (upper) S41.11-
  - with foreign body S41.12-
  - lower—*see* Laceration, forearm
- auditory canal (external) (meatus)—*see* Laceration, ear
- auricle, ear—*see* Laceration, ear
- axilla—*see* Laceration, arm
- back—*see also* Laceration, thorax, back
  - lower S31.010
    - with
      - ~ foreign body S31.020
- buttock S31.8-
  - with foreign body S31.8-
  - left S31.821
    - with foreign body S31.822
  - right S31.811
    - with foreign body S31.812
- calf—*see* Laceration, leg
- canaliculus lacrimalis—*see* Laceration, eyelid
- canthus, eye—*see* Laceration, eyelid
- capsule, joint—*see* Sprain
- cerebral

Laceration, *continued*
- left side S06.32-
- during birth P10.8
  - with hemorrhage P10.1
- right side S06.31-
- cheek (external) S01.41-
  - with foreign body S01.42-
  - internal—*see* Laceration, oral cavity
- chest wall—*see* Laceration, thorax
- chin—*see* Laceration, head, specified site NEC
- digit(s)
  - hand—*see* Laceration, finger
  - foot—*see* Laceration, toe
- ear (canal) (external) S01.31-
  - with foreign body S01.32-
  - drum S09.2-
- elbow S51.01-
  - with foreign body S51.02-
- epididymis—*see* Laceration, testis
- epigastric region—*see* Laceration, abdomen, wall, epigastric region
- esophagus K22.89
- eyebrow—*see* Laceration, eyelid
- eyelid S01.11-
  - with foreign body S01.12-
- face NEC—*see* Laceration, head, specified site NEC
- finger(s) S61.21-
  - with
    - damage to nail S61.31-
      - with
        - foreign body S61.32-
    - foreign body S61.22-
  - index S61.21-
    - with
      - damage to nail S61.31-
        - with
          - foreign body S61.32-
      - foreign body S61.22-
    - left S61.211
      - with
        - damage to nail S61.311
          - with
            - foreign body S61.221
    - right S61.210
      - with
        - damage to nail S61.310
          - with
            - foreign body S61.320
          - foreign body S61.220
  - little S61.218
    - with
      - damage to nail S61.31-
        - with
          - foreign body S61.32-
      - foreign body S61.22-
    - left S61.217
      - with
        - damage to nail S61.317
          - with
            - foreign body S61.327
          - foreign body S61.227
    - right S61.216
      - with
        - damage to nail S61.316
          - with
            - foreign body S61.326
          - foreign body S61.226
  - middle S61.218
    - with
      - damage to nail S61.31-
        - with
          - foreign body S61.32-
      - foreign body S61.22-
    - left S61.213
      - with
        - damage to nail S61.313
          - with
            - foreign body S61.323
          - foreign body S61.223
    - right S61.212
      - with
        - damage to nail S61.312

Laceration, *continued*
- with
  - foreign body S61.322
- foreign body S61.222
- ring S61.218
  - with
    - damage to nail S61.31-
      - with
        - foreign body S61.32-
    - foreign body S61.22-
  - left S61.215
    - with
      - damage to nail S61.315
        - with
          - foreign body S61.325
      - foreign body S61.225
  - right S61.214
    - with
      - damage to nail S61.314
        - with
          - foreign body S61.324
      - foreign body S61.224
- flank S31.119
  - with foreign body S31.129
- foot (except toe(s) alone) S91.31-
  - with foreign body S91.32-
  - left S91.312
    - with foreign body S91.322
  - right S91.311
    - with foreign body S91.321
  - toe—*see* Laceration, toe
- forearm S51.81-
  - with
    - foreign body S51.82-
  - elbow only—*see* Laceration
  - left S51.812
    - with
      - foreign body S51.822
  - right S51.811
    - with
      - foreign body S51.821
- forehead S01.81
  - with foreign body S01.82
- gum—*see* Laceration, oral cavity
- hand S61.41-
  - with
    - foreign body S61.42-
  - finger—*see* Laceration, finger
  - left S61.412
    - with
      - foreign body S61.422
  - right S61.411
    - with
      - foreign body S61.421
  - thumb—*see* Laceration, thumb
- head S01.91
  - with foreign body S01.92
  - cheek—*see* Laceration, cheek
  - ear—*see* Laceration, ear
  - eyelid—*see* Laceration, eyelid
  - lip—*see* Laceration, lip
  - nose—*see* Laceration, nose
  - oral cavity—*see* Laceration, oral cavity
  - scalp S01.01
    - with foreign body S01.02
  - specified site NEC S01.81
    - with foreign body S01.82
  - temporomandibular area—*see* Laceration, cheek
- heel—*see* Laceration, foot
- hip S71.01-
  - with foreign body S71.02-
  - left S71.012
    - with foreign body S71.022
  - right S71.011
    - with foreign body S71.021
- hypochondrium—*see* Laceration, abdomen, wall
- hypogastric region—*see* Laceration, abdomen, wall
- inguinal region—*see* Laceration, abdomen, wall
- instep—*see* Laceration, foot
- interscapular region—*see* Laceration, thorax, back
- jaw—*see* Laceration, head, specified site NEC
- joint capsule—*see* Sprain, by site

Laceration, *continued*
- knee S81.01-
  - with foreign body S81.02-
- labium (majus) (minus)—*see* Laceration, vulva
- lacrimal duct—*see* Laceration, eyelid
- leg (lower) S81.81-
  - with foreign body S81.82-
  - foot—*see* Laceration, foot
  - knee—*see* Laceration, knee
  - left S81.812
    - with foreign body S81.822
  - right S81.811
    - with foreign body S81.821
  - upper—*see* Laceration, thigh
- ligament—*see* Sprain
- lip S01.511
  - with foreign body S01.521
- loin—*see* Laceration, abdomen, wall
- lower back—*see* Laceration, back, lower
- lumbar region—*see* Laceration, back, lower
- malar region—*see* Laceration, head, specified site NEC
- mammary—*see* Laceration
- mastoid region—*see* Laceration, head, specified site NEC
- mouth—*see* Laceration, oral cavity
- muscle—*see* Injury, muscle, by site, laceration
- nail
  - finger—*see* Laceration, finger, with, damage to nail
  - toe—*see* Laceration, toe, with, damage to nail
- nasal (septum) (sinus)—*see* Laceration, nose
- nasopharynx—*see* Laceration, head, specified site NEC
- neck S11.91
  - with foreign body S11.92
- nerve—*see* Injury, nerve
- nose (septum) (sinus) S01.21
  - with foreign body S01.22
- ocular NOS
  - adnexa NOS S01.11-
- oral cavity S01.512
  - with foreign body S01.522
- palate—*see* Laceration, oral cavity
- palm—*see* Laceration, hand
- pelvic S31.010
  - with
    - foreign body S31.020
- penis S31.21
- perineum
  - female S31.41
    - with
      - foreign body S31.42
  - male S31.119
    - with foreign body S31.129
- periocular area (with or without lacrimal passages)— *see* Laceration, eyelid
- periumbilic region—*see* Laceration, abdomen, wall, periumbilic
- phalanges
  - finger—*see* Laceration, finger
  - toe—*see* Laceration, toe
- pinna—*see* Laceration, ear
- popliteal space—*see* Laceration, knee
- prepuce—*see* Laceration, penis
- pubic region S31.119
  - with foreign body S31.129
- pudendum—*see* Laceration
- rectovaginal septum—*see* Laceration, vagina
- rectum S36.63
- sacral region—*see* Laceration, back, lower
- sacroiliac region—*see* Laceration, back, lower
- salivary gland—*see* Laceration, oral cavity
- scalp S01.01
  - with foreign body S01.02
- scapular region—*see* Laceration, shoulder
- scrotum S31.31
- shin—*see* Laceration, leg
- shoulder S41.01-
  - with foreign body S41.02-
  - left S41.012
    - with foreign body S41.022
  - right S41.011
    - with foreign body S41.021
- spleen S36.03-
  - superficial (minor) S36.030

Laceration, *continued*
- submaxillary region—*see* Laceration, head, specified site NEC
- submental region—*see* Laceration, head, specified site NEC
- subungual
  - finger(s)—*see* Laceration, finger, with, damage to nail
  - toe(s)—*see* Laceration, toe, with, damage to nail
- temple, temporal region—*see* Laceration, head, specified site NEC
- temporomandibular area—*see* Laceration, cheek
- tendon—*see* Injury, muscle, by site, laceration
  - Achilles S86.02-
- testis S31.31
- thigh S71.11-
  - with foreign body S71.12-
- thorax, thoracic (wall) S21.91
  - with foreign body S21.92
    - back S21.22-
    - front S21.12-
  - back S21.21-
    - with
      - ~ foreign body S21.22-
  - front S21.11-
    - with
      - ~ foreign body S21.12-
- thumb S61.01-
  - with
    - damage to nail S61.11-
      - ~ with
        - ◊ foreign body S61.12-
    - foreign body S61.02-
  - left S61.012
    - with
      - ~ damage to nail S61.112
        - ◊ with
          - » foreign body S61.122
      - ~ foreign body S61.022
  - right S61.011
    - with
      - ~ damage to nail S61.111
        - ◊ with
          - » foreign body S61.121
      - ~ foreign body S61.021
- toe(s) S91.11-
  - with
    - damage to nail S91.21-
      - ~ with
        - ◊ foreign body S91.22-
    - foreign body S91.12-
  - great S91.11-
    - with
      - ~ damage to nail S91.21-
        - ◊ with
          - » foreign body S91.22-
      - ~ foreign body S91.12-
    - left S91.112
      - with
        - ◊ damage to nail S91.212
          - » with
            - ❖ foreign body S91.222
        - ◊ foreign body S91.122
    - right S91.111
      - with
        - ◊ damage to nail S91.211
          - » with
            - ❖ foreign body S91.221
        - ◊ foreign body S91.121
  - lesser S91.11-
    - with
      - ~ damage to nail S91.21-
        - ◊ with
          - » foreign body S91.22-
      - ~ foreign body S91.12-
    - left S91.115
      - with
        - ◊ damage to nail S91.215
          - » with
            - ❖ foreign body S91.225
        - ◊ foreign body S91.125
    - right S91.114
      - ~ with

Laceration, *continued*
- ◊ damage to nail S91.214
  - » with
    - ❖ foreign body S91.224
- ◊ foreign body S91.124
- tongue—*see* Laceration, oral cavity
- tunica vaginalis—*see* Laceration, testis
- tympanum, tympanic membrane—*see* Laceration, ear, drum
- umbilical region S31.115
  - with foreign body S31.125
- uvula—*see* Laceration, oral cavity
- vagina S31.41
  - with
    - foreign body S31.42
  - nonpuerperal, nontraumatic N89.8
  - old (postpartal) N89.8
- vulva S31.41
  - with
    - foreign body S31.42
- wrist S61.51-
  - with
    - foreign body S61.52-
  - left S61.512
    - with
      - ~ foreign body S61.522
  - right S61.511
    - with
      - ~ foreign body S61.521

Lack of
- adequate
  - food Z59.48
  - sleep Z72.820
- appetite (*see* Anorexia) R63.0
- care
  - in home Z74.2
  - of infant (at or after birth) T76.02
    - confirmed T74.02
- coordination R27.9
  - ataxia R27.0
  - specified type NEC R27.8
- development (physiological) R62.50
  - failure to thrive (child over 28 days old) R62.51
    - newborn P92.6
  - short stature R62.52
  - specified type NEC R62.59
- energy R53.83
- food Z59.48
- growth R62.52
- heating Z59.1
- housing (permanent) (temporary) Z59.00
  - adequate Z59.1
- ovulation N97.0
- person able to render necessary care Z74.2
- physical exercise Z72.3
- safe drinking water Z58.6
- shelter Z59.02
- water T73.1
  - safe drinking Z58.6

Lactation, lactating (breast) (puerperal, postpartum)
- associated
  - cracked nipple O92.13
  - retracted nipple O92.03
- defective O92.4
- disorder NEC O92.79
- excessive O92.6
- failed (complete) O92.3
  - partial O92.4
- mastitis NEC N61.1
- mother (care and/or examination) Z39.1
- nonpuerperal N64.3

Lacunar skull Q75.8

Lalling F80.0

Lambliasis, lambliosis A07.1

Landouzy-Déjérine dystrophy or facioscapulohumeral atrophy G71.02

Lapsed immunization schedule status Z28.3

Large
- baby (regardless of gestational age) (4000g-4499g) P08.1

Large-for-dates (infant) (4000g to 4499g) P08.1
- affecting management of pregnancy O36.6-
- exceptionally (4500g or more) P08.0

Larsen-Johansson disease or osteochondrosis—*see* Osteochondrosis, juvenile, patella

Laryngismus (stridulus) J38.5
- congenital P28.89

Laryngitis (acute) (edematous) (fibrinous) (infective) (infiltrative) (malignant) (membranous) (phlegmonous) (pneumococcal) (pseudomembranous) (septic) (subglottic) (suppurative) (ulcerative) J04.0
- with
  - influenza, flu, or grippe—*see* Influenza, laryngitis
  - tracheitis (acute)—*see* Laryngotracheitis
- atrophic J37.0
- catarrhal J37.0
- chronic J37.0
  - with tracheitis (chronic) J37.1
- Hemophilus influenzae J04.0
- H. influenzae J04.0
- hypertrophic J37.0
- influenzal—*see* Influenza, respiratory manifestations NEC
- obstructive J05.0
- sicca J37.0
- spasmodic J05.0
  - acute J04.0
- streptococcal J04.0
- stridulous J05.0

Laryngomalacia (congenital) Q31.5

Laryngopharyngitis (acute) J06.0
- chronic J37.0

Laryngoplegia J38.00
- bilateral J38.02
- unilateral J38.01

Laryngotracheitis (acute) (Infectional) (infective) (viral) J04.2
- atrophic J37.1
- catarrhal J37.1
- chronic J37.1
- Hemophilus influenzae J04.2
- hypertrophic J37.1
- influenzal—*see* Influenza, respiratory manifestations NEC
- sicca J37.1
- spasmodic J38.5
  - acute J05.0
- streptococcal J04.2

Laryngotracheobronchitis—*see* Bronchitis

Late
- talker R62.0
- walker R62.0

Late effects—*see* Sequela

Latent tuberculosis (LTBI) Z22.7

Launois' syndrome (pituitary gigantism) E22.0

Lax, laxity—*see also* Relaxation
- ligament(ous)—*see also* Disorder
  - familial M35.7
- skin congenital Q82.8

Lazy leukocyte syndrome D70.8

Leak, leakage
- air NEC J93.82
  - postprocedural J95.812
- cerebrospinal fluid G96.00
  - cranial
  - postoperative G96.08
    - specified NEC G96.08
    - spontaneous G96.01
    - traumatic G96.08
  - spinal
    - postoperative G96.09
    - post-traumatic G96.09
    - specified NEC G96.09
    - spontaneous G96.02
  - spontaneous
    - from
      - ~ skull base G96.01
      - ~ spine G96.02

Leak, leakage, *continued*
- device, implant or graft—*see also* Complications, by site and type, mechanical
  - persistent air J93.82

Leaky heart—*see* Endocarditis

Learning defect (specific) F81.9

Leber's
- congenital amaurosis H35.50

Lederer's anemia D59.19

Legg (-Calvé)-Perthes disease, syndrome or osteochondrosis M91.1-

Leiner's disease L21.1

Lenegre's disease I44.2

Lengthening, leg—*see* Deformity, limb

Lennox-Gastaut syndrome G40.812
- intractable G40.814
  - with status epilepticus G40.813
  - without status epilepticus G40.814
- not intractable G40.812
  - with status epilepticus G40.811
  - without status epilepticus G40.812

Lenticonus (anterior) (posterior) (congenital) Q12.8

Lentiglobus (posterior) (congenital) Q12.8

Lentigo (congenital) L81.4

Leptocytosis, hereditary D56.9

Leptomeningitis (chronic) (circumscribed) (hemorrhagic) (nonsuppurative)—*see* Meningitis

Leptomeningopathy G96.198

Leptus dermatitis B88.0

Leri-Weill syndrome Q77.8

Lesch-Nyhan syndrome E79.1

Lesion(s) (nontraumatic)
- angiocentric immunoproliferative D47.Z9
- anorectal K62.9
- aortic (valve) I35.9
- basal ganglion G25.9
- brain G93.9
  - congenital Q04.9
    - hypertensive I67.4
- buccal cavity K13.79
- cardiac (*see also* Disease, heart) I51.9
  - congenital Q24.9
- cerebrovascular I67.9
  - degenerative I67.9
  - hypertensive I67.4
- chorda tympani G51.8
- hypothalamic E23.7
- joint—*see* Disorder, joint
  - sacroiliac (old) M53.3
- lip K13.0
- maxillary sinus J32.0
- mitral I05.9
- motor cortex NEC G93.89
- mouth K13.79
- nervous system, congenital Q07.9
- nose (internal) J34.89
- oral mucosa K13.70
- peptic K27.9
- primary (*see also* Syphilis, primary) A51.0
- pulmonary J98.4
  - valve I37.9
- sacroiliac (joint) (old) M53.3
- sinus (accessory) (nasal) J34.89
- skin L98.9
  - suppurative L08.0
- tonsillar fossa J35.9
- tricuspid (valve) I07.9
  - nonrheumatic I36.9
- vascular I99.9
- vagina N89.8
- vulva N90.89

Lethargy R53.83

Leukemia, leukemic C95.9-
- acute lymphoblastic C91.0-
- acute myeloblastic (minimal differentiation) (with maturation) C92.0-
- AML (1/ETO) (M0) (M1) (M2) (without a FAB

Leukemia, leukemic, *continued*
  classification) NOS C92.0-
- chronic myelomonocytic C93.1-
- CMML (-1) (-2) (with eosinophilia) C93.1-
- juvenile myelomonocytic C93.3-
- lymphoid C91.9-
- monocytic (subacute) C93.9-
- myelogenous (*see also* Category C92) C92.9-
- myeloid C92.9-
- subacute lymphocytic C91.9-

Leukemoid reaction (*see also* Reaction, leukemoid) D72.823-

Leukocytopenia D72.819

Leukocytosis D72.829
- eosinophilic D72.19

Leukoencephalitis G04.81
- acute (subacute) hemorrhagic G36.1
  - postimmunization or postvaccinal G04.02
- postinfectious G04.01

Leukoencephalopathy (Encephalopathy) G93.49
- postimmunization and postvaccinal G04.02
- reversible, posterior G93.6

Leukomalacia, cerebral, newborn P91.2

Leukomelanopathy, hereditary D72.0
- periventricular P91.2

Leukonychia (punctata) (striata) L60.8
- congenital Q84.4

Leukopathia unguium L60.8
- congenital Q84.4

Leukopenia D72.819
- basophilic D72.818
- chemotherapy (cancer) induced D70.1
- congenital D70.0
- cyclic D70.0
- drug induced NEC D70.2
  - due to cytoreductive cancer chemotherapy D70.1
- eosinophilic D72.818
- familial D70.0
- infantile genetic D70.0
- malignant D70.9
- periodic D70.0
- transitory neonatal P61.5

Leukoplakia
- anus K62.89
- rectum K62.89

Leukorrhea N89.8
- due to Trichomonas (vaginalis) A59.00
- trichomonal A59.00

Leukosarcoma C85.9-

Levocardia (isolated) Q24.1
- with situs inversus Q89.3

Lev's disease or syndrome (acquired complete heart block) I44.2

Leyden-Moebius dystrophy G71.09

Liar, pathologic F60.2

Libman-Sacks disease M32.11

Lice (infestation) B85.2
- body (Pediculus corporis) B85.1
- crab B85.3
- head (Pediculus corporis) B85.0
- mixed (classifiable to more than one of the titles B85.0–B85.3) B85.4
- pubic (Phthirus pubis) B85.3

Lichen L28.0
- congenital Q82.8
- pilaris Q82.8
  - acquired L85.8

Light
- for gestational age—*see* Light for dates
- headedness R42

Light-for-dates (infant) P05.00
- with weight of
  - 499 grams or less P05.01
  - 500–749 grams P05.02
  - 750–999 grams P05.03
  - 1000–1249 grams P05.04
  - 1250–1499 grams P05.05

Light-for-dates, *continued*
  - 1500–1749 grams P05.06
  - 1750–1999 grams P05.07
  - 2000–2499 grams P05.08
  - 2500 g and over P05.09
- and small-for-dates—*see* Small for dates
- affecting management of pregnancy O36.59-

Ligneous thyroiditis E06.5

Lindau (-von Hippel) disease Q85.8

Line(s)
- Harris'—*see* Arrest, epiphyseal

Lingua
- geographica K14.1

Linguatulosis B88.8

Lipochondrodystrophy E76.01

Lipochrome histiocytosis (familial) D71

Lipodystrophy (progressive) E88.1
- intestinal K90.81

Lipoid—*see also* Disease, diseased
- histiocytosis D76.3
- nephrosis N04.9

Lipoma D17.9
- infiltrating D17.9
- intramuscular D17.9
- pleomorphic D17.9
- site classification
  - arms (skin) (subcutaneous) D17.2-
  - connective tissue D17.30
    - intra-abdominal D17.5
    - intrathoracic D17.4
    - peritoneum D17.79
    - retroperitoneum D17.79
    - specified site NEC D17.39
    - spermatic cord D17.6
  - face (skin) (subcutaneous) D17.0
  - genitourinary organ NEC D17.72
  - head (skin) (subcutaneous) D17.0
  - intra-abdominal D17.5
  - intrathoracic D17.4
  - kidney D17.71
  - legs (skin) (subcutaneous) D17.2-
  - neck (skin) (subcutaneous) D17.0
  - peritoneum D17.79
  - retroperitoneum D17.79
  - skin D17.30
    - specified site NEC D17.39
  - specified site NEC D17.79
  - spermatic cord D17.6
  - subcutaneous D17.30
    - specified site NEC D17.39
  - trunk (skin) (subcutaneous) D17.1
  - unspecified D17.9
- spindle cell D17.9

Lipoproteinemia E78.5
- broad-beta E78.2
- floating-beta E78.2

Lisping F80.0

Listeriosis, Listerellosis A32.9
- congenital (disseminated) P37.2
- cutaneous A32.0
- neonatal, newborn (disseminated) P37.2
- oculoglandular A32.81
- specified NEC A32.89

Lithemia E79.0

Little leaguer's elbow—*see* Epicondylitis, medial

Little's disease G80.9

Livedo (annularis) (racemosa) (reticularis) R23.1

Living alone (problems with) Z60.2
- with handicapped person Z74.2

Living in a shelter (motel) (scattered site housing) (temporary or transitional living situation) Z59.01

Lobstein (-Ekman) disease or syndrome Q78.0

Lone Star fever A77.0

Long
- COVID (-19) (*see also* COVID-19) U09.9
- QT syndrome I45.81

Long-term (current) (prophylactic) drug therapy (use of)
- antibiotics Z79.2
  - short-term use—omit code
- anti-inflammatory, non-steroidal (NSAID) Z79.1
- aspirin Z79.82
- drug, specified NEC Z79.899
- hypoglycemic, oral, drugs Z79.84
- insulin Z79.4
- non-insulin antidiabetic drug, injectable Z79.899
- non-steroidal anti-inflammatories (NSAID) Z79.1
- steroids
  - inhaled Z79.51
  - systemic Z79.52

Longitudinal stripes or grooves, nails L60.8
- congenital Q84.6

Lorain (-Levi) short stature syndrome E23.0

Lordosis M40.50
- acquired—see Lordosis, specified type NEC
- congenital Q76.429
  - lumbar region Q76.426
  - lumbosacral region Q76.427
  - sacral region Q76.428
  - sacrococcygeal region Q76.428
  - thoracolumbar region Q76.425
- lumbar region M40.56
- lumbosacral region M40.57
- postural—see Lordosis, specified type NEC
- specified type NEC M40.40
  - lumbar region M40.46
  - lumbosacral region M40.47
  - thoracolumbar region M40.45
- thoracolumbar region M40.55

Loss (of)
- appetite (see Anorexia) R63.0
  - hysterical F50.89
  - nonorganic origin F50.89
  - psychogenic F50.89
- blood—see Hemorrhage
- consciousness, transient R55
  - traumatic—see Injury, intracranial
- control, sphincter, rectum R15.9
  - nonorganic origin F98.1
- fluid (acute) E86.9
  - with
    - hypernatremia E87.0
    - hyponatremia E87.1
- hearing—see also Deafness
  - central NOS H90.5
  - conductive H90.2
    - bilateral H90.0
    - unilateral
      ~ with
        ◊ restricted hearing on the contralateral side H90.A1-
        ◊ unrestricted hearing on the contralateral side H90.1-
  - mixed conductive and sensorineural hearing loss H90.8
    - bilateral H90.6
    - unilateral
      ~ with
        ◊ restricted hearing on the contralateral side H90.A3-
        ◊ unrestricted hearing on the contralateral side H90.7-
  - neural NOS H90.5
  - perceptive NOS H90.5
  - sensorineural NOS H90.5
    - bilateral H90.3
    - unilateral
      ~ with
        ◊ restricted hearing on the contralateral side H90.A2-
        ◊ unrestricted hearing on the contralateral side H90.4-
  - sensory NOS H90.5
- parent in childhood Z63.4
- self-esteem, in childhood Z62.898
- sense of
  - smell—see Disturbance, sensation
  - taste—see Disturbance, sensation
  - touch R20.8

Loss, continued
- sensory R44.9
  - dissociative F44.6
- vision, visual H54.7
- weight (abnormal) (cause unknown) R63.4

Louis-Bar syndrome (ataxia-telangiectasia) G11.3

Louping ill (encephalitis) A84.89

Louse, lousiness—see Lice

Low
- achiever, school Z55.3
- back syndrome M54.50
- basal metabolic rate R94.8
- birthweight (2499 grams or less) P07.10
  - with weight of
    - 1000–1249 grams P07.14
    - 1250–1499 grams P07.15
    - 1500–1749 grams P07.16
    - 1750–1999 grams P07.17
    - 2000–2499 grams P07.18
  - extreme (999 grams or less) P07.00
    - with weight of
      ~ 499 grams or less P07.01
      ~ 500–749 grams P07.02
      ~ 750–999 grams P07.03
  - for gestational age—see Light for dates
- blood pressure—see also Hypotension
  - reading (incidental) (isolated) (nonspecific) R03.1
- cardiac reserve—see Disease, heart
- hematocrit D64.9
- hemoglobin D64.9
- salt syndrome E87.1
- self-esteem R45.81
- vision H54.2X-
  - one eye (other eye normal) H54.5-
    - left (normal vision on right) H54.52A-
    - other eye blind—see Blindness
    - right (normal vision on left) H54.511-

Low-density-lipoprotein-type (LDL) hyperlipoproteinemia E78.00

Lowe's syndrome E72.03

Lown-Ganong-Levine syndrome I45.6

Ludwig's angina or disease K12.2

Luetscher's syndrome E86.0

Lumbago, lumbalgia M54.50
- with sciatica M54.4-

Lumbermen's itch B88.0

Lump—see also Mass
- breast N63.0
  - axillary tail N63.3-
  - left N63.2-
  - right N63.1-
  - subareolar N63.4-

Lupoid (miliary) **of Boeck** D86.3

Lupus
- anticoagulant D68.62
  - with
    - hemorrhagic disorder D68.312
- erythematosus (discoid) (local)
  - disseminated M32.9
  - systemic M32.9
    - with organ or system involvement M32.10
      ~ endocarditis M32.11
      ~ lung M32.13
      ~ pericarditis M32.12
      ~ renal (glomerular) M32.14
        ◊ tubulo-interstitial M32.15
      ~ specified organ or system NEC M32.19
    - drug-induced M32.0
    - inhibitor (presence of) D68.62
      ~ with
        ◊ hemorrhagic disorder D68.312
- nephritis (chronic) M32.14

Lutembacher's disease or syndrome (atrial septal defect with mitral stenosis) Q21.1

Luxation—see also Dislocation
- eyeball (nontraumatic)
  - birth injury P15.3
- lens (old) (partial) (spontaneous)
  - congenital Q12.1

Lyell's syndrome L51.2
- due to drug L51.2
  - correct substance properly administered—see Table of Drugs and Chemicals, by drug, adverse effect
  - overdose or wrong substance given or taken—see Table of Drugs and Chemicals, by drug, poisoning

Lyme disease A69.20

Lymphadenitis I88.9
- acute L04.9
  - axilla L04.2
  - face L04.0
  - head L04.0
  - hip L04.3
  - limb
    - lower L04.3
    - upper L04.2
  - neck L04.0
  - shoulder L04.2
  - specified site NEC L04.8
  - trunk L04.1
- any site, except mesenteric I88.9
  - chronic I88.1
  - subacute I88.1
- chronic I88.1
  - mesenteric I88.0
- gonorrheal A54.89
- infective—see Lymphadenitis, acute
- mesenteric (acute) (chronic) (nonspecific) (subacute) I88.0
  - tuberculous A18.39
- mycobacterial A31.8
- purulent—see Lymphadenitis, acute
- pyogenic—see Lymphadenitis, acute
- regional, nonbacterial I88.8
- septic—see Lymphadenitis, acute
- subacute, unspecified site I88.1
- suppurative—see Lymphadenitis, acute
- syphilitic
  - late A52.79

Lymphadenoid goiter E06.3

Lymphadenopathy (generalized) R59.1
- due to toxoplasmosis (acquired) B58.89
  - congenital (acute) (subacute) (chronic) P37.1

Lymphadenosis R59.1

Lymphangitis I89.1
- with
  - abscess—code by site under Abscess
  - cellulitis—code by site under Cellulitis
- acute L03.91
  - abdominal wall L03.321
  - auricle (ear)—see Lymphangitis, acute
  - axilla L03.12-
  - back (any part) L03.322
  - buttock L03.327
  - cervical (meaning neck) L03.222
  - cheek (external) L03.212
  - chest wall L03.323
- digit
  - finger—see Cellulitis, finger
  - toe—see Cellulitis, toe
- ear (external) H60.1-
- eyelid—see Abscess, eyelid
- face NEC L03.212
- finger (intrathecal) (periosteal) (subcutaneous) (subcuticular) L03.02-
- gluteal (region) L03.327
- groin L03.324
- head NEC L03.891
  - face (any part, except ear, eye and nose) L03.212
- jaw (region) L03.212
- lower limb L03.12-
- navel L03.326
- neck (region) L03.222
- orbit, orbital—see Cellulitis, orbit
- pectoral (region) L03.323
- perineal, perineum L03.325
- scalp (any part) L03.891
- specified site NEC L03.898
- strumous tuberculous A18.2
- subacute (any site) I89.1
- toe (intrathecal) (periosteal) (subcutaneous) (subcuticular) L03.04-

Lymphangitis, *continued*
- trunk L03.329
  - abdominal wall L03.321
  - back (any part) L03.322
  - buttock L03.327
  - chest wall L03.323
  - groin L03.324
  - perineal, perineum L03.325
  - umbilicus L03.326
- umbilicus L03.326
- upper limb L03.12-

Lymphocytoma, benign cutis L98.8

Lymphocytopenia D72.810

Lymphocytosis (symptomatic) D72.820
- infectious (acute) B33.8

Lymphogranulomatosis (malignant)—*see also* Lymphoma, Hodgkin
- benign (Boeck's sarcoid) (Schaumann's) D86.1

Lymphohistiocytosis, hemophagocytic (familial) D76.1

Lymphoma (of) (malignant) C85.90
- diffuse large cell C83.3-
  - anaplastic C83.3-
  - B-cell C83.3-
  - CD30-positive C83.3-
  - centroblastic C83.3-
  - immunoblastic C83.3-
  - plasmablastic C83.3-
  - subtype not specified C83.3-
  - T-cell rich C83.3-
- histiocytic C85.9-
  - true C96.A
- Hodgkin C81.-
  - mixed cellularity classical C81.2-
    - nodular lymphocyte predominant C81.0-
- Lennert's C84.4-
- lymphoepithelioid C84.4-
- mature T-cell NEC C84.4-
- non-Hodgkin (*see also* Lymphoma, by type) C85.9-
- peripheral T-cell, not classified C84.4-

Lymphopenia D72.810

Lymphoproliferation, X-linked disease D82.3

Lymphosarcoma (diffuse) (*see also* Lymphoma) C85.9-

M

Macrocolon (*see also* Megacolon) Q43.1

Macrocornea Q15.8
- with glaucoma Q15.0

Macrocytosis D75.89

Macrodactylia, macrodactylism (fingers) (thumbs) Q74.0
- toes Q74.2

Macrogenitosomia (adrenal) (male) (praecox) E25.9
- congenital E25.0

Macrophthalmos Q11.3
- in congenital glaucoma Q15.0

Macrosigmoid K59.39
- congenital Q43.2
- toxic K59.31

Macrospondylitis, acromegalic E22.0

Maculae ceruleae B85.1

Madelung's
- deformity (radius) Q74.0
- disease
  - radial deformity Q74.0

Main en griffe (acquired)
- congenital Q74.0

Maintenance (encounter for)
- antineoplastic chemotherapy Z51.11
- antineoplastic radiation therapy Z51.0

Malabsorption K90.9
- calcium K90.89
- carbohydrate K90.49
- disaccharide E73.9
- fat K90.49
- intestinal K90.9
  - specified NEC K90.89
- lactose E73.9
- postgastrectomy K91.2

Malabsorption, *continued*
- postsurgical K91.2
- protein K90.49
- starch K90.49
- syndrome K90.9
  - postsurgical K91.2

Maladaptation—*see* Maladjustment

Maladie de Roger Q21.0

Maladjustment
- educational Z55.4
- family Z63.9
- social Z60.9
  - due to
    - acculturation difficulty Z60.3

Malaise R53.81

Malaria, malarial (fever) B54
- clinically diagnosed (without parasitological confirmation) B54
- congenital NEC P37.4
  - falciparum P37.3
- congestion, congestive B54
- hemorrhagic B54
- recurrent B54
- remittent B54
- specified type NEC (parasitologically confirmed) B53.8
- spleen B54
- typhoid B54

Malassimilation K90.9

Mal de mer T75.3

Maldescent, testis Q53.9
- bilateral Q53.20
  - abdominal Q53.211
  - perineal Q53.22
- unilateral Q53.10
  - abdominal Q53.111
  - perineal Q53.12

Maldevelopment—*see also* Anomaly
- brain Q07.9
- hip Q74.2
  - congenital dislocation Q65.2
    - bilateral Q65.1
    - unilateral Q65.0-
- mastoid process Q75.8
- toe Q74.2

Male type pelvis Q74.2

Malformation (congenital)—*see also* Anomaly
- alimentary tract Q45.9
  - specified type NEC Q45.8
  - upper Q40.9
    - specified type NEC Q40.8
- aorta Q25.40
  - absence Q25.41
  - aneurysm, congenital Q25.43
  - aplasia Q25.41
  - atresia Q25.29
    - aortic arch Q25.21
  - coarctation (preductal) (postductal) Q25.1
  - dilatation, congenital Q25.44
  - hypoplasia Q25.42
  - patent ductus arteriosus Q25.0
  - specified type NEC Q25.49
  - stenosis Q25.1
    - supravalvular Q25.3
- arteriovenous, aneurysmatic (congenital) Q27.3-
  - brain Q28.2
    - ruptured I60.8-
      - intracerebral I61.8
      - intraparenchymal I61.8
      - intraventricular I61.5
      - subarachnoid I60.8-
  - cerebral—*see also* Malformation, arteriovenous, brain Q28.2
  - peripheral Q27.3-
- bile duct Q44.5
- bone Q79.9
  - face Q75.9
    - specified type NEC Q75.8
  - skull Q75.9
    - specified type NEC Q75.8

Malformation, *continued*
- broad ligament Q50.6
- bursa Q79.9
- corpus callosum (congenital) Q04.0
- digestive system NEC, specified type NEC Q45.8
- dura Q07.9
  - brain Q04.9
  - spinal Q06.9
- ear Q17.9
  - causing impairment of hearing Q16.9
  - external Q17.9
    - accessory auricle Q17.0
      ~ absence of
        ◊ auditory canal Q16.1
        ◊ auricle Q16.0
    - macrotia Q17.1
    - microtia Q17.2
    - misplacement Q17.4
    - misshapen NEC Q17.3
    - prominence Q17.5
    - specified type NEC Q17.8
  - inner Q16.5
  - middle Q16.4
    - absence of eustachian tube Q16.2
    - ossicles (fusion) Q16.3
  - ossicles Q16.3
    - external Q17.9
- eye Q15.9
  - lid Q10.3
  - specified NEC Q15.8
- fallopian tube Q50.6
- great
  - vein Q26.9
    - anomalous
      ~ pulmonary venous connection Q26.4
        ◊ partial Q26.3
        ◊ total Q26.2
- heart Q24.9
  - specified type NEC Q24.8
- integument Q84.9
- joint Q74.9
  - ankle Q74.2
  - sacroiliac Q74.2
- kidney Q63.9
  - accessory Q63.0
  - giant Q63.3
  - horseshoe Q63.1
  - hydronephrosis (congenital) Q62.0
  - malposition Q63.2
  - specified type NEC Q63.8
- lacrimal apparatus Q10.6
- meninges or membrane (congenital) Q07.9
  - cerebral Q04.8
  - spinal (cord) Q06.9
- multiple types NEC Q89.7
- musculoskeletal system Q79.9
- nervous system (central) Q07.9
- ovary Q50.39
- parathyroid gland Q89.2
- penis Q55.69
  - aplasia Q55.5
  - curvature (lateral) Q55.61
  - hypoplasia Q55.62
- pulmonary
  - arteriovenous Q25.72
  - artery Q25.9
    - atresia Q25.5
    - specified type NEC Q25.79
- respiratory system Q34.9
- scrotum—*see* Malformation, testis and scrotal transposition
- sense organs NEC Q07.9
- specified NEC Q89.8
- tendon Q79.9
- testis and scrotum Q55.20
  - aplasia Q55.0
  - hypoplasia Q55.1
  - polyorchism Q55.21
  - retractile testis Q55.22
  - scrotal transposition Q55.23
  - specified NEC Q55.29
- thyroid gland Q89.2

Malformation, *continued*
- tongue (congenital) Q38.3
  - hypertrophy Q38.2
  - tie Q38.1
- urinary system Q64.9

Malibu disease L98.8

Malignancy—*see also* Neoplasm
- unspecified site (primary) C80.1

Malignant—*see* Disease, diseased

Malingerer, malingering Z76.5

Mallet finger (acquired) M20.01-
- congenital Q74.0

Malnutrition E46
- degree
  - first E44.1
  - mild (protein) E44.1
  - moderate (protein) E44.0
  - second E44.0
- following gastrointestinal surgery K91.2
- lack of care, or neglect (child) (infant) T76.02
  - confirmed T74.02
- protein E46
  - calorie E46
    - mild E44.1
    - moderate E44.0
  - energy E46
    - mild E44.1
    - moderate E44.0

Malocclusion (teeth) M26.4
- temporomandibular (joint) M26.69

Malposition
- arterial trunk Q20.0
- cervix—*see* Malposition
- congenital
  - alimentary tract Q45.8
    - lower Q43.8
    - upper Q40.8
  - aorta Q25.4
  - artery (peripheral) Q27.8
    - pulmonary Q25.79
  - biliary duct or passage Q44.5
  - clavicle Q74.0
  - digestive organ or tract NEC Q45.8
    - lower Q43.8
    - upper Q40.8
  - endocrine (gland) NEC Q89.2
  - fallopian tube Q50.6
  - finger(s) Q68.1
    - supernumerary Q69.0
  - gallbladder Q44.1
  - gastrointestinal tract Q45.8
  - genitalia, genital organ(s) or tract
    - female Q52.8
      - ~ external Q52.79
      - ~ internal NEC Q52.8
    - male Q55.8
  - heart Q24.8
    - dextrocardia Q24.0
      - ~ with complete transposition of viscera Q89.3
  - hepatic duct Q44.5
  - hip (joint) Q65.89
  - ovary Q50.39
  - parathyroid (gland) Q89.2
  - pituitary (gland) Q89.2
  - scapula Q74.0
  - shoulder Q74.0
  - symphysis pubis Q74.2
  - thymus (gland) Q89.2
  - thyroid (gland) (tissue) Q89.2
    - cartilage Q31.8
  - toe(s) Q66.9-
    - supernumerary Q69.2
- gastrointestinal tract, congenital Q45.8

Malposture R29.3

Malrotation
- cecum Q43.3
- colon Q43.3
- intestine Q43.3
- kidney Q63.2

Maltreatment
- child
  - abandonment
    - confirmed T74.02
    - suspected T76.02
  - bullying
    - confirmed T74.32
    - suspected T76.32
  - confirmed T74.92
  - history of—*see* History, personal (of), abuse
  - intimidation (through social media)
    - confirmed T74.32
    - suspected T76.32
  - neglect
    - confirmed T74.02
    - history of—*see* History, personal (of), abuse
    - suspected T76.02
  - physical abuse
    - confirmed T74.12
    - history of—*see* History, personal (of), abuse
    - suspected T76.12
  - psychological abuse
    - confirmed T74.32
    - history of—*see* History, personal (of), abuse
    - suspected T76.32
  - sexual abuse
    - confirmed T74.22
    - history of—*see* History, personal (of), abuse
    - suspected T76.22
  - suspected T76.92
- personal history of Z91.89

Mammillitis N61.0

Mammitis—*see* Mastitis

Mammogram (examination) Z12.39
- routine Z12.31

Mammoplasia N62

Manic depression F31.9

Mannosidosis E77.1

Maple-syrup-urine disease E71.0

Marchesani (-Weill) syndrome Q87.0

Marie's
- cerebellar ataxia (late-onset) G11.2
- disease or syndrome (acromegaly) E22.0

Marion's disease (bladder neck obstruction) N32.0

Mark
- port wine Q82.5
- raspberry Q82.5
- strawberry Q82.5
- tattoo L81.8

Maroteaux-Lamy syndrome (mild) (severe) E76.29

Marrow (bone)
- arrest D61.9

Masculinization (female) with adrenal hyperplasia E25.9
- congenital E25.0

Mass
- abdominal R19.00
  - epigastric R19.06
  - generalized R19.07
  - left lower quadrant R19.04
  - left upper quadrant R19.02
  - periumbilic R19.05
  - right lower quadrant R19.03
  - right upper quadrant R19.01
  - specified site NEC R19.09
- breast (*see also* Lump, breast) N63.0
- chest R22.2
- cystic—*see* Cyst
- ear H93.8-
- head R22.0
- intra-abdominal (diffuse) (generalized)—*see* Mass, abdominal
- kidney N28.89
- liver R16.0
- localized (skin) R22.9
  - chest R22.2
  - head R22.0
  - limb
    - lower R22.4-
    - upper R22.3-

Mass, *continued*
- neck R22.1
- trunk R22.2
- lung R91.8
- malignant—*see* Neoplasm, malignant, by site in Table of Neoplasms in the complete *ICD-10-CM* manual
- neck R22.1
- pelvic (diffuse) (generalized)—*see* Mass, abdominal
- specified organ NEC—*see* Disease, by site
- splenic R16.1
- substernal thyroid—*see* Goiter
- superficial (localized) R22.9
- umbilical (diffuse) (generalized) R19.09

Mast cell
- disease, systemic tissue D47.02
- leukemia C94.3-
- neoplasm
  - malignant C96.20
    - specified type NEC C96.29
  - of uncertain behavior NEC D47.09
- sarcoma C96.22
- tumor D47.09

Mastalgia N64.4

Mastitis (acute) (diffuse) (nonpuerperal) (subacute) N61.0
- infective N61.0
  - newborn P39.0
- neonatal (noninfective) P83.4
  - infective P39.0

Mastocytosis D47.09
- aggressive systemic C96.21
- cutaneous (diffuse) (maculopapular) D47.01
  - congenital Q82.2
  - of neonatal onset Q82.2
  - of newborn onset Q82.2
- indolent systemic D47.02
- isolated bone marrow D47.02
- malignant C96.29
- systemic (indolent) (smoldering)
  - with an associated hematological non-mast cell lineage disease (SM-AHNMD) D47.02

Mastodynia N64.4

Mastoidalgia—*see* subcategory H92.0

Mastoplasia, mastoplastia N62

Masturbation (excessive) F98.8

May (-Hegglin) anomaly or syndrome D72.0

McQuarrie's syndrome (idiopathic familial hypoglycemia) E16.2

Measles (black) (hemorrhagic) (suppressed) B05.9
- with
  - complications NEC B05.89
  - encephalitis B05.0
  - intestinal complications B05.4
  - keratitis (keratoconjunctivitis) B05.81
  - meningitis B05.1
  - otitis media B05.3
  - pneumonia B05.2
- French—*see* Rubella
- German—*see* Rubella
- Liberty—*see* Rubella

Meckel-Gruber syndrome Q61.9

Meckel's diverticulitis, diverticulum (displaced) (hypertrophic) Q43.0

Meconium
- ileus, newborn P76.0
  - in cystic fibrosis E84.11
  - meaning meconium plug (without cystic fibrosis) P76.0
- obstruction, newborn P76.0
  - due to fecaliths P76.0
  - in mucoviscidosis E84.11
- plug syndrome (newborn) NEC P76.0

Mediastinopericarditis—*see also* Pericarditis
- acute I30.9
- adhesive I31.0
- chronic I31.8
  - rheumatic I09.2

Medulloblastoma
- desmoplastic C71.6
- specified site—*see* Neoplasm, malignant, by site in Table of Neoplasms in the complete *ICD-10-CM* manual
- unspecified site C71.6

Medullomyoblastoma
- specified site—*see* Neoplasm, malignant, by site in Table of Neoplasms in the complete *ICD-10-CM* manual
- unspecified site C71.6

Meekeren-Ehlers-Danlos syndrome Q79.69
- classical Ehlers-Danlos syndrome Q79.61
- hypermobile Ehlers-Danlos syndrome Q79.62
- other Ehlers-Danlos syndromes Q79.69
- vascular Ehlers-Danlos syndrome Q79.63

Megacolon (acquired) (functional) (not Hirschsprung's disease) (in) K59.39
- congenital, congenitum (aganglionic) Q43.1
- Hirschsprung's (disease) Q43.1
- toxic K59.31

Megalerythema (epidemic) B08.3

Megalocornea Q15.8
- with glaucoma Q15.0

Megalodactylia (fingers) (thumbs) (congenital) Q74.0
- toes Q74.2

Megarectum K62.89

Megasigmoid K59.39
- congenital Q43.2
- toxic K59.31

Melancholia F32.A
- hypochondriac F45.29
- intermittent (single episode) F32.89
  - recurrent episode F33.9

Melanocytosis, neurocutaneous Q82.8

Melanoderma, melanodermia L81.4

Melanodontia, infantile K03.89

Melanodontoclasia K03.89

Melanoma (malignant) C43.9
- benign—*see* Nevus
- skin C43.-

Melanosis L81.4
- Riehl's L81.4
- tar L81.4
- toxic L81.4

MELAS syndrome E88.41

Melena K92.1
- with ulcer—*code by* site under Ulcer, with hemorrhage K27.4
- due to swallowed maternal blood P78.2
- newborn, neonatal P54.1
  - due to swallowed maternal blood P78.2

Membrane(s), membranous—*see also* Disease, diseased
- over face of newborn P28.9

Menarche
- delayed E30.0
- precocious E30.1

Meningism—*see* Meningismus

Meningismus (infectional) (pneumococcal) R29.1
- due to serum or vaccine R29.1
- influenzal—*see* Influenza

Meningitis (basal) (basic) (brain) (cerebral) (cervical) (congestive) (diffuse) (hemorrhagic) (infantile) (membranous) (metastatic) (nonspecific) (pontine) (progressive) (simple) (spinal) (subacute) (sympathetic) (toxic) G03.9
- abacterial G03.0
- arbovirus A87.8
- aseptic G03.0
- bacterial G00.9
  - Escherichia Coli (E. coli) G00.8
  - gram-negative G00.9
  - H. influenzae G00.0
  - pneumococcal G00.1
  - specified organism NEC G00.8
  - streptococcal (acute) G00.2
- candidal B37.5
- caseous (tuberculous) A17.0
- cerebrospinal A39.0
- clear cerebrospinal fluid NEC G03.0

Meningitis, *continued*
- coxsackievirus A87.0
- diplococcal (gram positive) A39.0
- echovirus A87.0
- enteroviral A87.0
- epidemic NEC A39.0
- Escherichia Coli (E. coli) G00.8
- fibrinopurulent G00.9
  - specified organism NEC G00.8
- gram-negative cocci G00.9
- gram-positive cocci G00.9
- Haemophilus (influenzae) G00.0
- H. influenzae G00.0
- in (due to)
  - bacterial disease NEC A48.8 *[G01]*
  - chickenpox B01.0
  - Diplococcus pneumoniae G00.1
  - enterovirus A87.0
  - herpes (simplex) virus B00.3
  - infectious mononucleosis B27.92
  - Lyme disease A69.21
  - measles B05.1
  - parasitic disease NEC B89 [G02}
  - Streptococcal pneumoniae G00.1
  - varicella B01.0
  - viral disease NEC A87.8
  - whooping cough A37.90
- infectious G00.9
- influenzal (H. influenzae) G00.0
- meningococcal A39.0
- monilial B37.5
- mycotic NEC B49 [G02]
- Neisseria A39.0
- nonbacterial G03.0
- nonpyogenic G03.0
- ossificans G96.198
- pneumococcal streptococcus pneumoniae G00.1
- postmeasles B05.1
- purulent G00.9
  - specified organism NEC G00.8
- pyogenic G00.9
  - specified organism NEC G00.8
- septic G00.9
  - specified organism NEC G00.8
- serosa circumscripta NEC G03.0
- serous NEC G93.2
- specified organism NEC G00.8
- sterile G03.0
- streptococcal (acute) G00.2
- suppurative G00.9
  - specified organism NEC G00.8
- tuberculous A17.0
- viral NEC A87.9

Meningocele (spinal) — *see also* Spina bifida
- acquired (traumatic) G96.198

Meningococcemia A39.4
- acute A39.2
- chronic A39.3

Meningococcus, meningococcal (*see also* Disease, diseased) A39.9
- carrier (suspected) of Z22.31
- meningitis (cerebrospinal) A39.0

Meningoencephalitis (*see also* Encephalitis) G04.90
- acute NEC (*see also* Encephalitis, viral) A86
  - disseminated G04.00
    - postimmunization or postvaccination G04.02
- California A83.5
- herpesviral, herpetic B00.4
  - due to herpesvirus 7 B10.09
  - specified NEC B10.09
- in (due to)
  - diseases classified elsewhere G05.3
  - Haemophilus influenzae (H. Influenzae) G00.0
  - herpes B00.4
    - due to herpesvirus 7 B10.09
    - specified NEC B10.09
  - H. influenzae G00.0
  - Lyme disease A69.22
  - toxoplasmosis (acquired) B58.2
    - congenital P37.1
- infectious (acute) (viral) A86
- parasitic NEC B89 *[G05.3]*

Meningoencephalitis, *continued*
- pneumococcal G04.2
- toxic NEC G92.8
- virus NEC A86

Meningoencephalomyelitis—*see also* Encephalitis
- acute NEC (viral) A86
  - disseminated G04.00
    - postimmunization or postvaccination G04.02
    - postinfectious G04.01
  - due to
    - Toxoplasma or toxoplasmosis (acquired) B58.2
      - congenital P37.1
- postimmunization or postvaccination G04.02

Meningomyelitis—*see also* Meningoencephalitis
- in diseases classified elsewhere G05.4

Menkes' disease or syndrome E83.09
- meaning maple-syrup-urine disease E71.0

Menometrorrhagia N92.1

Menorrhagia (primary) N92.0
- pubertal (menses retained) N92.2

Menostaxis N92.0

Menses, retention N94.89

Menstrual—*see* Menstruation

Menstruation
- absent—*see* Amenorrhea
- anovulatory N97.0
- cycle, irregular N92.6
- during pregnancy O20.8
- excessive (with regular cycle) N92.0
  - with irregular cycle N92.1
  - at puberty N92.2
- frequent N92.0
- irregular N92.6
  - specified NEC N92.5
- latent N92.5
- membranous N92.5
  - painful (*see also* Dysmenorrhea) N94.6 primary N94.4
  - psychogenic F45.8
  - secondary N94.5
- passage of clots N92.0
- precocious E30.1
- protracted N92.5
- retained N94.89
- retrograde N92.5
- suppression N94.89
- vicarious (nasal) N94.89

Mental—*see also* Disease, diseased
- observation without need for further medical care Z03.89

MERRF syndrome (myoclonic epilepsy associated with ragged-red fiber) E88.42

Metabolic syndrome E88.81

Metal
- pigmentation L81.8

Metaplasia
- gastric intestinal K31.A-

Metatarsus, metatarsal—*see also* Disease, diseased
- valgus (abductus), congenital Q66.6
- varus (adductus) (congenital) Q66.22-
  - primus Q66.21-

Methemoglobinemia D74.9
- congenital D74.0
- enzymatic (congenital) D74.0
- Hb M disease D74.0
- hereditary D74.0
- toxic D74.8

Metropathia hemorrhagica N93.8

Metrorrhagia N92.1
- psychogenic F45.8

Metrostaxis N93.8

Meyer-Schwickerath and Weyers syndrome Q87.0

Mibelli's disease (porokeratosis) Q82.8

Micrencephalon, micrencephaly Q02

Microalbuminuria R80.9

Microangiopathy (peripheral)
- thrombotic M31.10

Microcephalus, microcephalic, microcephaly Q02
- due to toxoplasmosis (congenital) P37.1

Microdeletions NEC Q93.88

Microdrepanocytosis D57.40
- with
  - acute chest syndrome D57.411
  - cerebral vascular involvement D57.413
  - crisis (painful) D57.419
    - with specified complication NEC D57.418
  - splenic sequestration D57.412
  - vasoocclusive pain D57.419

Microencephalon Q02

Microgenitalia, congenital
- female Q52.8
- male Q55.8

Microlentia (congenital) Q12.8

Microophthalmos, microphthalmia (congenital) Q11.2
- due to toxoplasmosis P37.1

Micropenis Q55.62

Microphakia (congenital) Q12.8

Microsporon furfur infestation B36.0

Micturition
- disorder NEC R39.198
  - psychogenic F45.8
- frequency R35.0
  - psychogenic F45.8
- hesitancy R39.11
- need to immediately re-void R39.191
- painful
  - dysuria R30.0
  - psychogenic F45.8
  - poor stream R39.12
- position dependent R39.192
- urgency R39.15

Migraine (idiopathic) G43.909
- with aura (acute-onset) (prolonged) (typical) (without headache) G43.109
  - with refractory migraine G43.119
    - with status migrainosus G43.111
    - without status migrainosus G43.119
  - not intractable G43.109
    - with status migrainosus G43.101
    - without status migrainosus G43.109
  - without mention of refractory migraine G43.109
    - with status migrainosus G43.101
    - without status migrainosus G43.109
- with refractory migraine G43.919
  - with status migrainosus G43.911
  - without status migrainosus G43.919
- basilar—see Migraine, with aura
- classical—see Migraine, with aura
- common—see Migraine, without aura
- complicated G43.109
- equivalents—see Migraine, with aura
- intractable G43.919
  - with status migrainosus G43.911
  - without status migrainosus G43.919
- menstrual G43.829
  - with refractory migraine G43.839
    - with status migrainosus G43.831
    - without status migrainosus G43.839
  - intractable G43.839
    - with status migrainosus G43.831
    - without status migrainosus G43.839
  - not intractable G43.829
    - with status migrainosus G43.821
    - without status migrainosus G43.829
  - without refractory migraine G43.829
    - with status migrainosus G43.821
    - without status migrainosus G43.829
- menstrually related—see Migraine, menstrual
- not intractable G43.909
  - with status migrainosus G43.901
  - without status migrainosus G43.919
- post-traumatic G44.309
  - acute G44.319
    - intractable G44.311
    - not intractable G44.319
  - chronic G44.329
    - intractable G44.321

Migraine, continued
- - not intractable G44.329
  - intractable G44.301
  - not intractable G44.309
- specified NEC G43.809
  - intractable G43.819
    - with status migrainosus G43.811
    - without status migrainosus G43.819
  - not intractable G43.809
    - with status migrainosus G43.801
    - without status migrainosus G43.809
- triggered seizures—see Migraine, with aura
- without aura G43.009
  - with refractory migraine G43.019
    - with status migrainosus G43.011
    - without status migrainosus G43.019
  - not intractable
    - with status migrainosus G43.001
    - without status migrainosus G43.009
  - without mention of refractory migraine G43.009
    - with status migrainosus G43.001
    - without status migrainosus G43.009
- without refractory migraine G43.909
  - with status migrainosus G43.901
  - without status migrainosus G43.919

Migrant, social Z59.00

Migration, anxiety concerning Z60.3

Migratory, migrating—see also Disease, diseased
- person Z59.00
- testis Q55.29

Miliaria L74.3
- alba L74.1
- crystallina L74.1
- rubra L74.0

Milk
- crust L21.0
- poisoning—see Poisoning, food, noxious
- sickness—see Poisoning, food, noxious
- spots I31.0

Milk-alkali disease or syndrome E83.52

Minot's disease (hemorrhagic disease), newborn P53

Mirror writing F81.0

Misadventure (of) (prophylactic) (therapeutic)—see also Complications T88.9
- administration of insulin (by accident)—see subcategory T38.3

Miscarriage O03.9

Misperception, sleep state F51.02

Missed
- delivery O36.4

Missing—see Absence

Mite(s) (infestation) B88.9
- diarrhea B88.0
- grain (itch) B88.0
- hair follicle (itch) B88.0
- in sputum B88.0

Mittelschmerz N94.0

Mixed—see Disease, diseased

MNGIE (Mitochondrial Neurogastrointestinal Encephalopathy) syndrome E88.49

Mobile, mobility
- gallbladder, congenital Q44.1

Mobitz heart block (atrioventricular) I44.1

Moebius, Möbius
- syndrome Q87.0
  - congenital oculofacial paralysis (with other anomalies) Q87.0

Moeller's glossitis K14.0

Mohr's syndrome (Types I and II) Q87.0

Molding, head (during birth)—omit code

Mole (pigmented)—see also Nevus
- tubal O00.10
  - with intrauterine pregnancy O00.11

Molimen, molimina (menstrual) N94.3

Molluscum contagiosum (epitheliale) B08.1

Moniliasis (see also Candidiasis) B37.9
- neonatal P37.5

Monitoring (encounter for)
- therapeutic drug level Z51.81

Monocytopenia D72.818

Monocytosis (symptomatic) D72.821

Mononeuropathy G58.9

Mononucleosis, infectious B27.90
- with
  - complication NEC B27.99
  - meningitis B27.92
  - polyneuropathy B27.91
- cytomegaloviral B27.10
  - with
    - complication NEC B27.19
    - meningitis B27.12
    - polyneuropathy B27.11
- Epstein-Barr (virus) B27.00
  - with
    - complication NEC B27.09
    - meningitis B27.02
    - polyneuropathy B27.01
- gammaherpesviral B27.00
  - with
    - complication NEC B27.09
    - meningitis B27.02
    - polyneuropathy B27.01
- specified NEC B27.80
  - with
    - complication NEC B27.89
    - meningitis B27.82
    - polyneuropathy B27.81

Monoplegia G83.3-
- hysterical (transient) F44.4
- psychogenic (conversion reaction) F44.4

Monorchism, monorchidism Q55.0

Monosomy (see also Deletion, chromosome) Q93.9
- specified NEC Q93.89
- X Q96.9

Monster, monstrosity (single) Q89.7

Monteggia's fracture (-dislocation) S52.27-

Morbidity not stated or unknown R69

Morbilli—see Measles

Morbus—see also Disease
- angelicus, anglorum E55.0
- celiacus K90.0
- hemorrhagicus neonatorum P53
- maculosus neonatorum P54.5

Morgagni's
- cyst, organ, hydatid, or appendage
  - female Q50.5
  - male (epididymal) Q55.4
    - testicular Q55.29

Morgagni-Stokes-Adams syndrome I45.9

Morgagni-Turner (-Albright) **syndrome** Q96.9

Moron (I.Q.50-69) F70

Morvan's disease or syndrome G60.8

Mosaicism, mosaic (autosomal) (chromosomal)
- 45,X/other cell lines NEC with abnormal sex chromosome Q96.4
- 45,X/46,XX Q96.3
- sex chromosome
  - female Q97.8
  - lines with various numbers of X chromosomes Q97.2
  - male Q98.7
- XY Q96.3

Motion sickness (from travel, any vehicle) (from roundabouts or swings) T75.3

Mountain
- sickness T70.29
  - with polycythemia, acquired (acute) D75.1
- tick fever A93.2

MRSA (Methicillin resistant Staphylococcus aureus)
- infection A49.02
  - as the cause of disease classified elsewhere B95.62
- sepsis A41.02

MSD (multiple sulfatase deficiency) E75.26

MSSA (Methicillin susceptible Staphylococcus aureus)
- infection A49.02
  - as the cause of disease classified elsewhere B95.61
- sepsis A41.01

Mucinosis (cutaneous) (focal) (papular) (reticular erythematous) (skin) L98.5
- oral K13.79

Mucocele
- buccal cavity K13.79
- nasal sinus J34.1
- nose J34.1
- sinus (accessory) (nasal) J34.1
- turbinate (bone) (middle) (nasal) J34.1

Mucolipidosis
- I E77.1
- II, III E77.0

Mucopolysaccharidosis E76.3
- beta-gluduronidase deficiency E76.29
- cardiopathy E76.3 [I52]
- Hunter's syndrome E76.1
- Hurler's syndrome E76.01
- Maroteaux-Lamy syndrome E76.29
- Morquio syndrome E76.219
  - A E76.210
  - B E76.211
  - classic E76.210
- Sanfilippo syndrome E76.22
- specified NEC E76.29
- type
  - I
    - Hurler's syndrome E76.01
    - Hurler-Scheie syndrome E76.02
    - Scheie's syndrome E76.03
  - II E76.1
  - III E76.22
  - IV E76.219
  - IVA E76.210
  - IVB E76.211
  - VI E76.29
  - VII E76.29

Mucositis (ulcerative) K12.30
- nasal J34.81

Mucoviscidosis E84.9
- with meconium obstruction E84.11

Mucus
- asphyxiation or suffocation—see Asphyxia
- in stool R19.5
- plug—see Asphyxia

Muguet B37.0

Multicystic kidney (development) Q61.4

Multisystem inflammatory syndrome (in adult) (in children) M35.81

Mumps B26.9

Murmur (cardiac) (heart) (organic) R01.1
- aortic (valve)—see Endocarditis, aortic
- benign R01.0
- diastolic—see Endocarditis
- Flint I35.1
- functional R01.0
- Graham Steell I37.1
- innocent R01.0
- mitral (valve)—see Insufficiency, mitral
- nonorganic R01.0
- presystolic, mitral—see Insufficiency, mitral
- pulmonic (valve) I37.8
- systolic R01.1
- tricuspid (valve) I07.9
- valvular—see Endocarditis

Muscle, muscular—see also Disease, diseased
- carnitine (palmityltransferase) deficiency E71.314

Mutation(s)
- surfactant, of lung J84.83

Mutism—see also Aphasia
- deaf (acquired) (congenital) NEC H91.3
- elective (adjustment reaction) (childhood) F94.0
- hysterical F44.4
- selective (childhood) F94.0

Myalgia M79.1-
- traumatic NEC T14.8

Myasthenia G70.9
- congenital G70.2
- cordis—see Failure, heart
- developmental G70.2
- gravis G70.00
  - with exacerbation (acute) G70.01
  - in crisis G70.01
  - neonatal, transient P94.0
  - pseudoparalytica G70.00
    - with exacerbation (acute) G70.01
    - in crisis G70.01
- stomach, psychogenic F45.8
- syndrome
  - in
    - diabetes mellitus—see E08-E13 with .44
    - neoplastic disease (see also Table of Neoplasms in the complete ICD-10-CM manual) D49.9 [G73.3]
    - thyrotoxicosis E05.90 [G73.3]
      ~ with thyroid storm E05.91 [G73.3]

Myasthenic M62.81

Mycoplasma (M.) pneumoniae, as cause of disease classified elsewhere B96.0

Mycosis, mycotic B49
- mouth B37.0
- nails B35.1
- stomatitis B37.0
- vagina, vaginitis (candidal) B37.3

Myelitis (acute) (ascending) (childhood) (chronic) (descending) (diffuse) (disseminated) (idiopathic) (pressure) (progressive) (spinal cord) (subacute) (see also Encephalitis) G04.91
- flaccid G04.82
- in diseases classified elsewhere G05.4
- post–chicken pox B01.12
- postimmunization G04.02
- postinfectious G04.89
- postvaccinal G04.02
- specified NEC G04.89
- toxic G92.9
- varicella B01.12

Myelogenous—see Disease, diseased

Myeloid—see Disease, diseased

Myelokathexis D70.9

Myelopathy (spinal cord) G95.9
- in (due to)
  - infection—see Encephalitis
  - mercury—see subcategory T56.1
  - neoplastic disease (see also Table of Neoplasms in the complete ICD-10-CM manual) D49.9 [G99.2]

Myelophthisis D61.82

Myelosclerosis D75.89
- disseminated, of nervous system G35

Myelosis
- acute C92.0-
- aleukemic C92.9-
- nonleukemic D72.828
- subacute C92.9-

Myocardiopathy (congestive) (constrictive) (familial) (hypertrophic nonobstructive) (idiopathic) (infiltrative) (obstructive) (primary) (restrictive) (sporadic) (see also Cardiomyopathy) I42.9
- hypertrophic obstructive I42.1
- in (due to)
  - Friedreich's ataxia G11.11 [I43]
  - progressive muscular dystrophy G71.09 [I43]
- secondary I42.9
- thyrotoxic E05.90 [I43]
  - with storm E05.91 [I43]

Myocarditis (with arteriosclerosis) (chronic) (fibroid) (interstitial) (old) (progressive) (senile) I51.4
- with
  - rheumatic fever (conditions in I00) I09.0
    - active—see Myocarditis, acute, rheumatic
    - inactive or quiescent (with chorea) I09.0
- active I40.9
  - rheumatic I01.2
    - with chorea (acute) (rheumatic) (Sydenham's) I02.0
- acute or subacute (interstitial) I40.9
  - due to

Myocarditis, continued
  - streptococcus (beta-hemolytic) I01.2
  - idiopathic I40.1
  - rheumatic I01.2
    - with chorea (acute) (rheumatic) (Sydenham's) I02.0
  - specified NEC I40.8
- bacterial (acute) I40.0
- eosinophilic I40.1
- epidemic of newborn (Coxsackie) B33.22
- Fiedler's (acute) (isolated) I40.1
- giant cell (acute) (subacute) I40.1
- granulomatous (idiopathic) (isolated) (nonspecific) I40.1
- idiopathic (granulomatous) I40.1
- in (due to)
  - Lyme disease A69.29
  - sarcoidosis D86.85
- infective I40.0
- influenzal—see Influenza, myocarditis
- isolated (acute) I40.1
- nonrheumatic, active I40.9
- parenchymatous I40.9
- pneumococcal I40.0
- rheumatic (chronic) (inactive) (with chorea) I09.0
  - active or acute I01.2
    - with chorea (acute) (rheumatic) (Sydenham's) I02.0
- septic I40.0
- staphylococcal I40.0
- suppurative I40.0
- toxic I40.8
- virus, viral I40.0
  - of newborn (Coxsackie) B33.22

Myoclonus, myoclonic, myoclonia (familial) (essential) (multifocal) (simplex) G25.3
- drug-induced G25.3
- epilepsy (see also Epilepsy, generalized, specified NEC) G40.4-
  - familial (progressive) G25.3
- familial progressive G25.3
- Friedreich's G25.3
- jerks G25.3
- massive G25.3
- palatal G25.3
- pharyngeal G25.3

Myofibromatosis
- infantile Q89.8

Myopathy G72.9
- autosomal (dominant) (recessive) G71.228
  - other specified NEC G71.228
- benign congenital G71.20
- central core G71.29
- centronuclear G71.228
- congenital (benign) G71.20
- distal G71.09
- facioscapulohumeral G71.02hyaline body G71.29
- in (due to)
  - Cushing's syndrome E24.9 [G73.7]
  - hyperadrenocorticism E24.9 [G73.7]
  - hypopituitarism E23.0 [G73.7]
  - hypothyroidism E03.9 [G73.7]
  - myxedema E03.9 [G73.7]
  - sarcoidosis D86.87
  - scarlet fever A38.1
  - systemic lupus erythematosus M32.19
  - thyrotoxicosis (hyperthyroidism) E05.90 [G73.7]
    - with thyroid storm E05.91 [G73.7]
- limb-girdle G71.09
- myosin storage G71.29
  - myotubular (centronuclear) G71.220
    - X-linked G71.220
- nemaline G71.21
- ocular G71.09
- oculopharyngeal G71.09
- rod (body) G71.21
- scapulohumeral G71.02

Myopia (axial) (congenital) H52.1-

Myositis M60.9
- in (due to)
  - sarcoidosis D86.87
- infective M60.009
  - arm
    - left M60.001

Myositis, *continued*
- ■ right M60.000
- – leg
  - ■ left M60.004
  - ■ right M60.003
- – lower limb
  - ■ ankle M60.07-
  - ■ foot M60.07-
  - ■ lower leg M60.06-
  - ■ thigh M60.05-
  - ■ toe M60.07-
- – multiple sites M60.09
- – specified site NEC M60.08
- – upper limb
  - ■ finger M60.04-
  - ■ forearm M60.03-
  - ■ hand M60.04-
  - ■ shoulder region M60.01-
  - ■ upper arm M60.02-

Myospasia impulsiva F95.2

Myotonia (acquisita) (intermittens) M62.89
- • congenita (acetazolamide responsive) (dominant) (recessive) G71.12
- • levior G71.12

Myriapodiasis B88.2

Myringitis H73.2-
- • with otitis media—*see* Otitis, media
- • acute H73.00-
  - – bullous H73.01-
- • bullous—*see* Myringitis, acute, bullous
- • chronic H73.1-

Myxadenitis labialis K13.0

Myxedema (adult) (idiocy) (infantile) (juvenile) (*see also* Hypothyroidism) E03.9
- • circumscribed E05.90
  - – with storm E05.91
- • congenital E00.1
- • cutis L98.5
- • localized (pretibial) E05.90
  - – with storm E05.91

Myxolipoma D17.9

N

Naegeli's
- • disease Q82.8

Nail—*see also* Disease, diseased
- • biting F98.8

Nanism, nanosomia—*see* Dwarfism

Napkin rash L22

Narcosis R06.89

Narcotism—*see* Dependence

NARP (Neuropathy, Ataxia and Retinitis pigmentosa) syndrome E88.49

Narrowness, abnormal, eyelid Q10.3

Nasopharyngeal—*see also* Disease, diseased
- • pituitary gland Q89.2
- • torticollis M43.6

Nasopharyngitis (acute) (infective) (streptococcal) (subacute) J00
- • chronic (suppurative) (ulcerative) J31.1

Nasopharynx, nasopharyngeal—*see* Disease, diseased

Natal tooth, teeth K00.6

Nausea (without vomiting) R11.0
- • with vomiting R11.2
- • marina T75.3
- • navalis T75.3

Near drowning T75.1

Nearsightedness—*see* Myopia

Near-syncope R55

Necrolysis, toxic epidermal L51.2
- • due to drug
  - – correct substance properly administered—*see* Table of Drugs and Chemicals, by drug, adverse effect
  - – overdose or wrong substance given or taken—*see* Table of Drugs and Chemicals, by drug, poisoning

Necrosis, necrotic (ischemic)—*see also* Gangrene
- • adrenal (capsule) (gland) E27.49
- • antrum J32.0
- • cortical (acute) (renal) N17.1
- • ethmoid (bone) J32.2
- • fat, fatty (generalized)—*see also* Disorder, specified type NEC
  - – skin (subcutaneous), newborn P83.0
  - – subcutaneous due to birth injury P15.6
- • kidney (bilateral) N28.0
  - – acute N17.9
  - – cortical (acute) (bilateral) N17.1
  - – medullary (bilateral) (in acute renal failure) (papillary) N17.2
  - – papillary (bilateral) (in acute renal failure) N17.2
  - – tubular N17.0
    - ■ medullary (acute) (renal) N17.2
- • papillary (acute) (renal) N17.2
- • pharynx J02.9
  - – in granulocytopenia—*see* Neutropenia
- • phosphorus—*see* subcategory T54.2
- • pituitary (gland) E23.0
- • subcutaneous fat, newborn P83.88
- • suprarenal (capsule) (gland) E27.49
- • tonsil J35.8
- • tubular (acute) (anoxic) (renal) (toxic) N17.0
  - – postprocedural N99.0

Need (for)
- • care provider because (of)
  - – assistance with personal care Z74.1
  - – continuous supervision required Z74.3
  - – impaired mobility Z74.09
  - – no other household member able to render care Z74.2
  - – specified reason NEC Z74.8
- • immunization—*see* Vaccination
- • vaccination—*see* Vaccination

Neglect
- • child (childhood)
  - – confirmed T74.02
  - – history of Z62.812
  - – suspected T76.02
- • emotional, in childhood Z62.898

Nelaton's syndrome G60.8

Neonatal—*see also* Newborn
- • acne L70.4
- • bradycardia P29.12
- • screening, abnormal findings on P09.-
- • tachycardia P29.11
- • tooth, teeth K00.6

Neonatorum—*see* Disease, diseased

Neoplasia
- • intraepithelial (histologically confirmed)
  - – anal (AIN) (histologically confirmed) K62.82
    - ■ grade I K62.82
    - ■ grade II K62.82

Neoplasm, neoplastic—*see also* Table of Neoplasms in the complete *ICD-10-CM* manual.
- • lipomatous, benign—*see* Lipoma

Nephralgia N23

Nephritis, nephritic (albuminuric) (azotemic) (congenital) (disseminated) (epithelial) (familial) (focal) (granulomatous) (hemorrhagic) (infantile) (nonsuppurative, excretory) (uremic) N05.9
- • with
  - – C3
    - ■ glomerulonephritis N05.A
    - ■ glomerulopathy N05.A
      - ~ with dense deposit disease N05.6
- • acute N00.9
  - – with
    - ■ C3
      - ~ glomerulonephritis N00.A
      - ~ glomerulopathy N00.A
        - ◊ with dense deposit disease N00.6
        - ◊ dense deposit disease N00.6
    - ■ diffuse
      - ~ crescentic glomerulonephritis N00.7
      - ~ endocapillary proliferative glomerulonephritis N00.4
      - ~ membranous glomerulonephritis N00.2

Nephritis, nephritic, *continued*
- - ~ mesangial proliferative glomerulonephritis N00.3
- - ~ mesangiocapillary glomerulonephritis N00.5
- - ■ focal and segmental glomerular lesions N00.1
- - ■ minor glomerular abnormality N00.0
- - ■ specified morphological changes NEC N00.8
- • chronic N03.9
  - – with
    - ■ C3
      - ~ glomerulonephritis N03.A
      - ~ glomerulopathy N03.A
        - ◊ with dense deposit disease N03.6
- • croupous N00.9
- • due to
  - – diabetes mellitus—*see* E08-E13 with .21
  - – subacute bacterial endocarditis I33.0
  - – systemic lupus erythematosus (chronic) M32.14
- • in
  - – diabetes mellitus—*see* E08–E13 with.21
- • polycystic Q61.3
  - – autosomal
    - ■ dominant Q61.2
    - ■ recessive NEC Q61.19
  - – childhood type NEC Q61.19
  - – infantile type NEC Q61.19
- • poststreptococcal N05.9
  - – acute N00.9
  - – chronic N03.9
- • rapidly progressive N01.-
  - – with
    - ■ C3
      - ~ glomerulonephritis N01.A
      - ~ glomerulopathy N01.A
        - ◊ with dense deposit disease N01.6
- • tubulo-interstitial (in) N12
  - – acute (infectious) N10
- • war N00.9

Nephroblastoma (epithelial) (mesenchymal) C64.-

Nephrocystitis, pustular—*see* Nephritis, tubulo-interstitial

Nephroma C64-

Nephronephritis—*see* Nephrosis

Nephronophthisis Q61.5

Nephropathy (*see also* Nephritis) N28.9
- • analgesic N14.0
  - – with medullary necrosis, acute N17.2
- • diabetic—*see* E08–E13 with .21
- • hereditary NEC N07.9
  - – with
    - ■ C3
      - ~ glomerulonephritis N07.A
      - ~ glomerulopathy N07.A
        - ◊ with dense deposit disease N07.6
- • obstructive N13.8
- • phenacetin N17.2
- • vasomotor N17.0

Nephrosis, nephrotic (Epstein's) (syndrome) (congenital) N04.9
- • with
  - – glomerular lesion N04.1
  - – hypocomplementemic N04.5
- • acute N04.9
- • anoxic—*see* Nephrosis, tubular
- • chemical—*see* Nephrosis, tubular
- • Finnish type (congenital) Q89.8
- • hemoglobin N10
- • hemoglobinuric—*see* Nephrosis, tubular
- • in
  - – diabetes mellitus—*see* E08–E13 with .21
- • lipoid N04.9
- • minimal change N04.0
- • myoglobin N10
- • radiation N04.9
- • toxic—*see* Nephrosis, tubular
- • tubular (acute) N17.0
  - – postprocedural N99.0
  - – radiation N04.9

Nerves R45.0

Nervous (*see also* Disease, diseased) R45.0
- • heart F45.8
- • stomach F45.8

Nervous, *continued*
- tension R45.0

Nervousness R45.0

Nettleship's syndrome—*see* Urticaria pigmentosa

Neuralgia, neuralgic (acute) M79.2
- ciliary G44.009
  - intractable G44.001
  - not intractable G44.009
- ear—*see* subcategory H92.0
- migrainous G44.009
  - intractable G44.001
  - not intractable G44.009
- perineum R10.2
- pubic region R10.2
- scrotum R10.2
- spermatic cord R10.2

Neurasthenia F48.8
- cardiac F45.8
- gastric F45.8
- heart F45.8

Neuritis (rheumatoid) M79.2
- cranial nerve
  - due to Lyme disease A69.22
  - fifth or trigeminal G51.0
  - seventh or facial G51.8
    - newborn (birth injury) P11.3
  - sixth or abducent—*see* Strabismus, paralytic, sixth nerve
- facial G51.8
  - newborn (birth injury) P11.3
- serum (*see also* Reaction, serum) T80.69

Neuroblastoma
- specified site—*see* Neoplasm, malignant, by site in Table of Neoplasms in the complete *ICD-10-CM* manual
- unspecified site C74.90

Neurocirculatory asthenia F45.8

Neurodermatitis (circumscribed) (circumscripta) (local) L28.0
- atopic L20.81
- diffuse (Brocq) L20.81
- disseminated L20.81

Neurofibromatosis (multiple) (nonmalignant) Q85.00
- acoustic Q85.02
- malignant—*see* Neoplasm, nerve, malignant in Table of Neoplasms in the complete *ICD-10-CM* manual
- specified NEC Q85.09
- type 1 (von Recklinghausen) Q85.01
- type 2 Q85.02

Neurogenic—*see also* Disease, diseased
- bladder (*see also* Dysfunction) N31.9
  - cauda equina syndrome G83.4
- bowel NEC K59.2
- heart F45.8

Neuromyopathy G70.9
- paraneoplastic D49.9 *[G13.0]*

Neuropathy, neuropathic G62.9
- hereditary G60.9
  - motor and sensory (types I–IV) G60.0
  - sensory G60.8
  - specified NEC G60.8
- idiopathic G60.9
  - progressive G60.3
  - specified NEC G60.8
- peripheral (nerve) (*see also* Polyneuropathy) G62.9
  - autonomic G90.9
    - in (due to)
      - hyperthyroidism E05.90 [G99.0]
        ◊ with thyroid storm E05.91 [G99.0]

Neurosis, neurotic F48.9
- anankastic F42.8
- anxiety (state) F41.1
  - panic type F41.0
- bladder F45.8
- cardiac (reflex) F45.8
- cardiovascular F45.8
- character F60.9
- colon F45.8
- compulsive, compulsion F42.9
- conversion F44.9
- cutaneous F45.8
- excoriation F42.4

Neurosis, neurotic, *continued*
- gastric F45.8
- gastrointestinal F45.8
- heart F45.8
- hysterical F44.9
- incoordination F45.8
  - larynx F45.8
  - vocal cord F45.8
- intestine F45.8
- larynx (sensory) F45.8
  - hysterical F44.4
- mixed NEC F48.8
- musculoskeletal F45.8
- obsessional F42.9
- obsessive-compulsive F42.9
- ocular NEC F45.8
- pharynx F45.8
- phobic F40.9
- posttraumatic (situational) F43.10
  - acute F43.11
  - chronic F43.12
- rectum F45.8
- respiratory F45.8
- rumination F45.8
- state F48.9
- stomach F45.8
- traumatic F43.10
  - acute F43.11
  - chronic F43.12
- vasomotor F45.8
- visceral F45.8

Neurospongioblastosis diffusa Q85.1

Neutropenia, neutropenic (chronic) (genetic) (idiopathic) (immune) (infantile) (malignant) (pernicious) (splenic) D70.9
- congenital (primary) D70.0
- cyclic D70.4
- cytoreductive cancer chemotherapy sequela D70.1
- drug-induced D70.2
  - due to cytoreductive cancer chemotherapy D70.1
- due to infection D70.3
- fever D70.9
- neonatal, transitory (isoimmune) (maternal transfer) P61.5
- periodic D70.4
- secondary (cyclic) (periodic) (splenic) D70.4
  - drug-induced D70.2
    - due to cytoreductive cancer chemotherapy D70.1
- toxic D70.8

Neutrophilia, hereditary giant D72.0

Nevus D22-
- achromic—*see* Neoplasm, skin, benign in Table of Neoplasms in the complete *ICD-10-CM* manual
- amelanotic—*see* Neoplasm, skin, benign in Table of Neoplasms in the complete *ICD-10-CM* manual
- angiomatous D18.00
  - skin D18.01
  - specified site NEC D18.09
- araneus I78.1
- blue—(*see* Neoplasm, skin, benign for blue, cellular, giant, or Jadassohn's or other than malignant in Table of Neoplasms in the complete *ICD-10-CM* manual)
  - malignant—*see* Melanoma
- capillary D18.00
  - skin D18.01
  - specified site NEC D18.09
- cavernous D18.00
  - skin D18.01
  - specified site NEC D18.09
- cellular—*see* Neoplasm, skin, benign in Table of Neoplasms in the complete *ICD-10-CM* manual
  - blue—*see* Neoplasm, skin, benign in Table of Neoplasms in the complete *ICD-10-CM* manual
- comedonicus Q82.5
- dermal—*see* Neoplasm, skin, benign in Table of Neoplasms in the complete *ICD-10-CM* manual
  - with epidermal nevus—*see* Neoplasm, skin, benign in Table of Neoplasms in the complete *ICD-10-CM* manual
- dysplastic—*see* Neoplasm, skin, benign in Table of Neoplasms in the complete *ICD-10-CM* manual
- flammeus Q82.5

Nevus, *continued*
- hemangiomatous D18.00
  - skin D18.01
  - specified site NEC D18.09
- lymphatic D18.1
- meaning hemangioma D18.00
  - skin D18.01
  - specified site NEC D18.09
- multiplex Q85.1
- non-neoplastic I78.1
- portwine Q82.5
- sanguineous Q82.5
- skin D22.9
  - abdominal wall D22.5
  - ala nasi D22.39
  - ankle D22.7-
  - anus, anal D22.5
  - arm D22.6-
  - auditory canal (external) D22.2-
  - auricle (ear) D22.2-
  - auricular canal (external) D22.2-
  - axilla, axillary fold D22.5
  - back D22.5
  - breast D22.5
  - brow D22.39
  - buttock D22.5
  - canthus (eye) D22.1-
  - cheek (external) D22.39
  - chest wall D22.5
  - chin D22.39
  - ear (external) D22.2-
    - external meatus (ear) D22.2-
  - eyebrow D22.39
  - eyelid (lower) (upper) D22.1-
  - face D22.3-
  - finger D22.6-
  - flank D22.5
  - foot D22.7-
  - forearm D22.6-
  - forehead D22.39
  - foreskin D29.0
  - genital organ (external) NEC
    - female D28.0
    - male D29.9
  - gluteal region D22.5
  - groin D22.5
  - hand D22.6-
  - heel D22.7-
  - helix D22.2-
  - hip D22.7-
  - interscapular region D22.5
  - jaw D22.39
  - knee D22.7-
  - leg D22.7-
  - lip (lower) (upper) D22.0
  - lower limb D22.7-
  - nail D22.9
    - finger D22.6-
    - toe D22.7-
  - nasolabial groove D22.39
  - nates D22.5
  - neck D22.4
  - nose (external) D22.39
  - palpebra D22.1-
  - penis D29.0
  - perianal skin D22.5
  - perineum D22.5
  - pinna D22.2-
  - popliteal fossa or space D22.7-
  - scalp D22.4
  - shoulder D22.6-
  - submammary fold D22.5
  - temple D22.39
  - thigh D22.7-
  - toe D22.7-
  - trunk NEC D22.5
  - umbilicus D22.5
  - upper limb D22.6-
  - vulva D28.0
  - specified site NEC -see Neoplasm, by site, benign in Table of Neoplasms in the complete *ICD-10-CM* manual

Nevus, *continued*
- – Sutton's benign D22.9
  - ■ spider I78.1
  - ■ stellar I78.1
  - ■ strawberry Q82.5
  - ■ unius lateris Q82.5
  - ■ Unna's Q82.5
  - ■ vascular Q82.5
  - ■ verrucous Q82.5

Newborn (infant) (liveborn) (singleton) Z38.2
- • abstinence syndrome P96.1
- • acne L70.4
- • affected by
  - – abruptio placenta P02.1
  - – amniocentesis (while in utero) P00.6
  - – amnionitis P02.78
  - – apparent life threatening event (ALTE) R68.13
  - – bleeding (into)
    - ■ cerebral cortex P52.22
    - ■ germinal matrix P52.0
    - ■ ventricles P52.1
  - – breech delivery P03.0
  - – cardiac arrest P29.81
  - – cerebral ischemia P91.0
  - – Cesarean delivery P03.4
  - – chemotherapy agents P04.1
  - – chorioamnionitis P02.78
  - – cocaine (crack) P04.41
  - – complications of labor and delivery P03.9
    - ■ specified NEC P03.89
  - – compression of umbilical cord NEC P02.5
  - – contracted pelvis P03.1
  - – cyanosis P28.2
  - – delivery P03.9
    - ■ Cesarean P03.4
    - ■ forceps P03.2
    - ■ vacuum extractor P03.3
  - – drugs of addiction P04.40
    - ■ cocaine P04.41
    - ■ hallucinogens P04.42
    - ■ specified drug NEC P04.49
  - – entanglement (knot) in umbilical cord P02.5
  - – fetal (intrauterine)
    - ■ growth retardation P05.9
    - ■ inflammatory response syndrome (FIRS) P02.70
  - – FIRS (fetal inflammatory response syndrome) P02.70
  - – forceps delivery P03.2
  - – heart rate abnormalities
    - ■ bradycardia P29.12
    - ■ intrauterine P03.819
      - ~ before onset of labor P03.810
      - ~ during labor P03.811
    - ■ tachycardia P29.11
  - – hemorrhage (antepartum) P02.1
    - ■ intraventricular (nontraumatic) P52.3
      - ~ grade 1 P52.0
      - ~ grade 2 P52.1
      - ~ grade 3 P52.21
      - ~ grade 4 P52.22
    - ■ subependymal P52.0
      - ~ with intracerebral extension P52.22
      - ~ with intraventricular extension P52.1
        - ◊ with enlargement of ventricles P52.21
      - ~ without intraventricular extension P52.0
  - – hypoxic ischemic encephalopathy [HIE] P91.60
    - ■ mild P91.61
    - ■ moderate P91.62
    - ■ severe P91.63
  - – induction of labor P03.89
  - – intrauterine (fetal) blood loss P50.9
  - – intrauterine (fetal) hemorrhage P50.9
  - – malpresentation (malposition) NEC P03.1
  - – maternal (complication of) (use of)
    - ■ alcohol P04.3
    - ■ amphetamines P04.16
    - ■ analgesia (maternal) P04.0
    - ■ anesthesia (maternal) P04.0
    - ■ anticonvulsants P04.13
    - ■ antidepressants P04.15
    - ■ antineoplastic chemotherapy P04.11
    - ■ anxiolytics P04.1A
    - ■ blood loss P02.1
    - ■ cannabis P04.81

Newborn, *continued*
- ■ circulatory disease P00.3
- ■ condition P00.9
  - ~ specified NEC P00.89
- ■ cytotoxic drugs P04.12
- ■ delivery P03.9
  - ~ Cesarean P03.4
  - ~ forceps P03.2
  - ~ vacuum extractor P03.3
- ■ diabetes mellitus (pre-existing) P70.1
- ■ disorder P00.9
  - ~ specified NEC P00.89
- ■ drugs (addictive) (illegal) NEC P04.49
- ■ group B streptococcus (GBS) colonization (positive) P00.82
- ■ hemorrhage P02.1
- ■ incompetent cervix P01.0
- ■ infectious disease P00.2
- ■ malpresentation before labor P01.7
- ■ medical procedure P00.7
- ■ medication (legal) (maternal use) (prescribed) P04.19
- ■ opiates P04.14
  - ~ administered for procedures during pregnancy or labor and delivery P04.0
- ■ parasitic disease P00.2
- ■ placenta previa P02.0
- ■ premature rupture of membranes P01.1
- ■ respiratory disease P00.3
- ■ sedative-hypnotics P04.17
  - ~ tranquilizers administered for procedures during pregnancy or labor and delivery P04.0
- ■ surgical procedure P00.6
- ■ medication (legal) (maternal use) (prescribed) P04.19
- ■ specified type NEC P04.18
- – membranitis P02.78
- – methamphetamine(s) P04.49
- – mixed metabolic and respiratory acidosis P84
- – neonatal abstinence syndrome P96.1
- – noxious substances transmitted via placenta or breast milk P04.9
  - ■ cannabis P04.81
  - ■ specified NEC P04.89
- – placenta previa P02.0
- – placental
  - ■ abnormality (functional) (morphological) P02.20
    - ~ specified NEC P02.29
  - ■ dysfunction P02.29
  - ■ infarction P02.29
  - ■ insufficiency P02.29
  - ■ separation NEC P02.1
  - ■ transfusion syndromes P02.3
- – placentitis P02.78
- – prolapsed cord P02.4
- – respiratory arrest P28.81
- – slow intrauterine growth P05.9
- – tobacco P04.2
- – twin to twin transplacental transfusion P02.3
- – umbilical cord (tightly) around neck P02.5
- – umbilical cord condition P02.60
  - ■ short cord P02.69
  - ■ specified NEC P02.69
- – uterine contractions (abnormal) P03.6
- – vasa previa P02.69
  - ■ from intrauterine blood loss P50.0
- • apnea P28.4
  - – primary P28.3
  - – obstructive P28.4
  - – sleep (central) (obstructive) (primary) P28.3
- • born in hospital Z38.00
  - – by cesarean Z38.01
- • born outside hospital Z38.1
- • breast buds P96.89
- • breast engorgement P83.4
- • check-up—*see* Newborn, examination
- • convulsion P90
- • dehydration P74.1
- • examination
  - – 8 to 28 days old Z00.111
  - – under 8 days old Z00.110
- • fever P81.9
  - – environmentally-induced P81.0

Newborn, *continued*
- • hyperbilirubinemia P59.9
  - – of prematurity P59.0
- • hypernatremia P74.21
- • hyponatremia P74.22
- • infection P39.9
  - – candidal P37.5
  - – specified NEC P39.8
  - – urinary tract P39.3
- • jaundice P59.9
  - – due to
    - ■ breast milk inhibitor P59.3
    - ■ hepatocellular damage P59.20
      - ~ specified NEC P59.29
    - ■ preterm delivery P59.0
  - – of prematurity P59.0
  - – specified NEC P59.8
- • mastitis P39.0
  - – infective P39.0
  - – noninfective P83.4
- • multiple born NEC Z38.8
  - – born in hospital Z38.68
    - ■ by cesarean Z38.69
  - – born outside hospital Z38.7
- • omphalitis P38.9
  - – with mild hemorrhage P38.1
  - – without hemorrhage P38.9
- • post-term P08.21
- • prolonged gestation (over 42 completed weeks) P08.22
- • quadruplet Z38.8
  - – born in hospital Z38.63
    - ■ by cesarean Z38.64
  - – born outside hospital Z38.7
- • quintuplet Z38.8
  - – born in hospital Z38.65
    - ■ by cesarean Z38.66
  - – born outside hospital Z38.7
- • seizure P90
- • sepsis (congenital) P36.9
  - – due to
    - ■ anaerobes NEC P36.5
    - ■ Escherichia coli P36.4
    - ■ Staphylococcus P36.30
      - ~ aureus P36.2
      - ~ specified NEC P36.39
    - ■ Streptococcus P36.10
      - ~ group B P36.0
      - ~ specified NEC P36.19
  - – specified NEC P36.8
- • triplet Z38.8
  - – born in hospital Z38.61
    - ■ by cesarean Z38.62
  - – born outside hospital Z38.7
- • twin Z38.5
  - – born in hospital Z38.30
    - ■ by cesarean Z38.31
  - – born outside hospital Z38.4
- • vomiting P92.09
  - – bilious P92.01
- • weight check Z00.111

Niemann-Pick disease or syndrome E75.249
- • specified NEC E75.248
- • type
  - – A E75.240
  - – A/B E75.244
  - – B E75.241
  - – C E75.242
  - – D E75.243

Night
- • sweats R61
- • terrors (child) F51.4

Nightmares (REM sleep type) F51.5

Nipple—*see* Disease, diseased

Nitrosohemoglobinemia D74.8

Nocturia R35.1
- • psychogenic F45.8

Nocturnal—*see* Disease, diseased

Node(s)—*see also* Nodule
- • Osler's I33.0

Nodule(s), nodular
- • breast NEC N63.0

Obstruction, obstructed, obstructive, *continued*
- ■ specified NEC P76.8
- – partial K56.600
- – reflex K56.0
- – specified NEC K56.699
  - ■ complete K56.691
  - ■ incomplete K56.690
  - ■ partial K56.690
- – volvulus K56.2
- kidney (calices) (see also Hydronephrosis) N28.89
- lacrimal (passages) (duct)
  - – by
    - ■ stenosis—*see* Stenosis, lacrimal
  - – congenital Q10.5
  - – neonatal H04.53-
- lacrimonasal duct—*see* Obstruction, lacrimal
- meconium (plug)
  - – newborn P76.0
    - ■ due to fecaliths P76.0
    - ■ in mucoviscidosis E84.11
- nasal J34.89
- nasolacrimal duct—*see also* Obstruction, lacrimal
  - – congenital Q10.5
- nose J34.89
- portal (circulation) (vein) I81
- pulmonary valve (heart) I37.0
- pylorus
  - – congenital or infantile Q40.0
- rectum K62.4
- renal N28.89
  - – outflow N13.8
  - – pelvis, congenital Q62.39
- sinus (accessory) (nasal) J34.89
- stomach NEC K31.89
  - – congenital Q40.2
  - – due to pylorospasm K31.3
- ureter (functional) (pelvic junction) NEC N13.5
  - – with
    - ■ hydronephrosis N13.1
    - ■ congenital Q62.39
    - ■ urinary (moderate) N13.9
  - – organ or tract (lower) N13.9
  - – specified NEC N13.8
- uropathy N13.9
- vagina N89.5
- vesical NEC N32.0
- vesicourethral orifice N32.0
  - – congenital Q64.31

Occlusion, occluded
- anus K62.4
  - – congenital Q42.3
    - ■ with fistula Q42.2
- aqueduct of Sylvius G91.1
  - – congenital Q03.0
    - ■ with spina bifida—*see* Spina bifida, by site, with hydrocephalus
- artery (*see also* Embolism, artery) I70.9
- choanal Q30.0
- fallopian tube N97.1
  - – congenital Q50.6
- gallbladder—*see also* Obstruction, gallbladder
  - – congenital (causing jaundice) Q44.1
- hymen N89.6
  - – congenital Q52.3
- nose J34.89
  - – congenital Q30.0
- oviduct N97.1
  - – congenital Q50.6
- posterior lingual, of mandibular teeth M26.29
- teeth (mandibular) (posterior lingual) M26.29
- ureter (complete) (partial) N13.5
  - – congenital Q62.10
- ureteropelvic junction N13.5
  - – congenital Q62.11
- ureterovesical orifice N13.5
  - – congenital Q62.12
- vagina N89.5
- ventricle (brain) NEC G91.1

Occult
- blood in feces (stools) R19.5

Oculogyric crisis or disturbance H51.8
- psychogenic F45.8

Odontoclasia K03.89

Oligoastrocytoma
- specified site—*see* Neoplasm, malignant, by site in Table of Neoplasms in the complete *ICD-10-CM* manual
- unspecified site C71.9

Oligocythemia D64.9

Oligodendroblastoma
- specified site—*see* Neoplasm, malignant in Table of Neoplasms in the complete *ICD-10-CM* manual
- unspecified site C71.9

Oligodendroglioma
- anaplastic type
  - – specified site—*see* Neoplasm, malignant, by site in Table of Neoplasms in the complete *ICD-10-CM* manual
  - – unspecified site C71.9
- specified site—*see* Neoplasm, malignant, by site in Table of Neoplasms in the complete *ICD-10-CM* manual
- unspecified site C71.9

Oligodontia—*see* Anodontia

Oligoencephalon Q02

Oligohydramnios O41.0-

Oligophrenia—*see also* Disability, intellectual
- phenylpyruvic E70.0

Oliguria R34
- postprocedural N99.0

Omphalitis (congenital) (newborn) P38.9
- with mild hemorrhage P38.1
- without hemorrhage P38.9

Omphalocele Q79.2

Omphalomesenteric duct, persistent Q43.0

Omphalorrhagia, newborn P51.9

Onanism (excessive) F98.8

Onychia—*see also* Cellulitis
- with lymphangitis—*see* Lymphangitis, acute
- candidal B37.2
- dermatophytic B35.1

Onychocryptosis L60.0

Onycholysis L60.1

Onychomadesis L60.8

Onychomycosis (finger) (toe) B35.1

Onychophagia F98.8

Onychophosis L60.8

Onychoptosis L60.8

Onyxis (finger) (toe) L60.0

Oophoritis (cystic) (infectional) (interstitial) N70.92
- with salpingitis N70.93

Ophthalmia (*see also* Conjunctivitis) H10.9
- blennorrhagic (gonococcal) (neonatorum) A54.31
- gonococcal (neonatorum) A54.31
- neonatorum, newborn P39.1
  - – gonococcal A54.31

Orchitis (gangrenous) (nonspecific) (septic) (suppurative) N45.2
- blennorrhagic (gonococcal) (acute) (chronic) A54.23
- chlamydial A56.19
- gonococcal (acute) (chronic) A54.23
- mumps B26.0
- syphilitic A52.76

Orotaciduria, oroticaciduria (congenital) (hereditary) (pyrimidine deficiency) E79.8
- anemia D53.0

Orthopnea R06.01

Osgood-Schlatter disease or osteochondrosis M92.52-

Osler (-Weber)-Rendu disease I78.0

Osler's nodes I33.0

Ossification
- diaphragm J98.6
- falx cerebri G96.198
- meninges (cerebral) (spinal) G96.198

Osteitis—*see also* Osteomyelitis
- deformans M88.9
- fragilitans Q78.0
  - – in (due to)
    - ■ malignant neoplasm of bone C41.9

Osteitis, *continued*
- ■ neoplastic disease (*see also* Table of Neoplasms in the complete *ICD-10-CM* manual) D49.9
  - ~ carpus D49.9
  - ~ clavicle D49.9
  - ~ femur D49.9
  - ~ fibula D49.9
  - ~ finger D49.9
  - ~ humerus D49.9
  - ~ ilium D49.9
  - ~ ischium D49.9
  - ~ metacarpus D49.9
  - ~ metatarsus D49.9
  - ~ multiple sites D49.9
  - ~ neck D49.9
  - ~ radius D49.9
  - ~ rib D49.9
  - ~ scapula D49.9
  - ~ skull D49.9
  - ~ tarsus D49.9
  - ~ tibia D49.9
  - ~ toe D49.9
  - ~ ulna D49.9
  - ~ vertebra D49.9
- – skull M88.0
- – specified NEC—*see* Paget's disease, bone, by site
- – vertebra M88.1
- tuberculosa A18.09
  - – cystica D86.89
  - – multiplex cystoides D86.89

Osteochondritis—*see also* Osteochondropathy
- juvenile M92.9
- patellar M92.4-

Osteochondrodysplasia Q78.9
- with defects of growth of tubular bones and spine Q77.9
- specified NEC Q78.8

Osteochondropathy M93.9-
- slipped upper femoral epiphysis—*see* Slipped, epiphysis, upper femoral

Osteochondrosis—*see also* Osteochondropathy
- acetabulum (juvenile) M91.0
- astragalus (juvenile) M92.6-
- Blount's M92.51-
- Buchanan's M91.0
- Burns' M92.1-
- calcaneus (juvenile) M92.6-
- capitular epiphysis (femur) (juvenile) M91.1-
- carpal (juvenile) (lunate) (scaphoid) M92.21-
- coxae juvenilis M91.1-
- deformans juvenilis, coxae M91.1-
- Diaz's M92.6-
- femoral capital epiphysis (juvenile) M91.1-
- femur (head), juvenile M91.1-
- fibula (juvenile) M92.5-
- foot NEC (juvenile) M92.8
- Freiberg's M92.7-
- Haas' (juvenile) M92.0-
- Haglund's M92.6-
- hip (juvenile) M91.1-
- humerus (capitulum) (head) (juvenile) M92.0-
- ilium, iliac crest (juvenile) M91.0
- ischiopubic synchondrosis M91.0
- Iselin's M92.7-
- juvenile, juvenilis M92.9
  - – after congenital dislocation of hip reduction M91.8-
  - – arm M92.3-
  - – capitular epiphysis (femur) M91.1-
  - – clavicle, sternal epiphysis M92.3-
  - – coxae M91.1-
  - – deformans M92.9
  - – fibula M92.50-
  - – foot NEC M92.8
  - – hand M92.20-
    - ■ carpal lunate M92.21-
    - ■ metacarpal head M92.22-
    - ■ specified site NEC M92.29-
  - – head of femur M91.1-
  - – hip and pelvis M91.9-
    - ■ femoral head M91.1-
    - ■ pelvis M91.0
    - ■ specified NEC M91.8-
  - – humerus M92.0-

Osteochondrosis, *continued*
- limb
  - lower NEC M92.8
  - upper NEC M92.3-
- medial cuneiform bone M92.6-
- metatarsus M92.7-
- patella M92.4-
- radius M92.1-
- specified site NEC M92.8
- tarsus M92.6-
- tibia M92.50-
  - proximal M92.51-
  - tubercle M92.52
- ulna M92.1-
- upper limb NEC M92.3-
- Kienböck's M92.21-
- Köhler's
  - patellar M92.4-
  - tarsal navicular M92.6-
- Legg-Perthes (-Calvé) (-Waldenström) M91.1-
- limb
  - lower NEC (juvenile) M92.8
  - tibia and fibula M92.59-
  - upper NEC (juvenile) M92.3-
- lunate bone (carpal) (juvenile) M92.21-
- Mauclaire's M92.22-
- metacarpal (head) (juvenile) M92.22-
- metatarsus (fifth) (head) (juvenile) (second) M92.7-
- navicular (juvenile) M92.6-
- os
  - calcis (juvenile) M92.6-
  - tibiale externum (juvenile) M92.6-
- Osgood-Schlatter M92.52-
- Panner's M92.0-
- patellar center (juvenile) (primary) (secondary) M92.4-
- pelvis (juvenile) M91.0
- Pierson's M91.0
- radius (head) (juvenile) M92.1-
- Sever's M92.6-
- Sinding-Larsen M92.4-
- symphysis pubis (juvenile) M91.0
- talus (juvenile) M92.6-
- tarsus (navicular) (juvenile) M92.6-
- tibia (proximal) (tubercle) (juvenile) M92.5-
- ulna (lower) (juvenile) M92.1-
- van Neck's M91.0

Osteogenesis imperfecta Q78.0

Osteomyelitis (general) (infective) (localized) (neonatal) (purulent) (septic) (staphylococcal) (streptococcal) (suppurative) (with periostitis) M86.9
- acute M86.10
  - carpus M86.14-
  - clavicle M86.11-
  - femur M86.15-
  - fibula M86.16-
  - finger M86.14-
  - humerus M86.12-
  - ilium M86.18
  - ischium M86.18
  - metacarpus M86.14-
  - metatarsus M86.17-
  - multiple sites M86.19
  - neck M86.18
  - radius M86.13-
  - rib M86.18
  - scapula M86.11-
  - skull M86.18
  - tarsus M86.17-
  - tibia M86.16-
  - toe M86.17-
  - ulna M86.13-

Osteonecrosis M87.9
- secondary
  - due to
    - hemoglobinopathy NEC D58.2 [M90.50]
      - carpus D58.2 [M90.54-]
      - clavicle D58.2 [M90.51-]
      - femur D58.2 [M90.55-]
      - fibula D58.2 [M90.56-]
      - finger D58.2 [M90.54-]
      - humerus D58.2 [M90.52-]
      - ilium D58.2 [M90.55-]

Osteonecrosis, *continued*
- ischium D58.2 [M90.55-]
- metacarpus D58.2 [M90.54-]
- metatarsus D58.2 [M90.57-]
- multiple sites D58.2 [M90.58]
- neck D58.2 [M90.58]
- radius D58.2 [M90.53-]
- rib D58.2 [M90.58]
- scapula D58.2 [M90.51-]
- skull D58.2 [M90.58]
- tarsus D58.2 [M90.57-]
- tibia D58.2 [M90.56-]
- toe D58.2 [M90.57-]
- ulna D58.2 [M90.53-]
- vertebra D58.2 [M90.58]

Osteophyte M25.70
- ankle M25.77-
- elbow M25.72-
- foot joint M25.77-
- hand joint M25.74-
- hip M25.75-
- knee M25.76-
- shoulder M25.71-
- spine M25.78
- vertebrae M25.78
- wrist M25.73-

Osteopsathyrosis (idiopathica) Q78.0

Osteosclerosis Q78.2
- acquired M85.8-
- congenita Q77.4
- fragilitas (generalisata) Q78.2
- myelofibrosis D75.81

Osteosis
- cutis L94.2

Ostium
- atrioventriculare commune Q21.2
- primum (arteriosum) (defect) (persistent) Q21.2
- secundum (arteriosum) (defect) (patent) (persistent) Q21.1

Ostrum-Furst syndrome Q75.8

Otalgia—*see* subcategory H92.0

Otitis (acute) H66.9-
- with effusion—*see also* Otitis, media, nonsuppurative
  - purulent—*see* Otitis, media
- chronic—*see also* Otitis, media, chronic
  - with effusion—*see also* Otitis, media, nonsuppurative
- externa H60.9-
  - abscess—*see also* Abscess, ear, external
  - acute (noninfective) H60.50-
    - infective—*see* Otitis, externa, infective
  - cellulitis—*see* Cellulitis, ear
  - in (due to)
    - aspergillosis B44.89
    - candidiasis B37.84
    - erysipelas A46 [H62.4-]
    - herpes (simplex) virus infection B00.1
    - impetigo L01.00 [H62.4-]
    - infectious disease NEC B99 [H62.4-]
    - mycosis NEC B36.9 [H62.4-]
    - parasitic disease NEC B89 [H62.4-]
    - viral disease NEC B34.9 [H62.4-]
  - infective NEC H60.39-
    - abscess—*see* Abscess, ear, external
    - cellulitis—*see* Cellulitis, ear
    - swimmer's ear H60.33-
  - mycotic NEC B36.9 [H62.4-]
    - in
      - aspergillosis B44.89
      - candidiasis B37.84
      - moniliasis B37.84
  - specified NEC—*see* subcategory H60.8-
  - tropical NEC B36.8
    - in
      - aspergillosis B44.89
      - candidiasis B37.84
      - moniliasis B37.84
- interna—*see* subcategory H83.0
- media (hemorrhagic) (staphylococcal) (streptococcal) H66.9-
  - with effusion (nonpurulent)—*see* Otitis, media, nonsuppurative

Otitis, *continued*
- acute, subacute H66.9-
  - allergic—*see* Otitis, media, nonsuppurative, acute or subacute NEC allergic
  - exudative—*see* Otitis, media, nonsuppurative, acute or subacute NEC allergic
  - mucoid—*see* Otitis, media, nonsuppurative, acute or subacute NEC allergic
  - necrotizing—*see also* Otitis, media, suppurative, acute
    - in
      - measles B05.3
      - scarlet fever A38.0
  - nonsuppurative NEC—*see* Otitis, media, nonsuppurative, acute or subacute NEC allergic
  - purulent—*see* Otitis, media, suppurative, acute
  - sanguinous—*see* Otitis, media, nonsuppurative, acute or subacute NEC allergic
  - secretory—*see* Otitis, media, nonsuppurative, acute or subacute NEC allergic, serous
  - seromucinous—*see* Otitis, media, nonsuppurative, acute or subacute NEC allergic
  - serous—*see* Otitis, media, nonsuppurative, acute or subacute NEC allergic, serous
  - suppurative—*see* Otitis, media, suppurative, acute
- allergic—*see* Otitis, media, nonsuppurative
- catarrhal—*see* Otitis, media, nonsuppurative
- chronic H66.9-
  - with effusion (nonpurulent)—*see* Otitis, media, nonsuppurative, chronic
  - allergic—*see* Otitis, media, nonsuppurative, chronic, allergic
  - benign suppurative—*see* Otitis, media, suppurative, chronic
  - catarrhal—*see* Otitis, media, nonsuppurative, chronic, serous
  - exudative—*see* Otitis, media, suppurative, chronic
  - mucinous—*see* Otitis, media, nonsuppurative, chronic, mucoid
  - mucoid—*see* Otitis, media, nonsuppurative, chronic, mucoid
  - nonsuppurative NEC—*see* Otitis, media, nonsuppurative, chronic
  - purulent—*see* Otitis, media, suppurative, chronic
  - secretory—*see* Otitis, media, nonsuppurative, chronic, mucoid
  - seromucinous—*see* Otitis, media, nonsuppurative, chronic
  - serous—*see* Otitis, media, nonsuppurative, chronic, serous
  - suppurative—*see* Otitis, media, suppurative, chronic
  - transudative—*see* Otitis, media, nonsuppurative, chronic, mucoid
- exudative—*see* Otitis, media, suppurative
- in (due to) (with)
  - influenza—*see* Influenza, with, otitis media
  - measles B05.3
  - scarlet fever A38.0
  - tuberculosis A18.6
  - viral disease NEC B34.- [H67.-]
- mucoid—*see* Otitis, media, nonsuppurative
- nonsuppurative H65.9-
  - acute or subacute NEC allergic H65.11- (6th characters 1—3, 9)
    - recurrent H65.11- (6th characters 4—7)
    - secretory—*see* Otitis, media, nonsuppurative, serous
    - serous H65.0- (6th characters 0—3)
      - recurrent H65.0- (6th characters 4—7)
  - chronic H65.49-
    - allergic H65.41-
    - mucoid H65.3-
    - serous H65.2-
- postmeasles B05.3
- purulent—*see* Otitis, media, suppurative
- secretory—*see* Otitis, media, nonsuppurative
- seromucinous—*see* Otitis, media, nonsuppurative
- serous—*see* Otitis, media, nonsuppurative
- suppurative H66.4-
  - acute H66.00- (6th characters 1—3, 9)
    - with rupture of ear drum H66.01- (6th characters 1—3, 9)
    - recurrent H66.00- (6th characters 4—7)

Otitis, *continued*
◊ with rupture of ear drum H66.01- (6th characters 4–7)
■ chronic (*see also* subcategory) H66.3
~ atticoantral H66.2-
~ tubotympanic (benign) H66.1-
– transudative—*see* Otitis, media, nonsuppurative
– tuberculous A18.6

Otomycosis (diffuse) NEC B36.9 [H62.4-]
● in
– aspergillosis B44.89
– candidiasis B37.84
– moniliasis B37.84

Otorrhea H92.1-
● cerebrospinal (fluid) G96.01
– postoperative G96.08
– specified NEC G96.08
– spontaneous G96.01
– traumatic G96.08

Ovary, ovarian—*see also* Disease, diseased
● vein syndrome N13.8

Overactive—*see also* Hyperfunction
● bladder N32.81
● hypothalamus E23.3

Overactivity R46.3
● child—*see* Disorder, attention-deficit hyperactivity

Overbite (deep) (excessive) (horizontal) (vertical) M26.29

Overconscientious personality F60.5

Overeating R63.2
● nonorganic origin F50.89
● psychogenic F50.89

Overlapping toe (acquired)—*see also* Deformity, toe
● congenital (fifth toe) Q66.89

Overload
● circulatory, due to transfusion (blood) (blood components) (TACO) E87.71
● fluid E87.70
– due to transfusion (blood) (blood components) E87.71
– specified NEC E87.79
● iron, due to repeated red blood cell transfusions E83.111
● potassium (K) E87.5
● sodium (Na) E87.0

Overnutrition—*see* Hyperalimentation

Overproduction—*see also* Hypersecretion
● growth hormone E22.0

Overriding
● toe (acquired)—*see also* Deformity, toe
– congenital Q66.89

Overstrained R53.83

Overweight E66.3

Overworked R53.83

Ovulation (cycle)
● failure or lack of N97.0
● pain N94.0

Oxyuriasis B80

Oxyuris vermicularis (infestation) B80

Ozena J31.0

P

Pachydermatocele (congenital) Q82.8

Paget's disease
● bone M88.9
– carpus M88.84-
– clavicle M88.81-
– femur M88.85-
– fibula M88.86-
– finger M88.84-
– humerus M88.82-
– ilium M88.85-
– in neoplastic disease D49.9 *[M90.6-]*
– ischium M88.85-
– metacarpus M88.84-
– metatarsus M88.87-
– multiple sites M88.89
– neck M88.88
– radius M88.83-
– rib M88.88

Paget's disease, *continued*
– scapula M88.81-
– skull M88.0
– specified NEC M88.88
– tarsus M88.87-
– tibia M88.86-
– toe M88.87-
– ulna M88.83-
– vertebra M88.1
● osteitis deformans—*see* Paget's disease, bone

Pain(s) (*see also* Painful) R52
● abdominal R10.9
– colic R10.83
– generalized R10.84
■ with acute abdomen R10.0
– lower R10.30
■ left quadrant R10.32
■ pelvic or perineal R10.2
■ periumbilical R10.33
■ right quadrant R10.31
– rebound—*see* Tenderness, abdominal, rebound
– severe with abdominal rigidity R10.0
– tenderness—*see* Tenderness, abdominal
– upper R10.10
■ epigastric R10.13
■ left quadrant R10.12
■ right quadrant R10.11
● acute R52
– due to trauma G89.11
– neoplasm related G89.3
– postprocedural NEC G89.18
● adnexa (uteri) R10.2
● anus K62.89
● axillary (axilla) M79.62-
● back (postural) M54.9
● bladder R39.89
– associated with micturition—*see* Micturition, painful
– chronic R39.82
● breast N64.4
● broad ligament R10.2
● cancer associated (acute) (chronic) G89.3
● chest (central) R07.9
● chronic G89.29
– neoplasm related G89.3
● coccyx M53.3
● due to cancer G89.3
● due to malignancy (primary) (secondary) G89.3
● ear—*see* subcategory H92.0
● epigastric, epigastrium R10.13
● face, facial R51.9
● female genital organs NEC N94.89
● gastric—*see* Pain, abdominal
● generalized NOS R52
● genital organ
– female N94.89
– male
■ scrotal N50.82
■ testicular N50.81-
● groin—*see* Pain, abdominal, lower
● hand M79.64-
– joints M25.54-
● head—*see* Headache
● intermenstrual N94.0
● jaw R68.84
● joint M25.50
– ankle M25.57-
– elbow M25.52-
– finger M25.54-
– foot M25.57-
– hand M79.64-
– hip M25.55-
– knee M25.56-
– shoulder M25.51-
– specified site NEC M25.59
– toe M25.57-
– wrist M25.53-
● kidney N23
● laryngeal R07.0
● limb M79.60-
– lower M79.60-
■ foot M79.67-
■ lower leg M79.66-
■ thigh M79.65-

Pain(s), *continued*
■ toe M79.67-
– upper M79.60-
■ axilla M79.62-
■ finger M79.64-
■ forearm M79.63-
■ hand M79.64-
■ upper arm M79.62-
● loin M54.50
● low back M54.5-
● lumbar region M54.50
● mandibular R68.84
● mastoid—*see* subcategory H92.0
● maxilla R68.84
● menstrual (*see also* Dysmenorrhea) N94.6
● mouth K13.79
● muscle—*see* Myalgia
● musculoskeletal (*see also* Pain, by site) M79.18
● myofascial M79.18
● nasal J34.89
● nasopharynx J39.2
● neck NEC M54.2
● nose J34.89
● ocular H57.1-
● ophthalmic H57.1-
● orbital region H57.1-
● ovary N94.89
● ovulation N94.0
● pelvic (female) R10.2
● perineal, perineum R10.2
● postoperative NOS G89.18
● postprocedural NOS G89.18
● premenstrual F32.81
● psychogenic (persistent) (any site) F45.41
● rectum K62.89
● round ligament (stretch) R10.2
● sacroiliac M53.3
● scrotal N50.82
● shoulder M25.51-
● spine M54.9
– cervical M54.2
– low back M54.0
■ with sciatica M54.4-
● temporomandibular (joint) M26.62-
● testicular N50.81-
● throat R07.0
● tibia M79.66-
● toe M79.67-
● tumor associated G89.3
● ureter N23
● urinary (organ) (system) N23
● uterus NEC N94.89
● vagina R10.2
● vesical R39.89
– associated with micturition—*see* Micturition, painful
● vulva R10.2

Painful—*see also* Pain
● menstruation—*see* Dysmenorrhea
– psychogenic F45.8
● micturition—*see* Micturition, painful
● scar NEC L90.5
● wire sutures T81.89

Painter's colic—*see* subcategory T56.0

Palate—*see* Disease, diseased

Palatoplegia K13.79

Palatoschisis—*see* Cleft, palate

Palliative care Z51.5

Pallor R23.1

Palpitations (heart) R00.2
● psychogenic F45.8

Palsy (*see also* Paralysis) G83.9
● Bell's—*see also* Palsy, facial
– newborn P11.3
● brachial plexus NEC G54.0
– newborn (birth injury) P14.3
● cerebral (congenital) G80.9
● cranial nerve—*see also* Disorder, nerve, cranial
– multiple G52.7

Palsy, *continued*
- ■ in
  - ~ neoplastic disease (*see also* Table of Neoplasms in the complete *ICD-10-CM* manual) D49.9 *[G53]*
  - ~ sarcoidosis D86.82
- Erb's P14.0
- facial G51.0
  - newborn (birth injury) P11.3
- Klumpke (-Déjérine) P14.1
- lead—*see* subcategory T56.0
- seventh nerve—*see also* Palsy, facial
  - newborn P11.3

Pancake heart R93.1
- with cor pulmonale (chronic) I27.81

Pancarditis (acute) (chronic) I51.89
- rheumatic I09.89
  - active or acute I01.8

Pancolitis, ulcerative (chronic) K51.00
- with
  - abscess K51.014
  - complication K51.019
  - fistula K51.013
  - obstruction K51.012
  - rectal bleeding K51.011
  - specified complication NEC K51.018

Pancreatitis (annular) (apoplectic) (calcareous) (edematous) (hemorrhagic) (malignant) (subacute) (suppurative) K85.90
- acute K85.90
- idiopathic K85.00
  - with infected necrosis K85.02
  - with uninfected necrosis K85.01
  - with infected necrosis K85.92
  - with uninfected necrosis K85.91

Pancytopenia (acquired) D61.818
- with
  - malformations D61.09
  - myelodysplastic syndrome—*see* Syndrome, myelodysplastic
- antineoplastic chemotherapy induced D61.810
- congenital D61.09
- drug-induced NEC D61.811

PANDAS (pediatric autoimmune neuropsychiatric disorders associated with streptococcal infections syndrome) D89.89

Panhematopenia D61.9
- congenital D61.09
- constitutional D61.09

Panhemocytopenia D61.9
- congenital D61.09
- constitutional D61.09

Panhypopituitarism E23.0
- prepubertal E23.0

Panic (attack) (state) F41.0
- reaction to exceptional stress (transient) F43.0

Panmyelopathy, familial, constitutional D61.09

Panmyelophthisis D61.82
- congenital D61.09

Pansinusitis (chronic) (hyperplastic) (nonpurulent) (purulent) J32.4
- acute J01.40
  - recurrent J01.41

Papanicolaou smear, cervix Z12.4
- as part of routine gynecological examination Z01.419
  - with abnormal findings Z01.411
- for suspected neoplasm Z12.4
- routine Z01.419
  - with abnormal findings Z01.411

Papilledema (choked disc) H47.10
- associated with
  - decreased ocular pressure H47.12
  - increased intracranial pressure H47.11
  - retinal disorder H47.13

Papillitis
- anus K62.89
- necrotizing, kidney N17.2
- renal, necrotizing N17.2
- tongue K14.0

Papilloma—*see also* Neoplasm, benign, by site in Table of Neoplasms in the complete *ICD-10-CM* manual
- acuminatum (female) (male) (anogenital) A63.0
- choroid plexus (lateral ventricle) (third ventricle)
  - anaplastic C71.5
  - malignant C71.5
- rectum K62.89

Papillomatosis—*see also* Neoplasm, benign, by site in Table of Neoplasms in the complete *ICD-10-CM* manual
- confluent and reticulated L83

Papillon-Léage and Psaume syndrome Q87.0

Para-albuminemia E88.09

Paracephalus Q89.7

Parageusia R43.2
- psychogenic F45.8

Paralysis, paralytic (complete) (incomplete) G83.9
- anus (sphincter) K62.89
- asthenic bulbar G70.00
  - with exacerbation (acute) G70.01
  - in crisis G70.01
- Bell's G51.0
  - newborn P11.3
- bowel, colon or intestine K56.0
- brachial plexus G54.0
  - birth injury P14.3
  - newborn (birth injury) P14.3
- brain G83.9
- bulbospinal G70.00
  - with exacerbation (acute) G70.01
  - in crisis G70.01
- cardiac (*see also* Failure, heart) I50.9
- Clark's G80.9
- colon K56.0
- conjugate movement (gaze) (of eye) H51.0
  - cortical (nuclear) (supranuclear) H51.0
- deglutition R13.0
  - hysterical F44.4
- diaphragm (flaccid) J98.6
  - due to accidental dissection of phrenic nerve during procedure—*see* Puncture
- Duchenne's
  - birth injury P14.0
  - due to or associated with
    - ■ muscular dystrophy G71.01
- due to intracranial or spinal birth injury—*see* Palsy, cerebral
- Erb (-Duchenne) (birth) (newborn) P14.0
- facial (nerve) G51.0
  - birth injury P11.3
  - congenital P11.3
  - following operation NEC—*see* Puncture, accidental complicating surgery
  - newborn (birth injury) P11.3
- gait R26.1
- glottis J38.00
  - bilateral J38.02
  - unilateral J38.01
- Hoppe-Goldflam G70.00
  - with exacerbation (acute) G70.01
  - in crisis G70.01
- hysterical F44.4
- ileus K56.0
- infantile A80.30
- infective A80.-
- inferior nuclear G83.9
- intestine K56.0
- Klumpke (-Déjérine) (birth) (newborn) P14.1
- laryngeal nerve (recurrent) (superior) (unilateral) J38.00
  - bilateral J38.02
  - unilateral J38.01
- larynx J38.00
  - bilateral J38.02
  - unilateral J38.01
- lead—*see* subcategory T56.0
- left side—*see* Hemiplegia
- leg G83.1-
  - both—*see* Paraplegia
  - hysterical F44.4
  - psychogenic F44.4
- lip K13.0
- monoplegic—*see* Monoplegia

Paralysis, paralytic, *continued*
- motor G83.9
- muscle, muscular NEC G72.89
- nerve—*see also* Disorder, nerve
  - facial G51.0
    - ■ birth injury P11.3
    - ■ congenital P11.3
    - ■ newborn (birth injury) P11.3
  - seventh or facial G51.0
    - ■ newborn (birth injury) P11.3
- oculofacial, congenital (Moebius) Q87.0
- palate (soft) K13.79
- progressive, spinal G12.25
- pseudohypertrophic (muscle) G71.09
- psychogenic F44.4
- radicular NEC
  - upper limbs, newborn (birth injury) P14.3
- recurrent isolated sleep G47.53
- respiratory (muscle) (system) (tract) R06.81
  - center NEC G93.89
  - congenital P28.89
  - newborn P28.89
- right side—*see* Hemiplegia
- saturnine—*see* subcategory T56.0
- sleep, recurrent isolated G47.53
- spastic G83.9
  - cerebral G80.-
  - congenital (cerebral) G80.-
- spinal (cord) G83.9
- spinal progressive G12.25
  - pseudohypertrophic G71.02
- syndrome G83.9
- uveoparotitic D86.89
- uvula K13.79
- velum palate K13.79
- vocal cords J38.00
  - bilateral J38.02
  - unilateral J38.01

Paramenia N92.6

Paramyoclonus multiplex G25.3

Paranoid
- personality F60.0
- traits F60.0
- trends F60.0
- type, psychopathic personality F60.0

Paraphimosis (congenital) N47.2

Paraplegia (lower) G82.20
- complete G82.21
- functional (hysterical) F44.4
- hysterical F44.4
- incomplete G82.22
- psychogenic F44.4

Parasitic—*see also* Disease, diseased
- disease NEC B89
- stomatitis B37.0
- sycosis (beard) (scalp) B35.0

Parasitism B89
- intestinal B82.9
- skin B88.9
- specified—*see* Infestation

Parasomnia G47.50
- in conditions classified elsewhere G47.54
- nonorganic origin F51.8
- organic G47.50
- specified NEC G47.59

Paraspadias Q54.9

Paraspasmus facialis G51.8

Parasuicide (attempt)
- history of (personal) Z91.51
  - in family Z81.8

Paratrachoma A74.0

Parencephalitis—*see also* Encephalitis
- sequelae G09

Parent-child conflict—*see* Conflict, parent-child
- estrangement NEC Z62.890

Paresis—*see also* Paralysis
- bowel, colon or intestine K56.0
- pseudohypertrophic G71.09

Paronychia—*see also* Cellulitis
- with lymphangitis—*see* Lymphangitis, digit
- candidal (chronic) B37.2

Parorexia (psychogenic) F50.89

Parosmia R43.1
- psychogenic F45.8

Parry-Romberg syndrome G51.8

Particolored infant Q82.8

Parulis K04.7

Parvovirus, as the cause of disease classified elsewhere B97.6

Passage
- meconium (newborn) during delivery P03.82
- of sounds or bougies—*see* Attention to, artificial, opening

Passive—*see* Disease, diseased
- smoking Z77.22

Past due on rent or mortgage Z59.81-

Pasteurella septica A28.0

PAT (paroxysmal atrial tachycardia) I47.1

Patent—*see also* Imperfect, closure
- ductus arteriosus or Botallo's Q25.0
- foramen
  - botalli Q21.1
  - ovale Q21.1
- interauricular septum Q21.1
- interventricular septum Q21.0
- omphalomesenteric duct Q43.0
- ostium secundum Q21.1
- vitelline duct Q43.0

Pathologic, pathological—*see also* Disease, diseased
- asphyxia R09.01

Pattern, sleep-wake, irregular G47.23

Patulous—*see also* Imperfect, closure (congenital)
- alimentary tract Q45.8
  - lower Q43.8
  - upper Q40.8

Pause, sinoatrial I49.5

Pectenosis K62.4

Pectus
- carinatum (congenital) Q67.7
- excavatum (congenital) Q67.6
- recurvatum (congenital) Q67.6

Pediculosis (infestation) B85.2
- capitis (head-louse) (any site) B85.0
- corporis (body-louse) (any site) B85.1
- eyelid B85.0
- mixed (classifiable to more than one of the titles B85.0–B85.3) B85.4
- pubis (pubic louse) (any site) B85.3
- vestimenti B85.1
- vulvae B85.3

Pediculus (infestation)—*see* Pediculosis

Pelger-Huët anomaly or syndrome D72.0

Pelvic—*see also* Disease, diseased
- examination (periodic) (routine) Z01.419
  - with abnormal findings Z01.411
- kidney, congenital Q63.2

Pelviperitonitis—*see also* Peritonitis, pelvic
- gonococcal A54.24

Pemphigus
- benign familial (chronic) Q82.8

Pentosuria (essential) E74.89

Perforation, perforated (nontraumatic) (of)
- accidental during procedure (blood vessel) (nerve) (organ)—*see* Complication
- antrum—*see* Sinusitis, maxillary
- appendix K35.32
- atrial septum, multiple Q21.1
- by
  - device, implant or graft (*see also* Complications, by site and type, mechanical) T85.628
    - catheter NEC T85.698
      - cystostomy T83.090
      - urinary—*see also* Complications, catheter, urinary T83.098
    - ventricular intracranial shunt T85.09

Perforation, perforated, *continued*
- instrument (any) during a procedure, accidental—*see* Puncture
- cecum K35.32
- ear drum—*see* Perforation, tympanum
- nasal
  - septum J34.89
    - congenital Q30.3
  - sinus J34.89
    - congenital Q30.8
    - due to sinusitis—*see* Sinusitis
- palate (*see also* Cleft, palate) Q35.9
- palatine vault (*see also* Cleft, palate, hard) Q35.1
- sinus (accessory) (chronic) (nasal) J34.89
- sphenoidal sinus—*see* Sinusitis, sphenoidal
- tympanum, tympanic (membrane) (persistent post-traumatic) (postinflammatory) H72.9-
  - attic H72.1-
    - multiple H72.81-
    - total H72.82-
  - central H72.0-
    - multiple H72.81-
    - total H72.82-
  - marginal NEC—*see* subcategory H72.2
  - multiple H72.81-
  - pars flaccida—*see* Perforation, tympanum, attic
  - total H72.82-
  - traumatic, current episode S09.2-
- uvula K13.79

Periadenitis mucosa necrotica recurrens K12.0

Pericarditis (with decompensation) (with effusion) I31.9
- with rheumatic fever (conditions in I00)
  - active—*see* Pericarditis, rheumatic
  - inactive or quiescent I09.2
- acute (hemorrhagic) (nonrheumatic) (Sicca) I30.9
  - with chorea (acute) (rheumatic) (Sydenham's) I02.0
  - benign I30.8
  - nonspecific I30.0
  - rheumatic I01.0
    - with chorea (acute) (Sydenham's) I02.0
- adhesive or adherent (chronic) (external) (internal) I31.0
  - acute—*see* Pericarditis, acute
  - rheumatic I09.2
- bacterial (acute) (subacute) (with serous or seropurulent effusion) I30.1
- calcareous I31.1
- cholesterol (chronic) I31.8
  - acute I30.9
- chronic (nonrheumatic) I31.9
  - rheumatic I09.2
- constrictive (chronic) I31.1
- coxsackie B33.23
- fibrinopurulent I30.1
- fibrinous I30.8
- fibrous I31.0
- idiopathic I30.0
- in systemic lupus erythematosus M32.12
- infective I30.1
- meningococcal A39.53
- neoplastic (chronic) I31.8
  - acute I30.9
- obliterans, obliterating I31.0
- plastic I31.0
- pneumococcal I30.1
- purulent I30.1
- rheumatic (active) (acute) (with effusion) (with pneumonia) I01.0
  - with chorea (acute) (rheumatic) (Sydenham's) I02.0
  - chronic or inactive (with chorea) I09.2
- septic I30.1
- serofibrinous I30.8
- staphylococcal I30.1
- streptococcal I30.1
- suppurative I30.1
- syphilitic A52.06
- tuberculous A18.84
- viral I30.1

Perichondritis
- auricle—*see* Perichondritis, ear
- bronchus J98.09
- ear (external) H61.00-
  - acute H61.01-

Perichondritis, *continued*
- chronic H61.02-
- nose J34.89

Periepididymitis N45.1

Perilabyrinthitis (acute)—*see* subcategory H83.0

Periods—*see also* Menstruation
- heavy N92.0
- irregular N92.6
- shortened intervals (irregular) N92.1

Periorchitis N45.2

Periproctitis K62.89

Peritonitis (adhesive) (bacterial) (fibrinous) (hemorrhagic) (idiopathic) (localized) (perforative) (primary) (with adhesions) (with effusion) K65.9
- with or following
  - abscess K65.1
  - appendicitis
    - with perforation or rupture K35.32
    - generalized K35.20
    - localized K35.30
- acute (generalized) K65.0
- chlamydial A74.81
- diaphragmatic K65.0
- diffuse K65.0
- disseminated K65.0
- eosinophilic K65.8
  - acute K65.0
- fibropurulent K65.0
- general (ized) K65.0
- meconium (newborn) P78.0
- neonatal P78.1
  - meconium P78.0
- pancreatic K65.0
- pelvic
  - female N73.5
    - acute N73.3
    - chronic N73.4
      - with adhesions N73.6
  - male K65.0
- purulent K65.0
- septic K65.0
- specified NEC K65.8
- spontaneous bacterial K65.2
- subdiaphragmatic K65.0
- subphrenic K65.0
- suppurative K65.0

Peritonsillitis J36

Perlèche NEC K13.0
- due to
  - candidiasis B37.83
  - moniliasis B37.83

Persistence, persistent (congenital)
- anal membrane Q42.3
  - with fistula Q42.2
- atrioventricular canal Q21.2
- branchial cleft NOS Q18.2
  - cyst Q18.0
  - fistula Q18.0
  - sinus Q18.0
- canal of Cloquet Q14.0
- capsule (opaque) Q12.8
- cilioretinal artery or vein Q14.8
- convolutions
  - aortic arch Q25.46
  - fallopian tube Q50.6
  - oviduct Q50.6
  - uterine tube Q50.6
- fetal
  - circulation P29.38
  - hemoglobin, hereditary (HPFH) D56.4
- foramen
  - Botalli Q21.1
  - ovale Q21.1
- hemoglobin, fetal (hereditary) (HPFH) D56.4
- Meckel's diverticulum Q43.0
- omphalomesenteric duct Q43.0
- ostium
  - atrioventriculare commune Q21.2
  - primum Q21.2
  - secundum Q21.1

Persistence, persistent, *continued*
- ovarian rests in fallopian tube Q50.6
- primary (deciduous)
  - teeth K00.6
- sinus
  - urogenitalis
    - female Q52.8
    - male Q55.8
- thyroglossal duct Q89.2
- thyrolingual duct Q89.2
- truncus arteriosus or communis Q20.0
- tunica vasculosa lentis Q12.2
- vitelline duct Q43.0

Person (with)
- concern (normal) about sick person in family Z63.6
- consulting on behalf of another Z71.0
- feigning illness Z76.5
- living (in)
  - without
    - adequate housing (heating) (space) Z59.1
    - housing (permanent) (temporary) Z59.00
    - person able to render necessary care Z74.2
    - shelter Z59.02

Personality (disorder) F60.9
- affective F34.0
- aggressive F60.3
- amoral F60.2
- anacastic, anankastic F60.5
- antisocial F60.2
- anxious F60.6
- asocial F60.2
- asthenic F60.7
- avoidant F60.6
- borderline F60.3
- compulsive F60.5
- cycloid F34.0
- cyclothymic F34.0
- depressive F34.1
- dissocial F60.2
- emotionally unstable F60.3
- expansive paranoid F60.0
- explosive F60.3
- fanatic F60.0
- histrionic F60.4
- hyperthymic F34.0
- hypothymic F34.1
- hysterical F60.4
- obsessional F60.5
- obsessive (-compulsive) F60.5
- organic F07.0
- overconscientious F60.5
- paranoid F60.0
- pathologic F60.9
- pattern defect or disturbance F60.9
- psychoinfantile F60.4
- psychopathic F60.2
- querulant F60.0
- schizoid F60.1
- sensitive paranoid F60.0
- sociopathic (amoral) (antisocial) (asocial) (dissocial) F60.2
- specified NEC F60.89

Perthes' disease M91.1-

Pertussis (*see also* Whooping cough) A37.90

Perversion, perverted
- appetite F50.89
  - psychogenic F50.89
- function
  - pituitary gland E23.2
    - posterior lobe E22.2
- sense of smell and taste R43.8
  - psychogenic F45.8
- sexual—*see* Deviation, sexual transvestism

Pervious, congenital—*see also* Imperfect, closure
- ductus arteriosus Q25.0

Pes (congenital)—*see also* Talipes
- adductus Q66.89
- cavus Q66.7-
- valgus Q66.6

Petechia, petechiae R23.3
- newborn P54.5

Petit mal seizure—*see* Epilepsy, generalized, specified NEC

Petit's hernia—*see* Hernia
- Peutz-Jeghers disease or syndrome Q85.8

Pfeiffer's disease—*see* Mononucleosis, infectious

Phagedena (dry) (moist) (sloughing)—*see also* Gangrene
- geometric L88

Phakomatosis Q85.9
- Bourneville's Q85.1
- specified NEC Q85.8

Pharyngeal pouch syndrome D82.1

Pharyngitis (acute) (catarrhal) (gangrenous) (infective) (malignant) (membranous) (phlegmonous) (pseudomembranous) (simple) (subacute) (suppurative) (ulcerative) (viral) J02.9
- aphthous B08.5
- atrophic J31.2
- chlamydial A56.4
- chronic (atrophic) (granular) (hypertrophic) J31.2
- coxsackievirus B08.5
- enteroviral vesicular B08.5
- follicular (chronic) J31.2
- granular (chronic) J31.2
- herpesviral B00.2
- hypertrophic J31.2
- infectional, chronic J31.2
- influenzal—*see* Influenza, with, respiratory manifestations NEC
- pneumococcal J02.8
- purulent J02.9
- putrid J02.9
- septic J02.0
- sicca J31.2
- specified organism NEC J02.8
- staphylococcal J02.8
- streptococcal J02.0
- vesicular, enteroviral B08.5
- viral NEC J02.8

Pharyngolaryngitis (acute) J06.0
- chronic J37.0

Pharyngotonsillitis, herpesviral B00.2

Phenomenon
- vasomotor R55
- vasovagal R55
- Wenckebach's I44.1

Phenylketonuria E70.1
- classical E70.0

Phimosis (congenital) (due to infection) N47.1

Phlebitis (infective) (pyemic) (septic) (suppurative) I80.9
- calf muscular vein (NOS) I80.25-
- femoral vein (superficial) I80.1-
- femoropopliteal vein I80.0-
- gastrocnemial vein I80.25-
- hepatic veins I80.8
- iliac vein (common) (external) (internal) I80.21-
- iliofemoral—*see* Phlebitis, femoral vein
- leg I80.3
  - deep (vessels) NEC I80.20-
    - iliac I80.21-
    - popliteal vein I80.22-
    - specified vessel NEC I80.29-
    - tibial vein I80.23-
  - femoral vein (superficial) I80.1-
  - superficial (vessels) I80.0-
- lower limb—*see* Phlebitis, leg
- peroneal vein I80.24-
- popliteal vein—*see* Phlebitis, leg
- saphenous (accessory) (great) (long) (small)—*see* Phlebitis, leg
- soleal vein I80.25-
- specified site NEC I80.8
- tibial vein—*see* Phlebitis, leg
- ulcerative I80.9
  - leg—*see* Phlebitis, leg
- umbilicus I80.8

Phobia, phobic F40.9
- reaction F40.9
- state F40.9

Photodermatitis (sun) L56.8
- chronic L57.8
- due to drug L56.8

Photosensitivity, photosensitization (sun) skin L56.8

Phthiriasis (pubis) B85.3
- with any infestation classifiable to B85.0–B85.2 B85.4

Physical restraint status Z78.1

Pica F50.89
- in adults F50.89
- infant or child F98.3

Picking, nose F98.8

Pickwickian syndrome E66.2

Pierre Robin deformity or syndrome Q87.0

Pig-bel A05.2

Pigeon
- breast or chest (acquired) M95.4
  - congenital Q67.7

Pigmentation (abnormal) (anomaly) L81.9
- iron L81.8
- lids, congenital Q82.8
- metals L81.8
- optic papilla, congenital Q14.2
- retina, congenital (grouped) (nevoid) Q14.1
- scrotum, congenital Q82.8
- tattoo L81.8

Piles (*see also* Hemorrhoids) K64.9

Pinhole meatus (*see also* Stricture, urethra) N35.919

Pink
- eye—*see* Conjunctivitis, acute, mucopurulent

Pinworm (disease) (infection) (infestation) B80

Pithecoid pelvis Q74.2

Pitting (*see also* Edema) R60.9
- lip R60.0
- nail L60.8

Pityriasis (capitis) L21.0
- alba L30.5
- circinata (et maculata) L42
- furfuracea L21.0
- maculata (et circinata) L30.5
- rosea L42
- simplex L30.5
- specified type NEC L30.5
- streptogenes L30.5
- versicolor (scrotal) B36.0

Plagiocephaly
- aquired M95.2
- congenital Q67.3

Plaque(s)
- epicardial I31.8

Planning, family
- contraception Z30.9
- procreation Z31.69

Plasmacytopenia D72.818

Plasmacytosis D72.822

Platybasia Q75.8

Platyonychia (congenital) Q84.6
- acquired L60.8

Platypelloid pelvis M95.5
- congenital Q74.2

Plethora R23.2
- newborn P61.1

Pleurisy (acute) (adhesive) (chronic) (costal) (diaphragmatic) (double) (dry) (fibrinous) (fibrous) (interlobar) (latent) (plastic) (primary) (residual) (sicca) (sterile) (subacute) (unresolved) R09.1
- with
  - adherent pleura J86.0
  - effusion J90
- pneumococcal J90
- purulent—*see* Pyothorax
- septic—*see* Pyothorax
- serofibrinous—*see* Pleurisy, with effusion
- seropurulent—*see* Pyothorax
- serous—*see* Pleurisy, with effusion
- staphylococcal J86.9
- streptococcal J90
- suppurative—*see* Pyothorax

Pleuropericarditis—*see also* Pericarditis
- acute I30.9

Pleuro-pneumonia-like organism (PPLO), as the cause of disease classified elsewhere B96.0

Plica
- polonica B85.0
- tonsil J35.8

Plug
- meconium (newborn) NEC syndrome P76.0
- mucus—*see* Asphyxia

Plumbism—*see* subcategory T56.0

PMEI (polymorphic epilepsy in infancy) G40.83-

Pneumatocele (lung) J98.4
- intracranial G93.89

Pneumaturia R39.89

Pneumocephalus G93.89

Pneumococcemia A40.3

Pneumococcus, pneumococcal—*see* Disease, diseased

Pneumohemopericardium I31.2

Pneumomediastinum J98.2
- congenital or perinatal P25.2

Pneumonia (acute) (double) (migratory) (purulent) (septic) (unresolved) J18.9
- with
  - due to specified organism—*see* Pneumonia, in (due to)
  - influenza—*see* Influenza, with, pneumonia
- 2019 (novel) coronavirus J12.82
- anaerobes J15.8
- anthrax A22.1
- Ascaris B77.81
- aspiration J69.0
  - due to
    - aspiration of microorganisms
      - ~ bacterial J15.9
      - ~ viral J12.9
    - food (regurgitated) J69.0
    - gastric secretions J69.0
    - milk (regurgitated) J69.0
    - oils, essences J69.1
    - solids, liquids NEC J69.8
    - vomitus J69.0
  - newborn P24.81
    - amniotic fluid (clear) P24.11
    - blood P24.21
    - food (regurgitated) P24.31
    - liquor (amnii) P24.11
    - meconium P24.01
    - milk P24.31
    - mucus P24.11
    - specified NEC P24.81
    - stomach contents P24.31
- atypical NEC J18.9
- bacillus J15.9
  - specified NEC J15.8
- bacterial J15.9
  - specified NEC J15.8
- Bacteroides (fragilis) (oralis) (melaninogenicus) J15.8
- broncho-, bronchial (confluent) (croupous) (diffuse) (disseminated) (hemorrhagic) (involving lobes) (lobar) (terminal) J18.0
  - aspiration—*see* Pneumonia, aspiration
  - bacterial J15.9
    - specified NEC J15.8
  - diplococcal J13
  - Eaton's agent J15.7
  - Escherichia coli (E. coli) J15.5
  - Friedländer's bacillus J15.0
  - Hemophilus influenzae J14
  - inhalation—*see also* Pneumonia, aspiration
    - of oils or essences J69.1
  - Klebsiella (pneumoniae) J15.0
  - lipid, lipoid J69.1
  - Mycoplasma (pneumoniae) J15.7
  - pleuro-pneumonia-like-organisms (PPLO) J15.7
  - pneumococcal J13
  - Proteus J15.6
  - Pseudomonas J15.1
  - Serratia marcescens J15.6
  - specified organism NEC J16.8
  - streptococcal NEC J15.4
    - group B J15.3

Pneumonia, *continued*
- pneumoniae J13
- Butyrivibrio (fibriosolvens) J15.8
- Candida B37.1
- chlamydial J16.0
  - congenital P23.1
- Clostridium (haemolyticum) (novyi) J15.8
- confluent—*see* Pneumonia, broncho
- congenital (infective) P23.9
  - due to
    - bacterium NEC P23.6
    - Chlamydia P23.1
    - Escherichia coli P23.4
    - Haemophilus influenzae P23.6
    - infective organism NEC P23.8
    - Klebsiella pneumoniae P23.6
    - Mycoplasma P23.6
    - Pseudomonas P23.5
    - Staphylococcus P23.2
    - Streptococcus (except group B) P23.6
      - ~ group B P23.3
    - viral agent P23.0
  - specified NEC P23.8
- coronavirus (novel) (disease) 2019 J12.82
- croupous—*see* Pneumonia, lobar
- cytomegalovirus (CMV) B25.0
- diplococcal, diplococcus (broncho-) (lobar) J13
- Eaton's agent J15.7
- Enterobacter J15.6
- Escherichia coli (E. coli) J15.5
- Eubacterium J15.8
- Friedländer's bacillus J15.0
- Fusobacterium (nucleatum) J15.8
- giant cell (measles) B05.2
- gram-negative bacteria NEC J15.6
  - anaerobic J15.8
- Hemophilus influenzae (broncho-) (lobar) J14
- human metapneumovirus (hMPV) J12.3
- in (due to)
  - actinomycosis A42.0
  - adenovirus J12.0
  - anthrax A22.1
  - ascariasis B77.81
  - aspergillosis B44.9
  - Bacillus anthracis A22.1
  - Bacterium anitratum J15.6
  - candidiasis B37.1
  - chickenpox B01.2
  - Chlamydia J16.0
    - neonatal P23.1
  - cytomegalovirus disease B25.0
  - Diplococcus (pneumoniae) J13
  - Eaton's agent J15.7
  - Enterobacter J15.6
  - Escherichia coli (E. coli) J15.5
  - Friedländer's bacillus J15.0
  - gonorrhea A54.84
  - Hemophilus influenzae (H. influenzae) J14
  - Herellea J15.6
  - human metapneumovirus (hMPV) J12.3
  - Klebsiella (pneumoniae) J15.0
  - measles B05.2
  - Mycoplasma (pneumoniae) J15.7
  - nocardiosis, nocardiasis A43.0
  - parainfluenza virus J12.2
  - pleuro-pneumonia-like-organism (PPLO) J15.7
  - pneumococcus J13
  - Proteus J15.6
  - Pseudomonas NEC J15.1
  - rheumatic fever I00 *[J17]*
  - Serratia marcescens J15.6
  - specified
    - bacterium NEC J15.8
    - organism NEC J16.8
  - Staphylococcus J15.20
    - aureus (methicillin susceptible) (MSSA) J15.211
      - ~ methicillin resistant (MRSA) J15.212
    - specified NEC J15.29
  - Streptococcus J15.4
    - group B J15.3
    - pneumoniae J13
    - specified NEC J15.4
  - varicella B01.2

Pneumonia, *continued*
- whooping cough A37.91
  - due to
    - Bordetella parapertussis A37.11
    - Bordetella pertussis A37.01
    - specified NEC A37.81
- inhalation of food or vomit—*see* Pneumonia, aspiration
- interstitial J84.9
  - pseudomonas J15.1
- Klebsiella (pneumoniae) J15.0
- lipid, lipoid (exogenous) J69.1
- lobar (disseminated) (double) (interstitial) J18.1
  - bacterial J15.9
    - specified NEC J15.8
  - Escherichia coli (E. coli) J15.5
  - Friedländer's bacillus J15.0
  - Hemophilus influenzae J14
  - Klebsiella (pneumoniae) J15.0
  - pneumococcal J13
  - Proteus J15.6
  - Pseudomonas J15.1
  - specified organism NEC J16.8
  - staphylococcal—*see* Pneumonia, staphylococcal
  - streptococcal NEC J15.4
  - Streptococcus pneumoniae J13
  - viral, virus—*see* Pneumonia, viral
- lobular—*see* Pneumonia, broncho
- massive—*see* Pneumonia, lobar
- meconium P24.01
- MRSA (methicillin resistant Staphylococcus aureus) J15.212
- MSSA (methicillin susceptible Staphylococcus aureus) J15.211
- multilobar—*see* Pneumonia, by type
- Mycoplasma (pneumoniae) J15.7
- neonatal P23.9
  - aspiration—*see* Aspiration, by substance, with pneumonia
- parainfluenza virus J12.2
- Peptococcus J15.8
- Peptostreptococcus J15.8
- pleuro-pneumonia-like organism (PPLO) J15.7
- pneumococcal (broncho-) (lobar) J13
- postinfectional NEC B99 *[J17]*
- postmeasles B05.2
- Proteus J15.6
- Pseudomonas J15.1
- respiratory syncytial virus (RSV) J12.1
- resulting from a procedure J95.89
- rheumatic I00 *[J17]*
- SARS-associated coronavirus J12.81
- Serratia marcescens J15.6
- specified NEC J18.8
  - bacterium NEC J15.8
  - organism NEC J16.8
  - virus NEC J12.89
- staphylococcal (broncho) (lobar) J15.20
  - aureus (methicillin susceptible) (MSSA) J15.211
    - methicillin resistant (MRSA) J15.212
  - specified NEC J15.29
- streptococcal NEC (broncho) (lobar) J15.4
  - group
    - A J15.4
    - B J15.3
  - specified NEC J15.4
- Streptococcus pneumoniae J13
- varicella B01.2
- Veillonella J15.8
- ventilator associated J95.851
- viral, virus (broncho) (interstitial) (lobar) J12.9
  - congenital P23.0
  - human metapneumovirus (hMPV) J12.3
  - parainfluenza J12.2
  - respiratory syncytial (RSV) J12.1
  - SARS-associated coronavirus J12.81
  - specified NEC J12.89

Pneumonitis (acute) (primary)—*see also* Pneumonia
- aspiration J69.0
- congenital rubella P35.0
- due to
  - detergent J69.8
  - food, vomit (aspiration) J69.0

Pneumonitis, *continued*
- – inhalation
  - ▪ blood J69.8
  - ▪ essences J69.1
  - ▪ food (regurgitated), milk, vomit J69.0
  - ▪ oils, essences J69.1
  - ▪ saliva J69.0
  - ▪ solids, liquids NEC J69.8
  - – oils, essences J69.1
  - – solids, liquids NEC J69.8
  - – toxoplasmosis (acquired) B58.3
    - ▪ congenital P37.1
  - – ventilator J95.851
- • meconium P24.01
- • rubella, congenital P35.0
- • ventilator associated J95.851

Pneumopathy NEC J98.4
- • alveolar J84.09
- • parietoalveolar J84.09

Pneumopericarditis—*see also* Pericarditis
- • acute I30.9

Pneumopericardium—*see also* Pericarditis
- • congenital P25.3
- • newborn P25.3

Pneumophagia (psychogenic) F45.8

Pneumopyopericardium I30.1

Pneumopyothorax—*see* Pyopneumothorax
- • with fistula J86.0

Pneumothorax NOS J93.9
- • acute J93.83
- • chronic J93.81
- • congenital P25.1
- • perinatal period P25.1
- • postprocedural J95.811
- • specified NEC J93.83
- • spontaneous NOS J93.83
  - – newborn P25.1
  - – primary J93.11
  - – secondary J93.12
  - – tension J93.0
- • tense valvular, infectional J93.0
- • tension (spontaneous) J93.0
- • traumatic S27.0

Podencephalus Q01.9

Poikiloderma L81.6
- • congenital Q82.8

Pointed ear (congenital) Q17.3

Poison ivy, oak, sumac or other plant dermatitis (allergic) (contact) L23.7

Poisoning (acute)—*see also* Table of Drugs and Chemicals
- • algae and toxins T65.82-
- • Bacillus B (aertrycke) (cholerae (suis)) (paratyphosus) (suipestifer) A02.9
  - – botulinus A05.1
- • bacterial toxins A05.9
- • berries, noxious—*see* Poisoning, food, noxious, berries
- • botulism A05.1
- • Clostridium botulinum A05.1
- • drug—*see* Table of Drugs and Chemicals, by drug, poisoning
- • epidemic, fish (noxious)—*see* Poisoning, food, noxious or naturally toxic, seafood
  - – bacterial A05.9
- • fava bean D55.0
- • food (acute) (diseased) (infected) (noxious) NEC A05.9
  - – bacterial—*see* Intoxication, foodborne, by agent
  - – due to
    - ▪ Bacillus (aertrycke) (choleraesuis) (paratyphosus) (suipestifer) A02.9
      - ~ botulinus A05.1
    - ▪ Clostridium (perfringens) (Welchii) A05.2
    - ▪ salmonella (aertrycke) (callinarum) (choleraesuis) (enteritidis) (paratyphi) (suipestifer) A02.9
      - ~ with
        - ◊ gastroenteritis A02.0
        - ◊ sepsis A02.1
    - ▪ staphylococcus A05.0
    - ▪ Vibrio
      - ~ parahaemolyticus A05.3
      - ~ vulnificus A05.5

Poisoning, *continued*
- – noxious or naturally toxic
  - ▪ berries—*see* subcategory T62.1-
  - ▪ fish—*see* Poisoning, food, noxious or naturally toxic, seafood
  - ▪ mushrooms—*see* subcategory T62.0X-
  - ▪ plants NEC—*see* subcategory T62.2X-
  - ▪ seafood—*see* Poisoning, food, noxious or naturally toxic, seafood
  - ▪ specified NEC—*see* subcategory T62.8X-
- • kreotoxism, food A05.9
- • lead T56.0-
- • mushroom—*see* Poisoning, food, noxious, mushroom
- • mussels—*see also* Poisoning
  - – bacterial—*see* Intoxication, foodborne, by agent
- • shellfish (amnesic) (azaspiracid) (diarrheic) (neurotoxic) (noxious) (paralytic) T61.78-
- • Staphylococcus, food A05.0

Poliomyelitis (acute) (anterior) (epidemic) A80.9
- • congenital P35.8 (if included in tabular list)
- • imported A80.1
- • indigenous A80.2
  - – spinal, acute A80.9
- • nonepidemic A80.9
- • paralytic
  - – specified NEC A80.39
  - – wild virus

Pollakiuria R35.0
- • psychogenic F45.8

Pollinosis J30.1

Pollitzer's disease L73.2

Polycystic (disease)
- • degeneration, kidney Q61.3
  - – autosomal recessive (infantile type) NEC Q61.19
- • kidney Q61.3
  - – autosomal
    - ▪ recessive NEC Q61.19
  - – autosomal recessive (childhood type) NEC Q61.19
  - – infantile type NEC Q61.19
- • ovary, ovaries E28.2

Polycythemia (secondary) D75.1
- • acquired D75.1
- • benign (familial) D75.0
- • due to
  - – donor twin P61.1
  - – erythropoietin D75.1
  - – fall in plasma volume D75.1
  - – high altitude D75.1
  - – maternal-fetal transfusion P61.1
  - – stress D75.1
- • emotional D75.1
- • erythropoietin D75.1
- • familial (benign) D75.0
- • Gaisböck's (hypertonica) D75.1
- • high altitude D75.1
- • hypertonica D75.1
- • hypoxemic D75.1
- • neonatorum P61.1
- • nephrogenous D75.1
- • relative D75.1
- • secondary D75.1
- • spurious D75.1
- • stress D75.1

Polycytosis cryptogenica D75.1

Polydactylism, polydactyly Q69.9
- • toes Q69.2

Polydipsia R63.1

Polydystrophy, pseudo-Hurler E77.0

Polyhydramnios O40.-

Polymenorrhea N92.0

Polyneuritis, polyneuritic—*see also* Polyneuropathy
- • cranialis G52.7
- • inflammatory G61.9

Polyneuropathy (peripheral) G62.9
- • hereditary G60.9
  - – specified NEC G60.8
- • in (due to)
  - – hypoglycemia E16.2 *[G63]*
  - – infectious

Polyneuropathy, *continued*
  - ▪ disease NEC B99 *[G63]*
  - ▪ mononucleosis B27.91
- – Lyme disease A69.22
- – neoplastic disease (*see also* Table of Neoplasms in the complete *ICD-10-CM* manual) D49.9 *[G63]*
- – sarcoidosis D86.89
- – systemic
  - ▪ lupus erythematosus M32.19
- • sensory (hereditary) (idiopathic) G60.8

Polyopia H53.8

Polyorchism, polyorchidism Q55.21

Polyp, polypus
- • accessory sinus J33.8
- • adenoid tissue J33.0
- • antrum J33.8
- • anus, anal (canal) K62.0
- • choanal J33.0
- • colon K63.5
  - – adenomatous D12.6
    - ▪ sigmoid D12.5
    - ▪ transverse D12.3
  - – ascending K63.5
  - – cecum K63.5
  - – descending K63.5
  - – inflammatory K51.40
    - ▪ with
      - ~ abscess K51.414
      - ~ complication K51.419
        - ◊ specified NEC K51.418
      - ~ fistula K51.413
      - ~ intestinal obstruction K51.412
      - ~ rectal bleeding K51.411
  - – sigmoid K63.5
  - – transverse K63.5
- • esophageal K22.81
- • esophagogastric junction K22.82
- • ethmoidal (sinus) J33.8
- • frontal (sinus) J33.8
- • maxillary (sinus) J33.8
- • nares
  - – anterior J33.9
  - – posterior J33.0
- • nasal (mucous) J33.9
  - – cavity J33.0
  - – septum J33.0
- • nasopharyngeal J33.0
- • nose (mucous) J33.9
- • rectum (nonadenomatous) K62.1
- • septum (nasal) J33.0
- • sinus (accessory) (ethmoidal) (frontal) (maxillary) (sphenoidal) J33.8
- • sphenoidal (sinus) J33.8
- • turbinate, mucous membrane J33.8
- • umbilical, newborn P83.6

Polyposis—*see also* Polyp
- • coli (adenomatous) D12.6
- • colon (adenomatous) D12.6
- • familial D12.6
- • intestinal (adenomatous) D12.6

Polyserositis
- • due to pericarditis I31.1
- • pericardial I31.1

Polysyndactyly (*see also* Syndactylism) Q70.4

Polyuria R35.89
- • nocturnal R35.81
- • psychogenic F45.8
- • specified NEC R35.89

Pomphylox L30.1

Poor
- • urinary stream R39.12
- • vision NEC H54.7

Porencephaly (congenital) (developmental) (true) Q04.6
- • acquired G93.0
- • nondevelopmental G93.0
- • traumatic (post) F07.89

Porocephaliasis B88.8

Porokeratosis Q82.8

Port wine nevus, mark, or stain Q82.5

Positive
- culture (nonspecific)
  - blood R78.81
  - bronchial washings R84.5
  - cerebrospinal fluid R83.5
  - nose R84.5
    - staphylococcus (Methicillin susceptible) Z22.321
      - Methicillin resistant Z22.322
  - urine R82.79
- PPD (skin test) R76.11
- serology for syphilis A53.0
  - false R76.8
  - with signs or symptoms—*code as* Syphilis, by site and stage
- skin test, tuberculin (without active tuberculosis) R76.11
- test, human immunodeficiency virus (HIV) R75
- VDRL A53.0
  - with signs and symptoms—*code by* site and stage under Syphilis A53.9
- Wassermann reaction A53.0

Postcardiotomy syndrome I97.0

Postcommissurotomy syndrome I97.0

Postconcussional syndrome F07.81

Postcontusional syndrome F07.81

Post COVID-19 condition, unspecified U09.9

Posthemorrhagic anemia (chronic) D50.0
- acute D62
- newborn P61.3

Postmaturity, postmature (over 42 weeks)
- newborn P08.22

Postmeasles complication NEC (*see also* Disease, diseased) B05.89

Postnasal drip R09.82
- due to
  - allergic rhinitis—*see* Rhinitis, allergic
  - common cold J00
  - gastroesophageal reflux—*see* Reflux, gastroesophageal
  - nasopharyngitis—*see* Nasopharyngitis
  - other known condition—*code to* condition
  - sinusitis—*see* Sinusitis

Postoperative (postprocedural)—*see* Complication, postprocedural
- state NEC Z98.890

Post-term (40-42 weeks) (pregnancy) (mother)
- infant P08.21

Post-traumatic brain syndrome, nonpsychotic F07.81

Postvaccinal reaction or complication—*see* Complications, vaccination

Postvalvulotomy syndrome I97.0

Potter's
- facies Q60.6
- syndrome (with renal agenesis) Q60.6

Poultrymen's itch B88.0

Poverty NEC Z59.6
- extreme Z59.5

Prader-Willi syndrome Q87.11

Precocious
- adrenarche E30.1
- menarche E30.1
- menstruation E30.1
- pubarche E30.1
- puberty E30.1
  - central E22.8
- sexual development NEC E30.1

Precocity, sexual (constitutional) (female) (idiopathic) (male) E30.1
- with adrenal hyperplasia E25.9
  - congenital E25.0

Prediabetes, prediabetic R73.03

Pre-eclampsia O14.9
- with pre-existing hypertension—*see* Hypertension, complicating, pregnancy, pre-existing, with, pre-eclampsia
- mild O14.0-
- moderate O14.0-

Pre-eclampsia, *continued*
- severe O14.1
  - with hemolysis, elevated liver enzymes and low platelet count (HELLP) O14.2-

Pre-excitation atrioventricular conduction I45.6

Pregnancy (single) (uterine)—*see also* Delivery

Note: The Tabular must be reviewed for assignment of the appropriate character indicating the trimester of the pregnancy

Note: The Tabular must be reviewed for assignment of appropriate seventh character for multiple gestation codes in Chapter 15
- abdominal (ectopic) O00.00
  - with uterine pregnancy O00.01
  - with viable fetus O36.7-
- ampullar O00.10-
- broad ligament O00.80
- cervical O00.80
- complicated by (care of) (management affected by)
  - abnormal, abnormality
    - findings on antenatal screening of mother O28.9
      - biochemical O28.1
      - chromosomal O28.5
      - cytological O28.2
      - genetic O28.5
      - hematological O28.0
      - radiological O28.4
      - specified NEC O28.8
      - ultrasonic O28.3
  - conjoined twins O30.02-
  - death of fetus (near term) O36.4
    - early pregnancy O02.1
  - decreased fetal movement O36.81-
  - diabetes (mellitus)
    - gestational (pregnancy induced—*see* Diabetes, gestational
      - type 1 O24.01-
      - type 2 O24.11-
  - edema
    - with
      - gestational hypertension, mild (*see also* Pre-eclampsia) O14.0-
  - fetal (maternal care for)
    - abnormality or damage O35.9
      - specified type NEC O35.8
    - anemia and thrombocytopenia O36.82-
    - anencephaly O35.0
    - bradycardia O36.83-
    - chromosomal abnormality (conditions in Q90 – Q99) O35.1
    - conjoined twins O30.02-
    - damage from
      - amniocentesis O35.7
      - biopsy procedures O35.7
      - drug addiction O35.5
      - hematological investigation O35.7
      - intrauterine contraceptive device O35.7
      - maternal
        - alcohol addiction O35.4
        - cytomegalovirus infection O35.3
        - disease NEC O35.8
        - drug addiction O35.5
        - listeriosis O35.8
        - rubella O35.3
        - toxoplasmosis O35.8
        - viral infection O35.3
      - medical procedure NEC O35.7
      - radiation O35.6
    - death (near term) O36.4
      - early pregnancy O02.1
    - decreased movement O36.81-
    - depressed heart rate tones O36.83-
    - excessive growth (large for dates) O36.6-
    - fetal heart rate or rhythm O36.83-
    - growth retardation O36.59-
      - light for dates O36.59-
      - small for dates O36.59-
    - heart rate irregularity (abnormal variability) (bradycardia) (decelerations) (tachycardia) O36.83-
    - hereditary disease O35.2
    - hydrocephalus O35.0

Pregnancy, *continued*
- intrauterine death O36.4
- non-reassuring heart rate or rhythm O36.83-
- poor growth O36.59-
  - light for dates O36.59-
  - small for dates O36.59-
- problem O36.9-
  - specified NEC O36.89-
- spina bifida O35.0
- thrombocytopenia O36.82-
  - HELLP syndrome (hemolysis, elevated liver enzymes and low platelet count) O14.2-
  - hemorrhage
    - before 20 completed weeks gestation O20.9
      - specified NEC O20.8
    - early O20.9
      - specified NEC O20.8
    - threatened abortion O20.0
  - hydramnios O40.-
  - hydrops
    - amnii O40.-
    - fetalis O36.2-
      - associated with isoimmunization (*see also* Pregnancy, complicated by, isoimmunization) O36.11-
  - hydrorrhea O42.90
  - inconclusive fetal viability O36.80
  - intrauterine fetal death (near term) O36.4
    - early pregnancy O02.1
  - isoimmunization O36.11-
    - anti-A sensitization O36.11-
    - anti-B sensitization O36.19-
    - Rh O36.09-
      - anti-D antibody O36.01-
    - specified NEC O36.19-
  - missed
    - abortion O02.1
    - delivery O36.4
  - multiple gestations
    - conjoined twins O30.02-
    - specified number of multiples NEC—*see* Pregnancy, multiple (gestation), specified NEC
    - quadruplet—*see* Pregnancy, quadruplet
    - specified complication NEC O31.8X-
    - triplet—*see* Pregnancy, triplet
    - twin—*see* Pregnancy, twin
  - oligohydramnios O41.0-
    - with premature rupture of membranes (*see also* Pregnancy, complicated by, premature rupture of membranes) O42.-
  - placental insufficiency O36.51-
  - polyhydramnios O40.-
  - pre-eclampsia O14.9-
    - mild O14.0-
    - moderate O14.0-
    - severe O14.1-
      - with hemolysis, elevated liver enzymes and low platelet count (HELLP) O14.2-
  - premature rupture of membranes O42.90
    - after 37 weeks gestation O42.92
    - full-term, unspec as to length of time between rupture and onset of labor O42.92
    - with onset of labor
      - within 24 hours O42.00
        - at or after 37 weeks gestation O42.02
        - pre-term (before 37 completed weeks of gestation) O42.01-
      - after 24 hours O42.10
        - at or after 37 weeks gestation O42.12
        - pre-term (before 37 completed weeks of gestation) O42.11-
    - pre-term (before 37 completed weeks of gestation) O42.91-
  - preterm labor
    - second trimester
      - without delivery O60.02
    - third trimester
      - without delivery O60.03
    - without delivery
      - second trimester O60.02
      - third trimester O60.03
  - Rh immunization, incompatibility or sensitization NEC O36.09-

Pregnancy, *continued*
- ■ anti-D antibody O36.01-
- – threatened
  - ■ abortion O20.0
- – young mother
  - ■ multigravida O09.62-
  - ■ primigravida O09.61-
- • cornual O00.8-
- • ectopic (ruptured) O00.9-
  - – abdominal O00.00
    - ■ with uterine pregnancy O00.01
    - ■ with viable fetus O36.7-
  - – cervical O00.8-
  - – cornual O00.8-
  - – intraligamentous O00.8-
  - – mural O00.8-
  - – ovarian O00.20-
  - – specified site NEC O00.8-
  - – tubal (ruptured) O00.10-
    - ■ with intrauterine pregnancy O00.11
- • fallopian O00.10-
  - – with intrauterine pregnancy O00.11
- • incidental finding Z33.1
- • interstitial O00.8-
- • intraligamentous O00.8-
- • intramural O00.8-
- • intraperitoneal O00.00
  - – with intrauterine pregnancy O00.01
- • isthmian O00.10-
- • mesometric (mural) O00.8-
- • multiple (gestation)
  - – greater than quadruplets—*see* Pregnancy, multiple (gestation), specified NEC
  - – specified NEC O30.80-
    - ■ number of chorions and amnions are both equal to the number of fetuses O30.83-
    - ■ two or more monoamniotic fetuses O30.82-
    - ■ two or more monochorionic fetuses O30.81-
    - ■ unable to determine number of placenta and number of amniotic sacs O30.89-
    - ■ unspecified number of placenta and unspecified number of amniotic sacs O30.80-
- • mural O00.8-
- • ovarian O00.2-
- • quadruplet O30.20-
  - – with
    - ■ two or more monoamniotic fetuses O30.22-
    - ■ two or more monochorionic fetuses O30.21-
  - – quadrachorionic/quadra-amniotic O30.23-
  - – two or more monoamniotic fetuses O30.22-
  - – two or more monochorionic fetuses O30.21-
  - – unable to determine number of placenta and number of amniotic sacs O30.29-
  - – unspecified number of placenta and unspecified number of amniotic sacs O30.20-
- • quintuplet—*see* Pregnancy, multiple (gestation), specified NEC
- • sextuplet—*see* Pregnancy, multiple (gestation), specified NEC
- • supervision of
  - – young mother
    - ■ multigravida O09.62-
    - ■ primigravida O09.61-
- • triplet O30.10-
  - – with
    - ■ two or more monoamniotic fetuses O30.12-
    - ■ two or more monochrorionic fetuses O30.11-
  - – trichorionic/triamniotic O30.13-
  - – two or more monoamniotic fetuses O30.12-
  - – two or more monochrorionic fetuses O30.11-
  - – unable to determine number of placenta and number of amniotic sacs O30.19-
  - – unspecified number of placenta and unspecified number of amniotic sacs O30.10-
- • tubal (with abortion) (with rupture) O00.10-
  - – with intrauterine pregnancy O00.11
- • twin O30.00-
  - – conjoined O30.02-
  - – dichorionic/diamniotic (two placentae, two amniotic sacs) O30.04-
  - – monochorionic/diamniotic (one placenta, two amniotic sacs) O30.03-

Pregnancy, *continued*
- – monochorionic/monoamniotic (one placenta, one amniotic sac) O30.01-
- – unable to determine number of placenta and number of amniotic sacs O30.09-
- – unspecified number of placenta and unspecified number of amniotic sacs O30.00-
- • unwanted Z64.0
- • weeks of gestation
  - – 8 weeks Z3A.08
  - – 9 weeks Z3A.09
  - – 10 weeks Z3A.10
  - – 11 weeks Z3A.11
  - – 12 weeks Z3A.12
  - – 13 weeks Z3A.13
  - – 14 weeks Z3A.14
  - – 15 weeks Z3A.15
  - – 16 weeks Z3A.16
  - – 17 weeks Z3A.17
  - – 18 weeks Z3A.18
  - – 19 weeks Z3A.19
  - – 20 weeks Z3A.20
  - – 21 weeks Z3A.21
  - – 22 weeks Z3A.22
  - – 23 weeks Z3A.23
  - – 24 weeks Z3A.24
  - – 25 weeks Z3A.25
  - – 26 weeks Z3A.26
  - – 27 weeks Z3A.27
  - – 28 weeks Z3A.28
  - – 29 weeks Z3A.29
  - – 30 weeks Z3A.30
  - – 31 weeks Z3A.31
  - – 32 weeks Z3A.32
  - – 33 weeks Z3A.33
  - – 34 weeks Z3A.34
  - – 35 weeks Z3A.35
  - – 36 weeks Z3A.36
  - – 37 weeks Z3A.37
  - – 38 weeks Z3A.38
  - – 39 weeks Z3A.39
  - – 40 weeks Z3A.40
  - – 41 weeks Z3A.41
  - – 42 weeks Z3A.42
  - – greater than 42 weeks Z3A.49
  - – less than 8 weeks Z3A.01
  - – not specified Z3A.00

Premature—*see also* Disease, diseased
- • beats I49.40
  - – atrial I49.1
  - – auricular I49.1
  - – supraventricular I49.1
- • birth NEC—*see* Preterm, newborn
- • closure, foramen ovale Q21.8
- • contraction
  - – atrial I49.1
  - – auricular I49.1
  - – auriculoventricular I49.49
  - – heart (extrasystole) I49.49
- • lungs P28.0
- • newborn
  - – extreme (less than 28 completed weeks)—*see* Immaturity, extreme
  - – less than 37 completed weeks—*see* Preterm, newborn
- • puberty E30.1

Premenstrual
- • dysphoric disorder (PMDD) F32.81
- • tension N94.3

Prenatal
- • teeth K00.6

Preponderance, left or right ventricular I51.7

Prescription of contraceptives (initial) Z30.019
- • barrier Z30.018
- • diaphragm Z30.018
- • emergency (postcoital) Z30.012
- • implantable subdermal Z30.017
- • injectable Z30.013
- • intrauterine contraceptive device Z30.014
- • pills Z30.011
- • postcoital (emergency) Z30.012

Prescription of contraceptives, *continued*
- • repeat Z30.40
  - – barrier Z30.49
  - – diaphragm Z30.49
  - – implantable subdermal Z30.46
  - – injectable Z30.42
  - – pills Z30.41
  - – specified type NEC Z30.49
  - – transdermal patch Z30.45
  - – vaginal ring Z30.44
- • specified type NEC Z30.018
- • transdermal patch Z30.016
- • vaginal ring Z30.015

Presence (of)
- • arterial-venous shunt (dialysis) Z99.2
- • artificial
  - – heart (fully implantable) (mechanical) Z95.812
    - ■ valve Z95.2
- • bladder implant (functional) Z96.0
- • cardiac
  - – pacemaker Z95.0
- • cardioverter-defibrillator Z95.810
- • cerebrospinal fluid drainage device Z98.2
- • contact lens(es) Z97.3
- • CSF shunt Z98.2
- • endocrine implant (functional) NEC Z96.49
- • external hearing-aid or device Z97.4
- • functional implant Z96.9
  - – specified NEC Z96.89
- • heart valve implant (functional) Z95.2
  - – prosthetic Z95.2
  - – specified type NEC Z95.4
  - – xenogenic Z95.3
- • implanted device (artificial) (functional) (prosthetic) Z96.9
  - – cardiac pacemaker Z95.0
  - – heart valve Z95.2
    - ■ prosthetic Z95.2
    - ■ specified NEC Z95.4
    - ■ xenogenic Z95.3
  - – neurostimulator Z96.82
  - – skin Z96.81

Prespondylolisthesis (congenital) Q76.2

Pressure
- • area, skin—*see* Ulcer, pressure, by site
- • increased
  - – intracranial (benign) G93.2
    - ■ injury at birth P11.0

Pre-syncope R55

Preterm
- • newborn (infant) P07.30
  - – gestational age
    - ■ 28 completed weeks (28 weeks, 0 days through 28 weeks, 6 days) P07.31
    - ■ 29 completed weeks (29 weeks, 0 days through 29 weeks, 6 days) P07.32
    - ■ 30 completed weeks (30 weeks, 0 days through 30 weeks, 6 days) P07.33
    - ■ 31 completed weeks (31 weeks, 0 days through 31 weeks, 6 days) P07.34
    - ■ 32 completed weeks (32 weeks, 0 days through 32 weeks, 6 days) P07.35
    - ■ 33 completed weeks (33 weeks, 0 days through 33 weeks, 6 days) P07.36
    - ■ 34 completed weeks (34 weeks, 0 days through 34 weeks, 6 days) P07.37
    - ■ 35 completed weeks (35 weeks, 0 days through 35 weeks, 6 days) P07.38
    - ■ 36 completed weeks (36 weeks, 0 days through 36 weeks, 6 days) P07.39

Priapism N48.30
- • due to
  - – disease classified elsewhere N48.32
  - – drug N48.33
  - – specified cause NEC N48.39
  - – trauma N48.31

Prickly heat L74.0

Primus varus (bilateral) Q66.21-

Pringle's disease (tuberous sclerosis) Q85.1

Problem (with) (related to)
- academic Z55.8
- acculturation Z60.3
- adopted child Z62.821
- alcoholism in family Z63.72
- atypical parenting situation Z62.9
- bankruptcy Z59.89
- behavioral (adult)
  - drug seeking Z76.5
- birth of sibling affecting child Z62.898
- care (of)
- child
  - abuse (affecting the child)—see Maltreatment, child
  - custody or support proceedings Z65.3
  - in care of non-parental family member Z62.21
  - in foster care Z62.21
  - in welfare custody Z62.21
  - living in orphanage or group home Z62.22
- conflict or discord (with)
  - classmates Z55.4
  - counselor Z64.4
  - family Z63.9
    - specified NEC Z63.8
  - probation officer Z64.4
  - social worker Z64.4
  - teachers Z55.4
- drug addict in family Z63.72
- economic Z59.9
- education Z55.9
  - specified NEC Z55.8
- enuresis, child F98.0
- failed examinations (school) Z55.2
- falling Z91.81
- family (see also Disruption, family) Z63.9-
  - specified NEC Z63.8
- feeding (elderly) (infant) R63.39
  - newborn P92.9
    - breast P92.5
    - overfeeding P92.4
    - slow P92.2
    - specified NEC P92.8
    - underfeeding P92.3
  - nonorganic F50.89
- finance Z59.-
- foster child Z62.822
- genital NEC
  - female N94.9
  - male N50.9
- homelessness Z59.00
- housing Z59.9
  - inadequate Z59.1
- identity (of childhood) F93.8
- intrafamilial communication Z63.8
  - isolated Z59.89
- jealousy, child F93.8
- language (developmental) F80.9
- learning (developmental) F81.9
- lifestyle Z72.9
  - gambling Z72.6
  - high-risk sexual behavior (heterosexual) Z72.51
    - bisexual Z72.53
    - homosexual Z72.5
  - inappropriate eating habits Z72.4
  - self-damaging behavior NEC Z72.89
  - specified NEC Z72.89
  - tobacco use Z72.0
- literacy Z55.9
  - low level Z55.0
  - specified NEC Z55.8
- mental F48.9
- presence of sick or disabled person in family or household Z63.79
  - needing care Z63.6
- primary support group (family) Z63.9
  - specified NEC Z63.8
- psychosocial Z65.9
  - specified NEC Z65.8
- relationship Z63.9
  - childhood F93.8
- seeking and accepting known hazardous and harmful
  - behavioral or psychological interventions Z65.8
  - chemical, nutritional or physical interventions Z65.8
- sight H54.7

Problem (with) (related to), *continued*
- speech R47.9
  - developmental F80.9
  - specified NEC R47.89
- swallowing—see Dysphagia
- taste—see Disturbance, sensation
- tic, child F95.0
- underachievement in school Z55.3
- voice production R47.89

Procedure (surgical)
- for purpose other than remedying health state Z41.9
  - specified NEC Z41.8
- not done Z53.9
  - because of
    - administrative reasons Z53.8
    - contraindication Z53.09
      ~ smoking Z53.01
    - patient's decision Z53.20
      ~ for reasons of belief or group pressure Z53.1
      ~ left against medical advice (AMA) Z53.29
      ~ left without being seen Z53.21
      ~ specified reason NEC Z53.29
    - specified reason NEC Z53.8

Proctalgia K62.89

Proctitis K62.89
- amebic (acute) A06.0
- chlamydial A56.3
- gonococcal A54.6
- granulomatous—see Enteritis, regional, large intestine
- herpetic A60
- ulcerative (chronic) K51.20
  - with
    - complication K51.219
      ~ abscess K51.214
      ~ fistula K51.213
      ~ obstruction K51.212
      ~ rectal bleeding K51.211
      ~ specified NEC K51.218

Proctocele
- male K62.3

Proctocolitis
- allergic K52.29
- food-induced eosinophilic K52.29
- food protein-induced K52.29
- milk protein-induced K52.29

Proctoptosis K62.3

Proctorrhagia K62.5

Proctospasm K59.4
- psychogenic F45.8

Prolapse, prolapsed
- anus, anal (canal) (sphincter) K62.2
- bladder (mucosa) (sphincter) (acquired)
  - congenital Q79.4
- rectum (mucosa) (sphincter) K62.3

Prolonged, prolongation (of)
- bleeding (time) (idiopathic) R79.1
- coagulation (time) R79.1
- gestation (over 42 completed weeks)
  - newborn P08.22
- interval I44.0
- partial thromboplastin time (PTT) R79.1
- prothrombin time R79.1
- QT interval R94.31

Pronation
- ankle—see Deformity, limb, foot, specified NEC
- foot—see also Deformity, limb, foot, specified NEC
  - congenital Q74.2

Prophylactic
- administration of
  - antibiotics, long-term Z79.2
  - antivenin Z29.12
    - short-term use—omit code
  - drug (see also Long-term (current) (prophylactic) drug therapy (use of)) Z79.899-
  - fluoride varnish application Z29.3
  - other specified Z29.8
  - rabies immune therapy Z29.14
  - respiratory syncytial virus (RSV) immune globulin Z29.11

Prophylactic, *continued*
  - Rho (D) immune globulin Z29.13
  - unspecified Z29.9
- medication Z79.899
- vaccination Z23

Prostatitis (congestive) (suppurative) (with cystitis) N41.9
- acute N41.0

Prostration R53.83
- heat—see also Heat, exhaustion
  - anhydrotic T67.3
  - due to
    - salt (and water) depletion T67.4
    - water depletion T67.3

Protein
- sickness (see also Reaction, serum) T80.69

Proteinuria R80.9
- Bence Jones R80.3
- isolated R80.0
- orthostatic R80.2
  - with glomerular lesion—see Proteinuria, isolated, with glomerular lesion
- postural R80.2
  - with glomerular lesion—see Proteinuria, isolated, with glomerular lesion
- specified type NEC R80.8

Proteolysis, pathologic D65

Proteus (mirabilis) (morganii), **as the cause of disease classified elsewhere** B96.4

Protrusion, protrusio
- device, implant or graft (see also Complications, by site and type, mechanical) T85.698
  - catheter NEC T85.698
    - cystostomy T83.090
    - urinary—see also Complications, catheter, urinary T83.098
  - ventricular intracranial shunt T85.09

Prune belly (syndrome) Q79.4

Prurigo (ferox) (gravis) (Hebrae) (Hebra's) (mitis) (simplex) L28.2
- Besnier's L20.0
- psychogenic F45.8

Pruritus, pruritic (essential) L29.9
- ani, anus L29.0
  - psychogenic F45.8
- anogenital L29.3
  - psychogenic F45.8
- hiemalis L29.8
- neurogenic (any site) F45.8
- perianal L29.0
- psychogenic (any site) F45.8
- scroti, scrotum L29.1
  - psychogenic F45.8
- specified NEC L29.8
  - psychogenic F45.8
- Trichomonas A59.9
- vulva, vulvae L29.2
  - psychogenic F45.8

Pseudo-Hurler's polydystrophy E77.0

Pseudoangioma I81

Pseudarthrosis, pseudoarthrosis (bone)
- clavicle, congenital Q74.0

Pseudocirrhosis, liver, pericardial I31.1

Pseudocyesis F45.8

Pseudohemophilia (Bernuth's) (hereditary) (type B) D68.0

Pseudohermaphroditism Q56.3
- adrenal E25.8
- female Q56.2
  - with adrenocortical disorder E25.8
  - without adrenocortical disorder Q56.2
  - adrenal, congenital E25.0
- male Q56.1
  - with
    - androgen resistance E34.51
    - feminizing testis E34.51

Pseudohydrocephalus G93.2

Pseudohypertrophic muscular dystrophy (Erb's) G71.02

Pseudohypertrophy, muscle G71.09

Pseudoinsomnia F51.03

Purpura, *continued*
- arthritic D69.0
- autoerythrocyte sensitization D69.2
- autoimmune D69.0
- bacterial D69.0
- Bateman's (senile) D69.2
- capillary fragility (hereditary) (idiopathic) D69.8
- Devil's pinches D69.2
- fibrinolytic—*see* Fibrinolysis
- fulminans, fulminous D65
- gangrenous D65
- hemorrhagic, hemorrhagica D69.3
  - not due to thrombocytopenia D69.0
- Henoch (-Schönlein) (allergic) D69.0
- idiopathic (thrombocytopenic) D69.3
  - nonthrombocytopenic D69.0
- immune thrombocytopenic D69.3
- infectious D69.0
- malignant D69.0
- neonatorum P54.5
- nervosa D69.0
- newborn P54.5
- nonthrombocytopenic D69.2
  - hemorrhagic D69.0
  - idiopathic D69.0
- nonthrombopenic D69.2
- peliosis rheumatica D69.0
- posttransfusion (post-transfusion) (from fresh) whole blood or blood products) D69.51
- primary D69.49
- red cell membrane sensitivity D69.2
- rheumatica D69.0
- Schönlein (-Henoch) (allergic) D69.0
- senile D69.2
- simplex D69.2
- symptomatica D69.0
- telangiectasia annularis L81.7
- thrombocytopenic D69.49
  - congenital D69.42
  - hemorrhagic D69.3
  - hereditary D69.42
  - idiopathic D69.3
  - immune D69.3
  - neonatal, transitory P61.0
  - thrombotic M31.19
- thrombohemolytic—*see* Fibrinolysis
- thrombolytic—*see* Fibrinolysis
- thrombopenic D69.49
- thrombotic, thrombocytopenic M31.19
- toxic D69.0
- vascular D69.0
- visceral symptoms D69.0

Purpuric spots R23.3

Purulent—*see* Disease, diseased

Pus
- in
  - stool R19.5
  - urine N39.0
- tube (rupture)—*see* Salpingo-oophoritis

Pustular rash L08.0

Pustule (nonmalignant) L08.9
- malignant A22.0

Pyelectasis—*see* Hydronephrosis

Pyelitis (congenital) (uremic)—*see also* Pyelonephritis
- with
  - calculus—*see* category N20
    - with hydronephrosis N13.6
- acute N10
- chronic N11.9
  - with calculus—*see* category N20
    - with hydronephrosis N13.6

Pyelonephritis—*see also* Nephritis, tubulo-interstitial
- with
  - calculus—*see* category N20
    - with hydronephrosis N13.6
- acute N10
- calculous—*see* category N20
  - with hydronephrosis N13.6
- chronic N11.9
  - with calculus—*see* category N20
    - with hydronephrosis N13.6

Pyelonephritis, *continued*
- in (due to)
  - lymphoma NEC C85.90 *[N16]*
  - sarcoidosis D86.84
  - sepsis A41.9 *[N16]*
  - transplant rejection T86.- *[N16]*

Pyelophlebitis I80.8

Pyemia, pyemic (fever) (infection) (purulent)—*see also* Sepsis
- pneumococcal
- specified organism NEC A41.89

Pyloritis K29.90
- with bleeding K29.91

Pylorospasm (reflex) NEC K31.3
- congenital or infantile Q40.0
- newborn Q40.0
- neurotic F45.8
- psychogenic F45.8

Pylorus, pyloric—*see* Disease, diseased

Pyoarthrosis—*see* Arthritis, pyogenic or pyemic

Pyocele
- sinus (accessory)—*see* Sinusitis
- turbinate (bone) J32.9

Pyoderma, pyodermia L08.0
- gangrenosum L88
- newborn P39.4
- phagedenic L88

Pyodermatitis L08.0

Pyopericarditis, pyopericardium I30.1

Pyopneumopericardium I30.1

Pyopneumothorax (infective) J86.9
- with fistula J86.0

Pyothorax J86.9
- with fistula J86.0

Pyrexia (of unknown origin) R50.9
- atmospheric T67.01
- heat T67.01
- newborn P81.9
  - environmentally-induced P81.0
- persistent R50.9

Pyroglobulinemia NEC E88.09

Pyrosis R12

Pyuria
- abnormal laboratory finding R82.81
- bacterial N39.0

Pityriasis (capitis) L21.0
- furfuracea L21.0

Q

Quadriparesis—*see* Quadriplegia
- meaning muscle weakness M62.81

Quadriplegia G82.50
- complete
  - C1–C4 level G82.51
  - C5–C7 level G82.53
- incomplete
  - C1–C4 level G82.52
  - C5–C7 level G82.54
- traumatic *code to* injury with seventh character S
  - current episode—*see* Injury, spinal (cord), cervical

Quervain's disease M65.4
- thyroid E06.1

Quincke's disease or edema T78.3

Quinsy (gangrenous) J36

R

Rabies A82.9
- contact Z20.3
- exposure to Z20.3
- inoculation reaction—*see* Complications, vaccination

Radiation
- therapy, encounter for Z51.0

Radiotherapy session Z51.0

Rag picker's disease A22.1

Rag sorter's disease A22.1

Rales R09.89

Ramsay-Hunt disease or syndrome (*see also* Hunt's)
- meaning dyssynergia cerebellaris myoclonica G11.19

Rape
- alleged, observation or examination, ruled out
  - child Z04.42
- child
  - confirmed T74.22
  - suspected T76.22

Rapid
- feeble pulse, due to shock, following injury T79.4
- heart (beat) R00.0
  - psychogenic F45.8

Rash (toxic) R21
- canker A38.9
- diaper L22
- drug (internal use) L27.0
  - contact (*see also* Dermatitis, due to, drugs and medicaments) L25.1
- following immunization T88.1-
- food—*see* Dermatitis, due to, food
- heat L74.0
- napkin (psoriasiform) L22
- nettle—*see* Urticaria
- pustular L08.0
- rose R21
  - epidemic B06.9
- scarlet A38.9
- serum (*see also* Reaction, serum) T80.69
- wandering tongue K14.1

Rat-bite fever A25.9
- due to Streptobacillus moniliformis A25.1
- spirochetal (morsus muris) A25.0

RDS (newborn) (type I) P22.0
- type II P22.1

Reaction—*see also* Disorder
- adverse
  - food (any) (ingested) NEC T78.1
    - anaphylactic—*see* Shock, anaphylactic, due to food
- allergic—*see* Allergy
- anaphylactic—*see* Shock, anaphylactic
- anaphylactoid—*see* Shock, anaphylactic
- antitoxin (prophylactic) (therapeutic)—*see* Complications, vaccination
- combat and operational stress F43.0
- compulsive F42.8
- conversion F44.9
- crisis, acute F43.0
- deoxyribonuclease (DNA) (DNase) hypersensitivity D69.2
- depressive (single episode) F32.9
  - psychotic F32.3
  - recurrent—*see* Disorder, depressive, recurrent
- dissociative F44.9
- drug NEC T88.7
  - allergic—*see* Allergy, drug
  - newborn P93.8
    - gray baby syndrome P93.0
  - overdose or poisoning (by accident)—*see* Table of Drugs and Chemicals, by drug, poisoning
  - photoallergic L56.1
  - phototoxic L56.0
  - withdrawal—*see* Dependence, by drug, with, withdrawal
    - infant of dependent mother P96.1
    - newborn P96.1
  - wrong substance given or taken (by accident)—*see* Table of Drugs and Chemicals, by drug, poisoning
- fear F40.9
  - child (abnormal) F93.8
- febrile nonhemolytic transfusion (FNHTR) R50.84
- hypoglycemic, due to insulin E16.0
  - therapeutic misadventure—*see* subcategory T38.3
- hysterical F44.9
- immunization—*see* Complications, vaccination
- insulin T38.3-
- leukemoid D72.823
  - basophilic D72.823
  - lymphocytic D72.823
  - monocytic D72.823

Reaction, *continued*
- – myelocytic D72.823
- – neutrophilic D72.823
- neurogenic—*see* Neurosis
- neurotic F48.9
- nonspecific
  - – to
    - ■ cell mediated immunity measurement of gamma interferon antigen response without active tuberculosis R76.12
    - ■ QuantiFERON-TB test (QFT) without active tuberculosis R76.12
    - ■ tuberculin test (*see also* Reaction) R76.11
- obsessive-compulsive F42.8
- phobic F40.9
- psychoneurotic—*see also* Neurosis
  - – compulsive F42
  - – obsessive F42
- psychophysiologic—*see* Disorder, somatoform
- psychosomatic—*see* Disorder, somatoform
- psychotic—*see* Psychosis
- scarlet fever toxin—*see* Complications, vaccination
- serum T80.69-
  - – anaphylactic (immediate) (*see also* Shock, anaphylactic) T80.59-
  - – specified reaction NEC
    - ■ due to
      - ~ administration of blood and blood products T80.61-
      - ~ immunization T80.62-
      - ~ serum specified NEC T80.69-
      - ~ vaccination T80.62-
- spinal puncture G97.1
  - – dural G97.1
- stress (severe) F43.9
  - – acute (agitation) ("daze") (disorientation) (disturbance of consciousness) (flight reaction) (fugue) F43.0
  - – specified NEC F43.8
- surgical procedure—*see* Complications, surgical procedure
- tetanus antitoxin—*see* Complications, vaccination
- toxic, to local anesthesia T81.89
- toxin-antitoxin—*see* Complications, vaccination
- tuberculin skin test, abnormal R76.11
- withdrawing, child or adolescent F93.8

Reactive airway disease—*see* Asthma

Reactive depression—*see* Reaction, depressive

Recklinghausen disease Q85.01

Rectalgia K62.89

Rectitis K62.89

Rectocele
- male K62.3

Rectosigmoiditis K63.89
- ulcerative (chronic) K51.30
  - – with
    - ■ complication K51.319
      - ~ abscess K51.314
      - ~ fistula K51.313
      - ~ obstruction K51.312
      - ~ rectal bleeding K51.311
      - ~ specified NEC K51.318

Red bugs B88.0

Reduced
- mobility Z74.09
- ventilatory or vital capacity R94.2

Redundant, redundancy
- foreskin (congenital) N47.8
- prepuce (congenital) N47.8

Reflex R29.2
- vasovagal R55

Reflux K21.9
- acid K21.9
- esophageal K21.9
  - – with esophagitis K21.0-
  - – newborn P78.83
- gastroesophageal K21.9
  - – with esophagitis K21.0-
- vesicoureteral (with scarring) N13.70
  - – without nephropathy N13.71

Refusal of
- food, psychogenic F50.89
- treatment (because of) Z53.20
  - – left against medical advice (AMA) Z53.29
  - – left without being seen Z53.21

Regurgitation R11.10
- aortic (valve)—*see* Insufficiency, aortic
- food—*see also* Vomiting
  - – with reswallowing—*see* Rumination
  - – newborn P92.1
- gastric contents—*see* Vomiting
- heart—*see* Endocarditis
- mitral (valve)—*see* Insufficiency, mitral
  - – congenital Q23.3
- myocardial—*see* Endocarditis
- pulmonary (valve) (heart) I37.1
  - – congenital Q22.2
  - – syphilitic A52.03
- tricuspid—*see* Insufficiency, tricuspid
- valve, valvular—*see* Endocarditis
  - – congenital Q24.8

Reifenstein syndrome E34.52

Reinsertion
- implantable subdermal contraceptive Z30.46
- intrauterine contraceptive device Z30.433

Rejection
- food, psychogenic F50.89
- transplant
  - – bone
    - ■ marrow T86.01
  - – heart T86.21
    - ■ with lung(s) T86.31
  - – kidney T86.11
  - – liver T86.41
  - – lung(s) T86.810
    - ■ with heart T86.31
  - – organ (immune or nonimmune cause) T86.-
  - – stem cell (peripheral blood) (umbilical cord) T86.5

Relapsing fever A68.9
- louse-borne (epidemic) A68.0
- Novy's (American) A68.1
- tick borne (endemic) A68.1

Relaxation
- anus (sphincter) K62.89
  - – psychogenic F45.8
- cardioesophageal K21.9
- diaphragm J98.6
- posture R29.3
- rectum (sphincter) K62.89

Remittent fever (malarial) B54

Remnant
- fingernail L60.8
  - – congenital Q84.6
- thyroglossal duct Q89.2
- tonsil J35.8
  - – infected (chronic) J35.01

Removal (from) (of)
- device
  - – contraceptive Z30.432
    - ■ implantable subdermal Z30.46
- dressing (nonsurgical) Z48.00
  - – surgical Z48.01
- home in childhood (to foster home or institution) Z62.29
- staples Z48.02
- suture Z48.02

Rendu-Osler-Weber disease or syndrome I78.0

Renon-Delille syndrome E23.3

Replacement by artificial or mechanical device or prosthesis of
- heart Z95.812
  - – valve Z95.2
    - ■ prosthetic Z95.2
    - ■ specified NEC Z95.4
    - ■ xenogenic Z95.3
- organ replacement
  - – by artificial or mechanical device or prosthesis of
    - ■ heart Z95.812
      - ~ valve Z95.2

Request for expert evidence Z04.89

Residing
- in place not meant for human habitation (abandoned building) (car) (park) (sidewalk) (street) Z59.02

Residual—*see also* Disease, diseased
- urine R39.198

Resistance, resistant (to)
- insulin E88.81
- organism(s)
  - – to
    - ■ drug Z16.30
      - ~ aminoglycosides Z16.29
      - ~ amoxicillin Z16.11
      - ~ ampicillin Z16.11
      - ~ antibiotic(s) Z16.20
        - ◊ multiple Z16.24
        - ◊ specified NEC Z16.29
      - ~ antimicrobial (single) Z16.30
        - ◊ multiple Z16.35
        - ◊ specified NEC Z16.39
      - ~ beta lactam antibiotics Z16.10
        - ◊ specified NEC Z16.19
      - ~ cephalosporins Z16.19
      - ~ extended beta lactamase (ESBL) Z16.12
      - ~ macrolides Z16.29
      - ~ methicillin—*see* MRSA
      - ~ multiple drugs (MDRO)
        - ◊ antibiotics Z16.24
        - ◊ antimycobacterial (single) Z16.341
      - ~ penicillins Z16.11
      - ~ sulfonamides Z16.29
      - ~ tetracyclines Z16.29
      - ~ vancomycin Z16.21
        - ◊ related antibiotics Z16.22

Respiration
- Cheyne-Stokes R06.3
- decreased due to shock, following injury T79.4
- disorder of, psychogenic F45.8
- insufficient, or poor R06.89
  - – newborn P28.5
- painful R07.1
- sighing, psychogenic F45.8

Respiratory—*see also* Disease, diseased
- distress syndrome (newborn) (type I) P22.0
  - – type II P22.1
- syncytial virus (RSV), as cause of disease classified elsewhere B97

Restless legs (syndrome) G25.81

Rests, ovarian, in fallopian tube Q50.6

Retained—*see also* Retention
- foreign body fragments (type of) Z18.9
  - – acrylics Z18.2
  - – animal quill(s) or spines Z18.31
  - – cement Z18.83
  - – concrete Z18.83
  - – crystalline Z18.83
  - – diethylhexylphthalates Z18.2
  - – glass Z18.81
  - – isocyanate Z18.2
  - – magnetic metal Z18.11
  - – metal Z18.10
  - – nonmagnetic metal Z18.12
  - – organic NEC Z18.39
  - – plastic Z18.2
  - – quill(s) (animal) Z18.31
  - – specified NEC Z18.89
  - – spine(s) (animal) Z18.31
  - – stone Z18.83
  - – tooth (teeth) Z18.32
  - – wood Z18.33
- fragments (type of) Z18.9
  - – acrylics Z18.2
  - – animal quill(s) or spines Z18.31
  - – cement Z18.83
  - – concrete Z18.83
  - – crystalline Z18.83
  - – diethylhexylphthalates Z18.2
  - – glass Z18.81
  - – isocyanate Z18.2
  - – magnetic metal Z18.11
  - – metal Z18.10
  - – nonmagnetic metal Z18.12

Retained, *continued*
- organic NEC Z18.39
- plastic Z18.2
- quill(s) (animal) Z18.31
- specified NEC Z18.89
- spine(s) (animal) Z18.31
- stone Z18.83
- tooth (teeth) Z18.32
- wood Z18.33

Retardation
- development, developmental, specific—*see* Disorder, developmental
- growth R62.50
  - due to malnutrition E45
- mental—*see* Disability, intellectual
- motor function, specific F82
- physical (child) R62.52
  - due to malnutrition E45
- reading (specific) F81.0
- spelling (specific) (without reading disorder) F81.81

Retching—*see* Vomiting

Retention—*see also* Retained
- cyst—*see* Cyst
- dead
  - fetus (at or near term) (mother) O36.4
- deciduous tooth K00.6
- fetus
  - dead O36.4
- fluid R60.9
- foreign body
  - current trauma—*code as* Foreign body, by site or type
- menses N94.89
- urine R33.9
  - psychogenic F45.8

Reticulocytosis R70.1

Reticulohistiocytoma (giant-cell) D76.3

Reticulosis (skin)
- hemophagocytic, familial D76.1

Retina, retinal—*see also* Disease, diseased

Retinoblastoma C69.2-
- differentiated C69.2-
- undifferentiated C69.2-

Retinopathy (background) H35.00
- of prematurity H35.10-
  - stage 0 H35.11-
  - stage 1 H35.12-
  - stage 2 H35.13-
  - stage 3 H35.14-
  - stage 4 H35.15-
  - stage 5 H35.16-

Retractile testis Q55.22

Retraction
- nipple N64.53
  - associated with
  - congenital Q83.8

Retrograde menstruation N92.5

Retrosternal thyroid (congenital) Q89.2

Retroversion, retroverted
- testis (congenital) Q55.29

Rett's disease or syndrome F84.2

Rh (factor)
- hemolytic disease (newborn) P55.0
- incompatibility, immunization or sensitization
  - affecting management of pregnancy NEC O36.09-
    - anti-D antibody O36.01-
  - newborn P55.0
  - transfusion reaction—*see* Complication(s), transfusion, incompatibility reaction
- negative mother affecting newborn P55.0
- titer elevated—*see* Complication(s), transfusion, incompatibility reaction
- transfusion reaction—*see* Complication(s), transfusion, incompatibility reaction

Rhabdomyolysis (idiopathic) **NEC** M62.82

Rheumatic (acute) (subacute)
- chronic I09.89
- coronary arteritis I01.8

Rheumatic, *continued*
- fever (acute)—*see* Fever, rheumatic
- heart—*see* Disease, heart, rheumatic
- myocardial degeneration—*see* Degeneration, myocardium
- myocarditis (chronic) (inactive) (with chorea) I09.0
  - active or acute I01.2
  - with chorea (acute) (rheumatic) (Sydenham's) I02.0
- pancarditis, acute I01.8
  - with chorea (acute (rheumatic) Sydenham's) I02.0
- pericarditis (active) (acute) (with effusion) (with pneumonia) I01.0
  - with chorea (acute) (rheumatic) (Sydenham's) I02.0
  - chronic or inactive I09.2
- pneumonia I00 *[J17]*
- torticollis M43.6

Rheumatism (articular) (neuralgic) (nonarticular) M79.0
- intercostal, meaning Tietze's disease M94.0
- sciatic M54.4-

Rhinitis (atrophic) (catarrhal) (chronic) (croupous) (fibrinous) (granulomatous) (hyperplastic) (hypertrophic) (membranous) (obstructive) (purulent) (suppurative) (ulcerative) J31.0
- with
  - sore throat—*see* Nasopharyngitis
- acute J00
- allergic J30.9
  - with asthma J45.909
    - with
      - ~ exacerbation (acute) J45.901
      - ~ status asthmaticus J45.902
  - due to
    - food J30.5
    - pollen J30.1
  - nonseasonal J30.89
  - perennial J30.89
  - seasonal NEC J30.2
  - specified NEC J30.89
- infective J00
- pneumococcal J00
- vasomotor J30.0

Rhinoantritis (chronic)—*see* Sinusitis, maxillary

Rhinolith (nasal sinus) J34.89

Rhinomegaly J34.89

Rhinopharyngitis (acute) (subacute)—*see also* Nasopharyngitis

Rhinorrhea J34.89
- cerebrospinal (fluid) G96.01
  - postoperative G96.08
  - specified NEC G96.08
  - spontaneous G96.01
  - traumatic G96.08
- paroxysmal—*see* Rhinitis, allergic
- spasmodic—*see* Rhinitis, allergic

Rhinovirus infection NEC B34.8

Rhizomelic chondrodysplasia punctata E71.540

Rhythm
- disorder I49.9
- escape I49.9
- heart, abnormal I49.9
- idioventricular I44.2
- sleep, inversion G47.2-

Rhytidosis facialis L98.8

Rickets (active) (acute) (adolescent) (chest wall) (congenital) (current) (infantile) (intestinal) E55.0
- celiac K90.0
- hypophosphatemic with nephrotic-glycosuric dwarfism E72.09

Rickettsial disease A79.9
- specified type NEC A79.89

Rickettsialpox (rickettsia akari) A79.1

Rickettsiosis A79.9
- due to
  - Rickettsia akari (rickettsialpox) A79.1
- specified type NEC A79.89
- tick-borne A77.9
- vesicular A79.1

Riedel's
- struma, thyroiditis or disease E06.5

Riehl's melanosis L81.4

Rietti-Greppi-Micheli anemia D56.9

Rieux's hernia—*see* Hernia

Riga (-Fede) **disease** K14.0

Right middle lobe syndrome J98.11

Rigid, rigidity—*see also* Disease, diseased
- abdominal R19.30
  - with severe abdominal pain R10.0
- nuchal R29.1

Rigors R68.89
- with fever R50.9

Ringworm B35.9
- beard B35.0
- black dot B35.0
- body B35.4
- corporeal B35.4
- foot B35.3
- groin B35.6
- hand B35.2
- honeycomb B35.0
- nails B35.1
- perianal (area) B35.6
- scalp B35.0
- specified NEC B35.8

Risk
- for
  - dental caries Z91.849
    - high Z91.843
    - low Z91.841
    - moderate Z91.842
  - homelessness, imminent Z59.811
- suicidal
  - meaning personal history of attempted suicide Z91.51
  - meaning suicidal ideation—*see* Ideation, suicidal

Ritter's disease L00

Robert's pelvis Q74.2

Robin (-Pierre) syndrome Q87.0

Robinow-Silvermann-Smith syndrome Q87.19

Rocky Mountain (spotted) **fever** A77.0

Roger's disease Q21.0

Rolando's fracture (displaced) S62.22-
- nondisplaced S62.22-

Romano-Ward (prolonged QT interval) **syndrome** I45.81

Romberg's disease or syndrome G51.8

Roof, mouth—*see* Disease, diseased

Rosary, rachitic E55.0

Rose
- cold J30.1
- fever J30.1
- rash R21
  - epidemic B06.9

Rosenthal's disease or syndrome D68.1

Roseola B09
- infantum B08.20
  - due to human herpesvirus 6 B08.21
  - due to human herpesvirus 7 B08.22

Rossbach's disease K31.89
- psychogenic F45.8

Rothmund (-Thomson) **syndrome** Q82.8

Rotor's disease or syndrome E80.6

Round
- worms (large) (infestation) NEC B82.0
  - Ascariasis (*see also* Ascariasis) B77.9

Rubella (German measles) B06.9
- complication NEC B06.09
  - neurological B06.00
- congenital P35.0
- contact Z20.4
- exposure to Z20.4
- maternal
  - care for (suspected) damage to fetus O35.3
  - manifest rubella in infant P35.0
  - suspected damage to fetus affecting management of pregnancy O35.3
- specified complications NEC B06.89

Rubeola (meaning measles)—*see* Measles
- meaning rubella—*see* Rubella

Rudimentary (congenital)—*see also* Agenesis
- bone Q79.9

Ruled out condition—*see* Observation, suspected

Rumination R11.10
- with nausea R11.2
- disorder of infancy F98.21
- neurotic F42.8
- newborn P92.1
- obsessional F42.8
- psychogenic F42.8

Runny nose R09.89

Rupture, ruptured
- abscess (spontaneous)—*code by* site under Abscess
- aorta, aortic I71.8
  – valve or cusp (*see also* Endocarditis, aortic) I35.8
- appendix (with peritonitis) K35.32
  – with localized peritonitis K35.32
- arteriovenous fistula, brain I60.8-
- cardiac (auricle) (ventricle) (wall) I23.3
  – with hemopericardium I23.0
  – infectional I40.9
- cecum (with peritonitis) K65.0
  – with peritoneal abscess K35.33
- cerebral aneurysm (congenital) (*see* Hemorrhage, intra-cranial, subarachnoid)
- circle of Willis I60.6
- corpus luteum (infected) (ovary) N83.1-
- cyst—*see* Cyst
- ear drum (nontraumatic)—*see also* Perforation, tympanum
  – traumatic S09.2-
- fallopian tube NEC (nonobstetric) (nontraumatic) N83.8
  – due to pregnancy O00.10
- gastric
  – vessel K92.2
- graafian follicle (hematoma) N83.0-
- hymen (nontraumatic) (nonintentional) N89.8
- kidney (traumatic) birth injury P15.8
- meningeal artery I60.8-
- ovary, ovarian N83.8
  – corpus luteum cyst N83.1-
  – follicle (graafian) N83.0-
- oviduct (nonobstetric) (nontraumatic) N83.8
  – due to pregnancy O00.10
- pulmonary
  – valve (heart) I37.8
- rotator cuff (nontraumatic) M75.10-
  – complete M75.12-
  – incomplete M75.11-
- spleen (traumatic) S36.03-
  – birth injury P15.1
- tonsil J35.8
- traumatic
  – spleen S36.03-
- tricuspid (heart) (valve) I07.8
- tube, tubal (nonobstetric) (nontraumatic) N83.8
  – abscess—*see* Salpingitis
  – due to pregnancy O00.10
- tympanum, tympanic (membrane) (nontraumatic) (*see also* Perforation, tympanic membrane) H72.9-
  – traumatic—*see* Rupture, ear drum, traumatic
- viscus R19.8

Russell-Silver syndrome Q87.19

Ruvalcaba-Myhre-Smith syndrome E71.440

Rytand-Lipsitch syndrome I44.2

S

Saccharomyces infection B37.9

Sachs' amaurotic familial idiocy or disease E75.02

Sachs-Tay disease E75.02

Sacks-Libman disease M32.11

Sacralgia M53.3

Sacrodynia M53.3

Saint
- Anthony's fire—*see* Erysipelas

Salmonella—*see* Infection, Salmonella

Salmonellosis A02.0

Salpingitis (catarrhal) (fallopian tube) (nodular) (pseudofollicular) (purulent) (septic) N70.91
- with oophoritis N70.93
- acute N70.01
  – with oophoritis N70.03
- chlamydial A56.11
- chronic N70.11
  – with oophoritis N70.13
- gonococcal (acute) (chronic) A54.24
- specific (gonococcal) (acute) (chronic) A54.24
- venereal (gonococcal) (acute) (chronic) A54.24

Salpingo-oophoritis (catarrhal) (purulent) (ruptured) (septic) (suppurative) N70.93
- acute N70.03
  – gonococcal A54.24
- chronic N70.13
- gonococcal (acute) (chronic) A54.24
- specific (gonococcal) (acute) (chronic) A54.24
- venereal (gonococcal) (acute) (chronic) A54.24

Sandhoff's disease E75.01

Sanfilippo (Type B) (Type C) (Type D) syndrome E76.22

Sanger-Brown ataxia G11.2

Sao Paulo fever or typhus A77.0

Sarcoepiplocele—*see* Hernia

Sarcoepiplomphalocele Q79.2

Sarcoid—*see also* Sarcoidosis
- arthropathy D86.86
- Boeck's D86.9
- Darier-Roussy D86.3
- iridocyclitis D86.83
- meningitis D86.81
- myocarditis D86.85
- myositis D86.87
- pyelonephritis D86.84

Sarcoidosis D86.9
- with
  – cranial nerve palsies D86.82
  – hepatic granuloma D86.89
  – polyarthritis D86.86
  – tubulo-interstitial nephropathy D86.84
- combined sites NEC D86.89
- lung D86.0
  – and lymph nodes D86.2
- lymph nodes D86.1
  – and lung D86.2
- meninges D86.81
- skin D86.3
- specified type NEC D86.89

Sarcoma (of)—*see also* Neoplasm, connective tissue, malignant in Table of Neoplasms in the complete *ICD-10-CM* manual
- cerebellar C71.6
  – circumscribed (arachnoidal) C71.6
- circumscribed (arachnoidal) cerebellar C71.6
- clear cell—*see also* Neoplasm, connective tissue, malignant in Table of Neoplasms in the complete *ICD-10-CM* manual
  – kidney C64.-
- monstrocellular
  – specified site—*see* Neoplasm, malignant, by site in Table of Neoplasms in the complete *ICD-10-CM* manual
  – unspecified site C71.9

SARS-CoV-2—*see also* COVID-19
- sequelae (post acute) U09.9

SBE (subacute bacterial endocarditis) I33.0

Scabies (any site) B86

Scaglietti-Dagnini syndrome E22.0

Scald—*see* Burn

Scapulohumeral myopathy G71.02

Scar, scarring (*see also* Cicatrix) L90.5
- adherent L90.5
- atrophic L90.5
- cheloid L91.0
- hypertrophic L91.0
- keloid L91.0
- painful L90.5

Scar, scarring, *continued*
- vagina N89.8
  – postoperative N99.2
- vulva N90.89

Scarabiasis B88.2

Scarlatina (anginosa) (maligna) A38.9
- myocarditis (acute) A38.1
  – old—*see* Myocarditis
- otitis media A38.0
- ulcerosa A38.8

Scarlet fever (albuminuria) (angina) A38.9

Schaumann's
- benign lymphogranulomatosis D86.1
- disease or syndrome—*see* Sarcoidosis

Schistosomiasis B65.9
- cutaneous B65.3

Schizencephaly Q04.6

Schizophrenia, schizophrenic
- childhood type F84.5
- syndrome of childhood F84.5

Schlatter-Osgood disease or osteochondrosis M92.52-

Schlatter's tibia M92.52-

Schmorl's disease or nodes
- sacrococcygeal region M53.3

Schönlein (-Henoch) disease or purpura (primary) (rheumatic) D69.0

Schultze's type acroparesthesia, simple I73.89

Schwannomatosis Q85.03

Schwartz-Bartter syndrome E22.2

Sciatica (infective)
- with lumbago M54.4-

Scleredema
- newborn P83.0

Sclerema (adiposum) (edematosum) (neonatorum) (newborn) P83.0

Sclerocystic ovary syndrome E28.2

Scleroderma, sclerodermia (acrosclerotic) (diffuse) (generalized) (progressive) (pulmonary) (*see also* Sclerosis)
- newborn P83.88

Sclérose en plaques G35

Sclerosis, sclerotic
- ascending multiple G35
- brain (generalized) (lobular) G37.9
  – disseminated G35
  – insular G35
  – miliary G35
  – multiple G35
  – stem, multiple G35
  – tuberous Q85.1
- bulbar, multiple G35
- cerebrospinal (disseminated) (multiple) G35
- disseminated G35
- dorsal G35
- extrapyramidal G25.9
- Friedreich's (spinal cord) G11.11
- hereditary
  – spinal (Friedreich's ataxia) G11.11
- hippocampal G93.81
- insular G35
- mesial temporal G93.81
- mitral I05.8
- multiple (brain stem) (cerebral) (generalized) (spinal cord) G35
- plaques G35
- pulmonary
  – artery I27.0
- spinal (cord) (progressive) G95.89
  – hereditary (Friedreich's) (mixed form) G11.11
- temporal (mesial) G93.81
- tricuspid (heart) (valve) I07.8
- tuberous (brain) Q85.1

Scoliosis (acquired) (postural) M41.9
- adolescent (idiopathic)—*see* Scoliosis, idiopathic, juvenile
- congenital Q67.5
  – due to bony malformation Q76.3
- idiopathic M41.20

Scoliosis, *continued*
- adolescent M41.129
  - cervical region M41.122
  - cervicothoracic region M41.123
  - lumbar region M41.126
  - lumbosacral region M41.127
  - thoracic region M41.124
  - thoracolumbar region M41.125
- cervical region M41.22
- cervicothoracic region M41.23
- infantile M41.00
  - cervical region M41.02
  - cervicothoracic region M41.03
  - lumbar region M41.06
  - lumbosacral region M41.07
  - sacrococcygeal region M41.08
  - thoracic region M41.04
  - thoracolumbar region M41.05
- juvenile M41.119
  - cervical region M41.112
  - cervicothoracic region M41.113
  - lumbar region M41.116
  - lumbosacral region M41.117
  - thoracic region M41.114
  - thoracolumbar region M41.115
- lumbar M41.26
  - lumbosacral M41.27
  - thoracic M41.24
  - thoracolumbar M41.25
- sciatic M54.4-

Scratch—*see* Abrasion

Scratchy throat R09.89

Screening (for) Z13.9
- alcoholism Z13.89
- anemia Z13.0
- autism Z13.41
- behavioral disorders Z13.30
- cardiovascular disorder Z13.6
- chlamydial diseases Z11.8
- chromosomal abnormalities (nonprocreative) NEC Z13.79
- congenital
  - dislocation of hip Z13.89
  - eye disorder Z13.5
  - malformation or deformation Z13.89
- cystic fibrosis Z13.228
- depression (adult) (adolescent) (child) Z13.31
  - maternal or perinatal Z13.32
- developmental
  - delays Z13.40
    - global (milestones) Z13.42
    - specified NEC Z13.49
  - handicap Z13.42
    - in early childhood Z13.42
- diabetes mellitus Z13.1
- disability, intellectual Z13.39
  - infant Z13.41
- disease or disorder Z13.9
  - bacterial NEC Z11.2
    - intestinal infectious Z11.0
    - respiratory tuberculosis Z11.1
  - behavioral Z13.30
    - specified NEC Z13.49
  - blood or blood-forming organ Z13.0
  - cardiovascular Z13.6
  - chlamydial Z11.8
  - coronavirus (novel) 2019 Z11.52
  - dental Z13.89
  - developmental delays Z13.40
    - global (milestones) Z13.42
    - specified NEC Z13.49
  - endocrine Z13.29
  - heart Z13.6
  - human immunodeficiency virus (HIV) infection Z11.4
  - immunity Z13.0
  - infectious Z11.9
  - mental health and behavioral Z13.30
  - metabolic Z13.228
  - neurological Z13.89
  - nutritional Z13.21
    - metabolic Z13.228
      ~ lipoid disorders Z13.220
  - respiratory Z13.83

Screening, *continued*
- rheumatic Z13.828
- rickettsial Z11.8
- sexually-transmitted NEC Z11.3
  - human immunodeficiency virus (HIV) Z11.4
- sickle cell trait Z13.0
- spirochetal Z11.8
- thyroid Z13.29
- venereal Z11.3
- viral NEC Z11.59
  - human immunodeficiency virus (HIV) Z11.4
- elevated titer Z13.89
- galactosemia Z13.228
- gonorrhea Z11.3
- hematopoietic malignancy Z12.89
- hemoglobinopathies Z13.0
- Hodgkin disease Z12.89
- human immunodeficiency virus (HIV) Z11.4
- human papillomavirus (HPV) Z11.51
- hypertension Z13.6
- immunity disorders Z13.0
- infant or child (over 28 days old) Z00.12-
- infection
  - mycotic Z11.8
  - parasitic Z11.8
- intellectual disability Z13.39
- leukemia Z12.89
- lymphoma Z12.89
- malaria Z11.6
- measles Z11.59
- mental health disorder Z13.30
- metabolic errors, inborn Z13.228
- musculoskeletal disorder Z13.828
- mycoses Z11.8
- neoplasm (malignant) (of) Z12.9
  - blood Z12.89
  - breast Z12.39
    - routine mammogram Z12.31
  - cervix Z12.4
  - hematopoietic system Z12.89
  - lymph (glands) Z12.89
  - nervous system Z12.82
- nephropathy Z13.89
- nervous system disorders NEC Z13.858
- neurological condition Z13.89
- parasitic infestation Z11.9
  - specified NEC Z11.8
- phenylketonuria Z13.228
- poisoning (chemical) (heavy metal) Z13.88
- postnatal, chromosomal abnormalities Z13.89
- rheumatoid arthritis Z13.828
- sexually-transmitted disease NEC Z11.3
  - human immunodeficiency virus (HIV) Z11.4
- sickle-cell disease or trait Z13.0
- special Z13.9
  - specified NEC Z13.89
- syphilis Z11.3
- traumatic brain injury Z13.850
- tuberculosis, respiratory
  - active Z11.1
  - latent Z11.7
- venereal disease Z11.3
- viral encephalitis (mosquito- or tick-borne) Z11.59
- whooping cough Z11.2

Scrofula, scrofulosis (tuberculosis of cervical lymph glands) A18.2

Scurvy, scorbutic
- anemia D53.2
- rickets E55.0 *[M90.80]*

Seasickness T75.3

Seatworm (infection) (infestation) B80

Seborrhea, seborrheic L21.9
- capillitii R23.8
- capitis L21.0
- dermatitis L21.9
  - infantile L21.1
- eczema L21.9
  - infantile L21.1
- sicca L21.0

Seckel's syndrome Q87.19

Second hand tobacco smoke exposure (acute) (chronic) Z77.22
- in the perinatal period P96.81

Secretion
- antidiuretic hormone, inappropriate E22.2
- hormone
  - antidiuretic, inappropriate (syndrome) E22.2
- urinary
  - excessive R35.89
  - suppression R34

Seitelberger's syndrome (infantile neuraxonal dystrophy) G31.89

Seizure(s) (*see also* Convulsions) R56.9
- akinetic—*see* Epilepsy, generalized, specified NEC
- atonic—*see* Epilepsy, generalized, specified NEC
- convulsive—*see* Convulsions
- disorder (*see also* Epilepsy) G40.909
- epileptic—*see* Epilepsy
- febrile (simple) R56.00
  - with status epilepticus G40.901
  - complex (atypical) (complicated) R56.01
    - with status epilepticus G40.901
- newborn P90
- nonspecific epileptic
  - atonic—*see* Epilepsy, generalized, specified NEC
  - clonic—*see* Epilepsy, generalized, specified NEC
  - myoclonic—*see* Epilepsy, generalized, specified NEC
  - tonic—*see* Epilepsy, generalized, specified NEC
  - tonic-clonic—*see* Epilepsy, generalized, specified NEC
- partial, developing into secondarily generalized seizures
  - complex—*see* Epilepsy, localization-related, symptomatic, with complex partial seizures
  - simple—*see* Epilepsy, localization-related, symptomatic
- petit mal G40.A-
  - intractable G40.A1-
    - with status epilepticus G40.A11
    - without status epilepticus G40.A19
  - not intractable G40.A0-
    - with status epilepticus G40.A01
    - without status epilepticus G40.A09
- post traumatic R56.1
- recurrent G40.909
- specified NEC G40.89

Self-damaging behavior (life-style) Z72.89

Self-harm (attempted)
- history (personal)
  - in family Z81.8
  - nonsuicidal Z91.52
  - suicidal Z91.51
- nonsuicidal R45.88

Self-injury, nonsuicidal R45.88
- personal history Z91.52

Self-mutilation (attempted)
- history (personal)
  - in family Z81.8
  - nonsuicidal Z91.52
  - suicidal Z91.51
- nonsuicidal R45.88

Self-poisoning
- history (personal) Z91.51
  - in family Z81.8
- observation following (alleged) attempt Z03.6

Semicoma R40.1

Sensitive, sensitivity—*see also* Allergy
- child (excessive) F93.8
- cold, autoimmune D59.12
- dentin K03.89
- gluten (non-celiac) K90.41
- methemoglobin D74.8
- tuberculin, without clinical or radiological symptoms R76.11

Sensitization, auto-erythrocytic D69.2

Separation
- anxiety, abnormal (of childhood) F93.0
- apophysis, traumatic—*code as* Fracture, by site
- epiphysis, epiphyseal

Separation, *continued*
- – nontraumatic—*see also* Osteochondropathy
  - ▪ upper femoral—*see* Slipped, epiphysis, upper femoral
- – traumatic—*code as* Fracture, by site

Sepsis (generalize) (unspecified organism) A41.9
- • with
  - – organ dysfunction (acute) (multiple) R65.20
    - ▪ with septic shock R65.21
- • anaerobic A41.4
- • candidal B37.7
- • cryptogenic A41.9
- • due to device, implant or graft T85.79
  - – catheter NEC T85.79
    - ▪ dialysis (renal) T82.7
    - ▪ infusion NEC T82.7
    - ▪ urethral indwelling T83.511
    - ▪ urinary T83.518
  - – vascular T82.7
- • Enterococcus A41.81
- • Escherichia coli (E. coli) A41.51
- • following
  - – immunization T88.0
  - – infusion, therapeutic injection or transfusion NEC T80.29
- • gangrenous A41.9
- • Gram-negative (organism) A41.5-
  - – anaerobic A41.4
- • Haemophilus influenzae A41.3
- • localized—code to specific localized infection
  - – in operation wound T81.49
  - – postprocedural T81.44
- • meningeal—*see* Meningitis
- • meningococcal A39.4
  - – acute A39.2
  - – chronic A39.3
- • MSSA (Methicillin susceptible Staphylococcus aureus) A41.01
- • newborn P36.9
  - – due to
    - ▪ anaerobes NEC P36.5
    - ▪ Escherichia coli P36.4
    - ▪ Staphylococcus P36.30
      - ~ aureus P36.2
      - ~ specified NEC P36.39
    - ▪ Streptococcus P36.10
      - ~ group B P36.0
      - ~ specified NEC P36.19
  - – specified NEC P36.8
- • Pasteurella multocida A28.0
- • pneumococcal A40.3
- • severe R65.20
  - – with septic shock R65.21
- • Shigella (*see also* Dysentery, bacillary) A03.9
- • skin, localized—*see* Abscess
- • specified organism NEC A41.89
- • Staphylococcus, staphylococcal A41.2
  - – aureus (methicillin susceptible) (MSSA) A41.01
    - ▪ methicillin resistant (MRSA) A41.02
  - – coagulase-negative A41.1
  - – specified NEC A41.1
- • Streptococcus, streptococcal A40.9
  - – group
    - ▪ D A41.81
  - – neonatal P36.10
    - ▪ group B P36.0
    - ▪ specified NEC P36.19
  - – pneumoniae A40.3

Septic—*see* Disease, diseased
- • gallbladder (acute) K81.0
- • sore—*see also* Abscess
  - – throat J02.0
    - ▪ streptococcal J02.0
- • tonsils, chronic J35.01
  - – with adenoiditis J35.03

Septicemia A41.9
- • meaning sepsis—*see* Sepsis

Septum, septate (congenital)—*see also* Anomaly, by site
- • anal Q42.3
  - – with fistula Q42.2
- • aqueduct of Sylvius Q03.0

Septum, septate, *continued*
- – with spina bifida—*see* Spina bifida, by site, with hydrocephalus
- • uterus Q51.2-
- • vaginal, longitudinal Q52.129
  - – microperforate
    - ▪ left side Q52.124
    - ▪ right side Q52.123
  - – nonobstructing Q52.120
  - – obstructing
    - ▪ left side Q52.122
    - ▪ right side Q52.121

Sequelae (of)—*see also* Disease, diseased
- • COVID-19 (post acute) U09.9
- • encephalitis or encephalomyelitis (conditions in G04) G09
  - – in infectious disease NEC B94.8
  - – viral B94.1
- • hepatitis, viral B94.2
- • infectious disease B94.9
  - – specified NEC B94.8
- • parasitic disease B94.9
- • SARS-CoV-2 (post acute) U09.9
- • viral
  - – encephalitis B94.1
  - – hepatitis B94.2

Serology for syphilis
- • doubtful
  - – with signs or symptoms—*code by* site and stage under Syphilis
- • reactivated A53.0
- • positive A53.0

Serositis, multiple K65.8
- • pericardial I31.1

Serum
- • allergy, allergic reaction (*see also* Reaction, serum) T80.69
  - – shock (*see also* Shock, anaphylactic) T80.59
- • arthritis (*see also* Reaction, serum) T80.69
- • complication or reaction NEC (*see also* Reaction, serum) T80.69
- • disease NEC (*see also* Reaction, serum) T80.69
- • hepatitis—*see also* Hepatitis, viral, type B
  - – carrier (suspected) of B18.1
- • intoxication (*see also* Reaction, serum) T80.69
- • neuritis (*see also* Reaction, serum) T80.69
- • poisoning NEC (*see also* Reaction, serum) T80.69
- • rash NEC (*see also* Reaction, serum) T80.69
- • reaction NEC (*see also* Reaction, serum) T80.69
- • sickness NEC (*see also* Reaction, serum) T80.69
- • urticaria (*see also* Reaction, serum) T80.69

Severe sepsis R65.20
- • with septic shock R65.21

Sexual
- • immaturity (female) (male) E30.0
- • precocity (constitutional) (cryptogenic) (female) (idiopathic) (male) E30.1

Shadow lung R91.8

Shedding
- • nail L60.8
- • premature, primary (deciduous) teeth K00.6

Sheehan's disease or syndrome E23.0

Shelf, rectal K62.89

Shellshock (current) F43.0
- • lasting state—*see* Disorder, post-traumatic stress

Shigellosis A03.9
- • Group A A03.0
- • Group B A03.1
- • Group C A03.2
- • Group D A03.3

Shock R57.9
- • adverse food reaction (anaphylactic)—*see* Shock, anaphylactic, due to food
- • allergic—*see* Shock, anaphylactic
- • anaphylactic T78.2
  - – chemical—*see* Table of Drugs and Chemicals
  - – due to drug or medicinal substance
    - ▪ correct substance properly administered T88.6-

Shock, *continued*
- ▪ overdose or wrong substance given or taken (by accident)—*see* Table of Drugs and Chemicals, by drug, poisoning
- – due to food (nonpoisonous) T78.00
  - ▪ additives T78.06
  - ▪ dairy products T78.07
  - ▪ eggs T78.08
  - ▪ fish T78.03
    - ~ shellfish T78.02
  - ▪ fruit T78.04
  - ▪ milk T78.07
  - ▪ nuts T78.05
    - ~ peanuts T78.01
  - ▪ peanuts T78.01
  - ▪ seeds T78.05
  - ▪ specified type NEC T78.09
  - ▪ vegetable T78.04
- – following sting(s)—*see* Table of Drugs and Chemicals, by animal or substance, poisoning
- – immunization T80.52-
- – serum T80.59-
  - ▪ blood and blood products T80.51-
  - ▪ immunization T80.52-
  - ▪ specified NEC T80.59-
  - ▪ vaccination T80.52-
- • anaphylactoid—*see* Shock, anaphylactic
- • cardiogenic R57.0
- • chemical substance—*see* Table of Drugs and Chemicals
- • culture—*see* Disorder, adjustment
- • drug
  - – due to correct substance properly administered T88.6
  - – overdose or wrong substance given or taken (by accident)—*see* Table of Drugs and Chemicals, by drug, poisoning
- • electric T75.4
  - – (taser) T75.4
- • endotoxic R65.21
  - – postprocedural (during or resulting from a procedure, not elsewhere classified) T81.12-
- • following
  - – injury (immediate) (delayed) T79.4
- • food (anaphylactic)—*see* Shock, anaphylactic, due to food
- • from electroshock gun (taser) T75.4
- • gram-negative R65.21
  - – postprocedural (during or resulting from a procedure, NEC) T81.12
- • hematologic R57.8
- • hemorrhagic R57.8
  - – surgery (intraoperative) (postoperative) T81.19
  - – trauma T79.4
- • hypovolemic R57.1
  - – surgical T81.19
  - – traumatic T79.4
- • insulin E15
  - – therapeutic misadventure—*see* subcategory T38.3
- • kidney N17.0
- • lung J80
- • pleural (surgical) T81.19
  - – due to trauma T79.4
- • postprocedural (postoperative) T81.10
  - – cardiogenic T81.11
  - – endotoxic T81.12-
  - – gram-negative T81.12-
  - – hypovolemic T81.19
  - – septic T81.12-
  - – specified type NEC T81.19
- • psychic F43.0
- • septic (due to severe sepsis) R65.21
- • specified NEC R57.8
- • surgical T81.10
- • taser gun (taser) T75.4
- • therapeutic misadventure NEC T81.10
- • toxic, syndrome A48.3
- • transfusion—*see* Complications, transfusion
- • traumatic (immediate) (delayed) T79.4

Short, shortening, shortness
- • arm (acquired)—*see also* Deformity, limb length
  - – congenital Q71.81-
- • breath R06.02
- • bowel syndrome K91.2
- • common bile duct, congenital Q44.5

Short, shortening, shortness, *continued*
- cystic duct, congenital Q44.5
- frenum, frenulum, linguae (congenital) Q38.1
- hip (acquired)—*see also* Deformity, limb
  - congenital Q65.89
- leg (acquired)—*see also* Deformity, limb
  - congenital Q72.81-
- lower limb (acquired)—*see also* Deformity, limb
  - congenital Q72.81-
- rib syndrome Q77.2
- stature (child) (hereditary) (idiopathic) NEC R62.52
  - constitutional E34.3
  - due to endocrine disorder E34.3
  - Laron-type E34.3
- tendon—*see also* Contraction
  - with contracture of joint—*see* Contraction, joint
  - Achilles (acquired) M67.0-
    - congenital Q66.89
  - congenital Q79.8

Shunt
- arterial-venous (dialysis) Z99.2
- arteriovenous, pulmonary (acquired) I28.0
  - congenital Q25.72
- cerebral ventricle (communicating) in situ Z98.2

Sialitis, silitis (any gland) (chronic) (suppurative)—*see* Sialoadenitis

Sialoadenitis (any gland) (periodic) (suppurative) K11.20
- acute K11.21
  - recurrent K11.22
- chronic K11.23

Sialidosis E77.1

Sibling rivalry Z62.891

Sicard's syndrome G52.7

Sick R69
- or handicapped person in family Z63.79
  - needing care at home Z63.6
- sinus (syndrome) I49.5

Sickle-cell
- anemia—*see* Disease, sickle-cell
- beta plus—*see* Disease, sickle-cell, thalassemia, beta plus
- beta zero—*see* Disease, sickle-cell, thalassemia, beta zero
- trait D57.3

Sicklemia—*see also* Disease, sickle-cell
- trait D57.3

Sickness
- air (travel) T75.3
- airplane T75.3
- car T75.3
- green D50.8
- milk—*see* Poisoning, food, noxious
- motion T75.3
- mountain T70.29
  - acute D75.1
- protein (*see also* Reaction, serum) T80.69
- roundabout (motion) T75.3
- sea T75.3
- serum NEC (*see also* Reaction, serum) T80.69
- swing (motion) T75.3
- train (railway) (travel) T75.3
- travel (any vehicle) T75.3

Siemens' syndrome (ectodermal dysplasia) Q82.8

Sighing R06.89
- psychogenic F45.8

Sigmoiditis (*see also* Enteritis) K52.9
- infectious A09
- noninfectious K52.9

Silver's syndrome Q87.19

Simple, simplex—*see* Disease, diseased

Simulation, conscious (of illness) Z76.5

Single
- atrium Q21.2
- umbilical artery Q27.0

Sinus—*see also* Fistula
- bradycardia R00.1
- dermal (congenital) Q06.8
  - with abscess Q06.8

Sinus, *continued*
- pilonidal (infected) (rectum) L05.92
  - with abscess L05.02
- preauricular Q18.1
- tachycardia R00.0
  - paroxysmal I47.1
- tarsi syndrome—M25.57-

Sinusitis (accessory) (chronic) (hyperplastic) (nasal) (nonpurulent) (purulent) J32.9
- acute J01.90
  - ethmoidal J01.20
    - recurrent J01.21
  - frontal J01.10
    - recurrent J01.11
  - involving more than one sinus, other than pansinusitis J01.80
    - recurrent J01.81
  - maxillary J01.00
    - recurrent J01.01
  - pansinusitis J01.40
    - recurrent J01.41
  - recurrent J01.91
  - specified NEC J01.80
    - recurrent J01.81
  - sphenoidal J01.30
    - recurrent J01.31
- allergic—*see* Rhinitis, allergic
- ethmoidal J32.2
  - acute J01.20
    - recurrent J01.21
- frontal J32.1
  - acute J01.10
    - recurrent J01.11
- influenzal—*see* Influenza, with, respiratory manifestations NEC
- involving more than one sinus but not pansinusitis J32.8
  - acute J01.80
    - recurrent J01.81
- maxillary J32.0
  - acute J01.00
    - recurrent J01.01
- sphenoidal J32.3
  - acute J01.30
    - recurrent J01.31

Sinusitis-bronchiectasis-situs inversus (syndrome) (triad) Q89.3

Siriasis T67.01

Situation, psychiatric F99

Situational
- disturbance (transient)—*see* Disorder, adjustment
  - acute F43.0
- maladjustment—*see* Disorder, adjustment
- reaction—*see* Disorder, adjustment
  - acute F43.0

Situs inversus or transversus (abdominalis) (thoracis) Q89.3

Sixth disease B08.20
- due to human herpesvirus 6 B08.21
- due to human herpesvirus 7 B08.22

Sjögren-Larsson syndrome Q87.19

Skin—*see also* Disease, diseased
- clammy R23.1
- dry L85.3

Sleep
- disorder or disturbance G47.9
  - child F51.9
  - nonorganic origin F51.9
  - specified NEC G47.8
- disturbance G47.9
  - nonorganic origin F51.9
- drunkenness F51.9
- rhythm inversion G47.2-
- terrors F51.4
- walking F51.3
  - hysterical F44.89

Sleep-wake schedule disorder G47.20

Slim disease (in HIV infection) B20

Slipped, slipping
- epiphysis (traumatic)—*see also* Osteochondropathy
  - capital femoral (traumatic)

Slipped, slipping, *continued*
- acute (on chronic) S79.01-
  - current traumatic—*code as* Fracture, by site
  - upper femoral (nontraumatic) M93.00-
    - acute M93.01-
      - ~ on chronic M93.03-
    - chronic M93.02-
- ligature, umbilical P51.8

Slow
- feeding, newborn P92.2
- heart (beat) R00.1

Slowing, urinary stream R39.198

Small(ness)
- for gestational age—*see* Small for dates
- introitus, vagina N89.6
- kidney (unknown cause)
  - bilateral N27.1
  - unilateral N27.0
- ovary (congenital) Q50.39
- uterus N85.8
- white kidney N03.9

Small-and-light-for-dates—*see* Small for dates

Small-for-dates (infant) P05.10
- with weight of
  - 499 grams or less P05.11
  - 500–749 grams P05.12
  - 750–999 grams P05.13
  - 1000–1249 grams P05.14
  - 1250–1499 grams P05.15
  - 1500–1749 grams P05.16
  - 1750–1999 grams P05.17
  - 2000–2499 grams P05.18
  - 2500 grams and over P05.19

Smearing, fecal R15.1

SMEI (severe myoclonic epilepsy in infancy) G40.83-

Smith's fracture S52.54-

Smoker—*see* Dependence, drug, nicotine

Smoking
- passive Z77.22

Smothering spells R06.81

Sneezing (intractable) R06.7

Sniffing
- cocaine
  - abuse—*see* Abuse, drug, cocaine
  - dependence—*see* Dependence, drug, cocaine
- gasoline
  - abuse—*see* Abuse, drug, inhalant
  - dependence—*see* Dependence, drug, inhalant
- glue (airplane)
  - abuse—*see* Abuse, drug, inhalant
  - drug dependence—*see* Dependence, drug, inhalant

Sniffles
- newborn P28.89

Snoring R06.83

Snuffles (non-syphilitic) R06.5
- newborn P28.89

Social
- exclusion Z60.4
- migrant Z59.0
  - acculturation difficulty Z60.3
- skills inadequacy NEC Z73.4
- transplantation Z60.3

Sodoku A25.0

Softening
- brain (necrotic) (progressive) G93.89
  - congenital Q04.8
- cartilage M94.2-
  - patella M22.4-

Soldier's
- heart F45.8
- patches I31.0

Solitary
- cyst, kidney N28.1
- kidney, congenital Q60.0

Soor B37.0

Sore
- mouth K13.79
  - canker K12.0
- muscle M79.10
- skin L98.9
- throat (acute)—*see also* Pharyngitis
  - with influenza, flu, or grippe—*see* Influenza, with, respiratory manifestations NEC
  - chronic J31.2
  - coxsackie (virus) B08.5
  - herpesviral B00.2
  - influenzal—*see* Influenza, with, respiratory manifestations NEC
  - septic J02.0
  - streptococcal (ulcerative) J02.0
  - viral NEC J02.8
    - coxsackie B08.5

Soto's syndrome (cerebral gigantism) Q87.3

Spading nail L60.8
- congenital Q84.6

Spanish collar N47.1

Spasm(s), spastic, spasticity (*see also* Disease, diseased) R25.2
- artery I73.9
  - cerebral G45.9
- anus, ani (sphincter) (reflex) K59.4
  - psychogenic F45.8
- bladder (sphincter, external or internal) N32.89
  - psychogenic F45.8
- bronchus, bronchiole J98.01
- cerebral (arteries) (vascular) G45.9
- colon K58.9
  - with constipation K58.1
  - with diarrhea K58.0
  - mixed K58.2
  - other K58.8
  - psychogenic F45.8
- diaphragm (reflex) R06.6
  - psychogenic F45.8
- esophagus (diffuse) K22.4
  - psychogenic F45.8
- gastrointestinal (tract) K31.89
  - psychogenic F45.8
- glottis J38.5
  - hysterical F44.4
  - psychogenic F45.8
    - conversion reaction F44.4
  - reflex through recurrent laryngeal nerve J38.5
- habit—*see* Tic
- hysterical F44.4
- intestinal (*see also* Syndrome, irritable, bowel) K58.9
  - psychogenic F45.8
- larynx, laryngeal J38.5
  - hysterical F44.4
  - psychogenic F45.8
    - conversion reaction F44.4
- muscle NEC M62.838
  - back M62.830
- nerve, trigeminal G51.0
- nervous F45.8
- nodding F98.4
- oculogyric H51.8
  - psychogenic F45.8
- perineal, female N94.89
- pharynx (reflex) J39.2
  - hysterical F45.8
  - psychogenic F45.8
- psychogenic F45.8
- pylorus NEC K31.3
  - congenital or infantile Q40.0
  - psychogenic F45.8
- rectum (sphincter) K59.4
  - psychogenic F45.8
- sigmoid (*see also* Syndrome, irritable, bowel) K58.9
  - psychogenic F45.8
- stomach K31.89
  - neurotic F45.8
- throat J39.2
  - hysterical F45.8
  - psychogenic F45.8

Spasm(s), spastic, spasticity, *continued*
- tic F95.9
  - chronic F95.1
  - transient of childhood F95.0
- urethra (sphincter) N35.919

Spasmodic—*see* Disease, diseased

Spasmus nutans F98.4

Spastic, spasticity—*see also* Spasm
- child (cerebral) (congenital) (paralysis) G80.1

Specific, specified—*see* Disease, diseased

Speech
- defect, disorder, disturbance, impediment R47.9
  - psychogenic, in childhood and adolescence F98.8
  - slurring R47.81
  - specified NEC R47.89

Spens' syndrome (syncope with heart block) I45.9

Spermatocele N43.40
- congenital Q55.4
- multiple N43.42
- single N43.41

Sphericity, increased, lens (congenital) Q12.4

Spherocytosis (congenital) (familial) (hereditary) D58.0
- hemoglobin disease D58.0
- sickle-cell (disease) D57.8-

Spherophakia Q12.4

Spider
- bite—*see* Table of Drugs and Chemicals, by animal or substance, poisoning
- fingers—*see* Syndrome, Marfan's
- nevus I78.1
- toes—*see* Syndrome, Marfan's
- vascular I78.1

Spiegler-Fendt
- benign lymphocytoma L98.8

Spina bifida (aperta) Q05.9
- with hydrocephalus NEC Q05.4
- cervical Q05.5
  - with hydrocephalus Q05.0
- dorsal Q05.6
  - with hydrocephalus Q05.1
- lumbar Q05.7
  - with hydrocephalus Q05.2
- lumbosacral Q05.7
  - with hydrocephalus Q05.2
- occulta Q76.0
- sacral Q05.8
  - with hydrocephalus Q05.3
- thoracic Q05.6
  - with hydrocephalus Q05.1
- thoracolumbar Q05.6
  - with hydrocephalus Q05.1

Spirillosis A25.0

Splenitis (interstitial) (malignant) (nonspecific) D73.89
- malarial (*see also* Malaria) B54 *[D77]*
- tuberculous A18.85

Splenomegaly, splenomegalia (Bengal) (cryptogenic) (idiopathic) (tropical) R16.1
- with hepatomegaly R16.2
- malarial (*see also* Malaria) B54 *[D77]*
- neutropenic D73.81

Spondylolisthesis (acquired) (degenerative) M43.1-
- congenital Q76.2

Spondylolysis (acquired) M43.0-
- congenital Q76.2

Spongioblastoma (any type)—*see* Neoplasm, malignant, by site in Table of Neoplasms in the complete *ICD-10-CM* manual
- specified site—*see* Neoplasm, malignant, by site in Table of Neoplasms in the complete *ICD-10-CM* manual
- unspecified site C71.9

Spongioneuroblastoma—*see* Neoplasm, malignant, by site in Table of Neoplasms in the complete *ICD-10-CM* manual

Sporadic—*see* Disease, diseased

Spots, spotting (in) (of)
- café au lait L81.3
- Cayenne pepper I78.1
- de Morgan's (senile angiomas) I78.1

Spots, spotting, *continued*
- intermenstrual (regular) N92.0
  - irregular N92.1
- liver L81.4
- purpuric R23.3
- ruby I78.1

Sprain (joint) (ligament)
- ankle S93.40-
  - calcaneofibular ligament S93.41-
  - deltoid ligament S93.42-
  - internal collateral ligament S93.49-
  - specified ligament NEC S93.49-
  - talofibular ligament S93.49-
  - tibiofibular ligament S93.43-
- anterior longitudinal, cervical S13.4
- atlas, atlanto-axial, atlanto-occipital S13.4
- cervical, cervicodorsal, cervicothoracic S13.4
- elbow S53.40-
  - radial collateral ligament S53.43-
  - radiohumeral S53.41-
  - specified type NEC S53.49-
  - ulnar collateral ligament S53.44-
  - ulnohumeral S53.42-
- finger(s) S63.61-
  - index S63.61-
  - interphalangeal (joint) S63.63-
    - index S63.63-
    - little S63.63-
    - middle S63.63-
    - ring S63.63-
  - little S63.61-
  - middle S63.61-
  - ring S63.61-
  - metacarpophalangeal (joint) S63.65-
  - specified site NEC S63.69-
    - index S63.69-
    - little S63.69-
    - middle S63.69-
    - ring S63.69-
- foot S93.60-
  - specified ligament NEC S93.69-
  - tarsal ligament S93.61-
  - tarsometatarsal ligament S93.62-
- hand S63.9-
  - specified site NEC—*see* subcategory S63.8
- innominate
  - sacral junction S33.6
- jaw (articular disc) (cartilage) (meniscus) S03.4-
  - old M26.69
- knee S83.9-
  - collateral ligament S83.40-
    - lateral (fibular) S83.42-
    - medial (tibial) S83.41-
  - cruciate ligament S83.50-
    - anterior S83.51-
    - posterior S83.52-
- lumbar (spine) S33.5
- lumbosacral S33.9
- mandible (articular disc) S03.4-
  - old M26.69
- meniscus
  - jaw S03.4-
    - old M26.69
  - mandible S03.4
    - old M26.69
- neck S13.9
  - anterior longitudinal cervical ligament S13.4
  - atlanto-axial joint S13.4
  - atlanto-occipital joint S13.4
  - cervical spine S13.4
- pelvis NEC S33.8
- rotator cuff (capsule) S43.42-
- sacroiliac (region)
  - joint S33.6
- spine
  - cervical S13.4
  - lumbar S33.5
- symphysis
  - jaw S03.4-
    - old M26.69
  - mandibular S03.4-
    - old M26.69

Sprain (joint) (ligament), *continued*
- talofibular S93.49-
- tarsal—*see* Sprain, foot, specified site NEC
- tarsometatarsal—*see* Sprain, foot, specified site NEC
- temporomandibular S03.4-
  - old M26.69
- thumb S63.60-
  - interphalangeal (joint) S63.62-
  - metacarpophalangeal (joint) S63.64-
  - specified site NEC S63.68-
- toe(s) S93.50-
  - great S93.50-
  - interphalangeal joint S93.51-
    - great S93.51-
    - lesser S93.51-
  - lesser S93.50-
  - metatarsophalangeal joint S93.52-
    - great S93.52-
    - lesser S93.52-
- wrist S63.50-
  - carpal S63.51-
  - radiocarpal S63.52-
  - specified site NEC S63.59-

Sprengel's deformity (congenital) Q74.0

Sprue (tropical) K90.1
- celiac K90.0
- idiopathic K90.49
- meaning thrush B37.0
- nontropical K90.0

Spur, bone—*see also* Enthesopathy
- iliac crest M76.2-
- nose (septum) J34.89

Spurway's syndrome Q78.0

Sputum
- abnormal (amount) (color) (odor) (purulent) R09.3
- blood-stained R04.2
- excessive (cause unknown) R09.3

Squashed nose M95.0
- congenital Q67.4

SSADHD (succinic semialdehyde dehydrogenase deficiency) E72.81

St. Hubert's disease A82.9

Staggering gait R26.0
- hysterical F44.4

Stain, staining
- meconium (newborn) P96.83
- port wine Q82.5

Stammering (*see also* Disorder, fluency) F80.81

Staphylitis (acute) (catarrhal) (chronic) (gangrenous) (membranous) (suppurative) (ulcerative) K12.2

Staphylococcal scalded skin syndrome L00

Staphylococcemia A41.2

Staphylococcus, staphylococcal—*see also* Disease, diseased
- as cause of disease classified elsewhere B95.8
  - aureus (methicillin susceptible) (MSSA) B95.61
    - methicillin resistant (MRSA) B95.62
- specified NEC, as the cause of disease classified elsewhere B95.7

Stasis
- renal N19
  - tubular N17.0

State (of)
- agitated R45.1
  - acute reaction to stress F43.0
- compulsive F42.8
  - mixed with obsessional thoughts F42.2
- crisis F43.0
- depressive F32.A
- dissociative F44.9
- neurotic F48.9
- obsessional F42.8
- panic F41.0
- persistent vegetative R40.3
- phobic F40.9
- pregnant, incidental Z33.1
- tension (mental) F48.9
  - specified NEC F48.8

State (of), *continued*
- vegetative, persistent R40.3
- withdrawal—*see* Withdrawal state

Status (post)—*see also* Presence (of)
- absence, epileptic—*see* Epilepsy, by type, with status epilepticus
- asthmaticus—*see* Asthma, by type, with, status asthmaticus
- awaiting organ transplant Z76.82
- colectomy (complete) (partial) Z90.49
- colonization—*see* Carrier (suspected) of
- delinquent immunization Z28.3
- dialysis (hemodialysis) (peritoneal) Z99.2
- do not resuscitate (DNR) Z66
- epileptic, epilepticus (*see also* Epilepsy, by type, with status epilepticus) G40.901
- gastrostomy Z93.1
- human immunodeficiency virus (HIV) infection, asymptomatic Z21
- lapsed immunization schedule Z28.3
- nephrectomy (unilateral) (bilateral) Z90.5
- pacemaker
  - cardiac Z95.0
- physical restraint Z78.1
- postcommotio cerebri F07.81
- postoperative (postprocedural) NEC Z98.890
- postsurgical (postprocedural) NEC Z98.890
- pregnant, incidental Z33.1
- renal dialysis (hemodialysis) (peritoneal) Z99.2
- retained foreign body—*see* Retained, foreign body fragments (type of)
- shunt
  - arteriovenous (for dialysis) Z99.2
  - cerebrospinal fluid Z98.2
- transplant—*see* Transplant
  - organ removed Z98.85
- underimmunization Z28.3
  - ventricular (communicating) (for drainage) Z98.2

Stealing
- child problem F91.8
  - in company with others Z72.810

Steam burn—*see* Burn

Steatoma L72.3
- eyelid (cystic)—*see* Dermatitis
- infected—*see* Hordeolum

Steatorrhea (chronic) K90.49
- idiopathic (adult) (infantile) K90.9
- primary K90.0

Stein-Leventhal syndrome E28.2

Stein's syndrome E28.2

Stenocephaly Q75.8

Stenosis, stenotic (cicatricial)—*see also* Stricture
- anus, anal (canal) (sphincter) K62.4
  - and rectum K62.4
  - congenital Q42.3
    - with fistula Q42.2
- aorta (ascending) (supraventricular) (congenital) Q25.1
- aortic (valve) I35.0
  - with insufficiency I35.2
  - congenital Q23.0
  - rheumatic I06.0
    - with
      - ~ incompetency, insufficiency or regurgitation I06.2
        - ◊ with mitral (valve) disease I08.0
          - » with tricuspid (valve) disease I08.3
      - ~ mitral (valve) disease I08.0
        - ◊ with tricuspid (valve) disease I08.3
      - ~ tricuspid (valve) disease I08.2
        - ◊ with mitral (valve) disease I08.3
  - specified cause NEC I35.0
- aqueduct of Sylvius (congenital) Q03.0
  - with spina bifida—*see* Spina bifida, by site, with hydrocephalus
  - acquired G91.1
- bile duct (common) (hepatic) K83.1
  - congenital Q44.3
- brain G93.89
- colon—*see also* Obstruction, intestine
  - congenital Q42.9
    - specified NEC Q42.8

Stenosis, stenotic, *continued*
- common (bile) duct K83.1
  - congenital Q44.3
- heart valve (see also endocarditis) I38
  - congenital Q24.8
    - pulmonary Q22.1
    - tricuspid Q22.4
- hypertrophic subaortic (idiopathic) I42.1
- intestine—*see also* Obstruction, intestine
  - congenital (small) Q41.9
    - large Q42.9
      - ~ specified NEC Q42.8
    - specified NEC Q41.8
- lacrimal (passage)
  - congenital Q10.5
  - duct H04.55-
  - sac H04.57-
- lacrimonasal duct—*see* Stenosis, lacrimal, duct
  - congenital Q10.5
- mitral (chronic) (inactive) (valve) I05.0
  - with
    - aortic valve disease I08.0
    - incompetency, insufficiency or regurgitation I05.2
  - active or acute I01.1
    - with rheumatic or Sydenham's chorea I02.0
  - congenital Q23.2
  - specified cause, except rheumatic I34.2
- myocardium, myocardial—*see also* Degeneration, myocardial
  - hypertrophic subaortic (idiopathic) I42.1
- nares (anterior) (posterior) J34.89
  - congenital Q30.0
- nasal duct—*see also* Stenosis, lacrimal, duct
  - congenital Q10.5
- nasolacrimal duct—*see also* Stenosis, lacrimal, duct
  - congenital Q10.5
- pulmonary (artery) (congenital) Q25.6
  - with ventricular septal defect, transposition of aorta, and hypertrophy of right ventricle Q21.3
  - in tetralogy of Fallot Q21.3
  - infundibular Q24.3
  - subvalvular Q24.3
  - supravalvular Q25.6
  - valve I37.0
    - with insufficiency I37.2
    - congenital Q22.1
    - rheumatic I09.89
      - ~ with aortic, mitral or tricuspid (valve) disease I08.8
- pulmonic (congenital) Q22.1
- pylorus (hypertrophic) (acquired) K31.1
  - congenital Q40.0
  - infantile Q40.0
- spinal M48.0-
- subaortic (congenital) Q24.4
  - hypertrophic (idiopathic) I42.1
- tricuspid (valve) I07.0
  - with
    - aortic (valve) disease I08.2
    - incompetency, insufficiency or regurgitation I07.2
      - ~ with aortic (valve) disease I08.2
        - ◊ with mitral (valve) disease I08.3
    - mitral (valve) disease I08.1
      - ~ with aortic (valve) disease I08.3
  - congenital Q22.4
  - nonrheumatic I36.0
    - with insufficiency I36.2
- ureteropelvic junction, congenital Q62.11
- ureterovesical orifice, congenital Q62.12
- vagina N89.5
  - congenital Q52.4
- valve (cardiac) (heart) (*see also* Endocarditis) I38
  - congenital Q24.8
    - aortic Q23.0
    - pulmonary Q22.1

Stercolith (impaction) K56.41

Stercoraceous, stercoral ulcer K63.3
- anus or rectum K62.6

Stereotypies NEC F98.4

Steroid
- effects (adverse) (adrenocortical) (iatrogenic)
  - cushingoid E24.2
    - correct substance properly administered—*see* Table of Drugs and Chemicals, by drug, adverse effect
    - overdose or wrong substance given or taken—*see* Table of Drugs and Chemicals, by drug, poisoning

Stevens-Johnson disease or syndrome L51.1
- toxic epidermal necrolysis overlap L51.3

Sticker's disease B08.3

Stiffness, joint NEC M25.60-
- ankle M25.67-
- contracture—*see* Contraction, joint
- elbow M25.62-
- foot M25.67-
- hand M25.64-
- hip M25.65-
- knee M25.66-
- shoulder M25.61-
- wrist M25.63-

Stillbirth P95

Still's disease or syndrome (juvenile) M08.20
- specified site NEC M08.2A

Stitch
- abscess T81.41

Stokes-Adams disease or syndrome I45.9

Stomatitis (denture) (ulcerative) K12.1
- angular K13.0
- aphthous K12.0
- candidal B37.0
- catarrhal K12.1
- due to
  - thrush B37.0
- follicular K12.1
- herpesviral, herpetic B00.2
- herpetiformis K12.0
- malignant K12.1
- membranous acute K12.1
- monilial B37.0
- mycotic B37.0
- parasitic B37.0
- septic K12.1
- suppurative (acute) K12.2
- vesicular K12.1
  - with exanthem (enteroviral) B08.4

Stomatocytosis D58.8

Stomatomycosis B37.0

Stomatorrhagia K13.79

Stovkis (-Talma) **disease** D74.8

Strabismus (congenital) (nonparalytic) H50.9
- concomitant H50.40
  - convergent—*see* Strabismus, convergent concomitant
  - divergent—*see* Strabismus, divergent concomitant
- convergent concomitant H50.00
  - accommodative component H50.43
  - alternating H50.05
    - with
      - ~ A pattern H50.06
      - ~ specified nonconcomitances NEC H50.08
      - ~ V pattern H50.07
  - monocular H50.01-
    - with
      - ~ A pattern H50.02-
      - ~ specified nonconcomitances NEC H50.04-
      - ~ V pattern H50.03-
    - intermittent H50.31-
      - ~ alternating H50.32
- cyclotropia H50.41
- divergent concomitant H50.10
  - alternating H50.15
    - with
      - ~ A pattern H50.16
      - ~ specified noncomitances NEC H50.18
      - ~ V pattern H50.17
  - monocular H50.11-
    - with
      - ~ A pattern H50.12-
      - ~ specified noncomitances NEC H50.14-

Strabismus, *continued*
  - ~ V pattern H50.13-
  - intermittent H50.33
    - ~ alternating H50.34
- Duane's syndrome H50.81-
- due to adhesions, scars H50.69
- heterophoria H50.50
  - alternating H50.55
  - cyclophoria H50.54
  - esophoria H50.51
  - exophoria H50.52
  - vertical H50.53
- heterotropia H50.40
  - intermittent H50.30
- hypertropia H50.2-
- hypotropia—*see* Strabismus, Hypertropia
- latent H50.50
- mechanical H50.60
  - Brown's sheath syndrome H50.61-
  - specified type NEC H50.69
- monofixation syndrome H50.42
- paralytic H49.9
  - abducens nerve H49.2-
  - fourth nerve H49.1-
  - Kearns-Sayre syndrome H49.81-
  - ophthalmoplegia (external)
    - progressive H49.4-
      - ~ with pigmentary retinopathy H49.81-
    - total H49.3-
  - sixth nerve H49.2-
  - specified type NEC H49.88-
  - third nerve H49.0-
  - trochlear nerve H49.1-
- specified type NEC H50.89
- vertical H50.2-

Strain
- cervical S16.1
- neck S16.1

Strangulation, strangulated—*see also* Asphyxia, traumatic
- bladder-neck N32.0
- bowel or colon K56.2
- intestine (large) (small) K56.2
  - with hernia—*see also* Hernia, by site, with, obstruction
    - with gangrene—*see* Hernia, by site, with, gangrene
- mesentery K56.2
- omentum K56.2
- organ or site, congenital NEC—*see* Atresia, by site
- vesicourethral orifice N32.0

Strangury R30.0

Strawberry
- mark Q82.5

Straw itch B88.0

Strephosymbolia F81.0
- secondary to organic lesion R48.8

Streptobacillary fever A25.1

Streptococcus, streptococcal—*see also* Disease, diseased
- as cause of disease classified elsewhere B95.5
- group
  - A, as cause of disease classified elsewhere B95.0
  - B, as cause of disease classified elsewhere B95.1
  - D, as cause of disease classified elsewhere B95.2
- pneumoniae, as cause of disease classified elsewhere B95.3
- specified NEC, as cause of disease classified elsewhere B95.4

Stress F43.9
- family—*see* Disruption, family
- fetal P84
- polycythemia D75.1
- reaction (*see also* Reaction, stress) F43.9

Stricture—*see also* Stenosis
- anus (sphincter) K62.4
  - congenital Q42.3
    - with fistula Q42.2
  - infantile Q42.3
    - with fistula Q42.3
- aorta (ascending) (congenital) Q25.1
- aortic (valve)—*see* Stenosis, aortic

Stricture, *continued*
- aqueduct of Sylvius (congenital) Q03.0
  - with spina bifida—*see* Spina bifida, by site, with hydrocephalus
  - acquired G91.1
- artery I77.1
  - congenital (peripheral) Q27.8
    - umbilical Q27.0
- bile duct (common) (hepatic) K83.1
  - congenital Q44.3
- bladder N32.89
  - neck N32.0
- brain G93.89
- colon—*see also* Obstruction, intestine
  - congenital Q42.9
    - specified NEC Q42.8
- digestive organs NEC, congenital Q45.8
- fallopian tube N97.1
  - gonococcal A54.24
- heart—*see also* Disease, heart
  - valve (*see also* Endocarditis) I38
    - aortic Q23.0
    - mitral Q23.4
    - pulmonary Q22.1
- intestine—*see also* Obstruction, intestine
  - congenital (small) Q41.9
    - large Q42.9
      - ~ specified NEC Q42.8
    - specified NEC Q41.8
  - ischemic K55.1
- myocardium, myocardial I51.5
  - hypertrophic subaortic (idiopathic) I42.1
- nares (anterior) (posterior) J34.89
  - congenital Q30.0
- nose J34.89
  - congenital Q30.0
- nostril (anterior) (posterior) J34.89
  - congenital Q30.0
- pelviureteric junction (congenital) Q62.11
- pulmonary, pulmonic
  - artery (congenital) Q25.6
  - infundibulum (congenital) Q24.3
  - valve I37.0
    - congenital Q22.1
- punctum lacrimale
  - congenital Q10.5
- pylorus (hypertrophic) K31.1
  - congenital Q40.0
  - infantile Q40.0
- rectum (sphincter) K62.4
  - congenital Q42.1
    - with fistula Q42.0
  - gonococcal A54.6
- subaortic Q24.4
  - hypertrophic (acquired) (idiopathic) I42.1
- ureter (postoperative) N13.5
  - with
    - hydronephrosis N13.1
- ureteropelvic junction N13.0
  - congenital Q62.11
- urethra (organic) (spasmodic) N35.9-
  - congenital Q64.39
    - valvular (posterior) Q64.2
  - female N35.92
  - gonococcal, gonorrheal A54.01
  - male N35.919
    - anterior urethra N35.914
    - bulbous urethra N35.912
    - meatal N35.911
    - membranous urethra N35.913
    - overlapping sites N35.116
  - postinfective NEC
    - female N35.12
    - male N35.119
      - ~ anterior urethra N35.114
      - ~ bulbous urethra N35.112
      - ~ meatal N35.111
      - ~ membranous urethra N35.113
      - ~ overlapping sites N35.116
  - post-traumatic
    - female N35.028
    - male N35.014
      - ~ anterior urethra N35.013

Stricture, *continued*
- ~ bulbous urethra N35.011
- ~ meatal N35.010
- ~ membranous urethra N35.012
- ~ overlapping sites N35.016
- – specified cause NEC
  - ■ female N35.82
  - ■ male N35.819
    - ~ anterior urethra N35.814
    - ~ bulbous urethra N35.812
    - ~ meatal N35.811
    - ~ membranous urethra N35.813
    - ~ overlapping sites N35.816
- • valve (cardiac) (heart)—*see also* Endocarditis
  - – congenital
    - ■ aortic Q23.0
    - ■ pulmonary Q22.1
- • vesicourethral orifice N32.0
  - – congenital Q64.31

Stridor R06.1
- • congenital (larynx) P28.89

Stroke (apoplectic) (brain) (embolic) (ischemic) (paralytic) (thrombotic)
- • cerebral, perinatal P91.82-
- • epileptic—*see* Epilepsy
- • heat T67.01
  - – exertional T67.02
  - – specified NEC T67.09
- • ischemic, perinatal arterial P91.82-
- • neonatal P91.82-
- • sun T67.01
  - – specified NEC T67.09

Struma—*see also* Goiter
- • Hashimoto E06.3
- • lymphomatosa E06.3
- • nodosa (simplex) E04.9
  - – endemic E01.2
    - ■ multinodular E01.1
- • Riedel's E06.5

Stupor (catatonic) R40.1
- • reaction to exceptional stress (transient) F43.0

Sturge (-Weber) (-Dimitri) (-Kalischer) **disease or syndrome** Q85.8

Stuttering F80.81
- • childhood onset F80.81
- • in conditions classified elsewhere R47.82

Sty, stye (external) (internal) (meibomian) (zeisian)—*see* Hordeolum

Subacidity, gastric K31.89
- • psychogenic F45.8

Subacute—*see* Disease, diseased

Subarachnoid—*see* Disease, diseased

Subcortical—*see* Disease, diseased

Subglossitis—*see* Glossitis

Subhemophilia D66

Subluxation—*see also* Dislocation
- • finger S63.20-
  - – index S63.20-
  - – interphalangeal S63.2-
    - ■ distal S63.24-
      - ~ index S63.24-
      - ~ little S63.24-
      - ~ middle S63.24-
      - ~ ring S63.24-
    - ■ index S63.2-
    - ■ little S63.2-
    - ■ middle S63.2-
    - ■ proximal S63.23-
      - ~ index S63.23-
      - ~ little S63.23-
      - ~ middle S63.23-
      - ~ ring S63.23-
    - ■ ring S63.2-
  - – little S63.20-
  - – metacarpophalangeal (joint) S63.21-
    - ■ index S63.26-
    - ■ little S63.26-
    - ■ middle S63.26-
    - ■ ring S63.26-

Subluxation, *continued*
- – middle S63.20-
- – ring S63.20
- • hip S73.0-
  - – anterior S73.03-
    - ■ obturator S73.02-
  - – central S73.04-
  - – posterior S73.01-
- • interphalangeal (joint)
  - – finger S63.2-
    - ■ distal joint S63.24-
      - ~ index S63.24-
      - ~ little S63.24-
      - ~ middle S63.24-
      - ~ ring S63.24-
    - ■ index S63.2-
    - ■ little S63.2-
    - ■ middle S63.2-
    - ■ proximal joint S63.23-
      - ~ index S63.23-
      - ~ little S63.23-
      - ~ middle S63.23-
      - ~ ring S63.23-
    - ■ ring S63.2-
  - – thumb S63.12-
- • knee S83.10-
  - – cap—*see* Subluxation, patella
  - – patella—*see* Subluxation, patella
  - – proximal tibia
    - ■ anteriorly S83.11-
    - ■ laterally S83.14-
    - ■ medially S83.13-
    - ■ posteriorly S83.12-
  - – specified type NEC S83.19-
- • metacarpal (bone)
  - – proximal end S63.06-
- • metacarpophalangeal (joint)
  - – finger S63.21-
    - ■ index S63.21-
    - ■ little S63.21-
    - ■ middle S63.21-
    - ■ ring S63.21-
  - – thumb S63.11-
- • patella S83.00-
  - – lateral S83.01-
  - – recurrent (nontraumatic) M22.1-
  - – specified type NEC S83.09-
- • radial head S53.00-
  - – nursemaid's elbow S53.03-
  - – specified type NEC S53.09-
- • thumb S63.10-
  - – interphalangeal joint—*see* Subluxation, interphalangeal (joint), thumb
  - – metacarpophalangeal joint S63.11-

Submersion (fatal) (nonfatal) T75.1

Substernal thyroid E04.9
- • congenital Q89.2

Substitution disorder F44.9

Subthyroidism (acquired)—*see also* Hypothyroidism
- • congenital E03.1

Sucking thumb, child (excessive) F98.8

Sudamen, sudamina L74.1

Sugar
- • blood
  - – high (transient) R73.9
  - – low (transient) E16.2
- • in urine R81

Suicide, suicidal (attempted) T14.91
- • by poisoning—*see* Table of Drugs and Chemicals
- • history of (personal) Z91.51
  - – in family Z81.8
- • ideation—*see* Ideation, suicidal
- • risk
  - – meaning personal history of attempted suicide Z91.51
  - – meaning suicidal ideation—*see* Ideation, suicidal
- • tendencies
  - – meaning personal history of attempted suicide Z91.51
  - – meaning suicidal ideation—*see* Ideation, suicidal
- • trauma—*see* nature of injury by site

Sulfhemoglobinemia, sulphemoglobinemia (acquired) (with methemoglobinemia) D74.8

Sunburn L55.9
- • due to
  - – tanning bed (acute) L56.8
- • first degree L55.0
- • second degree L55.1
- • third degree L55.2

Sunstroke T67.01

Supernumerary (congenital)
- • carpal bones Q74.0
- • fallopian tube Q50.6
- • finger Q69.0
- • lacrimonasal duct Q10.6
- • lobule (ear) Q17.0
- • nipple(s) Q83.3
- • ovary Q50.31
- • oviduct Q50.6.
- • ossicles, auditory Q16.3
- • tarsal bones Q74.2
- • testis Q55.29
- • thumb Q69.1
- • toe Q69.2
- • uterus Q51.28

Supervision (of)
- • contraceptive—*see* Prescription of contraceptives
- • dietary (for) Z71.3
  - – allergy (food) Z71.3
  - – colitis Z71.3
  - – diabetes mellitus Z71.3
  - – food allergy or intolerance Z71.3
  - – gastritis Z71.3
  - – hypercholesterolemia Z71.3
  - – hypoglycemia Z71.3
  - – intolerance (food) Z71.3
  - – obesity Z71.3
  - – specified NEC Z71.3
- • healthy infant or child Z76.2
  - – foundling Z76.1
- • lactation Z39.1

Suppression
- • menstruation N94.89
- • urine, urinary secretion R34

Suppuration, suppurative—*see also* Disease, diseased
- • accessory sinus (chronic)—*see* Sinusitis
- • antrum (chronic)—*see* Sinusitis, maxillary
- • bladder—*see* Cystitis
- • brain G06.0
  - – sequelae G09
- • breast N61.1
- • ear (middle)—*see also* Otitis, media
  - – external NEC—*see* Otitis, externa, infective
  - – internal—*see* subcategory H83.0
- • ethmoidal (chronic) (sinus)—*see* Sinusitis, ethmoidal
- • frontal (chronic) (sinus)—*see* Sinusitis, frontal
- • gallbladder (acute) K81.0
- • intracranial G06.0
- • joint—*see* Arthritis, pyogenic or pyemic
- • labyrinthine—*see* subcategory H83.0
- • mammary gland N61.1
- • maxilla, maxillary M27.2
  - – sinus (chronic)—*see* Sinusitis, maxillary
- • muscle—*see* Myositis, infective
- • nasal sinus (chronic)—*see* Sinusitis
- • pelvis, pelvic
  - – female—*see* Disease, pelvis, inflammatory
  - – male K65.0
- • sinus (accessory) (chronic) (nasal)—*see* Sinusitis
- • sphenoidal sinus (chronic)—*see* Sinusitis, sphenoidal
- • thyroid (gland) E06.0
- • tonsil—*see* Tonsillitis
- • uterus—*see* Endometritis

Supraglottitis J04.30
- • with obstruction J04.31

Surgical
- • shock T81.10

Surveillance (of) (for)—*see also* Observation
- • alcohol abuse Z71.41
- • contraceptive—*see* Prescription of contraceptives
- • dietary Z71.3
- • drug abuse Z71.51

Suspected condition, ruled out—*see also* Observation, suspected
- fetal anomaly Z03.73
- fetal growth Z03.74
- newborn—*see* Observation, newborn (for suspected condition, ruled out) Z05-

Suture
- burst (in operation wound) T81.31
  - external operation wound T81.31
- removal Z48.02

Swearing, compulsive F42.8
- in Gilles de la Tourette's syndrome F95.2

Sweat, sweats
- night R61

Sweating, excessive R61

Swelling (of) R60.9
- abdomen, abdominal (not referable to any particular organ)—*see* Mass, abdominal
- ankle—*see* Effusion, joint, ankle
- arm M79.89
  - forearm M79.89
- breast (*see also*, Lump, breast) N63.0
- chest, localized R22.2
- extremity (lower) (upper)—*see* Disorder
- finger M79.89
- foot M79.89
- glands R59.9
  - generalized R59.1
  - localized R59.0
- hand M79.89
- head (localized) R22.0
- inflammatory—*see* Inflammation
- intra-abdominal—*see* Mass, abdominal
- joint—*see* Effusion, joint
- leg M79.89
  - lower M79.89
- limb—*see* Disorder
- localized (skin) R22.9
  - chest R22.2
  - head R22.0
  - limb
    - lower—*see* Mass, localized, limb, lower
    - upper—*see* Mass, localized, limb, upper
  - neck R22.1
  - trunk R22.2
- neck (localized) R22.1
- pelvic—*see* Mass, abdominal
- scrotum N50.89
- splenic—*see* Splenomegaly
- testis N50.89
- toe M79.89
- umbilical R19.09

Swimmer's
- cramp T75.1
- ear H60.33-
- itch B65.3

Swimming in the head R42

Swollen—*see* Swelling

Sycocis L73.8
- barbae (not parasitic) L73.8
- contagiosa (mycotic) B35.0
- lupoides L73.8
- mycotic B35.0
- parasitic B35.0
- vulgaris L73.8

Symblepharon
- congenital Q10.3

Symond's syndrome G93.2

Sympathetic—*see* Disease, diseased

Sympathicoblastoma
- specified site—*see* Neoplasm, malignant, by site in Table of Neoplasms in the complete *ICD-10-CM* manual
- unspecified site C74.90

Sympathogonioma—*see* Sympathicoblastoma

Symphalangy (fingers) (toes) Q70.9

Symptoms NEC R68.89
- breast NEC N64.59
- cold J00
- development NEC R63.8

Symptoms NEC, *continued*
- genital organs, female R10.2
- involving
  - abdomen NEC R19.8
  - awareness R41.9
    - altered mental status R41.82
  - cardiovascular system NEC R09.89
  - chest NEC R09.89
  - circulatory system NEC R09.89
  - cognitive functions R41.9
    - altered mental status R41.82
  - development NEC R62.50
  - digestive system R19.8
  - food and fluid intake R63.8
  - general perceptions and sensations R44.9
    - specified NEC R44.8
  - musculoskeletal system R29.91
    - specified NEC R29.898
  - nervous system R29.90
    - specified NEC R29.818
  - pelvis R19.8
  - respiratory system NEC R09.89
- metabolism NEC R63.8
- of infancy R68.19
- pelvis NEC, female R10.2
- viral syndrome J00

Sympus Q74.2

Syncope (near) (pre-) R55
- bradycardia R00.1
- cardiac R55
- heart R55
- heat T67.1
- laryngeal R05.4
- psychogenic F48.8
- tussive R05.8
- vasoconstriction R55
- vasodepressor R55
- vasomotor R55
- vasovagal R55

Syndactylism, syndactyly Q70.9
- complex (with synostosis)
  - fingers Q70.0-
  - toes Q70.2-
- simple (without synostosis)
  - fingers Q70.1-
  - toes Q70.3-

Syndrome—*see also* Disease
- abdominal
  - acute R10.0
  - muscle deficiency Q79.4
- abstinence, neonatal P96.1
- acquired immunodeficiency—*see* Human, immuno-deficiency virus (HIV) disease
- acute abdominal R10.0
- acute respiratory distress (adult) (child) J80
- Adair-Dighton Q78.0
- Adams-Stokes (-Morgagni) I45.9
- adrenocortical—*see* Cushing's, syndrome
- adrenogenital E25.9
  - congenital, associated with enzyme deficiency E25.0
- Alder's D72.0
- Aldrich (-Wiskott) D82.0
- Alport Q87.81
- alveolar hypoventilation E66.2
- androgen insensitivity E34.50
  - complete E34.51
  - partial E34.52
- androgen resistance (*see also* Syndrome, androgen insensitivity) E34.50
- Angelman Q93.51
- ankyloglossia superior Q38.1
- antibody deficiency D80.9
  - agammaglobulinemic D80.1
    - hereditary D80.0
  - congenital D80.0
  - hypogammaglobulinemic D80.1
    - hereditary D80.0
- Arnold-Chiari—*see* Arnold-Chiari disease
- Arrillaga-Ayerza I27.0
- arterial tortuosity Q87.82

Syndrome, *continued*
- aspiration, of newborn—*see* Aspiration, by substance, with, pneumonia
  - meconium P24.01
- ataxia-telangiectasia G11.3
- autoerythrocyte sensitization (Gardner-Diamond) D69.2
- autoimmune lymphoproliferative *[ALPS]* D89.82
- Ayerza (-Arrillaga) I27.0
- Beals Q87.40
- bilateral polycystic ovarian E28.2
- black
  - widow spider bite—*see* Table of Drugs and Chemicals, by animal or substance, poisoning
- Blackfan-Diamond D61.01
- blind loop K90.2
  - congenital Q43.8
  - postsurgical K91.2
- blue sclera Q78.0
- Boder-Sedgewick G11.3
- Borjeson Forssman Lehmann Q89.8
- Bouillaud's I01.9
- Bourneville (-Pringle) Q85.1
- bradycardia-tachycardia I49.5
- brain (nonpsychotic) F09
  - with psychosis, psychotic reaction F09
  - acute or subacute—*see* Delirium
  - congenital—*see* Disability, intellectual
  - organic F09
    - post-traumatic (nonpsychotic) F07.81
  - postcontusional F07.81
  - post-traumatic, nonpsychotic F07.81
- Brock's J98.11
- bronze baby P83.88
- Burnett's (milk-alkali) E83.52
- carbohydrate-deficient glycoprotein (CDGS) E77.8
- cardiacos negros I27.0
- cardiopulmonary-obesity E66.2
- cardiorespiratory distress (idiopathic), newborn P22.0
- cat cry Q93.4
- celiac K90.0
- cerebral
  - gigantism E22.0
- CHARGE Q89.8
- child maltreatment—*see* Maltreatment, child
- chondrocostal junction M94.0
- chondroectodermal dysplasia Q77.6
- chromosome 5 short arm deletion Q93.4
- Clerambault's automatism G93.89
- clumsiness, clumsy child F82
- cluster headache G44.009
  - intractable G44.001
  - not intractable G44.009
- Coffin-Lowry Q89.8
- combined immunity deficiency D81.9
- concussion F07.81
- congenital
  - facial diplegia Q87.0
  - oculo-auriculovertebral Q87.0
  - oculofacial diplegia (Moebius) Q87.0
  - rubella (manifest) P35.0
- congestive dysmenorrhea N94.6
- Costen's (complex) M26.69
- costochondral junction M94.0
- costovertebral E22.0
- Cowden Q85.8
- cri-du-chat Q93.4
- crib death R99
- croup J05.0
- Cushing's E24.9
  - due to
    - drugs E24.2
    - overproduction of pituitary ACTH E24.0
  - drug-induced E24.2
  - overdose or wrong substance given or taken—*see* Table of Drugs and Chemicals, by drug, poisoning
  - pituitary-dependent E24.0
  - specified type NEC E24.8
- cryptophthalmos Q87.0
- cytokine release D89.839
  - grade 1 D89.831
  - grade 2 D89.832
  - grade 3 D89.833

Syndrome, *continued*
- – grade 4 D89.834
- – grade 5 D89.835
- Dandy-Walker Q03.1
  - – with spina bifida Q07.01
- defibrination—*see also* Fibrinolysis
  - – newborn P60
- dependence—*see* F10-F19 with fourth character .2
- De Quervain E34.51
- de Vivo syndrome E74.810
- diabetes mellitus in newborn infant P70.2
- Diamond-Blackfan D61.01
- Diamond-Gardener D69.2
- DIC (diffuse or disseminated intravascular coagulopathy) D65
- di George's D82.1
- Dighton's Q78.0
- disequilibrium E87.8
- Döhle body-panmyelopathic D72.0
- Down (*see also* Down syndrome) Q90.9
- Dravet (intractable) G40.834
  - – with status epilepticus G40.833
  - – without status epilepticus G40.834
- DRESS (drug rash with eosinophilia and systemic symptoms) D72.12
- Dressler's (postmyocardial infarction) I24.1
  - – postcardiotomy I97.0
- drug rash with eosinophilia and systemic symptoms (DRESS) D72.12
- drug withdrawal, infant of dependent mother P96.1
- dry eye H04.12-
- due to abnormality
  - – chromosomal Q99.9
    - ▪ sex
      - ~ female phenotype Q97.9
      - ~ male phenotype Q98.9
    - ▪ specified NEC Q99.8
- Dupré's (meningism) R29.1
- dysmetabolic X E88.81
- dyspraxia, developmental F82
- Eagle-Barrett Q79.4
- eczema-thrombocytopenia D82.0
- Eddowes' Q78.0
- effort (psychogenic) F45.8
- Ehlers-Danlos Q79.60
  - – classical Ehlers-Danlos syndrome Q79.61
  - – hypermobile Ehlers-Danlos syndrome Q79.62
  - – other Ehlers-Danlos syndromes Q79.69
  - – vascular Ehlers-Danlos syndrome Q79.63
- Eisenmenger's I27.83
- Ekman's Q78.0
- Ellis-van Creveld Q77.6
- eosinophilia-myalgia M35.8
- epileptic—*see* Epilepsy, by type
- Erdheim's E22.0
- Evans D69.41
- eye retraction—*see* Strabismus
- eyelid-malar-mandible Q87.0
- facet M47.89-
- Fallot's Q21.3
- familial eczema-thrombocytopenia (Wiskott-Aldrich) D82.0
- Fanconi's (anemia) (congenital pancytopenia) D61.09
- fatigue
  - – chronic R53.82
- faulty bowel habit K59.39
- fetal
  - – alcohol (dysmorphic) Q86.0
- Fiedler's I40.1
- first arch Q87.0
- fish odor E72.89
- floppy
  - – baby P94.2
- food protein-induced enterocolitis (FPIES) K52.21
- fragile X Q99.2
- Fukuhara E88.49
- functional
  - – bowel K59.9
- Gaisböck's D75.1
- Gardener-Diamond D69.2
- Gee-Herter-Heubner K90.0
- Gianotti-Crosti L44.4
- Gilles de la Tourette's F95.2

Syndrome, *continued*
- Gleich's D72.118
- Goldberg Q89.8
- Goldberg-Maxwell E34.51
- Good's D83.8
- Gouley's I31.1
- Gower's R55
- hand-foot L27.1
- Hegglin's D72.0
- hemolytic-uremic D59.3
- hemophagocytic, infection-associated D76.2
- Henoch-Schönlein D69.0
- hepatopulmonary K76.81
- hereditary alpha tryptasemia D89.44
- Herter (-Gee) (nontropical sprue) K90.0
- Heubner-Herter K90.0
- histamine-like (fish poisoning)—*see* Poisoning, food, noxious or naturally toxic, fish
- histiocytic D76.3
- histiocytosis NEC D76.3
- HIV infection, acute B20
- Hoffmann-Werdnig G12.0
- hypereosinophilic (HES) D72.119
  - – idiopathic (IHES) D72.110
  - – lymphocytic variant (LHES) D72.111
  - – myeloid D72.118
  - – specified NEC D72.118
- hyperkinetic—*see* Hyperkinesia
- hypermobility M35.7
- hypernatremia E87.0
- hyperosmolarity E87.0
- hypertransfusion, newborn P61.1
- hyperventilation F45.8
- hyperviscosity (of serum)
  - – polycythemic D75.1
- hypoglycemic (familial) (neonatal) E16.2
- hyponatremic E87.1
- hypoplastic left-heart Q23.4
- hyposmolality E87.1
- hypothenar hammer I73.89
- ICF (intravascular coagulation-fibrinolysis) D65
- idiopathic
  - – cardiorespiratory distress, newborn P22.0
  - – nephrotic (infantile) N04.9
- immune effector cell-associated neurotoxicity (ICANS) G92.00
  - – grade
    - ▪ 1 G92.01
    - ▪ 2 G92.02
    - ▪ 3 G92.03
    - ▪ 4 G92.04
    - ▪ 5 G92.05
    - ▪ unspecified G92.00
- immunity deficiency, combined D81.9
- immunodeficiency
  - – acquired—*see* Human, immunodeficiency virus (HIV) disease
  - – combined D81.9
- inappropriate secretion of antidiuretic hormone E22.2
- inspissated bile (newborn) P59.1
- intestinal
  - – knot K56.2
- intravascular coagulation-fibrinolysis (ICF) D65
- iodine-deficiency, congenital E00.-
- IRDS (idiopathic respiratory distress, newborn) P22.0
- irritable
  - – bowel K58.9
    - ▪ with constipation K58.1
    - ▪ with diarrhea K58.0
    - ▪ mixed K58.2
    - ▪ other K58.8
    - ▪ psychogenic F45.8
  - – heart (psychogenic) F45.8
- IVC (intravascular coagulopathy) D65
- Jervell-Lange-Nielsen I45.81
- Job's D71
- Joseph-Diamond-Blackfan D61.01
- jugular foramen G52.7
- Kabuki Q89.8
- Kanner's (autism) F84.0
- Kartagener's Q89.3
- Kostmann's D70.0

Syndrome, *continued*
- Lambert-E
  - – in neoplastic disease G73.1
- Launois' E22.0
- lazy
  - – leukocyte D70.8
- Lemiere I80.8
- Lennox-Gastaut G40.812
  - – intractable G40.814
    - ▪ with status epilepticus G40.813
    - ▪ without status epilepticus G40.814
  - – not intractable G40.812
    - ▪ with status epilepticus G40.811
    - ▪ without status epilepticus G40.812
- Leopold-Levi's E05.90
- Lev's I44.2
- long arm 18 or 21 deletion Q93.89
- long QT I45.81
- Louis-Barré G11.3
- low
  - – back M54.50
  - – output (cardiac) I50.9
- Luetscher's (dehydration) E86.0
- Lutembacher's Q21.1
- macrophage activation D76.1
  - – due to infection D76.2
- Mal de Debarquement R42
- malabsorption K90.9
  - – postsurgical K91.2
- malformation, congenital, due to
  - – alcohol Q86.0
- maple-syrup-urine E71.0
- Marfan's Q87.40
  - – with
    - ▪ cardiovascular manifestations Q87.418
      - ~ aortic dilation Q87.410
    - ▪ ocular manifestations Q87.42
    - ▪ skeletal manifestations Q87.43
- Marie's E22.0
- mast cell activation D89.40
  - – idiopathic D89.42
  - – monoclonal D89.41
  - – other D89.49
  - – secondary D89.43
- May (-Hegglin) D72.0
- McQuarrie's E16.2
- meconium plug (newborn) P76.0
- Meekeren-Ehlers-Danlos Q79.6-
- MELAS E88.41
- MERRF (myoclonic epilepsy associated with ragged-red fibers) E88.42
- metabolic E88.81
- micrognathia-glossoptosis Q87.0
- midbrain NEC G93.89
- migraine—*see also* Migraine G43.909
- milk-alkali E83.52
- Miller-Dieker Q93.88
- Minkowski-Chauffard D58.0
- MNGIE (Mitochondrial Neurogastrointestinal Encephalo-pathy) E88.49
- Morgagni-Adams-Stokes I45.9
- mucocutaneous lymph node (acute febrile) (MCLS) M30.3
- myasthenic G70.9
  - – in
    - ▪ diabetes mellitus—*see* Diabetes, type 1, with, amyotrophy
    - ▪ endocrine disease NEC E34.9 [G73.3]
    - ▪ neoplastic disease (*see also* Table of Neoplasms in the complete *ICD-10-CM* manual) D49.9 [G73.3]
    - ▪ thyrotoxicosis (hyperthyroidism) E05.90 [G73.3]
      - ~ with thyroid storm E05.91 [G73.3]
- myelodysplastic D46.9
  - – with
    - ▪ multilineage dysplasia D46.A
      - ~ with ringed sideroblasts D46.B
  - – myeloid hypereosinophilic D72.118
- myofascial pain M79.18
- NARP (Neuropathy, Ataxia and Retinitis pigmentosa) E88.49
- neonatal abstinence P96.1
- nephritic—*see also* Nephritis
  - – with edema—*see* Nephrosis

Syndrome, *continued*
- acute N00.9
- chronic N03.9
- nephrotic (congenital) (*see also* Nephrosis) N04.9
  - with
    - C3
      ~ glomerulonephritis N04.A
      ~ glomerulopathy N04.A
        ◊ with dense deposit disease N04.6
    - dense deposit disease N04.6
    - diffuse
      ~ crescentic glomerulonephritis N04.7
      ~ endocapillary proliferative glomerulonephritis N04.4
      ~ membranous glomerulonephritis N04.2
      ~ mesangial proliferative glomerulonephritis N04.3
      ~ mesangiocapillary glomerulonephritis N04.5
    - focal and segmental glomerular lesions N04.1
    - minor glomerular abnormality N04.0
    - specified morphological changes NEC N04.8
- Nothnagel's vasomotor acroparesthesia I73.89
- Ogilvie K59.81
- ophthalmoplegia-cerebellar ataxia—*see* Strabismus, paralytic, third nerve
- oral-facial-digital Q87.0
- oro-facial-digital Q87.0
- Osler-Weber-Rendu I78.0
- oto-palatal-digital Q87.0
- ovary
  - polycystic E28.2
  - sclerocystic E28.2
- pain—*see also* Pain
  - complex regional I G90.5-
    - lower limb G90.52-
    - specified site NEC G90.59
    - upper limb G90.51-
- painful
  - bruising D69.2
- paralytic G83.9
- pediatric autoimmune neuropsychiatric disorders associated with streptococcal infections (PANDAS) D89.89
- pharyngeal pouch D82.1
- Pick's (heart) (liver) I31.1
- Pickwickian E66.2
- pituitary E22.0
- pontine NEC G93.89
- postcardiac injury
  - postcardiotomy I97.0
- postcommissurotomy I97.0
- postconcussional F07.81
- postcontusional F07.81
- post-COVID (-19) U09.9
- postvalvulotomy I97.0
- prune belly Q79.4
- pseudoparalytica G70.00
  - with exacerbation (acute) G70.01
  - in crisis G70.01
- pseudo-Turner's Q87.19
- pulmonary
  - arteriosclerosis I27.0
  - dysmaturity (Wilson-Mikity) P27.0
  - hypoperfusion (idiopathic) P22.0
- QT interval prolongation I45.81
- RDS (respiratory distress syndrome, newborn) P22.0
- Reifenstein E34.52
- Rendu-Osler-Weber I78.0
- respiratory
  - distress
    - acute J80
      ~ child J80
    - newborn (idiopathic) (type I) P22.0
      ~ type II P22.1
- retinoblastoma (familial) C69.2
- retroviral seroconversion (acute) Z21
- Romano-Ward (prolonged QT interval) I45.81
- rubella (congenital) P35.0
- Ruvalcaba-Myhre-Smith E71.440
- Rytand-Lipsitch I44.2
- salt
  - depletion E87.1

Syndrome, *continued*
- due to heat NEC T67.8
  ~ causing heat exhaustion or prostration T67.4
- low E87.1
- Scaglietti-Dagnini E22.0
- scapuloperoneal G71.09
- schizophrenic, of childhood NEC F84.5
- Schwartz-Bartter E22.2
- sclerocystic ovary E28.2
- Seitelberger's G31.89
- seroconversion, retroviral (acute) Z21
- serous meningitis G93.2
- severe acute respiratory (SARS) J12.81
- shaken infant T74.4
- shock (traumatic) T79.4
  - kidney N17.0
  - toxic A48.3
- shock-lung J80
- short
  - bowel K91.2
  - rib Q77.2
- Shwachman's D70.4
- sick
  - cell E87.1
  - sinus I49.5
- sinus tarsi M25.57-
- sinusitis-bronchiectasis-situs inversus Q89.3
- Smith-Magenis Q93.88
- Soto's Q87.3
- Spen's I45.9
- splenic
  - neutropenia D73.81
- Spurway's Q78.0
- staphylococcal scalded skin L00
- Stein-Leventhal E28.2
- Stein's E28.2
- Stevens-Johnson syndrome L51.1
  - toxic epidermal necrolysis overlap L51.3
- Stickler Q89.8
- stiff baby Q89.8
- Stokes (-Adams) I45.9
- swallowed blood P78.2
- sweat retention L74.0
- Symond's G93.2
- systemic inflammatory response (SIRS), of non-infectious origin (without organ dysfunction) R65.10
  - with acute organ dysfunction R65.11
- tachycardia-bradycardia I49.5
- teething K00.7
- tegmental G93.89
- telangiectasia-pigmentation-cataract Q82.8
- temporal pyramidal apex—*see* Otitis, media, suppurative, acute
- temporomandibular joint-pain-dysfunction M26.62-
- testicular feminization (*see also* Syndrome, androgen insensitivity) E34.51
- Tietze's M94.0
- toxic shock A48.3
- triple X, female Q97.0
- trisomy Q92.9
  - 13 Q91.7
    - meiotic nondisjunction Q91.4
  - 18 Q91.3
    - meiotic nondisjunction Q91.0
  - 21 Q90.9
- tumor lysis (following antineoplastic chemotherapy) (spontaneous) NEC E88.3
- uremia, chronic (*see also* Disease, kidney, chronic) N18.9
- vago-hypoglossal G52.7
- van der Hoeve's Q78.0
- vasovagal R55
- velo-cardio-facial Q93.81
- visual disorientation H53.8
- von Willebrand (-Jürgens) D68.0
- Werdnig-Hoffman G12.0
- wet
  - lung, newborn P22.1
- whiplash S13.4
- whistling face Q87.0
- Willebrand (-Jürgens) D68.0
- Williams Q93.82
- Wiskott-Aldrich D82.0

Syndrome, *continued*
- withdrawal—*see* Withdrawal state
  - drug
    - infant of dependent mother P96.1
    - therapeutic use, newborn P96.2
- Yao M04.8
- Zahorsky's B08.5
- Zellweger syndrome E71.510
- Zellweger-like syndrome E71.541

Synostosis (congenital) Q78.8
- astragalo-scaphoid Q74.2
- radioulnar Q74.0

Syphilis, syphilitic (acquired) A52.79
- age under 2 years NOS—*see also* Syphilis, congenital, early
  - acquired A51.9
- anemia (late) A52.79 *[D63.8]*
- asymptomatic—*see* Syphilis, latent
- bubo (primary) A51.0
- chancre (multiple) A51.0
  - extragenital A51.2
  - Rollet's A51.0
- congenital A50.9
  - early, or less than 2 years after birth NEC A50.2
    - with manifestations—*see* Syphilis, congenital, early
- contact Z20.2
- cutaneous A51.39
- early A51.9
  - symptomatic A51.9
    - extragenital chancre A51.2
    - primary, except extragenital chancre A51.0
- exposure to Z20.2
- genital (primary) A51.0
- inactive—*see* Syphilis, latent
- infantum—*see* Syphilis, congenital
- inherited—*see* Syphilis, congenital
- latent A53.0
  - with signs or symptoms—*code by* site and stage under Syphilis
  - date of infection unspecified A53.0
  - early, or less than 2 years after infection A51.5
  - follow-up of latent syphilis A53.0
    - date of infection unspecified A53.0
    - late, or 2 years or more after infection A52.8
  - late, or 2 years or more after infection A52.8
  - positive serology (only finding) A53.0
    - date of infection unspecified A53.0
    - early, or less than 2 years after infection A51.5
    - late, or 2 years or more after infection A52.8
- lip A51.39
  - chancre (primary) A51.2
  - late A52.79
- penis (chancre) A51.0
- primary A51.0
  - extragenital chancre NEC A51.2
  - fingers A51.2
  - genital A51.0
  - lip A51.2
  - specified site NEC A51.2
  - tonsils A51.2
- skin (with ulceration) (early) (secondary) A51.39
- tonsil (lingual) (late) A52.76
  - primary A51.2
- vagina A51.0
  - late A52.76
- vulva A51.0
  - late A52.76
  - secondary A51.39

System, systemic—*see also* Disease, diseased
- inflammatory response syndrome (SIRS) of non-infectious origin (without organ dysfunction) R65.10
  - with acute organ dysfunction R65.11
- lupus erythematosus M32.9

T

Tachyalimentation K91.2

Tachyarrhythmia, tachyrhythmia—*see* Tachycardia

Tachycardia R00.0
- atrial (paroxysmal) I47.1
- auricular I47.1

Tachycardia, *continued*
- AV nodal re-entry (re-entrant) I47.1
- junctional (paroxysmal) I47.1
- newborn P29.11
- nodal (paroxysmal) I47.1
- paroxysmal (sustained) (nonsustained) I47.9
  - with sinus bradycardia I49.5
  - atrial (PAT) I47.1
  - atrioventricular (AV) (re-entrant) I47.1
    - psychogenic F54
  - junctional I47.1
    - ectopic I47.1
  - nodal I47.1
  - supraventricular (sustained) I47.1
- psychogenic F45.8
- sick sinus I49.5
- sinoauricular NOS R00.0
  - paroxysmal I47.1
- sinus [sinusal] NOS R00.0
  - paroxysmal I47.1
- supraventricular I47.1
- ventricular (paroxysmal) (sustained) I47.2

Tachypnea R06.82
- hysterical F45.8
- newborn (idiopathic) (transitory) P22.1
- psychogenic F45.8
- transitory, of newborn P22.1

TACO (transfusion associated circulatory overload) E87.71

Tag (hypertrophied skin) (infected) L91.8
- adenoid J35.8
- anus K64.4
- hemorrhoidal K64.4
- sentinel K64.4
- skin L91.8
  - accessory (congenital) Q82.8
  - anus K64.4
  - congenital Q82.8
  - preauricular Q17.0
- tonsil J35.8

Talipes (congenital) Q66.89
- acquired, planus—*see* Deformity, limb, flat foot
- asymmetric Q66.89
- calcaneovalgus Q66.4-
- calcaneovarus Q66.1-
- calcaneus Q66.89
- cavus Q66.7-
- equinovalgus Q66.6
- equinovarus Q66.0-
- equinus Q66.89
- percavus Q66.7-
- planovalgus Q66.6
- planus (acquired) (any degree)—*see also* Deformity, limb, flat foot
  - congenital Q66.5-
- valgus Q66.6
- varus Q66.3-

Tall stature, constitutional E34.4

Tamponade, heart I31.4

Tantrum, child problem F91.8

Tapeworm (infection) (infestation)—*see* Infestation, tapeworm

Tapia's syndrome G52.7

Tattoo (mark) L81.8

Tay-Sachs amaurotic familial idiocy or disease E75.02

TBI (traumatic brain injury) S06.9

Tear, torn (traumatic)—*see also* Laceration
- anus, anal (sphincter) S31.831
  - nontraumatic (healed) (old) K62.81
- rotator cuff (nontraumatic) M75.10-
  - complete M75.12-
  - incomplete M75.11-
  - traumatic S46.01-
    - capsule S43.42-
- vagina—*see* Laceration, vagina

Teeth—*see also* Disease, diseased
- grinding
  - psychogenic F45.8
  - sleep related G47.63

Teething (syndrome) K00.7

Telangiectasia, telangiectasis (verrucous) I78.1
- ataxic (cerebellar) (Louis-Bar) G11.3
- familial I78.0
- hemorrhagic, hereditary (congenital) (senile) I78.0
- hereditary, hemorrhagic (congenital) (senile) I78.0
- spider I78.1

Telescoped bowel or intestine K56.1
- congenital Q43.8

Temperature
- body, high (of unknown origin) R50.9
- cold, trauma from
  - newborn P80.0

Temporomandibular joint pain-dysfunction syndrome M26.62-

Tendency
- bleeding—*see* Defect, coagulation
- suicide
  - meaning personal history of attempted suicide Z91.51
  - meaning suicidal ideation—*see* Ideation, suicidal

Tenderness, abdominal R10.819
- epigastric R10.816
- generalized R10.817
- left lower quadrant R10.814
- left upper quadrant R10.812
- periumbilic R10.815
- right lower quadrant R10.813
- right upper quadrant R10.811
- rebound R10.829
  - epigastric R10.826
  - generalized R10.827
  - left lower quadrant R10.824
  - left upper quadrant R10.822
  - periumbilic R10.825
  - right lower quadrant R10.823
  - right upper quadrant R10.821

Tendinitis, tendonitis—*see also* Enthesopathy
- Achilles M76.6-

Tenesmus (rectal) R19.8

Tennis elbow—*see* Epicondylitis, lateral

Tenosynovitis M65.9
- adhesive—*see* Tenosynovitis, specified type NEC
- shoulder region M65.81-
  - adhesive—*see* Capsulitis, adhesive
- specified type NEC M65.88
  - ankle M65.87-
  - foot M65.87-
  - forearm M65.83-
  - hand M65.84-
  - lower leg M65.86-
  - multiple sites M65.89
  - pelvic region M65.85-
  - shoulder region M65.81-
  - specified site NEC M65.88
  - thigh M65.85-
  - upper arm M65.82-

Tension
- arterial, high—*see also* Hypertension
  - without diagnosis of hypertension R03.0
- headache G44.209
  - intractable G44.201
  - not intractable G44.209
- nervous R45.0
- pneumothorax J93.0
- state (mental) F48.9

Tentorium—*see* Disease, diseased

Teratencephalus Q89.8

Teratism Q89.7

Terror(s) night (child) F51.4

Test, tests, testing (for)
- blood-alcohol Z02.83
  - positive—*see* Findings
- blood-drug Z02.83
  - positive—*see* Findings
- hearing Z01.10
  - with abnormal findings NEC Z01.118
  - infant or child (over 28 days old) Z00.129
    - with abnormal findings Z00.121

Test, tests, testing, *continued*
- HIV (human immunodeficiency virus)
  - nonconclusive (in infants) R75
  - positive Z21
  - seropositive Z21
- immunity status Z01.84
- laboratory (as part of a general medical examination) Z00.00
  - with abnormal finding Z00.01
  - for medicolegal reason NEC Z04.89
- Mantoux (for tuberculosis) Z11.1
  - abnormal result R76.11
- skin, diagnostic
  - allergy Z01.82
    - special screening examination—*see* Screening, by name of disease
  - Mantoux Z11.1
  - tuberculin Z11.1
- specified NEC Z01.89
- tuberculin Z11.1
  - abnormal result R76.11
- vision Z01.00
  - with abnormal findings Z01.01
  - after failed exam Z01.02-
  - infant or child (over 28 days old) Z00.129
    - with abnormal findings Z00.121
- Wassermann Z11.3
  - positive—*see* Serology for syphilis

Testicle, testicular, testes—*see also* Disease, diseased
- feminization syndrome (*see also* Syndrome, androgen insensitivity) E34.51
- migrans Q55.29

Tetanus, tetanic (cephalic) (convulsions) A35

Tetany (due to) R29.0
- associated with rickets E55.0
- hyperpnea R06.4
  - hysterical F44.5
  - psychogenic F45.8
- hyperventilation (*see also* Hyperventilation) R06.4
  - hysterical F44.5
- neonatal (without calcium or magnesium deficiency) P71.3
- psychogenic (conversion reaction) F44.5

Tetralogy of Fallot Q21.3

Tetraplegia (chronic) (*see also* Quadriplegia) G82.50

Thalassemia (anemia) (disease) D56.9
- with other hemoglobinopathy D56.8
- alpha (major) (severe) (triple gene defect) D56.0
  - minor D56.3
  - silent carrier D56.3
  - trait D56.3
- beta (severe) D56.1
  - homozygous D56.1
  - major D56.1
  - minor D56.3
  - trait D56.3
- delta-beta (homozygous) D56.2
  - minor D56.3
  - trait D56.3
- dominant D56.8
- hemoglobin
  - C D56.8
  - E-beta D56.5
- intermedia D56.1
- major D56.1
- minor D56.3
- mixed D56.8
- sickle-cell—*see* Disease, sickle-cell, thalassemia
- specified type NEC D56.8
- trait D56.3
- variants D56.8

Thanatophoric dwarfism or short stature Q77.1

Thaysen-Gee disease (nontropical sprue) K90.0

Thaysen's disease K90.0

Thelitis N61.0

Therapy
- drug, long-term (current) (prophylactic)
  - antibiotics Z79.2
  - anti-inflammatory Z79.1
  - aspirin Z79.82

Therapy, *continued*
- drug, specified NEC Z79.899
- hypoglycemic drugs, oral Z79.84
- insulin Z79.4
- steroids
  - inhaled Z79.51
  - systemic Z79.52

Thermoplegia T67.0

Thickening
- breast N64.59

Thirst, excessive R63.1
- due to deprivation of water T73.1

Thomsen disease G71.12

Threadworm (infection) (infestation) B80

Threatened
- abortion O20.0
  - with subsequent abortion O03.9
- miscarriage O20.0

Thrombocythemia (essential) (hemorrhagic) (idiopathic) (primary) D47.3
- essential D47.3
- idiopathic D47.3
- primary D47.3

Thrombocytopenia, thrombocytopenic D69.6
- with absent radius (TAR) Q87.2
- congenital D69.42
- dilutional D69.59
- due to
  - drugs D69.59
    - heparin induced (HIT) D75.82
  - extracorporeal circulation of blood D69.59
  - (massive) blood transfusion D69.59
  - platelet alloimmunization D69.59
- essential D69.3
- heparin induced (HIT) D75.82
- hereditary D69.42
- idiopathic D69.3
- neonatal, transitory P61.0
  - due to
    - exchange transfusion P61.0
    - idiopathic maternal thrombocytopenia P61.0
    - isoimmunization P61.0
- primary NEC D69.49
  - idiopathic D69.3
- secondary D69.59
- transient neonatal P61.0

Thrombocytosis, essential D47.3
- essential D47.3
- idiopathic D47.3
- primary D47.3
- reactive D75.838
- secondary D75.838
- specified NEC D75.838

Thromboembolism—*see* Embolism

Thrombopathy (Bernard-Soulier) D69.1
- constitutional D68.0
- Willebrand-Jürgens D68.0

Thrombophlebitis I80.9
- calf muscular vein (NOS) I80.25-
- femoral vein (superficial) I80.1-
- femoropopliteal vein I80.0-
- gastrocnemial vein I80.25-
- hepatic (vein) I80.8
- iliac vein (common) (external) (internal) I80.21-
- iliofemoral I80.1-
- leg I80.3
  - superficial I80.0-
- lower extremity I80.299
- peroneal vein I80.24-
- popliteal vein—*see* Phlebitis, leg
- saphenous (greater) (lesser) I80.0-
- soleal vein I80.25-
- specified site NEC I80.8
- tibial vein (anterior) (posterior) I80.23-

Thrombosis, thrombotic (bland) (multiple) (progressive) (silent) (vessel) I82.90
- anus K64.5
- artery, arteries (postinfectional) I74.9
- genital organ
  - female NEC N94.89

Thrombosis, thrombotic, *continued*
- liver (venous) I82.0
  - artery I74.8
  - portal vein I81
- mesenteric (artery) (with gangrene) K55.0
  - vein (inferior) (superior) I81
- perianal venous K64.5
- portal I81
- renal (artery) N28.0
  - vein I82.3
- tricuspid I07.8
- vein (acute) I82.90
  - perianal K64.5
  - renal I82.3
- venous, perianal K64.5

Thrombus—*see* Thrombosis

Thrush—*see also* Candidiasis
- oral B37.0
- newborn P37.5
- vagina B37.3

Thumb—*see also* Disease, diseased
- sucking (child problem) F98.8

Thyroglossal—*see also* Disease, diseased
- cyst Q89.2
- duct, persistent Q89.2

Thyroid (gland) (body)—*see also* Disease, diseased
- lingual Q89.2

Thyroiditis E06.9
- acute (nonsuppurative) (pyogenic) (suppurative) E06.0
- autoimmune E06.3
- chronic (nonspecific) (sclerosing) E06.5
  - with thyrotoxicosis, transient E06.2
  - fibrous E06.5
  - lymphadenoid E06.3
  - lymphocytic E06.3
  - lymphoid E06.3
- de Quervain's E06.1
- drug-induced E06.4
- fibrous (chronic) E06.5
- giant-cell (follicular) E06.1
- granulomatous (de Quervain) (subacute) E06.1
- Hashimoto's (struma lymphomatosa) E06.3
- iatrogenic E06.4
- ligneous E06.5
- lymphocytic (chronic) E06.3
- lymphoid E06.3
- lymphomatous E06.3
- nonsuppurative E06.1
- pseudotuberculous E06.1
- pyogenic E06.0
- radiation E06.4
- Riedel's E06.5
- subacute (granulomatous) E06.1
- suppurative E06.0
- viral E06.1
- woody E06.5

Thyrolyngual duct, persistent Q89.2

Thyrotoxic
- crisis—*see* Thyrotoxicosis
- heart disease or failure (*see also* Thyrotoxicosis) E05.90 *[I43]*
  - with thyroid storm E05.91 *[I43]*
- storm—*see* Thyrotoxicosis

Thyrotoxicosis (recurrent) E05.90
- with
  - goiter (diffuse) E05.00
    - with thyroid storm E05.01
- heart E05.90 *[I43]*
  - with thyroid storm E05.91 *[I43]*
  - failure E05.90 *[I43]*
- neonatal (transient) P72.1
- transient with chronic thyroiditis E06.2

Tibia vara M92.51-

Tic (disorder) F95.9
- child problem F95.0
- compulsive F95.1
- de la Tourette F95.2
- disorder
  - chronic
    - motor F95.1

Tic, *continued*
- vocal F95.1
- combined vocal and multiple motor F95.2
- transient F95.0
- habit F95.9
  - transient of childhood F95.0
- lid, transient of childhood F95.0
- motor-verbal F95.2
- orbicularis F95.8
  - transient of childhood F95.0
- provisional F95.0
- spasm (motor or vocal) F95.9
  - chronic F95.1
  - transient of childhood F95.0

Tick-borne—*see* Disease, diseased

Tietze's disease or syndrome M94.0

Tight, tightness
- anus K62.89
- foreskin (congenital) N47.1
- rectal sphincter K62.89
- urethral sphincter N35.919

Timidity, child F93.8

Tinea (intersecta) (tarsi) B35.9
- asbestina B35.0
- barbae B35.0
- beard B35.0
- black dot B35.0
- capitis B35.0
- corporis B35.4
- cruris B35.6
- flava B36.0
- foot B35.3
- furfuracea B36.0
- imbricata (Tokelau) B35.5
- kerion B35.0
- microsporic—*see* Dermatophytosis
- nodosa B36.-
- pedis B35.3
- scalp B35.0
- specified NEC B35.8
- sycosis B35.0
- tonsurans B35.0
- trichophytic—*see* Dermatophytosis
- unguium B35.1
- versicolor B36.0

Tinnitus NOS H93.1-
- audible H93.1-
- aurium H93.1-
- pulsatile H93.A-
- subjective H93.1-

Tiredness R53.83

Tobacco (nicotine)
- abuse—*see* Tobacco, use
- dependence—*see* Dependence, drug, nicotine
- harmful use Z72.0
- heart—*see* Tobacco, toxic effect
- maternal use, affecting newborn P04.2
- toxic effect—*see* Table of Drugs and Chemicals, by substance, poisoning
  - chewing tobacco—*see* Table of Drugs and Chemicals, by substance, poisoning
  - cigarettes—*see* Table of Drugs and Chemicals, by substance, poisoning
- use Z72.0
  - counseling and surveillance Z71.6
  - history Z87.891
- withdrawal state—*see* Dependence, drug, nicotine F17.203

Tongue—*see also* Disease, diseased
- tie Q38.1

Tonsillitis (acute) (catarrhal) (croupous) (follicular) (gangrenous) (infective) (lacunar) (lingual) (malignant) (membranous) (parenchymatous) (phlegmonous) (pseudomembranous) (purulent) (septic) (subacute) (suppurative) (toxic) (ulcerative) (vesicular) (viral) J03.90
- chronic J35.01
  - with adenoiditis J35.03
- hypertrophic J35.01
  - with adenoiditis J35.03
- recurrent J03.91

Tonsillitis, *continued*
- specified organism NEC J03.80
  - recurrent J03.81
- staphylococcal J03.80
  - recurrent J03.81
- streptococcal J03.00
  - recurrent J03.01

Tooth, teeth—*see* Disease, teeth, diseased

TORCH infection—*see* Infection, congenital
- without active infection P00.2

Torsion
- appendix epididymis N44.04
- appendix testis N44.03
- bile duct (common) (hepatic) K83.8
  - congenital Q44.5
- bowel, colon or intestine K56.2
- epididymis (appendix) N44.04
- gallbladder K82.8
  - congenital Q44.1
- hydatid of Morgagni
  - male N44.03
- Meckel's diverticulum (congenital) Q43.0
- mesentery K56.2
- omentum K56.2
- organ or site, congenital NEC—*see* Anomaly, by site
- ovary (pedicle) N83.51-
  - with fallopian tube N83.53
  - congenital Q50.2
- penis (acquired) N48.82
  - congenital Q55.63
- spermatic cord N44.02
  - extravaginal N44.01
  - intravaginal N44.02
- testis, testicle N44.00
  - appendix N44.03
- tibia—*see* Deformity, limb, specified type NEC, lower leg

Torticollis (intermittent) (spastic) M43.6
- congenital (sternomastoid) Q68.0
- due to birth injury P15.8
- hysterical F44.4
- ocular R29.891
- psychogenic F45.8
  - conversion reaction F44.4
- rheumatic M43.6
- traumatic, current S13.4

Tortuous
- ureter N13.8

Tourette's syndrome F95.2

Tourniquet syndrome—*see* Constriction, external, by site

Tower skull Q75.0
- with exophthalmos Q87.0

Toxemia
- erysipelatous—*see* Erysipelas
- food—*see* Poisoning, food
- staphylococcal, due to food A05.0

Toxic (poisoning) (*see also* Disease, diseased) T65.91
- effect—*see* Table of Drugs and Chemicals, by substance, poisoning
- shock syndrome A48.3

Toxicity—*see* Table of Drugs and Chemicals, by substance, poisoning
- fava bean D55.0
- food, noxious—*see* Poisoning, food
- from drug or nonmedicinal substance—*see* Table of Drugs and Chemicals, by drug

Toxicosis—*see also* Toxemia
- capillary, hemorrhagic D69.0

Toxoplasma, toxoplasmosis (acquired) B58.9
- with
  - meningoencephalitis B58.2
  - ocular involvement B58.00
  - other organ involvement B58.89
  - pneumonia, pneumonitis B58.3
- congenital (acute) (subacute) (chronic) P37.1
- maternal, manifest toxoplasmosis in infant (acute) (subacute) (chronic) P37.1

Tracheitis (catarrhal) (infantile) (membranous) (plastic) (septal) (suppurative) (viral) J04.10
- with

Tracheitis, *continued*
  - bronchitis (15 years of age and above) J40
    - acute or subacute—*see* Bronchitis, acute
    - under 15 years of age J20.9
  - laryngitis (acute) J04.2
    - chronic J37.1
- acute J04.10
  - with obstruction J04.11
- chronic J42
  - with
    - laryngitis (chronic) J37.1

Tracheomalacia J39.8
- congenital Q32.0

Tracheopharyngitis (acute) J06.9
- chronic J42

Trachoma, trachomatous A71.9
- Türck's J37.0

Train sickness T75.3

Trait
- Hb-S D57.3
- hemoglobin
  - abnormal NEC D58.2
    - with thalassemia D56.3
  - C—*see* Disease, hemoglobin or Hb
  - S (Hb-S) D57.3
- Lepore D56.3
- sickle-cell D57.3
  - with elliptocytosis or spherocytosis D57.3

Transaminasemia R74.01

Transfusion
- associated (red blood cell) hemochromatosis E83.111
- reaction (adverse)—*see* Complications, transfusion
- related acute lung injury (TRALI) J95.84

Transient (meaning homeless) (*see also* Disease, diseased) Z59.00

Translocation
- balanced autosomal Q95.9
  - in normal individual Q95.0
- chromosomes NEC Q99.8
  - balanced and insertion in normal individual Q95.0
- Down syndrome Q90.2
- trisomy
  - 13 Q91.6
  - 18 Q91.2
  - 21 Q90.2

Transplant (ed) (status) Z94.9
- awaiting organ Z76.82
- bone Z94.6
  - marrow Z94.81
- candidate Z76.82
- heart Z94.1
  - valve Z95.2
    - prosthetic Z95.2
    - specified NEC Z95.4
    - xenogenic Z95.3
- intestine Z94.82
- kidney Z94.0
- liver Z94.4
- lung(s) Z94.2
  - and heart Z94.3
- organ (failure) (infection) (rejection) Z94.9
  - removal status Z98.85
- pancreas Z94.83
- skin Z94.5
- social Z60.3
- specified organ or tissue NEC Z94.89
- stem cells Z94.84
- tissue Z94.9

Transposition (congenital)—*see also* Malposition, congenital
- abdominal viscera Q89.3
- aorta (dextra) Q20.3
- great vessels (complete) (partial) Q20.3
- heart Q24.0
  - with complete transposition of viscera Q89.3
- scrotum Q55.23
- stomach Q40.2
  - with general transposition of viscera Q89.3
- vessels, great (complete) (partial) Q20.3
- viscera (abdominal) (thoracic) Q89.3

Transsexualism F64.0

Transvestism, transvestitism (dual-role) F64.1

Trauma, traumatism—*see also* Injury
- acoustic—*see* subcategory H83.3
- occlusal
  - primary K08.81
  - secondary K08.82

Tremor(s) R25.1
- hysterical F44.4
- psychogenic (conversion reaction) F44.4

Triad
- Kartagener's Q89.3

Trichocephaliasis, trichocephalosis B79

Trichocephalus infestation B79

Trichomoniasis A59.9
- bladder A59.03
- cervix A59.09
- seminal vesicles A59.09
- specified site NEC A59.8
- urethra A59.03
- urogenitalis A59.00
- vagina A59.01
- vulva A59.01

Trigger finger (acquired)
- congenital Q74.0

Triphalangeal thumb Q74.0

Triple—*see also* Anomaly
- X, female Q97.0

Trismus R25.2

Trisomy (syndrome) Q92.9
- 13 (partial) Q91.7
  - meiotic nondisjunction Q91.4
- 18 (partial) Q91.3
  - meiotic nondisjunction Q91.0
- 21 (partial) Q90.9

Trombiculosis, trombiculiasis, trombidiosis B88.0

Trophoneurosis NEC G96.89

Trouble—*see also* Disease
- nervous R45.0

Truancy, childhood
- from school Z72.810

Truncus
- arteriosus (persistent) Q20.0
- communis Q20.0

Trunk—*see* Disease, diseased

Tryptasemia, hereditary alpha D89.44

Tuberculoma—*see also* Tuberculosis
- brain A17.81
- meninges (cerebral) (spinal) A17.1
- spinal cord A17.81

Tuberculosis, tubercular, tuberculous (calcification) (calcified) (caseous) (chromogenic acid-fast bacilli) (degeneration) (fibrocaseous) (fistula) (interstitial) (isolated circumscribed lesions) (necrosis) (parenchymatous) (ulcerative) A15.9
- abscess (respiratory) A15.9
  - latent Z22.7
  - meninges (cerebral) (spinal) A17.0
  - scrofulous A18.2
- arachnoid A17.0
- axilla, axillary (gland) A18.2
- cachexia A15.9
- cerebrospinal A17.81
  - meninges A17.0
- cervical (lymph gland or node) A18.2
- contact Z20.1
- dura (mater) (cerebral) (spinal) A17.0
  - abscess (cerebral) (spinal) A17.81
- exposure (to) Z20.1
- glandular, general A18.2
- immunological findings only A15.7
- infection A15.9
  - without clinical manifestation A15.7
- infraclavicular gland A18.2
- inguinal gland A18.2
- inguinalis A18.2
- latent Z22.7
- leptomeninges, leptomeningitis (cerebral) (spinal) A17.0
- lymph gland or node (peripheral) A18.2

Tuberculosis, tubercular, tuberculous, *continued*
- – cervical A18.2
- • marasmus A15.9
- • neck gland A18.2
- • meninges, meningitis (basilar) (cerebral) (cerebrospinal) (spinal) A17.0
- • pachymeningitis A17.0
- • respiratory A15.9
  - – primary A15.7
  - – specified site NEC A15.8
- • scrofulous A18.2
- • senile A15.9
- • spine, spinal (column) A18.01
  - – cord A17.81
  - – medulla A17.81
  - – membrane A17.0
  - – meninges A17.0
- • supraclavicular gland A18.2
- • unspecified site A15.9

Tuberous sclerosis (brain) Q85.1

Tumefaction—*see also* Swelling
- • liver—*see* Hypertrophy, liver

Tumor—*see also* Neoplasm, unspecified behavior, by site in Table of Neoplasms in the complete *ICD-10-CM* manual
- • Cock's peculiar L72.3
- • glomus D18.00
  - – skin D18.01
  - – specified site NEC D18.09
- • Grawitz's C64.-
- • neuroectodermal (peripheral)—*see* Neoplasm, malignant, by site in Table of Neoplasms in the complete *ICD-10-CM* manual
  - – primitive
    - ■ specified site—*see* Neoplasm, malignant, by site in Table of Neoplasms in the complete *ICD-10-CM* manual
    - ■ unspecified site C71.9
- • phantom F45.8
- • sternomastoid (congenital) Q68.0
- • turban D23.4
- • Wilms' C64.-

Tumor lysis syndrome (following antineoplastic chemotherapy) (spontaneous) NEC E88.3

Tungiasis B88.1

Tunica vasculosa lentis Q12.2

Turban tumor D23.4

Türck's trachoma J37.0

Turner-like syndrome Q87.19

Turner's syndrome Q96.9

Turner-Ullrich syndrome Q96.9

Twist, twisted
- • bowel, colon or intestine K56.2
- • mesentery K56.2
- • omentum K56.2
- • organ or site, congenital NEC—*see* Anomaly, by site

Tylosis (acquired) L84
- • palmaris et plantaris (congenital) (inherited) Q82.8
  - – acquired L85.1

Tympanism R14.0

Tympanites (abdominal) (intestinal) R14.0

Tympanitis—*see* Myringitis

Tympany
- • abdomen R14.0
- • chest R09.89

Typhus (fever)
- • Sao Paulo A77.0

U

Ulcer, ulcerated, ulcerating, ulceration, ulcerative
- • anorectal K62.6
- • anus (sphincter) (solitary) K62.6
- • aphthous (oral) (recurrent) K12.0
- • bleeding K27.4
- • breast N61.1
- • buccal (cavity) (traumatic) K12.1
- • cervix (uteri) (decubitus) (trophic) N86
  - – with cervicitis N72
- • Dieulafoy's K25.0

Ulcer, ulcerated, ulcerating, ulceration, ulcerative, *continued*
- • duodenum, duodenal (eroded) (peptic) K26.9
  - – with
    - ■ hemorrhage K26.4
      - ~ and perforation K26.6
    - ■ perforation K26.5
  - – acute K26.3
    - ■ with
      - ~ hemorrhage K26.0
      - ◊ and perforation K26.2
      - ~ perforation K26.1
  - – chronic K26.7
    - ■ with
      - ~ hemorrhage K26.4
      - ◊ and perforation K26.6
      - ~ perforation K26.5
- • dysenteric A09
- • esophagus (peptic) K22.10
  - – due to
    - ■ gastrointestinal reflux disease K21.0-
- • frenum (tongue) K14.0
- • hemorrhoid (*see also* Hemorrhoids, by degree) K64.8
- • intestine, intestinal K63.3
  - – rectum K62.6
- • lip K13.0
- • meatus (urinarius) N34.2
- • Meckel's diverticulum Q43.0
- • oral mucosa (traumatic) K12.1
- • palate (soft) K12.1
- • peptic (site unspecified) K27.9
  - – with
    - ■ hemorrhage K27.4
      - ~ and perforation K27.6
    - ■ perforation K27.5
  - – acute K27.3
    - ■ with
      - ~ hemorrhage K27.0
      - ◊ and perforation K27.2
      - ~ perforation K27.1
  - – chronic K27.7
    - ■ with
      - ~ hemorrhage K27.4
      - ◊ and perforation K27.6
      - ~ perforation K27.5
  - – esophagus K22.10
    - ■ with bleeding K22.11
  - – newborn P78.82
- • perforating K27.5
- • peritonsillar J35.8
- • pressure (pressure area) L89.9-
  - – ankle L89.5-
  - – back L89.1-
  - – buttock L89.3-
  - – coccyx L89.15-
  - – contiguous site of back, buttock, hip L89.4-
  - – elbow L89.0-
  - – face L89.81-
  - – head L89.81-
  - – heel L89.6-
  - – hip L89.2-
  - – sacral region (tailbone) L89.15-
  - – specified site NEC L89.89-
  - – stage 1 (healing) (pre-ulcer skin changes limited to persistent focal edema)
    - ■ ankle L89.5-
    - ■ back L89.1-
    - ■ buttock L89.3-
    - ■ coccyx L89.15-
    - ■ contiguous site of back, buttock, hip L89.4-
    - ■ elbow L89.0-
    - ■ face L89.81-
    - ■ head L89.81-
    - ■ heel L89.6-
    - ■ hip L89.2-
    - ■ sacral region (tailbone) L89.15-
    - ■ specified site NEC L89.89-
  - – stage 2 (healing) (abrasion, blister, partial thickness skin loss involving epidermis and/or dermis)
    - ■ ankle L89.5-
    - ■ back L89.1-
    - ■ buttock L89.3-
    - ■ coccyx L89.15-

Ulcer, ulcerated, ulcerating, ulceration, ulcerative, *continued*
- ■ contiguous site of back, buttock, hip L89.4-
- ■ elbow L89.0-
- ■ face L89.81-
- ■ head L89.81-
- ■ heel L89.6-
- ■ hip L89.2-
- ■ sacral region (tailbone) L89.15-
- ■ specified site NEC L89.89-
  - – stage 3 (healing) (full thickness skin loss involving damage or necrosis of subcutaneous tissue)
    - ■ ankle L89.5-
    - ■ back L89.1-
    - ■ buttock L89.3-
    - ■ coccyx L89.15-
    - ■ contiguous site of back, buttock, hip L89.4-
    - ■ elbow L89.0-
    - ■ face L89.81-
    - ■ head L89.81-
    - ■ heel L89.6-
    - ■ hip L89.2-
    - ■ sacral region (tailbone) L89.15-
    - ■ specified site NEC L89.89-
  - – stage 4 (healing) (necrosis of soft tissues through to underlying muscle, tendon, or bone)
    - ■ ankle L89.5-
    - ■ back L89.1-
    - ■ buttock L89.3-
    - ■ coccyx L89.15-
    - ■ contiguous site of back, buttock, hip L89.4-
    - ■ elbow L89.0-
    - ■ face L89.81-
    - ■ head L89.81-
    - ■ heel L89.6-
    - ■ hip L89.2-
    - ■ sacral region (tailbone) L89.15-
    - ■ specified site NEC L89.89-
- • rectum (sphincter) (solitary) K62.6
  - – stercoraceous, stercoral K62.6
- • scrofulous (tuberculous) A18.2
- • scrotum N50.89
  - – varicose I86.1
- • solitary, anus or rectum (sphincter) K62.6
- • sore throat J02.9
  - – streptococcal J02.0
- • stercoraceous, stercoral K63.3
  - – anus or rectum K62.6
- • stomach (eroded) (peptic) (round) K25.9
  - – with
    - ■ hemorrhage K25.4
      - ~ and perforation K25.6
    - ■ perforation K25.5
  - – acute K25.3
    - ■ with
      - ~ hemorrhage K25.0
      - ◊ and perforation K25.2
      - ~ perforation K25.1
  - – chronic K25.7
    - ■ with
      - ~ hemorrhage K25.4
      - ◊ and perforation K25.6
      - ~ perforation K25.5
- • stomatitis K12.1
- • strumous (tuberculous) A18.2
- • tongue (traumatic) K14.0
- • tonsil J35.8
- • turbinate J34.89
- • uterus N85.8
  - – cervix N86
    - ■ with cervicitis N72
  - – neck N86
    - ■ with cervicitis N72
- • valve, heart I33.0
- • varicose (lower limb, any part)—*see also* Varix
  - – scrotum I86.1

Ulcerosa scarlatina A38.8

Ulcus—*see also* Ulcer
- • durum (syphilitic) A51.0
  - – extragenital A51.2

Ulerythema
- ophryogenes, congenital Q84.2
- sycosiforme L73.8

Ullrich (-Bonnevie) (-Turner) syndrome Q87.19

Ullrich-Feichtiger syndrome Q87.0

Unavailability (of)
- medical facilities (at) Z75.3
  - due to
    - lack of services at home Z75.0
  - home Z75.0

Underdevelopment—*see also* Undeveloped
- sexual E30.0

Underdosing (*see also* Table of Drugs and Chemicals, categories T36–T50, with final character 6) Z91.14
- intentional NEC Z91.128
  - due to financial hardship of patient Z91.120
- unintentional NEC Z91.138

Underimmunization status Z28.3

Underweight R63.6
- for gestational age—*see* Light for dates

Underwood's disease P83.0

Undeveloped, undevelopment—*see also* Hypoplasia
- brain (congenital) Q02
- cerebral (congenital) Q02
- heart Q24.8
- lung Q33.6
- uterus E30.0

Undiagnosed (disease) R69

Unguis incarnatus L60.0

Unstable
- hip (congenital) Q65.6

Unsteadiness on feet R26.81

Untruthfulness, child problem F91.8

Upbringing, institutional Z62.22
- away from parents NEC Z62.29
- in care of non-parental family member Z62.21
- in foster care Z62.21
- in orphanage or group home Z62.22
- in welfare custody Z62.21

Upper respiratory—*see* Disease, diseased

Upset
- gastric K30
- gastrointestinal K30
  - psychogenic F45.8
- intestinal (large) (small) K59.9
  - psychogenic F45.8
- mental F48.9
- stomach K30
  - psychogenic F45.8

Uremia, uremic N19
- chronic NOS (*see also* Disease, kidney, chronic) N18.9
  - due to hypertension—*see* Hypertensive, kidney
- congenital P96.0

Ureteralgia N23

Ureteritis N28.89
- due to calculus N20.1
  - with calculus, kidney N20.2
    - with hydronephrosis N13.2
- nonspecific N28.89

Ureterocele N28.89
- congenital (orthotopic) Q62.31

Urethralgia R39.89

Urethritis (anterior) (posterior) N34.2
- candidal B37.41
- chlamydial A56.01
- diplococcal (gonococcal) A54.01
  - with abscess (accessory gland) (periurethral) A54.1
- gonococcal A54.01
  - with abscess (accessory gland) (periurethral) A54.1
- nongonococcal N34.1
- nonspecific N34.1
- nonvenereal N34.1
- specified NEC N34.2
- trichomonal or due to Trichomonas (vaginalis) A59.03

Urethrorrhea R36.9

Urgency
- fecal R15.2
- urinary R39.15

Uric acid in blood (increased) E79.0

Uricacidemia (asymptomatic) E79.0

Uricemia (asymptomatic) E79.0

Uricosuria R82.998

Urination
- frequent R35.0

Urine
- blood in—*see* Hematuria
- discharge, excessive R35.89
- enuresis, nonorganic origin F98.0
- frequency R35.0
- incontinence R32
  - nonorganic origin F98.0
- intermittent stream R39.198
- pus in N39.0
- retention or stasis R33.9
  - psychogenic F45.8
- secretion
  - deficient R34
  - excessive R35.89
  - frequency R35.0
- stream
  - intermittent R39.198
  - slowing R39.198
  - weak R39.12

Urodialysis R34

Uropathy N39.9
- obstructive N13.9
  - specified NEC N13.8
- reflux N13.9
  - specified NEC N13.8

Urticaria L50.9
- with angioneurotic edema T78.3
- allergic L50.0
- cholinergic L50.5
- chronic L50.8
- due to
  - cold or heat L50.2
  - drugs L50.0
  - food L50.0
  - inhalants L50.0
  - plants L50.6
  - serum (*see also* Reaction, serum) T80.69
- factitial L50.3
- giant T78.3
- gigantea T78.3
- idiopathic L50.1
- larynx T78.3
- neonatorum P83.88
- pigmentosa D47.01
  - congenital Q82.2
  - of neonatal onset Q82.2
- nonallergic L50.1
- pigmentosa D47.01
  - congenital Q82.2
  - of neonatal onset Q82.2
- recurrent periodic L50.8
- serum (*see also* Reaction, serum) T80.69
- specified type NEC L50.8
- thermal (cold) (heat) L50.2
- vibratory L50.4

Use (of)
- alcohol Z72.89
  - harmful—*see* Abuse, alcohol
- caffeine—*see* Use, stimulant NEC
- cannabis F12.90
  - withdrawal F12.93
- inhalants F18.9-
- stimulant NEC F15.90
  - with
    - withdrawal F15.93
  - harmful—*see* Abuse, drug, stimulant NEC
- tobacco Z72.0
  - with dependence—*see* Dependence, drug, nicotine
- volatile solvents (*see also* Use, inhalant) F18.90
  - harmful—*see* Abuse, drug, inhalant

Uveitis (anterior)
- due to toxoplasmosis (acquired) B58.09
  - congenital P37.1

Uveoparotitis D86.89

Uvulitis (acute) (catarrhal) (chronic) (membranous) (suppurative) (ulcerative) K12.2

V

Vaccination (prophylactic)
- complication or reaction—*see* Complications, vaccination
- delayed Z28.9
- encounter for Z23
- not done—*see* Immunization, not done, because (of)

Vaccinia (generalized) (localized) T88.1
- congenital P35.8

Vacuum, in sinus (accessory) (nasal) J34.89

Vagabond's disease B85.1

Vaginitis (acute) (circumscribed) (diffuse) (emphysematous) (nonvenereal) (ulcerative) N76.0
- with abscess (accessory gland) (periurethral) A54.1
- bacterial N76.0
- blennorrhagic (gonococcal) A54.02
- candidal B37.3
- chlamydial A56.02
- chronic N76.1
- due to Trichomonas (vaginalis) A59.01
- gonococcal A54.02
- in (due to)
  - candidiasis B37.3
  - herpesviral (herpes simplex) infection A60.04
  - pinworm infection B80 [N77.1]
- monilial B37.3
- mycotic (candidal) B37.3
- syphilitic (early) A51.0
  - late A52.76
- trichomonal A59.01

Vaginosis—*see* Vaginitis

Valve, valvular (formation)—*see also* Disease, diseased
- cerebral ventricle (communicating) in situ Z98.2

Van der Hoeve (-de Kleyn) **syndrome** Q78.0

Vapor asphyxia or suffocation
- specified agent—*see* Table of Drugs and Chemicals

Variants, thalassemic D56.8

Varicella B01.9
- with
  - complications NEC B01.89
  - encephalitis B01.11
  - encephalomyelitis B01.11
  - meningitis B01.0
  - myelitis B01.12
  - pneumonia B01.2
- congenital P35.8

Varices—*see* Varix

Varicocele (scrotum) (thrombosed) I86.1
- spermatic cord (ulcerated) I86.1

Varicose
- ulcer
  - anus (*see also* Hemorrhoids) K64.8
  - scrotum I86.1

Varix (lower limb) I83.9-
- esophagus (idiopathic) (primary) (ulcerated) I85.00
  - bleeding I85.01
  - congenital Q27.8
- scrotum (ulcerated) I86.1

Vascular—*see also* Disease, diseased
- spider I78.1

Vasculitis I77.6
- allergic D69.0
- systemic M31.8

Vasovagal attack (paroxysmal) R55
- psychogenic F45.8

Vegetation, vegetative
- adenoid (nasal fossa) J35.8
- endocarditis (acute) (any valve) (subacute) I33.0
- heart (mycotic) (valve) I33.0

Venereal
- disease A64

Venom, venomous—*see* Table of Drugs and Chemicals, by animal or substance, poisoning

Ventriculitis (cerebral) (*see also* Encephalitis) G04.90

Ventriculostomy status Z98.2

Vernet's syndrome G52.7

Verruca (due to HPV) (filiformis) (simplex) (viral) (vulgaris) B07.9
- acuminata A63.0
- plana B07.8
- plantaris B07.0
- venereal A63.0

Vertigo R42
- aural H81.31-
- benign paroxysmal (positional) H81.1-
- central (origin) H81.4
- cerebral H81.4
- laryngeal R05.4
- peripheral NEC H81.39-
  - malignant H81.4

Vesiculitis (seminal) N49.0
- trichomonal A59.09

Vestibulitis (ear) (*see also* subcategory) H83.0
- nose (external) J34.89
- vulvar N94.810

Villaret's syndrome G52.7

Virilism (adrenal) E25.9
- congenital E25.0

Virilization (female) (suprarenal) E25.9
- congenital E25.0
- isosexual E28.2

Virus, viral—*see also* Disease, diseased
- as cause of disease classified elsewhere B97.89
- cytomegalovirus B25.9
- human immunodeficiency (HIV)—*see* Human, immunodeficiency virus (HIV) disease
- infection—*see* Infection, virus
- respiratory syncytial (RSV)
  - as cause of disease classified elsewhere B97.4
  - bronchiolitis J21.0
  - bronchitis J20.5
  - bronchopneumonia J12.1
  - otitis media H65.- [B97.4]
  - pneumonia J12.1
  - upper respiratory infection J06.9 [B97.4]
- specified NEC B34.8
- swine influenza (viruses that normally cause infections in pigs) (*see also* Influenza, due to, identified novel influenza A virus) J09.X2
- West Nile (fever) A92.30
  - with
    - complications NEC A92.39
    - cranial nerve disorders A92.32
    - encephalitis A92.31
    - encephalomyelitis A92.31
    - neurologic manifestation NEC A92.32
    - optic neuritis A92.32
    - polyradiculitis A92.32
- Zika virus disease A92.5

Vision, visual
- blurred, blurring H53.8
  - hysterical F44.6
- defect, defective NEC H54.7
- disorientation (syndrome) H53.8
- disturbance H53.9
  - hysterical F44.6
- double H53.2
- examination Z01.00
  - with abnormal findings Z01.01
  - after failed exam Z01.02-
- hallucinations R44.1

Vitality, lack or want of R53.83
- newborn P96.89

Vitamin deficiency—*see* Deficiency, vitamin

Vitelline duct, persistent Q43.0

Vitiligo L80

Volvulus (bowel) (colon) (intestine) K56.2
- with perforation K56.2
- congenital Q43.8
- duodenum K31.5
  - without refractory migraine G43.A0

Vomiting R11.10
- with nausea R11.2
- bilious (cause unknown) R11.14
  - in newborn P92.01
- cyclical, in migraine G43.A0
  - with refractory migraine G43.A1
  - intractable G43.A1
  - not intractable G43.A0
  - psychogenic F50.89
  - without refractory migraine G43.A0
- cyclical syndrome NOS (unrelated to migraine) R11.1
- fecal matter R11.13
- following gastrointestinal surgery K91.0
  - psychogenic F50.89
- functional K31.89
- hysterical F50.89
- nervous F50.89
- neurotic F50.89
- newborn NEC P92.09
  - bilious P92.01
- periodic R11.10
  - psychogenic F50.89
- projectile R11.12
- psychogenic F50.89
- without nausea R11.11

Von Hippel (-Lindau) **disease or syndrome** Q85.8

Von Recklinghausen
- disease (neurofibromatosis) Q85.01

Vrolik's disease Q78.0

Vulvitis (acute) (allergic) (atrophic) (hypertrophic) (intertriginous) (senile) N76.2
- adhesive, congenital Q52.79
- blennorrhagic (gonococcal) A54.02
- candidal B37.3
- chlamydial A56.02
- gonococcal A54.02
  - with abscess (accessory gland) (periurethral) A54.1
- monilial B37.3
- syphilitic (early) A51.0
  - late A52.76
- trichomonal A59.01

Vulvodynia N94.819
- specified NEC N94.818

Vulvorectal—*see* Disease, diseased

Vulvovaginitis (acute)—*see* Vaginitis

W

Waiting list
- for organ transplant Z76.82

Walking
- difficulty R26.2
  - psychogenic F44.4
- sleep F51.3
  - hysterical F44.89

Wall, abdominal—*see* Disease, diseased

Wandering
- gallbladder, congenital Q44.1
- in diseases classified elsewhere Z91.83

Wart (due to HPV) (filiform) (infectious) (viral) B07.9
- anogenital region (venereal) A63.0
- common B07.8
- external genital organs (venereal) A63.0
- flat B07.8
- plantar B07.0
- venereal A63.0

Water
- lack of T73.1
  - safe drinking Z58.6

Waterbrash R12

Weak, weakening, weakness (generalized) R53.1
- bladder (sphincter) R32
- mind F70
- muscle M62.81

Weak, weakening, weakness, *continued*
- newborn P96.89
- urinary stream R39.12

Weaver's syndrome Q87.3

Web, webbed (congenital)
- fingers Q70.1-
- toes Q70.3-

Weber-Cockayne syndrome (epidermolysis bullosa) Q81.8

Weber-Osler syndrome I78.0

Weight
- 1000–2499 grams at birth (low)—*see* Low, birthweight
- 999 grams or less at birth (extremely low)—*see* Low, birthweight, extreme
- and length below 10th percentile for gestational age P05.1-
- below 10th percentile but length above 10th percentile P05.0-
- gain (abnormal) (excessive) R63.5
- loss (abnormal) (cause unknown) R63.4

Weil (I)-Marchesani syndrome Q87.19

Wen—*see* Cyst, sebaceous

Wenckebach's block or phenomenon I44.1

Werdnig-Hoffmann syndrome (muscular atrophy) G12.0

Werlhof's disease D69.3

Wernicke's
- developmental aphasia F80.2

West's syndrome—*see* Epilepsy, spasms

Wet
- lung (syndrome), newborn P22.1

Wheal—*see* Urticaria

Wheezing R06.2

Whiplash injury S13.4

Whipple's disease (*see also* subcategory M14.8-) K90.81

Whistling face Q87.0

White—*see also* Disease, diseased
- kidney, small N03.9
- mouth B37.0

Whitehead L70.0

Whitlow—*see also* Cellulitis
- with lymphangitis—*see* Lymphangitis, digit
- herpesviral B00.89

Whooping cough A37.90
- with pneumonia A37.91

Williams syndrome Q93.82

Wilms' tumor C64.-

Wiskott-Aldrich syndrome D82.0

Withdrawal state—*see also* Dependence, drug by type, with withdrawal
- newborn
  - correct therapeutic substance properly administered P96.2
  - infant of dependent mother P96.1
- therapeutic substance, neonatal P96.2

Witts' anemia D50.8

Wolff-Parkinson-White syndrome I45.6

Wool sorter's disease A22.1

Word
- blindness (congenital) (developmental) F81.0
- deafness (congenital) (developmental) H93.25

Worries R45.82

Wound, open T14.8

See Bite, Laceration, or Puncture by site for types of wounds not referenced here.
- abdomen, abdominal
  - wall S31.109
- ankle S91.0-
- antecubital space S51.0-
- anterior chamber, eye—*see* Wound, open, ocular
- anus S31.83-
  - bite S31.835
- arm (upper) S41.1-
  - forearm S51.8-
- axilla S41.10-

Wound, open, *continued*
- back—*see also* Wound, open, thorax, back
  - lower S31.000
- buttock S31.8-
  - left S31.82-
  - right S31.81-
- calf S81.8-
- canaliculus lacrimalis S01.10-
- canthus, eye S01.10-
- cheek (external) S01.4-
- chest wall—*see* Wound, open, thorax
- chin S01.8-
- choroid—*see* Wound, open, ocular
- ciliary body (eye)—*see* Wound, open, ocular
- clitoris S31.4-
  - bite S31.45
- conjunctiva—*see* Wound, open, ocular
- cornea—*see* Wound, open, ocular
- costal region—*see* Wound, open, thorax
- Descemet's membrane—*see* Wound, open, ocular
- digit(s)
  - foot—*see* Wound, open, toe
  - hand—*see* Wound, open, finger
- ear (canal) (external)
  - with amputation—*see* Amputation, traumatic, ear
  - drum S09.2-
- elbow S51.0-
- epididymis—*see* Wound, open, testis
- epiglottis S11.80
- eye—*see* Wound, open, ocular
- eyeball—*see* Wound, open, ocular
- eyebrow S01.10-
- eyelid S01.10-
- face NEC—*see* Wound, open, head, specified site NEC
- finger(s) S61.2-
  - with
    - amputation—*see* Amputation, traumatic, finger
    - damage to nail S61.3-
  - index S61.2-
    - with
      - ~ damage to nail S61.3-
    - left S61.2-
      - ~ with
        - ◊ damage to nail S61.3-
    - right S61.2-
      - ~ with
        - ◊ damage to nail S61.3-
  - little S61.2-
    - with
      - ~ damage to nail S61.3-
    - left S61.2-
      - ~ with damage to nail S61.3-
    - right S61.2-
      - ~ with damage to nail S61.3-
  - middle S61.2-
    - with
      - ~ damage to nail S61.3-
    - left S61.2-
      - ~ with damage to nail S61.3-
    - right S61.2-
      - ~ with damage to nail S61.3-
  - ring S61.2-
    - with
      - ~ damage to nail S61.3-
    - left S61.2-
      - ~ with damage to nail S61.3-
    - right S61.2-
      - ~ with damage to nail S61.3-
- flank—*see* Wound, open
- foot (except toe(s) alone) S91.3-
  - toe—*see* Wound, open, toe
- forearm S51.8-
  - elbow only S51.0-
- forehead S01.8-
- genital organs, external
  - female
    - vagina S31.4-
    - vulva S31.4-
  - male
    - penis S31.2-
    - scrotum S31.3-
    - testes S31.3-

Wound, open, *continued*
- globe (eye)—*see* Wound, open, ocular
- groin—*see* Wound, open
- gum—*see* Wound, open, oral cavity
- hand S61.4-
  - finger(s)—*see* Wound, open, finger
  - thumb—*see* Wound, open, thumb
- head S01.90
  - cheek S01.4-
  - ear S01.3-
  - eyelid S01.10-
  - lip S01.5-
  - nose S01.2-
  - oral cavity—*see* Wound, open, oral cavity
  - scalp—*see* Wound, open, scalp
  - specified site NEC S01.8-
  - temporomandibular area S01.4-
- heel S91.3-
- hip S71.0-
- hymen S31.4-
- instep S91.3-
- interscapular region—*see* Wound, open, thorax, back
- intraocular—*see* Wound, open, ocular
- iris—*see* Wound, open, ocular
- jaw S01.8-
- knee S81.0-
- labium (majus) (minus)—*see* Wound, open, vulva
- lacrimal duct S01.10-
- leg (lower) S81.8-
  - ankle S91.0-
  - foot S91.3-
  - knee S81.0-
  - toe—*see* Wound, open, toe
  - upper S71.1-
- lip S01.5-
- lower back—*see* Wound, open, back, lower
- lumbar region—*see* Wound, open, back, lower
- malar region—*see* Wound, open, head, specified site NEC
- mastoid region—*see* Wound, open, head, specified site NEC
- mouth—*see* Wound, open, oral cavity
- nail
  - finger—*see* Wound, open, finger, with, damage to nail
  - toe—*see* Wound, open, toe, with, damage to nail
- nape (neck)—*see* Wound, open, neck
- nasal (septum) (sinus) S01.20
- nasopharynx S01.8-
- neck S11.9-
  - involving
  - specified site NEC S11.80
- nose (septum) (sinus) S01.20
- ocular S05.9-
  - periocular area S01.10-
  - specified NEC S05.8X-
- oral cavity S01.5-
  - bite S01.552
- orbit—*see* Wound, open, ocular, orbit
- palate—*see* Wound, open, oral cavity
- palm S61.4-
- pelvis, pelvic—*see also* Wound, open, back, lower
  - girdle—*see* Wound, open, hip
- penetrating—*see* Puncture, by site
- penis S31.2-
  - bite S31.25
- periocular area (with or without lacrimal passages) S01.10-
- phalanges
  - finger—*see* Wound, open, finger
  - toe—*see* Wound, open, toe
- pinna S01.3-
- popliteal space S81.0-
- prepuce—*see* Wound, open, penis
- pubic region—*see* Wound, open, back, lower
- pudendum—*see* Wound, open, genital organs, external
- rectovaginal septum—*see* Wound, open, vagina
- sacral region—*see* Wound, open, back, lower
- sacroiliac region—*see* Wound, open, back, lower
- salivary gland—*see* Wound, open, oral cavity
- scalp S01.0-
  - bite S01.05

Wound, open, *continued*
- scalpel, newborn (birth injury) P15.8
- scapular region S41.0-
- sclera—*see* Wound, open, ocular
- scrotum S31.3-
  - bite S31.35
- shin S81.80-
- shoulder S41.0-
- skin NOS T14.8
- spermatic cord—*see* Wound, open, testis
- sternal region—*see* Wound, open, thorax, front
- submaxillary region S01.8-
- submental region S01.8-
- subungual
  - finger(s)—*see* Wound, open, finger
  - toe(s)—*see* Wound, open, toe
- supraclavicular region—*see* Wound, open, neck, specified site NEC
- temple, temporal region S01.8-
- temporomandibular area—*see* Wound, open, cheek
- testis S31.3-
  - bite S31.35
- thigh S71.10-
- thorax, thoracic (wall) S21.9-
  - back S21.2-
  - front S21.1-
- throat—*see* Wound, open, neck
- thumb S61.0
  - with
    - damage to nail S61.1-
  - left S61.0-
    - with
      - ~ damage to nail S61.1-
  - right S61.0-
    - with
      - ~ damage to nail S61.1-
- toe(s) S91.1-
  - with
    - damage to nail S91.2-
  - bite—*see* Bite, toe
  - great S91.1-
    - with
    - damage to nail S91.2-
    - left S91.1-
      - ~ with
        - ◊ damage to nail S91.2-
    - right S91.1-
      - ~ with
        - ◊ damage to nail S91.2-
  - lesser S91.1-
    - with
      - ~ damage to nail S91.2-
    - left S91.1-
      - ~ with
        - ◊ damage to nail S91.2-
    - right S91.1-
      - ~ with
        - ◊ damage to nail S91.2-
- tongue—*see* Wound, open, oral cavity
- tunica vaginalis—*see* Wound, open, testis
- tympanum, tympanic membrane S09.2-
- umbilical region—*see* Wound, open, abdomen
- uvula—*see* Wound, open, oral cavity
- vagina S31.4-
  - bite S31.45
- vitreous (humor)—*see* Wound, open, ocular
- vulva S31.4-
  - bite S31.45
- wrist S61.5-

Wound, superficial—*see* Injury—*see also* specified injury type

X

Xanthelasmatosis (essential) E78.2

Xanthinuria, hereditary E79.8

Xanthoastrocytoma
- specified site—*see* Neoplasm, malignant, by in Table of Neoplasms in the complete *ICD-10-CM* manual
- unspecified site C71.9

Xanthogranuloma D76.3

Xanthoma(s), xanthomatosis (primary) (familial) (hereditary)
- with
  - hyperlipoproteinemia
    - Type III E78.2
- disseminatum (skin) E78.2
- eruptive E78.2
- hypercholesterinemic E78.00
- hypercholesterolemic E78.00
- hyperlipidemic E78.5
- multiple (skin) E78.2
- tuberosum E78.2
- tuberous E78.2
- tubo-eruptive E78.2

Xerosis
- cutis (dry skin) L85.3

XO syndrome Q96.9

X-ray (of)
- abnormal findings—Abnormal, diagnostic imaging
- breast (mammogram) (routine) Z12.31
- chest
  - routine (as part of a general medical examination) Z00.00
    - with abnormal findings Z00.01
- routine (as part of a general medical examination) Z00.00
  - with abnormal findings Z00.01

Y

Yawning R06.89
- psychogenic F45.8

Yeast infection (*see also* Candidiasis) B37.9

Z

Zahorsky's syndrome (herpangina) B08.5

Zika virus NOS A92.5
- congential P35.4

Chapter 1. Certain infectious and parasitic diseases (A00–B99)

GUIDELINES

COVID-19 Infection (Infection Due to SARS-CoV-2)
See category U07.

HIV Infections
See category B20.

Coding of Sepsis and Severe Sepsis

SEPSIS
For a diagnosis of sepsis, assign the appropriate code for the underlying systemic infection. If the type of infection or causal organism is not further specified, assign code A41.9, Sepsis, unspecified organism. A code from subcategory R65.2, Severe sepsis, should not be assigned unless severe sepsis or an associated acute organ dysfunction is documented.

Negative or inconclusive blood cultures and sepsis
Negative or inconclusive blood cultures do not preclude a diagnosis of sepsis in patients with clinical evidence of the condition, however, the provider should be queried.

Urosepsis
The term urosepsis is a nonspecific term. It is not to be considered synonymous with sepsis. It has no default code in the Alphabetic Index. Should a provider use this term they should be queried.

Sepsis with organ dysfunction
If a patient has sepsis and associated acute organ dysfunction or multiple organ dysfunction (MOD), follow the instructions for coding severe sepsis.

Acute organ dysfunction that is not clearly associated with the sepsis
If a patient has sepsis and an acute organ dysfunction, but the medical record documentation indicates that the acute organ dysfunction is related to a medical condition other than the sepsis, do not assign a code from subcategory R65.2, Severe sepsis. An acute organ dysfunction must be associated with the sepsis in order to assign the severe sepsis code. If the documentation is not clear as to whether an acute organ dysfunction is related to the sepsis or another medical condition, query the provider.

SEVERE SEPSIS
The coding of severe sepsis requires a minimum of 2 codes: first a code for the underlying systemic infection, followed by a code from subcategory R65.2, Severe sepsis. If the causal organism is not documented, assign code A41.9, Sepsis, unspecified organism, for the infection. Additional code(s) for the associated acute organ dysfunction are also required.

Due to the complex nature of severe sepsis, some cases may require querying the provider prior to assignment of the codes.

Septic shock
Septic shock generally refers to circulatory failure associated with severe sepsis, and therefore, it represents a type of acute organ dysfunction. For cases of septic shock, the code for the systemic infection should be sequenced first, followed by code R65.21, Severe sepsis with septic shock or code T81.12, Postprocedural septic shock. Any additional codes for the other acute organ dysfunctions should also be assigned. As noted in the sequencing instructions in the Tabular List, the code for septic shock cannot be assigned as a principal diagnosis.

Sequencing of severe sepsis
If severe sepsis is present on admission, and meets the definition of principal diagnosis, the underlying systemic infection should be assigned as principal diagnosis followed by the appropriate code from subcategory R65.2 as required by the sequencing rules in the Tabular List. A code from subcategory R65.2 can never be assigned as a principal diagnosis. When severe sepsis develops during an encounter (it was not present on admission) the underlying systemic infection and the appropriate code from subcategory R65.2 should be assigned as secondary diagnoses. Severe sepsis may be present on admission but the diagnosis may not be confirmed until sometime after admission. If the documentation is not clear whether severe sepsis was present on admission, the provider should be queried.

Sepsis *or* severe sepsis with a localized infection
If the reason for admission is both sepsis or severe sepsis and a localized infection, such as pneumonia or cellulitis, a code(s) for the underlying systemic infection should be assigned first and the code for the localized infection should be assigned as a secondary diagnosis. If the patient has severe sepsis, a code from subcategory R65.2 should also be assigned as a secondary diagnosis. If the patient is admitted with a localized infection, such as pneumonia, and sepsis/severe sepsis doesn't develop until after admission, the localized infection should be assigned first, followed by the appropriate sepsis/severe sepsis codes.

SEPSIS DUE TO A POSTPROCEDURAL INFECTION
Documentation of causal relationship
As with all postprocedural complications, code assignment is based on the provider's documentation of the relationship between the infection and the procedure.

Sepsis due to a postprocedural infection
For infections following a procedure, a code from T81.40, to T81.43 Infection following a procedure, or a code from O86.00 to O86.03, Infection of obstetric surgical wound, that identifies the site of the infection should be coded first, if known. Assign an additional code for sepsis following a procedure (T81.44) or sepsis following an obstetrical procedure (O86.04). Use an additional code to identify the infectious agent. If the patient has severe sepsis, the appropriate code from subcategory R65.2 should also be assigned with the additional code(s) for any acute organ dysfunction.

For infections following infusion, transfusion, therapeutic injection, or immunization, a code from subcategory T80.2, Infections following infusion, transfusion, and therapeutic injection, or code T88.0-, Infection following immunization, should be coded first, followed by the code for the specific infection. If the patient has severe sepsis, the appropriate code from subcategory R65.2 should also be assigned, with the additional codes(s) for any acute organ dysfunction.

Postprocedural infection and postprocedural septic shock
If a postprocedural infection has resulted in postprocedural septic shock, assign the codes indicated above for sepsis due to a postprocedural infection, followed by code T81.12-, Postprocedural septic shock. Do not assign code R65.21, Severe sepsis with septic shock. Additional code(s) should be assigned for any acute organ dysfunction.

SEPSIS AND SEVERE SEPSIS ASSOCIATED WITH A NONINFECTIOUS PROCESS (CONDITION)
In some cases a noninfectious process (condition), such as trauma, may lead to an infection which can result in sepsis or severe sepsis. If sepsis or severe sepsis is documented as associated with a noninfectious condition, such as a burn or serious injury, and this condition meets the definition for principal diagnosis, the code for the noninfectious condition should be sequenced first, followed by the code for the resulting infection. If severe sepsis, is present a code from subcategory R65.2 should also be assigned with any associated organ dysfunction(s) codes. It is not necessary to assign a code from subcategory R65.1, SIRS of non-infectious origin, for these cases.

If the infection meets the definition of principal diagnosis it should be sequenced before the non-infectious condition. When both the associated non-infectious condition and the infection meet the definition of principal diagnosis either may be assigned as principal diagnosis.

Only one code from category R65, Symptoms and signs specifically associated with systemic inflammation and infection, should be assigned. Therefore, when a non-infectious condition leads to an infection resulting in severe sepsis, assign the appropriate code from subcategory R65.2, Severe sepsis. Do not additionally assign a code from subcategory R65.1, SIRS of non-infectious origin.

Includes: diseases generally recognized as communicable or transmissible
Use additional code to identify resistance to antimicrobial drugs (Z16.-)
Excludes1: certain localized infections — see body system-related chapters
Excludes2: carrier or suspected carrier of infectious disease (Z22.-)
    infectious and parasitic diseases specific to the perinatal period (P35–P39)
    influenza and other acute respiratory infections (J00–J22)

(A00–A09) INTESTINAL INFECTIOUS DISEASES

A02   **OTHER SALMONELLA INFECTIONS**
`4th`   *Includes:* infection or foodborne intoxication due to any Salmonella species other than S. typhi and S. paratyphi

    A02.0   **Salmonella enteritis**
             Salmonellosis
    A02.1   **Salmonella sepsis**
    A02.2   **Localized salmonella infections**
    `5th`   **A02.20**   **Localized salmonella infection, unspecified**

`4th` `5th` `6th` `7th` Additional Character Required   ✔   3-character code

•=New Code   *Excludes1*—Not coded here, do not use together
▲=Revised Code   *Excludes2*—Not included here

CHAPTER 1. CERTAIN INFECTIOUS AND PARASITIC DISEASES (A02.21–A15.9)

A02.21   **Salmonella meningitis**
A02.22   **Salmonella pneumonia**
A02.23   **Salmonella arthritis**
A02.24   **Salmonella osteomyelitis**
A02.25   **Salmonella pyelonephritis**
         Salmonella tubulointerstitial nephropathy
A02.29   **Salmonella with other localized infection**
A02.8 **Other specified salmonella infections**
A02.9 **Salmonella infection, unspecified**

A03   **SHIGELLOSIS**
`4th`
A03.0 **Shigellosis due to Shigella dysenteriae**
     Group A shigellosis [Shiga-Kruse dysentery]
A03.1 **Shigellosis due to Shigella flexneri**
     Group B shigellosis
A03.2 **Shigellosis due to Shigella boydii**
     Group C shigellosis
A03.3 **Shigellosis due to Shigella sonnei**
     Group D shigellosis
A03.8 **Other shigellosis**
A03.9 **Shigellosis, unspecified**
     Bacillary dysentery NOS

A04   **OTHER BACTERIAL INTESTINAL INFECTIONS**
`4th`
Excludes1: bacterial foodborne intoxications, NEC (A05.-)
     tuberculous enteritis (A18.32)
A04.0 **Enteropathogenic E. coli infection**
A04.1 **Enterotoxigenic E. coli infection**
A04.2 **Enteroinvasive E. coli infection**
A04.3 **Enterohemorrhagic E. coli infection**
A04.4 **Other intestinal E. coli infections**
     E. coli enteritis NOS
A04.5 **Campylobacter enteritis**
A04.6 **Enteritis due to Yersinia enterocolitica**
     Excludes1: extraintestinal yersiniosis (A28.2)
A04.7 **Enterocolitis due to Clostridium difficile**
  `5th` Foodborne intoxication by Clostridium difficile
     Pseudomembraneous colitis
     A04.71   **Enterocolitis due to Clostridium difficile, recurrent**
     A04.72   **Enterocolitis due to Clostridium difficile, not specified as recurrent**
A04.8 **Other specified bacterial intestinal infections**
     H. pylori
A04.9 **Bacterial intestinal infection, unspecified**
     Bacterial enteritis NOS

A05   **OTHER BACTERIAL FOODBORNE INTOXICATIONS, NOT ELSEWHERE CLASSIFIED**
`4th`
Excludes1: Clostridium difficile foodborne intoxication and infection (A04.7-)
     E. coli infection (A04.0–A04.4)
     listeriosis (A32.-)
     salmonella foodborne intoxication and infection (A02.-)
     toxic effect of noxious foodstuffs (T61–T62)
A05.0 **Foodborne staphylococcal intoxication**
A05.1 **Botulism food poisoning**
     Botulism NOS
     Classical foodborne intoxication due to Clostridium botulinum
     Excludes1: infant botulism (A48.51)
          wound botulism (A48.52)
A05.2 **Foodborne Clostridium perfringens [Clostridium welchii] intoxication**
     Enteritis necroticans
     Pigbel
A05.3 **Foodborne Vibrio parahaemolyticus intoxication**
A05.4 **Foodborne Bacillus cereus intoxication**
A05.5 **Foodborne Vibrio vulnificus intoxication**
A05.8 **Other specified bacterial foodborne intoxications**
A05.9 **Bacterial foodborne intoxication, unspecified**

A06   **AMEBIASIS**
`4th`
Includes: infection due to Entamoeba histolytica
Excludes1: other protozoal intestinal diseases (A07.-)
Excludes2: acanthamebiasis (B60.1-)
     Naegleriasis (B60.2)

A06.0 **Acute amebic dysentery**
     Acute amebiasis
     Intestinal amebiasis NOS

A07   **OTHER PROTOZOAL INTESTINAL DISEASES**
`4th`
A07.1 **Giardiasis [lambliasis]**
A07.2 **Cryptosporidiosis**

A08   **VIRAL AND OTHER SPECIFIED INTESTINAL INFECTIONS**
`4th`
Excludes1: influenza with involvement of gastrointestinal tract (J09.X3, J10.2, J11.2)
A08.0 **Rotaviral enteritis**
A08.3 **Other viral enteritis**
  `5th` A08.39   **Other viral enteritis**
          Coxsackie virus enteritis
          Echovirus enteritis
          Enterovirus enteritis NEC
          Torovirus enteritis
A08.4 **Viral intestinal infection, unspecified**
     Viral enteritis NOS
     Viral gastroenteritis NOS
     Viral gastroenteropathy NOS
A08.8 **Other specified intestinal infections**

A09   **INFECTIOUS GASTROENTERITIS AND COLITIS, UNSPECIFIED**
`✓`
Infectious colitis NOS
Infectious enteritis NOS
Infectious gastroenteritis NOS
Excludes1: colitis NOS (K52.9)
     diarrhea NOS (R19.7)
     enteritis NOS (K52.9)
     gastroenteritis NOS (K52.9)
     noninfective gastroenteritis and colitis, unspecified (K52.9)

(A15–A19) TUBERCULOSIS

Includes: infections due to Mycobacterium tuberculosis and Mycobacterium bovis
Excludes1: congenital tuberculosis (P37.0)
     nonspecific reaction to test for tuberculosis without active tuberculosis (R76.1-)
     pneumoconiosis associated with tuberculosis, any type in A15 (J65)
     positive PPD (R76.11)
     positive tuberculin skin test without active tuberculosis (R76.11)
     sequelae of tuberculosis (B90.-)
     silicotuberculosis (J65)

A15   **RESPIRATORY TUBERCULOSIS**
`4th`
A15.0 **Tuberculosis of lung**
     Tuberculous bronchiectasis
     Tuberculous fibrosis of lung
     Tuberculous pneumonia
     Tuberculous pneumothorax
A15.4 **Tuberculosis of intrathoracic lymph nodes**
     Tuberculosis of hilar lymph nodes
     Tuberculosis of mediastinal lymph nodes
     Tuberculosis of tracheobronchial lymph nodes
     Excludes1: tuberculosis specified as primary (A15.7)
A15.5 **Tuberculosis of larynx, trachea and bronchus**
     Tuberculosis of bronchus
     Tuberculosis of glottis
     Tuberculosis of larynx
     Tuberculosis of trachea
A15.6 **Tuberculous pleurisy**
     Tuberculosis of pleura Tuberculous empyema
     Excludes1: primary respiratory tuberculosis (A15.7)
A15.7 **Primary respiratory tuberculosis**
A15.8 **Other respiratory tuberculosis**
     Mediastinal tuberculosis
     Nasopharyngeal tuberculosis
     Tuberculosis of nose
     Tuberculosis of sinus [any nasal]
A15.9 **Respiratory tuberculosis unspecified**

A17   **TUBERCULOSIS OF NERVOUS SYSTEM**
`4th`
   A17.0   **Tuberculous meningitis**
      Tuberculosis of meninges (cerebral)(spinal)
      Tuberculous leptomeningitis
      Excludes1: tuberculous meningoencephalitis (A17.82)
   A17.1   **Meningeal tuberculoma**
      Tuberculoma of meninges (cerebral) (spinal)
      Excludes2: tuberculoma of brain and spinal cord (A17.81)
   A17.8   **Other tuberculosis of nervous system**
     `5th`   **A17.81**   **Tuberculoma of brain and spinal cord**
          Tuberculous abscess of brain and spinal cord
        A17.82   **Tuberculous meningoencephalitis**
          Tuberculous myelitis
        A17.83   **Tuberculous neuritis**
          Tuberculous mononeuropathy
        A17.89   **Other tuberculosis of nervous system**
          Tuberculous polyneuropathy
   A17.9   **Tuberculosis of nervous system, unspecified**

A18   **TUBERCULOSIS OF OTHER ORGANS**
`4th`
   A18.0   **Tuberculosis of bones and joints**
     `5th`   **A18.01**   **Tuberculosis of spine**
          Pott's disease or curvature of spine
          Tuberculous arthritis
          Tuberculous osteomyelitis of spine
          Tuberculous spondylitis
        A18.02   **Tuberculous arthritis of other joints**
          Tuberculosis of hip (joint)
          Tuberculosis of knee (joint)
        A18.03   **Tuberculosis of other bones**
          Tuberculous mastoiditis
          Tuberculous osteomyelitis
        A18.09   **Other musculoskeletal tuberculosis**
          Tuberculous myositis
          Tuberculous synovitis
          Tuberculous tenosynovitis
   A18.2   **Tuberculous peripheral lymphadenopathy**
      Tuberculous adenitis
      Excludes2: tuberculosis of bronchial and mediastinal lymph nodes
         (A15.4)
        tuberculosis of mesenteric and retroperitoneal lymph nodes
         (A18.39)
        tuberculous tracheobronchial adenopathy (A15.4)
   A18.3   **Tuberculosis of intestines, peritoneum and mesenteric glands**
     `5th`   **A18.31**   **Tuberculous peritonitis**
          Tuberculous ascites
        A18.32   **Tuberculous enteritis**
          Tuberculosis of anus and rectum
          Tuberculosis of intestine (large) (small)
        A18.39   **Retroperitoneal tuberculosis**
          Tuberculosis of mesenteric glands
          Tuberculosis of retroperitoneal (lymph glands)
   A18.4   **Tuberculosis of skin and subcutaneous tissue**
      Erythema induratum, tuberculous
      Lupus excedens
      Lupus vulgaris NOS
      Lupus vulgaris of eyelid
      Scrofuloderma
      Tuberculosis of external ear
      Excludes2: lupus erythematosus (L93.-)
        lupus NOS (M32.9)
        systemic lupus erythematosus (M32.-)
   A18.6   **Tuberculosis of (inner) (middle) ear**
      Tuberculous otitis media
      Excludes2: tuberculosis of external ear (A18.4)
        tuberculous mastoiditis (A18.03)
   A18.8   **Tuberculosis of other specified organs**
     `5th`   **A18.84**   **Tuberculosis of heart**
          Tuberculous cardiomyopathy
          Tuberculous endocarditis
          Tuberculous myocarditis
          Tuberculous pericarditis
        A18.85   **Tuberculosis of spleen**

        A18.89   **Tuberculosis of other sites**
          Tuberculosis of muscle
          Tuberculous cerebral arteritis

A19   **MILIARY TUBERCULOSIS**
`4th`
   Includes: disseminated tuberculosis
      generalized tuberculosis
      tuberculous polyserositis
   A19.0   **Acute miliary tuberculosis of a single specified site**
   A19.1   **Acute miliary tuberculosis of multiple sites**
   A19.2   **Acute miliary tuberculosis, unspecified**
   A19.8   **Other miliary tuberculosis**
   A19.9   **Miliary tuberculosis, unspecified**

(A20–A28) CERTAIN ZOONOTIC BACTERIAL DISEASES

A22   **ANTHRAX**
`4th`
   Includes: infection due to Bacillus anthracis
   A22.0   **Cutaneous anthrax**
      Malignant carbuncle
      Malignant pustule
   A22.1   **Pulmonary anthrax**
      Inhalation anthrax
      Rag picker's disease
      Wool sorter's disease
   A22.2   **Gastrointestinal anthrax**
   A22.9   **Anthrax, unspecified**

A25   **RAT-BITE FEVERS**
`4th`
   A25.0   **Spirillosis**
   A25.1   **Streptobacillosis**
   A25.9   **Rat-bite fever, unspecified**

A26   **ERYSIPELOID**
`4th`
   A26.0   **Cutaneous erysipeloid**
   A26.7   **Erysipelothrix sepsis**
   A26.8   **Other forms of erysipeloid**
   A26.9   **Erysipeloid, unspecified**

A27   **LEPTOSPIROSIS**
`4th`
   A27.0   **Leptospirosis icterohemorrhagica**
   A27.8   **Other forms of leptospirosis**
     `5th`   **A27.81**   **Aseptic meningitis in leptospirosis**
        A27.89   **Other forms of leptospirosis**
   A27.9   **Leptospirosis, unspecified**

A28   **OTHER ZOONOTIC BACTERIAL DISEASES, NEC**
`4th`
   A28.0   **Pasteurellosis**
   A28.1   **Cat-scratch disease**
      Cat-scratch fever
   A28.2   **Extraintestinal yersiniosis**
      Excludes1: enteritis due to Yersinia enterocolitica (A04.6)

(A30–A49) OTHER BACTERIAL DISEASES

A31   **INFECTION DUE TO OTHER MYCOBACTERIA**
`4th`
   Excludes2: tuberculosis (A15–A19)
   A31.0   **Pulmonary mycobacterial infection**
   A31.1   **Cutaneous mycobacterial infection**
   A31.2   **Disseminated mycobacterium avium-intracellulare complex (DMAC)**
   A31.8   **Other mycobacterial infections**
   A31.9   **Mycobacterial infection, unspecified**

A32   **LISTERIOSIS**
`4th`
   Includes: listerial foodborne infection
   Excludes1: neonatal (disseminated) listeriosis (P37.2)
   A32.0   **Cutaneous listeriosis**
   A32.1   **Listerial meningitis and meningoencephalitis**
     `5th`   **A32.11**   **Listerial meningitis**
        A32.12   **Listerial meningoencephalitis**
   A32.7   **Listerial sepsis**
   A32.8   **Other forms of listeriosis**
     `5th`   **A32.81**   **Oculoglandular listeriosis**
        A32.82   **Listerial endocarditis**
        A32.89   **Other forms of listeriosis**
          Listerial cerebral arteritis

`4th` `5th` `6th` `7th`   Additional Character Required   ✔   3-character code

•=New Code   *Excludes1*—Not coded here, do not use together
▲=Revised Code   *Excludes2*—Not included here

A32.9 **Listeriosis, unspecified**

A35 OTHER TETANUS ✔

A36 DIPHTHERIA 4th

A36.0 **Pharyngeal diphtheria**

A36.1 **Nasopharyngeal diphtheria**

A36.2 **Laryngeal diphtheria**

A36.8 **Other diphtheria**

> 5th A36.89 **Other diphtheritic complications**

A36.9 **Diphtheria, unspecified**

A37 WHOOPING COUGH 4th

A37.0 **Whooping cough due to Bordetella pertussis;**

> 5th A37.00 **without pneumonia**
> Paroxysmal cough due to Bordetella pertussis without pneumonia
>
> A37.01 **with pneumonia**
> Paroxysmal cough due to Bordetella pertussis with pneumonia

A37.1 **Whooping cough due to Bordetella parapertussis;**

> 5th A37.10 **without pneumonia**
>
> A37.11 **with pneumonia**

A37.8 **Whooping cough due to other Bordetella species;**

> 5th A37.80 **without pneumonia**
>
> A37.81 **with pneumonia**

A37.9 **Whooping cough, unspecified species;**

> 5th A37.90 **without pneumonia**
>
> A37.91 **with pneumonia**

A38 SCARLET FEVER 4th

Includes: scarlatina

Excludes2: streptococcal sore throat (J02.0)

A38.0 **Scarlet fever with otitis media**

A38.1 **Scarlet fever with myocarditis**

A38.8 **Scarlet fever with other complications**

A38.9 **Scarlet fever, uncomplicated**
Scarlet fever, NOS

A39 MENINGOCOCCAL INFECTION 4th

A39.0 **Meningococcal meningitis**

A39.1 **Waterhouse-Friderichsen syndrome**
Meningococcal hemorrhagic adrenalitis
Meningococcic adrenal syndrome

A39.2 **Acute meningococcemia**

A39.3 **Chronic meningococcemia**

A39.4 **Meningococcemia, unspecified**

A39.5 **Meningococcal heart disease**

> 5th A39.50 **Meningococcal carditis, unspecified**
>
> A39.51 **Meningococcal endocarditis**
>
> A39.52 **Meningococcal myocarditis**
>
> A39.53 **Meningococcal pericarditis**

A39.8 **Other meningococcal infections**

> 5th A39.89 **Other meningococcal infections**
> Meningococcal conjunctivitis

A39.9 **Meningococcal infection, unspecified**
Meningococcal disease NOS

A40 STREPTOCOCCAL SEPSIS 4th

GUIDELINES

Refer to Chapter 1 guidelines for sepsis guidelines.

Code first: postprocedural streptococcal sepsis (T81.4-)
streptococcal sepsis following immunization (T88.0)
streptococcal sepsis following infusion, transfusion or therapeutic injection (T80.2-)

Excludes1: neonatal (P36.0–P36.1)
sepsis due to Streptococcus, group D (A41.81)

A40.0 **Sepsis due to streptococcus, group A**

A40.1 **Sepsis due to streptococcus, group B**

A40.3 **Sepsis due to Streptococcus pneumoniae**
Pneumococcal sepsis

A40.8 **Other streptococcal sepsis**

A40.9 **Streptococcal sepsis, unspecified**

A41 OTHER SEPSIS 4th

GUIDELINES

Refer to Chapter 1 guidelines for sepsis guidelines.

Code first: postprocedural sepsis (T81.4-)
sepsis following immunization (T88.0)
sepsis following infusion, transfusion or therapeutic injection (T80.2-)

Excludes1: bacteremia NOS (R78.81)
neonatal (P36.-)
puerperal sepsis (O85)
streptococcal sepsis (A40.-)

Excludes2: sepsis (due to) (in) actinomycotic (A42.7)
sepsis (due to) (in) anthrax (A22.7)
sepsis (due to) (in) candidal (B37.7)
sepsis (due to) (in) Erysipelothrix (A26.7)
sepsis (due to) (in) extraintestinal yersiniosis (A28.2)
sepsis (due to) (in) gonococcal (A54.86)
sepsis (due to) (in) herpesviral (B00.7)
sepsis (due to) (in) listerial (A32.7)
sepsis (due to) (in) melioidosis (A24.1)
sepsis (due to) (in) meningococcal (A39.2–A39.4)
sepsis (due to) (in) plague (A20.7)
sepsis (due to) (in) tularemia (A21.7)
toxic shock syndrome (A48.3)

A41.0 **Sepsis due to Staphylococcus aureus**

> 5th A41.01 **Sepsis due to**
> MSSA
> MSSA sepsis
> Staphylococcus aureus sepsis NOS
>
> A41.02 **Sepsis due to MRSA**

A41.1 **Sepsis due to other specified staphylococcus**
Coagulase negative staphylococcus sepsis

A41.2 **Sepsis due to unspecified staphylococcus**

A41.3 **Sepsis due to H. influenzae**

A41.4 **Sepsis due to anaerobes**
Excludes1: gas gangrene (A48.0)

A41.5 **Sepsis due to other Gram-negative organisms**

> 5th A41.50 **Gram-negative sepsis, unspecified**
> Gram-negative sepsis NOS
>
> A41.51 **Sepsis due to E. coli**
>
> A41.52 **Sepsis due to Pseudomonas**
> Pseudomonas aeroginosa
>
> A41.53 **Sepsis due to Serratia**
>
> A41.59 **Other Gram-negative sepsis**

A41.8 **Other specified sepsis**

> 5th A41.81 **Sepsis due to Enterococcus**
>
> A41.89 **Other specified sepsis**
> If the type of infection or causal organism is not further specified for sepsis, assign code A41.9

A41.9 **Sepsis, unspecified organism**
Septicemia NOS

A42 ACTINOMYCOSIS 4th

Excludes1: actinomycetoma (B47.1)

A42.0 **Pulmonary actinomycosis**

A42.1 **Abdominal actinomycosis**

A42.2 **Cervicofacial actinomycosis**

A42.7 **Actinomycotic sepsis**

A42.8 **Other forms of actinomycosis**

> 5th A42.81 **Actinomycotic meningitis**
>
> A42.82 **Actinomycotic encephalitis**
>
> A42.89 **Other forms of actinomycosis**

A42.9 **Actinomycosis, unspecified**

A43 NOCARDIOSIS 4th

A43.0 **Pulmonary nocardiosis**

A43.1 **Cutaneous nocardiosis**

A43.8 **Other forms of nocardiosis**

A43.9 **Nocardiosis, unspecified**

A44 BARTONELLOSIS 4th

A44.0 **Systemic bartonellosis**

A44.1 **Cutaneous and mucocutaneous bartonellosis**

A44.8 **Other forms of bartonellosis**

A44.9 **Bartonellosis, unspecified**

 4th 5th 6th 7th Additional Character Required ✔ 3-character code

•=New Code
▲=Revised Code

Excludes1—Not coded here, do not use together
Excludes2—Not included here

A46 ERYSIPELAS
☑ *Excludes1:* postpartum or puerperal erysipelas (O86.89)

A48 OTHER BACTERIAL DISEASES, NOT ELSEWHERE CLASSIFIED
(4th)
Excludes1: actinomycetoma (B47.1)
A48.1 Legionnaires' disease
A48.2 Nonpneumonic Legionnaires' disease [Pontiac fever]
A48.3 Toxic shock syndrome
    Use additional code to identify the organism (B95, B96)
    Excludes1: endotoxic shock NOS (R57.8)
       sepsis NOS (A41.9)
A48.5 Other specified botulism
(5th)   Non-foodborne intoxication due to toxins of Clostridium botulinum [C. botulinum]
    Excludes1: food poisoning due to toxins of Clostridium botulinum (A05.1)
    A48.51 Infant botulism
    A48.52 Wound botulism
       Non-foodborne botulism NOS
       Use additional code for associated wound
A48.8 Other specified bacterial diseases

A49 BACTERIAL INFECTION OF UNSPECIFIED SITE
(4th)
Excludes1: bacterial agents as the cause of diseases classified elsewhere (B95–B96)
    chlamydial infection NOS (A74.9)
    meningococcal infection NOS (A39.9)
    rickettsial infection NOS (A79.9)
    spirochetal infection NOS (A69.9)
A49.0 Staphylococcal infection, unspecified site
(5th)

> **GUIDELINES**
>
> The condition or state of being colonized or carrying MSSA or MRSA is called colonization or carriage, while an individual person is described as being colonized or being a carrier. Colonization means that MSSA or MSRA is present on or in the body without necessarily causing illness. A positive MRSA colonization test might be documented by the provider as "MRSA screen positive" or "MRSA nasal swab positive". Assign code Z22.322, Carrier or suspected carrier of MRSA, for patients documented as having MRSA colonization. Assign code Z22.321, Carrier or suspected carrier of MSSA, for patient documented as having MSSA colonization. Colonization is not necessarily indicative of a disease process or as the cause of a specific condition the patient may have unless documented as such by the provider. If a patient is documented as having both MRSA colonization and infection during a hospital admission, code Z22.322, and a code for the MRSA infection may both be assigned.

    A49.01 MSSA infection, unspecified site
       MSSA infection
       Staphylococcus aureus infection NOS
    A49.02 MRSA infection, unspecified site
       MRSA infection
A49.1 Streptococcal infection, unspecified site
A49.2 H. influenzae infection, unspecified site
A49.3 Mycoplasma infection, unspecified site
A49.8 Other bacterial infections of unspecified site
A49.9 Bacterial infection, unspecified
    Excludes1: bacteremia NOS (R78.81)

(A50–A64) INFECTIONS WITH A PREDOMINANTLY SEXUAL MODE OF TRANSMISSION

Excludes1: HIV disease (B20)
    nonspecific and nongonococcal urethritis (N34.1)
    Reiter's disease (M02.3-)

A50 CONGENITAL SYPHILIS
(4th)
A50.0 Early congenital syphilis, symptomatic
(5th)   Any congenital syphilitic condition specified as early or manifest less than two years after birth.
    A50.01 Early congenital syphilitic; oculopathy
    A50.02   osteochondropathy

    A50.03 pharyngitis
       Early congenital syphilitic laryngitis
    A50.04 pneumonia
    A50.05 rhinitis
    A50.06 Early cutaneous congenital syphilis
    A50.07 Early mucocutaneous congenital syphilis
    A50.08 Early visceral congenital syphilis
    A50.09 Other early congenital syphilis, symptomatic
A50.1 Early congenital syphilis, latent
    Congenital syphilis without clinical manifestations, with positive serological reaction and negative spinal fluid test, less than two years after birth.
A50.2 Early congenital syphilis, unspecified
    Congenital syphilis NOS less than two years after birth.
A50.3 Late congenital syphilitic oculopathy
(5th)   *Excludes1:* Hutchinson's triad (A50.53)
    A50.30 Late congenital syphilitic oculopathy, unspecified
    A50.31 Late congenital syphilitic interstitial keratitis
    A50.32 Late congenital syphilitic chorioretinitis
    A50.39 Other late congenital syphilitic oculopathy
A50.4 Late congenital neurosyphilis [juvenile neurosyphilis]
(5th)   **Use additional code** to identify any associated mental disorder
    Excludes1: Hutchinson's triad (A50.53)
    A50.40 Late congenital neurosyphilis, unspecified
       Juvenile neurosyphilis NOS
    A50.41 Late congenital syphilitic meningitis
    A50.42 Late congenital syphilitic encephalitis
    A50.43 Late congenital syphilitic polyneuropathy
    A50.44 Late congenital syphilitic optic nerve atrophy
    A50.45 Juvenile general paresis
       Dementia paralytica juvenilis
       Juvenile tabetoparetic neurosyphilis
    A50.49 Other late congenital neurosyphilis
       Juvenile tabes dorsalis
A50.5 Other late congenital syphilis, symptomatic
(5th)   Any congenital syphilitic condition specified as late or manifest two years or more after birth.
    A50.51 Clutton's joints
    A50.52 Hutchinson's teeth
    A50.53 Hutchinson's triad
    A50.54 Late congenital cardiovascular syphilis
    A50.55 Late congenital syphilitic arthropathy
    A50.56 Late congenital syphilitic osteochondropathy
    A50.57 Syphilitic saddle nose
    A50.59 Other late congenital syphilis, symptomatic
A50.6 Late congenital syphilis, latent
    Congenital syphilis without clinical manifestations, with positive serological reaction and negative spinal fluid test, two years or more after birth.
A50.7 Late congenital syphilis, unspecified
    Congenital syphilis NOS two years or more after birth.
A50.9 Congenital syphilis, unspecified

A51 EARLY SYPHILIS
(4th)
A51.0 Primary genital syphilis
    Syphilitic chancre NOS
A51.1 Primary anal syphilis
A51.2 Primary syphilis of other sites
A51.3 Secondary syphilis of skin and mucous membranes
(5th)   **A51.31** Condyloma latum
    A51.32 Syphilitic alopecia
    A51.39 Other secondary syphilis of skin
A51.5 Early syphilis, latent
    Syphilis (acquired) without clinical manifestations, with positive serological reaction and negative spinal fluid test, less than two years after infection.
A51.9 Early syphilis, unspecified

A52 LATE SYPHILIS
(4th)
A52.0 Cardiovascular and cerebrovascular syphilis
(5th)   **A52.00** Cardiovascular syphilis, unspecified
    A52.03 Syphilitic endocarditis
       Syphilitic aortic valve incompetence or stenosis
       Syphilitic mitral valve stenosis
       Syphilitic pulmonary valve regurgitation

CHAPTER 1. CERTAIN INFECTIOUS AND PARASITIC DISEASES (A46–A52.03)

(4th) *(5th)* *(6th)* *(7th)* Additional Character Required   ✓ 3-character code

•=New Code
▲=Revised Code

Excludes1—Not coded here, do not use together
Excludes2—Not included here

CHAPTER 1. CERTAIN INFECTIOUS AND PARASITIC DISEASES   (A52.06–A64)

A52.06 Other syphilitic heart involvement
Syphilitic coronary artery disease
Syphilitic myocarditis
Syphilitic pericarditis
A52.09 Other cardiovascular syphilis
A52.7 Other symptomatic late syphilis
5th A52.76 Other genitourinary symptomatic late syphilis
A52.79 Other symptomatic late syphilis
A52.8 Late syphilis, latent
Syphilis (acquired) without clinical manifestations, with positive serological reaction and negative spinal fluid test, two years or more after infection
A52.9 Late syphilis, unspecified

A53 OTHER AND UNSPECIFIED SYPHILIS
4th
A53.0 Latent syphilis, unspecified as early or late
Latent syphilis NOS
Positive serological reaction for syphilis
A53.9 Syphilis, unspecified
Infection due to Treponema pallidum NOS
Syphilis (acquired) NOS
Excludes1: syphilis NOS under two years of age (A50.2)

A54 GONOCOCCAL INFECTION
4th
A54.0 Gonococcal infection of lower genitourinary tract without
5th periurethral or accessory gland abscess
Excludes1: gonococcal infection with genitourinary gland abscess (A54.1)
gonococcal infection with periurethral abscess (A54.1)
A54.00 Gonococcal infection of lower genitourinary tract, unspecified
A54.01 Gonococcal cystitis and urethritis, unspecified
A54.02 Gonococcal vulvovaginitis, unspecified
A54.03 Gonococcal cervicitis, unspecified
A54.09 Other gonococcal infection of lower genitourinary tract
A54.1 Gonococcal infection of lower genitourinary tract with periurethral and accessory gland abscess
Gonococcal Bartholin's gland abscess
A54.2 Gonococcal pelviperitonitis and other gonococcal
5th genitourinary infection
A54.21 Gonococcal infection of kidney and ureter
A54.22 Gonococcal prostatitis
A54.23 Gonococcal infection of other male genital organs
Gonococcal epididymitis
Gonococcal orchitis
A54.24 Gonococcal female pelvic inflammatory disease
Gonococcal pelviperitonitis
Excludes1: gonococcal peritonitis (A54.85)
A54.29 Other gonococcal genitourinary infections
A54.3 Gonococcal infection of eye
5th A54.30 Gonococcal infection of eye, unspecified
A54.31 Gonococcal conjunctivitis
Ophthalmia neonatorum due to gonococcus
A54.32 Gonococcal iridocyclitis
A54.33 Gonococcal keratitis
A54.39 Other gonococcal eye infection
Gonococcal endophthalmia
A54.4 Gonococcal infection of musculoskeletal system
5th A54.40 Gonococcal infection of musculoskeletal system, unspecified
A54.41 Gonococcal spondylopathy
Excludes2: gonococcal infection of spine (A54.41)
A54.49 Gonococcal infection of other musculoskeletal tissue
Gonococcal bursitis
Gonococcal myositis
Gonococcal synovitis
Gonococcal tenosynovitis
A54.5 Gonococcal pharyngitis
A54.6 Gonococcal infection of anus and rectum
A54.8 Other gonococcal infections
5th A54.84 Gonococcal pneumonia
A54.85 Gonococcal peritonitis
Excludes1: gonococcal pelviperitonitis (A54.24)
A54.86 Gonococcal sepsis

A54.89 Other gonococcal infections
Gonococcal keratoderma
Gonococcal lymphadenitis
A54.9 Gonococcal infection, unspecified

A56 OTHER SEXUALLY TRANSMITTED CHLAMYDIAL
4th DISEASES
Includes: sexually transmitted diseases due to Chlamydia trachomatis
Excludes1: neonatal chlamydial conjunctivitis (P39.1)
neonatal chlamydial pneumonia (P23.1)
Excludes2: chlamydial lymphogranuloma (A55)
conditions classified to A74.-
A56.0 Chlamydial infection of lower genitourinary tract
5th A56.00 Chlamydial infection of lower genitourinary tract, unspecified
A56.01 Chlamydial cystitis and urethritis
A56.02 Chlamydial vulvovaginitis
A56.09 Other chlamydial infection of lower genitourinary tract
Chlamydial cervicitis
A56.1 Chlamydial infection of pelviperitoneum and other
5th genitourinary organs
A56.11 Chlamydial female pelvic inflammatory disease
A56.19 Other chlamydial genitourinary infection
Chlamydial epididymitis
Chlamydial orchitis
A56.2 Chlamydial infection of genitourinary tract, unspecified
A56.3 Chlamydial infection of anus and rectum
A56.4 Chlamydial infection of pharynx
A56.8 Sexually transmitted chlamydial infection of other sites

A59 TRICHOMONIASIS
4th
Excludes2: intestinal trichomoniasis (A07.8)
A59.0 Urogenital trichomoniasis
5th A59.00 Urogenital trichomoniasis, unspecified
Fluor (vaginalis) due to Trichomonas
Leukorrhea (vaginalis) due to Trichomonas
A59.01 Trichomonal vulvovaginitis
A59.02 Trichomonal prostatitis
A59.03 Trichomonal cystitis and urethritis
A59.09 Other urogenital trichomoniasis
Trichomonas cervicitis
A59.8 Trichomoniasis of other sites
A59.9 Trichomoniasis, unspecified

A60 ANOGENITAL HERPESVIRAL [HERPES SIMPLEX]
4th INFECTIONS
A60.0 Herpesviral infection of genitalia and urogenital tract
5th A60.00 Herpesviral infection of urogenital system, unspecified
A60.01 Herpesviral infection of penis
A60.02 Herpesviral infection of other male genital organs
A60.03 Herpesviral cervicitis
A60.04 Herpesviral vulvovaginitis
Herpesviral [herpes simplex] ulceration
Herpesviral [herpes simplex] vaginitis
Herpesviral [herpes simplex] vulvitis
A60.09 Herpesviral infection of other urogenital tract
A60.1 Herpesviral infection of perianal skin and rectum
A60.9 Anogenital herpesviral infection, unspecified

A63 OTHER PREDOMINANTLY SEXUALLY TRANSMITTED
4th DISEASES, NEC
Excludes2: molluscum contagiosum (B08.1)
papilloma of cervix (D26.0)
A63.0 Anogenital (venereal) warts
Anogenital warts due to (human) papillomavirus [HPV]
Condyloma acuminatum
A63.8 Other specified predominantly sexually transmitted diseases

A64 UNSPECIFIED SEXUALLY TRANSMITTED DISEASE
Other spirochetal diseases (A65–A69)
Excludes2: leptospirosis (A27.-)
syphilis (A50–A53)

4th **5th** **6th** **7th** Additional Character Required   ✔ 3-character code   •=New Code   *Excludes1*—Not coded here, do not use together
▲=Revised Code   *Excludes2*—Not included here

(A65–A69) OTHER SPIROCHETAL DISEASES

A68 **RELAPSING FEVERS**
4th
Includes: recurrent fever
Excludes2: Lyme disease (A69.2-)

A68.0 **Louse-borne relapsing fever**
Relapsing fever due to Borrelia recurrentis

A68.1 **Tick-borne relapsing fever**
Relapsing fever due to any Borrelia species other than Borrelia recurrentis

A68.9 **Relapsing fever, unspecified**

A69 **OTHER SPIROCHETAL INFECTIONS**
4th
A69.2 **Lyme disease**
5th Erythema chronicum migrans due to Borrelia burgdorferi

A69.20 **Lyme disease, unspecified**
A69.21 **Meningitis due to Lyme disease**
A69.22 **Other neurologic disorders in Lyme disease**
Cranial neuritis
Meningoencephalitis
Polyneuropathy
A69.23 **Arthritis due to Lyme disease**
A69.29 **Other conditions associated with Lyme disease**
Myopericarditis due to Lyme disease

A69.8 **Other specified spirochetal infections**
A69.9 **Spirochetal infection, unspecified**
Other diseases caused by chlamydiae (A70–A74)
Excludes1: sexually transmitted chlamydial diseases (A55–A56)

(A70–A74) OTHER DISEASES CAUSED BY CHLAMYDIAE

A71 **TRACHOMA**
4th
A71.0 **Initial stage of trachoma**
Trachoma dubium
A71.1 **Active stage of trachoma**
Granular conjunctivitis (trachomatous)
Trachomatous follicular conjunctivitis
Trachomatous pannus
A71.9 **Trachoma, unspecified**

A74 **OTHER DISEASES CAUSED BY CHLAMYDIAE**
4th
Excludes1: neonatal chlamydial conjunctivitis (P39.1)
neonatal chlamydial pneumonia (P23.1)
Reiter's disease (M02.3-)
sexually transmitted chlamydial diseases (A55–A56)
Excludes2: chlamydial pneumonia (J16.0)

A74.0 **Chlamydial conjunctivitis**
Paratrachoma
A74.8 **Other chlamydial diseases**
5th **A74.81** **Chlamydial peritonitis**
A74.89 **Other chlamydial diseases**
A74.9 **Chlamydial infection, unspecified**
Chlamydiosis NOS

(A75–A79) RICKETTSIOSES

A77 **SPOTTED FEVER [TICK-BORNE RICKETTSIOSES]**
4th
A77.0 **Spotted fever due to Rickettsia rickettsii**
Rocky Mountain spotted fever
Sao Paulo fever
A77.4 **Ehrlichiosis**
5th *Excludes1:* anaplasmosis [A. phagocytophilum] (A79.82)
rickettsiosis due to Ehrlichia sennetsu (A79.81)
A77.40 **Ehrlichiosis, unspecified**
A77.41 **Ehrlichiosis chaffeensis [E. chaffeensis]**
A77.49 **Other ehrlichiosis**
Ehrlichiosis due to E. ewingii
Ehrlichiosis due to E. muris euclairensis
A77.8 **Other spotted fevers**
Rickettsia 364D/R. philipii (Pacific Coast tick fever)
Spotted fever due to Rickettsia africae (African tick bite fever)
Spotted fever due to Rickettsia parkeri
A77.9 **Spotted fever, unspecified**
Tick-borne typhus NOS

A79 **OTHER RICKETTSIOSES**
4th
A79.1 **Rickettsialpox due to Rickettsia akari**
Kew Garden fever
Vesicular rickettsiosis
A79.8 **Other specified rickettsioses**
5th •**A79.82** **Anaplasmosis [A. phagocytophilum]**
Transfusion transmitted A. phagocytophilum
A79.89 **Other specified rickettsioses**
A79.9 **Rickettsiosis, unspecified**
Rickettsial infection NOS

(A80–A89) VIRAL AND PRION INFECTIONS OF THE CENTRAL NERVOUS SYSTEM

Excludes1: postpolio syndrome (G14)
sequelae of poliomyelitis (B91)
sequelae of viral encephalitis (B94.1)

A80 **ACUTE POLIOMYELITIS**
4th
Excludes1: acute flaccid myelitis (G04.82)
A80.1 **Acute paralytic poliomyelitis, wild virus, imported**
A80.2 **Acute paralytic poliomyelitis, wild virus, indigenous**
A80.3 **Acute paralytic poliomyelitis, other and unspecified**
5th **A80.30** **Acute paralytic poliomyelitis, unspecified**
A80.39 **Other acute paralytic poliomyelitis**
A80.9 **Acute poliomyelitis, unspecified**

A82 **RABIES**
4th
A82.0 **Sylvatic rabies**
A82.1 **Urban rabies**
A82.9 **Rabies, unspecified**

A83 **MOSQUITO-BORNE VIRAL ENCEPHALITIS**
4th
Includes: mosquito-borne viral meningoencephalitis
Excludes2: Venezuelan equine encephalitis (A92.2)
West Nile fever (A92.3-)
West Nile virus (A92.3-)
A83.2 **Eastern equine encephalitis**
A83.3 **St Louis encephalitis**
A83.5 **California encephalitis**
California meningoencephalitis
La Crosse encephalitis
A83.8 **Other mosquito-borne viral encephalitis**
A83.9 **Mosquito-borne viral encephalitis, unspecified**

A84 **TICK-BORNE VIRAL ENCEPHALITIS**
4th
Includes: tick-borne viral meningoencephalitis
A84.8 **Other tick-borne viral encephalitis**
5th **A84.81** **Powassan virus disease**
A84.89 **Other tick-borne viral encephalitis**
Louping ill
Code first, if applicable, transfusion related infection (T80.22-)
A84.9 **Tick-borne viral encephalitis, unspecified**

A85 **OTHER VIRAL ENCEPHALITIS, NEC**
4th
Includes: specified viral encephalomyelitis NEC
specified viral meningoencephalitis NEC
Excludes1: benign myalgic encephalomyelitis (G93.3)
encephalitis due to cytomegalovirus (B25.8)
encephalitis due to herpesvirus NEC (B10.0-)
encephalitis due to herpesvirus [herpes simplex] (B00.4)
encephalitis due to measles virus (B05.0)
encephalitis due to mumps virus (B26.2)
encephalitis due to poliomyelitis virus (A80.-)
encephalitis due to zoster (B02.0)
lymphocytic choriomeningitis (A87.2)
A85.0 **Enteroviral encephalitis**
Enteroviral encephalomyelitis
A85.1 **Adenoviral encephalitis**
Adenoviral meningoencephalitis
A85.2 **Arthropod-borne viral encephalitis, unspecified**
Excludes1: West nile virus with encephalitis (A92.31)
A85.8 **Other specified viral encephalitis**
Encephalitis lethargica
Von Economo-Cruchet disease

4th 5th 6th 7th Additional Character Required	✔ 3-character code

•=New Code　　*Excludes1*—Not coded here, do not use together
▲=Revised Code　　*Excludes2*—Not included here

CHAPTER 1. CERTAIN INFECTIOUS AND PARASITIC DISEASES　(A65–A85.8)

CHAPTER 1. CERTAIN INFECTIOUS AND PARASITIC DISEASES (A86–B00.51)

A86 ✔ **UNSPECIFIED VIRAL ENCEPHALITIS**
Viral encephalomyelitis NOS
Viral meningoencephalitis NOS

A87 4th **VIRAL MENINGITIS**
Excludes1: meningitis due to herpesvirus [herpes simplex] (B00.3)
meningitis due to herpesvirus [herpes simplex] (B00.3)
meningitis due to measles virus (B05.1)
meningitis due to mumps virus (B26.1)
meningitis due to poliomyelitis virus (A80.-)
meningitis due to zoster (B02.1)
A87.0 Enteroviral meningitis
Coxsackievirus meningitis
Echovirus meningitis
A87.1 Adenoviral meningitis
A87.8 Other viral meningitis
A87.9 Viral meningitis, unspecified

A88 4th **OTHER VIRAL INFECTIONS OF CENTRAL NERVOUS SYSTEM, NEC**
Excludes1: viral encephalitis NOS (A86)
viral meningitis NOS (A87.9)
A88.0 Enteroviral exanthematous fever [Boston exanthem]
A88.1 Epidemic vertigo
A88.8 Other specified viral infections of central nervous system

A89 ✔ **UNSPECIFIED VIRAL INFECTION OF CENTRAL NERVOUS SYSTEM**

(A90–A99) ARTHROPOD-BORNE VIRAL FEVERS AND VIRAL HEMORRHAGIC FEVERS

A92 4th **OTHER MOSQUITO-BORNE VIRAL FEVERS**
Excludes1: Ross River disease (B33.1)
A92.3 West Nile virus infection
5th West Nile fever
A92.30 West Nile virus infection, unspecified
West Nile fever NOS
West Nile fever without complications
West Nile virus NOS
A92.31 West Nile virus infection with encephalitis
West Nile encephalitis
West Nile encephalomyelitis
A92.32 West Nile virus infection with other neurologic manifestation
Use additional code to specify the neurologic manifestation
A92.39 West Nile virus infection with other complications
Use additional code to specify the other conditions
A92.5 Zika virus disease

> **GUIDELINE**
>
> **1) Code only confirmed cases**
> Code only a confirmed diagnosis of Zika virus (A92.5, Zika virus disease) as documented by the provider. This is an exception to the hospital inpatient guideline Section II, H. In this context, "confirmation" does not require documentation of the type of test performed; the provider's diagnostic statement that the condition is confirmed is sufficient. This code should be assigned regardless of the stated mode of transmission.
> If the provider documents "suspected", "possible" or "probable" Zika, do not assign code A92.5. Assign a code(s) explaining the reason for encounter (such as fever, rash, or joint pain) or Z20.821, Contact with and (suspected) exposure to Zika virus.
> Zika virus fever
> Zika virus infection
> Zika, NOS
> *Excludes1:* congenital Zika virus disease (P35.4)

A92.8 Other specified mosquito-borne viral fevers
A92.9 Mosquito-borne viral fever, unspecified

A93 4th **OTHER ARTHROPOD-BORNE VIRAL FEVERS, NOT ELSEWHERE CLASSIFIED**
A93.0 Oropouche virus disease
Oropouche fever

A93.1 Sandfly fever
Pappataci fever
Phlebotomus fever
A93.2 Colorado tick fever
A93.8 Other specified arthropod-borne viral fevers
Piry virus disease
Vesicular stomatitis virus disease [Indiana fever]

A94 ✔ **UNSPECIFIED ARTHROPOD-BORNE VIRAL FEVER**
Arboviral fever NOS
Arbovirus infection NOS

A95 4th **YELLOW FEVER**
A95.0 Sylvatic yellow fever
Jungle yellow fever
A95.1 Urban yellow fever
A95.9 Yellow fever, unspecified

A96 4th **ARENAVIRAL HEMORRHAGIC FEVER**
A96.0 Junin hemorrhagic fever
Argentinian hemorrhagic fever
A96.1 Machupo hemorrhagic fever
Bolivian hemorrhagic fever
A96.2 Lassa fever
A96.8 Other arenaviral hemorrhagic fevers
A96.9 Arenaviral hemorrhagic fever, unspecified

A98 4th **OTHER VIRAL HEMORRHAGIC FEVERS, NOT ELSEWHERE CLASSIFIED**
Excludes1: chikungunya hemorrhagic fever (A92.0)
dengue hemorrhagic fever (A91)
A98.4 Ebola virus disease
A98.5 Hemorrhagic fever with renal syndrome
Epidemic hemorrhagic fever
Korean hemorrhagic fever
Russian hemorrhagic fever
Hantaan virus disease
Hantavirus disease with renal manifestations
Nephropathia epidemica
Songo fever
Excludes1: hantavirus (cardio)-pulmonary syndrome (B33.4)
A98.8 Other specified viral hemorrhagic fevers

A99 ✔ **UNSPECIFIED VIRAL HEMORRHAGIC FEVER**

(B00–B09) VIRAL INFECTIONS CHARACTERIZED BY SKIN AND MUCOUS MEMBRANE LESIONS

B00 4th **HERPESVIRAL [HERPES SIMPLEX] INFECTIONS**
Excludes1: congenital herpesviral infections (P35.2)
Excludes2: anogenital herpesviral infection (A60.-)
gammaherpesviral mononucleosis (B27.0-)
herpangina (B08.5)
B00.0 Eczema herpeticum
Kaposi's varicelliform eruption
B00.1 Herpesviral vesicular dermatitis
Herpes simplex facialis
Herpes simplex labialis
Herpes simplex otitis externa
Vesicular dermatitis of ear
Vesicular dermatitis of lip
B00.2 Herpesviral gingivostomatitis and pharyngotonsillitis
Herpesviral pharyngitis
B00.3 Herpesviral meningitis
B00.4 Herpesviral encephalitis
Herpesviral meningoencephalitis
Simian B disease
Excludes1: herpesviral encephalitis due to herpesvirus 6 and 7 (B10.01, B10.09)
non-simplex herpesviral encephalitis (B10.0-)
B00.5 Herpesviral ocular disease
5th **B00.50 Herpesviral ocular disease, unspecified**
B00.51 Herpesviral iridocyclitis
Herpesviral iritis
Herpesviral uveitis, anterior

4th 5th 6th 7th Additional Character Required   ✔ 3-character code   •=New Code   *Excludes1*—Not coded here, do not use together
▲=Revised Code   *Excludes2*—Not included here

B00.52 Herpesviral keratitis
Herpesviral keratoconjunctivitis
B00.53 Herpesviral conjunctivitis
B00.59 Other herpesviral disease of eye
Herpesviral dermatitis of eyelid
B00.7 Disseminated herpesviral disease
Herpesviral sepsis
B00.8 Other forms of herpesviral infections
5th **B00.81 Herpesviral hepatitis**
B00.82 Herpes simplex myelitis
B00.89 Other herpesviral infection
Herpesviral whitlow
B00.9 Herpesviral infection, unspecified
Herpes simplex infection NOS

B01 VARICELLA [CHICKENPOX]
4th **B01.0 Varicella meningitis**
B01.1 Varicella encephalitis, myelitis and encephalomyelitis
5th Postchickenpox encephalitis, myelitis and encephalomyelitis
B01.11 Varicella encephalitis and encephalomyelitis
Postchickenpox encephalitis and encephalomyelitis
B01.12 Varicella myelitis
Postchickenpox myelitis
B01.2 Varicella pneumonia
B01.8 Varicella with other complications
5th **B01.81 Varicella keratitis**
B01.89 Other varicella complications
B01.9 Varicella without complication
Varicella NOS

B05 MEASLES
4th *Includes:* morbilli
Excludes1: subacute sclerosing panencephalitis (A81.1)
B05.0 Measles complicated by encephalitis
Postmeasles encephalitis
B05.1 Measles complicated by meningitis
Postmeasles meningitis
B05.2 Measles complicated by pneumonia
Postmeasles pneumonia
B05.3 Measles complicated by otitis media
Postmeasles otitis media
B05.4 Measles with intestinal complications
B05.8 Measles with other complications
5th **B05.81 Measles keratitis and keratoconjunctivitis**
B05.89 Other measles complications
B05.9 Measles without complication
Measles NOS

B06 RUBELLA [GERMAN MEASLES]
4th *Excludes1:* congenital rubella (P35.0)
B06.0 Rubella with neurological complications
5th **B06.00 Rubella with neurological complication, unspecified**
B06.09 Other neurological complications of rubella
B06.8 Rubella with other complications
5th **B06.81 Rubella pneumonia**
B06.89 Other rubella complications
B06.9 Rubella without complication
Rubella NOS

B07 VIRAL WARTS
4th *Includes:* verruca simplex
verruca vulgaris
viral warts due to human papillomavirus
Excludes2: anogenital (venereal) warts (A63.0)
papilloma of bladder (D41.4)
papilloma of cervix (D26.0)
papilloma larynx (D14.1)
B07.0 Plantar wart
Verruca plantaris
B07.8 Other viral warts
Common wart
Flat wart
Verruca plana
B07.9 Viral wart, unspecified

B08 OTHER VIRAL INFECTIONS CHARACTERIZED BY SKIN
4th **AND MUCOUS MEMBRANE LESIONS, NEC**
Excludes1: vesicular stomatitis virus disease (A93.8)
B08.1 Molluscum contagiosum
B08.2 Exanthema subitum [sixth disease]
5th Roseola infantum
B08.20 Exanthema subitum [sixth disease], unspecified
Roseola infantum, unspecified
B08.21 Exanthema subitum [sixth disease] due to human herpesvirus 6
Roseola infantum due to human herpesvirus 6
B08.22 Exanthema subitum [sixth disease] due to human herpesvirus 7
Roseola infantum due to human herpesvirus 7
B08.3 Erythema infectiosum [fifth disease]
B08.4 Enteroviral vesicular stomatitis with exanthem
Hand, foot and mouth disease
B08.5 Enteroviral vesicular pharyngitis
Herpangina
B08.8 Other specified viral infections characterized by skin and mucous membrane lesions
Enteroviral lymphonodular pharyngitis
Foot-and-mouth disease
Poxvirus NEC

B09 UNSPECIFIED VIRAL INFECTION CHARACTERIZED BY
✔ **SKIN AND MUCOUS MEMBRANE LESIONS**
Viral enanthema NOS
Viral exanthema NOS

(B10) OTHER HUMAN HERPESVIRUSES

B10 OTHER HUMAN HERPESVIRUSES
4th *Excludes2:* cytomegalovirus (B25.9)
Epstein-Barr virus (B27.0-)
herpes NOS (B00.9)
herpes simplex (B00.-)
herpes zoster (B02.-)
human herpesvirus NOS (B00.-)
human herpesvirus 1 and 2 (B00.-)
human herpesvirus 3 (B01.-, B02.-)
human herpesvirus 4 (B27.0-)
human herpesvirus 5 (B25.-)
varicella (B01.-)
zoster (B02.-)
B10.0 Other human herpesvirus encephalitis
5th *Excludes2:* herpes encephalitis NOS (B00.4)
herpes simplex encephalitis (B00.4)
human herpesvirus encephalitis (B00.4)
simian B herpes virus encephalitis (B00.4)
B10.01 Human herpesvirus 6 encephalitis
B10.09 Other human herpesvirus encephalitis
Human herpesvirus 7 encephalitis
B10.8 Other human herpesvirus infection
5th **B10.81 Human herpesvirus 6 infection**
B10.82 Human herpesvirus 7 infection
B10.89 Other human herpesvirus infection
Human herpesvirus 8 infection
Kaposi's sarcoma-associated herpesvirus infection

(B15–B19) VIRAL HEPATITIS

Excludes1: sequelae of viral hepatitis (B94.2)
Excludes2: cytomegaloviral hepatitis (B25.1)
herpesviral [herpes simplex] hepatitis (B00.81)

B15 ACUTE HEPATITIS A
4th **B15.9 Hepatitis A without hepatic coma**
Hepatitis A (acute)(viral) NOS

B16 ACUTE HEPATITIS B
4th **B16.9 Acute hepatitis B without delta-agent and without hepatic coma**
Hepatitis B (acute) (viral) NOS

4th 5th 6th 7th Additional Character Required   ✔ 3-character code   •=New Code   *Excludes1*—Not coded here, do not use together
▲=Revised Code   *Excludes2*—Not included here

B17 **OTHER ACUTE VIRAL HEPATITIS**
`4th`
    B17.1 **Acute hepatitis C**
      `5th`   **B17.10**   **Acute hepatitis C without hepatic coma**
                  Acute hepatitis C NOS
    B17.9 **Acute viral hepatitis, unspecified**
          Acute infectious hepatitis NOS

B18 **CHRONIC VIRAL HEPATITIS**
`4th`
    Includes: Carrier of viral hepatitis
    B18.1 **Chronic viral hepatitis B without delta-agent**
          Carrier of viral hepatits B
    B18.2 **Chronic viral hepatitis C**
          Carrier of viral hepatitis C
    B18.8 **Other chronic viral hepatitis**
          Carrier of other viral hepatitis
    B18.9 **Chronic viral hepatitis, unspecified**
          Carrier of unspecified viral hepatitis

B19 **UNSPECIFIED VIRAL HEPATITIS**
`4th`
    B19.1 **Unspecified viral hepatitis B**
      `5th`   **B19.10**   **Unspecified viral hepatitis B without hepatic coma**
                  Unspecified viral hepatitis B NOS
    B19.2 **Unspecified viral hepatitis C**
      `5th`   **B19.20**   **Unspecified viral hepatitis C without hepatic coma**
                  Viral hepatitis C NOS
    B19.9 **Unspecified viral hepatitis without hepatic coma**
          Viral hepatitis NOS

(B20) HIV DISEASE

GUIDELINES

Code only confirmed cases of HIV infection/illness

In this context, "confirmation" does not require documentation of positive serology or culture for HIV; the provider's diagnostic statement that the patient is HIV positive, or has an HIV-related illness is sufficient.

Asymptomatic HIV

Z21, Asymptomatic HIV infection status, is to be applied when the patient without any documentation of symptoms is listed as being "HIV positive," "known HIV," "HIV test positive," or similar terminology. Do not use this code if the term "AIDS" **or "HIV Disease"** is used or if the patient is treated for any HIV-related illness or is described as having any condition(s) resulting from his/her HIV positive status; use B20 in these cases.

Patients with inconclusive HIV serology

Patients with inconclusive HIV serology, but no definitive diagnosis or manifestations of the illness, may be assigned code R75, Inconclusive laboratory evidence of HIV.

Encounters for testing for HIV

If a patient is being seen to determine his/her HIV status, use code Z11.4, Encounter for screening for human immunodeficiency virus [HIV]. Use additional codes for any associated high-risk behavior, **if applicable.**

If a patient with signs or symptoms is being seen for HIV testing, code the signs and symptoms. An additional counseling code Z71.7, Human immunodeficiency virus [HIV] counseling, may be used if counseling is provided during the encounter for the test.

When a patient returns to be informed of his/her HIV test results and the test result is negative, use code Z71.7, Human immunodeficiency virus [HIV] counseling.

If the results are positive, see previous guidelines and assign codes as appropriate.

(i) History of HIV managed by medication

If a patient with documented history of HIV disease is currently managed on antiretroviral medications, assign code B20, Human immunodeficiency virus [HIV] disease. Code Z79.899, Other long term (current) drug therapy, may be assigned as an additional code to identify the long-term (current) use of antiretroviral medications.

B20 **HIV DISEASE**
✔
    Includes: acquired immune deficiency syndrome [AIDS]
          AIDS-related complex [ARC]
          HIV infection, symptomatic
    Use additional code(s) to identify all manifestations of HIV infection
    Excludes1: asymptomatic HIV infection status (Z21)
          exposure to HIV virus (Z20.6)
          inconclusive serologic evidence of HIV (R75)
          Other viral diseases (B25–B34)

(B25–B34) OTHER VIRAL DISEASES

B25 **CYTOMEGALOVIRAL DISEASE**
`4th`
    Excludes1: congenital cytomegalovirus infection (P35.1)
          cytomegaloviral mononucleosis (B27.1-)
    B25.0 **Cytomegaloviral pneumonitis**
    B25.8 **Other cytomegaloviral diseases**
          Cytomegaloviral encephalitis
    B25.9 **Cytomegaloviral disease, unspecified**

B26 **MUMPS**
`4th`
    Includes: epidemic parotitis
          infectious parotitis
    B26.0 **Mumps orchitis**
    B26.1 **Mumps meningitis**
    B26.2 **Mumps encephalitis**
    B26.8 **Mumps with other complications**
      `5th`   **B26.89**   **Other mumps complications**
    B26.9 **Mumps without complication**
          Mumps NOS
          Mumps parotitis NOS

B27 **INFECTIOUS MONONUCLEOSIS**
`4th`
    Includes: glandular fever
          monocytic angina
          Pfeiffer's disease
    B27.0 **Gammaherpesviral mononucleosis**
      `5th`   Mononucleosis due to Epstein-Barr virus
          B27.00   **Gammaherpesviral mononucleosis without complication**
          B27.01   **Gammaherpesviral mononucleosis with polyneuropathy**
          B27.02   **Gammaherpesviral mononucleosis with meningitis**
          B27.09   **Gammaherpesviral mononucleosis with other complications**
                 Hepatomegaly in gammaherpesviral mononucleosis
    B27.1 **Cytomegaloviral mononucleosis**
      `5th`   **B27.10**   **Cytomegaloviral mononucleosis without complications**
          B27.11   **Cytomegaloviral mononucleosis with polyneuropathy**
          B27.12   **Cytomegaloviral mononucleosis with meningitis**
          B27.19   **Cytomegaloviral mononucleosis with other complication**
                 Hepatomegaly in cytomegaloviral mononucleosis
    B27.8 **Other infectious mononucleosis**
      `5th`   **B27.80**   **Other infectious mononucleosis without complication**
          B27.81   **Other infectious mononucleosis with polyneuropathy**
          B27.82   **Other infectious mononucleosis with meningitis**
          B27.89   **Other infectious mononucleosis with other complication**
                 Hepatomegaly in other infectious mononucleosis
    B27.9 **Infectious mononucleosis, unspecified**
      `5th`   **B27.90**   **Infectious mononucleosis, unspecified without complication**
          B27.91   **Infectious mononucleosis, unspecified with polyneuropathy**
          B27.92   **Infectious mononucleosis, unspecified with meningitis**
          B27.99   **Infectious mononucleosis, unspecified with other complication**
                 Hepatomegaly in unspecified infectious mononucleosis

B30 **VIRAL CONJUNCTIVITIS**
`4th`
    Excludes1: herpesviral [herpes simplex] ocular disease (B00.5)
          ocular zoster (B02.3)

`4th` `5th` `6th` `7th` Additional Character Required   ✔   3-character code

•=New Code   *Excludes1*—Not coded here, do not use together
▲=Revised Code   *Excludes2*—Not included here

B30.0 Keratoconjunctivitis due to adenovirus
Epidemic keratoconjunctivitis
Shipyard eye

B30.1 Conjunctivitis due to adenovirus
Acute adenoviral follicular conjunctivitis
Swimming-pool conjunctivitis

B30.2 Viral pharyngoconjunctivitis

B30.3 Acute epidemic hemorrhagic conjunctivitis (enteroviral)
Conjunctivitis due to coxsackievirus 24
Conjunctivitis due to enterovirus 70
Hemorrhagic conjunctivitis (acute)(epidemic)

B30.8 Other viral conjunctivitis
Newcastle conjunctivitis

B30.9 Viral conjunctivitis, unspecified

B33 OTHER VIRAL DISEASES, NEC
`4th`
B33.2 Viral carditis
`5th`
Coxsackie (virus) carditis
B33.20 Viral carditis, unspecified
B33.21 Viral endocarditis
B33.22 Viral myocarditis
B33.23 Viral pericarditis
B33.24 Viral cardiomyopathy

B33.3 Retrovirus infections, NEC
Retrovirus infection NOS

B33.8 Other specified viral diseases
Excludes1: anogenital human papillomavirus infection (A63.0)
viral warts due to human papillomavirus infection (B07)

B34 VIRAL INFECTION OF UNSPECIFIED SITE
`4th`
Excludes1: anogenital human papillomavirus infection (A63.0)
cytomegaloviral disease NOS (B25.9)
herpesvirus [herpes simplex] infection NOS (B00.9)
retrovirus infection NOS (B33.3)
viral agents as the cause of diseases classified elsewhere (B97.-)
viral warts due to human papillomavirus infection (B07)

B34.0 Adenovirus infection, unspecified

B34.1 Enterovirus infection, unspecified
Coxsackievirus infection NOS
Echovirus infection NOS

B34.2 Coronavirus infection, unspecified
Excludes1: COVID-19 (U07.1)
pneumonia due to SARS-associated coronavirus (J12.81)

B34.3 Parvovirus infection, unspecified

B34.4 Papovavirus infection, unspecified

B34.8 Other viral infections of unspecified site

B34.9 Viral infection, unspecified
Viremia NOS

(B35–B49) MYCOSES

Excludes2: hypersensitivity pneumonitis due to organic dust (J67.-)
mycosis fungoides (C84.0-)

B35 DERMATOPHYTOSIS
`4th`
Includes: favus
infections due to species of Epidermophyton, Micro-sporum and Trichophyton
tinea, any type except those in B36.-

B35.0 Tinea barbae and tinea capitis
Beard ringworm
Kerion
Scalp ringworm
Sycosis, mycotic

B35.1 Tinea unguium
Dermatophytic onychia
Dermatophytosis of nail
Onychomycosis
Ringworm of nails

B35.2 Tinea manuum
Dermatophytosis of hand
Hand ringworm

B35.3 Tinea pedis
Athlete's foot
Dermatophytosis of foot
Foot ringworm

B35.4 Tinea corporis
Ringworm of the body

B35.5 Tinea imbricata
Tokelau

B35.6 Tinea cruris
Dhobi itch
Groin ringworm
Jock itch

B35.8 Other dermatophytoses
Disseminated dermatophytosis
Granulomatous dermatophytosis

B35.9 Dermatophytosis, unspecified
Ringworm NOS

B36 OTHER SUPERFICIAL MYCOSES
`4th`
B36.0 Pityriasis versicolor
Tinea flava
Tinea versicolor

B36.8 Other specified superficial mycoses

B36.9 Superficial mycosis, unspecified

B37 CANDIDIASIS
`4th`
Includes: candidosis
moniliasis
Excludes1: neonatal candidiasis (P37.5)

B37.0 Candidal stomatitis
Oral thrush

B37.1 Pulmonary candidiasis
Candidal bronchitis
Candidal pneumonia

B37.2 Candidiasis of skin and nail
Candidal onychia
Candidal paronychia
Excludes2: diaper dermatitis (L22)

B37.3 Candidiasis of vulva and vagina
Candidal vulvovaginitis
Monilial vulvovaginitis
Vaginal thrush

B37.4 Candidiasis of other urogenital sites
`5th`
B37.41 Candidal cystitis and urethritis
B37.42 Candidal balanitis
B37.49 Other urogenital candidiasis
Candidal pyelonephritis

B37.5 Candidal meningitis

B37.6 Candidal endocarditis

B37.7 Candidal sepsis
Disseminated candidiasis
Systemic candidiasis

B37.8 Candidiasis of other sites
`5th`
B37.81 Candidal esophagitis
B37.82 Candidal enteritis
Candidal proctitis
B37.83 Candidal cheilitis
B37.84 Candidal otitis externa
B37.89 Other sites of candidiasis
Candidal osteomyelitis

B37.9 Candidiasis, unspecified
Thrush NOS

B39 HISTOPLASMOSIS
`4th`
Code first associated AIDS (B20)
Use additional code for any associated manifestations, such as:
endocarditis (I39)
meningitis (G02)
pericarditis (I32)
retinitits (H32)

B39.0 Acute pulmonary histoplasmosis capsulati

B39.1 Chronic pulmonary histoplasmosis capsulati

B39.2 Pulmonary histoplasmosis capsulati, unspecified

B39.3 Disseminated histoplasmosis capsulati
Generalized histoplasmosis capsulati

B39.4 Histoplasmosis capsulati, unspecified
American histoplasmosis

B39.9 Histoplasmosis, unspecified

`4th` `5th` `6th` `7th` Additional Character Required   ✓ 3-character code   • =New Code   ▲=Revised Code   *Excludes1*—Not coded here, do not use together   *Excludes2*—Not included here

B40 BLASTOMYCOSIS
4th

Excludes1: Brazilian blastomycosis (B41.-)
 keloidal blastomycosis (B48.0)

B40.0 Acute pulmonary blastomycosis
B40.1 Chronic pulmonary blastomycosis
B40.2 Pulmonary blastomycosis, unspecified
B40.3 Cutaneous blastomycosis
B40.7 Disseminated blastomycosis
 Generalized blastomycosis
B40.8 Other forms of blastomycosis
 5th B40.81 Blastomycotic meningoencephalitis
  Meningomyelitis due to blastomycosis
  B40.89 Other forms of blastomycosis
B40.9 Blastomycosis, unspecified

B44 ASPERGILLOSIS
4th

Includes: aspergilloma

B44.8 Other forms of aspergillosis
 5th B44.81 Allergic bronchopulmonary aspergillosis
  B44.89 Other forms of aspergillosis
B44.9 Aspergillosis, unspecified

B49 UNSPECIFIED MYCOSIS
✔

Fungemia NOS

(B50–B64) PROTOZOAL DISEASES

Excludes1: amebiasis (A06.-)
 other protozoal intestinal diseases (A07.-)

B54 UNSPECIFIED MALARIA
✔

B58 TOXOPLASMOSIS
4th

Includes: infection due to Toxoplasma gondii
Excludes1: congenital toxoplasmosis (P37.1)

B58.0 Toxoplasma oculopathy
 5th B58.00 Toxoplasma oculopathy, unspecified
  B58.01 Toxoplasma chorioretinitis
  B58.09 Other toxoplasma oculopathy
   Toxoplasma uveitis
B58.2 Toxoplasma meningoencephalitis
B58.3 Pulmonary toxoplasmosis
B58.8 Toxoplasmosis with other organ involvement
 5th B58.83 Toxoplasma tubulo-interstitial nephropathy
   Toxoplasma pyelonephritis
  B58.89 Toxoplasmosis with other organ involvement
B58.9 Toxoplasmosis, unspecified

B60 OTHER PROTOZOAL DISEASES, NOT ELSEWHERE CLASSIFIED
4th

Excludes1: cryptosporidiosis (A07.2)
 intestinal microsporidiosis (A07.8)
 isosporiasis (A07.3)

B60.0 Babesiosis
 5th B60.00 Babesiosis, unspecified
   Babesiosis due to unspecified Babesia species
   Piroplasmosis, unspecified
  B60.01 Babesiosis due to Babesia microti
   Infection due to B. microti
  B60.02 Babesiosis due to Babesia duncani
   Infection due to B. duncani and B. duncani-type species
  B60.03 Babesiosis due to Babesia divergens
   Babesiosis due to Babesia MO-1
   Infection due to B. divergens and B. divergens-like strains
  B60.09 Other babesiosis
   Babesiosis due to Babesia KO-1
   Babesiosis due to Babesia venatorum
   Infection due to other Babesia species
   Infection due to other protozoa of the order Piroplasmida
   Other piroplasmosis
B60.1 Acanthamebiasis
 5th B60.10 Acanthamebiasis, unspecified
  B60.11 Meningoencephalitis due to Acanthamoeba (culbertsoni)
  B60.12 Conjunctivitis due to Acanthamoeba

  B60.13 Keratoconjunctivitis due to Acanthamoeba
  B60.19 Other acanthamebic disease

B64 UNSPECIFIED PROTOZOAL DISEASE
✔

(B65–B83) HELMINTHIASES

B65 SCHISTOSOMIASIS [BILHARZIASIS]
4th

Includes: snail fever

B65.3 Cercarial dermatitis
 Swimmer's itch
B65.8 Other schistosomiasis
 Infection due to Schistosoma intercalatum
 Infection due to Schistosoma mattheei
 Infection due to Schistosoma mekongi
B65.9 Schistosomiasis, unspecified

B66 OTHER FLUKE INFECTIONS
4th

B66.8 Other specified fluke infections
 Echinostomiasis
 Heterophyiasis
 Metagonimiasis
 Nanophyetiasis
 Watsoniasis
B66.9 Fluke infection, unspecified

B69 CYSTICERCOSIS
4th

Includes: cysticerciasis infection due to larval form of Taenia solium
B69.0 Cysticercosis of central nervous system
B69.8 Cysticercosis of other sites
 5th B69.89 Cysticercosis of other sites
B69.9 Cysticercosis, unspecified

B71 OTHER CESTODE INFECTIONS
4th

B71.0 Hymenolepiasis
 Dwarf tapeworm infection
 Rat tapeworm (infection)
B71.8 Other specified cestode infections
 Coenurosis
B71.9 Cestode infection, unspecified
 Tapeworm (infection) NOS

B76 HOOKWORM DISEASES
4th

Includes: uncinariasis
B76.9 Hookworm disease, unspecified
 Cutaneous larva migrans NOS

B77 ASCARIASIS
4th

Includes: ascaridiasis
 roundworm infection
B77.0 Ascariasis with intestinal complications
B77.8 Ascariasis with other complications
 5th B77.81 Ascariasis pneumonia
  B77.89 Ascariasis with other complications
B77.9 Ascariasis, unspecified

B79 TRICHURIASIS
✔

Includes: trichocephaliasis
 whipworm (disease)(infection)

B80 ENTEROBIASIS
✔

Includes: oxyuriasis
 pinworm infection
 threadworm infection

B82 UNSPECIFIED INTESTINAL PARASITISM
4th

B82.0 Intestinal helminthiasis, unspecified
B82.9 Intestinal parasitism, unspecified

(B85–B89) PEDICULOSIS, ACARIASIS AND OTHER INFESTATIONS

B85 PEDICULOSIS AND PHTHIRIASIS
4th

B85.0 Pediculosis due to Pediculus humanus capitis
 Head-louse infestation
B85.1 Pediculosis due to Pediculus humanus corporis
 Body-louse infestation

4th **5th** **6th** **7th** Additional Character Required	**✔** 3-character code	•=New Code ▲=Revised Code	**Excludes1**—Not coded here, do not use together **Excludes2**—Not included here

B85.2 **Pediculosis, unspecified**

B85.3 **Phthiriasis**
Infestation by crab-louse
Infestation by Phthirus pubis

B85.4 **Mixed pediculosis and phthiriasis**
Infestation classifiable to more than one of the categories
B85.0–B85.3

B86 SCABIES
✔ Sarcoptic itch

B88 OTHER INFESTATIONS
4th B88.0 **Other acariasis**
Acarine dermatitis
Dermatitis due to Demodex species
Dermatitis due to Dermanyssus gallinae
Dermatitis due to Liponyssoides sanguineus
Trombiculosis
Excludes2: scabies (B86)

B88.1 **Tungiasis [sandflea infestation]**

B88.2 **Other arthropod infestations**
Scarabiasis

B88.3 **External hirudiniasis**
Leech infestation NOS
Excludes2: internal hirudiniasis (B83.4)

B88.8 **Other specified infestations**
Ichthyoparasitism due to Vandellia cirrhosa
Linguatulosis
Porocephaliasis

B88.9 **Infestation, unspecified**
Infestation (skin) NOS
Infestation by mites NOS
Skin parasites NOS

B89 UNSPECIFIED PARASITIC DISEASE
✔

(B90–B94) SEQUELAE OF INFECTIOUS AND PARASITIC DISEASES

Note: Categories B90–B94 are to be used to indicate conditions in categories A00–B89 as the cause of sequelae, which are themselves classified elsewhere. The 'sequelae' include conditions specified as such; they also include residuals of diseases classifiable to the above categories if there is evidence that the disease itself is no longer present. Codes from these categories are not to be used for chronic infections. Code chronic current infections to active infectious disease as appropriate.

Code first condition resulting from (sequela) the infectious or parasitic disease

B90 SEQUELAE OF TUBERCULOSIS
4th B90.0 **Sequelae of central nervous system tuberculosis**

B90.1 **Sequelae of genitourinary tuberculosis**

B90.2 **Sequelae of tuberculosis of bones and joints**

B90.8 **Sequelae of tuberculosis of other organs**
Excludes2: sequelae of respiratory tuberculosis (B90.9)

B90.9 **Sequelae of respiratory and unspecified tuberculosis**
Sequelae of tuberculosis NOS

B94 SEQUELAE OF OTHER AND UNSPECIFIED INFECTIOUS AND PARASITIC DISEASES
4th B94.1 **Sequelae of viral encephalitis**

B94.2 **Sequelae of viral hepatitis**

B94.8 **Sequelae of other specified infectious and parasitic diseases**

B94.9 **Sequelae of unspecified infectious and parasitic disease**
Excludes2: post COVID-19 condition (U09.9)

(B95–B97) BACTERIAL AND VIRAL INFECTIOUS AGENTS

Note: These categories are provided for use as supplementary or additional codes to identify the infectious agent(s) in diseases classified elsewhere.

B95 STREPTOCOCCUS, STAPHYLOCOCCUS, AND ENTEROCOCCUS AS THE CAUSE OF DISEASES CLASSIFIED ELSEWHERE
4th B95.0 **Streptococcus, group A, as the cause of diseases classified elsewhere**

B95.1 **Streptococcus, group B, as the cause of diseases classified elsewhere**

B95.2 **Enterococcus as the cause of diseases classified elsewhere**

B95.3 **Streptococcus pneumoniae as the cause of diseases classified elsewhere**

B95.4 **Other streptococcus as the cause of diseases classified elsewhere**

B95.5 **Unspecified streptococcus as the cause of diseases classified elsewhere**

B95.6 **Staphylococcus aureus as the cause of diseases classified elsewhere**
5th

B95.61 **MSSA infection as the cause of diseases classified elsewhere**
MSSA infection as the cause of diseases classified elsewhere
Staphylococcus aureus infection NOS as the cause of diseases classified elsewhere

B95.62 **MRSA infection as the cause of diseases classified elsewhere**
MRSA infection as the cause of diseases classified elsewhere

B95.7 **Other staphylococcus as the cause of diseases classified elsewhere**

B95.8 **Unspecified staphylococcus as the cause of diseases classified elsewhere**

B96 OTHER BACTERIAL AGENTS AS THE CAUSE OF DISEASES CLASSIFIED ELSEWHERE
4th B96.0 **M. pneumoniae as the cause of diseases classified elsewhere**
Pleuro-pneumonia-like-organism [PPLO]

B96.1 **K. pneumoniae as the cause of diseases classified elsewhere**

B96.2 **E. coli as the cause of diseases classified elsewhere**
5th

B96.20 **Unspecified E. coli as the cause of diseases classified elsewhere**
E. coli NOS

B96.21 **STEC O157 as the cause of diseases classified elsewhere**
E. coli O157:H- (nonmotile) with confirmation of Shiga toxin
E. coli O157 with confirmation of Shiga toxin when H antigen is unknown, or is not H7
O157:H7 E. coli with or without confirmation of Shiga toxin-production
STEC O157:H7 with or without confirmation of Shiga toxin-production
STEC O157:H7 with or without confirmation of Shiga toxin-production

B96.22 **Other specified STEC as the cause of diseases classified elsewhere**
Non-O157 STEC
Non-O157 STEC with known O group

B96.23 **STEC as the cause of diseases classified elsewhere**
STEC with unspecified O group
STEC NOS

B96.29 **Other E. coli as the cause of diseases classified elsewhere**
Non-STEC

B96.3 **H. influenzae as the cause of diseases classified elsewhere**

B96.4 **Proteus (mirabilis) (morganii) as the cause of diseases classified elsewhere**

B96.5 **Pseudomonas (aeruginosa) (mallei) (pseudomallei) as the cause of diseases classified elsewhere**

B96.8 **Other specified bacterial agents as the cause of diseases classified elsewhere**
5th

B96.81 **H. pylori as the cause of diseases classified elsewhere**

B96.89 **Other specified bacterial agents as the cause of diseases classified elsewhere**

B97 VIRAL AGENTS AS THE CAUSE OF DISEASES CLASSIFIED ELSEWHERE
4th B97.0 **Adenovirus as the cause of diseases classified elsewhere**

B97.1 **Enterovirus as the cause of diseases classified elsewhere**
5th

B97.10 **Unspecified enterovirus as the cause of diseases classified elsewhere**

4th 5th 6th 7th Additional Character Required ✔ 3-character code

•=New Code ▲=Revised Code

Excludes1—Not coded here, do not use together
Excludes2—Not included here

B97.11   **Coxsackievirus as the cause of diseases classified elsewhere**

B97.12   **Echovirus as the cause of diseases classified elsewhere**

B97.19   **Other enterovirus as the cause of diseases classified elsewhere**

B97.2 **Coronavirus as the cause of diseases classified elsewhere**

`5th` **B97.21**   **SARS-associated coronavirus as the cause of diseases classified elsewhere**

Excludes1: pneumonia due to SARS-associated coronavirus (J12.81)

B97.29   **Other coronavirus as the cause of diseases classified elsewhere**

B97.4 **Respiratory syncytial virus as the cause of diseases classified elsewhere**

RSV as the cause of diseases classified elsewhere

Code first related disorders, such as:
   otitis media (H65.-)
   upper respiratory infection (J06.9)

Excludes1: acute bronchiolitis due to respiratory syncytial virus (RSV) (J21.0)
   acute bronchitis due to respiratory syncytial virus (RSV) (J20.5)
   respiratory syncytial virus (RSV) pneumonia (J12.1)

B97.6 **Parvovirus as the cause of diseases classified elsewhere**

`5th` **B97.8** **Other viral agents as the cause of diseases classified elsewhere**

B97.89   **Other viral agents as the cause of diseases classified elsewhere**

(B99) OTHER INFECTIOUS DISEASES

B99   **OTHER AND UNSPECIFIED INFECTIOUS DISEASES**

`4th` **B99.8** **Other infectious disease**

B99.9 **Unspecified infectious disease**

`4th` `5th` `6th` `7th` Additional Character Required   ✔ 3-character code   •=New Code   ▲=Revised Code   *Excludes1*—Not coded here, do not use together   *Excludes2*—Not included here

Chapter 2. Neoplasms (C00–D49)

GUIDELINES

Chapter 2 of the *ICD-10-CM* contains the codes for most benign and all malignant neoplasms. Certain benign neoplasms, such as prostatic adenomas, may be found in the specific body system chapters. To properly code a neoplasm it is necessary to determine from the record if the neoplasm is benign, in-situ, malignant, or of uncertain histologic behavior. If malignant, any secondary (metastatic) sites should also be determined.

Primary malignant neoplasms overlapping site boundaries

A primary malignant neoplasm that overlaps two or more contiguous (next to each other) sites should be classified to the subcategory/code .8 ('overlapping lesion'), unless the combination is specifically indexed elsewhere. For multiple neoplasms of the same site that are not contiguous such as tumors in different quadrants of the same breast, codes for each site should be assigned.

Malignant neoplasm of ectopic tissue

Malignant neoplasms of ectopic tissue are to be coded to the site of origin mentioned, e.g., ectopic pancreatic malignant neoplasms involving the stomach are coded to malignant neoplasm of pancreas, unspecified (C25.9).

The neoplasm table in the Alphabetic Index should be referenced first. However, if the histological term is documented, that term should be referenced first, rather than going immediately to the Neoplasm Table, in order to determine which column in the Neoplasm Table is appropriate. For example, if the documentation indicates "adenoma," refer to the term in the Alphabetic Index to review the entries under this term and the instructional note to "see also neoplasm, by site, benign." The table provides the proper code based on the type of neoplasm and the site. It is important to select the proper column in the table that corresponds to the type of neoplasm. The Tabular List should then be referenced to verify that the correct code has been selected from the table and that a more specific site code does not exist.

Refer to the *ICD-10-CM* manual for information regarding Z15.0, codes for genetic susceptibility to cancer.

TREATMENT DIRECTED AT THE MALIGNANCY

If the treatment is directed at the malignancy, designate the malignancy as the principal diagnosis.

The only exception to this guideline is if a patient admission/encounter is solely for the administration of chemotherapy, immunotherapy or external beam radiation therapy, assign the appropriate Z51.- code as the first-listed or principal diagnosis, and the diagnosis or problem for which the service is being performed as a secondary diagnosis.

TREATMENT OF SECONDARY SITE

When a patient is admitted because of a primary neoplasm with metastasis and treatment is directed toward the secondary site only, the secondary neoplasm is designated as the principal diagnosis even though the primary malignancy is still present.

CODING AND SEQUENCING OF COMPLICATIONS

Coding and sequencing of complications associated with the malignancies or with the therapy thereof are subject to the following guidelines:

Anemia associated with malignancy

When admission/encounter is for management of an anemia associated with the malignancy, and the treatment is only for anemia, the appropriate code for the malignancy is sequenced as the principal or first-listed diagnosis followed by the appropriate code for the anemia (such as code D63.0, Anemia in neoplastic disease).

Anemia associated with chemotherapy, immunotherapy and radiation therapy

When the admission/encounter is for management of an anemia associated with an adverse effect of the administration of chemotherapy or immunotherapy and the only treatment is for the anemia, the anemia code is sequenced first followed by the appropriate codes for the neoplasm and the adverse effect (T45.1X5, Adverse effect of antineoplastic and immunosuppressive drugs).

When the admission/encounter is for management of an anemia associated with an adverse effect of radiotherapy, the anemia code should be sequenced first, followed by the appropriate neoplasm code and code Y84.2, Radiological procedure and radiotherapy as the cause of abnormal reaction of the patient, or of later complication, without mention of misadventure at the time of the procedure.

Management of dehydration due to the malignancy

When the admission/encounter is for management of dehydration due to the malignancy and only the dehydration is being treated (intravenous rehydration), the dehydration is sequenced first, followed by the code(s) for the malignancy.

Treatment of a complication resulting from a surgical procedure

When the admission/encounter is for treatment of a complication resulting from a surgical procedure, designate the complication as the principal or first-listed diagnosis if treatment is directed at resolving the complication.

PRIMARY MALIGNANCY PREVIOUSLY EXCISED

When a primary malignancy has been previously excised or eradicated from its site and there is no further treatment directed to that site and there is no evidence of any existing primary malignancy at that site, a code from category Z85, Personal history of malignant neoplasm, should be used to indicate the former site of the malignancy. Any mention of extension, invasion, or metastasis to another site is coded as a secondary malignant neoplasm to that site. The secondary site may be the principal or first-listed a diagnosis with the Z85 code used as a secondary code.

ADMISSIONS/ENCOUNTERS INVOLVING CHEMOTHERAPY, IMMUNO-THERAPY AND RADIATION THERAPY

Episode of care involves surgical removal of neoplasm

When an episode of care involves the surgical removal of a neoplasm, primary or secondary site, followed by adjunct chemotherapy or radiation treatment during the same episode of care, the code for the neoplasm should be assigned as principal or first-listed diagnosis.

Patient admission/encounter solely for administration of chemo-therapy, immunotherapy and radiation therapy

If a patient admission/encounter is solely for the administration of chemotherapy, immunotherapy or external beam radiation therapy assign code Z51.0, Encounter for antineoplastic radiation therapy, or Z51.11, Encounter for antineoplastic chemotherapy, or Z51.12, Encounter for antineoplastic immunotherapy as the first-listed or principal diagnosis. If a patient receives more than one of these therapies during the same admission more than one of these codes may be assigned, in any sequence. The malignancy for which the therapy is being administered should be assigned as a secondary diagnosis.

If a patient admission/encounter is for the insertion or implantation of radioactive elements (e.g., brachytherapy) the appropriate code for the malignancy is sequenced as the principal or first-listed diagnosis. Code Z51.0 should not be assigned.

Patient admitted for radiation therapy, chemotherapy or immuno-therapy and develops complications

When a patient is admitted for the purpose of external beam radiotherapy, immunotherapy or chemotherapy and develops complications such as uncontrolled nausea and vomiting or dehydration, the principal or first-listed diagnosis is Z51.0, Encounter for antineoplastic radiation therapy, or Z51.11, Encounter for antineoplastic chemotherapy, or Z51.12, Encounter for antineoplastic immunotherapy followed by any codes for the complications. When a patient is admitted for the purpose of insertion or implantation of radioactive elements (e.g., brachytherapy) and develops complications such as uncontrolled nausea and vomiting or dehydration, the principal or first-listed diagnosis is the appropriate code for the malignancy followed by any codes for the complications.

ADMISSION/ENCOUNTER TO DETERMINE EXTENT OF MALIGNANCY

When the reason for admission/encounter is to determine the extent of the malignancy, or for a procedure such as paracentesis or thoracentesis, the primary malignancy or appropriate metastatic site is designated as the principal or first-listed diagnosis, even though chemotherapy or radiotherapy is administered.

SYMPTOMS, SIGNS, AND ABNORMAL FINDINGS LISTED IN CHAPTER 18 ASSOCIATED WITH NEOPLASMS

Symptoms, signs, and ill-defined conditions listed in Chapter 18 characteristic of, or associated with, an existing primary or secondary site malignancy cannot be used to replace the malignancy as principal or first-listed diagnosis, regardless of the number of admissions or encounters for treatment and care of the neoplasm.

ADMISSION/ENCOUNTER FOR PAIN CONTROL/MANAGEMENT

Refer to category G89 for information on coding admission/encounter for pain control/management.

CHAPTER 2. NEOPLASMS

  Additional Character Required   3-character code

Unspecified laterality codes were excluded here.   •=New Code   ▲=Revised Code   ***Excludes1***—Not coded here, do not use together   ***Excludes2***—Not included here

MALIGNANCY IN TWO OR MORE NONCONTIGUOUS SITES

A patient may have more than one malignant tumor in the same organ. These tumors may represent different primaries or metastatic disease, depending on the site. Should the documentation be unclear, the provider should be queried as to the status of each tumor so that the correct codes can be assigned.

DISSEMINATED MALIGNANT NEOPLASM, UNSPECIFIED

See code C80.0.

MALIGNANT NEOPLASM WITHOUT SPECIFICATION OF SITE

See code C80.1.

SEQUENCING OF NEOPLASM CODES

Encounter for treatment of primary malignancy

If the reason for the encounter is for treatment of a primary malignancy, assign the malignancy as the principal/first-listed diagnosis. The primary site is to be sequenced first, followed by any metastatic sites.

Encounter for treatment of secondary malignancy

When an encounter is for a primary malignancy with metastasis and treatment is directed toward the metastatic (secondary) site(s) only, the metastatic site(s) is designated as the principal/first-listed diagnosis. The primary malignancy is coded as an additional code.

Encounter for complication associated with a neoplasm

When an encounter is for management of a complication associated with a neoplasm, such as dehydration, and the treatment is only for the complication, the complication is coded first, followed by the appropriate code(s) for the neoplasm.

The exception to this guideline is anemia. When the admission/encounter is for management of an anemia associated with the malignancy, and the treatment is only for anemia, the appropriate code for the malignancy is sequenced as the principal or first-listed diagnosis followed by code D63.0, Anemia in neoplastic disease.

Complication from surgical procedure for treatment of a neoplasm

When an encounter is for treatment of a complication resulting from a surgical procedure performed for the treatment of the neoplasm, designate the complication as the principal/first-listed diagnosis. See the guideline regarding the coding of a current malignancy versus personal history to determine if the code for the neoplasm should also be assigned.

Pathologic fracture due to a neoplasm

When an encounter is for a pathological fracture due to a neoplasm, and the focus of treatment is the fracture, a code from subcategory M84.5, should be sequenced first, followed by the code for the neoplasm.

If the focus of treatment is the neoplasm with an associated pathological fracture, the neoplasm code should be sequenced first, followed by a code from M84.5 for the pathological fracture.

CURRENT MALIGNANCY VERSUS PERSONAL HISTORY OF MALIGNANCY

When a primary malignancy has been excised but further treatment, such as additional surgery for the malignancy, radiation therapy or chemotherapy is directed to that site, the primary malignancy code should be used until treatment is completed.

When a primary malignancy has been previously excised or eradicated from its site, there is no further treatment (of the malignancy) directed to that site, and there is no evidence of any existing primary malignancy at that site, a code from category Z85, Personal history of malignant neoplasm, should be used to indicate the former site of the malignancy.

Subcategories Z85.0 – Z85.7 should only be assigned for the former site of a primary malignancy, not the site of a secondary malignancy. Codes from subcategory Z85.8-, may be assigned for the former site(s) of either a primary or secondary malignancy included in this subcategory.

Refer to Chapter 21, Factors influencing health status and contact with health services, History (of).

LEUKEMIA, MULTIPLE MYELOMA, AND MALIGNANT PLASMA CELL NEOPLASMS IN REMISSION VERSUS PERSONAL HISTORY

The categories for leukemia, and category C90, have codes indicating whether or not the leukemia has achieved remission. There are also codes Z85.6, Personal history of leukemia, and Z85.79, Personal history of other malignant neoplasms of lymphoid, hematopoietic and related tissues. If the documentation is unclear, as to whether the leukemia has achieved remission, the provider should be queried.

Refer to Chapter 21, Factors influencing health status and contact with health services, History (of)

AFTERCARE FOLLOWING SURGERY FOR NEOPLASM

Refer to Chapter 21, Factors influencing health status and contact with health services, Aftercare

FOLLOW-UP CARE FOR COMPLETED TREATMENT OF A MALIGNANCY

Refer to Chapter 21, Factors influencing health status and contact with health services, Follow-up

PROPHYLACTIC ORGAN REMOVAL FOR PREVENTION OF MALIGNANCY

Refer to Chapter 21, Factors influencing health

MALIGNANT NEOPLASM ASSOCIATED WITH TRANSPLANTED ORGAN

A malignant neoplasm of a transplanted organ should be coded as a transplant complication. Assign first the appropriate code from category T86.-, Complications of transplanted organs and tissue, followed by code C80.2, Malignant neoplasm associated with transplanted organ. Use an additional code for the specific malignancy.

BREAST IMPLANT ASSOCIATED ANAPLASTIC LARGE CELL LYMPHOMA

Breast implant associated anaplastic large cell lymphoma (BIA-ALCL) is a type of lymphoma that can develop around breast implants. Assign code C84.7A, Anaplastic large cell lymphoma, ALK-negative, breast, for BIA-ALCL. Do not assign a complication code from chapter 19.

NEOPLASMS (C00–D49)

Note: Functional activity

All neoplasms are classified in this chapter, whether they are functionally active or not. An additional code from Chapter 4 may be used, to identify functional activity associated with any neoplasm.

Morphology [Histology]

Chapter 2 classifies neoplasms primarily by site (topography), with broad groupings for behavior, malignant, in situ, benign, etc. The Table of Neoplasms should be used to identify the correct topography code. In a few cases, such as for malignant melanoma and certain neuroendocrine tumors, the morphology (histologic type) is included in the category and codes.

Primary malignant neoplasms overlapping site boundaries

A primary malignant neoplasm that overlaps two or more contiguous (next to each other) sites should be classified to the subcategory/code .8 ('overlapping lesion'), unless the combination is specifically indexed elsewhere. For multiple neoplasms of the same site that are not contiguous, such as tumors in different quadrants of the same breast, codes for each site should be assigned.

Malignant neoplasm of ectopic tissue

Malignant neoplasms of ectopic tissue are to be coded to the site mentioned, e.g., ectopic pancreatic malignant neoplasms are coded to pancreas, unspecified (C25.9).

(C00–C96) MALIGNANT NEOPLASMS

Includes: Malignant neoplasms, stated or presumed to be primary (of specified sites), and certain specified histologies, except neuroendocrine, and of lymphoid, hematopoietic and related tissue (C00–C75)

(C00–C14) MALIGNANT NEOPLASMS OF LIP, ORAL CAVITY AND PHARYNX

(C15–C26) MALIGNANT NEOPLASMS OF DIGESTIVE ORGANS

Excludes1: Kaposi's sarcoma of gastrointestinal sites (C46.4)

(C30–C39) MALIGNANT NEOPLASMS OF RESPIRATORY AND INTRATHORACIC ORGANS

Includes: malignant neoplasm of middle ear
Excludes1: mesothelioma (C45.-)

(C40–C41) MALIGNANT NEOPLASMS OF BONE AND ARTICULAR CARTILAGE

Includes: malignant neoplasm of cartilage (articular) (joint)
    malignant neoplasm of periosteum
Excludes1: malignant neoplasm of bone marrow NOS (C96.9)
    malignant neoplasm of synovia (C49.-)

  4th 5th 6th 7th Additional Character Required   3-character code

Unspecified laterality codes were excluded here. •=New Code ▲=Revised Code ***Excludes1***—Not coded here, do not use together ***Excludes2***—Not included here

C40 **MALIGNANT NEOPLASM OF BONE AND ARTICULAR**
`4th` **CARTILAGE OF LIMBS**

Use additional code to identify major osseous defect, if applicable (M89.7-)

C40.0 **Malignant neoplasm of scapula and long bones of upper limb**
`5th`   **C40.01**   **right upper limb**
     C40.02   **left upper limb**

C40.1 **Malignant neoplasm of short bones of; upper limb**
`5th`   **C40.11**   **right upper limb**
     C40.12   **left upper limb**

C40.2 **Malignant neoplasm of long bones of; lower limb**
`5th`   **C40.21**   **right lower limb**
     C40.22   **left lower limb**

C40.3 **Malignant neoplasm of short bones of; lower limb**
`5th`   **C40.31**   **right lower limb**
     C40.32   **left lower limb**

C40.8 **Malignant neoplasm of overlapping sites of bone and articular**
`5th` **cartilage of; limb**
     C40.81   **right limb**
     C40.82   **left limb**

C40.9 **Malignant neoplasm of unspecified bones and articular**
`5th` **cartilage of; limb**
     C40.91   **right limb**
     C40.92   **left limb**

C41 **MALIGNANT NEOPLASM OF BONE AND ARTICULAR**
`4th` **CARTILAGE OF OTHER AND UNSPECIFIED SITES**

Excludes1: malignant neoplasm of bones of limbs (C40.-)
   malignant neoplasm of cartilage of ear (C49.0)
   malignant neoplasm of cartilage of eyelid (C49.0)
   malignant neoplasm of cartilage of larynx (C32.3)
   malignant neoplasm of cartilage of limbs (C40.-)
   malignant neoplasm of cartilage of nose (C30.0)

C41.0 **Malignant neoplasm of bones of skull and face**
   Malignant neoplasm of maxilla (superior)
   Malignant neoplasm of orbital bone
   Excludes2: carcinoma, any type except intraosseous or
     odontogenic of:
     maxillary sinus (C31.0)
     upper jaw (C03.0)
     malignant neoplasm of jaw bone (lower) (C41.1)

C41.1 **Malignant neoplasm of mandible**
   Malignant neoplasm of inferior maxilla
   Malignant neoplasm of lower jaw bone
   Excludes2: carcinoma, any type except intraosseous or
     odontogenic of:
     jaw NOS (C03.9)
     lower (C03.1)
     malignant neoplasm of upper jaw bone (C41.0)

C41.2 **Malignant neoplasm of vertebral column**
   Excludes1: malignant neoplasm of sacrum and coccyx (C41.4)

C41.3 **Malignant neoplasm of ribs, sternum and clavicle**

C41.4 **Malignant neoplasm of pelvic bones, sacrum and coccyx**

C41.9 **Malignant neoplasm of bone and articular cartilage, unspecified**

(C43–C44) MELANOMA AND OTHER MALIGNANT NEOPLASMS OF SKIN

C43 **MALIGNANT MELANOMA OF SKIN**
`4th` *Excludes1:* melanoma in situ (D03.-)

Excludes2: malignant melanoma of skin of genital organs (C51-C52,
   C60.-, C63.-)
   Merkel cell carcinoma (C4A.-)
   sites other than skin-code to malignant neoplasm of the site

C43.0 **Malignant melanoma of lip**
   Excludes1: malignant neoplasm of vermilion border of lip
     (C00.0-C00.2)

C43.1 **Malignant melanoma of eyelid, including canthus**
`5th`   **C43.10**   **Malignant melanoma of unspecified eyelid, including canthus**
     C43.11   **Malignant melanoma of right eyelid, including**
     `6th` **canthus**

     C43.111   **Malignant melanoma of right upper eyelid, including canthus**
     C43.112   **Malignant melanoma of right lower eyelid, including canthus**
   C43.12   **Malignant melanoma of left eyelid, including canthus**
   `6th`   **C43.121**   **Malignant melanoma of left upper eyelid, including canthus**
     C43.122   **Malignant melanoma of left lower eyelid, including canthus**

C43.2 **Malignant melanoma of ear and external auricular canal**
`5th`   **C43.21**   **Malignant melanoma of right ear and external auricular canal**
     C43.22   **Malignant melanoma of left ear and external auricular canal**

C43.3 **Malignant melanoma of other and unspecified parts of face**
`5th`   **C43.30**   **Malignant melanoma of unspecified part of face**
     C43.31   **Malignant melanoma of nose**
     C43.39   **Malignant melanoma of other parts of face**

C43.4 **Malignant melanoma of scalp and neck**

C43.5 **Malignant melanoma of trunk**
`5th`   *Excludes2:* malignant neoplasm of anus NOS (C21.0)
     malignant neoplasm of scrotum (C63.2)
     C43.51   **Malignant melanoma of anal skin**
       Malignant melanoma of anal margin
       Malignant melanoma of perianal skin
     C43.52   **Malignant melanoma of skin of breast**
     C43.59   **Malignant melanoma of other part of trunk**

C43.6 **Malignant melanoma of upper limb, including shoulder**
`5th`   **C43.61**   **Malignant melanoma of right upper limb, including shoulder**
     C43.62   **Malignant melanoma of left upper limb, including shoulder**

C43.7 **Malignant melanoma of lower limb, including hip**
`5th`   **C43.71**   **Malignant melanoma of right lower limb, including hip**
     C43.72   **Malignant melanoma of left lower limb, including hip**

C43.8 **Malignant melanoma of overlapping sites of skin**

C43.9 **Malignant melanoma of skin, unspecified**
   Malignant melanoma of unspecified site of skin
   Melanoma (malignant) NOS

C4A **MERKEL CELL CARCINOMA**
`4th`   **C4A.0** **Merkel cell carcinoma of lip**
     Excludes1: malignant neoplasm of vermilion border of lip
       (C00.0-C00.2)

C4A.1 **Merkel cell carcinoma of eyelid, including canthus**
`5th`   **C4A.10**   **Merkel cell carcinoma of unspecified eyelid, including canthus**
     C4A.11   **Merkel cell carcinoma of right eyelid, including**
     `6th` **canthus**
       C4A.111   **Merkel cell carcinoma of right upper eyelid, including canthus**
       C4A.112   **Merkel cell carcinoma of right lower eyelid, including canthus**
     C4A.12   **Merkel cell carcinoma of left eyelid, including**
     `6th` **canthus**
       C4A.121   **Merkel cell carcinoma of left upper eyelid, including canthus**
       C4A.122   **Merkel cell carcinoma of left lower eyelid, including canthus**

C4A.2 **Merkel cell carcinoma of ear and external auricular canal**
`5th`   **C4A.20**   **Merkel cell carcinoma of unspecified ear and external auricular canal**
     C4A.21   **Merkel cell carcinoma of right ear and external auricular canal**
     C4A.22   **Merkel cell carcinoma of left ear and external auricular canal**

C4A.3 **Merkel cell carcinoma of other and unspecified parts of face**
`5th`   **C4A.30**   **Merkel cell carcinoma of unspecified part of face**
     C4A.31   **Merkel cell carcinoma of nose**
     C4A.39   **Merkel cell carcinoma of other parts of face**

C4A.4 **Merkel cell carcinoma of scalp and neck**

CHAPTER 2. NEOPLASMS   (C40–C4A.4)

`4th` `5th` `6th` `7th` Additional Character Required   ✔ 3-character code

Unspecified laterality codes were excluded here.   •=New Code   ▲=Revised Code

Excludes1—Not coded here, do not use together
Excludes2—Not included here

C4A.5   **Merkel cell carcinoma of trunk**
[5th]
     Excludes2: malignant neoplasm of anus NOS (C21.0)
       malignant neoplasm of scrotum (C63.2)

     C4A.51   **Merkel cell carcinoma of anal skin**
         Merkel cell carcinoma of anal margin
         Merkel cell carcinoma of perianal skin

     C4A.52   **Merkel cell carcinoma of skin of breast**
     C4A.59   **Merkel cell carcinoma of other part of trunk**

C4A.6   **Merkel cell carcinoma of upper limb, including shoulder**
[5th]
     C4A.61   **Merkel cell carcinoma of right upper limb, including shoulder**
     C4A.62   **Merkel cell carcinoma of left upper limb, including shoulder**

C4A.7   **Merkel cell carcinoma of lower limb, including hip**
[5th]
     C4A.71   **Merkel cell carcinoma of right lower limb, including hip**
     C4A.72   **Merkel cell carcinoma of left lower limb, including hip**

C4A.8   **Merkel cell carcinoma of overlapping sites**

C4A.9   **Merkel cell carcinoma, unspecified**
     Merkel cell carcinoma of unspecified site
     Merkel cell carcinoma NOS

C44   **OTHER AND UNSPECIFIED MALIGNANT NEOPLASM**
[4th]   **OF SKIN**
     Includes: malignant neoplasm of sebaceous glands
       malignant neoplasm of sweat glands
     Excludes1: Kaposi's sarcoma of skin (C46.0)
       malignant melanoma of skin (C43.-)
       malignant neoplasm of skin of genital organs (C51-C52, C60.-, C63.2)
       Merkel cell carcinoma (C4A.-)

C44.0   **Other and unspecified malignant neoplasm of skin of lip**
[5th]
     Excludes1: malignant neoplasm of lip (C00.-)
     C44.00   **Unspecified malignant neoplasm of skin of lip**
     C44.01   **Basal cell carcinoma of skin of lip**
     C44.02   **Squamous cell carcinoma of skin of lip**
     C44.09   **Other specified malignant neoplasm of skin of lip**

C44.1   **Other and unspecified malignant neoplasm of skin of eyelid,**
[5th]   **including canthus**
     Excludes1: connective tissue of eyelid (C49.0)
     C44.10   **Unspecified malignant neoplasm of skin of eyelid,**
     [6th]   **including canthus**
         C44.101   **Unspecified malignant neoplasm of skin of unspecified eyelid, including canthus**
         C44.102   **Unspecified malignant neoplasm of skin of**
         [7th]   **right eyelid, including canthus**
             C44.1021   **Unspecified malignant neoplasm of skin of right upper eyelid, including canthus**
             C44.1022   **Unspecified malignant neoplasm of skin of right lower eyelid, including canthus**
         C44.109   **Unspecified malignant neoplasm of skin of**
         [7th]   **left eyelid, including canthus**
             C44.1091   **Unspecified malignant neoplasm of skin of left upper eyelid, including canthus**
             C44.1092   **Unspecified malignant neoplasm of skin of left lower eyelid, including canthus**

     C44.11   **Basal cell carcinoma of skin of eyelid, including**
     [6th]   **canthus**
         C44.111   **Basal cell carcinoma of skin of unspecified eyelid, including canthus**
         C44.112   **Basal cell carcinoma of skin of right**
         [7th]   **eyelid, including canthus**
             C44.1121   **Basal cell carcinoma of skin of right upper eyelid, including canthus**
             C44.1122   **Basal cell carcinoma of skin of right lower eyelid, including canthus**
         C44.119   **Basal cell carcinoma of skin of left eyelid,**
         [7th]   **including canthus**

             C44.1191   **Basal cell carcinoma of skin of left upper eyelid, including canthus**
             C44.1192   **Basal cell carcinoma of skin of left lower eyelid, including canthus**

     C44.12   **Squamous cell carcinoma of skin of eyelid, including**
     [6th]   **canthus**
         C44.121   **Squamous cell carcinoma of skin of unspecified eyelid, including canthus**
         C44.122   **Squamous cell carcinoma of skin of right**
         [7th]   **eyelid, including canthus**
             C44.1221   **Squamous cell carcinoma of skin of right upper eyelid, including canthus**
             C44.1222   **Squamous cell carcinoma of skin of right lower eyelid, including canthus**
         C44.129   **Squamous cell carcinoma of skin of left**
         [7th]   **eyelid, including canthus**
             C44.1291   **Squamous cell carcinoma of skin of left upper eyelid, including canthus**
             C44.1292   **Squamous cell carcinoma of skin of left lower eyelid, including canthus**

     C44.13   **Sebaceous cell carcinoma of skin of eyelid, including**
     [6th]   **canthus**
         C44.131   **Sebaceous cell carcinoma of skin of unspecified eyelid, including canthus**
         C44.132   **Sebaceous cell carcinoma of skin of**
         [7th]   **specified lower eyelid**
             C44.1321   **Sebaceous cell carcinoma of skin of right upper eyelid, including canthus**
             C44.1322   **Sebaceous cell carcinoma of skin of right lower eyelid, including canthus**
         C44.139   **Sebaceous cell carcinoma of skin of**
         [7th]   **specified lower eyelid, including canthus**
             C44.1391   **Sebaceous cell carcinoma of skin of left upper eyelid, including canthus**
             C44.1392   **Sebaceous cell carcinoma of skin of left lower eyelid, including canthus**

     C44.19   **Other specified malignant neoplasm of skin of eyelid,**
     [6th]   **including canthus**
         C44.191   **Other specified malignant neoplasm of skin of unspecified eyelid, including canthus**
         C44.192   **Other specified malignant neoplasm of**
         [7th]   **skin of right eyelid, including canthus**
             C44.1921   **Other specified malignant neoplasm of skin of right upper eyelid, including canthus**
             C44.1922   **Other specified malignant neoplasm of skin of right lower eyelid, including canthus**
         C44.199   **Other specified malignant neoplasm of**
         [7th]   **skin of left eyelid, including canthus**
             C44.1991   **Other specified malignant neoplasm of skin of left upper eyelid, including canthus**
             C44.1992   **Other specified malignant neoplasm of skin of left lower eyelid, including canthus**

C44.2   **Other and unspecified malignant neoplasm of skin of ear and**
[5th]   **external auricular canal**
     Excludes1: connective tissue of ear (C49.0)
     C44.20   **Unspecified malignant neoplasm of skin of ear and**
     [6th]   **external auricular canal**

[4th] [5th] [6th] [7th] Additional Character Required   ✔   3-character code

Unspecified laterality codes were excluded here.   •=New Code   ▲=Revised Code   *Excludes1*—Not coded here, do not use together   *Excludes2*—Not included here

144   **PEDIATRIC ICD-10-CM 2022: A MANUAL FOR PROVIDER-BASED CODING**

C44.201   Unspecified malignant neoplasm of skin of unspecified ear and external auricular canal

C44.202   Unspecified malignant neoplasm of skin of right ear and external auricular canal

C44.209   Unspecified malignant neoplasm of skin of left ear and external auricular canal

C44.21 `6th`   Basal cell carcinoma of skin of ear and external auricular canal

C44.212   Basal cell carcinoma of skin of right ear and external auricular canal

C44.219   Basal cell carcinoma of skin of left ear and external auricular canal

C44.22 `6th`   Squamous cell carcinoma of skin of ear and external auricular canal

C44.222   Squamous cell carcinoma of skin of right ear and external auricular canal

C44.229   Squamous cell carcinoma of skin of left ear and external auricular canal

C44.29 `6th`   Other specified malignant neoplasm of skin of ear and external auricular canal

C44.292   Other specified malignant neoplasm of skin of right ear and external auricular canal

C44.299   Other specified malignant neoplasm of skin of left ear and external auricular canal

C44.3 `5th`   Other and unspecified malignant neoplasm of skin of other and unspecified parts of face

C44.30 `6th`   Unspecified malignant neoplasm of skin of other and unspecified parts of face

C44.300   Unspecified malignant neoplasm of skin of unspecified part of face

C44.301   Unspecified malignant neoplasm of skin of nose

C44.309   Unspecified malignant neoplasm of skin of other parts of face

C44.31 `6th`   Basal cell carcinoma of skin of other and unspecified parts of face

C44.310   Basal cell carcinoma of skin of unspecified parts of face

C44.311   Basal cell carcinoma of skin of nose

C44.319   Basal cell carcinoma of skin of other parts of face

C44.32 `6th`   Squamous cell carcinoma of skin of other and unspecified parts of face

C44.320   Squamous cell carcinoma of skin of unspecified parts of face

C44.321   Squamous cell carcinoma of skin of nose

C44.329   Squamous cell carcinoma of skin of other parts of face

C44.39 `6th`   Other specified malignant neoplasm of skin of other and unspecified parts of face

C44.390   Other specified malignant neoplasm of skin of unspecified parts of face

C44.391   Other specified malignant neoplasm of skin of nose

C44.399   Other specified malignant neoplasm of skin of other parts of face

C44.4 `5th`   Other and unspecified malignant neoplasm of skin of scalp and neck

C44.40   Unspecified malignant neoplasm of skin of scalp and neck

C44.41   Basal cell carcinoma of skin of scalp and neck

C44.42   Squamous cell carcinoma of skin of scalp and neck

C44.49   Other specified malignant neoplasm of skin of scalp and neck

C44.5 `5th`   Other and unspecified malignant neoplasm of skin of trunk

Excludes1: anus NOS (C21.0)
          scrotum (C63.2)

C44.50 `6th`   Unspecified malignant neoplasm of skin of trunk

C44.500   Unspecified malignant neoplasm of anal skin

Unspecified malignant neoplasm of anal margin

Unspecified malignant neoplasm of perianal skin

C44.501   Unspecified malignant neoplasm of skin of breast

C44.509   Unspecified malignant neoplasm of skin of other part of trunk

C44.51 `6th`   Basal cell carcinoma of skin of trunk

C44.510   Basal cell carcinoma of anal skin

Basal cell carcinoma of anal margin

Basal cell carcinoma of perianal skin

C44.511   Basal cell carcinoma of skin of breast

C44.519   Basal cell carcinoma of skin of other part of trunk

C44.52 `6th`   Squamous cell carcinoma of skin of trunk

C44.520   Squamous cell carcinoma of anal skin

Squamous cell carcinoma of anal margin

Squamous cell carcinoma of perianal skin

C44.521   Squamous cell carcinoma of skin of breast

C44.529   Squamous cell carcinoma of skin of other part of trunk

C44.59 `6th`   Other specified malignant neoplasm of skin of trunk

C44.590   Other specified malignant neoplasm of anal skin

Other specified malignant neoplasm of anal margin

Other specified malignant neoplasm of perianal skin

C44.591   Other specified malignant neoplasm of skin of breast

C44.599   Other specified malignant neoplasm of skin of other part of trunk

C44.6 `5th`   Other and unspecified malignant neoplasm of skin of upper limb, including shoulder

C44.60 `6th`   Unspecified malignant neoplasm of skin of upper limb, including shoulder

C44.602   Unspecified malignant neoplasm of skin of right upper limb, including shoulder

C44.609   Unspecified malignant neoplasm of skin of left upper limb, including shoulder

C44.61 `6th`   Basal cell carcinoma of skin of upper limb, including shoulder

C44.612   Basal cell carcinoma of skin of right upper limb, including shoulder

C44.619   Basal cell carcinoma of skin of left upper limb, including shoulder

C44.62 `6th`   Squamous cell carcinoma of skin of upper limb, including shoulder

C44.622   Squamous cell carcinoma of skin of right upper limb, including shoulder

C44.629   Squamous cell carcinoma of skin of left upper limb, including shoulder

C44.69 `6th`   Other specified malignant neoplasm of skin of upper limb, including shoulder

C44.692   Other specified malignant neoplasm of skin of right upper limb, including shoulder

C44.699   Other specified malignant neoplasm of skin of left upper limb, including shoulder

C44.7 `5th`   Other and unspecified malignant neoplasm of skin of lower limb, including hip

C44.70 `6th`   Unspecified malignant neoplasm of skin of lower limb, including hip

C44.702   Unspecified malignant neoplasm of skin of right lower limb, including hip

C44.709   Unspecified malignant neoplasm of skin of left lower limb, including hip

C44.71 `6th`   Basal cell carcinoma of skin of lower limb, including hip

C44.712   Basal cell carcinoma of skin of right lower limb, including hip

---

`4th` `5th` `6th` `7th` Additional Character Required   ✔ 3-character code   Unspecified laterality codes were excluded here.   •=New Code   ▲=Revised Code   *Excludes1*—Not coded here, do not use together   *Excludes2*—Not included here

C44.719 Basal cell carcinoma of skin of left lower limb, including hip

C44.72 Squamous cell carcinoma of skin of lower limb, including hip

C44.722 Squamous cell carcinoma of skin of right lower limb, including hip

C44.729 Squamous cell carcinoma of skin of left lower limb, including hip

C44.79 Other specified malignant neoplasm of skin of lower limb, including hip

C44.792 Other specified malignant neoplasm of skin of right lower limb, including hip

C44.799 Other specified malignant neoplasm of skin of left lower limb, including hip

C44.8 Other and unspecified malignant neoplasm of overlapping sites of skin

C44.80 Unspecified malignant neoplasm of overlapping sites of skin

C44.81 Basal cell carcinoma of overlapping sites of skin

C44.82 Squamous cell carcinoma of overlapping sites of skin

C44.89 Other specified malignant neoplasm of overlapping sites of skin

C44.9 Other and unspecified malignant neoplasm of skin, unspecified

C44.90 Unspecified malignant neoplasm of skin, unspecified
Malignant neoplasm of unspecified site of skin

C44.91 Basal cell carcinoma of skin, unspecified

C44.92 Squamous cell carcinoma of skin, unspecified

C44.99 Other specified malignant neoplasm of skin, unspecified

(C45–C49) MALIGNANT NEOPLASMS OF MESOTHELIAL AND SOFT TISSUE

(C50) MALIGNANT NEOPLASMS OF BREAST

(C51–C58) MALIGNANT NEOPLASMS OF FEMALE GENITAL ORGANS

Includes: malignant neoplasm of skin of female genital organs

(C60–C63) MALIGNANT NEOPLASMS OF MALE GENITAL ORGANS

Includes: malignant neoplasm of skin of male genital organs

(C64–C68) MALIGNANT NEOPLASMS OF URINARY TRACT

C64 MALIGNANT NEOPLASM OF KIDNEY, EXCEPT RENAL PELVIS
Excludes1: malignant carcinoid tumor of the kidney (C7A.093)
malignant neoplasm of renal calyces (C65.-)
malignant neoplasm of renal pelvis (C65.-)

C64.1 Malignant neoplasm of right kidney, except renal pelvis

C64.2 Malignant neoplasm of left kidney, except renal pelvis

(C69–C72) MALIGNANT NEOPLASMS OF EYE, BRAIN AND OTHER PARTS OF CENTRAL NERVOUS SYSTEM

C69 MALIGNANT NEOPLASM OF EYE AND ADNEXA
Excludes1: malignant neoplasm of connective tissue of eyelid (C49.0)
malignant neoplasm of eyelid (skin) (C43.1-, C44.1-)
malignant neoplasm of optic nerve (C72.3-)

C69.2 Malignant neoplasm of retina
Excludes1: dark area on retina (D49.81)
neoplasm of unspecified behavior of retina and choroid (D49.81)
retinal freckle (D49.81)

C69.21 Malignant neoplasm of right retina

C69.22 Malignant neoplasm of left retina

C71 MALIGNANT NEOPLASM OF BRAIN
Excludes1: malignant neoplasm of cranial nerves (C72.2–C72.5)
retrobulbar malignant neoplasm (C69.6-)

C71.0 Malignant neoplasm of; cerebrum, except lobes and ventricles
Malignant neoplasm of supratentorial NOS

C71.1 frontal lobe

C71.2 temporal lobe

C71.3 parietal lobe

C71.4 occipital lobe

C71.5 cerebral ventricle
Excludes1: malignant neoplasm of fourth cerebral ventricle (C71.7)

C71.6 cerebellum

C71.7 brain stem
Malignant neoplasm of fourth cerebral ventricle
Infratentorial malignant neoplasm NOS

C71.8 overlapping sites of brain

C71.9 brain, unspecified

(C73–C75) MALIGNANT NEOPLASMS OF THYROID AND OTHER ENDOCRINE GLANDS

C74 MALIGNANT NEOPLASM OF ADRENAL GLAND

C74.0 Malignant neoplasm of cortex of; adrenal gland

C74.01 right adrenal gland

C74.02 left adrenal gland

C74.1 Malignant neoplasm of medulla of; adrenal gland

C74.11 right adrenal gland

C74.12 left adrenal gland

C74.9 Malignant neoplasm of unspecified part of; adrenal gland

C74.91 right adrenal gland

C74.92 left adrenal gland

(C7A) MALIGNANT NEUROENDOCRINE TUMORS

(C7B) SECONDARY NEUROENDOCRINE TUMORS

(C76–C80) MALIGNANT NEOPLASMS OF ILL-DEFINED, OTHER SECONDARY AND UNSPECIFIED SITES

C80 MALIGNANT NEOPLASM WITHOUT SPECIFICATION OF SITE
Excludes1: malignant carcinoid tumor of unspecified site (C7A.00)
malignant neoplasm of specified multiple sites- code to each site

C80.0 Disseminated malignant neoplasm, unspecified
Use only in those cases where the patient has advanced metastatic disease and no known primary or secondary sites are specified. It should not be used in place of assigning codes for the primary site and all known secondary sites.
Carcinomatosis NOS
Generalized cancer, unspecified site (primary) (secondary)
Generalized malignancy, unspecified site (primary) (secondary)

C80.1 Malignant (primary) neoplasm, unspecified
Use only be used when no determination can be made as to the primary site of a malignancy.
Cancer NOS
Cancer unspecified site (primary)
Carcinoma unspecified site (primary)
Malignancy unspecified site (primary)
Excludes1: secondary malignant neoplasm of unspecified site (C79.9)

C80.2 Malignant neoplasm associated with transplanted organ
Code first complication of transplanted organ (T86.-)
Use additional code to identify the specific malignancy

(C81–C96) MALIGNANT NEOPLASMS OF LYMPHOID, HEMATOPOIETIC AND RELATED TISSUE

Excludes2: Kaposi's sarcoma of lymph nodes (C46.3)
secondary and unspecified neoplasm of lymph nodes (C77.-)
secondary neoplasm of bone marrow (C79.52)
secondary neoplasm of spleen (C78.89)

4th **5th** **6th** **7th** Additional Character Required ✔ 3-character code | Unspecified laterality codes were excluded here. | •=New Code ▲=Revised Code | ***Excludes1***—Not coded here, do not use together ***Excludes2***—Not included here

C81 HODGKIN LYMPHOMA

4th *Excludes1:* personal history of Hodgkin lymphoma (Z85.71)

C81.0 Nodular lymphocyte predominant Hodgkin lymphoma

5th
- **C81.00** Nodular lymphocyte predominant Hodgkin lymphoma, unspecified site
- **C81.01** Nodular lymphocyte predominant Hodgkin lymphoma, lymph nodes of head, face, and neck
- **C81.02** Nodular lymphocyte predominant Hodgkin lymphoma, intrathoracic lymph nodes
- **C81.03** Nodular lymphocyte predominant Hodgkin lymphoma, intra-abdominal lymph nodes
- **C81.04** Nodular lymphocyte predominant Hodgkin lymphoma, lymph nodes of axilla and upper limb
- **C81.05** Nodular lymphocyte predominant Hodgkin lymphoma, lymph nodes of inguinal region and lower limb
- **C81.06** Nodular lymphocyte predominant Hodgkin lymphoma, intrapelvic lymph nodes
- **C81.07** Nodular lymphocyte predominant Hodgkin lymphoma, spleen
- **C81.08** Nodular lymphocyte predominant Hodgkin lymphoma, lymph nodes of multiple sites
- **C81.09** Nodular lymphocyte predominant Hodgkin lymphoma, extranodal and solid organ sites

C81.2 Mixed cellularity Hodgkin lymphoma

5th Mixed cellularity classical Hodgkin lymphoma
- **C81.20** Mixed cellularity Hodgkin lymphoma, unspecified site
- **C81.21** lymph nodes of head, face, and neck
- **C81.22** intrathoracic lymph nodes
- **C81.23** intra-abdominal lymph nodes
- **C81.24** lymph nodes of axilla and upper limb
- **C81.25** lymph nodes of inguinal region and lower limb
- **C81.26** intrapelvic lymph nodes
- **C81.27** spleen
- **C81.28** lymph nodes of multiple sites
- **C81.29** extranodal and solid organ sites

C81.9 Hodgkin lymphoma, unspecified

5th
- **C81.91** Hodgkin lymphoma, unspecified; lymph nodes of head, face, and neck
- **C81.92** intrathoracic lymph nodes
- **C81.93** intra-abdominal lymph nodes
- **C81.94** lymph nodes of axilla and upper limb
- **C81.95** lymph nodes of inguinal region and lower limb
- **C81.96** intrapelvic lymph nodes
- **C81.97** spleen
- **C81.98** lymph nodes of multiple sites
- **C81.99** extranodal and solid organ sites

C83 NON-FOLLICULAR LYMPHOMA

4th *Excludes1:* personal history of non-Hodgkin lymphoma (Z85.72)

C83.3 Diffuse large B-cell lymphoma

5th Anaplastic diffuse large B-cell lymphoma
CD30-positive diffuse large B-cell lymphoma
Centroblastic diffuse large B-cell lymphoma
Diffuse large B-cell lymphoma, subtype not specified
Immunoblastic diffuse large B-cell lymphoma
Plasmablastic diffuse large B-cell lymphoma
Diffuse large B-cell lymphoma, subtype not specified
T-cell rich diffuse large B-cell lymphoma

Excludes1: mediastinal (thymic) large B-cell lymphoma (C85.2-)
mature T/NK-cell lymphomas (C84.-)
- **C83.30** Diffuse large B-cell lymphoma; unspecified site
- **C83.31** lymph nodes of head, face, and neck
- **C83.32** intrathoracic lymph nodes
- **C83.33** intra-abdominal lymph nodes
- **C83.34** lymph nodes of axilla and upper limb
- **C83.35** lymph nodes of inguinal region and lower limb
- **C83.36** intrapelvic lymph nodes
- **C83.37** spleen
- **C83.38** lymph nodes of multiple sites
- **C83.39** extranodal and solid organ sites

C83.7 Burkitt lymphoma

5th Atypical Burkitt lymphoma
Burkitt-like lymphoma

Excludes1: mature B-cell leukemia Burkitt type (C91.A-)
- **C83.70** Burkitt lymphoma, unspecified site
- **C83.71** Burkitt lymphoma, lymph nodes of head, face, and neck
- **C83.72** Burkitt lymphoma, intrathoracic lymph nodes
- **C83.73** Burkitt lymphoma, intra-abdominal lymph nodes
- **C83.74** Burkitt lymphoma, lymph nodes of axilla and upper limb
- **C83.75** Burkitt lymphoma, lymph nodes of inguinal region and lower limb
- **C83.76** Burkitt lymphoma, intrapelvic lymph nodes
- **C83.77** Burkitt lymphoma, spleen
- **C83.78** Burkitt lymphoma, lymph nodes of multiple sites
- **C83.79** Burkitt lymphoma, extranodal and solid organ sites

C84 MATURE T/NK-CELL LYMPHOMAS

4th *Excludes1:* personal history of non-Hodgkin lymphoma (Z85.72)

C84.4 Peripheral T-cell lymphoma, not classified

5th Lennert's lymphoma
Lymphoepithelioid lymphoma
Mature T-cell lymphoma, not elsewhere classified
- **C84.41** Peripheral T-cell lymphoma, not classified; lymph nodes of head, face, and neck
- **C84.42** intrathoracic lymph nodes
- **C84.43** intra-abdominal lymph nodes
- **C84.44** lymph nodes of axilla and upper limb
- **C84.45** lymph nodes of inguinal region and lower limb
- **C84.46** intrapelvic lymph nodes
- **C84.47** spleen
- **C84.48** lymph nodes of multiple sites
- **C84.49** extranodal and solid organ sites

C85 OTHER SPECIFIED AND UNSPECIFIED TYPES OF NON-HODGKIN LYMPHOMA

4th *Excludes1:* other specified types of T/NK-cell lymphoma (C86.-)
personal history of non-Hodgkin lymphoma (Z85.72)

C85.9 Non-Hodgkin lymphoma, unspecified

5th Lymphoma NOS
Malignant lymphoma NOS
Non-Hodgkin lymphoma NOS
- **C85.90** Non-Hodgkin lymphoma, unspecified, unspecified site
- **C85.91** Non-Hodgkin lymphoma, unspecified; lymph nodes of head, face, and neck
- **C85.92** intrathoracic lymph nodes
- **C85.93** intra-abdominal lymph nodes
- **C85.94** lymph nodes of axilla and upper limb
- **C85.95** lymph nodes of inguinal region and lower limb
- **C85.96** intrapelvic lymph nodes
- **C85.97** spleen
- **C85.98** lymph nodes of multiple sites
- **C85.99** extranodal and solid organ sites

C91 LYMPHOID LEUKEMIA

4th *Excludes1:* personal history of leukemia (Z85.6)

C91.0 Acute lymphoblastic leukemia [ALL]

5th **Note:** Codes in subcategory C91.0- should only be used for T-cell and B-cell precursor leukemia
- **C91.00** ALL, not having achieved remission
  ALL with failed remission
  ALL NOS
- **C91.01** ALL, in remission
- **C91.02** ALL, in relapse

C91.9 Lymphoid leukemia, unspecified

5th
- **C91.90** Lymphoid leukemia, unspecified; not having achieved remission
  Lymphoid leukemia with failed remission
  Lymphoid leukemia NOS
- **C91.91** in remission
- **C91.92** in relapse

  6th **7th** Additional Character Required   3-character code

Unspecified laterality codes were excluded here.   •=New Code   ▲=Revised Code   ***Excludes1***—Not coded here, do not use together   ***Excludes2***—Not included here

CHAPTER 2. NEOPLASMS (C92–D09)

C92 `4th` **MYELOID LEUKEMIA**
Includes: granulocytic leukemia
   myelogenous leukemia
Excludes1: personal history of leukemia (Z85.6)
C92.0 `5th` **Acute myeloblastic leukemia**
   Acute myeloblastic leukemia, minimal differentiation
   Acute myeloblastic leukemia (with maturation)
   Acute myeloblastic leukemia 1/ETO
   Acute myeloblastic leukemia M0 or M1 or M2
   Acute myeloblastic leukemia with t(8;21)
   Acute myeloblastic leukemia (without a FAB classification) NOS
   Refractory anemia with excess blasts in transformation [RAEB T]
   Excludes1: acute exacerbation of chronic myeloid leukemia (C92.10)
     refractory anemia with excess of blasts not in transformation (D46.2-)
   C92.00 **Acute myeloblastic leukemia; not having achieved remission**
     Acute myeloblastic leukemia with failed remission
     Acute myeloblastic leukemia NOS
   C92.01 **in remission**
   C92.02 **in relapse**
C92.1 `5th` **Chronic myeloid leukemia, BCR/ABL-positive**
   Chronic myelogenous leukemia, Philadelphia chromosome (Ph1) positive
   Chronic myelogenous leukemia, t(9;22) (q34;q11)
   Chronic myelogenous leukemia with crisis of blast cells
   Excludes1: atypical chronic myeloid leukemia BCR/ABL-negative (C92.2-)
     CMML (C93.1-)
     chronic myeloproliferative disease (D47.1)
   C92.10 **Chronic myeloid leukemia, BCR/ABL-positive; not having achieved remission**
     Chronic myeloid leukemia, BCR/ABL-positive with failed remission
     Chronic myeloid leukemia, BCR/ABL-positive NOS
   C92.11 **in remission**
   C92.12 **in relapse**
C92.2 `5th` **Atypical chronic myeloid leukemia, BCR/ABL-negative**
   C92.20 **Atypical chronic myeloid leukemia, BCR/ABL-negative; not having achieved remission**
     Atypical chronic myeloid leukemia, BCR/ABL-negative with failed remission
     Atypical chronic myeloid leukemia, BCR/ABL-negative NOS
   C92.21 **in remission**
   C92.22 **in relapse**
C92.9 `5th` **Myeloid leukemia, unspecified**
   C92.90 **Myeloid leukemia, unspecified; not having achieved remission**
     Myeloid leukemia, unspecified with failed remission
     Myeloid leukemia, unspecified NOS
   C92.91 **in remission**
   C92.92 **unspecified in relapse**

C93 `4th` **MONOCYTIC LEUKEMIA**
Includes: monocytoid leukemia
Excludes1: personal history of leukemia (Z85.6)
C93.0 `5th` **Acute monoblastic/monocytic leukemia**
   AML M5 or AML M5a or AML M5b
   C93.00 **Acute monoblastic/monocytic leukemia; not having achieved remission**
     Acute monoblastic/monocytic leukemia with failed remission
     Acute monoblastic/monocytic leukemia NOS
   C93.01 **in remission**
   C93.02 **in relapse**
C93.1 `5th` **Chronic myelomonocytic leukemia [CMML]**
   Chronic monocytic leukemia
   CMML-1 or CMML-2
   CMML with eosinophilia
   Code also, if applicable, eosinophilia (D72.18)
   C93.10 **CMML not having achieved remission**
     CMML with failed remission
     CMML NOS

   C93.11 **CMML, in remission**
   C93.12 **CMML, in relapse**
C93.3 **Juvenile myelomonocytic leukemia**
   `5th` **C93.30** **Juvenile myelomonocytic leukemia; not having achieved remission**
     Juvenile myelomonocytic leukemia with failed remission
     Juvenile myelomonocytic leukemia NOS
   C93.31 **in remission**
   C93.32 **in relapse**
C93.Z **Other monocytic leukemia**
   `5th` **C93.Z0** **Other monocytic leukemia; not having achieved remission**
     Other monocytic leukemia NOS
   C93.Z1 **in remission**
   C93.Z2 **in relapse**
C93.9 **Monocytic leukemia, unspecified**
   `5th` **C93.90** **Monocytic leukemia, unspecified; not having achieved remission**
     Monocytic leukemia, unspecified with failed remission
     leukemia, unspecified NOS
   C93.91 **in remission**
   C93.92 **in relapse**

C94 `4th` **OTHER LEUKEMIAS OF SPECIFIED CELL TYPE**
Excludes1: leukemic reticuloendotheliosis (C91.4-)
   myelodysplastic syndromes (D46.-)
   personal history of leukemia (Z85.6)
   plasma cell leukemia (C90.1-)
C94.0 `5th` **Acute erythroid leukemia**
   Acute myeloid leukemia M6(a)(b)
   Erythroleukemia
   C94.00 **Acute erythroid leukemia, not having achieved remission**
     Acute erythroid leukemia with failed remission
     Acute erythroid leukemia NOS
   C94.01 **Acute erythroid leukemia, in remission**
   C94.02 **Acute erythroid leukemia, in relapse**
C94.3 **Mast cell leukemia**
   `5th` **C94.30** **Mast cell leukemia not having achieved remission**
     Mast cell leukemia with failed remission
     Mast cell leukemia NOS
   C94.31 **Mast cell leukemia, in remission**
   C94.32 **Mast cell leukemia, in relapse**

C95 `4th` **LEUKEMIA OF UNSPECIFIED CELL TYPE**
Excludes1: personal history of leukemia (Z85.6)
C95.9 **Leukemia, unspecified**
   `5th` **C95.90** **Leukemia, unspecified not having achieved remission**
     Leukemia, unspecified with failed remission
     Leukemia NOS
   C95.91 **Leukemia, unspecified, in remission**
   C95.92 **Leukemia, unspecified, in relapse**

C96 `4th` **OTHER AND UNSPECIFIED MALIGNANT NEOPLASMS OF LYMPHOID, HEMATOPOIETIC AND RELATED TISSUE**
Excludes1: personal history of other malignant neoplasms of lymphoid, hematopoietic and related tissues (Z85.79)
C96.2 `5th` **Malignant mast cell neoplasm**
   Excludes1: indolent mastocytosis (D47.02)
   mast cell leukemia (C94.30)
   mastocytosis (congenital) (cutaneous) (Q82.2)
   C96.20 **Malignant mast cell neoplasm, unspecified**
   C96.21 **Aggressive systemic mastocytosis**
   C96.22 **Mast cell sarcoma**
   C96.29 **Other malignant mast cell neoplasm**
C96.A **Histiocytic sarcoma**
   Malignant histiocytosis

(D00–D09) IN SITU NEOPLASMS

Includes: Bowen's disease
   erythroplasia
   grade III intraepithelial neoplasia
   Queyrat's erythroplasia

`4th` `5th` `6th` `7th` Additional Character Required   ✔ 3-character code

Unspecified laterality codes were excluded here.   •=New Code   ▲=Revised Code   **Excludes1**—Not coded here, do not use together   **Excludes2**—Not included here

(D10–D36) BENIGN NEOPLASMS, EXCEPT BENIGN NEUROENDOCRINE TUMORS

D12 **BENIGN NEOPLASM OF COLON, RECTUM, ANUS AND**
`4th` **ANAL CANAL**

Excludes1: benign carcinoid tumors of the large intestine, and rectum (D3A.02-)

polyp of colon NOS (K63.5)

D12.0 **Benign neoplasm of; cecum**
Benign neoplasm of ileocecal valve

D12.1 **appendix**
Excludes1: benign carcinoid tumor of the appendix (D3A.020)

D12.2 **ascending colon**

D12.3 **transverse colon**
Benign neoplasm of hepatic flexure or splenic flexure

D12.4 **descending colon**

D12.5 **sigmoid colon**

D12.6 **colon, unspecified**
Adenomatosis of colon
Benign neoplasm of large intestine NOS
Polyposis (hereditary) of colon
Excludes1: inflammatory polyp of colon (K51.4-)

D12.7 **rectosigmoid junction**

D12.8 **rectum**
Excludes1: benign carcinoid tumor of the rectum (D3A.026)

D12.9 **Benign neoplasm of anus and anal canal**
Benign neoplasm of anus NOS
Excludes1: benign neoplasm of anal margin (D22.5, D23.5)
benign neoplasm of anal skin (D22.5, D23.5)
benign neoplasm of perianal skin (D22.5, D23.5)

D15 **BENIGN NEOPLASM OF OTHER AND UNSPECIFIED**
`4th` **INTRATHORACIC ORGANS**

Excludes1: benign neoplasm of mesothelial tissue (D19.-)

D15.1 **Benign neoplasm of heart**
Excludes1: benign neoplasm of great vessels (D21.3)

D17 **BENIGN LIPOMATOUS NEOPLASM**
`4th`

D17.0 **Benign lipomatous neoplasm of skin and subcutaneous tissue of; head, face and neck**

D17.1 **trunk**

D17.2 **Benign lipomatous neoplasm of skin and subcutaneous tissue**
`5th` **of; limb**
D17.21 **right arm**
D17.22 **left arm**
D17.23 **right leg**
D17.24 **left leg**

D17.3 **Benign lipomatous neoplasm of skin and subcutaneous tissue**
`5th` **of; other and unspecified sites**
D17.30 **unspecified sites**
D17.39 **other sites**

D17.4 **Benign lipomatous neoplasm of intrathoracic organs**

D17.5 **Benign lipomatous neoplasm of intra-abdominal organs**
Excludes1: benign lipomatous neoplasm of peritoneum and retroperitoneum (D17.79)

D17.6 **Benign lipomatous neoplasm of spermatic cord**

D17.7 **Benign lipomatous neoplasm of other sites**
`5th` **D17.71** **Benign lipomatous neoplasm of; kidney**
D17.72 **other genitourinary organ**
D17.79 **other sites**
Benign lipomatous neoplasm of peritoneum or retroperitoneum

D17.9 **Benign lipomatous neoplasm, unspecified**
Lipoma NOS

D18 **HEMANGIOMA AND LYMPHANGIOMA, ANY SITE**
`4th` *Excludes1:* benign neoplasm of glomus jugulare (D35.6)
blue or pigmented nevus (D22.-)
nevus NOS (D22.-)
vascular nevus (Q82.5)

D18.0 **Hemangioma**
`5th` Angioma NOS
Cavernous nevus
D18.00 **Hemangioma unspecified site**

D18.01 **Hemangioma of skin and subcutaneous tissue**
D18.02 **Hemangioma of intracranial structures**
D18.03 **Hemangioma of intra-abdominal structures**
D18.09 **Hemangioma of other sites**

D18.1 **Lymphangioma, any site**

D22 **MELANOCYTIC NEVI**
`4th` *Includes:* atypical nevus
blue hairy pigmented nevus
nevus NOS

D22.0 **Melanocytic nevi of lip**

D22.1 **Melanocytic nevi of eyelid, including canthus**
`5th` **D22.10** **Melanocytic nevi of unspecified eyelid, including canthus**
D22.11 **Melanocytic nevi of right eyelid, including canthus**
`6th` **D22.111** **Melanocytic nevi of right upper eyelid, including canthus**
D22.112 **Melanocytic nevi of right lower eyelid, including canthus**
D22.12 **Melanocytic nevi of left eyelid, including canthus**
`6th` **D22.121** **Melanocytic nevi of left upper eyelid, including canthus**
D22.122 **Melanocytic nevi of left lower eyelid, including canthus**

D22.2 **Melanocytic nevi of ear and external auricular canal**
`5th` **D22.21** **Melanocytic nevi of right ear and external auricular canal**
D22.22 **Melanocytic nevi of left ear and external auricular canal**

D22.3 **Melanocytic nevi of other and unspecified parts of face**
`5th` **D22.30** **Melanocytic nevi of unspecified part of face**
D22.39 **Melanocytic nevi of other parts of face**

D22.4 **Melanocytic nevi of scalp and neck**

D22.5 **Melanocytic nevi of trunk**
Melanocytic nevi of anal margin
Melanocytic nevi of anal skin
Melanocytic nevi of perianal skin
Melanocytic nevi of skin of breast

D22.6 **Melanocytic nevi of upper limb, including shoulder**
`5th` **D22.61** **Melanocytic nevi of right upper limb, including shoulder**
D22.62 **Melanocytic nevi of left upper limb, including shoulder**

D22.7 **Melanocytic nevi of lower limb, including hip**
`5th` **D22.71** **Melanocytic nevi of right lower limb, including hip**
D22.72 **Melanocytic nevi of left lower limb, including hip**

D22.9 **Melanocytic nevi, unspecified**

D23 **OTHER BENIGN NEOPLASMS OF SKIN**
`4th` *Includes:* benign neoplasm of hair follicles or sebaceous glands or sweat glands
Excludes1: benign lipomatous neoplasms of skin (D17.0-D17.3)
Excludes 2: melanocytic nevi (D22.-)

D23.0 **Other benign neoplasm of skin of lip**
Excludes1: benign neoplasm of vermilion border of lip (D10.0)

D23.1 **Other benign neoplasm of skin of; eyelid, including canthus**
`5th` **D23.11** **right eyelid, including canthus**
`6th` **D23.111** **Other benign neoplasm of skin of right upper eyelid, including canthus**
D23.112 **Other benign neoplasm of skin of right lower eyelid, including canthus**
D23.12 **left eyelid, including canthus**
`6th` **D23.121** **Other benign neoplasm of skin of left upper eyelid, including canthus**
D23.122 **Other benign neoplasm of skin of left lower eyelid, including canthus**

D23.2 **Other benign neoplasm of skin of; ear and external auricular**
`5th` **canal**
D23.21 **right ear and external auricular canal**
D23.22 **left ear and external auricular canal**

D23.3 **Other benign neoplasm of skin of; other and unspecified parts**
`5th` **of face**
D23.30 **unspecified part of face**
D23.39 **other parts of face**

(sidebar) CHAPTER 2. NEOPLASMS   (D10–D23.39)

`4th` `5th` `6th` `7th` Additional Character Required   ✔ 3-character code

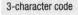

D23.4   Other benign neoplasm of skin of scalp and neck

D23.5   Other benign neoplasm of skin of trunk
> Other benign neoplasm of anal margin or anal skin or perianal skin
> Other benign neoplasm of skin of breast
> *Excludes1:* benign neoplasm of anus NOS (D12.9)

D23.6   **5th**   Other benign neoplasm of skin of; upper limb, including shoulder
> **D23.61**   right upper limb, including shoulder
> **D23.62**   left upper limb, including shoulder

D23.7   **5th**   Other benign neoplasm of skin of; lower limb, including hip
> **D23.71**   right lower limb, including hip
> **D23.72**   left lower limb, including hip

D23.9   Other benign neoplasm of skin, unspecified

D24   **4th**   BENIGN NEOPLASM OF BREAST
Includes: benign neoplasm of connective tissue of breast
> benign neoplasm of soft parts of breast
> fibroadenoma of breast

Excludes2: adenofibrosis of breast (N60.2)
> benign cyst of breast (N60.-)
> benign mammary dysplasia (N60.-)
> benign neoplasm of skin of breast (D22.5, D23.5)
> fibrocystic disease of breast (N60.-)

D24.1   Benign neoplasm of right breast

D24.2   Benign neoplasm of left breast

(D3A) BENIGN NEUROENDOCRINE TUMORS

(D37–D48) NEOPLASMS OF UNCERTAIN BEHAVIOR, POLYCYTHEMIA VERA AND MYELODYSPLASTIC SYNDROMES

Note: Categories D37–D44, and D48 classify by site neoplasms of uncertain behavior, i.e., histologic confirmation whether the neoplasm is malignant or benign cannot be made.
Excludes1: neoplasms of unspecified behavior (D49.-)

D47   **4th**   OTHER NEOPLASMS OF UNCERTAIN BEHAVIOR OF LYMPHOID, HEMATOPOIETIC AND RELATED TISSUE

D47.0   **5th**   Mast cell neoplasms of uncertain behavior
> *Excludes1:*
> congenital cutaneous mastocytosis (Q82.2)
> histiocytic neoplasms of uncertain behavior (D47.Z9)
> malignant mast cell neoplasm (C96.2-)

> **D47.01**   **Cutaneous mastocytosis**
> > Diffuse cutaneous mastocytosis
> > Maculopapular cutaneous mastocytosis
> > Solitary mastocytoma
> > Telangiectasia macularis eruptiva perstans
> > Urticaria pigmentosa
> > *Excludes1:* congenital (diffuse) (maculopapular) cutaneous mastocytosis (Q82.2)
> > > congenital urticaria pigmentosa (Q82.2)
> > > extracutaneous mastocytoma (D47.09)

> **D47.02**   **Systemic mastocytosis**
> > Indolent systemic mastocytosis
> > Isolated bone marrow mastocytosis
> > Smoldering systemic mastocytosis
> > Systemic mastocytosis, with an associated hematological non-mast cell lineage disease (SM-AHNMD)
> > Code also, if applicable, any associated hematological non-mast cell lineage disease
> > *Excludes1:* aggressive systemic mastocytosis (C96.21)
> > > mast cell leukemia (C94.3-)

> **D47.09**   **Other mast cell neoplasms of uncertain behavior**
> > Extracutaneous mastocytoma
> > Mast cell tumor NOS
> > Mastocytoma NOS
> > Mastocytosis NOS
> > Mastocytosis NOS

D47.3   Essential (hemorrhagic) thrombocythemia
> Essential thrombocytosis
> Idiopathic hemorrhagic thrombocythemia
> Primary thrombocytosis
> *Excludes2:* reactive thrombocytosis (D75.838)
> > secondary thrombocytosis (D75.838)
> > thrombocythemia NOS (D75.839)
> > thrombocytosis NOS (D75.839)

D47.Z   **5th**   Other specified neoplasms of uncertain behavior of lymphoid, hematopoietic and related tissue
> **D47.Z1**   **Post-transplant lymphoproliferative disorder (PTLD)**
> > **Code first** complications of transplanted organs and tissue (T86.-)

> **D47.Z9**   **Other specified neoplasms of uncertain behavior of lymphoid, hematopoietic and related tissue**
> > Histiocytic tumors of uncertain behavior
> > Use for kaposiform lymphangiomatosis

D47.9   Neoplasm of uncertain behavior of lymphoid, hematopoietic and related tissue, unspecified
> Lymphoproliferative disease NOS

(D49) NEOPLASMS OF UNSPECIFIED BEHAVIOR

D49   **4th**   NEOPLASMS OF UNSPECIFIED BEHAVIOR

Note: Category D49 classifies by site neoplasms of unspecified morphology and behavior. *The term 'mass', unless otherwise stated, is not to be regarded as a neoplastic growth.*
Includes: 'growth' NOS or neoplasm NOS or new growth NOS or tumor NOS
Excludes1: neoplasms of uncertain behavior (D37–D44, D48)

D49.0   Neoplasm of unspecified behavior of; digestive system
> *Excludes1:* neoplasm of unspecified behavior of margin of anus or perianal skin or skin of anus (D49.2)

D49.1   respiratory system

D49.2   bone, soft tissue, and skin
> *Excludes1:* neoplasm of unspecified behavior of anal canal or anus NOS (D49.0)
> > bone marrow (D49.89)
> > cartilage of larynx or nose (D49.1)
> > connective tissue of breast (D49.3)
> > skin of genital organs (D49.59)
> > vermilion border of lip (D49.0)

D49.3   breast
> *Excludes1:* neoplasm of unspecified behavior of skin of breast (D49.2)

D49.4   bladder

D49.5   other genitourinary organs
> **5th**   **D49.51**   **Neoplasm of unspecified behavior of kidney**
> > **6th**   **D49.511**   right kidney
> > **D49.512**   left kidney

> **D49.59**   **Neoplasm unspecified behavior of other genitourinary organ**

D49.6   brain
> *Excludes1:* neoplasm of unspecified behavior of cerebral meninges (D49.7)
> > neoplasm of unspecified behavior of cranial nerves (D49.7)

D49.7   endocrine glands and other parts of nervous system
> *Excludes1:* neoplasm of unspecified behavior of peripheral, sympathetic, and parasympathetic nerves and ganglia (D49.2)

D49.8   other specified sites
> *Excludes1:* neoplasm of unspecified behavior of eyelid (skin) (D49.2)

D49.9   unspecified site

4th   **5th**   **6th**   **7th**   Additional Character Required   3-character code

Unspecified laterality codes were excluded here.   •=New Code   ▲=Revised Code

Excludes1—Not coded here, do not use together
Excludes2—Not included here

Chapter 3. Diseases of the blood and blood-forming organs and certain disorders involving the immune mechanism (D50–D89)

GUIDELINES

None currently. Reserved for future guideline expansion.

Excludes2: autoimmune disease (systemic) NOS (M35.9)
    certain conditions originating in the perinatal period (P00–P96)
    complications of pregnancy, childbirth and the puerperium (O00–O9A)
    congenital malformations, deformations and chromosomal abnormalities
      (Q00–Q99)
    endocrine, nutritional and metabolic diseases (E00–E88)
    HIV disease (B20)
    injury, poisoning and certain other consequences of external causes (S00–T88)
    neoplasms (C00–D49)
    symptoms, signs and abnormal clinical and laboratory findings, NEC (R00–R94)

(D50–D53) NUTRITIONAL ANEMIAS

D50 IRON DEFICIENCY ANEMIA
[4th] **Includes:** asiderotic anemia
    hypochromic anemia
  D50.0 Iron deficiency anemia secondary to blood loss (chronic)
    Posthemorrhagic anemia (chronic)
    Excludes1: acute posthemorrhagic anemia (D62)
      congenital anemia from fetal blood loss (P61.3)
  D50.1 Sideropenic dysphagia
    Kelly-Paterson syndrome
    Plummer-Vinson syndrome
  D50.8 Other iron deficiency anemias
    Iron deficiency anemia due to inadequate dietary iron intake
  D50.9 Iron deficiency anemia, unspecified

D51 VITAMIN B12 DEFICIENCY ANEMIA
[4th] **Excludes1:** vitamin B12 deficiency (E53.8)
  D51.0 Vitamin B12 deficiency anemia due to intrinsic factor deficiency
    Addison anemia
    Biermer anemia
    Pernicious (congenital) anemia
    Congenital intrinsic factor deficiency
  D51.1 Vitamin B12 deficiency anemia due to selective vitamin B12 malabsorption with proteinuria
    Imerslund (Gräsbeck) syndrome
    Megaloblastic hereditary anemia
  D51.2 Transcobalamin II deficiency
  D51.3 Other dietary vitamin B12 deficiency anemia
    Vegan anemia
  D51.8 Other vitamin B12 deficiency anemias
  D51.9 Vitamin B12 deficiency anemia, unspecified

D52 FOLATE DEFICIENCY ANEMIA
[4th] **Excludes1:** folate deficiency without anemia (E53.8)
  D52.0 Dietary folate deficiency anemia
    Nutritional megaloblastic anemia
  D52.1 Drug-induced folate deficiency anemia
    Use additional code for adverse effect, if applicable, to identify
      drug (T36–T50 with fifth or sixth character 5)
  D52.8 Other folate deficiency anemias
  D52.9 Folate deficiency anemia, unspecified
    Folic acid deficiency anemia NOS

D53 OTHER NUTRITIONAL ANEMIAS
[4th] **Includes:** megaloblastic anemia unresponsive to vitamin B12 or folate
    therapy
  D53.0 Protein deficiency anemia
    Amino-acid deficiency anemia
    Orotaciduric anemia
    Excludes1: Lesch-Nyhan syndrome (E79.1)
  D53.1 Other megaloblastic anemias, NEC
    Megaloblastic anemia NOS
    Excludes1: Di Guglielmo's disease (C94.0)
  D53.2 Scorbutic anemia
    Excludes1: scurvy (E54)

  D53.8 Other specified nutritional anemias
    Anemia associated with deficiency of copper
    Anemia associated with deficiency of molybdenum
    Anemia associated with deficiency of zinc
    Excludes1: nutritional deficiencies without anemia, such as:
      copper deficiency NOS (E61.0)
      molybdenum deficiency NOS (E61.5)
      zinc deficiency NOS (E60)
  D53.9 Nutritional anemia, unspecified
    Simple chronic anemia
    Excludes1: anemia NOS (D64.9)

(D55–D59) HEMOLYTIC ANEMIAS

D55 ANEMIA DUE TO ENZYME DISORDERS
[4th] **Excludes1:** drug-induced enzyme deficiency anemia (D59.2)
  D55.0 Anemia due to glucose-6-phosphate dehydrogenase [G6PD] deficiency
    Excludes1: G6PD deficiency without anemia (D75.A)
    Favism
    G6PD deficiency anemia
  D55.1 Anemia due to other disorders of glutathione metabolism
    Anemia (due to) enzyme deficiencies, except G6PD, related to the
      hexose monophosphate [HMP] shunt pathway
    Anemia (due to) hemolytic nonspherocytic (hereditary), type I
  ▲**D55.2 Anemia due to disorders of glycolytic enzymes**
  [5th] **Excludes1:** disorders of glycolysis not associated with anemia
    (E74.81-)
    •**D55.21 Anemia due to pyruvate kinase deficiency**
      PK deficiency anemia
      Pyruvate kinase deficiency anemia
    •**D55.29 Anemia due to other disorders of glycolytic enzymes**
      Hexokinase deficiency anemia
      Triose-phosphate isomerase deficiency anemia
  D55.3 Anemia due to disorders of nucleotide metabolism
  D55.8 Other anemias due to enzyme disorders
  D55.9 Anemia due to enzyme disorder, unspecified

D56 THALASSEMIA
[4th] **Excludes1:** sickle-cell thalassemia (D57.4-)
  D56.0 Alpha thalassemia
    Alpha thalassemia major
    Hemoglobin H Constant Spring
    Hemoglobin H disease
    Hydrops fetalis due to alpha thalassemia
    Severe alpha thalassemia
    Triple gene defect alpha thalassemia
    Use additional code, if applicable, for hydrops fetalis due to alpha
      thalassemia (P56.99)
    Excludes1: alpha thalassemia trait or minor (D56.3)
      asymptomatic alpha thalassemia (D56.3)
      hydrops fetalis due to isoimmunization (P56.0)
      hydrops fetalis not due to immune hemolysis (P83.2)
  D56.1 Beta thalassemia
    Beta thalassemia major
    Cooley's anemia
    Homozygous beta thalassemia
    Severe beta thalassemia
    Thalassemia intermedia
    Thalassemia major
    Excludes1: beta thalassemia minor (D56.3)
      beta thalassemia trait (D56.3)
      delta-beta thalassemia (D56.2)
      hemoglobin E-beta thalassemia (D56.5)
      sickle-cell beta thalassemia (D57.4-)
  D56.2 Delta-beta thalassemia
    Homozygous delta-beta thalassemia
    Excludes1: delta-beta thalassemia minor (D56.3)
      delta-beta thalassemia trait (D56.3)

[4th] [5th] [6th] [7th] Additional Character Required   ✓ 3-character code   •=New Code   **Excludes1**—Not coded here, do not use together
    ▲=Revised Code   **Excludes2**—Not included here

D56.3 Thalassemia minor
Alpha thalassemia minor
Alpha thalassemia silent carrier
Alpha thalassemia trait
Beta thalassemia minor
Beta thalassemia trait
Delta-beta thalassemia minor
Delta-beta thalassemia trait
Thalassemia trait NOS
Excludes1: alpha thalassemia (D56.0)
   beta thalassemia (D56.1)
   delta-beta thalassemia (D56.2)
   hemoglobin E-beta thalassemia (D56.5)
   sickle-cell trait (D57.3)

D56.4 Hereditary persistence of fetal hemoglobin [HPFH]
D56.5 Hemoglobin E-beta thalassemia
Excludes1: beta thalassemia (D56.1)
   beta thalassemia minor (D56.3)
   beta thalassemia trait (D56.3)
   delta-beta thalassemia (D56.2)
   delta-beta thalassemia trait (D56.3)
   hemoglobin E disease (D58.2)
   other hemoglobinopathies (D58.2)
   sickle-cell beta thalassemia (D57.4-)

D56.8 Other thalassemias
Dominant thalassemia
Hemoglobin C thalassemia
Mixed thalassemia
Thalassemia with other hemoglobinopathy
Excludes1: hemoglobin C disease (D58.2)
   hemoglobin E disease (D58.2)
   other hemoglobinopathies (D58.2)
   sickle-cell anemia (D57.-)
   sickle-cell thalassemia (D57.4)

D56.9 Thalassemia, unspecified
Mediterranean anemia (with other hemoglobinopathy)

D57 SICKLE-CELL DISORDERS
`4th`
Use additional code for any associated fever (R50.81)
Excludes1: other hemoglobinopathies (D58.-)

D57.0 Hb-SS disease with crisis
`5th` Sickle-cell disease with crisis
Hb-SS disease with vaso-occlusive pain
   D57.00 Hb-SS disease with crisis, unspecified
         Hb-SS disease with (painful) crisis NOS
         Hb-SS disease with vasoocclusive pain NOS
   D57.01 Hb-SS disease with acute chest syndrome
   D57.02 Hb-SS disease with splenic sequestration
   D57.03 Hb-SS disease with cerebral vascular involvement
         Code also, if applicable, cerebral infarction (I63.-)
   D57.09 Hb-SS disease with crisis with other specified complication
         Use additional code to identify complications, such as:
            cholelithiasis (K80.-)
            priapism (N48.32)

D57.1 Sickle-cell disease without crisis
Hb-SS disease without crisis
Sickle-cell anemia NOS
Sickle-cell disease NOS
Sickle-cell disorder NOS

D57.2 Sickle-cell/Hb-C disease
`5th` Hb-SC disease
Hb-S/Hb-C disease
   D57.20 Sickle-cell/Hb-C disease without crisis
   D57.21 Sickle-cell/Hb-C disease with crisis
   `6th`   **D57.211 Sickle-cell/Hb-C disease with acute chest syndrome**
            D57.212 Sickle-cell/Hb-C disease with splenic sequestration
            D57.213 Sickle-cell/Hb-C disease with cerebral vascular involvement
                  Code also, if applicable, cerebral infarction (I63.-)

D57.218 Sickle-cell/Hb-C disease with crisis with other specified complication
      Use additional code to identify complications, such as:
         cholelithiasis (K80.-)
         priapism (N48.32)
D57.219 Sickle-cell/Hb-C disease with crisis, unspecified
      Sickle-cell/Hb-C disease with vasoocclusive pain NOS

D57.3 Sickle-cell trait
Hb-S trait
Heterozygous hemoglobin S

D57.4 Sickle-cell thalassemia
`5th` Sickle-cell beta thalassemia
Thalassemia Hb-S disease
   D57.40 Sickle-cell thalassemia without crisis
         Microdrepanocytosis
         Sickle-cell thalassemia NOS
   D57.41 Sickle-cell thalassemia, unspecified, with crisis
   `6th` Sickle-cell thalassemia with (painful) crisis NOS
         Sickle-cell thalassemia with vasoocclusive pain NOS
      D57.411 Sickle-cell thalassemia, unspecified, with acute chest syndrome
      D57.412 Sickle-cell thalassemia, unspecified, with splenic sequestration
      D57.413 Sickle-cell thalassemia, unspecified, with cerebral vascular involvement
            Code also, if applicable, cerebral infarction (I63.-)
      D57.418 Sickle-cell thalassemia, unspecified, with crisis with other specified complication
            Use additional code to identify complications, such as:
               cholelithiasis (K80.-)
               priapism (N48.32)
      D57.419 Sickle-cell thalassemia, unspecified, with crisis
            Sickle-cell thalassemia with (painful) crisis NOS
            Sickle-cell thalassemia with vasoocclusive pain NOS

   D57.42 Sickle-cell thalassemia beta zero without crisis
         HbS-beta zero without crisis
         Sickle-cell beta zero without crisis
   D57.43 Sickle-cell thalassemia beta zero
   `6th` HbS-beta zero with crisis
         Sickle-cell beta zero with crisis
      D57.431 Sickle-cell thalassemia beta zero with acute chest syndrome
            HbS-beta zero with acute chest syndrome
            Sickle-cell beta zero with acute chest syndrome
      D57.432 Sickle-cell thalassemia beta zero with splenic sequestration
            HbS-beta zero with splenic sequestration
            Sickle-cell beta zero with splenic sequestration
      D57.433 Sickle-cell thalassemia beta zero with cerebral vascular involvement
            HbS-beta zero with cerebral vascular involvement
            Sickle-cell beta zero with cerebral vascular involvement
            Code also, if applicable, cerebral infarction (I63.-)
      D57.438 Sickle-cell thalassemia beta zero with crisis with other specified complication
            HbS-beta zero with other specified complication
            Sickle-cell beta zero with other specified complication

`4th` `5th` `6th` `7th` Additional Character Required   ✔ 3-character code

•=New Code
▲=Revised Code

Excludes1—Not coded here, do not use together
Excludes2—Not included here

Use additional code to identify
complications, such as:
cholelithiasis (K80.-)
priapism (N48.32)

D57.439 Sickle-cell thalassemia beta zero with crisis, unspecified
HbS-beta zero with other specified complication
Sickle-cell beta zero with crisis unspecified
Sickle-cell thalassemia beta zero with (painful) crisis NOS
Sickle-cell thalassemia beta zero with vasoocclusive pain NOS

D57.44 Sickle-cell thalassemia beta plus without crisis
HbS-beta plus without crisis
Sickle-cell beta plus without crisis

D57.45 Sickle-cell thalassemia beta plus `6th`
HbS-beta plus with crisis
Sickle-cell beta plus with crisis

D57.451 Sickle-cell thalassemia beta plus with acute chest syndrome
HbS-beta plus with acute chest syndrome
Sickle-cell beta plus with acute chest syndrome

D57.452 Sickle-cell thalassemia beta plus with splenic sequestration
HbS-beta plus with splenic sequestration
Sickle-cell beta plus with splenic sequestration

D57.453 Sickle-cell thalassemia beta plus with cerebral vascular involvement
HbS-beta plus with cerebral vascular involvement
Sickle-cell beta plus with cerebral vascular involvement
Code also, if applicable, cerebral infarction (I63.-)

D57.458 Sickle-cell thalassemia beta plus with crisis with other specified complication
HbS-beta plus with crisis with other specified complication
Sickle-cell beta plus with crisis with other specified complication
Use additional code to identify complications, such as:
cholelithiasis (K80.-)
priapism (N48.32)

D57.459 Sickle-cell thalassemia beta plus with crisis, unspecified
HbS-beta plus with crisis with unspecified complication
Sickle-cell beta plus with crisis with unspecified complication
Sickle-cell thalassemia beta plus with (painful) crisis NOS
Sickle-cell thalassemia beta plus with vasoocclusive pain NOS

D57.8 Other sickle-cell disorders `5th`
Hb-SD disease
Hb-SE disease

D57.80 Other sickle-cell disorders without crisis
D57.81 Other sickle-cell disorders with crisis `6th`

D57.811 Other sickle-cell disorders with acute chest syndrome
D57.812 Other sickle-cell disorders with splenic sequestration
D57.813 Other sickle-cell disorders with cerebral vascular involvement
Code also, if applicable: cerebral infarction (I63.-)

D57.818 Other sickle-cell disorders with crisis with other specified complication
Use additional code to identify complications, such as:
cholelithiasis (K80.-)
priapism (N48.32)

D57.819 Other sickle-cell disorders with crisis, unspecified
Other sickle-cell disorders with (vasoocclusive pain) crisis NOS

D58 OTHER HEREDITARY HEMOLYTIC ANEMIAS `4th`
Excludes1: hemolytic anemia of the newborn (P55.-)

D58.0 Hereditary spherocytosis
Acholuric (familial) jaundice
Congenital (spherocytic) hemolytic icterus
Minkowski-Chauffard syndrome

D58.1 Hereditary elliptocytosis
Elliptocytosis (congenital)
Ovalocytosis (congenital) (hereditary)

D58.2 Other hemoglobinopathies
Abnormal hemoglobin NOS
Congenital Heinz body anemia
Hb-C disease
Hb-D disease
Hb-E disease
Hemoglobinopathy NOS
Unstable hemoglobin hemolytic disease
Excludes1: familial polycythemia (D75.0)
Hb-M disease (D74.0)
hemoglobin E-beta thalassemia (D56.5)
hereditary persistence of fetal hemoglobin [HPFH] (D56.4)
high-altitude polycythemia (D75.1)
methemoglobinemia (D74.-)
other hemoglobinopathies with thalassemia (D56.8)

D58.8 Other specified hereditary hemolytic anemias
Stomatocytosis

D58.9 Hereditary hemolytic anemia, unspecified

D59 ACQUIRED HEMOLYTIC ANEMIA `4th`
D59.0 Drug-induced autoimmune hemolytic anemia
Use additional code for adverse effect, if applicable, to identify drug (T36-T50 with fifth or sixth character 5)

D59.1 Other autoimmune hemolytic anemias `5th`
Excludes2: Evans syndrome (D69.41)
hemolytic disease of newborn (P55.-)
paroxysmal cold hemoglobinuria (D59.6)

D59.10 Autoimmune hemolytic anemia, unspecified
D59.11 Warm autoimmune hemolytic anemia
Warm type (primary) (secondary) (symptomatic) autoimmune hemolytic anemia
Warm type autoimmune hemolytic disease

D59.12 Cold autoimmune hemolytic anemia
Chronic cold hemagglutinin disease
Cold agglutinin disease
Cold agglutinin hemoglobinuria
Cold type (primary) (secondary) (symptomatic) autoimmune hemolytic anemia
Cold type autoimmune hemolytic disease

D59.13 Mixed type autoimmune hemolytic anemia
Mixed type autoimmune hemolytic disease
Mixed type, cold and warm, (primary) (secondary) (symptomatic) autoimmune hemolyticanemia

D59.19 Other autoimmune hemolytic anemia
D59.2 Drug-induced nonautoimmune hemolytic anemia
Drug-induced enzyme deficiency anemia
Use additional code for adverse effect, if applicable, to identify drug (T36-T50 with fifth or sixth character 5)

D59.3 Hemolytic-uremic syndrome
Use additional code to identify associated:
E. coli infection (B96.2-)
Pneumococcal pneumonia (J13)
Shigella dysenteriae (A03.9)

    `4th` `5th` `6th` `7th` Additional Character Required   ✓ 3-character code   •=New Code   *Excludes1*—Not coded here, do not use together
▲=Revised Code   *Excludes2*—Not included here

D59.4 Other nonautoimmune hemolytic anemias
Mechanical hemolytic anemia
Microangiopathic hemolytic anemia
Toxic hemolytic anemia

D59.5 Paroxysmal nocturnal hemoglobinuria [Marchiafava-Micheli]
Excludes1: hemoglobinuria NOS (R82.3)

D59.6 Hemoglobinuria due to hemolysis from other external causes
Hemoglobinuria from exertion
March hemoglobinuria
Paroxysmal cold hemoglobinuria
Use additional code (Chapter 20) to identify external cause
Excludes1: hemoglobinuria NOS (R82.3)

D59.8 Other acquired hemolytic anemias

D59.9 Acquired hemolytic anemia, unspecified
Idiopathic hemolytic anemia, chronic

(D60–D64) APLASTIC AND OTHER ANEMIAS AND OTHER BONE MARROW FAILURE SYNDROMES

D60 `4th` **ACQUIRED PURE RED CELL APLASIA [ERYTHROBLASTOPENIA]**
Includes: red cell aplasia (acquired) (adult) (with thymoma)
Excludes1: congenital red cell aplasia (D61.01)

D60.0 Chronic acquired pure red cell aplasia

D60.1 Transient acquired pure red cell aplasia

D60.8 Other acquired pure red cell aplasias

D60.9 Acquired pure red cell aplasia, unspecified

D61 `4th` **OTHER APLASTIC ANEMIAS AND OTHER BONE MARROW FAILURE SYNDROMES**
Excludes2: neutropenia (D70.-)

D61.0 Constitutional aplastic anemia

`5th` **D61.01 Constitutional (pure) red blood cell aplasia**
Blackfan-Diamond syndrome
Congenital (pure) red cell aplasia
Familial hypoplastic anemia
Primary (pure) red cell aplasia
Red cell (pure) aplasia of infants
Excludes1: acquired red cell aplasia (D60.9)

D61.09 Other constitutional aplastic anemia
Fanconi's anemia
Pancytopenia with malformations

D61.1 Drug-induced aplastic anemia
Use additional code for adverse effect, if applicable, to identify drug (T36–T50 with fifth or sixth character 5)

D61.2 Aplastic anemia due to other external agents
Code first, if applicable, toxic effects of substances chiefly nonmedicinal as to source (T51–T65)

D61.3 Idiopathic aplastic anemia

D61.8 Other specified aplastic anemias and other bone marrow
`5th` **failure syndromes**

D61.81 Pancytopenia
`6th` *Excludes1:* pancytopenia (due to) (with) aplastic anemia (D61.9)
pancytopenia (due to) (with) bone marrow infiltration (D61.82)
pancytopenia (due to) (with) congenital (pure) red cell aplasia (D61.01)
pancytopenia (due to) (with) hairy cell leukemia (C91.4-)
pancytopenia (due to) (with) HIV disease (B20.-)
pancytopenia (due to) (with) leukoerythroblastic anemia (D61.82)
pancytopenia (due to) (with) myeloproliferative disease (D47.1)
Excludes2: pancytopenia (due to) (with) myelodysplastic syndromes (D46.-)

D61.810 Antineoplastic chemotherapy induced pancytopenia
Excludes2: aplastic anemia due to antineoplastic chemotherapy (D61.1)

D61.811 Other drug-induced pancytopenia
Excludes2: aplastic anemia due to drugs (D61.1)

D61.818 Other pancytopenia

D61.82 Myelophthisis
Leukoerythroblastic anemia
Myelophthisic anemia
Panmyelophthisis
Code also the underlying disorder, such as: malignant neoplasm of breast (C50.-)
tuberculosis (A15.-)
Excludes1: idiopathic myelofibrosis (D47.1)
myelofibrosis NOS (D75.81)
myelofibrosis with myeloid metaplasia (D47.4)
primary myelofibrosis (D47.1)
secondary myelofibrosis (D75.81)

D61.89 Other specified aplastic anemias and other bone marrow failure syndromes

D61.9 Aplastic anemia, unspecified
Hypoplastic anemia NOS
Medullary hypoplasia

D62 `✔` **ACUTE POSTHEMORRHAGIC ANEMIA**
Excludes1: anemia due to chronic blood loss (D50.0)
blood loss anemia NOS (D50.0)
congenital anemia from fetal blood loss (P61.3)

D63 `4th` **ANEMIA IN CHRONIC DISEASES CLASSIFIED ELSEWHERE**

D63.0 Anemia in neoplastic disease
Code first neoplasm (C00–D49)
Excludes1: aplastic anemia due to antineoplastic chemotherapy (D61.1)
Excludes2: anemia due to antineoplastic chemotherapy (D64.81)

D63.1 Anemia in chronic kidney disease
Erythropoietin-resistant anemia (EPO-resistant anemia)
Code first underlying chronic kidney disease (CKD) (N18.-)

D63.8 Anemia in other chronic diseases classified elsewhere
Code first underlying disease

D64 `4th` **OTHER ANEMIAS**
Excludes1: refractory anemia (D46.-)
refractory anemia with excess blasts in transformation [RAEB T] (C92.0-)

D64.0 Hereditary sideroblastic anemia
Sex-linked hypochromic sideroblastic anemia

D64.1 Secondary sideroblastic anemia due to disease
Code first underlying disease

D64.2 Secondary sideroblastic anemia due to drugs and toxins
Code first poisoning due to drug or toxin, if applicable (T36 –T65 with fifth or sixth character 1-4 or 6)
Use additional code for adverse effect, if applicable, to identify drug (T36-T50 with fifth or sixth character 5)

D64.3 Other sideroblastic anemias
Sideroblastic anemia NOS
Pyridoxine-responsive sideroblastic anemia NEC

D64.4 Congenital dyserythropoietic anemia
Dyshematopoietic anemia (congenital)
Excludes1: Blackfan-Diamond syndrome (D61.01)
Di Guglielmo's disease (C94.0)

D64.8 Other specified anemias
`5th` **D64.81 Anemia due to antineoplastic chemotherapy**
Antineoplastic chemotherapy induced anemia
Excludes2: aplastic anemia due to antineoplastic chemotherapy (D61.1)
anemia in neoplastic disease (D63.0)

D64.89 Other specified anemias
Infantile pseudoleukemia

D64.9 Anemia, unspecified

`4th` `5th` `6th` `7th` Additional Character Required   `✔` 3-character code

•=New Code   *Excludes1*—Not coded here, do not use together
▲=Revised Code   *Excludes2*—Not included here

(D65–D69) COAGULATION DEFECTS, PURPURA AND OTHER HEMORRHAGIC CONDITIONS

D65 ✔ **DISSEMINATED INTRAVASCULAR COAGULATION [DEFIBRINATION SYNDROME]**
Afibrinogenemia, acquired
Consumption coagulopathy
Diffuse or disseminated intravascular coagulation [DIC]
Fibrinolytic hemorrhage, acquired
Fibrinolytic purpura
Purpura fulminans
Excludes1: disseminated intravascular coagulation (complicating):
  abortion or ectopic or molar pregnancy (O00–O07, O08.1)
  in newborn (P60)
  pregnancy, childbirth and the puerperium (O45.0, O46.0, O67.0, O72.3)

D66 ✔ **HEREDITARY FACTOR VIII DEFICIENCY**
Classical hemophilia
Deficiency factor VIII (with functional defect)
Hemophilia NOS
Hemophilia A
Excludes1: factor VIII deficiency with vascular defect (D68.0)

D67 ✔ **HEREDITARY FACTOR IX DEFICIENCY**
Christmas disease
Factor IX deficiency (with functional defect)
Hemophilia B
Plasma thromboplastin component [PTC] deficiency

D68 4th **OTHER COAGULATION DEFECTS**
Excludes1: abnormal coagulation profile (R79.1)
  coagulation defects complicating abortion or ectopic or molar pregnancy (O00–O07, O08.1)
  coagulation defects complicating pregnancy, childbirth and the puerperium (O45.0, O46.0, O67.0, O72.3)

  D68.0 Von Willebrand's disease
    Angiohemophilia
    Factor VIII deficiency with vascular defect
    Vascular hemophilia
    Excludes1: capillary fragility (hereditary) (D69.8)
      factor VIII deficiency NOS (D66)
      factor VIII deficiency with functional defect (D66)

  D68.1 Hereditary factor XI deficiency
    Hemophilia C
    Plasma thromboplastin antecedent [PTA] deficiency
    Rosenthal's disease

  D68.2 Hereditary deficiency of other clotting factors
    AC globulin deficiency
    Congenital afibrinogenemia
    Deficiency of factor I [fibrinogen]
    Deficiency of factor II [prothrombin]
    Deficiency of factor V [labile]
    Deficiency of factor VII [stable]
    Deficiency of factor X [Stuart-Prower]
    Deficiency of factor XII [Hageman]
    Deficiency of factor XIII [fibrin stabilizing]
    Dysfibrinogenemia (congenital)
    Hypoproconvertinemia
    Owren's disease
    Proaccelerin deficiency

  D68.3 Hemorrhagic disorder due to circulating anticoagulants
    5th **D68.31 Hemorrhagic disorder due to intrinsic circulating anticoagulants, antibodies, or inhibitors**
      6th
        D68.311 Acquired hemophilia
          Autoimmune hemophilia
          Autoimmune inhibitors to clotting factors
          Secondary hemophilia
        D68.312 Antiphospholipid antibody with hemorrhagic disorder
          LAC with hemorrhagic disorder
          SLE inhibitor with hemorrhagic disorder

        Excludes1: antiphospholipid antibody, finding without diagnosis (R76.0)
          antiphospholipid antibody syndrome (D68.61)
          antiphospholipid antibody with hypercoagulable state (D68.61)
          LAC finding without diagnosis (R76.0)
          LAC with hypercoagulable state (D68.62)
          SLE inhibitor finding without diagnosis (R76.0)
          SLE inhibitor with hypercoagulable state (D68.62)

        D68.318 Other hemorrhagic disorder due to intrinsic circulating anticoagulants, antibodies, or inhibitors
          Antithromboplastinemia
          Antithromboplastinogenemia
          Hemorrhagic disorder due to intrinsic increase in antithrombin
          Hemorrhagic disorder due to intrinsic increase in anti-VIIIa
          Hemorrhagic disorder due to intrinsic increase in anti-IXa
          Hemorrhagic disorder due to intrinsic increase in anti-Xia

    D68.32 Hemorrhagic disorder due to extrinsic circulating anticoagulants
      Drug-induced hemorrhagic disorder
      Hemorrhagic disorder due to increase in anti-IIa
      Hemorrhagic disorder due to increase in anti-Xa
      Hyperheparinemia
      Use additional code for adverse effect, if applicable, to identify drug (T45.515, T45.525)

  D68.4 Acquired coagulation factor deficiency
    Deficiency of coagulation factor due to liver disease
    Deficiency of coagulation factor due to vitamin K deficiency
    Excludes1: vitamin K deficiency of newborn (P53)

  D68.5 Primary thrombophilia
  5th
    Primary hypercoagulable states
    Excludes1: antiphospholipid syndrome (D68.61)
      LAC (D68.62)
      secondary activated protein C resistance (D68.69)
      secondary antiphospholipid antibody syndrome (D68.69)
      secondary LAC with hypercoagulable state (D68.69)
      SLE inhibitor with hypercoagulable state (D68.69)
      SLE inhibitor finding without diagnosis (R76.0)
      SLE inhibitor with hemorrhagic disorder (D68.312)
      thrombotic thrombocytopenic purpura (M31.19)

    D68.51 Activated protein C resistance
      Factor V Leiden mutation

    D68.52 Prothrombin gene mutation

    D68.59 Other primary thrombophilia
      Antithrombin III deficiency
      Hypercoagulable state NOS
      Primary hypercoagulable state NEC
      Primary thrombophilia NEC
      Protein C deficiency
      Protein S deficiency
      Thrombophilia NOS

  D68.6 Other thrombophilia
  5th
    Other hypercoagulable states
    Excludes1: diffuse or disseminated intravascular coagulation [DIC] (D65)
      heparin induced thrombocytopenia (HIT) (D75.82)
      hyperhomocysteinemia (E72.11)

    D68.61 Antiphospholipid syndrome
      Anticardiolipin syndrome
      Antiphospholipid antibody syndrome
      Excludes1: anti-phospholipid antibody, finding without diagnosis (R76.0)
        anti-phospholipid antibody with hemorrhagic disorder (D68.312)
        LAC syndrome (D68.62)

 | 4th | 5th | 6th | 7th | Additional Character Required   ✔ 3-character code   •=New Code   ▲=Revised Code   *Excludes1*—Not coded here, do not use together   *Excludes2*—Not included here

D68.62   **LAC syndrome**
LAC
Presence of SLE inhibitor
Excludes1: anticardiolipin syndrome (D68.61)
    antiphospholipid syndrome (D68.61)
    LAC finding without diagnosis (R76.0)
    LAC with hemorrhagic disorder (D68.312)

D68.69   **Other thrombophilia**
Hypercoagulable states NEC
Secondary hypercoagulable state NOS

D68.8   **Other specified coagulation defects**
Excludes1: hemorrhagic disease of newborn (P53)

D68.9   **Coagulation defect, unspecified**

D69   **PURPURA AND OTHER HEMORRHAGIC CONDITIONS**
4th   *Excludes1:* benign hypergammaglobulinemic purpura (D89.0)
    cryoglobulinemic purpura (D89.1)
    essential (hemorrhagic) thrombocythemia (D47.3)
    hemorrhagic thrombocythemia (D47.3)
    purpura fulminans (D65)
    thrombotic thrombocytopenic purpura (M31.19)
    Waldenström hypergammaglobulinemic purpura (D89.0)

D69.0   **Allergic purpura**
Allergic vasculitis
Nonthrombocytopenic hemorrhagic purpura
Nonthrombocytopenic idiopathic purpura
Purpura anaphylactoid
Purpura Henoch(-Schönlein)
Purpura rheumatica
Vascular purpura
Excludes1: thrombocytopenic hemorrhagic purpura (D69.3)

D69.1   **Qualitative platelet defects**
Bernard-Soulier [giant platelet] syndrome
Glanzmann's disease
Grey platelet syndrome
Thromboasthenia (hemorrhagic) (hereditary)
Thrombocytopathy
Excludes1: von Willebrand's disease (D68.0)

D69.2   **Other nonthrombocytopenic purpura**
Purpura NOS
Purpura simplex
Senile purpura

D69.3   **Immune thrombocytopenic purpura**
Hemorrhagic (thrombocytopenic) purpura
Idiopathic thrombocytopenic purpura
Tidal platelet dysgenesis

D69.4   **Other primary thrombocytopenia**
5th   *Excludes1:* transient neonatal thrombocytopenia (P61.0)
    Wiskott-Aldrich syndrome (D82.0)

    D69.41   **Evans syndrome**

    D69.42   **Congenital and hereditary thrombocytopenia purpura**
       Congenital thrombocytopenia
       Hereditary thrombocytopenia
       Code first congenital or hereditary disorder, such as:
          TAR syndrome (Q87.2)

    D69.49   **Other primary thrombocytopenia**
       Megakaryocytic hypoplasia
       Primary thrombocytopenia NOS

D69.5   **Secondary thrombocytopenia**
5th   *Excludes1:* heparin induced thrombocytopenia (HIT) (D75.82)
    transient thrombocytopenia of newborn (P61.0)

    D69.51   **Posttransfusion purpura**
       Posttransfusion purpura from whole blood (fresh) or
          blood products
       PTP

    D69.59   **Other secondary thrombocytopenia**

D69.6   **Thrombocytopenia, unspecified**

D69.8   **Other specified hemorrhagic conditions**
Capillary fragility (hereditary)
Vascular pseudohemophilia

D69.9   **Hemorrhagic condition, unspecified**

(D70–D77) OTHER DISORDERS OF BLOOD AND BLOOD-FORMING ORGANS

D70   **NEUTROPENIA**
4th   *Includes:* agranulocytosis
    decreased absolute neutrophil count (ANC)
Use additional code for any associated: fever (R50.81)
    mucositis (J34.81, K12.3-, K92.81, N76.81)
Excludes1: neutropenic splenomegaly (D73.81)
    transient neonatal neutropenia (P61.5)

D70.0   **Congenital agranulocytosis**
Congenital neutropenia
Infantile genetic agranulocytosis
Kostmann's disease

D70.1   **Agranulocytosis secondary to cancer chemotherapy**
Use additional code for adverse effect, if applicable, to identify
    drug (T45.1X5)
Code also underlying neoplasm

D70.2   **Other drug-induced agranulocytosis**
Use additional code for adverse effect, if applicable, to identify
    drug (T36–T50 with fifth or sixth character 5)

D70.3   **Neutropenia due to infection**

D70.4   **Cyclic neutropenia**
Cyclic hematopoiesis
Periodic neutropenia

D70.8   **Other neutropenia**

D70.9   **Neutropenia, unspecified**

D71   **FUNCTIONAL DISORDERS OF POLYMORPHONUCLEAR NEUTROPHILS**
✓   Cell membrane receptor complex [CR3] defect
Chronic (childhood) granulomatous disease
Congenital dysphagocytosis
Progressive septic granulomatosis

D72   **OTHER DISORDERS OF WHITE BLOOD CELLS**
4th   *Excludes1:* basophilia (D72.824)
    immunity disorders (D80–D89)
    neutropenia (D70)
    preleukemia (syndrome) (D46.9)

D72.0   **Genetic anomalies of leukocytes**
Alder syndrome
Hereditary leukocytic hyper/hypo segmentation
Hereditary leukomelanopathy
May-Hegglin syndrome
Pelger-Huët syndrome

D72.1   **Eosinophilia**
5th   *Excludes2:* Löffler's syndrome (J82.89)
    pulmonary eosinophilia (J82.-)

    D72.10   **Eosinophilia, unspecified**
6th

       D72.110   **Idiopathic hypereosinophilic syndrome [IHES]**

       D72.111   **Lymphocytic Variant Hypereosinophilic Syndrome [LHES]**
          Lymphocyte variant hypereosinophilia
          Code also, if applicable, any associated
             lymphocytic neoplastic disorder

       D72.118   **Other hypereosinophilic syndrome**
          Episodic angioedema with eosinophilia
          Gleich's syndrome

       D72.119   **Hypereosinophilic syndrome [HES], unspecified**

    D72.12   **Drug rash with eosinophilia and systemic symptoms syndrome**
       DRESS syndrome
       Use additional code for adverse effect, if applicable, to
          identify drug (T36–T50 with fifth or sixth character 5)

    D72.18   **Eosinophilia in diseases classified elsewhere**
       Code first underlying disease, such as:
          chronic myelomonocytic leukemia (C93.1-)

    D72.19   **Other eosinophilia**
       Familial eosinophilia
       Hereditary eosinophilia

4th   5th   6th   7th   Additional Character Required   ✓   3-character code   •=New Code   ▲=Revised Code   *Excludes1*—Not coded here, do not use together   *Excludes2*—Not included here

D72.8 **Other specified disorders of white blood cells**
[5th]   ***Excludes1:*** leukemia (C91–C95)
  D72.81 **Decreased white blood cell count**
[6th]   ***Excludes1:*** neutropenia (D70.-)
    D72.810 **Lymphocytopenia**
      Decreased lymphocytes
    D72.818 **Other decreased white blood cell count**
      Basophilic leukopenia
      Eosinophilic leukopenia
      Monocytopenia
      Other decreased leukocytes
      Plasmacytopenia
    D72.819 **Decreased white blood cell count, unspecified**
      Decreased leukocytes, unspecified
      Leukocytopenia, unspecified
      Leukopenia
      Excludes1: malignant leukopenia (D70.9)
  D72.82 **Elevated white blood cell count**
[6th]   ***Excludes1:*** eosinophilia (D72.1)
    D72.820 **Lymphocytosis (symptomatic)**
      Elevated lymphocytes
    D72.821 **Monocytosis (symptomatic)**
      Excludes1: infectious mononucleosis (B27.-)
    D72.822 **Plasmacytosis**
    D72.823 **Leukemoid reaction**
      Basophilic leukemoid reaction
      Leukemoid reaction NOS
      Lymphocytic leukemoid reaction
      Monocytic leukemoid reaction
      Myelocytic leukemoid reaction
      Neutrophilic leukemoid reaction
    D72.824 **Basophilia**
    D72.825 **Bandemia**
      Bandemia without diagnosis of specific infection
      Excludes1: confirmed infection—code to infection
        leukemia (C91.-, C92.-, C93.-, C94.-, C95.-)
    D72.828 **Other elevated white blood cell count**
    D72.829 **Elevated white blood cell count, unspecified**
      Elevated leukocytes, unspecified
      Leukocytosis, unspecified
  D72.89 **Other specified disorders of white blood cells**
    Abnormality of white blood cells NEC
D72.9 **Disorder of white blood cells, unspecified**
  Abnormal leukocyte differential NOS

D73 **DISEASES OF SPLEEN**
[4th] **D73.0** **Hyposplenism**
  Atrophy of spleen
  Excludes1: asplenia (congenital) (Q89.01)
    postsurgical absence of spleen (Z90.81)
D73.1 **Hypersplenism**
  Excludes1: neutropenic splenomegaly (D73.81)
    primary splenic neutropenia (D73.81)
    splenitis, splenomegaly in late syphilis (A52.79)
    splenitis, splenomegaly in tuberculosis (A18.85)
    splenomegaly NOS (R16.1)
    splenomegaly congenital (Q89.0)
D73.2 **Chronic congestive splenomegaly**
D73.3 **Abscess of spleen**
D73.4 **Cyst of spleen**
D73.5 **Infarction of spleen**
  Splenic rupture, nontraumatic
  Torsion of spleen
  Excludes1: rupture of spleen due to Plasmodium vivax malaria (B51.0)
    traumatic rupture of spleen (S36.03-)
D73.8 **Other diseases of spleen**
[5th]   **D73.81** **Neutropenic splenomegaly**
    Werner-Schultz disease

D73.89 **Other diseases of spleen**
  Fibrosis of spleen NOS
  Perisplenitis
  Splenitis NOS

D74 **METHEMOGLOBINEMIA**
[4th] **D74.0** **Congenital methemoglobinemia**
  Congenital NADH-methemoglobin reductase deficiency
  Hemoglobin-M [Hb-M] disease
  Methemoglobinemia, hereditary
D74.8 **Other methemoglobinemias**
  Acquired methemoglobinemia (with sulfhemoglobinemia)
  Toxic methemoglobinemia
D74.9 **Methemoglobinemia, unspecified**

D75 **OTHER AND UNSPECIFIED DISEASES OF BLOOD AND**
[4th] **BLOOD-FORMING ORGANS**
  Excludes2: acute lymphadenitis (L04.-)
    chronic lymphadenitis (I88.1)
    enlarged lymph nodes (R59.-)
    hypergammaglobulinemia NOS (D89.2)
    lymphadenitis NOS (I88.9)
    mesenteric lymphadenitis (acute) (chronic) (I88.0)
D75.0 **Familial erythrocytosis**
  Benign polycythemia
  Familial polycythemia
  Excludes1: hereditary ovalocytosis (D58.1)
D75.1 **Secondary polycythemia**
  Acquired polycythemia
  Emotional polycythemia
  Erythrocytosis NOS
  Hypoxemic polycythemia
  Nephrogenous polycythemia
  Polycythemia due to erythropoietin
  Polycythemia due to fall in plasma volume
  Polycythemia due to high altitude
  Polycythemia due to stress
  Polycythemia NOS
  Relative polycythemia
  Excludes1: polycythemia neonatorum (P61.1)
    polycythemia vera (D45)
D75.8 **Other specified diseases of blood and blood-forming organs**
[5th]   **D75.81** **Myelofibrosis**
    Myelofibrosis NOS
    Secondary myelofibrosis NOS
    Code first the underlying disorder
    Use additional code, if applicable, for associated therapy-related myelodysplastic syndrome (D46.-)
    Use additional code for adverse effect, if applicable, to identify drug (T45.1X5)
    Excludes1: acute myelofibrosis (C94.4-)
      idiopathic myelofibrosis (D47.1)
      leukoerythroblastic anemia (D61.82)
      myelofibrosis with myeloid metaplasia (D47.4)
      myelophthisic anemia (D61.82)
      myelophthisis (D61.82)
      primary myelofibrosis (D47.1)
  D75.82 **Heparin-induced thrombocytopenia (HIT)**
  • **D75.83** **Thrombocytosis**
[6th]   ***Excludes2:*** essential thrombocythemia (D47.3)
  • **D75.838** **Other thrombocytosis**
    Reactive thrombocytosis
    Secondary thrombocytosis
    Code also underlying condition, if known and applicable
  • **D75.839** **Thrombocytosis, unspecified**
    Thrombocythemia NOS
    Thrombocytosis NOS
  D75.89 **Other specified diseases of blood and blood-forming organs**
D75.9 **Disease of blood and blood-forming organs, unspecified**
D75.A **Glucose-6-phosphate dehydrogenase (G6PD) deficiency without anemia**
  Excludes1: G6PD deficiency with anemia (D55.0)

[4th] [5th] [6th] [7th] Additional Character Required   ✓ 3-character code   •=New Code   ***Excludes1***—Not coded here, do not use together
▲=Revised Code   ***Excludes2***—Not included here

D76 OTHER SPECIFIED DISEASES WITH PARTICIPATION OF
4th LYMPHORETICULAR AND RETICULOHISTIOCYTIC TISSUE

Excludes1: (Abt-) Letterer-Siwe disease (C96.0)
eosinophilic granuloma (C96.6)
Hand-Schüller-Christian disease (C96.5)
histiocytic medullary reticulosis (C96.9)
histiocytic sarcoma (C96.A)
histiocytosis X, multifocal (C96.5)
histiocytosis X, unifocal (C96.6)
Langerhans-cell histiocytosis, multifocal (C96.5)
Langerhans-cell histiocytosis NOS (C96.6)
Langerhans-cell histiocytosis, unifocal (C96.6)
leukemic reticuloendotheliosis (C91.4-)
lipomelanotic reticulosis (I89.8)
malignant histiocytosis (C96.A)
malignant reticulosis (C86.0)
nonlipid reticuloendotheliosis (C96.0)

D76.1 **Hemophagocytic lymphohistiocytosis**
Familial hemophagocytic reticulosis
Histiocytoses of mononuclear phagocytes

D76.2 **Hemophagocytic syndrome, infection-associated**
Use additional code to identify infectious agent or disease.

D76.3 **Other histiocytosis syndromes**
Reticulohistiocytoma (giant-cell)
Sinus histiocytosis with massive lymphadenopathy
Xanthogranuloma

D77 OTHER DISORDERS OF BLOOD AND BLOOD-FORMING
✓ ORGANS IN DISEASES CLASSIFIED ELSEWHERE

Code first underlying disease, such as:
amyloidosis (E85.-)
congenital early syphilis (A50.0)
echinococcosis (B67.0–B67.9)
malaria (B50.0–B54)
schistosomiasis [bilharziasis] (B65.0–B65.9)
vitamin C deficiency (E54)

Excludes1: rupture of spleen due to Plasmodium vivax malaria (B51.0)
splenitis, splenomegaly in late syphilis (A52.79)
splenitis, splenomegaly in tuberculosis (A18.85)

(D78) INTRAOPERATIVE AND POSTPROCEDURAL COMPLICATIONS OF THE SPLEEN

(D80–D89) CERTAIN DISORDERS INVOLVING THE IMMUNE MECHANISM

Includes: defects in the complement system
immunodeficiency disorders, except HIV disease
sarcoidosis

Excludes1: autoimmune disease (systemic) NOS (M35.9)
functional disorders of polymorphonuclear neutrophils (D71)
HIV disease (B20)

D80 IMMUNODEFICIENCY WITH PREDOMINANTLY ANTIBODY
4th DEFECTS

D80.0 **Hereditary hypogammaglobulinemia**
Autosomal recessive agammaglobulinemia (Swiss type)
X-linked agammaglobulinemia [Bruton] (with growth hormone deficiency)

D80.1 **Nonfamilial hypogammaglobulinemia**
Agammaglobulinemia with immunoglobulin-bearing B-lymphocytes
Common variable agammaglobulinemia [CVAgamma]
Hypogammaglobulinemia NOS

D80.2 **Selective deficiency of immunoglobulin A [IgA]**
D80.3 **Selective deficiency of immunoglobulin G [IgG] subclasses**
D80.4 **Selective deficiency of immunoglobulin M [IgM]**
D80.5 **Immunodeficiency with increased immunoglobulin M [IgM]**
D80.6 **Antibody deficiency with near-normal immunoglobulins or with hypogammaglobulinemia**
D80.7 **Transient hypogammaglobulinemia of infancy**
D80.8 **Other immunodeficiencies with predominantly antibody defects**
Kappa light chain deficiency
D80.9 **Immunodeficiency with predominantly antibody defects, unspecified**

D81 COMBINED IMMUNODEFICIENCIES
4th

Excludes1: autosomal recessive agammaglobulinemia (Swiss type) (D80.0)

D81.0 **SCID with reticular dysgenesis**
D81.1 **SCID with low T- and B-cell numbers**
D81.2 **SCID with low or normal B-cell numbers**
D81.3 **Adenosine deaminase [ADA] deficiency**

5th **D81.30** **Adenosine deaminase deficiency, unspecified**
ADA deficiency NOS

D81.31 **SCID due to adenosine deaminase deficiency**
ADA deficiency with SCID
Adenosine deaminase [ADA] deficiency with SCID

D81.32 **Adenosine deaminase 2 deficiency**
ADA2 deficiency
Adenosine deaminase deficiency type 2
Code also, if applicable, any associated manifestations, such as:
polyarteritis nodosa (M30.0)
stroke (I63.-)

D81.39 **Other adenosine deaminase deficiency**
Adenosine deaminase [ADA] deficiency type 1, NOS
Adenosine deaminase [ADA] deficiency type 1, without SCID
Partial adenosine deaminase deficiency (type 1)

D81.4 **Nezelof's syndrome**
D81.5 **Purine nucleoside phosphorylase [PNP] deficiency**
D81.6 **Major histocompatibility complex class I deficiency**
Bare lymphocyte syndrome
D81.7 **Major histocompatibility complex class II deficiency**
D81.8 **Other combined immunodeficiencies**

5th **D81.81** **Biotin-dependent carboxylase deficiency**
6th Multiple carboxylase deficiency
Excludes1: biotin-dependent carboxylase deficiency due to dietary deficiency of biotin (E53.8)

D81.810 **Biotinidase deficiency**
D81.818 **Other biotin-dependent carboxylase deficiency**
Holocarboxylase synthetase deficiency
Other multiple carboxylase deficiency

D81.819 **Biotin-dependent carboxylase deficiency, unspecified**
Multiple carboxylase deficiency, unspecified

D81.89 **Other combined immunodeficiencies**

D81.9 **Combined immunodeficiency, unspecified**
SCID NOS

D82 IMMUNODEFICIENCY ASSOCIATED WITH OTHER
4th MAJOR DEFECTS

Excludes1: ataxia telangiectasia [Louis-Bar] (G11.3)

D82.0 **Wiskott-Aldrich syndrome**
Immunodeficiency with thrombocytopenia and eczema

D82.1 **Di George's syndrome**
Pharyngeal pouch syndrome
Thymic alymphoplasia
Thymic aplasia or hypoplasia with immunodeficiency

D82.2 **Immunodeficiency with short-limbed stature**
D82.3 **Immunodeficiency following hereditary defective response to Epstein-Barr virus**
X-linked lymphoproliferative disease
D82.4 **Hyperimmunoglobulin E [IgE] syndrome**
D82.9 **Immunodeficiency associated with major defect, unspecified**

D83 COMMON VARIABLE IMMUNODEFICIENCY
4th

D83.0 **Common variable immunodeficiency with predominant abnormalities of B-cell numbers and function**
D83.1 **Common variable immunodeficiency with predominant immunoregulatory T-cell disorders**
Code first underlying condition, such as:
chromosomal abnormalities (Q90–Q99)
diabetes mellitus (E08–E13)
malignant neoplasms (C00–C96)
Excludes1: certain disorders involving the immune mechanism (D80-D83, D84.0, D84.1,D84.9)
human immunodeficiency virus [HIV] disease (B20)
D83.2 **Common variable immunodeficiency with autoantibodies to B- or T-cells**

  Additional Character Required   ✓ 3-character code

•=New Code   *Excludes1*—Not coded here, do not use together
▲=Revised Code   *Excludes2*—Not included here

D83.8 Other common variable immunodeficiencies
D83.9 Common variable immunodeficiency, unspecified

D84 OTHER IMMUNODEFICIENCIES
`4th`
  D84.0 Lymphocyte function antigen-1 [LFA-1] defect
  D84.1 Defects in the complement system
    C1 esterase inhibitor [C1-INH] deficiency
  D84.8 Other specified immunodeficiencies
    `5th` **D84.81 Immunodeficiency due to conditions classified elsewhere**
      Code first underlying condition, such as:
        chromosomal abnormalities (Q90–Q99)
        diabetes mellitus (E08–E13)
        malignant neoplasms (C00–C96)
      Excludes1: certain disorders involving the immune
        mechanism (D80–D83, D84.0, D84.1,D84.9)
        human immunodeficiency virus [HIV] disease (B20)
    D84.82 Immunodeficiency due to other causes
      `6th` **D84.821 Immunodeficiency due to drugs**
        Immunodeficiency due to (current or past) medication
        Use additional code for adverse effect, if applicable, to identify adverse effect ofdrug (T36–T50 with fifth or six character 5)
        Use additional code, if applicable, for associated long term (current) drug therapy drug or medication such as:
        long term (current) drug therapy systemic steroids (Z79.52)
        other long term (current) drug therapy (Z79.899)
      D84.822 Immunodeficiency due to external causes
        Code also, if applicable, radiological procedure and radiotherapy (Y84.2)
        Use additional code for external cause such as:
        exposure to ionizing radiation (W88)
    D84.89 Other immunodeficiencies
  D84.9 Immunodeficiency, unspecified
    Immunocompromised NOS
    Immunodeficient NOS
    Immunosuppressed NOS

D86 SARCOIDOSIS
`4th`
  D86.0 Sarcoidosis of lung
  D86.1 Sarcoidosis of lymph nodes
  D86.2 Sarcoidosis of lung with sarcoidosis of lymph nodes
  D86.3 Sarcoidosis of skin
  D86.8 Sarcoidosis of other sites
    `5th` **D86.81 Sarcoid meningitis**
    D86.82 Multiple cranial nerve palsies in sarcoidosis
    D86.83 Sarcoid iridocyclitis
    D86.84 Sarcoid pyelonephritis
      Tubulo-interstitial nephropathy in sarcoidosis
    D86.85 Sarcoid myocarditis
    D86.86 Sarcoid arthropathy
      Polyarthritis in sarcoidosis
    D86.87 Sarcoid myositis
    D86.89 Sarcoidosis of other sites
      Hepatic granuloma
      Uveoparotid fever [Heerfordt]
  D86.9 Sarcoidosis, unspecified

D89 OTHER DISORDERS INVOLVING THE IMMUNE MECHANISM, NEC
`4th`
  Excludes1: hyperglobulinemia NOS (R77.1)
    monoclonal gammopathy (of undetermined significance) (D47.2)
  Excludes2: transplant failure and rejection (T86.-)
  D89.0 Polyclonal hypergammaglobulinemia
    Benign hypergammaglobulinemic purpura
    Polyclonal gammopathy NOS

D89.1 Cryoglobulinemia
  Cryoglobulinemic purpura
  Cryoglobulinemic vasculitis
  Essential cryoglobulinemia
  Idiopathic cryoglobulinemia
  Mixed cryoglobulinemia
  Primary cryoglobulinemia
  Secondary cryoglobulinemia
D89.2 Hypergammaglobulinemia, unspecified
D89.3 Immune reconstitution syndrome
  Immune reconstitution inflammatory syndrome [IRIS]
    Use additional code for adverse effect, if applicable, to identify drug (T36-T50 with fifth or sixth character 5)
D89.4 Mast cell activation syndrome and related disorders
  `5th` *Excludes1:* aggressive systemic mastocytosis (C96.21)
    congenital cutaneous mastocytosis (Q82.2)
    indolent systemic mastocytosis (D47.02)
    malignant mast cell neoplasm (C96.2-)
    mast cell leukemia (C94.3-)
    malignant mastocytoma (C96.29)
    systemic mastocytosis associated with a clonal hematologic non-mast cell lineage disease (SM-AHNMD) (D47.02)
    mast cell sarcoma (C96.22)
    mastocytoma NOS (D47.09)
    other mast cell neoplasms of uncertain behavior (D47.09)
  D89.40 Mast cell activation disorder, unspecified or NOS
  D89.41 Monoclonal mast cell activation syndrome
  D89.42 Idiopathic mast cell activation syndrome
  D89.43 Secondary mast cell activation syndrome
    Secondary mast cell activation syndrome
    Code also underlying etiology, if known
  •**D89.44 Hereditary alpha tryptasemia**
    Use additional code, if applicable, for:
      allergy status, other than to drugs and biological substances (Z91.0-)
      personal history of anaphylaxis (Z87.892)
  D89.49 Other mast cell activation disorder
D89.8 Other specified disorders involving the immune mechanism, NEC
  `5th` **D89.81 Graft-versus-host disease**
    `6th` **Code first** underlying cause, such as:
      complications of transplanted organs and tissue (T86.-)
      complications of blood transfusion (T80.89)
    Use additional code to identify associated manifestations, such as:
      desquamative dermatitis (L30.8)
      diarrhea (R19.7)
      elevated bilirubin (R17)
      hair loss (L65.9)
    D89.810 Acute graft-versus-host disease
    D89.811 Chronic graft-versus-host disease
    D89.812 Acute on chronic graft-versus-host disease
    D89.813 Graft-versus-host disease, unspecified
  D89.82 Autoimmune lymphoproliferative syndrome [ALPS]
  D89.83 Cytokine release syndrome
    `6th` **Code first** underlying cause, such as:
      complications following infusion, transfusion and therapeutic injection (T80.89-)
      complications of transplanted organs and tissue (T86.-)
    Use additional code to identify associated manifestations
    D89.831 Cytokine release syndrome, grade 1
    D89.832 Cytokine release syndrome, grade 2
    D89.833 Cytokine release syndrome, grade 3
    D89.834 Cytokine release syndrome, grade 4
    D89.835 Cytokine release syndrome, grade 5
    D89.839 Cytokine release syndrome, grade unspecified
  D89.89 Other specified disorders involving the immune mechanism, NEC
    Excludes1: HIV disease (B20)
D89.9 Disorder involving the immune mechanism, unspecified
  Immune disease NOS

  > PANDAS code to D89.89 plus manifestations

`4th` `5th` `6th` `7th` Additional Character Required   ✓ 3-character code

• =New Code
▲ =Revised Code

Excludes1—Not coded here, do not use together
Excludes2—Not included here

Chapter 4. Endocrine, nutritional and metabolic diseases (E00–E89)

GUIDELINES

Diabetes Mellitus (DM)

Refer to categories E08–E13 for guidelines.
Note: All neoplasms, whether functionally active or not, are classified in Chapter 2. Appropriate codes in this chapter (ie, E05.8, E07.0, E16–E31, E34.-) may be used as additional codes to indicate either functional activity by neoplasms and ectopic endocrine tissue or hyperfunction and hypofunction of endocrine glands associated with neoplasms and other conditions classified elsewhere.
Excludes1: transitory endocrine and metabolic disorders specific to newborn (P70–P74)

(E00–E07) DISORDERS OF THYROID GLAND

E00 **CONGENITAL IODINE-DEFICIENCY SYNDROME**
`4th`   **Use additional code** (F70–F79) to identify associated intellectual disabilities.
    Excludes1: subclinical iodine-deficiency hypothyroidism (E02)
    E00.0 **Congenital iodine-deficiency syndrome, neurological type**
       Endemic cretinism, neurological type
    E00.1 **Congenital iodine-deficiency syndrome, myxedematous type**
       Endemic hypothyroid cretinism
       Endemic cretinism, myxedematous type
    E00.2 **Congenital iodine-deficiency syndrome, mixed type**
       Endemic cretinism, mixed type
    E00.9 **Congenital iodine-deficiency syndrome, unspecified**
       Congenital iodine-deficiency hypothyroidism NOS
       Endemic cretinism NOS

E01 **IODINE-DEFICIENCY RELATED THYROID DISORDERS**
`4th`   **AND ALLIED CONDITIONS**
    Excludes1: congenital iodine-deficiency syndrome (E00.-)
       subclinical iodine-deficiency hypothyroidism (E02)
    E01.0 **Iodine-deficiency related diffuse (endemic) goiter**
    E01.1 **Iodine-deficiency related multinodular (endemic) goiter**
       Iodine-deficiency related nodular goiter
    E01.2 **Iodine-deficiency related (endemic) goiter, unspecified**
       Endemic goiter NOS
    E01.8 **Other iodine-deficiency related thyroid disorders and allied conditions**
       Acquired iodine-deficiency hypothyroidism NOS

E02 **SUBCLINICAL IODINE-DEFICIENCY HYPOTHYROIDISM**
`✔`

E03 **OTHER HYPOTHYROIDISM**
`4th`   ***Excludes1:*** iodine-deficiency related hypothyroidism (E00–E02)
       postprocedural hypothyroidism (E89.0)
    E03.0 **Congenital hypothyroidism with diffuse goiter**
       Congenital parenchymatous goiter (nontoxic)
       Congenital goiter (nontoxic) NOS
       Excludes1: transitory congenital goiter with normal function (P72.0)
    E03.1 **Congenital hypothyroidism without goiter**
       Aplasia of thyroid (with myxedema)
       Congenital atrophy of thyroid
       Congenital hypothyroidism NOS
    E03.2 **Hypothyroidism due to medicines/drugs and other exogenous substances**
       Code first poisoning due to drug or toxin, if applicable (T36–T65 with fifth or sixth character 1–4 or 6)
       Use additional code for adverse effect, if applicable, to identify drug (T36–T50 with fifth or sixth character 5)
    E03.3 **Postinfectious hypothyroidism**
    E03.4 **Atrophy of thyroid (acquired)**
       Excludes1: congenital atrophy of thyroid (E03.1)
    E03.8 **Other specified hypothyroidism**
    E03.9 **Hypothyroidism, unspecified**
       Myxedema NOS

E04 **OTHER NONTOXIC GOITER**
`4th`   ***Excludes1:*** congenital goiter (NOS) (diffuse) (parenchymatous) (E03.0)
       iodine-deficiency related goiter (E00–E02)
    E04.0 **Nontoxic diffuse goiter**
       Diffuse (colloid) nontoxic goiter
       Simple nontoxic goiter
    E04.1 **Nontoxic single thyroid nodule**
       Colloid nodule (cystic) (thyroid)
       Nontoxic uninodular goiter
       Thyroid (cystic) nodule NOS
    E04.2 **Nontoxic multinodular goiter**
       Cystic goiter NOS
       Multinodular (cystic) goiter NOS
    E04.8 **Other specified nontoxic goiter**
    E04.9 **Nontoxic goiter, unspecified**
       Goiter NOS
       Nodular goiter (nontoxic) NOS

E05 **THYROTOXICOSIS [HYPERTHYROIDISM]**
`4th`   ***Excludes1:*** chronic thyroiditis with transient thyrotoxicosis (E06.2)
       neonatal thyrotoxicosis (P72.1)
    E05.0 **Thyrotoxicosis with diffuse goiter**
    `5th`   Exophthalmic or toxic goiter NOS
       Graves' disease
       Toxic diffuse goiter
       E05.00 **Thyrotoxicosis with diffuse goiter without thyrotoxic crisis or storm**
       E05.01 **Thyrotoxicosis with diffuse goiter with thyrotoxic crisis or storm**
    E05.9 **Thyrotoxicosis, unspecified**
    `5th`   Hyperthyroidism NOS
       E05.90 **Thyrotoxicosis, unspecified without thyrotoxic crisis or storm**
       E05.91 **Thyrotoxicosis, unspecified with thyrotoxic crisis or storm**

E06 **THYROIDITIS**
`4th`   ***Excludes1:*** postpartum thyroiditis (O90.5)
    E06.0 **Acute thyroiditis**
       Abscess of thyroid
       Pyogenic thyroiditis
       Suppurative thyroiditis
       Use additional code (B95–B97) to identify infectious agent.
    E06.1 **Subacute thyroiditis**
       de Quervain thyroiditis
       Giant-cell thyroiditis
       Granulomatous thyroiditis
       Nonsuppurative thyroiditis
       Viral thyroiditis
       Excludes1: autoimmune thyroiditis (E06.3)
    E06.2 **Chronic thyroiditis with transient thyrotoxicosis**
       Excludes1: autoimmune thyroiditis (E06.3)
    E06.3 **Autoimmune thyroiditis**
       Hashimoto's thyroiditis
       Hashitoxicosis (transient)
       Lymphadenoid goiter
       Lymphocytic thyroiditis
       Struma lymphomatosa
    E06.4 **Drug-induced thyroiditis**
       Use additional code for adverse effect, if applicable, to identify drug (T36-T50 with fifth or sixth character 5)
    E06.5 **Other chronic thyroiditis**
       Chronic fibrous thyroiditis
       Chronic thyroiditis NOS
       Ligneous thyroiditis
       Riedel thyroiditis
    E06.9 **Thyroiditis, unspecified**

E07 **OTHER DISORDERS OF THYROID**
`4th`   **E07.8** **Other specified disorders of thyroid**
    `5th`

E07.89   **Other specified disorders of thyroid**
Abnormality of thyroid-binding globulin
Hemorrhage of thyroid
Infarction of thyroid
E07.9   **Disorder of thyroid, unspecified**

(E08–E13) DIABETES MELLITUS

GUIDELINES

The DM codes are combination codes that include the type of DM, the body system affected, and the complications affecting that body system. As many codes within a particular category as are necessary to describe all of the complications of the disease may be used. They should be sequenced based on the reason for a particular encounter. Assign as many codes from categories E08–E13 as needed to identify all of the associated conditions that the patient has.

Type of diabetes

The age of a patient is not the sole determining factor, though most type 1 diabetics develop the condition before reaching puberty. For this reason type 1 DM is also referred to as juvenile diabetes.

Type of DM not documented

If the type of DM is not documented in the medical record the default is E11.-, Type 2 DM.

DM and the use of insulin and oral hypoglycemics

If the documentation in a medical record does not indicate the type of diabetes but does indicate that the patient uses insulin, code E11-, Type 2 DM, should be assigned. Additional codes should be assigned from category Z79 to identify the long-term (current) use of insulin or oral hypoglycemic drugs **or injectable non-insulin antidiabetic, as follows:** If the patient is treated with both oral medications and insulin, **both code Z79.4, Long term (current) use of insulin, and code Z79.84, Long term (current) use of oral hypoglycemic drugs,** should be assigned. If the patient is treated with both oral medications and insulin, only the code for long-term (current) use of insulin should be assigned. If the patient is treated with both insulin and an injectable non-insulin antidiabetic drug, assign codes Z79.4, Long-term (current) use of insulin, and Z79.899, Other long term (current) drug therapy. If the patient is treated with both oral hypoglycemic drugs and an injectable non-insulin antidiabetic drug, assign codes Z79.84, Long-term (current) use of oral hypoglycemic drugs, and Z79.899, Other long-term (current) drug therapy. Code Z79.4 should not be assigned if insulin is given temporarily to bring a type 2 patient's blood sugar under control during an encounter.

Complications due to insulin pump malfunction

UNDERDOSE OF INSULIN DUE TO INSULIN PUMP FAILURE

An underdose of insulin due to an insulin pump failure should be assigned to a code from subcategory T85.6, Mechanical complication of other specified internal and external prosthetic devices, implants and grafts, that specifies the type of pump malfunction, as the principal or first-listed code, followed by code T38.3x6-, Underdosing of insulin and oral hypoglycemic [antidiabetic] drugs. Additional codes for the type of DM and any associated complications due to the underdosing should also be assigned.

OVERDOSE OF INSULIN DUE TO INSULIN PUMP FAILURE

The principal or first-listed code for an encounter due to an insulin pump malfunction resulting in an overdose of insulin, should also be T85.6-, Mechanical complication of other specified internal and external prosthetic devices, implants and grafts, followed by code T38.3x1-, Poisoning by insulin and oral hypoglycemic [antidiabetic] drugs, accidental (unintentional).

Secondary DM

Codes under categories E08, DM due to underlying condition, E09, Drug or chemical induced DM, and E13, Other specified DM, identify complications/manifestations associated with secondary DM. Secondary diabetes is always caused by another condition or event (e.g., cystic fibrosis, malignant neoplasm of pancreas, pancreatectomy, adverse effect of drug, or poisoning).

SECONDARY DM AND THE USE OF INSULIN OR ORAL HYPOGLYCEMICS

For patients with secondary diabetes mellitus who routinely use insulin or oral hypoglycemic drugs, **or injectable non-insulin drugs,** an additional code from category Z79 should be assigned to identify the long-term (current) use of insulin or oral hypoglycemic drugs **or non-injectable non-insulin drugs as follows:**

If the patient is treated with both oral medications and insulin, **both code Z79.4, Long term (current) use of insulin, and code Z79.84, Long term (current) use of oral hypoglycemic drugs,** should be assigned.

If the patient is treated with both oral medications and insulin, only the code for long-term (current) use of insulin should be assigned. If the patient is treated with both insulin and an injectable non-insulin antidiabetic drug, assign codes Z79.4, Long-term (current) use of insulin, and Z79.899, Other long term (current) drug therapy. If the patient is treated with both oral hypoglycemic drugs and an injectable non-insulin antidiabetic drug, assign codes Z79.84, Long-term (current) use of oral hypoglycemic drugs, and Z79.899, Other long-term (current) drug therapy. Code Z79.4 should not be assigned if insulin is given temporarily to bring a type 2 patient's blood sugar under control during an encounter.

ASSIGNING AND SEQUENCING SECONDARY DIABETES CODES AND ITS CAUSES

The sequencing of the secondary diabetes codes in relationship to codes for the cause of the diabetes is based on the Tabular List instructions for categories E08, E09 and E13.

Secondary DM due to pancreatectomy

For postpancreatectomy DM (lack of insulin due to the surgical removal of all or part of the pancreas), assign code E89.1, Postprocedural hypoinsulinemia. Assign a code from category E13 and a code from subcategory Z90.41-, Acquired absence of pancreas, as additional codes.

Secondary diabetes due to drugs

Secondary diabetes may be caused by an adverse effect of correctly administered medications, poisoning or sequela of poisoning.

Refer to categories T36–T50 for coding of adverse effects and poisoning.

Note for hyperglycemia not caused by DM or for transient hyperglycemia, refer to code R73.9, hyperglycemia, NOS

E08   **DM DUE TO UNDERLYING CONDITION**
`4th`   **Code first** the underlying condition, such as:
congenital rubella (P35.0)
Cushing's syndrome (E24.-)
cystic fibrosis (E84.-)
malignant neoplasm (C00–C96)
malnutrition (E40–E46)
pancreatitis and other diseases of the pancreas (K85-K86.-)
Use additional code to identify control using:
insulin (Z79.4)
oral antidiabetic drugs (Z79.84)
oral hypoglycemic drugs (Z79.84)
Excludes1: drug or chemical induced DM (E09.-)
gestational diabetes (O24.4-)
neonatal DM (transient) (P70.2)
postpancreatectomy DM (E13.-)
postprocedural DM (E13.-)
secondary DM NEC (E13.-)
type 1 DM (E10.-)
type 2 DM (E11.-)

E08.0   **DM due to underlying condition with hyperosmolarity;**
`5th`   **E08.00**   **without NKHHC**
        E08.01   **with coma**
E08.1   **DM due to underlying condition with ketoacidosis;**
`5th`   **E08.10**   **without coma**
        E08.11   **with coma**
E08.2   **DM due to underlying condition with; kidney complications**
`5th`   **E08.21**   **diabetic nephropathy or intercapillary**
                 glomerulosclerosis or intracapillary glomerulonephrosis or Kimmelstiel-Wilson disease
        E08.22   **diabetic CKD**
                 Use additional code to identify stage of CKD (N18.1–N18.6)
        E08.29   **other diabetic kidney complication**
                 Renal tubular degeneration in DM due to underlying condition

 `4th` `5th` `6th` `7th`   Additional Character Required   ✔   3-character code

•=New Code
▲=Revised Code

Excludes1—Not coded here, do not use together
Excludes2—Not included here

E08.3　DM due to underlying condition with ophthalmic complications

5th　E08.31　DM due to underlying condition with unspecified
6th　　diabetic retinopathy;
　　　E08.311　with macular edema
　　　7th
　　　E08.319　without macular edema
　　　7th

E08.32　DM due to underlying
6th　　condition with mild
　　nonproliferative
　　diabetic retinopathy
　　(NOS);

| 7th characters for subcategories E08.31, E08.32, E08.33, E08.34, E08.35 |
| 1—left eye |
| 2—right eye |
| 3—bilateral |

　　　E08.321　with macular
　　　7th　　　edema
　　　E08.329　without macular edema
　　　7th

E08.33　DM due to underlying condition with moderate
6th　　nonproliferative diabetic retinopathy;
　　　E08.331　with macular edema
　　　7th
　　　E08.339　without macular edema
　　　7th

E08.34　DM due to underlying condition with severe
6th　　nonproliferative diabetic retinopathy;
　　　E08.341　with macular edema
　　　7th
　　　E08.349　without macular edema
　　　7th

E08.35　DM due to underlying condition with proliferative
6th　　diabetic retinopathy;
　　　E08.351　with macular edema
　　　7th
　　　E08.359　without macular edema
　　　7th

E08.36　DM due to underlying condition with diabetic
　　cataract

E08.39　DM due to underlying condition with other diabetic
　　ophthalmic complication
　　Use additional code to identify manifestation, such as:
　　　diabetic glaucoma (H40–H42)

E08.4　DM due to underlying condition with; neurological
5th　complications
　　E08.40　diabetic neuropathy, unspecified
　　E08.41　diabetic mononeuropathy
　　E08.42　diabetic polyneuropathy
　　　diabetic neuralgia
　　E08.43　diabetic autonomic (poly)neuropathy
　　　diabetic gastroparesis
　　E08.44　diabetic amyotrophy
　　E08.49　other diabetic neurological complication

E08.5　DM due to underlying condition with; circulatory complications
5th
　　E08.51　diabetic peripheral angiopathy without gangrene
　　E08.52　diabetic peripheral angiopathy with gangrene
　　　diabetic gangrene
　　E08.59　other circulatory complications

E08.6　DM due to underlying condition with other specified
5th　complications
　　E08.61　DM due to underlying condition with; diabetic
　　6th　　arthropathy
　　　E08.610　diabetic neuropathic arthropathy
　　　　Charcôt's joints
　　　E08.618　other diabetic arthropathy
　　E08.62　DM due to underlying condition with; skin
　　6th　　complications
　　　E08.620　diabetic dermatitis
　　　　diabetic necrobiosis lipoidica
　　　E08.621　foot ulcer
　　　　Use additional code to identify site of ulcer
　　　　　(L97.4-, L97.5-)
　　　E08.622　other skin ulcer
　　　　Use additional code to identify site of ulcer
　　　　　(L97.1–L97.9, L98.41–L98.49)
　　　E08.628　other skin complications

E08.63　DM due to underlying condition with; oral
6th　　complications
　　　E08.630　periodontal disease
　　　E08.638　other oral complications
E08.64　DM due to underlying condition with hypoglycemia;
6th
　　　E08.641　with coma
　　　E08.649　without coma
E08.65　DM due to underlying condition with hyperglycemia
E08.69　DM due to underlying condition with other specified
　　complication
　　Use additional code to identify complication

E08.8　DM due to underlying condition with unspecified
　　complications

E08.9　DM due to underlying condition without complications

E09　DRUG OR CHEMICAL INDUCED DM
4th
　Refer to category E08 for guidelines
　Code first poisoning due to drug or toxin, if applicable (T36–T65 with fifth
　　or sixth character 1–4 or 6)
　Use additional code for adverse effect, if applicable, to identify drug
　　(T36–T50 with fifth or sixth character 5)
　Use additional code to identify control using:
　　insulin (Z79.4)
　　oral antidiabetic drugs (Z79.84)
　　oral hypoglycemic drugs (Z79.84)
　Excludes1: DM due to underlying condition (E08.-)
　　gestational diabetes (O24.4-)
　　neonatal DM (P70.2)
　　postpancreatectomy DM (E13.-)
　　postprocedural DM (E13.-)
　　secondary DM NEC (E13.-)
　　type 1 DM (E10.-)
　　type 2 DM (E11.-)

E09.0　Drug or chemical induced DM with hyperosmolarity
5th　E09.00　Drug or chemical induced DM with hyperosmolarity
　　　　without NKHHC
　　E09.01　Drug or chemical induced DM with hyperosmolarity
　　　　with coma

E09.1　Drug or chemical induced DM with ketoacidosis;
5th　E09.10　without coma
　　E09.11　with coma

E09.2　Drug or chemical induced DM with; kidney complications
5th　E09.21　diabetic nephropathy
　　　　Drug or chemical induced DM with intercapillary
　　　　　glomerulosclerosis or
　　　　intracapillary glomerulonephrosis or Kimmelstiel-Wilson
　　　　　disease
　　E09.22　diabetic CKD
　　　　Use additional code to identify stage of CKD
　　　　　(N18.1–N18.6)
　　E09.29　other diabetic kidney complication
　　　　Drug or chemical induced DM with renal tubular
　　　　　degeneration

E09.3　Drug or chemical induced DM with ophthalmic complications
5th　E09.31　Drug or chemical induced DM with unspecified
6th　　diabetic retinopathy;
　　　E09.311　with macular edema
　　　E09.319　without macular edema

E09.32　Drug or chemical
6th　induced DM with
　　mild nonproliferative
　　diabetic retinopathy;
　　Drug or chemical
　　　induced DM with
　　　nonproliferative
　　　diabetic retinopathy NOS

| 7th characters for subcategory E09.32, E09.33, E09.34, E09.35 |
| 1—left eye |
| 2—right eye |
| 3—bilateral |

　　E09.321　with macular edema
　　7th
　　E09.329　without macular edema
　　7th

E09.33　Drug or chemical induced DM with moderate
6th　　nonproliferative diabetic retinopathy;
　　E09.331　with macular edema
　　7th

CHAPTER 4. ENDOCRINE, NUTRITIONAL AND METABOLIC DISEASES　(E08.3–E09.331)

4th　5th　6th　7th　Additional Character Required　　✔　3-character code

•=New Code
▲=Revised Code

Excludes1—Not coded here, do not use together
Excludes2—Not included here

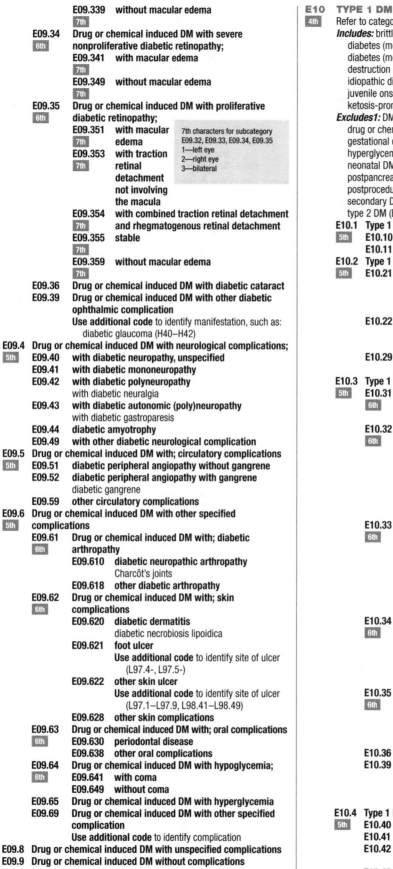

E09.339 without macular edema
7th

E09.34 Drug or chemical induced DM with severe nonproliferative diabetic retinopathy;
6th
    E09.341 with macular edema
    7th
    E09.349 without macular edema
    7th

E09.35 Drug or chemical induced DM with proliferative diabetic retinopathy;
6th
    E09.351 with macular edema
    7th
    E09.353 with traction retinal detachment not involving the macula
    7th
    E09.354 with combined traction retinal detachment and rhegmatogenous retinal detachment
    E09.355 stable
    7th
    E09.359 without macular edema
    7th

> 7th characters for subcategory E09.32, E09.33, E09.34, E09.35
> 1—left eye
> 2—right eye
> 3—bilateral

E09.36 Drug or chemical induced DM with diabetic cataract
E09.39 Drug or chemical induced DM with other diabetic ophthalmic complication
    Use additional code to identify manifestation, such as: diabetic glaucoma (H40–H42)

E09.4 Drug or chemical induced DM with neurological complications;
5th
    E09.40 with diabetic neuropathy, unspecified
    E09.41 with diabetic mononeuropathy
    E09.42 with diabetic polyneuropathy
        with diabetic neuralgia
    E09.43 with diabetic autonomic (poly)neuropathy
        with diabetic gastroparesis
    E09.44 diabetic amyotrophy
    E09.49 with other diabetic neurological complication

E09.5 Drug or chemical induced DM with; circulatory complications
5th
    E09.51 diabetic peripheral angiopathy without gangrene
    E09.52 diabetic peripheral angiopathy with gangrene
        diabetic gangrene
    E09.59 other circulatory complications

E09.6 Drug or chemical induced DM with other specified complications
5th
    E09.61 Drug or chemical induced DM with; diabetic arthropathy
    6th
        E09.610 diabetic neuropathic arthropathy
            Charcôt's joints
        E09.618 other diabetic arthropathy
    E09.62 Drug or chemical induced DM with; skin complications
    6th
        E09.620 diabetic dermatitis
            diabetic necrobiosis lipoidica
        E09.621 foot ulcer
            Use additional code to identify site of ulcer (L97.4-, L97.5-)
        E09.622 other skin ulcer
            Use additional code to identify site of ulcer (L97.1–L97.9, L98.41–L98.49)
        E09.628 other skin complications
    E09.63 Drug or chemical induced DM with; oral complications
    6th
        E09.630 periodontal disease
        E09.638 other oral complications
    E09.64 Drug or chemical induced DM with hypoglycemia;
    6th
        E09.641 with coma
        E09.649 without coma
    E09.65 Drug or chemical induced DM with hyperglycemia
    E09.69 Drug or chemical induced DM with other specified complication
        Use additional code to identify complication

E09.8 Drug or chemical induced DM with unspecified complications
E09.9 Drug or chemical induced DM without complications

E10 **TYPE 1 DM**
4th
Refer to category E08 for guidelines
Includes: brittle diabetes (mellitus)
    diabetes (mellitus) due to autoimmune process
    diabetes (mellitus) due to immune mediated pancreatic islet beta-cell destruction
    idiopathic diabetes (mellitus)
    juvenile onset diabetes (mellitus)
    ketosis-prone diabetes (mellitus)
Excludes1: DM due to underlying condition (E08.-)
    drug or chemical induced DM (E09.-)
    gestational diabetes (O24.4-)
    hyperglycemia NOS (R73.9)
    neonatal DM (P70.2)
    postpancreatectomy DM (E13.-)
    postprocedural DM (E13.-)
    secondary DM NEC (E13.-)
    type 2 DM (E11.-)

E10.1 Type 1 DM with ketoacidosis;
5th
    E10.10 Type 1 DM with ketoacidosis without coma
    E10.11 Type 1 DM with ketoacidosis with coma

E10.2 Type 1 DM with kidney complications
5th
    E10.21 Type 1 DM with diabetic nephropathy
        Type 1 DM with intercapillary glomerulosclerosis or intracapillary glomerulonephrosis or Kimmelstiel-Wilson disease
    E10.22 Type 1 DM with diabetic CKD
        Use additional code to identify stage of CKD (N18.1–N18.6)
    E10.29 Type 1 DM with other diabetic kidney complication
        Type 1 DM with renal tubular degeneration

E10.3 Type 1 DM with ophthalmic complications
5th
    E10.31 Type 1 DM with unspecified diabetic retinopathy;
    6th
        E10.311 with macular edema
        E10.319 without macular edema
    E10.32 Type 1 DM with mild nonproliferative diabetic retinopathy;
    6th
        diabetic retinopathy NOS
        E10.321 with macular edema
        7th
        E10.329 without macular edema
        7th

> 7th characters for subcategory E10.32, E10.33, E10.34, E10.35
> 1—left eye
> 2—right eye
> 3—bilateral

    E10.33 Type 1 DM with moderate nonproliferative diabetic retinopathy;
    6th
        E10.331 with macular edema
        7th
        E10.339 without macular edema
        7th
    E10.34 Type 1 DM with severe nonproliferative diabetic retinopathy;
    6th
        E10.341 with macular edema
        7th
        E10.349 without macular edema
        7th
    E10.35 Type 1 DM with proliferative diabetic retinopathy;
    6th
        E10.351 with macular edema
        7th
        E10.359 without macular edema
        7th
    E10.36 Type 1 DM with diabetic cataract
    E10.39 Type 1 DM with other diabetic ophthalmic complication
        Use additional code to identify manifestation, such as: diabetic glaucoma (H40–H42)

E10.4 Type 1 DM with neurological complications
5th
    E10.40 Type 1 DM with diabetic neuropathy, unspecified
    E10.41 Type 1 DM with diabetic mononeuropathy
    E10.42 Type 1 DM with diabetic polyneuropathy
        Type 1 DM with diabetic neuralgia
    E10.43 Type 1 DM with diabetic autonomic (poly)neuropathy

---

4th   5th   6th   7th   Additional Character Required   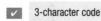 3-character code

•=New Code   ***Excludes1***—Not coded here, do not use together
▲=Revised Code   ***Excludes***—Not included here

E10.44   Type 1 DM with diabetic amyotrophy
E10.49   Type 1 DM with other diabetic neurological complication

E10.5   Type 1 DM with circulatory complications
5th E10.51   Type 1 DM with diabetic peripheral angiopathy without gangrene
E10.52   Type 1 DM with diabetic peripheral angiopathy with gangrene
Type 1 DM with diabetic gangrene
E10.59   Type 1 DM with other circulatory complications

E10.6   Type 1 DM with other specified complications
5th E10.61   Type 1 DM with diabetic arthropathy
6th   E10.610   Type 1 DM with diabetic neuropathic arthropathy
Type 1 DM with Charcôt's joints
E10.618   Type 1 DM with other diabetic arthropathy
E10.62   Type 1 DM with skin complications
6th   E10.620   Type 1 DM with diabetic dermatitis
Type 1 DM with diabetic necrobiosis lipoidica
E10.621   Type 1 DM with foot ulcer
Use additional code to identify site of ulcer (L97.4-, L97.5-)
E10.622   Type 1 DM with other skin ulcer
Use additional code to identify site of ulcer (L97.1–L97.9, L98.41–L98.49)
E10.628   Type 1 DM with other skin complications
E10.63   Type 1 DM with oral complications
6th   E10.630   Type 1 DM with periodontal disease
E10.638   Type 1 DM with other oral complications
E10.64   Type 1 DM with hypoglycemia
6th   E10.641   Type 1 DM with hypoglycemia with coma
E10.649   Type 1 DM with hypoglycemia without coma
E10.65   Type 1 DM with hyperglycemia
E10.69   Type 1 DM with other specified complication
Use additional code to identify complication

E10.8   Type 1 DM with unspecified complications
E10.9   Type 1 DM without complications

✓ **E11   TYPE 2 DM**
4th
Refer to category E08 for guidelines
If the type of DM is not documented in the medical record the default is E11.-, Type 2 DM.
Includes: diabetes (mellitus) due to insulin secretory defect
diabetes NOS
insulin resistant diabetes (mellitus)
Use additional code to identify control using:
insulin (Z79.4)
oral antidiabetic drugs (Z79.84)
oral hypoglycemic drugs (Z79.84)
Excludes1: DM due to underlying condition (E08.-)
drug or chemical induced DM (E09.-)
gestational diabetes (O24.4-)
neonatal DM (P70.2)
postpancreatectomy DM (E13.-)
postprocedural DM (E13.-)
secondary DM NEC (E13.-)
type 1 DM (E10.-)

E11.0   Type 2 DM with hyperosmolarity;
5th E11.00   without NKHHC
E11.01   with coma
E11.1   Type 2 diabetes mellitus with ketoacidosis
5th E11.10   Type 2 diabetes mellitus with ketoacidosis without coma
E11.11   Type 2 diabetes mellitus with ketoacidosis with coma
E11.2   Type 2 DM with kidney complications
5th E11.21   Type 2 DM with diabetic nephropathy or intercapillary glomerulosclerosis or intracapillary glomerulonephrosis or Kimmelstiel-Wilson disease
E11.22   Type 2 DM with diabetic CKD
Use additional code to identify stage of CKD (N18.1–N18.6)
E11.29   Type 2 DM with other diabetic kidney complication
Type 2 DM with renal tubular degeneration

E11.3   Type 2 DM with ophthalmic complications
5th E11.31   Type 2 DM with unspecified diabetic retinopathy;
6th   E11.311   with macular edema
E11.319   without macular edema
E11.32   Type 2 DM with mild nonproliferative diabetic retinopathy;
6th
Type 2 DM with nonproliferative diabetic retinopathy NOS

7th character for subcategories E11.32, E11.33, E11.34, E11.35
1—right eye
2—left eye
3—bilateral

E11.321   with macular edema
7th

E11.329   without macular edema
7th

E11.33   Type 2 DM with moderate nonproliferative diabetic retinopathy;
6th   E11.331   with macular edema
7th
E11.339   without macular edema
7th
E11.34   Type 2 DM with severe nonproliferative diabetic retinopathy;
6th   E11.341   with macular edema
7th
E11.349   without macular edema
7th
E11.35   Type 2 DM with proliferative diabetic retinopathy;
6th   E11.351   with macular edema
7th
E11.359   without macular edema
7th
E11.36   Type 2 DM with diabetic cataract
E11.39   Type 2 DM with other diabetic ophthalmic complication
Use additional code to identify manifestation, such as:
diabetic glaucoma (H40–H42)

E11.4   Type 2 DM with neurological complications
5th E11.40   Type 2 DM with diabetic neuropathy, unspecified
E11.41   Type 2 DM with diabetic mononeuropathy
E11.42   Type 2 DM with diabetic polyneuropathy
Type 2 DM with diabetic neuralgia
E11.43   Type 2 DM with diabetic autonomic (poly)neuropathy
Type 2 DM with diabetic gastroparesis
E11.44   Type 2 DM with diabetic amyotrophy
E11.49   Type 2 DM with other diabetic neurological complication

E11.5   Type 2 DM with circulatory complications
5th E11.51   Type 2 DM with diabetic peripheral angiopathy without gangrene
E11.52   Type 2 DM with diabetic peripheral angiopathy with gangrene
Type 2 DM with diabetic gangrene
E11.59   Type 2 DM with other circulatory complications

E11.6   Type 2 DM with other specified complications
5th E11.61   Type 2 DM with diabetic arthropathy
6th   E11.610   Type 2 DM with diabetic neuropathic arthropathy
Type 2 DM with Charcôt's joints
E11.618   Type 2 DM with other diabetic arthropathy
E11.62   Type 2 DM with skin complications
6th   E11.620   Type 2 DM with diabetic dermatitis
Type 2 DM with diabetic necrobiosis lipoidica
E11.621   Type 2 DM with foot ulcer
Use additional code to identify site of ulcer (L97.4-, L97.5-)
E11.622   Type 2 DM with other skin ulcer
Use additional code to identify site of ulcer (L97.1–L97.9, L98.41–L98.49)
E11.628   Type 2 DM with other skin complications
E11.63   Type 2 DM with oral complications
6th   E11.630   Type 2 DM with periodontal disease
E11.638   Type 2 DM with other oral complications

4th 5th 6th 7th   Additional Character Required   ✔ 3-character code

•=New Code
▲=Revised Code

Excludes1—Not coded here, do not use together
Excludes2—Not included here

E11.64 **Type 2 DM with hypoglycemia**
> 6th   **E11.641** **Type 2 DM with hypoglycemia with coma**
>   **E11.649** **Type 2 DM with hypoglycemia without coma**

E11.65 **Type 2 DM with hyperglycemia**

E11.69 **Type 2 DM with other specified complication**
> **Use additional code** to identify complication

E11.8 **Type 2 DM with unspecified complications**

E11.9 **Type 2 DM without complications**

(E15–E16) OTHER DISORDERS OF GLUCOSE REGULATION AND PANCREATIC INTERNAL SECRETION

E15 NONDIABETIC HYPOGLYCEMIC COMA
✔
> ***Includes:*** drug-induced insulin coma in nondiabetic
> hyperinsulinism with hypoglycemic coma
> hypoglycemic coma NOS

E16 OTHER DISORDERS OF PANCREATIC INTERNAL
4th **SECRETION**
E16.0 **Drug-induced hypoglycemia without coma**
> **Use additional code** for adverse effect, if applicable, to identify drug (T36–T50 with fifth or sixth character 5)
> ***Excludes 1:*** diabetes with hypoglycemia without coma (E09.649)

E16.1 **Other hypoglycemia**
> Functional hyperinsulinism
> Functional nonhyperinsulinemic hypoglycemia
> Hyperinsulinism NOS
> Hyperplasia of pancreatic islet beta cells NOS
> ***Excludes1:*** diabetes with hypoglycemia (E08.649, E10.649, E11.649)
> hypoglycemia in infant of diabetic mother (P70.1)
> neonatal hypoglycemia (P70.4)

E16.2 **Hypoglycemia, unspecified**
> ***Excludes 1:*** diabetes with hypoglycemia (E08.649, E10.649, E11.649)

E16.8 **Other specified disorders of pancreatic internal secretion**
> Increased secretion from endocrine pancreas of growth hormone-releasing hormone or pancreatic polypeptide or somatostatin or vasoactive-intestinal polypeptide

E16.9 **Disorder of pancreatic internal secretion, unspecified**
> Islet-cell hyperplasia NOS
> Pancreatic endocrine cell hyperplasia NOS

(E20–E35) DISORDERS OF OTHER ENDOCRINE GLANDS

Excludes1: galactorrhea (N64.3)
> gynecomastia (N62)

E20 HYPOPARATHYROIDISM
4th
> ***Excludes1:*** Di George's syndrome (D82.1)
> postprocedural hypoparathyroidism (E89.2)
> tetany NOS (R29.0)
> transitory neonatal hypoparathyroidism (P71.4)

E20.0 **Idiopathic hypoparathyroidism**

E20.1 **Pseudohypoparathyroidism**

E20.8 **Other hypoparathyroidism**

E20.9 **Hypoparathyroidism, unspecified**
> Parathyroid tetany

E22 HYPERFUNCTION OF PITUITARY GLAND
4th
> ***Excludes1:*** Cushing's syndrome (E24.-)
> Nelson's syndrome (E24.1)
> overproduction of ACTH not associated with Cushing's disease (E27.0)
> overproduction of pituitary ACTH (E24.0)
> overproduction of thyroid-stimulating hormone (E05.8-)

E22.0 **Acromegaly and pituitary gigantism**
> Overproduction of growth hormone
> ***Excludes1:*** constitutional gigantism (E34.4)
> constitutional tall stature (E34.4)
> increased secretion from endocrine pancreas of growth hormone-releasing hormone (E16.8)

E22.2 **Syndrome of inappropriate secretion of antidiuretic hormone**

E22.8 **Other hyperfunction of pituitary gland**
> Central precocious puberty

E22.9 **Hyperfunction of pituitary gland, unspecified**

E23 HYPOFUNCTION AND OTHER DISORDERS OF THE
4th **PITUITARY GLAND**
> **Includes:** the listed conditions whether the disorder is in the pituitary or the hypothalamus
> ***Excludes1:*** postprocedural hypopituitarism (E89.3)

E23.0 **Hypopituitarism**

E23.1 **Drug-induced hypopituitarism**
> **Use additional code** for adverse effect, if applicable, to identify drug (T36-T50 with fifth or sixth character 5)

E23.2 **Diabetes insipidus**
> ***Excludes1:*** nephrogenic diabetes insipidus (N25.1)

E23.3 **Hypothalamic dysfunction, not elsewhere classified**
> ***Excludes1:*** Prader-Willi syndrome (Q87.11)
> Russell-Silver syndrome (Q87.1)

E23.6 **Other disorders of pituitary gland**
> Abscess of pituitary
> Adiposogenital dystrophy

E24.8 **Other Cushing's syndrome**

E23.7 **Disorder of pituitary gland, unspecified**

E24 CUSHING'S SYNDROME
4th
> ***Excludes1:*** congenital adrenal hyperplasia (E25.0)

E24.0 **Pituitary-dependent Cushing's disease**
> Overproduction of pituitary ACTH
> Pituitary-dependent hypercorticalism

E24.2 **Drug-induced Cushing's syndrome**
> **Use additional code** for adverse effect, if applicable, to identify drug (T36-T50 with fifth or sixth character 5)

E24.8 **Other Cushing's syndrome**

E24.9 **Cushing's syndrome, unspecified**

E25 ADRENOGENITAL DISORDERS
4th
> ***Includes:*** adrenogenital syndromes, virilizing or feminizing, whether acquired or due to adrenal hyperplasia consequent on inborn enzyme defects in hormone synthesis
> Female adrenal pseudohermaphroditism
> Female heterosexual precocious pseudopuberty
> Male isosexual precocious pseudopuberty
> Male macrogenitosomia praecox
> Male sexual precocity with adrenal hyperplasia
> Male virilization (female)
> ***Excludes1:*** indeterminate sex and pseudohermaphroditism (Q56)
> chromosomal abnormalities (Q90–Q99)

E25.0 **Congenital adrenogenital disorders associated with enzyme deficiency**
> Congenital adrenal hyperplasia
> 21-Hydroxylase deficiency
> Salt-losing congenital adrenal hyperplasia

E25.8 **Other adrenogenital disorders**
> Idiopathic adrenogenital disorder
> **Use additional code** for adverse effect, if applicable, to identify drug (T36-T50 with fifth or sixth character 5)

E25.9 **Adrenogenital disorder, unspecified**
> Adrenogenital syndrome NOS

E27 OTHER DISORDERS OF ADRENAL GLAND
4th
> Refer to code C74, Malignant neoplasm of adrenal gland, to report neuroblastomas

E27.0 **Other adrenocortical overactivity**
> Overproduction of ACTH, not associated with Cushing's disease
> Premature adrenarche
> ***Excludes1:*** Cushing's syndrome (E24.-)

E27.1 **Primary adrenocortical insufficiency**
> Addison's disease
> Autoimmune adrenalitis
> ***Excludes1:*** Addison only phenotype adrenoleukodystrophy (E71.528)
> amyloidosis (E85.-)
> tuberculous Addison's disease (A18.7)
> Waterhouse-Friderichsen syndrome (A39.1)

E27.2 **Addisonian crisis**
> Adrenal crisis
> Adrenocortical crisis

| 4th | 5th | 6th | 7th | Additional Character Required | | ✔ | 3-character code |

•=New Code   ***Excludes1***—Not coded here, do not use together
▲=Revised Code   ***Excludes2***—Not included here

E27.3 Drug-induced adrenocortical insufficiency
Use additional code for adverse effect, if applicable, to identify drug (T36–T50 with fifth or sixth character 5)

E27.4 Other and unspecified adrenocortical insufficiency
> **[5th] E27.40 Unspecified adrenocortical insufficiency**
> Adrenocortical insufficiency NOS
> **E27.49 Other adrenocortical insufficiency**
> Adrenal hemorrhage
> Adrenal infarction

E27.8 Other specified disorders of adrenal gland
Abnormality of cortisol-binding globulin

E27.9 Disorder of adrenal gland, unspecified
Excludes1: adrenoleukodystrophy [Addison-Schilder] (E71.528)
Waterhouse-Friderichsen syndrome (A39.1)

E28 OVARIAN DYSFUNCTION
[4th]
Excludes1: isolated gonadotropin deficiency (E23.0)
postprocedural ovarian failure (E89.4-)

E28.0 Estrogen excess
Use additional code for adverse effect, if applicable, to identify drug (T36–T50 with fifth or sixth character 5)

E28.1 Androgen excess
Hypersecretion of ovarian androgens
Use additional code for adverse effect, if applicable, to identify drug (T36–T50 with fifth or sixth character 5)

E28.2 Polycystic ovarian syndrome
Sclerocystic ovary syndrome
Stein-Leventhal syndrome

E28.3 Primary ovarian failure
> **[5th]** *Excludes1:* pure gonadal dysgenesis (Q99.1)
> Turner's syndrome (Q96.-)
> **E28.39 Other primary ovarian failure**
> Decreased estrogen
> Resistant ovary syndrome

E30 DISORDERS OF PUBERTY, NEC
[4th]
E30.0 Delayed puberty
Constitutional delay of puberty
Delayed sexual development

E30.1 Precocious puberty
Precocious menstruation
Excludes1: Albright (-McCune) (-Sternberg) syndrome (Q78.1)
central precocious puberty (E22.8)
congenital adrenal hyperplasia (E25.0)
female heterosexual precocious pseudopuberty (E25.-)
male isosexual precocious pseudopuberty (E25.-)

E30.8 Other disorders of puberty
Premature thelarche

E30.9 Disorder of puberty, unspecified

E31 POLYGLANDULAR DYSFUNCTION
[4th]
Excludes1: ataxia telangiectasia [Louis-Bar] (G11.3)
dystrophia myotonica [Steinert] (G71.11)
pseudohypoparathyroidism (E20.1)

E31.2 Multiple endocrine neoplasia [MEN] syndromes
> **[5th]** Multiple endocrine adenomatosis
> **Code also** any associated malignancies and other conditions associated with the syndromes
> **E31.20 Multiple endocrine neoplasia [MEN] syndrome, unspecified**
> Multiple endocrine adenomatosis NOS
> Multiple endocrine neoplasia [MEN] syndrome NOS
> **E31.21 Multiple endocrine neoplasia [MEN] type I**
> Wermer's syndrome
> **E31.22 Multiple endocrine neoplasia [MEN] type IIA**
> Sipple's syndrome
> **E31.23 Multiple endocrine neoplasia [MEN] type IIB**

E34 OTHER ENDOCRINE DISORDERS
[4th]
Excludes1: pseudohypoparathyroidism (E20.1)

E34.0 Carcinoid syndrome
Note: May be used as an additional code to identify functional activity associated with a carcinoid tumor.

E34.3 Short stature due to endocrine disorder
Constitutional short stature
Laron-type short stature
Excludes1: achondroplastic short stature (Q77.4)
hypochondroplastic short stature (Q77.4)
nutritional short stature (E45)
pituitary short stature (E23.0)
progeria (E34.8)
renal short stature (N25.0)
Russell-Silver syndrome (Q87.19)
short-limbed stature with immunodeficiency (D82.2)
short stature in specific dysmorphic syndromes — **code to** syndrome — **see** Alphabetical Index
short stature NOS (R62.52)

E34.4 Constitutional tall stature

E34.5 Androgen insensitivity syndrome
> **[5th] E34.50 Androgen insensitivity syndrome, unspecified**
> Androgen insensitivity NOS
> **E34.51 Complete androgen insensitivity syndrome**
> Complete androgen insensitivity
> de Quervain syndrome
> Goldberg-Maxwell syndrome
> **E34.52 Partial androgen insensitivity syndrome**
> Partial androgen insensitivity
> Reifenstein syndrome

E34.8 Other specified endocrine disorders
Pineal gland dysfunction
Progeria
Excludes2: pseudohypoparathyroidism (E20.1)

E34.9 Endocrine disorder, unspecified
Endocrine disturbance NOS
Hormone disturbance NOS

(E36) INTRAOPERATIVE COMPLICATIONS OF ENDOCRINE SYSTEM

(E40–E46) MALNUTRITION

E40 KWASHIORKOR
[✔]
Severe malnutrition with nutritional edema with dyspigmentation of skin and hair
Excludes1: marasmic kwashiorkor (E42)

E44 PROTEIN-CALORIE MALNUTRITION OF MODERATE AND MILD DEGREE
[4th]
E44.0 Moderate protein-calorie malnutrition
E44.1 Mild protein-calorie malnutrition
Nutritional short stature
Nutritional stunting
Physical retardation due to malnutrition

E45 RETARDED DEVELOPMENT FOLLOWING PROTEIN-CALORIE MALNUTRITION
[✔]

E46 UNSPECIFIED PROTEIN-CALORIE MALNUTRITION
[✔]
Malnutrition NOS
Protein-calorie imbalance NOS
Excludes1: nutritional deficiency NOS (E63.9)

(E50–E64) OTHER NUTRITIONAL DEFICIENCIES

E55 VITAMIN D DEFICIENCY
[4th]
Excludes1: adult osteomalacia (M83.-)
osteoporosis (M80.-)
sequelae of rickets (E64.3)

E55.0 Rickets, active
Infantile osteomalacia
Juvenile osteomalacia
Excludes1: celiac rickets (K90.0)
Crohn's rickets (K50.-)
hereditary vitamin D-dependent rickets (E83.32)
inactive rickets (E64.3)
renal rickets (N25.0)
sequelae of rickets (E64.3)
vitamin D-resistant rickets (E83.31)

[4th] [5th] [6th] [7th] Additional Character Required   **[✔]** 3-character code

•=New Code   *Excludes1*—Not coded here, do not use together
▲=Revised Code   *Excludes2*—Not included here

E55.9 **Vitamin D deficiency, unspecified**
Avitaminosis D

E56 **OTHER VITAMIN DEFICIENCIES**
`4th` *Excludes1:* sequelae of other vitamin deficiencies (E64.8)
E56.0 **Deficiency of vitamin E**
E56.1 **Deficiency of vitamin K**
Excludes1: deficiency of coagulation factor due to vitamin K deficiency (D68.4)
vitamin K deficiency of newborn (P53)
E56.8 **Deficiency of other vitamins**
E56.9 **Vitamin deficiency, unspecified**

E58 **DIETARY CALCIUM DEFICIENCY**
`✓` *Excludes1:* disorders of calcium metabolism (E83.5-)
sequelae of calcium deficiency (E64.8)

E63 **OTHER NUTRITIONAL DEFICIENCIES**
`4th` *Excludes2:* dehydration (E86.0)
failure to thrive, adult (R62.7)
failure to thrive, child (R62.51)
feeding problems in newborn (P92.-)
sequelae of malnutrition and other nutritional deficiencies (E64.-)
E63.0 **Essential fatty acid [EFA] deficiency**
E63.1 **Imbalance of constituents of food intake**
E63.8 **Other specified nutritional deficiencies**
E63.9 **Nutritional deficiency, unspecified**

(E65–E68) OVERWEIGHT, OBESITY AND OTHER HYPERALIMENTATION

E66 **OVERWEIGHT AND OBESITY**
`4th` **Use additional code** to identify body mass index (BMI), if known (Z68.-)
Excludes1: adiposogenital dystrophy (E23.6)
lipomatosis NOS (E88.2)
lipomatosis dolorosa [Dercum] (E88.2)
Prader-Willi syndrome (Q87.11)
E66.0 **Obesity due to excess calories**
`5th` E66.01 **Morbid (severe) obesity due to excess calories**
Excludes1: morbid (severe) obesity with alveolar hypoventilation (E66.2)
E66.09 **Other obesity due to excess calories**
E66.1 **Drug-induced obesity**
Use additional code for adverse effect, if applicable, to identify drug (T36-T50 with fifth or sixth character 5)
E66.2 **Morbid (severe) obesity with alveolar hypoventilation**
obesity hypoventilation syndrome (OHS)
Use with Z68.30–Z68.45 (adults) or Z68.53 (pediatrics, 2–20 yrs)
Pickwickian syndrome
E66.3 **Overweight**
Use with Z68.25–Z68.29 (adults) or Z68.53 (pediatrics, 2–20 yrs)
E66.8 **Other obesity**
Use with Z68.30–Z68.45 (adults) or Z68.53 (pediatrics, 2–20 yrs)
E66.9 **Obesity, unspecified**
Use with Z68.30–Z68.45 (adults) or Z68.53 (pediatrics, 2–20 yrs)
Obesity NOS

(E70–E88) METABOLIC DISORDERS

Excludes1: androgen insensitivity syndrome (E34.5-)
congenital adrenal hyperplasia (E25.0)
hemolytic anemias attributable to enzyme disorders (D55.-)
Marfan's syndrome (Q87.4)
5-alpha-reductase deficiency (E29.1)
Excludes2: Ehlers-Danlos syndromes (Q79.6-)

E70 **DISORDERS OF AROMATIC AMINO-ACID METABOLISM**
`4th` E70.0 **Classical phenylketonuria**
E70.1 **Other hyperphenylalaninemias**
E70.8 **Disorders of aromatic amino-acid metabolism**
`5th` E70.81 **Aromatic L-amino acid decarboxylase deficiency**
AADC deficiency
E70.89 **Other disorders of aromatic amino-acid metabolism**

E71 **DISORDERS OF BRANCHED-CHAIN AMINO-ACID**
`4th` **METABOLISM AND FATTY-ACID METABOLISM**
E71.0 **Maple-syrup-urine disease**

E71.1 **Other disorders of branched-chain amino-acid metabolism**
`5th` E71.11 **Branched-chain organic acidurias**
`6th` E71.110 **Isovaleric acidemia**
E71.111 **3-methylglutaconic aciduria**
E71.118 **Other branched-chain organic acidurias**
E71.12 **Disorders of propionate metabolism**
`6th` E71.120 **Methylmalonic acidemia**
E71.121 **Propionic acidemia**
E71.128 **Other disorders of propionate metabolism**
E71.19 **Other disorders of branched-chain amino-acid metabolism**
Hyperleucine-isoleucinemia
Hypervalinemia
E71.2 **Disorder of branched-chain amino-acid metabolism, unspecified**
E71.3 **Disorders of fatty-acid metabolism**
`5th` *Excludes1:* peroxisomal disorders (E71.5)
Refsum's disease (G60.1)
Schilder's disease (G37.0)
Excludes2: carnitine deficiency due to inborn error of metabolism (E71.42)
E71.30 **Disorder of fatty-acid metabolism, unspecified**
E71.31 **Disorders of fatty-acid oxidation**
`6th` E71.310 **Long chain/very long chain acyl CoA dehydrogenase deficiency**
LCAD
VLCAD
E71.311 **Medium chain acyl CoA dehydrogenase deficiency**
MCAD
E71.312 **Short chain acyl CoA dehydrogenase deficiency**
SCAD
E71.313 **Glutaric aciduria type II**
Glutaric aciduria type II A
Glutaric aciduria type II B
Glutaric aciduria type II C
Excludes1: glutaric aciduria (type 1) NOS (E72.3)
E71.314 **Muscle carnitine palmitoyltransferase deficiency**
E71.318 **Other disorders of fatty-acid oxidation**
E71.32 **Disorders of ketone metabolism**
E71.39 **Other disorders of fatty-acid metabolism**
E71.4 **Disorders of carnitine metabolism**
`5th` *Excludes1:* Muscle carnitine palmitoyltransferase deficiency (E71.314)
E71.40 **Disorder of carnitine metabolism, unspecified**
E71.41 **Primary carnitine deficiency**
E71.42 **Carnitine deficiency due to inborn errors of metabolism**
Code also associated inborn error or metabolism
E71.43 **Iatrogenic carnitine deficiency**
Carnitine deficiency due to hemodialysis
Carnitine deficiency due to Valproic acid therapy
E71.44 **Other secondary carnitine deficiency**
`6th` E71.440 **Ruvalcaba-Myhre-Smith syndrome**
E71.448 **Other secondary carnitine deficiency**
E71.5 **Peroxisomal disorders**
`5th` *Excludes1:* Schilder's disease (G37.0)
E71.50 **Peroxisomal disorder, unspecified**
E71.51 **Disorders of peroxisome biogenesis**
`6th` Group 1 peroxisomal disorders
Excludes1: Refsum's disease (G60.1)
E71.510 **Zellweger syndrome**
E71.511 **Neonatal adrenoleukodystrophy**
Excludes1: X-linked adrenoleukodystrophy (E71.42-)
E71.518 **Other disorders of peroxisome biogenesis**
E71.52 **X-linked adrenoleukodystrophy**
`6th` E71.520 **Childhood cerebral X-linked adrenoleukodystrophy**
E71.521 **Adolescent X-linked adrenoleukodystrophy**

`4th` `5th` `6th` `7th` Additional Character Required   `✓` 3-character code

•=New Code
▲=Revised Code

Excludes1—Not coded here, do not use together
Excludes2—Not included here

E71.522   **Adrenomyeloneuropathy**
E71.528   **Other X-linked adrenoleukodystrophy**
     Addison only phenotype
       adrenoleukodystrophy
     Addison-Schilder adrenoleukodystrophy
E71.529   **X-linked adrenoleukodystrophy, unspecified type**
E71.53   **Other group 2 peroxisomal disorders**
E71.54   **Other peroxisomal disorders**
[6th]   E71.540   **Rhizomelic chondrodysplasia punctata**
     Excludes1: chondrodysplasia punctata NOS (Q77.3)
E71.541   **Zellweger-like syndrome**
E71.542   **Other group 3 peroxisomal disorders**
E71.548   **Other peroxisomal disorders**

E72   **OTHER DISORDERS OF AMINO-ACID METABOLISM**
[4th]   ***Excludes1:*** disorders of aromatic amino-acid metabolism (E70.-)
     branched-chain amino-acid metabolism (E71.0–E71.2)
     fatty-acid metabolism (E71.3)
     purine and pyrimidine metabolism (E79.-)
     gout (M1A.-, M10.-)
E72.0   **Disorders of amino-acid transport**
[5th]   ***Excludes1:*** disorders of tryptophan metabolism (E70.5)
E72.00   **Disorders of amino-acid transport, unspecified**
E72.01   **Cystinuria**
E72.02   **Hartnup's disease**
E72.03   **Lowe's syndrome**
     Use additional code for associated glaucoma (H42)
E72.04   **Cystinosis**
E72.09   **Other disorders of amino-acid transport**
     Fanconi (-de Toni) (-Debré) syndrome, unspecified
E72.5   **Disorders of glycine metabolism**
[5th]   E72.50   **Disorder of glycine metabolism, unspecified**
E72.51   **Non-ketotic hyperglycinemia**
E72.52   **Trimethylaminuria**
E72.53   **Primary hyperoxaluria**
     Oxalosis
     Oxaluria
E72.59   **Other disorders of glycine metabolism**
     D-glycericacidemia
     Hyperhydroxyprolinemia
     Hyperprolinemia (types I, II)
     Sarcosinemia
E72.8   **Other specified disorders of amino-acid metabolism**
[5th]   E72.81   **Disorders of gamma aminobutyric acid metabolism**
     4-hydroxybutyric aciduria
     Disorders of GABA metabolism
     GABA metabolic defect
     GABA transaminase deficiency
     GABA-T deficiency
     Gamma-hydroxybutyric aciduria
     SSADHD
     Succinic semialdehyde dehydrogenase deficiency
E72.89   **Other specified disorders of amino-acid metabolism**
     Disorders of beta-amino-acid metabolism
     Disorders of gamma-glutamyl cycle
E72.9   **Disorder of amino-acid metabolism, unspecified**

E73   **LACTOSE INTOLERANCE**
[4th]   **E73.0**   **Congenital lactase deficiency**
E73.1   **Secondary lactase deficiency**
E73.8   **Other lactose intolerance**
E73.9   **Lactose intolerance, unspecified**

E74   **OTHER DISORDERS OF CARBOHYDRATE METABOLISM**
[4th]   ***Excludes1:*** DM (E08–E13)
     hypoglycemia NOS (E16.2)
     increased secretion of glucagon (E16.3)
     mucopolysaccharidosis (E76.0–E76.3) E74.1
E74.1   **Disorders of fructose metabolism**
[5th]   ***Excludes1:*** muscle phosphofructokinase deficiency (E74.09)
E74.10   **Disorder of fructose metabolism, unspecified**
E74.11   **Essential fructosuria**
     Fructokinase deficiency

E74.12   **Hereditary fructose intolerance**
     Fructosemia
E74.19   **Other disorders of fructose metabolism**
     Fructose-1, 6-diphosphatase deficiency
E74.2   **Disorders of galactose metabolism**
[5th]   E74.20   **Disorders of galactose metabolism, unspecified**
E74.21   **Galactosemia**
E74.29   **Other disorders of galactose metabolism**
     Galactokinase deficiency
E74.3   **Other disorders of intestinal carbohydrate absorption**
[5th]   ***Excludes2:*** lactose intolerance (E73.-)
E74.31   **Sucrase-isomaltase deficiency**
E74.39   **Other disorders of intestinal carbohydrate absorption**
     Disorder of intestinal carbohydrate absorption NOS
     Glucose-galactose malabsorption
     Sucrase deficiency
E74.4   **Disorders of pyruvate metabolism and gluconeogenesis**
     Deficiency of phosphoenolpyruvate carboxykinase
     Deficiency of pyruvate carboxylase
     Deficiency of pyruvate dehydrogenase
     Excludes1: disorders of pyruvate metabolism and gluconeogenesis with anemia (D55.-)
     Leigh's syndrome (G31.82)
E74.8   **Disorders of carbohydrate metabolism**
[5th]   E74.81   **Disorders of glucose transport**
[6th]   E74.810   **Glucose transporter protein type 1 deficiency**
     De Vivo syndrome
     Glucose transport defect, blood-brain barrier
     Glut1 deficiency
     GLUT1 deficiency syndrome 1, infantile onset
     GLUT1 deficiency syndrome 2, childhood onset
E74.818   **Other disorders of glucose transport**
     (Familial) renal glycosuria
E74.819   **Disorders of glucose transport, unspecified**
E74.89   **Other specified disorders of carbohydrate metabolism**
     Essential pentosuria

E75   **DISORDERS OF SPHINGOLIPID METABOLISM AND OTHER LIPID STORAGE DISORDERS**
[4th]   ***Excludes1:*** mucolipidosis, types I-III (E77.0-E77.1)
     Refsum's disease (G60.1)
E75.0   **GM2 gangliosidosis**
[5th]   E75.00   **GM2 gangliosidosis, unspecified**
E75.01   **Sandhoff disease**
E75.02   **Tay-Sachs disease**
E75.2   **Other sphingolipidosis**
[5th]   ***Excludes1:*** adrenoleukodystrophy [Addison-Schilder] (E71.528)
E75.21   **Fabry (-Anderson) disease**
E75.22   **Gaucher disease**
E75.23   **Krabbe disease**
E75.24   **Niemann-Pick disease**
[6th]   E75.240   **Niemann-Pick disease type A**
     Acid sphingomyelinase deficiency type A (ASMD type A)
     Infantile neurovisceral acid sphingomyelinase deficiency
E75.241   **Niemann-Pick disease type B**
     Acid sphingomyelinase deficiency type B (ASMD type B)
     Chronic visceral acid sphingomyelinase deficiency
E75.242   **Niemann-Pick disease type C**
E75.243   **Niemann-Pick disease type D**
• E75.244   **Niemann-Pick disease type A/B**
     Acid sphingomyelinase deficiency type A/B (ASMD type A/B)
     Chronic neurovisceral acid sphingomyelinase deficiency
E75.248   **Other Niemann-Pick disease**

[4th] **[5th]** **[6th]** **[7th]** Additional Character Required   ✓   3-character code   •=New Code   ▲=Revised Code   ***Excludes1***—Not coded here, do not use together   ***Excludes2***—Not included here

CHAPTER 4. ENDOCRINE, NUTRITIONAL AND METABOLIC DISEASES (E75.249–E80.2)

E75.249 **Niemann-Pick disease, unspecified**
    Acid sphingomyelinase deficiency (ASMD) NOS
E75.25 **Metachromatic leukodystrophy**
E75.26 **Sulfatase deficiency**
    Multiple sulfatase deficiency (MSD)
E75.29 **Other sphingolipidosis**
    Farber's syndrome
    Sulfatide lipidosis

E76 [4th] **DISORDERS OF GLYCOSAMINOGLYCAN METABOLISM**
  E76.0 **Mucopolysaccharidosis, type I**
    [5th] E76.01 **Hurler's syndrome**
    E76.02 **Hurler-Scheie syndrome**
    E76.03 **Scheie's syndrome**
  E76.1 **Mucopolysaccharidosis, type II**
    Hunter's syndrome
  E76.2 **Other mucopolysaccharidoses**
    [5th] E76.21 **Morquio mucopolysaccharidosis**
      [6th] E76.210 **Morquio A mucopolysaccharidoses**
        Classic Morquio syndrome
        Morquio syndrome A
        Mucopolysaccharidosis, type IVA
      E76.211 **Morquio B mucopolysaccharidoses**
        Morquio-like mucopolysaccharidoses
        Morquio-like syndrome
        Morquio syndrome B
        Mucopolysaccharidosis, type IVB
      E76.219 **Morquio mucopolysaccharidoses, unspecified**
        Morquio syndrome
        Mucopolysaccharidosis, type IV
    E76.22 **Sanfilippo mucopolysaccharidoses**
      Mucopolysaccharidosis, type III (A) (B) (C) (D)
      Sanfilippo A syndrome
      Sanfilippo B syndrome
      Sanfilippo C syndrome
      Sanfilippo D syndrome
    E76.29 **Other mucopolysaccharidoses**
      beta-Glucuronidase deficiency
      Maroteaux-Lamy (mild) (severe) syndrome
      Mucopolysaccharidosis, types VI, VII
  E76.3 **Mucopolysaccharidosis, unspecified**
  E76.8 **Other disorders of glucosaminoglycan metabolism**
  E76.9 **Glucosaminoglycan metabolism disorder, unspecified**

E77 [4th] **DISORDERS OF GLYCOPROTEIN METABOLISM**
  E77.0 **Defects in post-translational modification of lysosomal enzymes**
    Mucolipidosis II [I-cell disease]
    Mucolipidosis III [pseudo-Hurler polydystrophy]
  E77.1 **Defects in glycoprotein degradation**
    Aspartylglucosaminuria
    Fucosidosis
    Mannosidosis
    Sialidosis [mucolipidosis I]
  E77.8 **Other disorders of glycoprotein metabolism**
  E77.9 **Disorder of glycoprotein metabolism, unspecified**

E78 [4th] **DISORDERS OF LIPOPROTEIN METABOLISM AND OTHER LIPIDEMIAS**
  Excludes1: sphingolipidosis (E75.0–E75.3)
  E78.0 **Pure hypercholesterolemia**
    [5th] E78.00 **Pure hypercholesterolemia, unspecified**
      Fredrickson's hyperlipoproteinemia, type IIa
      Hyperbetalipoproteinemia
      (Pure) hypercholesterolemia NOS
    E78.01 **Familial hypercholesterolemia**
  E78.1 **Pure hyperglyceridemia**
    Elevated fasting triglycerides
    Endogenous hyperglyceridemia
    Fredrickson's hyperlipoproteinemia, type IV
    Hyperlipidemia, group B
    Hyperprebetalipoproteinemia
    Very-low-density-lipoprotein-type [VLDL] hyperlipoproteinemia

E78.2 **Mixed hyperlipidemia**
  Broad- or floating-betalipoproteinemia
  Combined hyperlipidemia NOS
  Elevated cholesterol with elevated triglycerides NEC
  Fredrickson's hyperlipoproteinemia, type IIb or III
  Hyperbetalipoproteinemia with prebetalipoproteinemia
  Hypercholesteremia with endogenous hyperglyceridemia
  Hyperlipidemia, group C
  Tubo-eruptive xanthoma
  Xanthoma tuberosum
  Excludes1: cerebrotendinous cholesterosis [van Bogaert-Scherer-Epstein] (E75.5)
    familial combined hyperlipidemia (E78.49)
E78.3 **Hyperchylomicronemia**
  Chylomicron retention disease
  Fredrickson's hyperlipoproteinemia, type I or V
  Hyperlipidemia, group D
  Mixed hyperglyceridemia
E78.4 **Other hyperlipidemia**
  [5th] E78.41 **Elevated Lipoprotein(a)**
    Elevated Lp(a)
  E78.49 **Other hyperlipidemia**
    Familial combined hyperlipidemia
E78.5 **Hyperlipidemia, unspecified**
E78.6 **Lipoprotein deficiency**
  Abetalipoproteinemia
  Depressed HDL cholesterol
  High-density lipoprotein deficiency
  Hypoalphalipoproteinemia
  Hypobetalipoproteinemia (familial)
  Lecithin cholesterol acyltransferase deficiency
  Tangier disease
E78.7 **Disorders of bile acid and cholesterol metabolism**
  [5th] ***Excludes1:*** *Niemann-Pick disease type C (E75.242)*
    E78.70 **Disorder of bile acid and cholesterol metabolism, unspecified**
    E78.71 **Barth syndrome**
    E78.72 **Smith-Lemli-Opitz syndrome**
    E78.79 **Other disorders of bile acid and cholesterol metabolism**
E78.8 **Other disorders of lipoprotein metabolism**
  [5th] E78.81 **Lipoid dermatoarthritis**
  E78.89 **Other lipoprotein metabolism disorders**
E78.9 **Disorder of lipoprotein metabolism, unspecified**

E79 [4th] **DISORDERS OF PURINE AND PYRIMIDINE METABOLISM**
  Excludes1: Ataxia-telangiectasia (Q87.19)
    Bloom's syndrome (Q82.8)
    Cockayne's syndrome (Q87.19)
    calculus of kidney (N20.0)
    combined immunodeficiency disorders (D81.-)
    Fanconi's anemia (D61.09)
    gout (M1A.-, M10.-)
    orotaciduric anemia (D53.0)
    progeria (E34.8)
    Werner's syndrome (E34.8)
    xeroderma pigmentosum (Q82.1)
  E79.0 **Hyperuricemia without signs of inflammatory arthritis and tophaceous disease**
    Asymptomatic hyperuricemia
  E79.1 **Lesch-Nyhan syndrome**
    HGPRT deficiency
  E79.2 **Myoadenylate deaminase deficiency**
  E79.8 **Other disorders of purine and pyrimidine metabolism**
    Hereditary xanthinuria
  E79.9 **Disorder of purine and pyrimidine metabolism, unspecified**

E80 [4th] **DISORDERS OF PORPHYRIN AND BILIRUBIN METABOLISM**
  Includes: defects of catalase and peroxidase
  E80.0 **Hereditary erythropoietic porphyria**
    Congenital erythropoietic porphyria
    Erythropoietic protoporphyria
  E80.2 **Other and unspecified porphyria**
    [5th]

[4th] [5th] [6th] [7th] Additional Character Required   ☑ 3-character code

• =New Code   ***Excludes1***—Not coded here, do not use together
▲ =Revised Code   ***Excludes2***—Not included here

E80.20 Unspecified porphyria
Porphyria NOS
E80.21 Acute intermittent (hepatic) porphyria
E80.29 Other porphyria
Hereditary coproporphyria
E80.4 Gilbert syndrome
E80.5 Crigler-Najjar syndrome
E80.6 Other disorders of bilirubin metabolism
Dubin-Johnson syndrome
Rotor's syndrome
E80.7 Disorder of bilirubin metabolism, unspecified

E83 DISORDERS OF MINERAL METABOLISM `4th`
Excludes1: dietary mineral deficiency (E58–E61)
parathyroid disorders (E20–E21)
vitamin D deficiency (E55.-)
E83.0 Disorders of copper metabolism `5th`
     E83.00 Disorder of copper metabolism, unspecified
     E83.01 Wilson's disease
         Code also associated Kayser Fleischer ring (H18.04-)
     E83.09 Other disorders of copper metabolism
         Menkes' (kinky hair) (steely hair) disease
E83.1 Disorders of iron metabolism `5th`
Excludes1: iron deficiency anemia (D50.-)
sideroblastic anemia (D64.0–D64.3)
     E83.10 Disorder of iron metabolism, unspecified
     E83.11 Hemochromatosis `6th`
         Excludes1: Gestational alloimmune liver disease/GALD (P78.84)
         Neonatal hemochromatosis (P78.84)
         E83.110 Hereditary hemochromatosis
            Bronzed diabetes
            Pigmentary cirrhosis (of liver)
            Primary (hereditary) hemochromatosis
         E83.111 Hemochromatosis due to repeated red blood cell transfusions
            Iron overload due to repeated red blood cell transfusions
            Transfusion (red blood cell) associated hemochromatosis
         E83.118 Other hemochromatosis
         E83.119 Hemochromatosis, unspecified
     E83.19 Other disorders of iron metabolism
         Use additional code, if applicable, for idiopathic pulmonary hemosiderosis (J84.03)
E83.2 Disorders of zinc metabolism
Acrodermatitis enteropathica
E83.3 Disorders of phosphorus metabolism and phosphatases `5th`
Excludes1: adult osteomalacia (M83.-)
osteoporosis (M80.-)
     E83.30 Disorder of phosphorus metabolism, unspecified
     E83.31 Familial hypophosphatemia
         Vitamin D-resistant osteomalacia
         Vitamin D-resistant rickets
         Excludes1: vitamin D-deficiency rickets (E55.0)
     E83.32 Hereditary vitamin D-dependent rickets (type 1) (type 2)
         25-hydroxyvitamin D 1-alpha-hydroxylase deficiency
         Pseudovitamin D deficiency
         Vitamin D receptor defect
     E83.39 Other disorders of phosphorus metabolism
         Acid phosphatase deficiency
         Hyperphosphatemia
         Hypophosphatasia
E83.4 Disorders of magnesium metabolism `5th`
Refer to Category P71 for transitory neonatal disorders of magnesium metabolism
     E83.40 Disorders of magnesium metabolism, unspecified
     E83.41 Hypermagnesemia
     E83.42 Hypomagnesemia
     E83.49 Other disorders of magnesium metabolism

E83.5 Disorders of calcium metabolism `5th`
Excludes1: chondrocalcinosis (M11.1–M11.2)
Refer to Category P71 for transitory neonatal disorders of calcium metabolism
hungry bone syndrome (E83.81) hyperparathyroidism (E21.0–E21.3)
     E83.50 Unspecified disorder of calcium metabolism
     E83.51 Hypocalcemia
         For associated tetany report R29.0
     E83.52 Hypercalcemia
         Familial hypocalciuric hypercalcemia
     E83.59 Other disorders of calcium metabolism
E83.8 Other disorders of mineral metabolism `5th`
     E83.81 Hungry bone syndrome
     E83.89 Other disorders of mineral metabolism
E83.9 Disorder of mineral metabolism, unspecified

E84 CYSTIC FIBROSIS `4th`
Includes: mucoviscidosis
Code also exocrine pancreatic insufficiency (K86.81)
E84.0 Cystic fibrosis with pulmonary manifestations
     Use additional code to identify any infectious organism present, such as: Pseudomonas (B96.5)
E84.1 Cystic fibrosis with intestinal manifestations `5th`
     E84.11 Meconium ileus in cystic fibrosis
         Excludes1: meconium ileus not due to cystic fibrosis (P76.0)
     E84.19 Cystic fibrosis with other intestinal manifestations
         Distal intestinal obstruction syndrome
E84.8 Cystic fibrosis with other manifestations
E84.9 Cystic fibrosis, unspecified

E86 VOLUME DEPLETION `4th`
Use additional code(s) for any associated disorders of electrolyte and acid-base balance (E87.-)
Excludes1: dehydration of newborn (P74.1)
postprocedural hypovolemic shock (T81.19)
traumatic hypovolemic shock (T79.4)
Excludes 2: hypovolemic shock NOS (R57.1)
E86.0 Dehydration
E86.1 Hypovolemia
Depletion of volume of plasma
E86.9 Volume depletion, unspecified

E87 OTHER DISORDERS OF FLUID, ELECTROLYTE AND ACID-BASE BALANCE `4th`
Excludes1: diabetes insipidus (E23.2)
electrolyte imbalance associated with hyperemesis gravidarum (O21.1)
electrolyte imbalance following ectopic or molar pregnancy (O08.5)
familial periodic paralysis (G72.3)
E87.0 Hyperosmolality and hypernatremia
Refer to code P74.2 for transitory neonatal sodium imbalance
Sodium [Na] excess
Sodium [Na] overload
E87.1 Hypo-osmolality and hyponatremia
Sodium [Na] deficiency
Excludes1: syndrome of inappropriate secretion of antidiuretic hormone (E22.2)
E87.2 Acidosis
Acidosis NOS
Lactic acidosis
Metabolic acidosis
Respiratory acidosis
Excludes1: diabetic acidosis — see categories E08–E10, E11, E13 with ketoacidosis
E87.3 Alkalosis
Alkalosis NOS
Metabolic alkalosis
Respiratory alkalosis
E87.4 Mixed disorder of acid-base balance
E87.5 Hyperkalemia
Refer to code P74.3 for transitory neonatal potassium imbalance
Potassium [K] excess
Potassium [K] overload

`4th` `5th` `6th` `7th` Additional Character Required   3-character code   •=New Code   ▲=Revised Code   ***Excludes1***—Not coded here, do not use together   ***Excludes2***—Not included here

E87.6 Hypokalemia
Potassium [K] deficiency

E87.7 Fluid overload
`5th`
Excludes1: edema NOS (R60.9)
    fluid retention (R60.9)

  E87.70 Fluid overload, unspecified

  E87.71 Transfusion associated circulatory overload
    Fluid overload due to transfusion (blood) (blood
        components)
    TACO

  E87.79 Other fluid overload

E87.8 Other disorders of electrolyte and fluid balance, NEC
Electrolyte imbalance NOS
Hyperchloremia
Hypochloremia

E88 OTHER AND UNSPECIFIED METABOLIC DISORDERS
`4th`
Use additional codes for associated conditions

E88.0 Disorders of plasma-protein metabolism, NEC
`5th`
Excludes1: monoclonal gammopathy (of undetermined
    significance) (D47.2)
    polyclonal hypergammaglobulinemia (D89.0)
    Waldenström macroglobulinemia (C88.0)
Excludes2: disorder of lipoprotein metabolism (E78.-)

  E88.01 Alpha-1-antitrypsin deficiency
    AAT deficiency

  E88.02 Plasminogen deficiency
    Dysplasminogenemia
    Hypoplasminogenemia
    Type 1 plasminogen deficiency
    Type 2 plasminogen deficiency
    Code also, if applicable, ligneous conjunctivitis (H10.51)
    Use additional code for associated findings, such as:
      hydrocephalus (G91.4)
      ligneous conjunctivitis (H10.51)
      otitis media (H67.-)
      respiratory disorder related to plasminogen deficiency
        (J99)

  E88.09 Other disorders of plasma-protein metabolism, NEC
    Bisalbuminemia

E88.1 Lipodystrophy, NEC
Lipodystrophy NOS

E88.2 Lipomatosis, NEC
Lipomatosis NOS
Lipomatosis (Check) dolorosa [Dercum]

E88.3 Tumor lysis syndrome
Tumor lysis syndrome (spontaneous)
Tumor lysis syndrome following antineoplastic drug chemotherapy
Use additional code for adverse effect, if applicable, to identify
    drug (T45.1X5)

E88.4 Mitochondrial metabolism disorders
`5th`
Excludes1: disorders of pyruvate metabolism (E74.4)
    Kearns-Sayre syndrome (H49.81)
    Leber's disease (H47.22)
    Leigh's encephalopathy (G31.82)
    Mitochondrial myopathy, NEC (G71.3)
    Reye's syndrome (G93.7)

  E88.40 Mitochondrial metabolism disorder, unspecified

  E88.41 MELAS syndrome
    Mitochondrial myopathy, encephalopathy, lactic acidosis
      and stroke-like episodes

  E88.42 MERRF syndrome
    Myoclonic epilepsy associated with ragged-red fibers
    Code also progressive myoclonic epilepsy (G40.3-)

  E88.49 Other mitochondrial metabolism disorders

E88.8 Other specified metabolic disorders
`5th`
  E88.81 Metabolic syndrome
    Dysmetabolic syndrome X
    Use additional codes for associated manifestations,
      such as: obesity (E66.-)

  E88.89 Other specified metabolic disorders
    Launois-Bensaude adenolipomatosis
    Excludes1: adult pulmonary Langerhans cell
      histiocytosis (J84.82)

E88.9 Metabolic disorder, unspecified

(E89) POSTPROCEDURAL ENDOCRINE AND METABOLIC COMPLICATIONS AND DISORDERS, NOT ELSEWHERE CLASSIFIED

E89 POSTPROCEDURAL ENDOCRINE AND METABOLIC
`4th`
COMPLICATIONS AND DISORDERS, NOT ELSEWHERE CLASSIFIED
Excludes2: intraoperative complications of endocrine system organ or
    structure (E36.0-, E36.1-, E36.8)

E89.0 Postprocedural hypothyroidism
Postirradiation hypothyroidism
Postsurgical hypothyroidism

E89.1 Postprocedural hypoinsulinemia
Postpancreatectomy hyperglycemia
Postsurgical hypoinsulinemia
Use additional code, if applicable, to identify:
    acquired absence of pancreas (Z90.41-)
    diabetes mellitus (postpancreatectomy) (postprocedural) (E13.-)
    insulin use (Z79.4)
Excludes1: transient postprocedural hyperglycemia (R73.9)
    transient postprocedural hypoglycemia (E16.2)

E89.2 Postprocedural hypoparathyroidism
Parathyroprival tetany

E89.3 Postprocedural hypopituitarism
Postirradiation hypopituitarism

E89.8 Other postprocedural endocrine and metabolic complications
`5th` **and disorders**
  E89.89 Other postprocedural endocrine and metabolic
    complications and disorders
    Use additional code, if applicable, to further specify
      disorder

    Additional Character Required   3-character code   •=New Code   *Excludes1*—Not coded here, do not use together
▲=Revised Code   *Excludes2*—Not included here

172   **PEDIATRIC ICD-10-CM 2022: A MANUAL FOR PROVIDER-BASED CODING**

Chapter 5. Mental, behavioral, and neurodevelopmental disorders (F01–F99)

GUIDELINES

Pain disorders related to psychological factors

Refer to category F45.

Mental and behavioral disorders due to psychoactive substance use

Refer to categories F10–F19
Includes: disorders of psychological development
Excludes2: symptoms, signs and abnormal clinical laboratory findings, not elsewhere classified (R00–R99)

(F01–F09) MENTAL DISORDERS DUE TO KNOWN PHYSIOLOGICAL CONDITIONS

Note: This block comprises a range of mental disorders grouped together on the basis of their having in common a demonstrable etiology in cerebral disease, brain injury, or other insult leading to cerebral dysfunction. The dysfunction may be primary, as in diseases, injuries, and insults that affect the brain directly and selectively; or secondary, as in systemic diseases and disorders that attack the brain only as one of the multiple organs or systems of the body that are involved.

F02   **DEMENTIA IN OTHER DISEASES CLASSIFIED ELSEWHERE**
`4th`   **Code first** the underlying physiological condition, such as:
     cerebral lipidosis (E75.4)
     Creutzfeldt-Jakob disease (A81.0-)
     dementia with Lewy bodies (G31.83)
     dementia with Parkinsonism (G31.83)
     epilepsy and recurrent seizures (G40.-)
     frontotemporal dementia (G31.09)
     hepatolenticular degeneration (E83.0)
     HIV disease (B20)
     Huntington's disease (G10)
     hypercalcemia (E83.52)
     hypothyroidism, acquired (E00-E03.-)
     intoxications (T36-T65)
     Jakob-Creutzfeldt disease (A81.0-)
     multiple sclerosis (G35)
     neurosyphilis (A52.17)
     niacin deficiency [pellagra] (E52)
     Parkinson's disease (G20)
     Pick's disease (G31.01)
     polyarteritis nodosa (M30.0)
     SLE (M32.-)
     traumatic brain injury (S06.-)
     trypanosomiasis (B56.-, B57.-)
     vitamin B deficiency (E53.8)
Includes: major neurocognitive disorders in other diseases classified elsewhere
Excludes2: dementia in alcohol and psychoactive substance disorders (F10–F19, with .17, .27, .97)
     vascular dementia (F01.5-)

F02.8   **Dementia in other diseases classified elsewhere**
`5th`   **F02.80**   **Dementia in other diseases classified elsewhere without behavioral disturbance**
     Dementia in other diseases classified elsewhere NOS
     Major neurocognitive disorder in other diseases classified elsewhere

     F02.81   **Dementia in other diseases classified elsewhere with behavioral disturbance**
     Use additional code, if applicable, to identify wandering in dementia in conditions classified elsewhere (Z91.83)
     Dementia in other diseases classified elsewhere with:
         aggressive behavior
         combative behavior
         violent behavior
     Major neurocognitive disorder in other diseases classified elsewhere with:
         aggressive behavior
         combative behavior
         violent behavior

F07   **PERSONALITY AND BEHAVIORAL DISORDERS DUE TO**
`4th`   **KNOWN PHYSIOLOGICAL CONDITION**
     Code first the underlying physiological condition
     F07.8   **Other personality and behavioral disorders due to known**
`5th`   **physiological condition**
         F07.81   **Postconcussional syndrome**
         Postcontusional syndrome (encephalopathy)
         Post-traumatic brain syndrome, nonpsychotic
         Use additional code to identify associated post-traumatic headache, if applicable (G44.3-)
         Excludes1: current concussion (brain) (S06.0-)
         postencephalitic syndrome (F07.89)
         F07.89   **Other personality and behavioral disorders due to known physiological condition**
         Postencephalitic syndrome
         Right hemispheric organic affective disorder
     F07.9   **Unspecified personality and behavioral disorder due to known physiological condition**
     Organic p syndrome

F09   **UNSPECIFIED MENTAL DISORDER DUE TO KNOWN**
`✔`   **PHYSIOLOGICAL CONDITION**
     Mental disorder NOS due to known physiological condition
     Organic brain syndrome NOS
     Organic mental disorder NOS
     Organic psychosis NOS
     Symptomatic psychosis NOS
     Code first the underlying physiological condition
     Excludes1: psychosis NOS (F29)

(F10–F19) MENTAL AND BEHAVIORAL DISORDERS DUE TO PSYCHOACTIVE SUBSTANCE USE

GUIDELINES

Mental and behavioral disorders due to psychoactive substance use

IN REMISSION

Selection of codes for "in remission" for categories F10–F19, Mental and behavioral disorders due to psychoactive substance use (categories F10–F19 with -.21) requires the provider's clinical judgment. The appropriate codes for "in remission" are assigned only on the basis of provider documentation (as defined inthe Official Guidelines for Coding and Reporting) unless otherwise instructed by the classification. Mild substance use disorders in early or sustained remission are classified to the appropriate codes for substance abuse in remission, and moderate or severe substance use disorders in early or sustained remission are classified to the appropriate codes for substance dependence in remission.

PSYCHOACTIVE SUBSTANCE USE, ABUSE, AND DEPENDENCE

When the provider documentation refers to use, abuse and dependence of the same substance (e.g. alcohol, opioid, cannabis, etc.), only one code should be assigned to identify the pattern of use based on the following hierarchy:
* If both use and abuse are documented, assign only the code for abuse
* If both abuse and dependence are documented, assign only the code for dependence
* If use, abuse and dependence are all documented, assign only the code for dependence
* If both use and dependence are documented, assign only the code for dependence.

PSYCHOACTIVE SUBSTANCE USE, UNSPECIFIED

As with all other unspecified diagnoses, the codes for unspecified psychoactive substance use (F10.9-, F11.9-, F12.9-, F13.9-, F14.9-, F15.9-, F16.9-, F18.9-, F19.9-) should only be assigned based on provider documentation and when they meet the definition of a reportable diagnosis (see Section III, Reporting Additional Diagnoses). The codes are to be used only when the psychoactive substance use is associated with a **substance related** disorder (chapter 5 **disorders** such as sexual dysfunction, sleep disorder, or a mental or behavioral disorder) **or medical condition,** and when such a relationship is documented by the provider.

`4th` `5th` `6th` `7th`   Additional Character Required   `✔`   3-character code   •=New Code   ▲=Revised Code   ***Excludes1***—Not coded here, do not use together   ***Excludes2***—Not included here

 PEDIATRIC ICD-10-CM 2022: A MANUAL FOR PROVIDER-BASED CODING   173

CHAPTER 5. MENTAL, BEHAVIORAL, AND NEURODEVELOPMENTAL DISORDERS   (F10–F12.23)

MEDICAL CONDITIONS DUE TO PSYCHOACTIVE SUBSTANCE USE, ABUSE AND DEPENDENCE

Medical conditions due to substance use, abuse, and dependence are not classified as substance-induced disorders. Assign the diagnosis code for the medical condition as directed by the Alphabetical Index along with the appropriate psychoactive substance use, abuse or dependence code. For example, for alcoholic pancreatitis due to alcohol dependence, assign the appropriate code from subcategory K85.2, Alcohol induced acute pancreatitis, and the appropriate code from subcategory F10.2, such as code F10.20, Alcohol dependence, uncomplicated. It would not be appropriate to assign code F10.288, Alcohol dependence with other alcohol-induced disorder.

BLOOD ALCOHOL LEVEL

A code from category Y90, Evidence of alcohol involvement determined by blood alcohol level, may be assigned when this information is documented and the patient's provider has documented a condition classifiable to category F10, Alcohol related disorders. The blood alcohol level does not need to be documented by the patient's provider in order for it to be coded.

F10   **ALCOHOL RELATED DISORDERS**
`4th`
   Use additional code for blood alcohol level, if applicable (Y90.-)
   F10.1   **Alcohol abuse**
    `5th`   **Excludes1:** alcohol dependence (F10.2-)
       alcohol use, unspecified (F10.9-)
     F10.10   **Alcohol abuse, uncomplicated**
       Alcohol use disorder, mild
     F10.11   **Alcohol abuse, in remission**
       Alcohol use disorder, mild, in early remission
       Alcohol use disorder, mild, in sustained remission
     F10.12   **Alcohol abuse with intoxication**
      `6th`   **F10.120**   **Alcohol abuse with intoxication, uncomplicated**
        F10.121   **Alcohol abuse with intoxication delirium**
        F10.129   **Alcohol abuse with intoxication, unspecified**
     F10.13   **Alcohol abuse with withdrawal**
      `6th`   **F10.130**   **Alcohol abuse with withdrawal, uncomplicated**
        F10.131   **Alcohol abuse with withdrawal delirium**
        F10.132   **Alcohol abuse with withdrawal with perceptual disturbance**
        F10.139   **Alcohol abuse with withdrawal, unspecified**
   F10.2   **Alcohol dependence**
    `5th`   **Excludes1:** alcohol abuse (F10.1-)
       alcohol use, unspecified (F10.9-)
    Excludes2: toxic effect of alcohol (T51.0-)
     F10.20   **Alcohol dependence, uncomplicated**
       Alcohol use disorder, moderate
       Alcohol use disorder, severe
     F10.21   **Alcohol dependence, in remission**
       Alcohol use disorder, moderate or severe, in early remission
       Alcohol use disorder, moderate or severe, in sustained remission
     F10.22   **Alcohol dependence with intoxication**
      `6th`   Acute drunkenness (in alcoholism)
      Excludes2: alcohol dependence with withdrawal (F10.23-)
       F10.220   **Alcohol dependence with intoxication, uncomplicated**
       F10.221   **Alcohol dependence with intoxication delirium**
       F10.229   **Alcohol dependence with intoxication, unspecified**
     F10.23   **Alcohol dependence with withdrawal**
      `6th`   **Excludes2:** Alcohol dependence with intoxication (F10.22-)
       F10.230   **Alcohol dependence with withdrawal, uncomplicated**
       F10.231   **Alcohol dependence with withdrawal delirium**
       F10.232   **Alcohol dependence with withdrawal with perceptual disturbance**

       F10.239   **Alcohol dependence with withdrawal, unspecified**
     F10.24   **Alcohol dependence with alcohol-induced mood disorder**
       Alcohol use disorder, moderate or severe, with alcohol-induced bipolar or related disorder
       Alcohol use disorder, moderate or severe, with alcohol-induced depressive disorder
     F10.28   **Alcohol dependence with other alcohol-induced disorders**
      `6th`
       F10.280   **Alcohol dependence with alcohol-induced anxiety disorder**
       F10.282   **Alcohol dependence with alcohol-induced sleep disorder**
       F10.288   **Alcohol dependence with other alcohol-induced disorder**
        Alcohol use disorder, moderate or severe, with alcohol-induced mild neurocognitive disorder
   F10.9   **Alcohol use, unspecified**
    `5th`   **Excludes1:** alcohol abuse (F10.1-)
       alcohol dependence (F10.2-)
     F10.92   **Alcohol use, unspecified with intoxication;**
      `6th`   **F10.920**   **uncomplicated**
       F10.921   **delirium**
       F10.929   **unspecified**
     F10.93   **Alcohol use, unspecified with withdrawal**
      `6th`   **F10.930**   **Alcohol use, unspecified with withdrawal, uncomplicated**
       F10.931   **Alcohol use, unspecified with withdrawal delirium**
       F10.932   **Alcohol use, unspecified with withdrawal with perceptual disturbance**
       F10.939   **Alcohol use, unspecified with withdrawal, unspecified**

F11   **OPIOID RELATED DISORDERS**
`4th`
   F11.1   **Opioid abuse**
    `5th`   **Excludes1:** opioid dependence (F11.2-)
       opioid use, unspecified (F11.9-)
     F11.10   **Opioid abuse, uncomplicated**
       Opioid use disorder, mild
     F11.11   **Opioid abuse, in remission**
       Opioid use disorder, mild, in early or sustained remission
     F11.13   **Opioid abuse with withdrawal**

F12   **CANNABIS RELATED DISORDERS**
`4th`
   Includes: marijuana
   F12.1   **Cannabis abuse**
    `5th`   **Excludes1:** cannabis dependence (F12.2-)
       cannabis use, unspecified (F12.9-)
     F12.10   **Cannabis abuse, uncomplicated**
       cannabis use disorder, mild
     F12.11   **Cannabis abuse, in remission**
       Cannabis use disorder, mild, in early or sustained remission
     F12.13   **Cannabis abuse with withdrawal**
   F12.2   **Cannabis dependence**
    `5th`   **Excludes1:** cannabis abuse (F12.1-)
       cannabis use, unspecified (F12.9-)
    Excludes2: cannabis poisoning (T40.7-)
     F12.20   **Cannabis dependence, uncomplicated**
     F12.21   **Cannabis dependence, in remission**
       Cannabis use disorder, moderate or severe, in early remission
       Cannabis use disorder, moderate or severe, in sustained remission
     F12.22   **Cannabis dependence with intoxication;**
      `6th`   **F12.220**   **uncomplicated**
       Cannabis use disorder, moderate
       Cannabis use disorder, severe
       F12.221   **delirium**
       F12.222   **with perceptual disturbance**
       F12.229   **unspecified**
     F12.23   **Cannabis dependence with withdrawal**

`4th`   `5th`   `6th`   `7th`   Additional Character Required   ✔   3-character code

•=New Code   ▲=Revised Code

Excludes1—Not coded here, do not use together
Excludes2—Not included here

F12.9 Cannabis use, unspecified
`5th` *Excludes1:* cannabis abuse (F12.1-)
cannabis dependence (F12.2-)

F12.90 Cannabis use, unspecified, uncomplicated
Amphetamine type substance use disorder, moderate or severe, in early or sustained remission
Other or unspecified stimulant use disorder, moderate or severe, in early or sustained remission

F12.93 Cannabis use, unspecified with withdrawal

F13 SEDATIVE, HYPNOTIC, OR ANIOLYTIC RELATED DISORDERS
`4th`

F13.1 Sedative, hypnotic or anxiolytic-related abuse
`5th` *Excludes1:* sedative, hypnotic or anxiolytic-related dependence (F13.2-)
sedative, hypnotic, or anxiolytic use, unspecified (F13.9-)

F13.10 Sedative, hypnotic or anxiolytic abuse, uncomplicated
Sedative, hypnotic, or anxiolytic use disorder, mild

F13.11 Sedative, hypnotic or anxiolytic abuse, in remission
Sedative, hypnotic or anxiolytic use disorder, mild, in early or sustained remission

F13.13 Sedative, hypnotic or anxiolytic abuse with withdrawal
`6th`
    F13.130 Sedative, hypnotic or anxiolytic abuse with withdrawal, uncomplicated
    F13.131 Sedative, hypnotic or anxiolytic abuse with withdrawal delirium
    F13.132 Sedative, hypnotic or anxiolytic abuse with withdrawal with perceptual disturbance
    F13.139 Sedative, hypnotic or anxiolytic abuse with withdrawal, unspecified

F14 COCAINE RELATED DISORDERS
`4th`
Excludes2: other stimulant-related disorders (F15.-)

F14.1 Cocaine abuse
`5th` *Excludes1:* cocaine dependence (F14.2-)
cocaine use, unspecified (F14.9-)

F14.10 Cocaine abuse, uncomplicated
Cocaine use disorder, mild

F14.11 Cocaine abuse, in remission
Cocaine use disorder, mild, in early or sustained remission

F14.12 Cocaine abuse with intoxication;
`6th`
    F14.120 uncomplicated
    F14.121 delirium
    F14.122 with perceptual disturbance
    F14.129 unspecified

F14.13 Cocaine abuse, unspecified with withdrawal

F14.2 Cocaine dependence
`5th` *Excludes1:* cocaine abuse (F14.1-)
cocaine use, unspecified (F14.9-)
Excludes2: cocaine poisoning (T40.5-)

F14.20 Cocaine dependence, uncomplicated
Cocaine use disorder, moderate
Cocaine use disorder, severe

F14.21 Cocaine dependence, in remission
Cocaine use disorder, moderate, in early or sustained remission
Cocaine use disorder, severe, in early or sustained remission

F14.22 Cocaine dependence with intoxication;
`6th` *Excludes1:* cocaine dependence with withdrawal (F14.23)
    F14.220 uncomplicated
    F14.221 delirium
    F14.222 with perceptual disturbance
    F14.229 unspecified

F14.23 Cocaine dependence with withdrawal
Excludes1: cocaine dependence with intoxication (F14.22-)

F14.9 Cocaine use, unspecified
`5th` *Excludes1:* cocaine abuse (F14.1-)
cocaine dependence (F14.2-)

F14.90 Cocaine use, unspecified, uncomplicated

F14.92 Cocaine use, unspecified with intoxication;
`6th`
    F14.920 uncomplicated
    F14.921 delirium
    F14.922 with perceptual disturbance
    F14.929 unspecified

F14.93 Cocaine use, unspecified with withdrawal

F15 OTHER STIMULANT RELATED DISORDERS
`4th`
Includes: amphetamine-related disorders
caffeine
Excludes2: cocaine-related disorders (F14.-)

F15.1 Other stimulant abuse
`5th` *Excludes1:* other stimulant dependence (F15.2-)
other stimulant use, unspecified (F15.9-)

F15.10 Other stimulant abuse, uncomplicated
Amphetamine type substance use disorder, mild
Other or unspecified stimulant use disorder, mild
Cocaine use disorder, moderate, in early or sustained remission
Cocaine use disorder, severe, in early or sustained remission

F15.11 Other stimulant abuse, in remission
Amphetamine type substance use disorder, mild, in early or sustained remission
Other or unspecified stimulant use disorder, mild, in early or sustained remission

F15.12 Other stimulant abuse with intoxication;
`6th`
    F15.120 uncomplicated
    F15.121 delirium
    F15.122 perceptual disturbance
    Amphetamine or other stimulant use disorder, mild, with amphetamine or other stimulant intoxication, with perceptual disturbances
    F15.129 unspecified
    Amphetamine or other stimulant use disorder, mild, with amphetamine or other stimulant intoxication, without perceptual disturbances

F15.13 Other stimulant abuse with withdrawal

F15.2 Other stimulant dependence
`5th` *Excludes1:* other stimulant abuse (F15.1-)
other stimulant use, unspecified (F15.9-)

F15.20 Other stimulant dependence, uncomplicated
Amphetamine type substance use disorder, moderate or severe
Other or unspecified stimulant use disorder, moderate or severe

F15.21 Other stimulant dependence, in remission
Amphetamine type substance use disorder, moderate or severe, in early or sustained remission
Other or unspecified stimulant use disorder, moderate or severe, in early or sustained remission

F15.22 Other stimulant dependence with intoxication;
`6th` *Excludes1:* other stimulant dependence with withdrawal (F15.23)
    F15.220 uncomplicated
    F15.221 delirium
    F15.222 with perceptual disturbance
    Amphetamine or other stimulant use disorder, moderate, with amphetamine or other stimulant intoxication, with perceptual disturbances
    F15.229 unspecified
    Amphetamine or other stimulant use disorder, severe, with amphetamine or other stimulant intoxication, with perceptual disturbances

F15.23 Other stimulant dependence with withdrawal
Amphetamine or other stimulant withdrawal
Excludes1: other stimulant dependence with intoxication (F15.22-)

F15.9 Other stimulant use, unspecified
`5th` *Excludes1:* other stimulant abuse (F15.1-)
other stimulant dependence (F15.2-)

`4th` `5th` `6th` `7th` Additional Character Required   ✔ 3-character code

•=New Code   *Excludes1*—Not coded here, do not use together
▲=Revised Code   *Excludes2*—Not included here

F15.90   **Other stimulant use, unspecified, uncomplicated**
F15.93   **Other stimulant use, unspecified with withdrawal**
     Caffeine withdrawal

F16   **HALLUCINOGEN RELATED DISORDERS**
`4th`
    Includes: ecstasy
      PCP
      phencyclidine
   F16.1   **Hallucinogen abuse**
   `5th`   ***Excludes1:*** hallucinogen dependence (F16.2-)
        hallucinogen use, unspecified (F16.9-)
     F16.10   **Hallucinogen abuse, uncomplicated**
        Other hallucinogen use disorder, mild
        Phencyclidine use disorder, mild
     F16.11   **Hallucinogen abuse, in remission**
        Other hallucinogen use disorder, mild, in early or
          sustained remission
        Phencyclidine use disorder, mild, in early or sustained
          remission
   F16.2   **Hallucinogen dependence**
   `5th`   ***Excludes1:*** hallucinogen abuse (F16.1-)
        hallucinogen use, unspecified (F16.9-)
     F16.20   **Hallucinogen dependence, uncomplicated**
        Other hallucinogen use disorder, moderate
        Other hallucinogen use disorder, severe
        Phencyclidine use disorder, moderate
        Phencyclidine use disorder, severe

F17   **NICOTINE DEPENDENCE**
`4th`
    Excludes1: history of tobacco dependence (Z87.891)
        tobacco use NOS (Z72.0)
    Excludes2: tobacco use (smoking) during pregnancy, childbirth and the
        puerperium (O99.33-)
        toxic effect of nicotine (T65.2-)
   F17.2   **Nicotine dependence**
   `5th`   **F17.20**   **Nicotine dependence, unspecified**
       `6th`   **F17.200**   **Nicotine dependence, unspecified;**
           uncomplicated
           Tobacco use disorder, mild
           Tobacco use disorder, moderate
           Tobacco use disorder, severe
       F17.201   **in remission**
           Tobacco use disorder, mild, in early or
             sustained remission
           Tobacco use disorder, moderate, in early or
             sustained remission
           Tobacco use disorder, severe, in early or
             sustained remission
       F17.203   **with withdrawal**
           Tobacco withdrawal
       F17.208   **with other nicotine-induced disorders**
       F17.209   **with unspecified nicotine-induced**
           disorders
     F17.21   **Nicotine dependence, cigarettes**
     `6th`   **F17.210**   **Nicotine dependence, cigarettes;**
           uncomplicated
       F17.211   **in remission**
           Tobacco use disorder, cigarettes, mild or
             moderate or severe in early or sustained
             remission
       F17.213   **with withdrawal**
       F17.218   **with other nicotine-induced disorders**
       F17.219   **with unspecified nicotine-induced**
           disorders
     F17.22   **Nicotine dependence, chewing tobacco**
     `6th`   **F17.220**   **Nicotine dependence, chewing tobacco;**
           uncomplicated
       F17.221   **in remission**
           Tobacco use disorder, chewing tobacco,
             mild or moderate or severe in early or
             sustained remission
       F17.223   **with withdrawal**
       F17.228   **with other nicotine-induced disorders**
       F17.229   **with unspecified nicotine-induced**
           disorders

     F17.29   **Nicotine dependence, other tobacco product**
     `6th`   **F17.290**   **Nicotine dependence, other tobacco**
           product; uncomplicated
       F17.291   **in remission**
           Tobacco use disorder, other product, mild
             or moderate or severe in early or
             sustained remission
       F17.293   **with withdrawal**
       F17.298   **with other nicotine-induced disorders**
       F17.299   **with unspecified nicotine-induced**
           disorders

F18   **INHALANT RELATED DISORDERS**
`4th`
    Includes: volatile solvents
   F18.1   **Inhalant abuse**
   `5th`   ***Excludes1:*** inhalant dependence (F18.2-)
        inhalant use, unspecified (F18.9-)
     F18.10   **Inhalant abuse, uncomplicated**
        Inhalant use disorder, mild
     F18.11   **Inhalant abuse, in remission**
        Inhalant use disorder, mild, in early or sustained
          remission
     F18.12   **Inhalant abuse with intoxication**
     `6th`   **F18.120**   **Inhalant abuse with intoxication;**
           uncomplicated
       F18.121   **delirium**
       F18.129   **unspecified**
   F18.2   **Inhalant dependence**
   `5th`   ***Excludes1:*** inhalant abuse (F18.1-)
        inhalant use, unspecified (F18.9-)
     F18.20   **Inhalant dependence, uncomplicated**
        Inhalant use disorder, moderate
        Inhalant use disorder, severe
     F18.21   **Inhalant dependence, in remission**
     F18.22   **Inhalant dependence with intoxication**
     `6th`   **F18.220**   **Inhalant dependence with intoxication;**
           uncomplicated
       F18.221   **delirium**
       F18.229   **unspecified**
   F18.9   **Inhalant use, unspecified**
   `5th`   ***Excludes1:*** inhalant abuse (F18.1-)
        inhalant dependence (F18.2-)
     F18.90   **Inhalant use, unspecified, uncomplicated**
     F18.92   **Inhalant use, unspecified with intoxication**
     `6th`   **F18.920**   **Inhalant use, unspecified with**
           intoxication, uncomplicated
       F18.921   **Inhalant use, unspecified with intoxication**
           with delirium
       F18.929   **Inhalant use, unspecified with**
           intoxication, unspecified

F19   **OTHER PSYCHOACTIVE SUBSTANCE RELATED**
`4th`   **DISORDERS**
    Includes: polysubstance drug use (indiscriminate drug use)
   F19.1   **Other psychoactive substance abuse**
   `5th`   ***Excludes1:*** other psychoactive substance dependence (F19.2-)
        other psychoactive substance use, unspecified (F19.9-)
     F19.10   **Other psychoactive substance abuse, uncomplicated**
        Other (or unknown) substance use disorder, mild
     F19.12   **Other psychoactive substance abuse with**
     `6th`   **intoxication**
       F19.120   **Other psychoactive substance abuse with**
           intoxication; uncomplicated
       F19.121   **delirium**
       F19.122   **with perceptual disturbances**
       F19.129   **unspecified**
     F19.13   **Other psychoactive substance abuse**
     `6th`   **F19.130**   **Other psychoactive substance abuse with**
           withdrawal, uncomplicated
       F19.131   **Other psychoactive substance abuse with**
           withdrawal delirium
       F19.132   **Other psychoactive substance abuse with**
           withdrawal with perceptual disturbance
       F19.139   **Other psychoactive substance abuse with**
           withdrawal, unspecified

`4th`   `5th`   `6th`   `7th`   Additional Character Required   ✓   3-character code   •=New Code   ▲=Revised Code   ***Excludes1***—Not coded here, do not use together   ***Excludes2***—Not included here

F19.2   **Other psychoactive substance dependence**
> `5th`   *Excludes1:* other psychoactive substance abuse (F19.1-)
>> other psychoactive substance use, unspecified (F19.9-)

> **F19.20**   **Other psychoactive substance dependence, uncomplicated**
>> Other (or unknown) substance use disorder, moderate
>> Other (or unknown) substance use disorder, severe

> **F19.21**   **Other psychoactive substance dependence, in remission**
>> Other (or unknown) substance use disorder, moderate, in early remission or in sustained remission
>> Other (or unknown) substance use disorder, severe, in early remission or in sustained remission

> **F19.22**   **Other psychoactive substance dependence with**
> `6th`   **intoxication**
>> *Excludes1:* psychoactive other substance dependence with withdrawal (F19.23-)

>> **F19.220**   **Other psychoactive substance dependence with intoxication; uncomplicated**
>> **F19.221**   **delirium**
>> **F19.222**   **with perceptual disturbance**
>> **F19.229**   **unspecified**

> **F19.23**   **Other psychoactive substance dependence with**
> `6th`   **withdrawal**
>> *Excludes1:* other psychoactive substance dependence with intoxication (F19.22-)

>> **F19.230**   **Other psychoactive substance dependence with withdrawal; uncomplicated**
>> **F19.231**   **delirium**
>> **F19.232**   **with perceptual disturbance**
>> **F19.239**   **unspecified**

F19.9   **Other psychoactive substance use, unspecified**
> `5th`   *Excludes1:* other psychoactive substance abuse (F19.1-)
>> other psychoactive substance dependence (F19.2-)

> **F19.90**   **Other psychoactive substance use, unspecified, uncomplicated**

> **F19.92**   **Other psychoactive substance use, unspecified with**
> `6th`   **intoxication**
>> *Excludes1:* other psychoactive substance use, unspecified with withdrawal (F19.93)

>> **F19.920**   **Other psychoactive substance use, unspecified with intoxication; uncomplicated**
>> **F19.921**   **with delirium**
>>> Other (or unknown) substance-induced delirium
>> **F19.922**   **with perceptual disturbance**
>> **F19.929**   **unspecified**

(F20–F29) SCHIZOPHRENIA, SCHIZOTYPAL, DELUSIONAL, AND OTHER NON-MOOD PSYCHOTIC DISORDERS

(F30–F39) MOOD [AFFECTIVE] DISORDERS

F31   **BIPOLAR DISORDER**
> `4th`   *Includes:* bipolar I disorder
>> bipolar type I disorder manic-depressive illness manic-depressive psychosis manic-depressive reaction
> *Excludes1:* bipolar disorder, single manic episode (F30.-)
>> major depressive disorder, single episode (F32.-)
>> major depressive disorder, recurrent (F33.-)

F31.0   **Bipolar disorder, current episode hypomanic**

F31.1   **Bipolar disorder, current episode manic without psychotic**
> `5th`   **features**

> **F31.10**   **Bipolar disorder, current episode manic without psychotic features, unspecified**
> **F31.11**   **Bipolar disorder, current episode manic without psychotic features, mild**
> **F31.12**   **Bipolar disorder, current episode manic without psychotic features, moderate**
> **F31.13**   **Bipolar disorder, current episode manic without psychotic features, severe**

F31.3   **Bipolar disorder, current episode depressed, mild or moderate**
> `5th`   **severity**

> **F31.30**   **Bipolar disorder, current episode depressed, mild or moderate severity, unspecified**
> **F31.31**   **Bipolar disorder, current episode depressed, mild**
> **F31.32**   **Bipolar disorder, current episode depressed, moderate**

F31.4   **Bipolar disorder, current episode depressed, severe, without psychotic features**

F31.6   **Bipolar disorder, current episode mixed**
> `5th`   **F31.60**   **Bipolar disorder, current episode mixed, unspecified**
> **F31.61**   **Bipolar disorder, current episode mixed, mild**
> **F31.62**   **Bipolar disorder, current episode mixed, moderate**
> **F31.63**   **Bipolar disorder, current episode mixed, severe, without psychotic features**

F31.8   **Other bipolar disorders**
> `5th`   **F31.81**   **Bipolar II disorder**
>> Bipolar disorder, type 2
> **F31.89**   **Other bipolar disorder**
>> Recurrent manic episodes NOS

F31.9   **Bipolar disorder, unspecified**
> Manic depression

F32   **DEPRESSIVE EPISODE**
> `4th`   *Includes:* single episode of agitated depression
>> single episode of depressive reaction
>> single episode of major depression
>> single episode of psychogenic depression
>> single episode of reactive depression
>> single episode of vital depression
> *Excludes1:* bipolar disorder (F31.-)
>> manic episode (F30.-)
>> recurrent depressive disorder (F33.-)
> *Excludes2:* adjustment disorder (F43.2)

F32.0   **Major depressive disorder, single episode, mild**

F32.1   **Major depressive disorder, single episode, moderate**

F32.2   **Major depressive disorder, single episode, severe without psychotic features**

F32.3   **Major depressive disorder, single episode, severe with psychotic features**
> Single episode of major depression with mood-congruent psychotic symptoms
> Single episode of major depression with mood-incongruent psychotic symptoms
> Single episode of major depression with psychotic symptoms
> Single episode of psychogenic depressive psychosis
> Single episode of psychotic depression
> Single episode of reactive depressive psychosis

F32.4   **Major depressive disorder, single episode, in partial remission**

F32.5   **Major depressive disorder, single episode, in full remission**

F32.8   **Other depressive episodes**
> `5th`   **F32.81**   **Premenstrual dysphoric disorder**
>> *Excludes1:* premenstrual tension syndrome (N94.3)
> **F32.89**   **Other specified depressive episodes**
>> Atypical depression
>> Post-schizophrenic depression
>> Single episode of 'masked' depression NOS

F32.9   **Major depressive disorder, single episode, unspecified**
> Major depression NOS

•F32.A   **Depression, unspecified**
> Depression NOS
> Depressive disorder NOS

F33   **MAJOR DEPRESSIVE DISORDER, RECURRENT**
> `4th`   *Includes:* recurrent episodes of depressive reaction
>> recurrent episodes of endogenous depression
>> recurrent episodes of major depression
>> recurrent episodes of psychogenic depression
>> recurrent episodes of reactive depression
>> recurrent episodes of seasonal depressive disorder
>> recurrent episodes of vital depression
> *Excludes1:* bipolar disorder (F31.-)
>> manic episode (F30.-)

F33.0   **Major depressive disorder, recurrent, mild**

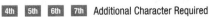 `4th`   `5th`   `6th`   `7th`   Additional Character Required   3-character code

•=New Code   *Excludes1*—Not coded here, do not use together
▲=Revised Code   *Excludes2*—Not included here

CHAPTER 5. MENTAL, BEHAVIORAL, AND NEURODEVELOPMENTAL DISORDERS   **(F33.1–F43.9)**

F33.1   **Major depressive disorder, recurrent, moderate**

F33.2   **Major depressive disorder, recurrent severe without psychotic features**

F33.3   **Major depressive disorder, recurrent, severe with psychotic symptoms**
Major depressive disorder, recurrent, with psychotic features
Endogenous depression with psychotic symptoms
Recurrent severe episodes of major depression with mood-congruent psychotic symptoms
Major depression with mood-incongruent psychotic symptoms
Major depression with psychotic symptoms
Psychogenic depressive psychosis
Psychotic depression
Reactive depressive psychosis

F33.4   **Major depressive disorder, recurrent, in remission**
> **5th**   **F33.40**   **Major depressive disorder, recurrent, in remission, unspecified**
> **F33.41**   **in partial remission**
> **F33.42**   **in full remission**

F33.8   **Other recurrent depressive disorders**
Recurrent brief depressive episodes

F33.9   **Major depressive disorder, recurrent, unspecified**
Monopolar depression NOS

F34   **PERSISTENT MOOD [AFFECTIVE] DISORDERS**
> **4th**

F34.0   **Cyclothymic disorder**
Affective personality disorder
Cycloid personality
Cyclothymia
Cyclothymic personality

F34.1   **Dysthymic disorder**
Depressive neurosis
Depressive personality disorder
Dysthymia
Neurotic depression
Persistent anxiety depression
Persistent depressive disorder
Excludes2: anxiety depression (mild or not persistent) (F41.8)

F34.8   **Other persistent mood [affective] disorders**
> **5th**   **F34.81**   **Disruptive mood dysregulation disorder**
> **F34.89**   **Other specified persistent mood disorders**

F34.9   **Persistent mood [affective] disorder, unspecified**

F39   **UNSPECIFIED MOOD [AFFECTIVE] DISORDER**
> ✔
Affective psychosis NOS

(F40–F48) ANXIETY, DISSOCIATIVE, STRESS-RELATED, SOMATOFORM AND OTHER NONPSYCHOTIC MENTAL DISORDERS

F40   **PHOBIC ANXIETY DISORDERS**
> **4th**

F40.0   **Agoraphobia**
> **5th**   **F40.00**   **Agoraphobia, unspecified**
> **F40.01**   **Agoraphobia with panic disorder**
> Panic disorder with agoraphobia
> *Excludes1:* panic disorder without agoraphobia (F41.0)
> **F40.02**   **Agoraphobia without panic disorder**

F40.1   **Social phobias**
> **5th**
Anthropophobia
Social anxiety disorder
Social anxiety disorder of childhood
Social neurosis
> **F40.10**   **Social phobia, unspecified**
> **F40.11**   **Social phobia, generalized**

F40.8   **Other phobic anxiety disorders**
Phobic anxiety disorder of childhood

F40.9   **Phobic anxiety disorder, unspecified**
Phobia NOS
Phobic state NOS

F41   **OTHER ANXIETY DISORDERS**
> **4th**   *Excludes2:* anxiety in: acute stress reaction (F43.0)
> transient adjustment reaction (F43.2)
> neurasthenia (F48.8)
> psychophysiologic disorders (F45.-)
> separation anxiety (F93.0)

F41.0   **Panic disorder [episodic paroxysmal anxiety]**
Panic attack
Panic state
Excludes1: panic disorder with agoraphobia (F40.01)

F41.1   **Generalized anxiety disorder**
Anxiety neurosis
Anxiety reaction
Anxiety state
Overanxious disorder
Excludes2: neurasthenia (F48.8)

F41.3   **Other mixed anxiety disorders**

F41.8   **Other specified anxiety disorders**
Anxiety depression (mild or not persistent)
Anxiety hysteria
Mixed anxiety and depressive disorder

F41.9   **Anxiety disorder, unspecified**
Anxiety NOS

F42   **OBSESSIVE-COMPULSIVE DISORDER**
> **4th**   *Excludes2:* obsessive-compulsive personality (disorder) (F60.5)
> obsessive-compulsive symptoms occurring in depression (F32–F33)
> obsessive-compulsive symptoms occurring in schizophrenia (F20.-)

F42.2   **Mixed obsessional thoughts and acts**

F42.3   **Hoarding disorder**

F42.4   **Excoriation (skin-picking) disorder**
Excludes1: factitial dermatitis (L98.1)
other specified behavioral and emotional disorders with onset usually occurring in early childhood and adolescence (F98.8)

F42.8   **Other obsessive compulsive disorder**
Anancastic neurosis
Obsessive-compulsive neurosis

F42.9   **Obsessive-compulsive disorder, unspecified**

F43   **REACTION TO SEVERE STRESS, AND ADJUSTMENT DISORDERS**
> **4th**

F43.0   **Acute stress reaction**
Acute crisis reaction
Acute reaction to stress
Combat and operational stress reaction
Combat fatigue
Crisis state
Psychic shock

F43.1   **Post-traumatic stress disorder (PTSD)**
> **5th**
Traumatic neurosis
> **F43.10**   **Post-traumatic stress disorder, unspecified**
> **F43.11**   **Post-traumatic stress disorder, acute**
> **F43.12**   **Post-traumatic stress disorder, chronic**

F43.2   **Adjustment disorders**
> **5th**
Culture shock
Grief reaction
Hospitalism in children
Excludes2: separation anxiety disorder of childhood (F93.0)
> **F43.20**   **Adjustment disorder, unspecified**
> **F43.21**   **Adjustment disorder with depressed mood**
> **F43.22**   **Adjustment disorder with anxiety**
> **F43.23**   **Adjustment disorder with mixed anxiety and depressed mood**
> **F43.24**   **Adjustment disorder with disturbance of conduct**
> **F43.25**   **Adjustment disorder with mixed disturbance of emotions and conduct**
> **F43.29**   **Adjustment disorder with other symptoms**

F43.8   **Other reactions to severe stress**
Other specified trauma and stressor-related disorder

F43.9   **Reaction to severe stress, unspecified**
Trauma and stressor-related disorder, NOS

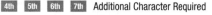

4th   **5th**   **6th**   **7th**   Additional Character Required   ✔   3-character code

•=New Code
▲=Revised Code

Excludes1—Not coded here, do not use together
Excludes2—Not included here

F44 **DISSOCIATIVE AND CONVERSION DISORDERS**
`4th`
Includes: conversion hysteria
    conversion reaction
    hysteria
    hysterical psychosis
Excludes2: malingering [conscious simulation] (Z76.5)

F44.4 Conversion disorder with motor symptom or deficit
    Conversion disorder with abnormal movement
    Conversion disorder with speech symptoms
    Conversion disorder with swallowing symptoms
    Conversion disorder with weakness/paralysis
    Psychogenic aphonia
    Psychogenic dysphonia

F44.5 Conversion disorder with seizures or convulsions
    Conversion disorder with attacks or seizures
    Dissociative convulsions

F44.6 Conversion disorder with sensory symptom or deficit
    Conversion disorder with anesthesia or sensory loss or with special sensory symptoms
    Dissociative anesthesia and sensory loss
    Psychogenic deafness

F44.7 Conversion disorder with mixed symptom presentation

F44.8 Other dissociative and conversion disorders
`5th` **F44.81 Dissociative identity disorder**
    Multiple personality disorder
F44.89 Other dissociative and conversion disorders
    Ganser's syndrome
    Psychogenic confusion
    Psychogenic twilight state
    Trance and possession disorders

F44.9 Dissociative and conversion disorder, unspecified
    Dissociative disorder NOS

F45 **SOMATOFORM DISORDERS**
`4th`

GUIDELINES

Pain disorders related to psychological factors
    Assign code F45.41, for pain that is exclusively related to psychological disorders. As indicated by the *Excludes1* note under category G89, a code from category G89 should not be assigned with code F45.41
    Code F45.42, Pain disorders with related psychological factors, should be used with a code from category G89, Pain, not elsewhere classified, if there is documentation of a psychological component for a patient with acute or chronic pain.
    See Chapter 6

Excludes2: dissociative and conversion disorders (F44.-)
    factitious disorders (F68.1-, F68.A)
    hair-plucking (F63.3)
    lalling (F80.0)
    lisping (F80.0)
    malingering [conscious simulation] (Z76.5)
    nail-biting (F98.8)
    psychological or behavioral factors associated with disorders or diseases classified elsewhere (F54)
    sexual dysfunction, not due to a substance or known physiological condition (F52.-)
    thumb-sucking (F98.8)
    tic disorders (in childhood and adolescence) (F95.-)
    Tourette's syndrome (F95.2)
    trichotillomania (F63.3)

F45.0 Somatization disorder
    Briquet's disorder
    Multiple psychosomatic disorders

F45.1 Undifferentiated somatoform disorder
    Somatic symptom disorder
    Undifferentiated psychosomatic disorder

F45.2 Hypochondriacal disorders
`5th` *Excludes2:* delusional dysmorphophobia (F22)
    fixed delusions about bodily functions or shape (F22)
F45.20 Hypochondriacal disorder, unspecified
F45.21 Hypochondriasis
    Hypochondriacal neurosis
    Illness anxiety disorder

F45.22 Body dysmorphic disorder
    Dysmorphophobia (nondelusional)
    Nosophobia
F45.29 Other hypochondriacal disorders

F45.4 Pain disorders related to psychological factors
`5th` *Excludes1:* pain NOS (R52)
F45.41 Pain disorder exclusively related to psychological factors
    Somatoform pain disorder (persistent)
F45.42 Pain disorder with related psychological factors
    Code also associated acute or chronic pain (G89.-)

F45.8 Other somatoform disorders
    Psychogenic dysmenorrhea
    Psychogenic dysphagia, including 'globus hystericus'
    Psychogenic pruritus
    Psychogenic torticollis
    Somatoform autonomic dysfunction
    Teeth grinding
    Excludes1: sleep related teeth grinding (G47.63)

F45.9 Somatoform disorder, unspecified
    Psychosomatic disorder NOS

F48 **OTHER NONPSYCHOTIC MENTAL DISORDERS**
`4th`
F48.8 Other specified nonpsychotic mental disorders
    Dhat syndrome
    Neurasthenia
    Occupational neurosis, including writer's cramp
    Psychasthenia
    Psychasthenic neurosis
    Psychogenic syncope

F48.9 Nonpsychotic mental disorder, unspecified
    Neurosis NOS

(F50–F59) BEHAVIORAL SYNDROMES ASSOCIATED WITH PHYSIOLOGICAL DISTURBANCES AND PHYSICAL FACTORS

F50 **EATING DISORDERS**
`4th`
Excludes1: anorexia NOS (R63.0)
    polyphagia (R63.2)
    Excludes2: feeding difficulties (R63.3)
Excludes2: feeding disorder in infancy or childhood (F98.2-)

F50.0 Anorexia nervosa
`5th` *Excludes1:* loss of appetite (R63.0)
    psychogenic loss of appetite (F50.89)
F50.00 Anorexia nervosa, unspecified
F50.01 Anorexia nervosa, restricting type
F50.02 Anorexia nervosa, binge eating/purging type
    Excludes1: bulimia nervosa (F50.2)

F50.2 Bulimia nervosa
    Bulimia NOS
    Hyperorexia nervosa
    Excludes1: anorexia nervosa, binge eating/purging type (F50.02)

F50.8 Other eating disorders
`5th` **F50.81 Binge eating disorder**
F50.82 Avoidant/restrictive food intake disorder
F50.89 Other specified eating disorder
    Pica in adults
    Psychogenic loss of appetite
    Excludes2: pica of infancy and childhood (F98.3)

F50.9 Eating disorder, unspecified
    Atypical anorexia nervosa
    Atypical bulimia nervosa
    Feeding or eating disorder, unspecified
    Other specified feeding disorder

> For picky eaters see R63.3

F51 **SLEEP DISORDERS NOT DUE TO A SUBSTANCE OR KNOWN PHYSIOLOGICAL CONDITION**
`4th`
Excludes2: organic sleep disorders (G47.-)

`4th` `5th` `6th` `7th` Additional Character Required   ✔ 3-character code

•=New Code   *Excludes1*—Not coded here, do not use together
▲=Revised Code   *Excludes2*—Not included here

F51.0 **Insomnia not due to a substance or known physiological**
5th **condition**
Excludes2: alcohol related insomnia
drug-related insomnia
insomnia NOS (G47.0-)
insomnia due to known physiological condition (G47.0-)
organic insomnia (G47.0-)
sleep deprivation (Z72.820)

F51.01 **Primary insomnia**
Idiopathic insomnia
F51.02 **Adjustment insomnia**
F51.03 **Paradoxical insomnia**
F51.04 **Psychophysiological insomnia**
F51.05 **Insomnia due to other mental disorder**
Code also associated mental disorder
F51.09 **Other insomnia not due to a substance or known**
physiological condition

F51.3 **Sleepwalking [somnambulism]**
Non-rapid eye movement sleep arousal disorders, sleepwalking
type
F51.4 **Sleep terrors [night terrors]**
Non-rapid eye movement sleep arousal disorders, sleep terror type
F51.5 **Nightmare disorder**
Dream anxiety disorder
F51.8 **Other sleep disorders not due to a substance or known**
physiological condition
F51.9 **Sleep disorder not due to a substance or known physiological**
condition, unspecified
Emotional sleep disorder NOS

F54 **PSYCHOLOGICAL AND BEHAVIORAL FACTORS**
✔ **ASSOCIATED WITH DISORDERS OR DISEASES**
CLASSIFIED ELSEWHERE
Psychological factors affecting physical conditions
Code first the associated physical disorder, such as:
asthma (J45.-)
dermatitis (L23-L25)
gastric ulcer (K25.-)
mucous colitis (K58.-)
ulcerative colitis (K51.-)
urticaria (L50.-)
Excludes2: tension-type headache (G44.2)

F55 **ABUSE OF NON-PSYCHOACTIVE SUBSTANCES**
4th *Excludes2:* abuse of psychoactive substances (F10-F19)
F55.0 **Abuse of antacids**
F55.1 **Abuse of herbal or folk remedies**
F55.2 **Abuse of laxatives**
F55.3 **Abuse of steroids or hormones**
F55.4 **Abuse of vitamins**
F55.8 **Abuse of other non-psychoactive substances**

F59 **UNSPECIFIED BEHAVIORAL SYNDROMES ASSOCIATED**
✔ **WITH PHYSIOLOGICAL DISTURBANCES AND PHYSICAL**
FACTORS
Psychogenic physiological dysfunction NOS

(F60–F69) DISORDERS OF ADULT PERSONALITY AND BEHAVIOR

F60 **SPECIFIC PERSONALITY DISORDERS**
4th **F60.0** **Paranoid personality disorder**
Expansive paranoid personality (disorder)
Fanatic personality (disorder)
Paranoid personality (disorder)
Sensitive paranoid personality (disorder)
Excludes2: paranoia (F22)
paranoid schizophrenia (F20.0)
F60.1 **Schizoid personality disorder**
Excludes2: Asperger's syndrome (F84.5)
delusional disorder (F22)
schizoid disorder of childhood (F84.5)
schizophrenia (F20.-)
schizotypal disorder (F21)

F60.2 **Antisocial personality disorder**
Dissocial personality disorder
Excludes1: conduct disorders (F91.-)
Excludes2: borderline personality disorder (F60.3)
F60.3 **Borderline personality disorder**
Aggressive personality (disorder)
Explosive personality (disorder)
Excludes2: antisocial personality disorder (F60.2)
F60.4 **Histrionic personality disorder**
F60.5 **Obsessive-compulsive personality disorder**
Excludes2: obsessive-compulsive disorder (F42.-)
F60.6 **Avoidant personality disorder**
Anxious personality disorder
F60.9 **Personality disorder, unspecified**
Character disorder NOS
Character neurosis NOS
Pathological personality NOS

F63 **IMPULSE DISORDERS**
4th *Excludes2:* habitual excessive use of alcohol or psychoactive substances
(F10–F19)
impulse disorders involving sexual behavior (F65.-)
F63.0 **Pathological gambling**
Compulsive gambling
Excludes1: gambling and betting NOS (Z72.6)
Excludes2: excessive gambling by manic patients (F30, F31)
gambling in antisocial personality disorder (F60.2)
F63.1 **Pyromania**
Pathological fire-setting
Excludes2: fire-setting (by) (in):
adult with antisocial personality disorder (F60.2)
alcohol or psychoactive substance intoxication (F10–F19)
conduct disorders (F91.-)
mental disorders due to known physiological condition
(F01–F09)
schizophrenia (F20.-)
F63.2 **Kleptomania**
Pathological stealing
Excludes1: shoplifting as the reason for observation for suspected
mental disorder (Z03.8)
Excludes2: depressive disorder with stealing (F31–F33)
stealing due to underlying mental condition-code to mental
condition
stealing in mental disorders due to known physiological
condition (F01–F09)
F63.3 **Trichotillomania**
Hair plucking
Excludes2: other stereotyped movement disorder (F98.4)
F63.8 **Other impulse disorders**
5th **F63.81** **Intermittent explosive disorder**
F63.89 **Other impulse disorders**
F63.9 **Impulse disorder, unspecified**
Impulse control disorder NOS

F64 **GENDER IDENTITY DISORDERS**
4th **F64.0** **Transsexualism**
Gender identity disorder in adolescence and adulthood
Gender dysphoria in adolescents and adults
F64.1 **Dual role transvestism**
Use additional code to identify sex reassignment status (Z87.890)
Excludes1: gender identity disorder in childhood (F64.2)
Excludes2: fetishistic transvestism (F65.1)
F64.2 **Gender identity disorder of childhood**
Gender dysphoria in children
Excludes1: gender identity disorder in adolescence and adulthood
(F64.0)
Excludes2: sexual maturation disorder (F66)
F64.8 **Other gender identity disorders**
F64.9 **Gender identity disorder, unspecified**
Gender dysphoria, unspecified
Gender-role disorder NOS

4th **5th** **6th** **7th** Additional Character Required   **✔** 3-character code

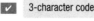

•=New Code   *Excludes1*—Not coded here, do not use together
▲=Revised Code   *Excludes2*—Not included here

F66   OTHER SEXUAL DISORDERS
✔
    Sexual maturation disorder
    Sexual relationship disorder

(F70–F79) INTELLECTUAL DISABILITIES

Code first any associated physical or developmental disorders
Excludes1: borderline intellectual functioning, IQ above 70 to 84 (R41.83)

F70   MILD INTELLECTUAL DISABILITIES
✔
    IQ level 50–55 to approximately 70
    Mild mental subnormality

F71   MODERATE INTELLECTUAL DISABILITIES
✔
    IQ level 35–40 to 50–55
    Moderate mental subnormality

F72   SEVERE INTELLECTUAL DISABILITIES
✔
    IQ 20–25 to 35–40
    Severe mental subnormality

F73   PROFOUND INTELLECTUAL DISABILITIES
✔
    IQ level below 20–25
    Profound mental subnormality

▲**F78   OTHER INTELLECTUAL DISABILITIES**
[4th] •**F78.A   Genetic related intellectual disability**
     [5th] •**F78.A1   SYNGAP1-related intellectual disability**
          Code also, if applicable, any associated:
           autism spectrum disorder (F84.0)
           autistic disorder (F84.0)
           encephalopathy (G93.4-)
           epilepsy and recurrent seizures (G40.-)
           other pervasive developmental disorders (F84.8)
           pervasive developmental disorder, NOS (F84.9)
    •**F78.A9   Other genetic related intellectual disability**
          Code also, if applicable, any associated disorders

F79   UNSPECIFIED INTELLECTUAL DISABILITIES
✔
    Mental deficiency NOS
    Mental subnormality NOS

(F80–F89) PERVASIVE AND SPECIFIC DEVELOPMENTAL DISORDERS

F80   SPECIFIC DEVELOPMENTAL DISORDERS OF SPEECH
[4th] **AND LANGUAGE**
   F80.0   Phonological disorder
      Dyslalia
      Functional speech articulation disorder
      Lalling
      Lisping
      Phonological developmental disorder
      Speech articulation developmental disorder
      Speech-sound disorder
      Excludes1: speech articulation impairment due to aphasia NOS
         (R47.01)
         speech articulation impairment due to apraxia (R48.2)
      Excludes2: speech articulation impairment due to hearing loss
         (F80.4)
         speech articulation impairment due to intellectual disabilities
         (F70–F79)
         speech articulation impairment with expressive language
         developmental disorder (F80.1)
         speech articulation impairment with mixed receptive expressive
         language developmental disorder (F80.2)
   F80.1   Expressive language disorder
      Developmental dysphasia or aphasia, expressive type
      Excludes1: mixed receptive-expressive language disorder (F80.2)
         dysphasia and aphasia NOS (R47.-)
      Excludes2: acquired aphasia with epilepsy [Landau-Kleffner]
         (G40.80-)
         selective mutism (F94.0)
         intellectual disabilities (F70–F79)
         pervasive developmental disorders (F84.-)

F80.2   Mixed receptive-expressive language disorder
    Developmental dysphasia or aphasia, receptive type
    Developmental Wernicke's aphasia
    Excludes1: central auditory processing disorder (H93.25)
       dysphasia or aphasia NOS (R47.-)
       expressive language disorder (F80.1)
       expressive type dysphasia or aphasia (F80.1)
       word deafness (H93.25)
    Excludes2: acquired aphasia with epilepsy [Landau-Kleffner]
       (G40.80-)
       pervasive developmental disorders (F84.-)
       selective mutism (F94.0)
       intellectual disabilities (F70–F79)
F80.4   Speech and language development delay due to hearing loss
    Code also type of hearing loss (H90.-, H91.-)
F80.8   Other developmental disorders of speech and language
   [5th] **F80.81   Childhood onset fluency disorder**
        Cluttering NOS
        Stuttering NOS
        Excludes1: adult onset fluency disorder (F98.5)
          fluency disorder in conditions classified elsewhere
          (R47.82)
          fluency disorder (stuttering) following cerebrovascular
          disease (I69. with final characters -23)
     F80.82   Social pragmatic communication disorder
        Excludes1: Asperger's syndrome (F84.5)
          autistic disorder (F84.0)
     F80.89   Other developmental disorders of speech and
          language
F80.9   Developmental disorder of speech and language, unspecified
    Communication disorder NOS
    Language disorder NOS

F81   SPECIFIC DEVELOPMENTAL DISORDERS OF
[4th] **SCHOLASTIC SKILLS**
   F81.0   Specific reading disorder
      'Backward reading'
      Developmental dyslexia
      Specific learning disorder, with impairment in reading
      Excludes1: alexia NOS (R48.0)
         dyslexia NOS (R48.0)
   F81.2   Mathematics disorder
      Developmental acalculia
      Developmental arithmetical disorder
      Developmental Gerstmann's syndrome
      Specific learning disorder, with impairment in mathematics
      Excludes1: acalculia NOS (R48.8)
      Excludes2: arithmetical difficulties associated with a reading
         disorder (F81.0)
         arithmetical difficulties associated with a spelling disorder
         (F81.81)
         arithmetical difficulties due to inadequate teaching (Z55.8)
   F81.8   Other developmental disorders of scholastic skills
   [5th] **F81.81   Disorder of written expression**
        Specific spelling disorder
        Specific learning disorder, with impairment in written
        expression
     F81.89   Other developmental disorders of scholastic skills
   F81.9   Developmental disorder of scholastic skills, unspecified
      Knowledge acquisition disability NOS
      Learning disability NOS
      Learning disorder NOS

F82   SPECIFIC DEVELOPMENTAL DISORDER OF
✔ **MOTOR FUNCTION**
   Clumsy child syndrome
   Developmental coordination disorder
   Developmental dyspraxia
   Excludes1: abnormalities of gait and mobility (R26.-)
     lack of coordination (R27.-)
   Excludes2: lack of coordination secondary to intellectual disabilities
     (F70–F79)

F84   PERVASIVE DEVELOPMENTAL DISORDERS
[4th] **Code also** to identify any associated medical condition and intellectual
    disabilities.

[4th] [5th] [6th] [7th]   Additional Character Required   ✔   3-character code

•=New Code   ***Excludes1***—Not coded here, do not use together
▲=Revised Code   ***Excludes2***—Not included here

CHAPTER 5. MENTAL, BEHAVIORAL, AND NEURODEVELOPMENTAL DISORDERS (F84.0–F95.9)

F84.0 **Autistic disorder**
Autism spectrum disorder
Infantile autism
Infantile psychosis
Kanner's syndrome
Excludes1: Asperger's syndrome (F84.5)

F84.2 **Rett's syndrome**
Excludes1: Asperger's syndrome (F84.5)
Autistic disorder (F84.0)
Other childhood disintegrative disorder (F84.3)

F84.3 **Other childhood disintegrative disorder**
Dementia infantilis
Disintegrative psychosis
Heller's syndrome
Symbiotic psychosis
Use additional code to identify any associated neurological condition.
Excludes1: Asperger's syndrome (F84.5)
Autistic disorder (F84.0)
Rett's syndrome (F84.2)

F84.5 **Asperger's syndrome**
Asperger's disorder
Autistic psychopathy
Schizoid disorder of childhood

F84.8 **Other pervasive developmental disorders**
Overactive disorder associated with intellectual disabilities and stereotyped movements

F84.9 **Pervasive developmental disorder, unspecified**
Atypical autism

F88   ✔ **OTHER DISORDERS OF PSYCHOLOGICAL DEVELOPMENT**
Developmental agnosia
Global developmental delay
Other specified neurodevelopmental disorder

F89   ✔ **UNSPECIFIED DISORDER OF PSYCHOLOGICAL DEVELOPMENT**
Developmental disorder NOS
Neurodevelopmental disorder NOS

(F90–F98) BEHAVIORAL AND EMOTIONAL DISORDERS WITH ONSET USUALLY OCCURRING IN CHILDHOOD AND ADOLESCENCE

Note: Codes within categories F90–F98 may be used regardless of the age of a patient. These disorders generally have onset within the childhood or adolescent years, but may continue throughout life or not be diagnosed until adulthood

F90   4th **ATTENTION-DEFICIT HYPERACTIVITY DISORDERS**
Includes: attention deficit disorder with hyperactivity
attention deficit syndrome with hyperactivity
Excludes2: anxiety disorders (F40.-, F41.-)
mood [affective] disorders (F30–F39)
pervasive developmental disorders (F84.-)
schizophrenia (F20.-)

F90.0 **Attention-deficit hyperactivity disorder, predominantly inattentive type**
ADD without hyperactivity

F90.1 **Attention-deficit hyperactivity disorder, predominantly hyperactive type**

F90.2 **Attention-deficit hyperactivity disorder, combined type**

F90.8 **Attention-deficit hyperactivity disorder, other type**

F90.9 **Attention-deficit hyperactivity disorder, unspecified type**
Attention-deficit hyperactivity disorder of childhood or adolescence NOS
Attention-deficit hyperactivity disorder NOS

F91   4th **CONDUCT DISORDERS**
Excludes1: antisocial behavior (Z72.81-)
antisocial personality disorder (F60.2)
Excludes2: conduct problems associated with attention-deficit hyperactivity disorder (F90.-)
mood [affective] disorders (F30–F39)
pervasive developmental disorders (F84.-)
schizophrenia (F20.-)

F91.0 **Conduct disorder confined to family context**

F91.1 **Conduct disorder, childhood-onset type**
Unsocialized conduct disorder
Conduct disorder, solitary aggressive type
Unsocialized aggressive disorder

F91.2 **Conduct disorder, adolescent-onset type**
Socialized conduct disorder
Conduct disorder, group type

F91.3 **Oppositional defiant disorder**

F91.8 **Other conduct disorders**
Other specified conduct disorder
Other specified disruptive disorder

F91.9 **Conduct disorder, unspecified**
Behavioral disorder NOS
Conduct disorder NOS
Disruptive behavior disorder NOS

F93   4th **EMOTIONAL DISORDERS WITH ONSET SPECIFIC TO CHILDHOOD**

F93.0 **Separation anxiety disorder of childhood**
Excludes2: mood [affective] disorders (F30–F39)
nonpsychotic mental disorders (F40–F48)
phobic anxiety disorder of childhood (F40.8)
social phobia (F40.1)

F93.8 **Other childhood emotional disorders**
Identity disorder
Excludes2: gender identity disorder of childhood (F64.2)

F93.9 **Childhood emotional disorder, unspecified**

F94   4th **DISORDERS OF SOCIAL FUNCTIONING WITH ONSET SPECIFIC TO CHILDHOOD AND ADOLESCENCE**

F94.0 **Selective mutism**
Elective mutism
Excludes2: pervasive developmental disorders (F84.-)
schizophrenia (F20.-)
specific developmental disorders of speech and language (F80.-)
transient mutism as part of separation anxiety in young children (F93.0)

F94.1 **Reactive attachment disorder of childhood**
Use additional code to identify any associated failure to thrive or growth retardation
Excludes1: disinhibited attachment disorder of childhood (F94.2)
normal variation in pattern of selective attachment
Excludes2: Asperger's syndrome (F84.5)
maltreatment syndromes (T74.-)
sexual or physical abuse in childhood, resulting in psychosocial problems (Z62.81-)

F94.2 **Disinhibited attachment disorder of childhood**
Affectionless psychopathy
Institutional syndrome
Excludes1: reactive attachment disorder of childhood (F94.1)
Excludes2: Asperger's syndrome (F84.5)
attention-deficit hyperactivity disorders (F90.-)
hospitalism in children (F43.2-)

F94.8 **Other childhood disorders of social functioning**

F94.9 **Childhood disorder of social functioning, unspecified**

F95   4th **TIC DISORDER**

F95.0 **Transient tic disorder**
Provisional tic disorder

F95.1 **Chronic motor or vocal tic disorder**

F95.2 **Tourette's disorder**
Combined vocal and multiple motor tic disorder [de la Tourette]
Tourette's syndrome

F95.8 **Other tic disorders**

F95.9 **Tic disorder, unspecified**
Tic NOS

 4th 5th 6th 7th   Additional Character Required   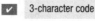 ✔   3-character code

•=New Code   *Excludes1*—Not coded here, do not use together
▲=Revised Code   *Excludes2*—Not included here

F98 **OTHER BEHAVIORAL AND EMOTIONAL DISORDERS**
4th **WITH ONSET USUALLY OCCURRING IN CHILDHOOD AND ADOLESCENCE**

Excludes2: breath-holding spells (R06.89)
    gender identity disorder of childhood (F64.2)
    Kleine-Levin syndrome (G47.13)
    obsessive-compulsive disorder (F42.-)
    sleep disorders not due to a substance or known physiological condition (F51.-)

F98.0 **Enuresis not due to a substance or known physiological condition**
    Enuresis (primary) (secondary) of nonorganic origin
    Functional enuresis
    Psychogenic enuresis
    Urinary incontinence of nonorganic origin
    Excludes1: enuresis NOS (R32)

F98.1 **Encopresis not due to a substance or known physiological condition**
    Functional encopresis
    Incontinence of feces of nonorganic origin
    Psychogenic encopresis
    Use additional code to identify the cause of any coexisting constipation.
    Excludes1: encopresis NOS (R15.-)

F98.2 **Other feeding disorders of infancy and childhood**
5th   *Excludes2:* feeding difficulties (R63.3)
        anorexia nervosa and other eating disorders (F50.-)
        feeding problems of newborn (P92.-)
        pica of infancy or childhood (F98.3)

    F98.21 **Rumination disorder of infancy**

    F98.29 **Other feeding disorders of infancy and early childhood**

F98.3 **Pica of infancy and childhood**

F98.4 **Stereotyped movement disorders**
    Stereotype/habit disorder
    Excludes1: abnormal involuntary movements (R25.-)
    Excludes2: compulsions in obsessive-compulsive disorder (F42.-)
        hair plucking (F63.3)
        movement disorders of organic origin (G20–G25)
        nail-biting (F98.8)
        nose-picking (F98.8)
        stereotypies that are part of a broader psychiatric condition (F01–F95)
        thumb-sucking (F98.8)
        tic disorders (F95.-)
        trichotillomania (F63.3)

F98.8 **Other specified behavioral and emotional disorders with onset usually occurring in childhood and adolescence**
    Excessive masturbation Nail-biting
    Nose-picking
    Thumb-sucking

F98.9 **Unspecified behavioral and emotional disorders with onset usually occurring in childhood and adolescence**

(F99) UNSPECIFIED MENTAL DISORDER

F99 **MENTAL DISORDER, NOT OTHERWISE SPECIFIED**
✔ Mental illness NOS
    Excludes1: unspecified mental disorder due to known physiological condition (F09)

4th 5th 6th 7th   Additional Character Required   ✔ 3-character code   •=New Code   *Excludes1*—Not coded here, do not use together
▲=Revised Code   *Excludes2*—Not included here

PEDIATRIC ICD-10-CM 2022: A MANUAL FOR PROVIDER-BASED CODING   183

Chapter 6. Diseases of the nervous system (G00–G99)

Dominant/nondominant side

Refer to category G81 and subcategories G83.1 and G83.2.

Pain

Refer to category G89.

Excludes2: certain conditions originating in the perinatal period (P04–P96)
certain infectious and parasitic diseases (A00–B99)
complications of pregnancy, childbirth and the puerperium (O00–O9A)
congenital malformations, deformations, and chromosomal abnormalities (Q00–Q99)
endocrine, nutritional and metabolic diseases (E00–E88)
injury, poisoning and certain other consequences of external causes (S00–T88)
neoplasms (C00–D49)
symptoms, signs and abnormal clinical and laboratory findings, not elsewhere classified (R00–R94)

(G00–G09) INFLAMMATORY DISEASES OF THE CENTRAL NERVOUS SYSTEM

G00 **BACTERIAL MENINGITIS, NOT ELSEWHERE CLASSIFIED**
`4th`
Includes: bacterial arachnoiditis
bacterial leptomeningitis
bacterial meningitis
bacterial pachymeningitis
Excludes1: bacterial meningoencephalitis (G04.2)
bacterial meningomyelitis (G04.2)
G00.0 **Hemophilus meningitis**
Meningitis due to H. influenzae
G00.1 **Pneumococcal meningitis**
Meningitis due to streptococcus pneumoniae
G00.2 **Streptococcal meningitis**
Use additional code to further identify organism (B95.0–B95.5)
G00.3 **Staphylococcal meningitis**
Use additional code to further identify organism (B95.61–B95.8)
G00.8 **Other bacterial meningitis**
Meningitis due to E. coli
Meningitis due to Friedländer's bacillus
Meningitis due to Klebsiella
Use additional code to further identify organism (B96.-)
G00.9 **Bacterial meningitis, unspecified**
Meningitis due to gram-negative bacteria, unspecified
Purulent meningitis NOS
Pyogenic meningitis NOS
Suppurative meningitis NOS

G01 **MENINGITIS IN BACTERIAL DISEASES CLASSIFIED**
`✔` **ELSEWHERE**
Code first underlying disease
Excludes1: meningitis (in): gonococcal (A54.81)
leptospirosis (A27.81)
listeriosis (A32.11)
Lyme disease (A69.21)
meningococcal (A39.0)
neurosyphilis (A52.13)
tuberculosis (A17.0)
meningoencephalitis and meningomyelitis in bacterial diseases classified elsewhere (G05)

G02 **MENINGITIS IN OTHER INFECTIOUS AND PARASITIC**
`✔` **DISEASES CLASSIFIED ELSEWHERE**
Code first underlying disease, such as: African trypanosomiasis (B56.-)
poliovirus infection (A80.-)
Excludes1: candidal meningitis (B37.5)
coccidioidomycosis meningitis (B38.4)
cryptococcal meningitis (B45.1)
herpesviral [herpes simplex] meningitis (B00.3)
infectious mononucleosis complicated by meningitis (B27.- with 5th character 2)

measles complicated by meningitis (B05.1)
meningoencephalitis and meningomyelitis in other infectious and parasitic diseases classified elsewhere (G05)
mumps meningitis (B26.1)
rubella meningitis (B06.02)
varicella [chickenpox] meningitis (B01.0)
zoster meningitis (B02.1)

G03 **MENINGITIS DUE TO OTHER AND UNSPECIFIED CAUSES**
`4th`
Includes: arachnoiditis NOS
leptomeningitis NOS
meningitis NOS
pachymeningitis NOS
Excludes1: meningoencephalitis (G04.-)
meningomyelitis (G04.-)
G03.0 **Nonpyogenic meningitis**
Aseptic meningitis
Nonbacterial meningitis
G03.1 **Chronic meningitis**
G03.2 **Benign recurrent meningitis [Mollaret]**
G03.8 **Meningitis due to other specified causes**
G03.9 **Meningitis, unspecified**
Arachnoiditis (spinal) NOS

G04 **ENCEPHALITIS, MYELITIS AND ENCEPHALOMYELITIS**
`4th`
Includes: acute ascending myelitis
meningoencephalitis
meningomyelitis
Excludes1: encephalopathy NOS (G93.40)
Excludes2: acute transverse myelitis (G37.3-)
alcoholic encephalopathy (G31.2)
benign myalgic encephalomyelitis (G93.3)
multiple sclerosis (G35)
subacute necrotizing myelitis (G37.4)
toxic encephalitis (G92.8)
toxic encephalopathy (G92.8)
G04.0 **Acute disseminated encephalitis and encephalomyelitis**
`5th` **(ADEM)**
Excludes1: acute necrotizing hemorrhagic encephalopathy (G04.3-)
other noninfectious acute disseminated encephalomyelitis (noninfectious ADEM) (G04.81)
G04.00 **Acute disseminated encephalitis and encephalomyelitis, unspecified**
G04.01 **Postinfectious acute disseminated encephalitis and encephalomyelitis (postinfectious ADEM)**
Excludes1: post chickenpox encephalitis (B01.1)
post measles encephalitis (B05.0)
post measles myelitis (B05.1)
G04.02 **Postimmunization acute disseminated encephalitis, myelitis and encephalomyelitis**
Encephalitis, post immunization
Encephalomyelitis, post immunization
Use additional code to identify the vaccine (T50.A-, T50.B-, T50.Z-)
G04.2 **Bacterial meningoencephalitis and meningomyelitis, not elsewhere classified**
G04.3 **Acute necrotizing hemorrhagic encephalopathy**
`5th` **Excludes1:** acute disseminated encephalitis and encephalomyelitis (G04.0-)
G04.30 **Acute necrotizing hemorrhagic encephalopathy, unspecified**
G04.31 **Postinfectious acute necrotizing hemorrhagic encephalopathy**
G04.32 **Postimmunization acute necrotizing hemorrhagic encephalopathy**
Use additional code to identify the vaccine (T50.A-, T50.B-, T50.Z-)
G04.39 **Other acute necrotizing hemorrhagic encephalopathy**
Code also underlying etiology, if applicable
G04.8 **Other encephalitis, myelitis and encephalomyelitis**
`5th` **Code also** any associated seizure (G40.-, R56.9)

•=New Code   **Excludes1**—Not coded here, do not use together
▲=Revised Code   **Excludes2**—Not included here

G04.81 Other encephalitis and encephalomyelitis
Noninfectious acute disseminated encephalomyelitis (noninfectious ADEM)

•**G04.82 Acute flaccid myelitis**
Excludes1: transverse myelitis (G37.3)

G04.89 Other myelitis

G04.9 Encephalitis, myelitis and encephalomyelitis, unspecified

5th **G04.90 Encephalitis and encephalomyelitis, unspecified**
Ventriculitis (cerebral) NOS

G04.91 Myelitis, unspecified

G05 **ENCEPHALITIS, MYELITIS AND ENCEPHALOMYELITIS IN**
4th **DISEASES CLASSIFIED ELSEWHERE**
Code first underlying disease, such as:
congenital toxoplasmosis encephalitis, myelitis and encephalomyelitis (P37.1)
cytomegaloviral encephalitis, myelitis and encephalomyelitis (B25.8)
encephalitis, myelitis and encephalomyelitis (in) SLE (M32.19)
eosinophilic meningoencephalitis (B83.2)
HIV disease (B20)
poliovirus (A80.-)
suppurative otitis media (H66.01–H66.4)
trichinellosis (B75)
Excludes1: adenoviral encephalitis, myelitis and encephalomyelitis (A85.1)
encephalitis, myelitis and encephalomyelitis (in) measles (B05.0)
enteroviral encephalitis, myelitis and encephalomyelitis (A85.0)
herpesviral [herpes simplex] encephalitis, myelitis and encephalomyelitis (B00.4)
listerial encephalitis, myelitis and encephalomyelitis (A32.12)
meningococcal encephalitis, myelitis and encephalomyelitis (A39.81)
mumps encephalitis, myelitis and encephalomyelitis (B26.2)
postchickenpox encephalitis, myelitis and encephalomyelitis (B01.1-)
rubella encephalitis, myelitis and encephalomyelitis (B06.01)
toxoplasmosis encephalitis, myelitis and encephalomyelitis (B58.2)
zoster encephalitis, myelitis and encephalomyelitis (B02.0)

G05.3 Encephalitis and encephalomyelitis in diseases classified elsewhere
Meningoencephalitis in diseases classified elsewhere

G05.4 Myelitis in diseases classified elsewhere
Meningomyelitis in diseases classified elsewhere

G06 **INTRACRANIAL AND INTRASPINAL ABSCESS AND**
4th **GRANULOMA**
Use additional code (B95–B97) to identify infectious agent.

G06.0 Intracranial abscess and granuloma
Brain [any part] abscess (embolic)
Cerebellar abscess (embolic)
Cerebral abscess (embolic)
Intracranial epidural abscess or granuloma
Intracranial extradural abscess or granuloma
Intracranial subdural abscess or granuloma
Otogenic abscess (embolic)
Excludes1: tuberculous intracranial abscess and granuloma (A17.81)

G06.1 Intraspinal abscess and granuloma
Abscess (embolic) of spinal cord [any part]
Intraspinal epidural abscess or granuloma
Intraspinal extradural abscess or granuloma
Intraspinal subdural abscess or granuloma
Excludes1: tuberculous intraspinal abscess and granuloma (A17.81)

G06.2 Extradural and subdural abscess, unspecified

G08 **INTRACRANIAL AND INTRASPINAL PHLEBITIS AND**
✔ **THROMBOPHLEBITIS**
Septic embolism of intracranial or intraspinal venous sinuses and veins
Septic endophlebitis of intracranial or intraspinal venous sinuses and veins
Septic phlebitis of intracranial or intraspinal venous sinuses and veins
Septic thrombophlebitis of intracranial or intraspinal venous sinuses and veins
Septic thrombosis of intracranial or intraspinal venous sinuses and veins
Excludes1: intracranial phlebitis and thrombophlebitis complicating:
abortion, ectopic or molar pregnancy (O00–O07, O08.7)
pregnancy, childbirth and the puerperium (O22.5, O87.3)
nonpyogenic intracranial phlebitis and thrombophlebitis (I67.6)

Excludes2: intracranial phlebitis and thrombophlebitis complicating nonpyogenic intraspinal phlebitis and thrombophlebitis (G95.1)

G09 **SEQUELAE OF INFLAMMATORY DISEASES OF CENTRAL**
✔ **NERVOUS SYSTEM**
Note: Category G09 is to be used to indicate conditions whose primary classification is to G00-G08 as the cause of sequelae, themselves classifiable elsewhere. The 'sequelae' include conditions specified as residuals.
Code first condition resulting from (sequela) of inflammatory diseases of central nervous system

(G10–G14) SYSTEMIC ATROPHIES PRIMARILY AFFECTING THE CENTRAL NERVOUS SYSTEM

G11 **HEREDITARY ATAXIA**
4th *Excludes2:* cerebral palsy (G80.-)
hereditary and idiopathic neuropathy (G60.-)
metabolic disorders (E70–E88)

G11.0 Congenital nonprogressive ataxia

G11.1 Early-onset cerebellar ataxia

5th **G11.10 Early-onset cerebellar ataxia, unspecified**

G11.11 Friedreich ataxia
Autosomal recessive Friedreich ataxia
Friedreich ataxia with retained reflexes

G11.19 Other early-onset cerebellar ataxia
Early-onset cerebellar ataxia with essential tremor
Early-onset cerebellar ataxia with myoclonus [Hunt's ataxia]
Early-onset cerebellar ataxia with retained tendon reflexes
X-linked recessive spinocerebellar ataxia

G11.2 Late-onset cerebellar ataxia

G11.3 Cerebellar ataxia with defective DNA repair
Ataxia telangiectasia [Louis-Bar]
Excludes2: Cockayne's syndrome (Q87.19)
other disorders of purine and pyrimidine metabolism (E79.-)
xeroderma pigmentosum (Q82.1)

G11.9 Hereditary ataxia, unspecified
Hereditary cerebellar ataxia NOS
Hereditary cerebellar degeneration
Hereditary cerebellar disease
Hereditary cerebellar syndrome

G12 **SPINAL MUSCULAR ATROPHY AND RELATED**
4th **SYNDROMES**

G12.0 Infantile spinal muscular atrophy, type I [Werdnig-Hoffman]

G12.2 Motor neuron disease

5th **G12.20 Motor neuron disease, unspecified**

G12.21 Amyotrophic lateral sclerosis

G12.22 Progressive bulbar palsy

G12.25 Progressive spinal muscle atrophy

G12.29 Other motor neuron disease

G12.9 Spinal muscular atrophy, unspecified

G13 **SYSTEMIC ATROPHIES PRIMARILY AFFECTING**
4th **CENTRAL NERVOUS SYSTEM IN DISEASES CLASSIFIED**
ELSEWHERE

G13.0 Paraneoplastic neuromyopathy and neuropathy
Carcinomatous neuromyopathy
Sensorial paraneoplastic neuropathy [Denny Brown]
Code first underlying neoplasm (C00-D49)

G13.1 Other systemic atrophy primarily affecting central nervous system in neoplastic disease
Paraneoplastic limbic encephalopathy
Code first underlying neoplasm (C00-D49)

G13.2 Systemic atrophy primarily affecting the central nervous system in myxedema
Code first underlying disease, such as:
hypothyroidism (E03.-)
myxedematous congenital iodine deficiency (E00.1)

G13.8 Systemic atrophy primarily affecting central nervous system in other diseases classified elsewhere
Code first underlying disease

4th	5th	6th	7th	Additional Character Required		✔	3-character code

•=New Code
▲=Revised Code

Excludes1—Not coded here, do not use together
Excludes2—Not included here

(G20–G26) EXTRAPYRAMIDAL AND MOVEMENT DISORDERS

G24 **DYSTONIA**
4th
Includes: dyskinesia
Excludes2: athetoid cerebral palsy (G80.3)

G24.0 **Drug induced dystonia**
5th **Use additional code** for adverse effect, if applicable, to identify drug (T36-T50 with fifth or sixth character 5)

G24.01 **Drug induced subacute dyskinesia**
Drug induced blepharospasm
Drug induced orofacial dyskinesia
Neuroleptic induced tardive dyskinesia
Tardive dyskinesia

G24.02 **Drug induced acute dystonia**
Acute dystonic reaction to drugs
Neuroleptic induced acute dystonia

G24.09 **Other drug induced dystonia**

G24.1 **Genetic torsion dystonia**
Dystonia deformans progressiva
Dystonia musculorum deformans
Familial torsion dystonia
Idiopathic familial dystonia
Idiopathic (torsion) dystonia NOS
(Schwalbe-) Ziehen-Oppenheim disease

G24.2 **Idiopathic nonfamilial dystonia**

G24.8 **Other dystonia**
Acquired torsion dystonia NOS

G24.9 **Dystonia, unspecified**
Dyskinesia NOS

G25 **OTHER EXTRAPYRAMIDAL AND MOVEMENT DISORDERS**
4th
Excludes2: sleep related movement disorders (G47.6-)

G25.0 **Essential tremor**
Familial tremor
Excludes1: tremor NOS (R25.1)

G25.1 **Drug-induced tremor**
Use additional code for adverse effect, if applicable, to identify drug (T36-T50 with fifth or sixth character 5)

G25.2 **Other specified forms of tremor**
Intention tremor

G25.3 **Myoclonus**
Drug-induced myoclonus
Palatal myoclonus
Use additional code for adverse effect, if applicable, to identify drug (T36–T50 with fifth or sixth character 5)
Excludes1: facial myokymia (G51.4)
myoclonic epilepsy (G40.-)

G25.4 **Drug-induced chorea**
Use additional code for adverse effect, if applicable, to identify drug (T36-T50 with fifth or sixth character 5)

G25.5 **Other chorea**
Chorea NOS
Excludes1: chorea NOS with heart involvement (I02.-)
Huntington's chorea (G10)

G25.6 **Drug induced tics and other tics of organic origin**
5th **G25.61** **Drug induced tics**
Use additional code for adverse effect, if applicable, to identify drug (T36-T50 with fifth or sixth character 5)

G25.69 **Other tics of organic origin**
Excludes1: habit spasm (F95.9)
tic NOS (F95.9)
Tourette's syndrome (F95.2)

G25.7 **Other and unspecified drug induced movement disorders**
5th **Use additional code** for adverse effect, if applicable, to identify drug (T36-T50 with fifth or sixth character 5)

G25.70 **Drug induced movement disorder, unspecified**

G25.71 **Drug induced akathisia**
Drug induced acathisia
Neuroleptic induced acute akathisia
Tardive akathisia

G25.79 **Other drug induced movement disorders**

G25.8 **Other specified extrapyramidal and movement disorders**
5th **G25.81** **Restless legs syndrome**
G25.83 **Benign shuddering attacks**

G25.89 **Other specified extrapyramidal and movement disorders**

G25.9 **Extrapyramidal and movement disorder, unspecified**

(G30–G32) OTHER DEGENERATIVE DISEASES OF THE NERVOUS SYSTEM

G31 **OTHER DEGENERATIVE DISEASES OF NERVOUS SYSTEM, NOT ELSEWHERE CLASSIFIED**
4th
For codes G31.0-G31.83, G31.85-G31.9, **use additional code** to identify:
dementia with behavioral disturbance (F02.81)
dementia without behavioral disturbance (F02.80)
Excludes2: Reye's syndrome (G93.7)

G31.8 **Other specified degenerative diseases of nervous system**
5th **G31.89** **Other specified degenerative diseases of nervous system**

G31.9 **Degenerative disease of nervous system, unspecified**

G32 **OTHER DEGENERATIVE DISORDERS OF NERVOUS SYSTEM IN DISEASES CLASSIFIED ELSEWHERE**
4th
G32.0 **Subacute combined degeneration of spinal cord in diseases classified elsewhere**
Dana-Putnam syndrome
Sclerosis of spinal cord (combined) (dorsolateral) (posterolateral)
Code first underlying disease, such as:
anemia (D51.9)
dietary (D51.3)
pernicious (D51.0)
vitamin B12 deficiency (E53.8)
Excludes1: syphilitic combined degeneration of spinal cord (A52.11)

G32.8 **Other specified degenerative disorders of nervous system in diseases classified elsewhere**
5th
Code first underlying disease, such as:
amyloidosis cerebral degeneration (E85.-)
cerebral degeneration (due to) hypothyroidism (E00.0-E03.9)
cerebral degeneration (due to) neoplasm (C00-D49)
cerebral degeneration (due to) vitamin B deficiency, except thiamine (E52-E53.-)
Excludes1: superior hemorrhagic polioencephalitis [Wernicke's encephalopathy] (E51.2)

G32.81 **Cerebellar ataxia in diseases classified elsewhere**
Code first underlying disease, such as:
celiac disease (with gluten ataxia) (K90.0)
cerebellar ataxia (in) neoplastic disease (paraneoplastic cerebellar degeneration) (C00-D49)
non-celiac gluten ataxia (M35.9)
Excludes1: systemic atrophy primarily affecting the central nervous system in alcoholic cerebellarataxia (G31.2)
systemic atrophy primarily affecting the central nervous system in myxedema (G13.2)

G32.89 **Other specified degenerative disorders of nervous system in diseases classified elsewhere**
Degenerative encephalopathy in diseases classified elsewhere

(G35–G37) DEMYELINATING DISEASES OF THE CENTRAL NERVOUS SYSTEM

G35 **MULTIPLE SCLEROSIS**
✔
Disseminated multiple sclerosis
Generalized multiple sclerosis
Multiple sclerosis NOS
Multiple sclerosis of brain stem
Multiple sclerosis of cord

G36 **OTHER ACUTE DISSEMINATED DEMYELINATION**
4th
Excludes1: postinfectious encephalitis and encephalomyelitis NOS (G04.01)

G36.0 **Neuromyelitis optica [Devic]**
Demyelination in optic neuritis
Excludes1: optic neuritis NOS (H46)

G36.1 **Acute and subacute hemorrhagic leukoencephalitis [Hurst]**

4th	5th	6th	7th	Additional Character Required		✔	3-character code

•=New Code
▲=Revised Code

Excludes1—Not coded here, do not use together
Excludes2—Not included here

G36.8 Other specified acute disseminated demyelination
G36.9 Acute disseminated demyelination, unspecified

G37 **OTHER DEMYELINATING DISEASES OF CENTRAL NERVOUS SYSTEM**
`4th`
   G37.1 Central demyelination of corpus callosum
   G37.8 Other specified demyelinating diseases of central nervous system
   G37.9 Demyelinating disease of central nervous system, unspecified

(G40–G47) EPISODIC AND PAROXYSMAL DISORDERS

G40 **EPILEPSY AND RECURRENT SEIZURES**
`4th`
   Note: the following terms are to be considered equivalent to intractable: pharmacoresistant (pharmacologically resistant), treatment resistant, refractory (medically) and poorly controlled

   Excludes1: conversion disorder with seizures (F44.5)
      convulsions NOS (R56.9)
      post traumatic seizures (R56.1)
      seizure (convulsive) NOS (R56.9)
      seizure of newborn (P90)

   Excludes2: hippocampal sclerosis (G93.81)
      mesial temporal sclerosis (G93.81)
      temporal sclerosis (G93.81)
      Todd's paralysis (G83.8)

> G40.0-, G40.1-, G40.2-, G40.3-, G40.A-, G40.B-, G40.40-, G40.41-, G40.91- Codes require a 6th character:
> 1 — with status epilepticus
> 9 — without status epilepticus or NOS

   G40.0 **Localization-related (focal) (partial) idiopathic epilepsy and epileptic syndromes with seizures of localized onset**
`5th`
      Benign childhood epilepsy with centrotemporal EEG spikes
      Childhood epilepsy with occipital EEG paroxysms
      Excludes1: adult onset localization-related epilepsy (G40.1-, G40.2-)
      G40.00 **Localization-related (focal) (partial) idiopathic epilepsy and epileptic syndromes with seizures of alcohol of localized onset, not intractable (without intractability)**
`6th`
      G40.01 **Localization-related (focal) (partial) idiopathic epilepsy and epileptic syndromes with seizures of localized onset, intractable**
`6th`

   G40.1 **Localization-related (focal) (partial) symptomatic epilepsy and epileptic syndromes with simple partial seizures**
`5th`
      Attacks without alteration of consciousness
      Epilepsia partialis continua [Kozhevnikof]
      Simple partial seizures developing into secondarily generalized seizures
      G40.10 **Localization-related (focal) (partial) symptomatic epilepsy and epileptic sydromes with simple partial seizures, not intractable (without intractability)**
`6th`
      G40.11 **Localization-related (focal) (partial) symptomatic epilepsy and epileptic syndromes with simple partial seizures, intractable**
`6th`

   G40.2 **Localization-related (focal) (partial) symptomatic epilepsy and epileptic syndromes with complex partial seizures**
`5th`
      Attacks with alteration of consciousness, often with automatisms
      Complex partial seizures developing into secondarily generalized seizures
      G40.20 **Localization-related (focal) (partial) symptomatic epilepsy and epileptic syndromes with complex partial seizures, not intractable (without intractability)**
`6th`
      G40.21 **Localization-related (focal) (partial) symptomatic epilepsy and epileptic sydromes with complex partial seizures, intractable**
`6th`

   G40.3 **Generalized idiopathic epilepsy and epileptic syndromes**
`5th`
      Code also MERRF syndrome, if applicable (E88.42)
      G40.30 **Generalized idiopathic epilepsy and epileptic syndromes, not intractable (without intractability)**
`6th`
      G40.31 **Generalized idiopathic epilepsy and epileptic syndromes, intractable**
`6th`

   G40.A **Absence epileptic syndrome**
`5th`
      Childhood absence epilepsy [pyknolepsy]
      Juvenile absence epilepsy
      Absence epileptic syndrome, NOS

G40.A0 **Absence epileptic syndrome, not intractable**
`6th`
G40.A1 **Absence epileptic syndrome, intractable**
`6th`

G40.B **Juvenile myoclonic epilepsy [impulsive petit mal]**
`5th`
   G40.B0 **Juvenile myoclonic epilepsy, not intractable**
`6th`
   G40.B1 **Juvenile myoclonic epilepsy, intractable**
`6th`

G40.4 **Other generalized epilepsy and epileptic syndromes**
`5th`
   Epilepsy with grand mal seizures on awakening
   Epilepsy with myoclonic absences
   Epilepsy with myoclonic-astatic seizures
   Grand mal seizure NOS
   Nonspecific atonic epileptic seizures
   Nonspecific clonic epileptic seizures
   Nonspecific myoclonic epileptic seizures
   Nonspecific tonic epileptic seizures
   Nonspecific tonic-clonic epileptic seizures
   Symptomatic early myoclonic encephalopathy
   G40.40 **Other generalized epilepsy and epileptic syndromes, not intractable**
`6th`
      Other generalized epilepsy and epileptic syndromes without intractability
      Other generalized epilepsy and epileptic syndromes NOS
   G40.41 **Other generalized epilepsy and epileptic syndromes, intractable**
`6th`
   G40.42 **Cyclin-Dependent Kinase-Like 5 Deficiency Disorder**
      CDKL5
      Use additional code, if known, to identify associated manifestations, such as:
         cortical blindness (H47.61-)
         global developmental delay (F88)

G40.5 **Epileptic seizures related to external causes**
`5th`
   Epileptic seizures related to alcohol
   Epileptic seizures related to drugs
   Epileptic seizures related to hormonal changes
   Epileptic seizures related to sleep deprivation
   Epileptic seizures related to stress
   Code also, if applicable, associated epilepsy and recurrent seizures (G40.-)
   Use additional code for adverse effect, if applicable, to identify drug (T36–T50 with fifth or sixth character 5)
   G40.50 **Epileptic seizures related to external causes, not intractable**
`6th`
      G40.501 **Epileptic seizures related to external causes, not intractable, with status epilepticus**
      G40.509 **Epileptic seizures related to external causes, not intractable, without status epilepticus**
         Epileptic seizures related to external causes, NOS

G40.8 **Other epilepsy and recurrent seizures**
`5th`
   Epilepsies and epileptic syndromes undetermined as to whether they are focal or generalized
   Landau-Kleffner syndrome
   G40.80 **Other epilepsy**
`6th`
      G40.801 **Other epilepsy, not intractable, with status epilepticus**
         Other epilepsy without intractability with status epilepticus
      G40.802 **Other epilepsy, not intractable, without status epilepticus**
         Other epilepsy NOS
         Other epilepsy without intractability without status epilepticus
      G40.803 **Other epilepsy, intractable, with status epilepticus**
      G40.804 **Other epilepsy, intractable, without status epilepticus**
   G40.81 **Lennox-Gastaut syndrome**
`6th`

`4th` `5th` `6th` `7th` Additional Character Required   ✔ 3-character code

•=New Code
▲=Revised Code

Excludes1—Not coded here, do not use together
Excludes2—Not included here

188   PEDIATRIC ICD-10-CM 2022: A MANUAL FOR PROVIDER-BASED CODING
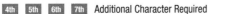

G40.811   **Lennox-Gastaut syndrome, not intractable, with status epilepticus**

G40.812   **Lennox-Gastaut syndrome, not intractable, without status epilepticus**

G40.813   **Lennox-Gastaut syndrome, intractable, with status epilepticus**

G40.814   **Lennox-Gastaut syndrome, intractable, without status epilepticus**

G40.82   **Epileptic spasms**
`6th`
Infantile spasms
Salaam attacks
West's syndrome

G40.821   **Epileptic spasms, not intractable, with status epilepticus**

G40.822   **Epileptic spasms, not intractable, without status epilepticus**

G40.823   **Epileptic spasms, intractable, with status epilepticus**

G40.824   **Epileptic spasms, intractable, without status epilepticus**

G40.83   **Dravet syndrome**
`6th`
Polymorphic epilepsy in infancy (PMEI)
Severe myoclonic epilepsy in infancy (SMEI)

G40.833   **Dravet syndrome, intractable, with status epilepticus**

G40.834   **Dravet syndrome, intractable, without status epilepticus**
Dravet syndrome NOS

G40.89   **Other seizures**
Excludes1: post traumatic seizures (R56.1)
recurrent seizures NOS (G40.909)
seizure NOS (R56.9)

G40.9   **Epilepsy, unspecified**
`5th`

G40.90   **Epilepsy, unspecified, not intractable**
`6th`
Epilepsy, unspecified, without intractability

G40.901   **Epilepsy, unspecified, not intractable, with status epilepticus**

G40.909   **Epilepsy, unspecified, not intractable, without status epilepticus**
Epilepsy NOS
Epileptic convulsions NOS
Epileptic fits NOS
Epileptic seizures NOS
Recurrent seizures NOS
Seizure disorder NOS

G40.91   **Epilepsy, unspecified, intractable**
`6th`
Intractable seizure disorder NOS

G43   **MIGRAINE**
`4th`
Note: the following terms are to be considered equivalent to intractable: pharmacoresistant (pharmacologically resistant), treatment resistant, refractory (medically) and poorly controlled
Use additional code for adverse effect, if applicable, to identify drug (T36–T50 with fifth or sixth character 5)
Excludes1: headache NOS (R51.9)
lower half migraine (G44.00)
Excludes2: headache syndromes (G44.-)

G43.0   **Migraine without aura**
`5th`
Common migraine
Excludes1: chronic migraine without aura (G43.7-)

G43.00   **Migraine without aura, not intractable**
`6th`
Migraine without aura without mention of refractory migraine

G43.001   **Migraine without aura, not intractable, with status migrainosus**

G43.009   **Migraine without aura, not intractable, without status migrainosus**
Migraine without aura NOS

G43.01   **Migraine without aura, intractable**
`6th`
Migraine without aura with refractory migraine

G43.011   **Migraine without aura, intractable, with status migrainosus**

G43.019   **Migraine without aura, intractable, without status migrainosus**

G43.1   **Migraine with aura**
`5th`
Basilar migraine
Classical migraine
Migraine equivalents
Migraine preceded or accompanied by transient focal neurological phenomena
Migraine triggered seizures
Migraine with acute-onset aura
Migraine with aura without headache (migraine equivalents)
Migraine with prolonged aura
Migraine with typical aura
Retinal migraine
Code also any associated seizure (G40.-, R56.9)
Excludes1: persistent migraine aura (G43.5-, G43.6-)

G43.10   **Migraine with aura, not intractable**
`6th`
Migraine with aura without mention of refractory migraine

G43.101   **Migraine with aura, not intractable, with status migrainosus**

G43.109   **Migraine with aura, not intractable, without status migrainosus**
Migraine with aura NOS

G43.11   **Migraine with aura, intractable**
`6th`
Migraine with aura with refractory migraine

G43.111   **Migraine with aura, intractable, with status migrainosus**

G43.119   **Migraine with aura, intractable, without status migrainosus**

G43.A   **Cyclical vomiting**
`5th`
Excludes 1: cyclical vomiting syndrome unrelated to migraine (R11.15)

G43.A0   **Cyclical vomiting, in migraine not intractable**
Cyclical vomiting, without refractory migraine

G43.A1   **Cyclical vomiting, in migraine intractable**
Cyclical vomiting, with refractory migraine

G43.C   **Periodic headache syndromes in child or adult**
`5th`

G43.C0   **Periodic headache syndromes in child or adult, not intractable**
Periodic headache syndromes in child or adult, without refractory migraine

G43.C1   **Periodic headache syndromes in child or adult, intractable**
Periodic headache syndromes in child or adult, with refractory migraine

G43.8   **Other migraine**
`5th`

G43.80   **Other migraine, not intractable**
`6th`
Other migraine, without refractory migraine

G43.801   **Other migraine, not intractable, with status migrainosus**

G43.809   **Other migraine, not intractable, without status migrainosus**

G43.81   **Other migraine, intractable**
`6th`
Other migraine, with refractory migraine

G43.811   **Other migraine, intractable, with status migrainosus**

G43.819   **Other migraine, intractable, without status migrainosus**

G43.82   **Menstrual migraine, not intractable**
`6th`
Menstrual migraine, without refractory migraine
Menstrually related migraine, not intractable
Pre-menstrual migraine/headache, not intractable
Pure menstrual migraine, not intractable
Code also associated premenstrual tension syndrome (N94.3)

G43.821   **Menstrual migraine, not intractable, with status migrainosus**

G43.829   **Menstrual migraine, not intractable, without status migrainosus**
Menstrual migraine NOS

`4th` `5th` `6th` `7th` Additional Character Required	✔ 3-character code	•=New Code	***Excludes1***—Not coded here, do not use together
		▲=Revised Code	***Excludes2***—Not included here

G43.83 **Menstrual migraine, intractable**
`6th`
Menstrual headache, intractable
Menstrual migraine, with refractory migraine
Menstrually related migraine, intractable
Pre-menstrual migraine/headache, intractable
Pure menstrual migraine, intractable
Code also associated premenstrual tension syndrome (N94.3)
    G43.831 **Menstrual migraine, intractable, with status migrainosus**
    G43.839 **Menstrual migraine, intractable, without status migrainosus**

G43.9 **Migraine, unspecified**
`5th`
  G43.90 **Migraine, unspecified, not intractable**
  `6th`
Migraine, unspecified, without refractory migraine
    G43.901 **Migraine, unspecified, not intractable, with status migrainosus**
    Status migrainosus NOS
    G43.909 **Migraine, unspecified, not intractable, without status migrainosus**
    Migraine NOS
  G43.91 **Migraine, unspecified, intractable**
  `6th`
Migraine, unspecified, with refractory migraine
    G43.911 **Migraine, unspecified, intractable, with status migrainosus**
    G43.919 **Migraine, unspecified, intractable, without status migrainosus**

G44 **OTHER HEADACHE SYNDROMES**
`4th`
Excludes1: headache NOS (R51.9)
Excludes2: atypical facial pain (G50.1)
headache due to lumbar puncture (G97.1)
migraines (G43.-)
trigeminal neuralgia (G50.0)

G44.0 **Cluster headaches and other trigeminal autonomic cephalgias (TAC)**
`5th`
  G44.00 **Cluster headache syndrome, unspecified**
  `6th`
Ciliary neuralgia
Cluster headache NOS
Histamine cephalgia
Lower half migraine
Migrainous neuralgia
    G44.001 **Cluster headache syndrome, unspecified, intractable**
    G44.009 **Cluster headache syndrome, unspecified, not intractable**
    Cluster headache syndrome NOS

G44.2 **Tension-type headache**
`5th`
  G44.20 **Tension-type headache, unspecified**
  `6th`
    G44.201 **Tension-type headache, unspecified, intractable**
    G44.209 **Tension-type headache, unspecified, not intractable**
    Tension headache NOS
  G44.21 **Episodic tension-type headache**
  `6th`
    G44.211 **Episodic tension-type headache, intractable**
    G44.219 **Episodic tension-type headache, not intractable**
    Episodic tension-type headache NOS
  G44.22 **Chronic tension-type headache**
  `6th`
    G44.221 **Chronic tension-type headache, intractable**
    G44.229 **Chronic tension-type headache, not intractable**
    Chronic tension-type headache NOS

G44.3 **Post-traumatic headache**
`5th`
  G44.30 **Post-traumatic headache, unspecified**
  `6th`
    G44.301 **Post-traumatic headache, unspecified, intractable**
    G44.309 **Post-traumatic headache, unspecified, not intractable**
    Post-traumatic headache NOS

  G44.31 **Acute post-traumatic headache**
  `6th`
    G44.311 **Acute post-traumatic headache, intractable**
    G44.319 **Acute post-traumatic headache, not intractable**
    Acute post-traumatic headache NOS
  G44.32 **Chronic post-traumatic headache**
  `6th`
    G44.321 **Chronic post-traumatic headache, intractable**
    G44.329 **Chronic post-traumatic headache, not intractable**
    Chronic post-traumatic headache NOS

G44.8 **Other specified headache syndromes**
`5th`
Excludes2: headache with orthostatic or positional component, not elsewhere classified (R51.0)
  G44.81 **Hypnic headache**
  G44.83 **Primary cough headache**
  G44.84 **Primary exertional headache**
  G44.85 **Primary stabbing headache**
  •**G44.86** **Cervicogenic headache**
  Code also associated cervical spinal condition, if known
  G44.89 **Other headache syndrome**

G45 **TRANSIENT CEREBRAL ISCHEMIC ATTACKS AND RELATED SYNDROMES**
`4th`
Excludes1: neonatal cerebral ischemia (P91.0)
transient retinal artery occlusion (H34.0-)

G45.8 **Other transient cerebral ischemic attacks and related syndromes**
G45.9 **Transient cerebral ischemic attack, unspecified**
Spasm of cerebral artery
TIA
Transient cerebral ischemia NOS

G47 **SLEEP DISORDERS**
`4th`
Excludes2: nightmares (F51.5)
nonorganic sleep disorders (F51.-)
sleep terrors (F51.4)
sleepwalking (F51.3)

G47.0 **Insomnia**
`5th`
Excludes2: alcohol or drug-related insomnia
idiopathic insomnia (F51.01)
insomnia due to a mental disorder (F51.05)
insomnia not due to a substance or known physiological condition (F51.0-)
nonorganic insomnia (F51.0-)
primary insomnia (F51.01)
sleep apnea (G47.3-)
  G47.00 **Insomnia, unspecified**
  Insomnia NOS
  G47.01 **Insomnia due to medical condition**
  Code also associated medical condition
  G47.09 **Other insomnia**

G47.2 **Circadian rhythm sleep disorders**
`5th`
Disorders of the sleep wake schedule
Inversion of nyctohemeral rhythm
Inversion of sleep rhythm
  G47.20 **Circadian rhythm sleep disorder, unspecified type**
  Sleep wake schedule disorder NOS
  G47.21 **Circadian rhythm sleep disorder, delayed sleep phase type**
  Delayed sleep phase syndrome
  G47.22 **Circadian rhythm sleep disorder, advanced sleep phase type**
  G47.23 **Circadian rhythm sleep disorder, irregular sleep wake type**
  Irregular sleep-wake pattern
  G47.24 **Circadian rhythm sleep disorder, free running type**
  Circadian rhythm sleep disorder, non-24-hour sleep-wake type
  G47.25 **Circadian rhythm sleep disorder, jet lag type**
  G47.27 **Circadian rhythm sleep disorder in conditions classified elsewhere**
  Code first underlying condition

`4th` `5th` `6th` `7th` Additional Character Required   ✔ 3-character code

•=New Code   *Excludes1*—Not coded here, do not use together
▲=Revised Code   *Excludes2*—Not included here

G47.29 Other circadian rhythm sleep disorder

G47.3 Sleep apnea

5th **Code also** any associated underlying condition

Excludes1: apnea NOS (R06.81)
Cheyne-Stokes breathing (R06.3)
pickwickian syndrome (E66.2)
sleep apnea of newborn (P28.3)

G47.30 Sleep apnea, unspecified
Sleep apnea NOS

G47.31 Primary central sleep apnea
Idiopathic central sleep apnea

G47.32 High altitude periodic breathing

G47.33 Obstructive sleep apnea (adult) (pediatric)
Obstructive sleep apnea hypopnea
Excludes1: obstructive sleep apnea of newborn (P28.3)

G47.37 Central sleep apnea in conditions classified elsewhere
Code first underlying condition

G47.39 Other sleep apnea

G47.5 Parasomnia

5th *Excludes1:* alcohol induced parasomnia
drug induced parasomnia
parasomnia not due to a substance or known physiological condition

G47.50 Parasomnia, unspecified
Parasomnia NOS

G47.51 Confusional arousals

G47.52 REM sleep behavior disorder

G47.53 Recurrent isolated sleep paralysis

G47.54 Parasomnia in conditions classified elsewhere
Code first underlying condition

G47.59 Other parasomnia

G47.6 Sleep related movement disorders

5th *Excludes2:* restless legs syndrome (G25.81)

G47.61 Periodic limb movement disorder

G47.62 Sleep related leg cramps

G47.63 Sleep related bruxism
Excludes1: psychogenic bruxism (F45.8)

G47.69 Other sleep related movement disorders

G47.8 Other sleep disorders
Other specified sleep-wake disorder

G47.9 Sleep disorder, unspecified
Sleep disorder NOS

(G50–G59) NERVE, NERVE ROOT AND PLEXUS DISORDERS

Excludes1: current traumatic nerve, nerve root and plexus disorders — see Injury, nerve by body region
neuralgia NOS (M79.2)
neuritis NOS (M79.2)
peripheral neuritis in pregnancy (O26.82-)
radiculitis NOS (M54.1-)

G51 FACIAL NERVE DISORDERS

4th *Includes:* disorders of 7th cranial nerve

G51.0 Bell's palsy
Facial palsy

G51.8 Other disorders of facial nerve

G51.9 Disorder of facial nerve, unspecified

G52 DISORDERS OF OTHER CRANIAL NERVES

4th *Excludes2:* disorders of acoustic [8th] nerve (H93.3)
disorders of optic [2nd] nerve (H46, H47.0)
paralytic strabismus due to nerve palsy (H49.0–H49.2)

G52.2 Disorders of vagus nerve
Disorders of pneumogastric [10th] nerve

G52.7 Disorders of multiple cranial nerves
Polyneuritis cranialis

G52.9 Cranial nerve disorder, unspecified

G53 CRANIAL NERVE DISORDERS IN DISEASES CLASSIFIED ELSEWHERE

✓ **Code first** underlying disease, such as:
neoplasm (C00-D49)
Excludes1: multiple cranial nerve palsy in sarcoidosis (D86.82)
multiple cranial nerve palsy in syphilis (A52.15)
postherpetic geniculate ganglionitis (B02.21)
postherpetic trigeminal neuralgia (B02.22)

G54 NERVE ROOT AND PLEXUS DISORDERS

4th *Excludes1:* current traumatic nerve root and plexus disorders—see nerve injury by body region
intervertebral disc disorders (M50-M51)
neuralgia or neuritis NOS (M79.2)
neuritis or radiculitis brachial NOS (M54.13)
neuritis or radiculitis lumbar NOS (M54.16)
neuritis or radiculitis lumbosacral NOS (M54.17)
neuritis or radiculitis thoracic NOS (M54.14)
radiculitis NOS (M54.10)
radiculopathy NOS (M54.10)
spondylosis (M47.-)

G54.0 Brachial plexus disorders
Thoracic outlet syndrome

G54.1 Lumbosacral plexus disorders

G54.9 Nerve root and plexus disorder, unspecified

G55 NERVE ROOT AND PLEXUS COMPRESSIONS IN DISEASES CLASSIFIED ELSEWHERE

✓ **Code first** underlying disease, such as:
neoplasm (C00-D49)
Excludes1: nerve root compression (due to) (in) ankylosing spondylitis (M45.-)
nerve root compression (due to) (in) dorsopathies (M53.-, M54.-)
nerve root compression (due to) (in) intervertebral disc disorders (M50.1-, M51.1.-)
nerve root compression (due to) (in) spondylopathies (M46.-, M48.-)
nerve root compression (due to) (in) spondylosis (M47.0–M47.2.-)

G58 OTHER MONONEUROPATHIES

4th **G58.9 Mononeuropathy, unspecified**

(G60–G65) POLYNEUROPATHIES AND OTHER DISORDERS OF THE PERIPHERAL NERVOUS SYSTEM

Excludes1: neuralgia NOS (M79.2)
neuritis NOS (M79.2)
peripheral neuritis in pregnancy (O26.82-)
radiculitis NOS (M54.10)

G60 HEREDITARY AND IDIOPATHIC NEUROPATHY

4th **G60.0 Hereditary motor and sensory neuropathy**
Charcot-Marie-Tooth disease
Déjérine-Sottas disease
Hereditary motor and sensory neuropathy, types I-IV
Hypertrophic neuropathy of infancy
Peroneal muscular atrophy (axonal type) (hypertrophic type)
Roussy-Levy syndrome

G60.3 Idiopathic progressive neuropathy

G60.8 Other hereditary and idiopathic neuropathies
Dominantly inherited sensory neuropathy
Morvan's disease
Nelaton's syndrome
Recessively inherited sensory neuropathy

G60.9 Hereditary and idiopathic neuropathy, unspecified

G61 INFLAMMATORY POLYNEUROPATHY

4th **G61.0 Guillain-Barre syndrome**
Acute (post-) infective polyneuritis
Miller Fisher Syndrome

G61.9 Inflammatory polyneuropathy, unspecified

G62 OTHER AND UNSPECIFIED POLYNEUROPATHIES

4th **G62.9 Polyneuropathy, unspecified**
Neuropathy NOS

CHAPTER 6. DISEASES OF THE NERVOUS SYSTEM (G47.29–G62.9)

    4th **5th** **6th** **7th** Additional Character Required

✓ 3-character code

•=New Code
▲=Revised Code

Excludes1—Not coded here, do not use together
Excludes2—Not included here

G63 ✓ **POLYNEUROPATHY IN DISEASES CLASSIFIED ELSEWHERE**

Code first underlying disease, such as:
amyloidosis (E85.-)
endocrine disease, except diabetes (E00-E07, E15-E16, E20-E34)
metabolic diseases (E70-E88)
neoplasm (C00-D49)
nutritional deficiency (E40-E64)
Excludes1: polyneuropathy (in):
diabetes mellitus (E08-E13 with .42)
diphtheria (A36.83)
infectious mononucleosis (B27.0-B27.9 with 5th character 1)
Lyme disease (A69.22)
mumps (B26.84)
postherpetic (B02.23)
rheumatoid arthritis (M05.5-)
scleroderma (M34.83)
systemic lupus erythematosus (M32.19)

(G70–G73) DISEASES OF MYONEURAL JUNCTION AND MUSCLE

G70 4th **MYASTHENIA GRAVIS AND OTHER MYONEURAL DISORDERS**

Excludes1: botulism (A05.1, A48.51–A48.52)
transient neonatal myasthenia gravis (P94.0)

G70.0 Myasthenia gravis
5th   **G70.00   Myasthenia gravis without (acute) exacerbation**
Myasthenia gravis NOS
G70.01   Myasthenia gravis with (acute) exacerbation
Myasthenia gravis in crisis

G70.1 Toxic myoneural disorders
Code first (T51–T65) to identify toxic agent

G70.2 Congenital and developmental myasthenia

G70.8 Other specified myoneural disorders
5th   **G70.80   Lambert-Eaton syndrome, unspecified**
Lambert-Eaton syndrome NOS
G70.81   Lambert-Eaton syndrome in disease classified elsewhere
Code first underlying disease
Excludes1: Lambert-Eaton syndrome in neoplastic disease (G73.1)
G70.89   Other specified myoneural disorders

G70.9 Myoneural disorder, unspecified

G71 4th **PRIMARY DISORDERS OF MUSCLES**

Excludes2: arthrogryposis multiplex congenita (Q74.3)
metabolic disorders (E70–E88)
myositis (M60.-)

G71.0 Muscular dystrophy
5th   **G71.00   Muscular dystrophy, unspecified**
G71.01   Duchenne or Becker muscular dystrophy
Autosomal recessive, childhood type, muscular dystrophy resembling Duchenne or Becker muscular dystrophy
Benign [Becker] muscular dystrophy
Severe [Duchenne] muscular dystrophy
G71.02   Facioscapulohumeral muscular dystrophy
Scapulohumeral muscular dystrophy
G71.09   Other specified muscular dystrophies
Benign scapuloperoneal muscular dystrophy with early contractures [Emery-Dreifuss]
Congenital muscular dystrophy NOS
Congenital muscular dystrophy with specific morphological abnormalities of the muscle fiber
Distal muscular dystrophy
Limb-girdle muscular dystrophy
Ocular muscular dystrophy
Oculopharyngeal muscular dystrophy
Scapuloperoneal muscular dystrophy

G71.1 Myotonic disorders
5th   **G71.11   Myotonic muscular dystrophy**
Dystrophia myotonica [Steinert]
Myotonia atrophica

G71.12   Myotonia congenita
Acetazolamide responsive myotonia congenita
Dominant myotonia congenita [Thomsen disease]
Myotonia levior
Recessive myotonia congenita [Becker disease]
G71.13   Myotonic chondrodystrophy
Chondrodystrophic myotonia
Congenital myotonic chondrodystrophy
Schwartz-Jampel disease

G71.2 Congenital myopathies
5th   *Excludes2:* arthrogryposis multiplex congenita (Q74.3)
G71.20   Congenital myopathy, unspecified
G71.21   Nemaline myopathy
G71.22   Centronuclear myopathy
6th   **G71.220   X-linked myotubular myopathy**
Myotubular (centronuclear) myopathy
G71.228   Other centronuclear myopathy
Autosomal centronuclear myopathy
Autosomal dominant centronuclear myopathy
Autosomal recessive centronuclear myopathy
Centronuclear myopathy, NOS
G71.29   Other congenital myopathy
Central core disease
Minicore disease
Multicore disease
Multiminicore disease

G71.9 Primary disorder of muscle, unspecified
Hereditary myopathy NOS

G72 4th **OTHER AND UNSPECIFIED MYOPATHIES**

Excludes1: arthrogryposis multiplex congenita (Q74.3)
dermatopolymyositis (M33.-)
ischemic infarction of muscle (M62.2-)
myositis (M60.-)
polymyositis (M33.2.-)

G72.8 Other specified myopathies
5th   **G72.81   Critical illness myopathy**
Acute necrotizing myopathy
Acute quadriplegic myopathy
Intensive care (ICU) myopathy
Myopathy of critical illness
G72.89   Other specified myopathies

G72.9 Myopathy, unspecified

G73 4th **DISORDERS OF MYONEURAL JUNCTION AND MUSCLE IN DISEASES CLASSIFIED ELSEWHERE**

G73.1 Lambert-Eaton syndrome in neoplastic disease
Code first underlying neoplasm (C00–D49)
Excludes1: Lambert-Eaton syndrome not associated with neoplasm (G70.80–G70.81)

G73.3 Myasthenic syndromes in other diseases classified elsewhere
Code first underlying disease, such as:
neoplasm (C00-D49)
thyrotoxicosis (E05.-)

G73.7 Myopathy in diseases classified elsewhere
Code first underlying disease, such as:
hyperparathyroidism (E21.0, E21.3)
hypoparathyroidism (E20.-)
glycogen storage disease (E74.0)
lipid storage disorders (E75.-)
Excludes1: myopathy in:
rheumatoid arthritis (M05.32)
sarcoidosis (D86.87)
scleroderma (M34.82)
Sjögren syndrome (M35.03)
systemic lupus erythematosus (M32.19)

(G80–G83) CEREBRAL PALSY AND OTHER PARALYTIC SYNDROMES

G80 4th **CEREBRAL PALSY**

Excludes1: hereditary spastic paraplegia (G11.4)
G80.0 Spastic quadriplegic cerebral palsy
Congenital spastic paralysis (cerebral)

| 4th | 5th | 6th | 7th | Additional Character Required | ✓ | 3-character code |

•=New Code
▲=Revised Code

Excludes1—Not coded here, do not use together
Excludes2—Not included here

G80.1 Spastic diplegic cerebral palsy
Spastic cerebral palsy NOS
G80.2 Spastic hemiplegic cerebral palsy
G80.3 Athetoid cerebral palsy
Double athetosis (syndrome)
Dyskinetic cerebral palsy
Dystonic cerebral palsy
Vogt disease
G80.4 Ataxic cerebral palsy
G80.8 Other cerebral palsy
Mixed cerebral palsy syndromes
G80.9 Cerebral palsy, unspecified
Cerebral palsy NOS

G81 HEMIPLEGIA AND HEMIPARESIS
`4th`

> **GUIDELINES**
>
> Codes from category G81, identify whether the dominant or nondominant side is affected. Should the affected side be documented, but not specified as dominant or nondominant, and the classification system does not indicate a default, code selection is as follows:
> For ambidextrous patients, the default should be dominant.
> If the left side is affected, the default is non-dominant.
> If the right side is affected, the default is dominant.
> **Note:** This category is to be used only when hemiplegia (complete) (incomplete) is reported without further specification, or is stated to be old or longstanding but of unspecified cause. The category is also for use in multiple coding to identify these types of hemiplegia resulting from any cause.
> ***Excludes1:*** congenital cerebral palsy (G80.-)
> hemiplegia and hemiparesis due to sequela of cerebrovascular disease (I69.05-, I69.15-, I69.25-, I69.35-, I69.85-, I69.95-)

G81.0 Flaccid hemiplegia
`5th`   **G81.01 Flaccid hemiplegia affecting right dominant side**
     G81.02 Flaccid hemiplegia affecting left dominant side
     G81.03 Flaccid hemiplegia affecting right nondominant side
     G81.04 Flaccid hemiplegia affecting left nondominant side
G81.1 Spastic hemiplegia
`5th`   **G81.11 Spastic hemiplegia affecting right dominant side**
     G81.12 Spastic hemiplegia affecting left dominant side
     G81.13 Spastic hemiplegia affecting right nondominant side
     G81.14 Spastic hemiplegia affecting left nondominant side
G81.9 Hemiplegia, unspecified
`5th`   **G81.91 Hemiplegia, unspecified affecting right dominant side**
     G81.92 Hemiplegia, unspecified affecting left dominant side
     G81.93 Hemiplegia, unspecified affecting right nondominant side
     G81.94 Hemiplegia, unspecified affecting left nondominant side

G82 PARAPLEGIA (PARAPARESIS) AND QUADRIPLEGIA (QUADRIPARESIS)
`4th`

> **Note:** This category is to be used only when the listed conditions are reported without further specification, or are stated to be old or longstanding but of unspecified cause. The category is also for use in multiple coding to identify these conditions resulting from any cause
> ***Excludes1:*** congenital cerebral palsy (G80.-)
> functional quadriplegia (R53.2)
> hysterical paralysis (F44.4)

G82.2 Paraplegia
`5th`   Paralysis of both lower limbs NOS
     Paraparesis (lower) NOS
     Paraplegia (lower) NOS
     G82.20 Paraplegia, unspecified
     G82.21 Paraplegia, complete
     G82.22 Paraplegia, incomplete
G82.5 Quadriplegia
`5th`   **G82.50 Quadriplegia, unspecified**
     G82.51 Quadriplegia, C1-C4 complete
     G82.52 Quadriplegia, C1-C4 incomplete
     G82.53 Quadriplegia, C5-C7 complete
     G82.54 Quadriplegia, C5-C7 incomplete

G83 OTHER PARALYTIC SYNDROMES
`4th`

> **GUIDELINES**
>
> Codes from subcategories, G83.1, G83.2, and G83.3, identify whether the dominant or nondominant side is affected. Should the affected side be documented, but not specified as dominant or nondominant, and the classification system does not indicate a default, code selection is as follows:
> For ambidextrous patients, the default should be dominant.
> If the left side is affected, the default is non-dominant.
> If the right side is affected, the default is dominant.
> **Note:** This category is to be used only when the listed conditions are reported without further specification, or are stated to be old or longstanding but of unspecified cause. The category is also for use in multiple coding to identify these conditions resulting from any cause.
> ***Includes:*** paralysis (complete) (incomplete), except as in G80–G82

G83.0 Diplegia of upper limbs
Diplegia (upper)
Paralysis of both upper limbs
G83.1 Monoplegia of lower limb
`5th`   Paralysis of lower limb
     Excludes1: monoplegia of lower limbs due to sequela of cerebrovascular disease (I69.04-, I69.14-, I69.24-, I69.34-, I69.84-, I69.94-)
     G83.10 Monoplegia of lower limb affecting; unspecified side
     G83.11 right dominant side
     G83.12 left dominant side
     G83.13 right nondominant side
     G83.14 left nondominant side
G83.2 Monoplegia of upper limb
`5th`   Paralysis of upper limb
     Excludes1: monoplegia of upper limbs due to sequela of cerebrovascular disease (I69.03-, I69.13-, I69.23-, I69.33-, I69.83-, I69.93-)
     G83.21 Monoplegia of upper limb affecting; right dominant side
     G83.22 left dominant side
     G83.23 right nondominant side
     G83.24 left nondominant side
G83.3 Monoplegia, unspecified
`5th`   **G83.31 Monoplegia, unspecified affecting; right dominant side**
     G83.32 left dominant side
     G83.33 right nondominant side
     G83.34 left nondominant side
G83.4 Cauda equina syndrome
Neurogenic bladder due to cauda equina syndrome
Excludes1: cord bladder NOS (G95.89)
neurogenic bladder NOS (N31.9)
G83.9 Paralytic syndrome, unspecified

(G89–G99) OTHER DISORDERS OF THE NERVOUS SYSTEM

G89 PAIN, NOT ELSEWHERE CLASSIFIED
`4th`

> **GUIDELINES**

General coding information
Codes in category G89, Pain, not elsewhere classified, may be used in conjunction with codes from other categories and chapters to provide more detail about acute or chronic pain and neoplasm-related pain, unless otherwise indicated below.

If the pain is not specified as acute or chronic, post-thoracotomy, post-procedural, or neoplasm-related, do not assign codes from category G89.

A code from category G89 should not be assigned if the underlying (definitive) diagnosis is known, unless the reason for the encounter is pain control/management and not management of the underlying condition.

When an admission or encounter is for a procedure aimed at treating the underlying condition (e.g., spinal fusion, kyphoplasty), a code for the underlying condition (e.g., vertebral fracture, spinal stenosis) should be assigned as the principal diagnosis. No code from category G89 should be assigned.

`4th` `5th` `6th` `7th` Additional Character Required   ✔ 3-character code   •=New Code   ***Excludes1***—Not coded here, do not use together
                                                                     ▲=Revised Code   ***Excludes2***—Not included here

(margin) CHAPTER 6. DISEASES OF THE NERVOUS SYSTEM   (G89.1–G90)

CATEGORY G89 CODES AS PRINCIPAL OR FIRST-LISTED DIAGNOSIS

Category G89 codes are acceptable as principal diagnosis or the first-listed code:

- When pain control or pain management is the reason for the admission/encounter. The underlying cause of the pain should be reported as an additional diagnosis, if known.
- When a patient is admitted for the insertion of a neurostimulator for pain control. When an admission or encounter is for a procedure aimed at treating the underlying condition and a neurostimulator is inserted for pain control during the same admission/encounter, a code for the underlying condition should be assigned as the principal diagnosis and the appropriate pain code should be assigned as a secondary diagnosis.

USE OF CATEGORY G89 CODES IN CONJUNCTION WITH SITE-SPECIFIC PAIN CODES

Assigning Category G89 and Site-Specific Pain Codes

Codes from category G89 may be used in conjunction with codes that identify the site of pain (including codes from Chapter 18) if the category G89 code provides additional information. For example, if the code describes the site of the pain, but does not fully describe whether the pain is acute or chronic, then both codes should be assigned.

Sequencing of Category G89 Codes with Site-Specific Pain Codes

The sequencing of category G89 codes with site-specific pain codes (including Chapter 18 codes), is dependent on the circumstances of the encounter/admission as follows:

- If the encounter is for pain control or pain management, assign the code from category G89 followed by the code identifying the specific site of pain (e.g., encounter for pain management for acute neck pain from trauma is assigned code G89.11, Acute pain due to trauma, followed by code M54.2, Cervicalgia, to identify the site of pain).
- If the encounter is for any other reason except pain control or pain management, and a related definitive diagnosis has not been established (confirmed) by the provider, assign the code for the specific site of pain first, followed by the appropriate code from category G89.

Pain due to devices, implants, and grafts

Refer to Chapter 19 for pain due to medical devices.

Postoperative Pain

The provider's documentation should be used to guide the coding of postoperative pain, as well as Section IV. Diagnostic Coding and Reporting in the Outpatient Setting (page XIX).

The default for post-thoracotomy and other postoperative pain not specified as acute or chronic is the code for the acute form.

Routine or expected postoperative pain immediately after surgery should not be coded.

- Postoperative pain not associated with a specific postoperative complication is assigned to the appropriate postoperative pain code in category G89.
- Postoperative pain associated with a specific postoperative complication (such as painful wire sutures) is assigned to the appropriate code(s) found in Chapter 19. If appropriate, use additional code(s) from category G89 to identify acute or chronic pain (G89.18 or G89.28).

Chronic Pain

Chronic pain is classified to subcategory G89.2. There is no time frame defining when pain becomes chronic pain. The provider's documentation should be used to guide use of these codes.

Neoplasm Related Pain

Code G89.3 is assigned to pain documented as being related, associated or due to cancer, primary or secondary malignancy, or tumor. This code is assigned regardless of whether the pain is acute or chronic. This code may be assigned as the principal or first-listed code when the stated reason for the admission/encounter is documented as pain control/pain management. The underlying neoplasm should be reported as an additional diagnosis.

When the reason for the admission/encounter is management of the neoplasm and the pain associated with the neoplasm is also documented, code G89.3 may be assigned as an additional diagnosis. It is not necessary to assign an additional code for the site of the pain.

Refer to Chapter 2 for instructions on the sequencing of neoplasms for all other stated reasons for the admission/encounter (except for pain control/pain management).

Chronic Pain Syndrome

Central pain syndrome (G89.0) and chronic pain syndrome (G89.4) are different than the term "chronic pain," and therefore codes should only be used when the provider has specifically documented this condition.

See Chapter 5 for pain disorders related to psychological factors

Code also related psychological factors associated with pain (F45.42)

Excludes1: generalized pain NOS (R52)
    pain disorders exclusively related to psychological factors (F45.41)
    pain NOS (R52)

Excludes2: atypical face pain (G50.1)
    headache syndromes (G44.-)
    localized pain, unspecified type — code to pain by site, such as:
    abdomen pain (R10.-)
    back pain (M54.9)
    breast pain (N64.4)
    chest pain (R07.1–R07.9)
    ear pain (H92.0-)
    eye pain (H57.1)
    headache (R51.9)
    joint pain (M25.5-)
    limb pain (M79.6-)
    lumbar region pain (M54.5-)
    painful urination (R30.9)
    pelvic and perineal pain (R10.2)
    shoulder pain (M25.51-)
    spine pain (M54.-)
    throat pain (R07.0)
    tongue pain (K14.6)
    tooth pain (K08.8)
    renal colic (N23)
    migraines (G43.-)
    myalgia (M79.1-)
    pain from prosthetic devices, implants, and grafts (T82.84, T83.84, T84.84, T85.84-)
    phantom limb syndrome with pain (G54.6)
    vulvar vestibulitis (N94.810)
    vulvodynia (N94.81-)

G89.1   Acute pain, not elsewhere classified
- `5th` **G89.11   Acute pain due to trauma**
- **G89.12   Acute post-thoracotomy pain**
    Post-thoracotomy pain NOS
- **G89.18   Other acute postprocedural pain**
    Postoperative pain NOS
    Postprocedural pain NOS

G89.2   Chronic pain, NEC
- `5th` **Excludes1:** causalgia, lower limb (G57.7-)
    causalgia, upper limb (G56.4-)
    central pain syndrome (G89.0)
    chronic pain syndrome (G89.4)
    complex regional pain syndrome II, lower limb (G57.7-)
    complex regional pain syndrome II, upper limb (G56.4-)
    neoplasm related chronic pain (G89.3)
    reflex sympathetic dystrophy (G90.5-)
- **G89.21   Chronic pain due to trauma**
- **G89.22   Chronic post-thoracotomy pain**
- **G89.28   Other chronic postprocedural pain**
    Other chronic postoperative pain

G89.3   Neoplasm related pain (acute) (chronic)
    Cancer associated pain
    Pain due to malignancy (primary) (secondary)
    Tumor associated pain

G90   DISORDERS OF AUTONOMIC NERVOUS SYSTEM
- `4th` **Excludes1:** dysfunction of the autonomic nervous system due to alcohol (G31.2)

  `4th` `5th` `6th` `7th` Additional Character Required   ✔ 3-character code   •=New Code   ▲=Revised Code   **Excludes1**—Not coded here, do not use together   **Excludes2**—Not included here

194   PEDIATRIC ICD-10-CM 2022: A MANUAL FOR PROVIDER-BASED CODING

G90.5 **Complex regional pain syndrome I (CRPS I)**
`5th`   Reflex sympathetic dystrophy
   Excludes1: causalgia of lower limb (G57.7-)
     causalgia of upper limb (G56.4-)
     complex regional pain syndrome II of lower limb (G57.7-)
     complex regional pain syndrome II of upper limb (G56.4-)
   G90.51 **Complex regional pain syndrome I of upper limb**
     `6th` **G90.511** **Complex regional pain syndrome I of; right upper limb**
       G90.512 **left upper limb**
       G90.513 **bilateral**
       G90.519 **unspecified upper limb**
   G90.52 **Complex regional pain syndrome I of lower limb**
     `6th` **G90.521** **Complex regional pain syndrome I of; right lower limb**
       G90.522 **left lower limb**
       G90.523 **bilateral**
       G90.529 **unspecified lower limb**
   G90.59 **Complex regional pain syndrome I of other specified site**
G90.8 **Other disorders of autonomic nervous system**
G90.9 **Disorder of the autonomic nervous system, unspecified**

G91 **HYDROCEPHALUS**
`4th`   *Includes:* acquired hydrocephalus
   Excludes1: Arnold-Chiari syndrome with hydrocephalus (Q07.-)
     congenital hydrocephalus (Q03.-)
     spina bifida with hydrocephalus (Q05.-)
G91.0 **Communicating hydrocephalus**
   Secondary normal pressure hydrocephalus
G91.1 **Obstructive hydrocephalus**
G91.2 **(Idiopathic) normal pressure hydrocephalus**
   Normal pressure hydrocephalus NOS
G91.3 **Post-traumatic hydrocephalus, unspecified**
G91.4 **Hydrocephalus in diseases classified elsewhere**
   Code first underlying condition, such as:
   plasminogen deficiency E88.02
   Excludes1: hydrocephalus due to congenital toxoplasmosis (P37.1)
G91.8 **Other hydrocephalus**
G91.9 **Hydrocephalus, unspecified**

▲**G92** **TOXIC ENCEPHALOPATHY**
`4th` •**G92.0** **Immune effector cell-associated neurotoxicity syndrome (ICANS)**
`5th`   **Code first** if applicable, drug induced (T36–T50) or use (T51–T65) to identify toxic agent
   Code also associated signs and symptoms, such as seizures and cerebral edema
   Code also, if applicable:
     cerebral edema (G93.6)
     unspecified convulsions (R56.9)
   •**G92.00** **ICANS, grade unspecified**
   •**G92.01** **ICANS, grade 1**
   •**G92.02** **ICANS, grade 2**
   •**G92.03** **ICANS, grade 3**
   •**G92.04** **ICANS, grade 4**
   •**G92.05** **ICANS, grade 5**
•**G92.8** **Other toxic encephalopathy**
   Toxic encephalitis
   Toxic metabolic encephalopathy
   Code first poisoning due to drug or toxin, if applicable, (T36–T65 with 5th or 6th character 1–4 or 6)
   Use Additional code for adverse effect, if applicable, to identify drug (T36–T50 with 5th or 6th character 5)
•**G92.9** **Unspecified toxic encephalopathy**
   Code first poisoning due to drug or toxin, if applicable, (T36–T65 with 5th or 6th character 1–4 or 6)
   Use Additional code for adverse effect, if applicable, to identify drug (T36–T50 with 5th or 6th character 5)

G93 **OTHER DISORDERS OF BRAIN**
`4th` **G93.0** **Cerebral cysts**
   Arachnoid cyst
   Porencephalic cyst, acquired
   Excludes1: acquired periventricular cysts of newborn (P91.1)
     congenital cerebral cysts (Q04.6)
G93.1 **Anoxic brain damage, not elsewhere classified**
   Excludes1: cerebral anoxia due to anesthesia during labor and delivery (O74.3)
     cerebral anoxia due to anesthesia during the puerperium (O89.2)
     neonatal anoxia (P84)
G93.2 **Benign intracranial hypertension**
   Pseudotumor
   Excludes1: hypertensive encephalopathy (I67.4)
     obstructive hydrocephalus (G91.1)
G93.4 **Other and unspecified encephalopathy**
`5th`   *Excludes1:* alcoholic encephalopathy (G31.2)
     encephalopathy in diseases classified elsewhere (G94)
     hypertensive encephalopathy (I67.4)
   Excludes2: toxic (metabolic) encephalopathy (G92.8)
   G93.40 **Encephalopathy, unspecified**
   G93.41 **Metabolic encephalopathy**
     Septic encephalopathy
   G93.49 **Other encephalopathy**
     Encephalopathy NEC
G93.5 **Compression of brain**
   Arnold-Chiari type 1 compression of brain
   Compression of brain (stem)
   Herniation of brain (stem)
   Excludes1: traumatic compression of brain (S06.A-)
G93.6 **Cerebral edema**
   Excludes1: cerebral edema due to birth injury (P11.0)
     traumatic cerebral edema (S06.1-)
G93.7 **Reye's syndrome**
   Code first poisoning due to salicylates, if applicable (T39.0-, with 6th character 1–4)
   Use additional code for adverse effect due to salicylates, if applicable (T39.0-, with 6th character 5)
G93.8 **Other specified disorders of brain**
`5th`   **G93.81** **Temporal sclerosis**
     Hippocampal sclerosis
     Mesial temporal sclerosis
   G93.82 **Brain death**
   G93.89 **Other specified disorders of brain**
     Post-radiation encephalopathy
G93.9 **Disorder of brain, unspecified**

G94 **OTHER DISORDERS OF BRAIN IN DISEASES CLASSIFIED ELSEWHERE**
`✔`   **Code first** underlying disease

G95 **OTHER AND UNSPECIFIED DISEASES OF SPINAL CORD**
`4th`   *Excludes2:* myelitis (G04.-)
G95.1 **Vascular myelopathies**
`5th`   *Excludes2:* intraspinal phlebitis and thrombophlebitis, except non-pyogenic (G08)
   G95.11 **Acute infarction of spinal cord (embolic) (nonembolic)**
     Anoxia of spinal cord
     Arterial thrombosis of spinal cord
   G95.19 **Other vascular myelopathies**
     Edema of spinal cord
     Hematomyelia
     Nonpyogenic intraspinal phlebitis and thrombophlebitis
     Subacute necrotic myelopathy
G95.8 **Other specified diseases of spinal cord**
`5th`   *Excludes1:* neurogenic bladder NOS (N31.9)
     neurogenic bladder due to cauda equina syndrome (G83.4)
     neuromuscular dysfunction of bladder without spinal cord lesion (N31.-)

 `4th` `5th` `6th` `7th` Additional Character Required   `✔` 3-character code

•=New Code   ▲=Revised Code

Excludes1—Not coded here, do not use together
Excludes2—Not included here

G95.89 **Other specified diseases of spinal cord**
Cord bladder NOS
Drug-induced myelopathy
Radiation-induced myelopathy
Excludes1: myelopathy NOS (G95.9)

G95.9 **Disease of spinal cord, unspecified**
Myelopathy NOS

G96 **OTHER DISORDERS OF THE CENTRAL NERVOUS SYSTEM**

G96.0 **Cerebrospinal fluid leak**
Excludes1: cerebrospinal fluid leak from spinal puncture (G97.0)
Code also, if applicable:
intracranial hypotension (G96.81-)

G96.00 **Cerebrospinal fluid leak, unspecified**
Code also, if applicable:
head injury (S00.- to S09.-)

G96.01 **Cranial cerebrospinal fluid leak, spontaneous**
Otorrhea due to spontaneous cerebrospinal fluid CSF leak
Rhinorrhea due to spontaneous cerebrospinal fluid CSF leak
Spontaneous cerebrospinal fluid leak from skull base

G96.02 **Spinal cerebrospinal fluid leak, spontaneous**
Spontaneous cerebrospinal fluid leak from spine

G96.08 **Other cranial cerebrospinal fluid leak**
Postoperative cranial cerebrospinal fluid leak
Traumatic cranial cerebrospinal fluid leak
Code also, if applicable:
head injury (S00.- to S09.-)

G96.09 **Other spinal cerebrospinal fluid leak**
Other spinal CSF leak
Postoperative spinal cerebrospinal fluid leak
Traumatic spinal cerebrospinal fluid leak
Code also, if applicable:
head injury (S00.- to S09.-)

G96.1 **Disorders of meninges, not elsewhere classified**

G96.11 **Dural tear**
Excludes1: accidental puncture or laceration of dura during a procedure (G97.41)
Code also intracranial hypotension, if applicable (G96.81-)

G96.12 **Meningeal adhesions (cerebral) (spinal)**

G96.19 **Other disorders of meninges, NEC**

G96.191 **Perineural cyst**
Cervical nerve root cyst
Lumbar nerve root cyst
Sacral nerve root cyst
Tarlov cyst
Thoracic nerve root cyst

G96.198 **Other disorders of meninges, not elsewhere classified**

G96.8 **Other specified disorders of central nervous system**

G96.81 **Intracranial hypotension**
Code also any associated diagnoses, such as:
Brachial amyotrophy (G54.5)
Cerebrospinal fluid leak from spine (G96.02)
Cranial nerve disorders in diseases classified elsewhere (G53)
Nerve root and compressions in diseases classified elsewhere (G55)
Nonpyogenic thrombosis of intracranial venous system (I67.6)
Nontraumatic intracerebral hemorrhage (I61.-)
Nontraumatic subdural hemorrhage (I62.0-)
Other and unspecified cord compression (G95.2-)
Other secondary parkinsonism (G21.8)
Reversible cerebrovascular vasoconstriction syndrome (I67.841)
Spinal cord herniation (G95.89)
Stroke (I63.-)
Syringomyelia (G95.0)

G96.810 **Intracranial hypotension, unspecified**
G96.811 **Intracranial hypotension, spontaneous**
G96.819 **Other intracranial hypotension**

G96.89 **Other specified disorders of central nervous system**

G96.9 **Disorder of central nervous system, unspecified**

G98 **OTHER DISORDERS OF NERVOUS SYSTEM NOT ELSEWHERE CLASSIFIED**
Includes: nervous system disorder NOS

G98.0 **Neurogenic arthritis, not elsewhere classified**
Nonsyphilitic neurogenic arthropathy NEC
Nonsyphilitic neurogenic spondylopathy NEC
Excludes1: spondylopathy (in):
syringomyelia and syringobulbia (G95.0)
tabes dorsalis (A52.11)

G98.8 **Other disorders of nervous system**
Nervous system disorder NOS

G99 **OTHER DISORDERS OF NERVOUS SYSTEM IN DISEASES CLASSIFIED ELSEWHERE**

G99.0 **Autonomic neuropathy in diseases classified elsewhere**
Code first underlying disease, such as:
amyloidosis (E85.-)
gout (M1A.-, M10.-)
hyperthyroidism (E05.-)
Excludes1: diabetic autonomic neuropathy (E08-E13 with .43)

G99.2 **Myelopathy in diseases classified elsewhere**
Code first underlying disease, such as:
neoplasm (C00-D49)
Excludes1: myelopathy in:
intervertebral disease (M50.0-, M51.0-)
spondylosis (M47.0-, M47.1-)

4th 5th 6th 7th Additional Character Required   ✓ 3-character code   •=New Code   ▲=Revised Code   *Excludes1*—Not coded here, do not use together   *Excludes2*—Not included here

Chapter 7. Diseases of the eye and adnexa (H00–H59)

GUIDELINES

Refer to ICD-10-CM Official Guidelines for Coding and Reporting for reporting adult glaucoma
Note: Use an external cause code following the code for the eye condition, if applicable, to identify the cause of the eye condition
Excludes2: certain conditions originating in the perinatal period (P04–P96)
   certain infectious and parasitic diseases (A00–B99)
   complications of pregnancy, childbirth and the puerperium (O00–O9A)
   congenital malformations, deformations, and chromosomal abnormalities (Q00–Q99)
   DM related eye conditions (E09.3-, E10.3-, E11.3-, E13.3-)
   endocrine, nutritional and metabolic diseases (E00–E88)
   injury (trauma) of eye and orbit (S05.-)
   injury, poisoning and certain other consequences of external causes (S00–T88)
   neoplasms (C00–D49)
   symptoms, signs and abnormal clinical and laboratory findings, not elsewhere classified (R00–R94)
   syphilis related eye disorders (A50.01, A50.3-, A51.43, A52.71)

(H00–H05) DISORDERS OF EYELID, LACRIMAL SYSTEM AND ORBIT

H00   **HORDEOLUM AND CHALAZION**
`4th`
   H00.0   **Hordeolum (externum) (internum) of eyelid**
     `5th`   **H00.01**   **Hordeolum externum**
        `6th`   Hordeolum NOS
          Stye
          H00.011   **Hordeolum externum right upper eyelid**
          H00.012   **Hordeolum externum right lower eyelid**
          H00.013   **Hordeolum externum right eye, unspecified eyelid**
          H00.014   **Hordeolum externum left upper eyelid**
          H00.015   **Hordeolum externum left lower eyelid**
          H00.016   **Hordeolum externum left eye, unspecified eyelid**
     H00.02   **Hordeolum internum**
        `6th`   Infection of meibomian gland
          H00.021   **Hordeolum internum right upper eyelid**
          H00.022   **Hordeolum internum right lower eyelid**
          H00.023   **Hordeolum internum right eye, unspecified eyelid**
          H00.024   **Hordeolum internum left upper eyelid**
          H00.025   **Hordeolum internum left lower eyelid**
          H00.026   **Hordeolum internum left eye, unspecified eyelid**
     H00.03   **Abscess of eyelid**
        `6th`   Furuncle of eyelid
          H00.031   **Abscess of right upper eyelid**
          H00.032   **Abscess of right lower eyelid**
          H00.033   **Abscess of eyelid right eye, unspecified eyelid**
          H00.034   **Abscess of left upper eyelid**
          H00.035   **Abscess of left lower eyelid**
          H00.036   **Abscess of eyelid left eye, unspecified eyelid**
   H00.1   **Chalazion**
     `5th`   Meibomian (gland) cyst
        Excludes2: infected meibomian gland (H00.02-)
        H00.11   **Chalazion right upper eyelid**
        H00.12   **Chalazion right lower eyelid**
        H00.13   **Chalazion right eye, unspecified eyelid**
        H00.14   **Chalazion left upper eyelid**
        H00.15   **Chalazion left lower eyelid**
        H00.16   **Chalazion left eye, unspecified eyelid**

H01   **OTHER INFLAMMATION OF EYELID**
`4th`
   H01.0   **Blepharitis**
     `5th`   ***Excludes1:*** blepharoconjunctivitis (H10.5-)
        H01.00   **Unspecified blepharitis**
          `6th`   **H01.001**   **Unspecified blepharitis right upper eyelid**
             H01.002   **Unspecified blepharitis right lower eyelid**

             H01.003   **Unspecified blepharitis right eye, unspecified eyelid**
             H01.004   **Unspecified blepharitis left upper eyelid**
             H01.005   **Unspecified blepharitis left lower eyelid**
             H01.006   **Unspecified blepharitis left eye, unspecified eyelid**
             H01.00A   **Unspecified blepharitis right eye, upper and lower eyelids**
             H01.00B   **Unspecified blepharitis left eye, upper and lower eyelids**
   H01.1   **Noninfectious dermatoses of eyelid**
     `5th`   **H01.11**   **Allergic dermatitis of eyelid**
        `6th`   Contact dermatitis of eyelid
          H01.111   **Allergic dermatitis of right upper eyelid**
          H01.112   **Allergic dermatitis of right lower eyelid**
          H01.113   **Allergic dermatitis of right eye, unspecified eyelid**
          H01.114   **Allergic dermatitis of left upper eyelid**
          H01.115   **Allergic dermatitis of left lower eyelid**
          H01.116   **Allergic dermatitis of left eye, unspecified eyelid**
   H01.8   **Other specified inflammations of eyelid**
   H01.9   **Unspecified inflammation of eyelid**
        Inflammation of eyelid NOS

H02   **OTHER DISORDERS OF EYELID**
`4th`   ***Excludes1:*** congenital malformations of eyelid (Q10.0–Q10.3)
   H02.4   **Ptosis of eyelid**
     `5th`   **H02.40**   **Unspecified ptosis of eyelid**
        `6th`   **H02.401**   **Unspecified ptosis of right eyelid**
          H02.402   **Unspecified ptosis of left eyelid**
          H02.403   **Unspecified ptosis of bilateral eyelids**
          H02.409   **Unspecified ptosis of unspecified eyelid**
   H02.8   **Other specified disorders of eyelid**
     `5th`   **H02.82**   **Cysts of eyelid**
        `6th`   Sebaceous cyst of eyelid
          H02.821   **Cysts of right upper eyelid**
          H02.822   **Cysts of right lower eyelid**
          H02.823   **Cysts of right eye, unspecified eyelid**
          H02.824   **Cysts of left upper eyelid**
          H02.825   **Cysts of left lower eyelid**
          H02.826   **Cysts of left eye, unspecified eyelid**
     H02.84   **Edema of eyelid**
        `6th`   Hyperemia of eyelid
          H02.841   **Edema of right upper eyelid**
          H02.842   **Edema of right lower eyelid**
          H02.843   **Edema of right eye, unspecified eyelid**
          H02.844   **Edema of left upper eyelid**
          H02.845   **Edema of left lower eyelid**
          H02.846   **Edema of left eye, unspecified eyelid**
     H02.88   **Meibomian gland dysfunction**
        `6th`   **H02.881**   **Meibomian gland dysfunction right upper eyelid**
          H02.882   **Meibomian gland dysfunction right lower eyelid**
          H02.883   **Meibomian gland dysfunction of right eye, unspecified eyelid**
          H02.884   **Meibomian gland dysfunction left upper eyelid**
          H02.885   **Meibomian gland dysfunction left lower eyelid**
          H02.886   **Meibomian gland dysfunction of left eye, unspecified eyelid**
          H02.889   **Meibomian gland dysfunction of unspecified eye, unspecified eyelid**
          H02.88A   **Meibomian gland dysfunction right eye, upper and lower eyelids**
          H02.88B   **Meibomian gland dysfunction left eye, upper and lower eyelids**
     H02.89   **Other specified disorders of eyelid**
        Hemorrhage of eyelid

`4th` `5th` `6th` `7th`   Additional Character Required   ✓   3-character code   Unspecified laterality codes were excluded here.   •=New Code   ▲=Revised Code   ***Excludes1***—Not coded here, do not use together   ***Excludes2***—Not included here

H02.9 Unspecified disorder of eyelid
Disorder of eyelid NOS

H04 DISORDERS OF LACRIMAL SYSTEM
`4th`
Excludes1: congenital malformations of lacrimal system (Q10.4-Q10.6)

H04.1 Other disorders of lacrimal gland
`5th`
    H04.12 Dry eye syndrome
    `6th`
      Tear film insufficiency, NOS
      H04.121 Dry eye syndrome of right lacrimal gland
      H04.122 Dry eye syndrome of left lacrimal gland
      H04.123 Dry eye syndrome of bilateral lacrimal glands

H04.5 Stenosis and insufficiency of lacrimal passages
`5th`
    H04.53 Neonatal obstruction of nasolacrimal duct
    `6th`
      Excludes1: congenital stenosis and stricture of lacrimal duct (Q10.5)
      H04.531 Neonatal obstruction of right nasolacrimal duct
      H04.532 Neonatal obstruction of left nasolacrimal duct
      H04.533 Neonatal obstruction of bilateral nasolacrimal duct
    H04.55 Acquired stenosis of nasolacrimal duct
    `6th`
      H04.551 Acquired stenosis of right nasolacrimal duct
      H04.552 Acquired stenosis of left nasolacrimal duct
      H04.553 Acquired stenosis of bilateral nasolacrimal duct
    H04.57 Stenosis of lacrimal sac
    `6th`
      H04.571 Stenosis of right lacrimal sac
      H04.572 Stenosis of left lacrimal sac
      H04.573 Stenosis of bilateral lacrimal sac

H04.9 Disorder of lacrimal system, unspecified

H05 DISORDERS OF ORBIT
`4th`
Excludes1: congenital malformation of orbit (Q10.7)

H05.0 Acute inflammation of orbit
`5th`
    H05.00 Unspecified acute inflammation of orbit
    H05.01 Cellulitis of orbit
    `6th`
      Abscess of orbit
      H05.011 Cellulitis of right orbit
      H05.012 Cellulitis of left orbit
      H05.013 Cellulitis of bilateral orbits
    H05.11 Granuloma of orbit
    `6th`
      Pseudotumor (inflammatory) of orbit
      H05.111 Granuloma of right orbit
      H05.112 Granuloma of left orbit
      H05.113 Granuloma of bilateral orbits

(H10–H11) DISORDERS OF CONJUNCTIVA

H10 CONJUNCTIVITIS
`4th`
Excludes1: keratoconjunctivitis (H16.2-)

H10.0 Mucopurulent conjunctivitis
`5th`
    H10.01 Acute follicular conjunctivitis
    `6th`
      H10.011 Acute follicular conjunctivitis, right eye
      H10.012 Acute follicular conjunctivitis, left eye
      H10.013 Acute follicular conjunctivitis, bilateral
    H10.02 Other mucopurulent conjunctivitis
    `6th`
      H10.021 Other mucopurulent conjunctivitis, right eye
      H10.022 Other mucopurulent conjunctivitis, left eye
      H10.023 Other mucopurulent conjunctivitis, bilateral

H10.1 Acute atopic conjunctivitis
`5th`
    Acute papillary conjunctivitis
    H10.11 Acute atopic conjunctivitis, right eye
    H10.12 Acute atopic conjunctivitis, left eye
    H10.13 Acute atopic conjunctivitis, bilateral

H10.2 Other acute conjunctivitis
`5th`
    H10.21 Acute toxic conjunctivitis
    `6th`
      Acute chemical conjunctivitis
      Code first (T51–T65) to identify chemical and intent
      Excludes1: burn and corrosion of eye and adnexa (T26.-)

      H10.211 Acute toxic conjunctivitis, right eye
      H10.212 Acute toxic conjunctivitis, left eye
      H10.213 Acute toxic conjunctivitis, bilateral
    H10.22 Pseudomembranous conjunctivitis
    `6th`
      H10.221 Pseudomembranous conjunctivitis, right eye
      H10.222 Pseudomembranous conjunctivitis, left eye
      H10.223 Pseudomembranous conjunctivitis, bilateral
    H10.23 Serous conjunctivitis, except viral
    `6th`
      Excludes1: viral conjunctivitis (B30.-)
      H10.231 Serous conjunctivitis, except viral, right eye
      H10.232 Serous conjunctivitis, except viral, left eye
      H10.233 Serous conjunctivitis, except viral, bilateral
      H10.239 Serous conjunctivitis, except viral, unspecified eye

H10.3 Unspecified acute conjunctivitis
`5th`
    Excludes1: ophthalmia neonatorum NOS (P39.1)
    H10.31 Unspecified acute conjunctivitis, right eye
    H10.32 Unspecified acute conjunctivitis, left eye
    H10.33 Unspecified acute conjunctivitis, bilateral

H10.5 Blepharoconjunctivitis
`5th`
    H10.50 Unspecified blepharoconjunctivitis
    `6th`
      H10.501 Unspecified blepharoconjunctivitis, right eye
      H10.502 Unspecified blepharoconjunctivitis, left eye
      H10.503 Unspecified blepharoconjunctivitis, bilateral

H10.8 Other conjunctivitis
`5th`
    H10.82 Rosacea conjunctivitis
    `6th`
      Code first underlying rosacea dermatitis (L71.-)
      H10.821 Rosacea conjunctivitis, right eye
      H10.822 Rosacea conjunctivitis, left eye
      H10.823 Rosacea conjunctivitis, bilateral

H10.9 Unspecified conjunctivitis

H11 OTHER DISORDERS OF CONJUNCTIVA
`4th`
Excludes1: keratoconjunctivitis (H16.2-)

H11.3 Conjunctival hemorrhage
`5th`
    Subconjunctival hemorrhage
    H11.31 Conjunctival hemorrhage, right eye
    H11.32 Conjunctival hemorrhage, left eye
    H11.33 Conjunctival hemorrhage, bilateral

H11.4 Other conjunctival vascular disorders and cysts
`5th`
    H11.42 Conjunctival edema
    `6th`
      H11.421 Conjunctival edema, right eye
      H11.422 Conjunctival edema, left eye
      H11.423 Conjunctival edema, bilateral

H11.9 Unspecified disorder of conjunctiva

(H15–H22) DISORDERS OF SCLERA, CORNEA, IRIS AND CILIARY BODY

H16 KERATITIS
`4th`
H16.2 Keratoconjunctivitis
`5th`
    H16.20 Unspecified keratoconjunctivitis
    `6th`
      Superficial keratitis with conjunctivitis NOS
      H16.201 Unspecified keratoconjunctivitis, right eye
      H16.202 Unspecified keratoconjunctivitis, left eye
      H16.203 Unspecified keratoconjunctivitis, bilateral

H16.9 Unspecified keratitis

H18 OTHER DISORDERS OF CORNEA
`4th`
H18.5 Hereditary corneal dystrophies
`5th`
    H18.50 Unspecified hereditary corneal dystrophies
    `6th`
      H18.501 Unspecified hereditary corneal dystrophies, right eye
      H18.502 Unspecified hereditary corneal dystrophies, left eye

---

`4th` `5th` `6th` `7th` Additional Character Required   ✓ 3-character code

Unspecified laterality codes were excluded here.   *=New Code   ▲=Revised Code   ***Excludes1***—Not coded here, do not use together   ***Excludes2***—Not included here

H18.503   **Unspecified hereditary corneal dystrophies, bilateral**

H18.51   **Endothelial corneal dystrophy**
`6th`   Fuchs' dystrophy

H18.511   **Endothelial corneal dystrophy, right eye**
H18.512   **Endothelial corneal dystrophy, left eye**
H18.513   **Endothelial corneal dystrophy, bilateral**

H18.52   **Epithelial (juvenile) corneal dystrophy**
`6th`
H18.521   **Epithelial (juvenile) corneal dystrophy, right eye**
H18.522   **Epithelial (juvenile) corneal dystrophy, left eye**
H18.523   **Epithelial (juvenile) corneal dystrophy, bilateral**

H18.59   **Other hereditary corneal dystrophies**
`6th`
H18.591   **Other hereditary corneal dystrophies, right eye**
H18.592   **Other hereditary corneal dystrophies, left eye**
H18.593   **Other hereditary corneal dystrophies, bilateral**

H18.79   **Other corneal deformities**
`6th`
H18.791   **Other corneal deformities, right eye**
H18.792   **Other corneal deformities, left eye**
H18.793   **Other corneal deformities, bilateral**

H18.8   **Other specified disorders of cornea**
`5th`
H18.82   **Corneal disorder due to contact lens**
`6th`   *Excludes2:* corneal edema due to contact lens (H18.21-)

H18.821   **Corneal disorder due to contact lens, right eye**
H18.822   **Corneal disorder due to contact lens, left eye**
H18.823   **Corneal disorder due to contact lens, bilateral**

H18.9   **Unspecified disorder of cornea**

(H25–H28) DISORDERS OF LENS

H26   **OTHER CATARACT**
`4th`   *Excludes1:* congenital cataract (Q12.0)

H26.0   **Infantile and juvenile cataract**
`5th`
H26.00   **Unspecified infantile and juvenile cataract**
`6th`
H26.001   **Unspecified infantile and juvenile cataract, right eye**
H26.002   **Unspecified infantile and juvenile cataract, left eye**
H26.003   **Unspecified infantile and juvenile cataract, bilateral**

H26.01   **Infantile and juvenile cortical, lamellar, or zonular cataract**
`6th`
H26.011   **Infantile and juvenile cortical, lamellar, or zonular cataract, right eye**
H26.012   **Infantile and juvenile cortical, lamellar, or zonular cataract, left eye**
H26.013   **Infantile and juvenile cortical, lamellar, or zonular cataract, bilateral**

H26.03   **Infantile and juvenile nuclear cataract**
`6th`
H26.031   **Infantile and juvenile nuclear cataract, right eye**
H26.032   **Infantile and juvenile nuclear cataract, left eye**
H26.033   **Infantile and juvenile nuclear cataract, bilateral**

H26.04   **Anterior subcapsular polar infantile and juvenile cataract**
`6th`
H26.041   **Anterior subcapsular polar infantile and juvenile cataract, right eye**
H26.042   **Anterior subcapsular polar infantile and juvenile cataract, left eye**
H26.043   **Anterior subcapsular polar infantile and juvenile cataract, bilateral**

H26.05   **Posterior subcapsular polar infantile and juvenile cataract**
`6th`

H26.051   **Posterior subcapsular polar infantile and juvenile cataract, right eye**
H26.052   **Posterior subcapsular polar infantile and juvenile cataract, left eye**
H26.053   **Posterior subcapsular polar infantile and juvenile cataract, bilateral**

H26.06   **Combined forms of infantile and juvenile cataract**
`6th`
H26.061   **Combined forms of infantile and juvenile cataract, right eye**
H26.062   **Combined forms of infantile and juvenile cataract, left eye**
H26.063   **Combined forms of infantile and juvenile cataract, bilateral**

H26.09   **Other infantile and juvenile cataract**

H26.9   **Unspecified cataract**

H27   **OTHER DISORDERS OF LENS**
`4th`   *Excludes1:* congenital lens malformations (Q12.-)
    mechanical complications of intraocular lens implant (T85.2)
    pseudophakia (Z96.1)

H27.0   **Aphakia**
`5th`   Acquired absence of lens
    Acquired aphakia
    Aphakia due to trauma
    Excludes1: cataract extraction status (Z98.4-)
      congenital absence of lens (Q12.3)
      congenital aphakia (Q12.3)

H27.01   **Aphakia, right eye**
H27.02   **Aphakia, left eye**
H27.03   **Aphakia, bilateral**

H27.1   **Dislocation of lens**
`5th`
H27.10   **Unspecified dislocation of lens**
H27.11   **Subluxation of lens**
`6th`
H27.111   **Subluxation of lens, right eye**
H27.112   **Subluxation of lens, left eye**
H27.113   **Subluxation of lens, bilateral**

H27.12   **Anterior dislocation of lens**
`6th`
H27.121   **Anterior dislocation of lens, right eye**
H27.122   **Anterior dislocation of lens, left eye**
H27.123   **Anterior dislocation of lens, bilateral**

H27.13   **Posterior dislocation of lens**
`6th`
H27.131   **Posterior dislocation of lens, right eye**
H27.132   **Posterior dislocation of lens, left eye**
H27.133   **Posterior dislocation of lens, bilateral**

H27.8   **Other specified disorders of lens**
H27.9   **Unspecified disorder of lens**

H28   **CATARACT IN DISEASES CLASSIFIED ELSEWHERE**
`✔`   **Code first** underlying disease, such as:
    hypoparathyroidism (E20.-)
    myotonia (G71.1-)
    myxedema (E03.-)
    protein-calorie malnutrition (E40-E46)
    Excludes1: cataract in diabetes mellitus

(H30–H36) DISORDERS OF CHOROID AND RETINA

H32   **CHORIORETINAL DISORDERS IN DISEASES CLASSIFIED ELSEWHERE**
`✔`   **Code first** underlying disease, such as:
    congenital toxoplasmosis (P37.1)
    histoplasmosis (B39.-)
    leprosy (A30.-)
    Excludes1: chorioretinitis (in):
    toxoplasmosis (acquired) (B58.01)
    tuberculosis (A18.53)

H35   **OTHER RETINAL DISORDERS**
`4th`   *Excludes2:* diabetic retinal disorders (E08.311–E08.359, E09.311–E09.359, E10.311–E10.359, E11.311–E11.359, E13.311–E13.359)

H35.1   **Retinopathy of prematurity [ROP]**
`5th`
H35.10   **Retinopathy of prematurity, unspecified**
`6th`   Retinopathy of prematurity NOS
H35.101   **ROP, unspecified, right eye**

`4th` `5th` `6th` `7th`   Additional Character Required   `✔`   3-character code   Unspecified laterality codes were excluded here.   •=New Code   ▲=Revised Code   *Excludes1*—Not coded here, do not use together   *Excludes2*—Not included here

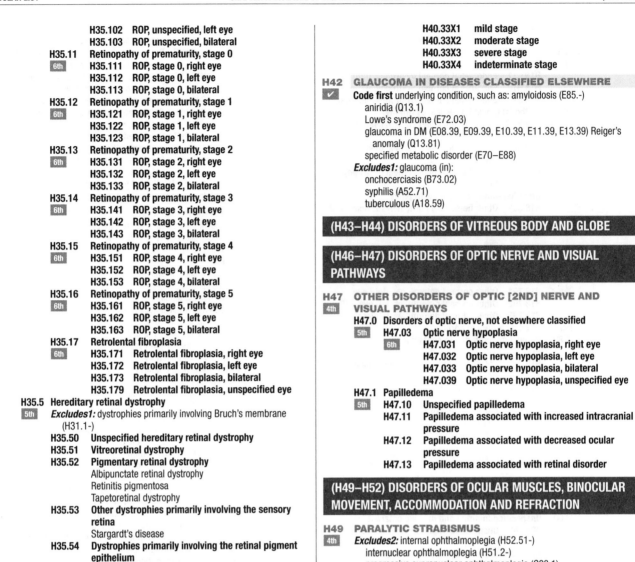

	H35.102	ROP, unspecified, left eye	
	H35.103	ROP, unspecified, bilateral	

H35.11 Retinopathy of prematurity, stage 0
- H35.111   ROP, stage 0, right eye
- H35.112   ROP, stage 0, left eye
- H35.113   ROP, stage 0, bilateral

H35.12 Retinopathy of prematurity, stage 1
- H35.121   ROP, stage 1, right eye
- H35.122   ROP, stage 1, left eye
- H35.123   ROP, stage 1, bilateral

H35.13 Retinopathy of prematurity, stage 2
- H35.131   ROP, stage 2, right eye
- H35.132   ROP, stage 2, left eye
- H35.133   ROP, stage 2, bilateral

H35.14 Retinopathy of prematurity, stage 3
- H35.141   ROP, stage 3, right eye
- H35.142   ROP, stage 3, left eye
- H35.143   ROP, stage 3, bilateral

H35.15 Retinopathy of prematurity, stage 4
- H35.151   ROP, stage 4, right eye
- H35.152   ROP, stage 4, left eye
- H35.153   ROP, stage 4, bilateral

H35.16 Retinopathy of prematurity, stage 5
- H35.161   ROP, stage 5, right eye
- H35.162   ROP, stage 5, left eye
- H35.163   ROP, stage 5, bilateral

H35.17 Retrolental fibroplasia
- H35.171   Retrolental fibroplasia, right eye
- H35.172   Retrolental fibroplasia, left eye
- H35.173   Retrolental fibroplasia, bilateral
- H35.179   Retrolental fibroplasia, unspecified eye

H35.5 Hereditary retinal dystrophy
Excludes1: dystrophies primarily involving Bruch's membrane (H31.1-)

H35.50 Unspecified hereditary retinal dystrophy

H35.51 Vitreoretinal dystrophy

H35.52 Pigmentary retinal dystrophy
Albipunctate retinal dystrophy
Retinitis pigmentosa
Tapetoretinal dystrophy

H35.53 Other dystrophies primarily involving the sensory retina
Stargardt's disease

H35.54 Dystrophies primarily involving the retinal pigment epithelium
Vitelliform retinal dystrophy

(H40–H42) GLAUCOMA

H40   GLAUCOMA
Excludes1: absolute glaucoma (H44.51-)
congenital glaucoma (Q15.0)
traumatic glaucoma due to birth injury (P15.3)

H40.3 Glaucoma secondary to eye trauma
Code also underlying condition

H40.31X Glaucoma secondary to eye trauma, right eye
- H40.31X0   Glaucoma secondary to eye trauma, right eye; stage unspecified
- H40.31X1   mild stage
- H40.31X2   moderate stage
- H40.31X3   severe stage
- H40.31X4   indeterminate stage

H40.32X Glaucoma secondary to eye trauma, left eye
- H40.32X0   Glaucoma secondary to eye trauma, left eye; stage unspecified
- H40.32X1   mild stage
- H40.32X2   moderate stage
- H40.32X3   severe stage
- H40.32X4   indeterminate stage

H40.33X Glaucoma secondary to eye trauma, bilateral
- H40.33X0   Glaucoma secondary to eye trauma, bilateral; stage unspecified

- H40.33X1   mild stage
- H40.33X2   moderate stage
- H40.33X3   severe stage
- H40.33X4   indeterminate stage

H42   GLAUCOMA IN DISEASES CLASSIFIED ELSEWHERE
✔   **Code first** underlying condition, such as: amyloidosis (E85.-)
aniridia (Q13.1)
Lowe's syndrome (E72.03)
glaucoma in DM (E08.39, E09.39, E10.39, E11.39, E13.39) Reiger's anomaly (Q13.81)
specified metabolic disorder (E70–E88)
Excludes1: glaucoma (in):
onchocerciasis (B73.02)
syphilis (A52.71)
tuberculous (A18.59)

(H43–H44) DISORDERS OF VITREOUS BODY AND GLOBE

(H46–H47) DISORDERS OF OPTIC NERVE AND VISUAL PATHWAYS

H47   OTHER DISORDERS OF OPTIC [2ND] NERVE AND VISUAL PATHWAYS

H47.0 Disorders of optic nerve, not elsewhere classified

H47.03 Optic nerve hypoplasia
- H47.031   Optic nerve hypoplasia, right eye
- H47.032   Optic nerve hypoplasia, left eye
- H47.033   Optic nerve hypoplasia, bilateral
- H47.039   Optic nerve hypoplasia, unspecified eye

H47.1 Papilledema
- **H47.10**   Unspecified papilledema
- **H47.11**   Papilledema associated with increased intracranial pressure
- **H47.12**   Papilledema associated with decreased ocular pressure
- **H47.13**   Papilledema associated with retinal disorder

(H49–H52) DISORDERS OF OCULAR MUSCLES, BINOCULAR MOVEMENT, ACCOMMODATION AND REFRACTION

H49   PARALYTIC STRABISMUS
Excludes2: internal ophthalmoplegia (H52.51-)
internuclear ophthalmoplegia (H51.2-)
progressive supranuclear ophthalmoplegia (G23.1)

H49.0 Third [oculomotor] nerve palsy
- **H49.00**   Third [oculomotor] nerve palsy, unspecified eye
- **H49.01**   Third [oculomotor] nerve palsy, right eye
- **H49.02**   Third [oculomotor] nerve palsy, left eye
- **H49.03**   Third [oculomotor] nerve palsy, bilateral

H49.1 Fourth [trochlear] nerve palsy
- **H49.11**   Fourth [trochlear] nerve palsy, right eye
- **H49.12**   Fourth [trochlear] nerve palsy, left eye
- **H49.13**   Fourth [trochlear] nerve palsy, bilateral

H49.2 Sixth [abducent] nerve palsy
- **H49.21**   Sixth [abducent] nerve palsy, right eye
- **H49.22**   Sixth [abducent] nerve palsy, left eye
- **H49.23**   Sixth [abducent] nerve palsy, bilateral

H49.3 Total (external) ophthalmoplegia
- **H49.31**   Total (external) ophthalmoplegia, right eye
- **H49.32**   Total (external) ophthalmoplegia, left eye
- **H49.33**   Total (external) ophthalmoplegia, bilateral

H49.4 Progressive external ophthalmoplegia
Excludes1: Kearns-Sayre syndrome (H49.81-)
- **H49.41**   Progressive external ophthalmoplegia, right eye
- **H49.42**   Progressive external ophthalmoplegia, left eye
- **H49.43**   Progressive external ophthalmoplegia, bilateral

H49.8 Other paralytic strabismus
- **H49.81**   Kearns-Sayre syndrome
Progressive external ophthalmoplegia with pigmentary retinopathy
Use additional code for other manifestation, such as: heart block (I45.9)

4th 5th 6th 7th   Additional Character Required   ✔   3-character code   Unspecified laterality codes were excluded here.   •=New Code   ▲=Revised Code   *Excludes1*—Not coded here, do not use together   *Excludes2*—Not included here

H49.811 Kearns-Sayre syndrome, right eye
H49.812 Kearns-Sayre syndrome, left eye
H49.813 Kearns-Sayre syndrome, bilateral
H49.88 Other paralytic strabismus
6th   External ophthalmoplegia NOS
H49.881 Other paralytic strabismus, right eye
H49.882 Other paralytic strabismus, left eye
H49.883 Other paralytic strabismus, bilateral
H49.9 Unspecified paralytic strabismus

H50   **OTHER STRABISMUS**
4th
H50.0 Esotropia
5th   Convergent concomitant strabismus
Excludes1: intermittent esotropia (H50.31-, H50.32)
H50.00 Unspecified esotropia
H50.01 Monocular esotropia
6th   **H50.011** Monocular esotropia, right eye
H50.012 Monocular esotropia, left eye
H50.02 Monocular esotropia with A pattern
6th   **H50.021** Monocular esotropia with A pattern, right eye
H50.022 Monocular esotropia with A pattern, left eye
H50.03 Monocular esotropia with V pattern
6th   **H50.031** Monocular esotropia with V pattern, right eye
H50.032 Monocular esotropia with V pattern, left eye
H50.04 Monocular esotropia with other noncomitancies
6th   **H50.041** Monocular esotropia with other noncomitancies, right eye
H50.042 Monocular esotropia with other noncomitancies, left eye
H50.05 Alternating esotropia
H50.06 Alternating esotropia with A pattern
H50.07 Alternating esotropia with V pattern
H50.08 Alternating esotropia with other noncomitancies
H50.1 Exotropia
5th   Divergent concomitant strabismus
Excludes1: intermittent exotropia (H50.33-, H50.34)
H50.10 Unspecified exotropia
H50.11 Monocular exotropia
6th   **H50.111** Monocular exotropia, right eye
H50.112 Monocular exotropia, left eye
H50.12 Monocular exotropia with A pattern
6th   **H50.121** Monocular exotropia with A pattern, right eye
H50.122 Monocular exotropia with A pattern, left eye
H50.13 Monocular exotropia with V pattern
6th   **H50.131** Monocular exotropia with V pattern, right eye
H50.132 Monocular exotropia with V pattern, left eye
H50.14 Monocular exotropia with other noncomitancies
6th   **H50.141** Monocular exotropia with other noncomitancies, right eye
H50.142 Monocular exotropia with other noncomitancies, left eye
H50.15 Alternating exotropia
H50.16 Alternating exotropia with A pattern
H50.17 Alternating exotropia with V pattern
H50.18 Alternating exotropia with other noncomitancies
H50.2 Vertical strabismus
5th   Hypertropia
H50.21 Vertical strabismus, right eye
H50.22 Vertical strabismus, left eye
H50.3 Intermittent heterotropia
5th   **H50.30** Unspecified intermittent heterotropia
H50.31 Intermittent monocular esotropia
6th   **H50.311** Intermittent monocular esotropia, right eye
H50.312 Intermittent monocular esotropia, left eye

H50.32 Intermittent alternating esotropia
H50.33 Intermittent monocular exotropia
6th   **H50.331** Intermittent monocular exotropia, right eye
H50.332 Intermittent monocular exotropia, left eye
H50.34 Intermittent alternating exotropia
H50.4 Other and unspecified heterotropia
5th   **H50.40** Unspecified heterotropia
H50.41 Cyclotropia
6th   **H50.411** Cyclotropia, right eye
H50.412 Cyclotropia, left eye
H50.42 Monofixation syndrome
H50.43 Accommodative component in esotropia
H50.5 Heterophoria
5th   **H50.50** Unspecified heterophoria
H50.51 Esophoria
H50.52 Exophoria
H50.53 Vertical heterophoria
H50.54 Cyclophoria
H50.55 Alternating heterophoria
H50.6 Mechanical strabismus
5th   **H50.60** Mechanical strabismus, unspecified
H50.61 Brown's sheath syndrome
6th   **H50.611** Brown's sheath syndrome, right eye
H50.612 Brown's sheath syndrome, left eye
H50.69 Other mechanical strabismus
     Strabismus due to adhesions
     Traumatic limitation of duction of eye muscle
H50.8 Other specified strabismus
5th   **H50.81** Duane's syndrome
6th   **H50.811** Duane's syndrome, right eye
H50.812 Duane's syndrome, left eye
H50.89 Other specified strabismus
H50.9 Unspecified strabismus

H51   **OTHER DISORDERS OF BINOCULAR MOVEMENT**
4th
H51.0 Palsy (spasm) of conjugate gaze
H51.8 Other specified disorders of binocular movement
H51.9 Unspecified disorder of binocular movement

H52   **DISORDERS OF REFRACTION AND ACCOMMODATION**
4th
H52.0 Hypermetropia
5th   **H52.01** Hypermetropia, right eye
H52.02 Hypermetropia, left eye
H52.03 Hypermetropia, bilateral
H52.1 Myopia
5th   *Excludes1:* degenerative myopia (H44.2-)
H52.11 Myopia, right eye
H52.12 Myopia, left eye
H52.13 Myopia, bilateral
H52.2 Astigmatism
5th   **H52.20** Unspecified astigmatism
6th   **H52.201** Unspecified astigmatism, right eye
H52.202 Unspecified astigmatism, left eye
H52.203 Unspecified astigmatism, bilateral
H52.21 Irregular astigmatism
6th   **H52.211** Irregular astigmatism, right eye
H52.212 Irregular astigmatism, left eye
H52.213 Irregular astigmatism, bilateral
H52.22 Regular astigmatism
6th   **H52.221** Regular astigmatism, right eye
H52.222 Regular astigmatism, left eye
H52.223 Regular astigmatism, bilateral
H52.3 Anisometropia and aniseikonia
5th   **H52.31** Anisometropia
H52.32 Aniseikonia
H52.4 Presbyopia
H52.5 Disorders of accommodation
5th   **H52.51** Internal ophthalmoplegia (complete) (total)
6th   **H52.511** right eye
H52.512 left eye
H52.513 bilateral
H52.52 Paresis of accommodation
6th   **H52.521** Paresis of accommodation, right eye

CHAPTER 7. DISEASES OF THE EYE AND ADNEXA   (H52.522–H54.42A3)

H52.522	Paresis of accommodation, left eye
H52.523	Paresis of accommodation, bilateral

H52.53   Spasm of accommodation   [6th]
- H52.531   Spasm of accommodation, right eye
- H52.532   Spasm of accommodation, left eye
- H52.533   Spasm of accommodation, bilateral

H52.6   Other disorders of refraction

H52.7   Unspecified disorder of refraction

(H53–H54) VISUAL DISTURBANCES AND BLINDNESS

H53 [4th]   **VISUAL DISTURBANCES**

H53.0   Amblyopia ex anopsia   [5th]
> *Excludes1:* amblyopia due to vitamin A deficiency (E50.5)

H53.00   Unspecified amblyopia   [6th]
- H53.001   Unspecified amblyopia, right eye
- H53.002   Unspecified amblyopia, left eye
- H53.003   Unspecified amblyopia, bilateral

H53.01   Deprivation amblyopia   [6th]
- H53.011   Deprivation amblyopia, right eye
- H53.012   Deprivation amblyopia, left eye
- H53.013   Deprivation amblyopia, bilateral

H53.02   Refractive amblyopia   [6th]
- H53.021   Refractive amblyopia, right eye
- H53.022   Refractive amblyopia, left eye
- H53.023   Refractive amblyopia, bilateral

H53.04   Amblyopia suspect   [6th]
- H53.041   Amblyopia suspect, right eye
- H53.042   Amblyopia suspect, left eye
- H53.043   Amblyopia suspect, bilateral eye

H53.2   Diplopia
> Double vision

H53.3   Other and unspecified disorders of binocular vision   [5th]
- H53.30   Unspecified disorder of binocular vision
- H53.31   Abnormal retinal correspondence

H53.8   Other visual disturbances

H53.9   Unspecified visual disturbance

H54 [4th]   **BLINDNESS AND LOW VISION**

> **GUIDELINES**
>
> If "blindness" or "low vision" of both eyes is documented but the visual impairment category is not documented, assign code H54.3, Unqualified visual loss, both eyes. If "blindness" or "low vision" in one eye is documented but the visual impairment category is not documented, assign a code from H54.6-, Unqualified visual loss, one eye. If "blindness" or "visual loss" is documented without any information about whether one or both eyes are affected, assign code H54.7, Unspecified visual loss. **Note:** For definition of visual impairment categories see table below
> **Code first** any associated underlying cause of the blindness
> *Excludes1:* amaurosis fugax (G45.3)

H54.0   Blindness, both eyes   [5th]
> Visual impairment categories 3, 4, 5 in both eyes.

H54.0X   Blindness, both eyes, different category levels   [6th]

H54.0X3   Blindness right eye, category 3   [7th]
- H54.0X33   Blindness right eye category 3, blindness left eye category 3
- H54.0X34   Blindness right eye category 3, blindness left eye category 4
- H54.0X35   Blindness right eye category 3, blindness left eye category 5

H54.0X4   Blindness right eye, category 4   [7th]
- H54.0X43   Blindness right eye category 4, blindness left eye category 3
- H54.0X44   Blindness right eye category 4, blindness left eye category 4
- H54.0X45   Blindness right eye category 4, blindness left eye category 5

H54.0X5   Blindness right eye, category 5   [7th]
- H54.0X53   Blindness right eye category 5, blindness left eye category 3
- H54.0X54   Blindness right eye category 5, blindness left eye category 4
- H54.0X55   Blindness right eye category 5, blindness left eye category 5

H54.1   Blindness, one eye, low vision other eye   [5th]
> Visual impairment categories 3, 4, 5 in one eye, with categories 1 or 2 in the other eye.

H54.11   Blindness, right eye, low vision left eye   [6th]

H54.113   Blindness right eye category 3, low vision left eye   [7th]
- H54.1131   Blindness right eye category 3, low vision left eye category 1
- H54.1132   Blindness right eye category 3, low vision left eye category 2

H54.114   Blindness right eye category 4, low vision left eye   [7th]
- H54.1141   Blindness right eye category 4, low vision left eye category 1
- H54.1142   Blindness right eye category 4, low vision left eye category 2

H54.115   Blindness right eye category 5, low vision left eye   [7th]
- H54.1151   Blindness right eye category 5, low vision left eye category 1
- H54.1152   Blindness right eye category 5, low vision left eye category 2

H54.12   Blindness, left eye, low vision right eye   [6th]

H54.121   Low vision right eye category 1, blindness left eye   [7th]
- H54.1213   Low vision right eye category 1, blindness left eye category 3
- H54.1214   Low vision right eye category 1, blindness left eye category 4
- H54.1215   Low vision right eye category 1, blindness left eye category 5

H54.122   Low vision right eye category 2, blindness left eye   [7th]
- H54.1223   Low vision right eye category 2, blindness left eye category 3
- H54.1224   Low vision right eye category 2, blindness left eye category 4
- H54.1225   Low vision right eye category 2, blindness left eye category 5

H54.2   Low vision, both eyes   [5th]
> Visual impairment categories 1 or 2 in both eyes.

H54.2X   Low vision, both eyes, different category levels   [6th]

H54.2X1   Low vision, right eye, category 1   [7th]
- H54.2X11   Low vision right eye category 1, low vision left eye category 1
- H54.2X12   Low vision right eye category 1, low vision left eye category 2

H54.2X2   Low vision, right eye, category 2   [7th]
- H54.2X21   Low vision right eye category 2, low vision left eye category 1
- H54.2X22   Low vision right eye category 2, low vision left eye category 2

H54.3   Unqualified visual loss, both eyes
> Visual impairment category 9 in both eyes.

H54.4   Blindness, one eye   [5th]
> Visual impairment categories 3, 4, 5 in one eye [normal vision in other eye].

H54.41   Blindness, right eye, normal vision left eye   [6th]

H54.413   Blindness, right eye, category 3   [7th]
- H54.413A   Blindness right eye category 3, normal vision left eye

H54.414   Blindness, right eye, category 4   [7th]
- H54.414A   Blindness right eye category 4, normal vision left eye

H54.415   Blindness, right eye, category 5   [7th]
- H54.415A   Blindness right eye category 5, normal vision left eye

H54.42   Blindness, left eye, normal vision right eye   [6th]

H54.42A   Blindness, left eye, category 3-5   [7th]
- H54.42A3   Blindness left eye category 3, normal vision right eye

---

[4th] [5th] [6th] [7th] Additional Character Required   ✓ 3-character code

Unspecified laterality codes were excluded here.   •=New Code   ▲=Revised Code   ***Excludes1***—Not coded here, do not use together   ***Excludes2***—Not included here

| | H54.42A4 | **Blindness left eye category 4, normal vision right eye** |
| | H54.42A5 | **Blindness left eye category 5, normal vision right eye** |

H54.5 **Low vision, one eye**

`5th` Visual impairment categories 1 or 2 in one eye [normal vision in other eye].

     H54.51   **Low vision, right eye, normal vision left eye**

       `6th`   H54.511   **Low vision, right eye, category 1-2**

          `7th`   H54.511A   **Low vision right eye category 1, normal vision left eye**

              H54.512A   **Low vision right eye category 2, normal vision left eye**

     H54.52   **Low vision, left eye, normal vision right eye**

       `6th`   H54.52A   **Low vision, left eye, category 1-2**

          `7th`   H54.52A1   **Low vision left eye category 1, normal vision right eye**

              H54.52A2   **Low vision left eye category 2, normal vision right eye**

H54.6 **Unqualified visual loss, one eye**

`5th` Visual impairment category 9 in one eye [normal vision in other eye].

     H54.61   **Unqualified visual loss, right eye, normal vision left eye**

     H54.62   **Unqualified visual loss, left eye, normal vision right eye**

H54.7 **Unspecified visual loss**

     Visual impairment category 9 NOS

H54.8 **Legal blindness, as defined in USA**

     Blindness NOS according to USA definition

     Excludes1: legal blindness with specification of impairment level (H54.0–H54.7)

     Note: The term 'low vision' in category H54 comprises categories 1 and 2 of the table, the term 'blindness' categories 3, 4, and 5, and the term 'unqualified visual loss' category 9.

     If the extent of the visual field is taken into account, patients with a field no greater than 10 but greater than 5 around central fixation should be placed in category 3 and patients with a field no greater than 5 around central fixation should be placed in category 4, even if the central acuity is not impaired.

Category of visual impairment	Visual acuity with best possible correction	
	Maximum less than:	**Minimum equal to or better than:**
	6/18	6/60
3/10 (0.3)	1/10 (0.1)	
20/70	20/200	
	6/60	3/60
1/10 (0.1)	1/20 (0.05)	
20/200	20/400	
	3/60	1/60 (finger counting at one meter)
1/20 (0.05)	1/50 (0.02)	
20/400	5/300 (20/1200)	
	1/60 (finer counting at one meter)	Light perception
1/50 (0.02)		
5/300		
	No light perception	
	Undetermined or unspecified	

(H55–H57) OTHER DISORDERS OF EYE AND ADNEXA

H55   **NYSTAGMUS AND OTHER IRREGULAR EYE MOVEMENTS**

`4th`   **H55.0**   **Nystagmus**

     `5th`   H55.00   **Unspecified nystagmus**

         H55.01   **Congenital nystagmus**

         H55.02   **Latent nystagmus**

         H55.03   **Visual deprivation nystagmus**

         H55.04   **Dissociated nystagmus**

         H55.09   **Other forms of nystagmus**

H57   **OTHER DISORDERS OF EYE AND ADNEXA**

`4th`   **H57.0**   **Anomalies of pupillary function**

     `5th`   H57.00   **Unspecified anomaly of pupillary function**

           Excludes1: syphilitic Argyll Robertson pupil (A52.19)

         H57.02   **Anisocoria**

         H57.09   **Other anomalies of pupillary function**

     H57.1   **Ocular pain**

     `5th`   H57.11   **Ocular pain, right eye**

         H57.12   **Ocular pain, left eye**

         H57.13   **Ocular pain, bilateral**

     H57.8   **Other specified disorders of eye and adnexa**

     `5th`   H57.81   **Brow ptosis acquired**

       `6th`   H57.811   **Brow ptosis, right**

              H57.812   **Brow ptosis, left**

              H57.813   **Brow ptosis, bilateral**

              H57.819   **Brow ptosis, unspecified**

         H57.89   **Other specified disorders of eye and adnexa**

     H57.9   **Unspecified disorder of eye and adnexa**

(H59) INTRAOPERATIVE AND POSTPROCEDURAL COMPLICATIONS AND DISORDERS OF EYE AND ADNEXA, NOT ELSEWHERE CLASSIFIED

CHAPTER 7. DISEASES OF THE EYE AND ADNEXA   (H54.42A4–H59)

`4th` `5th` `6th` `7th` Additional Character Required   ✓   3-character code

Unspecified laterality codes were excluded here.

•=New Code
▲=Revised Code

Excludes1—Not coded here, do not use together
Excludes2—Not included here

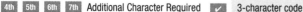

Chapter 8. Diseases of the ear and mastoid process (H60–H95)

GUIDELINES

Note: Use an external cause code following the code for the ear condition, if applicable, to identify the cause of the ear condition

Excludes2: certain conditions originating in the perinatal period (P04–P96)
    certain infectious and parasitic diseases (A00–B99)
    complications of pregnancy, childbirth and the puerperium (O00–O9A)
    congenital malformations, deformations and chromosomal abnormalities (Q00–Q99)
    endocrine, nutritional and metabolic diseases (E00–E88)
    injury, poisoning and certain other consequences of external causes (S00–T88)
    neoplasms (C00–D49)
    symptoms, signs and abnormal clinical and laboratory findings, not elsewhere classified (R00–R94)

(H60–H62) DISEASES OF EXTERNAL EAR

H60   **OTITIS EXTERNA**
  [4th]

H60.0   **Abscess of external ear**
  [5th]   Boil of external ear
     Carbuncle of auricle or external auditory canal
     Furuncle of external ear
     H60.01   **Abscess of right external ear**
     H60.02   **Abscess of left external ear**
     H60.03   **Abscess of external ear, bilateral**

H60.1   **Cellulitis of external ear**
  [5th]   Cellulitis of auricle
     Cellulitis of external auditory canal
     H60.11   **Cellulitis of right external ear**
     H60.12   **Cellulitis of left external ear**
     H60.13   **Cellulitis of external ear, bilateral**

H60.3   **Other infective otitis externa**
  [5th]   **H60.31**   **Diffuse otitis externa**
     [6th]   **H60.311**   **Diffuse otitis externa, right ear**
       H60.312   **Diffuse otitis externa, left ear**
       H60.313   **Diffuse otitis externa, bilateral**
     H60.32   **Hemorrhagic otitis externa**
     [6th]   **H60.321**   **Hemorrhagic otitis externa, right ear**
       H60.322   **Hemorrhagic otitis externa, left ear**
       H60.323   **Hemorrhagic otitis externa, bilateral**
     H60.33   **Swimmer's ear**
     [6th]   **H60.331**   **Swimmer's ear, right ear**
       H60.332   **Swimmer's ear, left ear**
       H60.333   **Swimmer's ear, bilateral**
     H60.39   **Other infective otitis externa**
     [6th]   **H60.391**   **Other infective otitis externa, right ear**
       H60.392   **Other infective otitis externa, left ear**
       H60.393   **Other infective otitis externa, bilateral**

H60.5   **Acute noninfective otitis externa**
  [5th]   **H60.50**   **Unspecified acute noninfective otitis externa**
     [6th]   Acute otitis externa NOS
       H60.501   **Unspecified acute noninfective otitis externa, right ear**
       H60.502   **Unspecified acute noninfective otitis externa, left ear**
       H60.503   **Unspecified acute noninfective otitis externa, bilateral**

H60.8   **Other otitis externa**
  [5th]   **H60.8X**   **Other otitis externa**
     [6th]   **H60.8X1**   **Other otitis externa, right ear**
       H60.8X2   **Other otitis externa, left ear**
       H60.8X3   **Other otitis externa, bilateral**
       H60.8X9   **Other otitis externa, unspecified ear**

H60.9   **Unspecified otitis externa**
  [5th]   **H60.91**   **Unspecified otitis externa, right ear**
     H60.92   **Unspecified otitis externa, left ear**
     H60.93   **Unspecified otitis externa, bilateral**

H61   **OTHER DISORDERS OF EXTERNAL EAR**
  [4th]   **H61.0**   **Chondritis and perichondritis of external ear**
     [5th]   Chondrodermatitis nodularis chronica helicis
     Perichondritis of auricle
     Perichondritis of pinna
     H61.00   **Unspecified perichondritis of external ear**
     [6th]   **H61.001**   **Unspecified perichondritis of right external ear**
       H61.002   **Unspecified perichondritis of left external ear**
       H61.003   **Unspecified perichondritis of external ear, bilateral**
     H61.01   **Acute perichondritis of external ear**
     [6th]   **H61.011**   **Acute perichondritis of right external ear**
       H61.012   **Acute perichondritis of left external ear**
       H61.013   **Acute perichondritis of external ear, bilateral**
     H61.02   **Chronic perichondritis of external ear**
     [6th]   **H61.021**   **Chronic perichondritis of right external ear**
       H61.022   **Chronic perichondritis of left external ear**
       H61.023   **Chronic perichondritis of external ear, bilateral**

H61.1   **Noninfective disorders of pinna**
  [5th]   ***Excludes2:*** cauliflower ear (M95.1-)
     gouty tophi of ear (M1A.-)
     H61.10   **Unspecified noninfective disorders of pinna**
     [6th]   Disorder of pinna NOS
       H61.101   **Unspecified noninfective disorders of pinna, right ear**
       H61.102   **Unspecified noninfective disorders of pinna, left ear**
       H61.103   **Unspecified noninfective disorders of pinna, bilateral**
     H61.11   **Acquired deformity of pinna**
     [6th]   Acquired deformity of auricle
     Excludes2: cauliflower ear (M95.1-)
       H61.111   **Acquired deformity of pinna, right ear**
       H61.112   **Acquired deformity of pinna, left ear**
       H61.113   **Acquired deformity of pinna, bilateral**
     H61.12   **Hematoma of pinna**
     [6th]   Hematoma of auricle
       H61.121   **Hematoma of pinna, right ear**
       H61.122   **Hematoma of pinna, left ear**
       H61.123   **Hematoma of pinna, bilateral**
     H61.19   **Other noninfective disorders of pinna**
     [6th]   **H61.191**   **Noninfective disorders of pinna, right ear**
       H61.192   **Noninfective disorders of pinna, left ear**
       H61.193   **Noninfective disorders of pinna, bilateral**

H61.2   **Impacted cerumen**
  [5th]   Wax in ear
     H61.21   **Impacted cerumen, right ear**
     H61.22   **Impacted cerumen, left ear**
     H61.23   **Impacted cerumen, bilateral**

H62   **DISORDERS OF EXTERNAL EAR IN DISEASES**
  [4th]   **CLASSIFIED ELSEWHERE**
   H62.4   **Otitis externa in other diseases classified elsewhere**
     [5th]   **Code first** underlying disease, such as: erysipelas (A46)
     impetigo (L01.0)
     Excludes1: otitis externa (in):
     candidiasis (B37.84)
     herpes viral [herpes simplex] (B00.1)
     herpes zoster (B02.8)
     H62.41   **Otitis externa in other diseases classified elsewhere, right ear**
     H62.42   **Otitis externa in other diseases classified elsewhere, left ear**
     H62.43   **Otitis externa in other diseases classified elsewhere, bilateral**

      [4th] [5th] [6th] [7th]   Additional Character Required   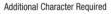   3-character code   Unspecified laterality codes were excluded here.   •=New Code   ▲=Revised Code   ***Excludes1***—Not coded here, do not use together   ***Excludes2***—Not included here

(H65–H75) DISEASES OF MIDDLE EAR AND MASTOID

H65 **NONSUPPURATIVE OTITIS MEDIA**

`4th`

Includes: nonsuppurative otitis media with myringitis

Use additional code for any associated perforated tympanic membrane (H72.-)

Use additional code, if applicable, to identify:
exposure to environmental tobacco smoke (Z77.22)
exposure to tobacco smoke in the perinatal period (P96.81)
history of tobacco dependence (Z87.891)
infectious agent (B95–B97)
occupational exposure to environmental tobacco smoke (Z57.31)
tobacco dependence (F17.-)
tobacco use (Z72.0)

H65.0 **Acute serous otitis media**

`5th` Acute and subacute secretory otitis

H65.01 **Acute serous otitis media, right ear**
H65.02 **Acute serous otitis media, left ear**
H65.03 **Acute serous otitis media, bilateral**
H65.04 **Acute serous otitis media, recurrent, right ear**
H65.05 **Acute serous otitis media, recurrent, left ear**
H65.06 **Acute serous otitis media, recurrent, bilateral**

H65.1 **Other acute nonsuppurative otitis media**

`5th` *Excludes1:* otitic barotrauma (T70.0)
otitis media (acute) NOS (H66.9)

H65.11 **Acute and subacute allergic otitis media (mucoid)**
`6th` **(sanguinous) (serous)**
H65.111 **Acute and subacute allergic otitis media (mucoid) (sanguinous) (serous), right ear**
H65.112 **Acute and subacute allergic otitis media (mucoid) (sanguinous) (serous), left ear**
H65.113 **Acute and subacute allergic otitis media (mucoid) (sanguinous) (serous), bilateral**
H65.114 **Acute and subacute allergic otitis media (mucoid) (sanguinous) (serous), recurrent, right ear**
H65.115 **Acute and subacute allergic otitis media (mucoid) (sanguinous) (serous), recurrent, left ear**
H65.116 **Acute and subacute allergic otitis media (mucoid) (sanguinous) (serous), recurrent, bilateral**

H65.2 **Chronic serous otitis media**

`5th` Chronic tubotympanal catarrh

H65.21 **Chronic serous otitis media, right ear**
H65.22 **Chronic serous otitis media, left ear**
H65.23 **Chronic serous otitis media, bilateral**

H65.3 **Chronic mucoid otitis media**

`5th` Chronic mucinous otitis media
Chronic secretory otitis media
Chronic transudative otitis media
Glue ear
Excludes1: adhesive middle ear disease (H74.1)

H65.31 **Chronic mucoid otitis media, right ear**
H65.32 **Chronic mucoid otitis media, left ear**
H65.33 **Chronic mucoid otitis media, bilateral**

H65.4 **Other chronic nonsuppurative otitis media**

`5th`

H65.41 **Chronic allergic otitis media**
`6th` **H65.411** **Chronic allergic otitis media, right ear**
H65.412 **Chronic allergic otitis media, left ear**
H65.413 **Chronic allergic otitis media, bilateral**

H65.49 **Other chronic nonsuppurative otitis media**
`6th` Chronic exudative otitis media
Chronic nonsuppurative otitis media NOS
Chronic otitis media with effusion (nonpurulent)
Chronic seromucinous otitis media
H65.491 **Other chronic nonsuppurative otitis media, right ear**
H65.492 **Other chronic nonsuppurative otitis media, left ear**
H65.493 **Other chronic nonsuppurative otitis media, bilateral**

H65.9 **Unspecified nonsuppurative otitis media**

`5th` Allergic otitis media NOS
Catarrhal otitis media NOS
Exudative otitis media NOS
Mucoid otitis media NOS
Otitis media with effusion (nonpurulent) NOS
Secretory otitis media NOS
Seromucinous otitis media NOS
Serous otitis media NOS
Transudative otitis media NOS

H65.91 **Unspecified nonsuppurative otitis media, right ear**
H65.92 **Unspecified nonsuppurative otitis media, left ear**
H65.93 **Unspecified nonsuppurative otitis media, bilateral**

H66 **SUPPURATIVE AND UNSPECIFIED OTITIS MEDIA**

`4th`

Includes: suppurative and unspecified otitis media with myringitis

Use additional code to identify: exposure to environmental tobacco smoke (Z77.22)
exposure to tobacco smoke in the perinatal period (P96.81)
history of tobacco dependence (Z87.891)
occupational exposure to environmental tobacco smoke (Z57.31)
tobacco dependence (F17.-)
tobacco use (Z72.0)

H66.0 **Acute suppurative otitis media**

`5th` **H66.00** **Acute suppurative otitis media without spontaneous**
`6th` **rupture of; ear drum**
H66.001 **right ear drum**
H66.002 **left ear drum**
H66.003 **bilateral ear drums**
H66.004 **recurrent, right ear drum**
H66.005 **recurrent, left ear drum**
H66.006 **recurrent, bilateral ear drums**

H66.01 **Acute suppurative otitis media with spontaneous**
`6th` **rupture of; ear drum**
H66.011 **right ear drum**
H66.012 **left ear drum**
H66.013 **bilateral ear drums**
H66.014 **recurrent, right ear drum**
H66.015 **recurrent, left ear drum**
H66.016 **recurrent, bilateral ear drums**

H66.1 **Chronic tubotympanic suppurative otitis media**

`5th` Benign chronic suppurative otitis media
Chronic tubotympanic disease
Use additional code for any associated perforated tympanic membrane (H72.-)
H66.11 **Chronic tubotympanic suppurative otitis media, right ear**
H66.12 **Chronic tubotympanic suppurative otitis media, left ear**
H66.13 **Chronic tubotympanic suppurative otitis media, bilateral**

H66.2 **Chronic atticoantral suppurative otitis media**

`5th` Chronic atticoantral disease
Use additional code for any associated perforated tympanic membrane(H72.-)
H66.21 **Chronic atticoantral suppurative otitis media, right ear**
H66.22 **Chronic atticoantral suppurative otitis media, left ear**
H66.23 **Chronic atticoantral suppurative otitis media, bilateral**

H66.3 **Other chronic suppurative otitis media**

`5th` Chronic suppurative otitis media NOS
Use additional code for any associated perforated tympanic membrane (H72.-)
Excludes1: tuberculous otitis media (A18.6)
H66.3X **Other chronic suppurative otitis media**
`6th` **H66.3X1** **Other chronic suppurative otitis media, right ear**
H66.3X2 **Other chronic suppurative otitis media, left ear**
H66.3X3 **Other chronic suppurative otitis media, bilateral**

    `4th` `5th` `6th` `7th` Additional Character Required ✔ 3-character code | Unspecified laterality codes were excluded here. | •=New Code ▲=Revised Code | *Excludes1*—Not coded here, do not use together *Excludes2*—Not included here

H66.4 **Suppurative otitis media, unspecified**
`5th` Purulent otitis media NOS

Use additional code for any associated perforated tympanic membrane (H72.-)

H66.41 **Suppurative otitis media, unspecified, right ear**
H66.42 **Suppurative otitis media, unspecified, left ear**
H66.43 **Suppurative otitis media, unspecified, bilateral**

H66.9 **Otitis media, unspecified**
`5th` Otitis media NOS
Acute otitis media NOS
Chronic otitis media NOS

Use additional code for any associated perforated tympanic membrane (H72.-)

H66.91 **Otitis media, unspecified, right ear**
H66.92 **Otitis media, unspecified, left ear**
H66.93 **Otitis media, unspecified, bilateral**

H67 **OTITIS MEDIA IN DISEASES CLASSIFIED ELSEWHERE**
`4th`
Code first underlying disease, such as:
plasminogen deficiency (E88.02)
viral disease NEC (B00–B34)

Use additional code for any associated perforated tympanic membrane (H72.-)

Excludes1: otitis media in: influenza (J09.X9, J10.83, J11.83)
measles (B05.3)
scarlet fever (A38.0)
tuberculosis (A18.6)

H67.1 **Otitis media in diseases classified elsewhere, right ear**
H67.2 **Otitis media in diseases classified elsewhere, left ear**
H67.3 **Otitis media in diseases classified elsewhere, bilateral**

H69 **OTHER AND UNSPECIFIED DISORDERS OF EUSTACHIAN TUBE**
`4th`
H69.8 **Other specified disorders of Eustachian tube**
`5th` Use for Eustachian tube dysfunction

H69.81 **Other specified disorders of Eustachian tube, right ear**
H69.82 **Other specified disorders of Eustachian tube, left ear**
H69.83 **Other specified disorders of Eustachian tube, bilateral**

H69.9 **Unspecified Eustachian tube disorder**
`5th`
H69.91 **Unspecified Eustachian tube disorder, right ear**
H69.92 **Unspecified Eustachian tube disorder, left ear**
H69.93 **Unspecified Eustachian tube disorder, bilateral**

H72 **PERFORATION OF TYMPANIC MEMBRANE**
`4th`
Includes: persistent post-traumatic perforation of ear drum
postinflammatory perforation of ear drum

Code first any associated otitis media

Excludes1: acute suppurative otitis media with rupture of the tympanic membrane
traumatic rupture of ear drum

H72.0 **Central perforation of tympanic membrane**
`5th`
H72.01 **Central perforation of tympanic membrane, right ear**
H72.02 **Central perforation of tympanic membrane, left ear**
H72.03 **Central perforation of tympanic membrane, bilateral**

H72.1 **Attic perforation of tympanic membrane**
`5th` Perforation of pars flaccida

H72.11 **Attic perforation of tympanic membrane, right ear**
H72.12 **Attic perforation of tympanic membrane, left ear**
H72.13 **Attic perforation of tympanic membrane, bilateral**

H72.2 **Other marginal perforations of tympanic membrane**
`5th` **H72.2X** **Other marginal perforations of tympanic membrane**
`6th` **H72.2X1** **Other marginal perforations of tympanic membrane, right ear**
H72.2X2 **Other marginal perforations of tympanic membrane, left ear**
H72.2X3 **Other marginal perforations of tympanic membrane, bilateral**

H72.8 **Other perforations of tympanic membrane**
`5th` **H72.81** **Multiple perforations of tympanic membrane**
`6th` **H72.811** **Multiple perforations of tympanic membrane, right ear**
H72.812 **Multiple perforations of tympanic membrane, left ear**

H72.813 **Multiple perforations of tympanic membrane, bilateral**

H72.82 **Total perforations of tympanic membrane**
`6th` **H72.821** **Total perforations of tympanic membrane, right ear**
H72.822 **Total perforations of tympanic membrane, left ear**
H72.823 **Total perforations of tympanic membrane, bilateral**

H72.9 **Unspecified perforation of tympanic membrane**
`5th` **H72.91** **Unspecified perforation of tympanic membrane, right ear**
H72.92 **Unspecified perforation of tympanic membrane, left ear**
H72.93 **Unspecified perforation of tympanic membrane, bilateral**

H73 **OTHER DISORDERS OF TYMPANIC MEMBRANE**
`4th`
H73.0 **Acute myringitis**
`5th` **Excludes1:** acute myringitis with otitis media (H65, H66)

H73.00 **Unspecified acute myringitis**
`6th` Acute tympanitis NOS
H73.001 **Acute myringitis, right ear**
H73.002 **Acute myringitis, left ear**
H73.003 **Acute myringitis, bilateral**

H73.01 **Bullous myringitis**
`6th` **H73.011** **Bullous myringitis, right ear**
H73.012 **Bullous myringitis, left ear**
H73.013 **Bullous myringitis, bilateral**

H73.1 **Chronic myringitis**
`5th` Chronic tympanitis
Excludes1: chronic myringitis with otitis media (H65, H66)
H73.11 **Chronic myringitis, right ear**
H73.12 **Chronic myringitis, left ear**
H73.13 **Chronic myringitis, bilateral**

H73.2 **Unspecified myringitis**
`5th` **H73.21** **Unspecified myringitis, right ear**
H73.22 **Unspecified myringitis, left ear**
H73.23 **Unspecified myringitis, bilateral**

H73.8 **Other specified disorders of tympanic membrane**

(H80–H83) DISEASES OF INNER EAR

H81 **DISORDERS OF VESTIBULAR FUNCTION**
`4th`
Excludes1: epidemic vertigo (A88.1)
vertigo NOS (R42)

H81.0 **Ménière's disease**
`5th` Labyrinthine hydrops
Ménière's syndrome or vertigo
H81.01 **Ménière's disease, right ear**
H81.02 **Ménière's disease, left ear**
H81.03 **Ménière's disease, bilateral**

H81.1 **Benign paroxysmal vertigo**
`5th` **H81.11** **Benign paroxysmal vertigo, right ear**
H81.12 **Benign paroxysmal vertigo, left ear**
H81.13 **Benign paroxysmal vertigo, bilateral**

H81.3 **Other peripheral vertigo**
`5th` **H81.31** **Aural vertigo**
`6th` **H81.311** **Aural vertigo, right ear**
H81.312 **Aural vertigo, left ear**
H81.313 **Aural vertigo, bilateral**

H81.39 **Other peripheral vertigo**
`6th` Lermoyez' syndrome
Otogenic vertigo
Peripheral vertigo NOS
H81.391 **Other peripheral vertigo, right ear**
H81.392 **Other peripheral vertigo, left ear**
H81.393 **Other peripheral vertigo, bilateral**

H81.4 **Vertigo of central origin**
Central positional nystagmus

H81.8 **Other disorders of vestibular function**
`5th` **H81.8X** **Other disorders of vestibular function**
`6th` **H81.8X1** **Other disorders of vestibular function, right ear**

`4th` `5th` `6th` `7th` Additional Character Required   ✓ 3-character code

Unspecified laterality codes were excluded here.

•=New Code
▲=Revised Code

Excludes1—Not coded here, do not use together
Excludes2—Not included here

CHAPTER 8. DISEASES OF THE EAR AND MASTOID PROCESS   (H81.8X2–H93.2)

H81.8X2   Other disorders of vestibular function, left ear
H81.8X3   Other disorders of vestibular function, bilateral

H81.9   Unspecified disorder of vestibular function
    5th
    Vertiginous syndrome NOS
    H81.91   Unspecified disorder of vestibular function, right ear
    H81.92   Unspecified disorder of vestibular function, left ear
    H81.93   Unspecified disorder of vestibular function, bilateral

H83   OTHER DISEASES OF INNER EAR
  4th
H83.0   Labyrinthitis
    5th
    H83.01   Labyrinthitis, right ear
    H83.02   Labyrinthitis, left ear
    H83.03   Labyrinthitis, bilateral
    H83.09   Labyrinthitis, unspecified ear
H83.3   Noise effects on inner ear
    5th
    Acoustic trauma of inner ear
    Noise-induced hearing loss of inner ear
    H83.3X   Noise effects on inner ear
      6th
      H83.3X1   Noise effects on right inner ear
      H83.3X2   Noise effects on left inner ear
      H83.3X3   Noise effects on inner ear, bilateral

(H90–H94) OTHER DISORDERS OF EAR

H90   CONDUCTIVE AND SENSORINEURAL HEARING LOSS
  4th
    Excludes1: deaf nonspeaking NEC (H91.3)
      deafness NOS (H91.9-)
      hearing loss NOS (H91.9-)
      noise-induced hearing loss (H83.3-)
      ototoxic hearing loss (H91.0-)
      sudden (idiopathic) hearing loss (H91.2-)
H90.0   Conductive hearing loss, bilateral
H90.1   Conductive hearing loss, unilateral with unrestricted hearing on the contralateral side
    5th
    H90.11   Conductive hearing loss, unilateral, right ear, with unrestricted hearing on the contralateral side
    H90.12   Conductive hearing loss, unilateral, left ear, with unrestricted hearing on the contralateral side
H90.2   Conductive hearing loss, unspecified
    Conductive deafness NOS
H90.3   Sensorineural hearing loss, bilateral
H90.4   Sensorineural hearing loss, unilateral with unrestricted hearing on the contralateral side
    5th
    H90.41   Sensorineural hearing loss, unilateral, right ear, with unrestricted hearing on the contralateral side
    H90.42   Sensorineural hearing loss, unilateral, left ear, with unrestricted hearing on the contralateral side
H90.5   Unspecified sensorineural hearing loss
    Central hearing loss NOS
    Congenital deafness NOS
    Neural hearing loss NOS
    Perceptive hearing loss NOS
    Sensorineural deafness NOS
    Sensory hearing loss NOS
    Excludes1: abnormal auditory perception (H93.2-)
      psychogenic deafness (F44.6)
H90.6   Mixed conductive and sensorineural hearing loss, bilateral
H90.7   Mixed conductive and sensorineural hearing loss, unilateral with unrestricted hearing on the contralateral side
    5th
    H90.71   Mixed conductive and sensorineural hearing loss, unilateral, right ear, with unrestricted hearing on the contralateral side
    H90.72   Mixed conductive and sensorineural hearing loss, unilateral, left ear, with unrestricted hearing on the contralateral side
H90.8   Mixed conductive and sensorineural hearing loss, unspecified
H90.A   Hearing loss, unilateral, with restricted hearing on the contralateral side
    5th
    H90.A1   Conductive hearing loss, unilateral, with restricted hearing on the contralateral side
      6th

      H90.A11   Conductive hearing loss, unilateral, right ear with restricted hearing on the contralateral side
      H90.A12   Conductive hearing loss, unilateral, left ear with restricted hearing on the contralateral side
    H90.A2   Sensorineural hearing loss, unilateral, with restricted hearing on the contralateral side
      6th
      H90.A21   Sensorineural hearing loss, unilateral, right ear, with restricted hearing on the contralateral side
      H90.A22   Sensorineural hearing loss, unilateral, left ear, with restricted hearing on the contralateral side
    H90.A3   Mixed conductive and sensorineural hearing loss, unilateral, with restricted hearing on the contralateral side
      6th
      H90.A31   Mixed conductive and sensorineural hearing loss, unilateral, right ear with restricted hearing on the contralateral side
      H90.A32   Mixed conductive and sensorineural hearing, unilateral, left ear with restricted hearing on the contralateral side

H91   OTHER AND UNSPECIFIED HEARING LOSS
  4th
    Excludes1: abnormal auditory perception (H93.2-)
      hearing loss as classified in H90.-
      impacted cerumen (H61.2-)
      noise-induced hearing loss (H83.3-)
      psychogenic deafness (F44.6)
      transient ischemic deafness (H93.01-)
H91.2   Sudden idiopathic hearing loss
    5th
    Sudden hearing loss NOS
    H91.21   Sudden idiopathic hearing loss, right ear
    H91.22   Sudden idiopathic hearing loss, left ear
    H91.23   Sudden idiopathic hearing loss, bilateral
H91.3   Deaf nonspeaking, not elsewhere classified
H91.8   Other specified hearing loss
    5th
    H91.8X   Other specified hearing loss
      6th
      H91.8X1   Other specified hearing loss, right ear
      H91.8X2   Other specified hearing loss, left ear
      H91.8X3   Other specified hearing loss, bilateral
H91.9   Unspecified hearing loss
    5th
    Deafness NOS
    High frequency deafness
    Low frequency deafness
    H91.91   Unspecified hearing loss, right ear
    H91.92   Unspecified hearing loss, left ear
    H91.93   Unspecified hearing loss, bilateral

H92   OTALGIA AND EFFUSION OF EAR
  4th
H92.0   Otalgia
    5th
    H92.01   Otalgia, right ear
    H92.02   Otalgia, left ear
    H92.03   Otalgia, bilateral
H92.1   Otorrhea
    5th
    Excludes1: leakage of cerebrospinal fluid through ear (G96.0)
    H92.11   Otorrhea, right ear
    H92.12   Otorrhea, left ear
    H92.13   Otorrhea, bilateral

H93   OTHER DISORDERS OF EAR, NOT ELSEWHERE CLASSIFIED
  4th
H93.1   Tinnitus
    5th
    H93.11   Tinnitus, right ear
    H93.12   Tinnitus, left ear
    H93.13   Tinnitus, bilateral
H93.A   Pulsatile tinnitus
    5th
    H93.A1   Pulsatile tinnitus, right ear
    H93.A2   Pulsatile tinnitus, left ear
    H93.A3   Pulsatile tinnitus, bilateral
H93.2   Other abnormal auditory perceptions
    5th
    auditory hallucinations (R44.0)

4th   5th   6th   7th   Additional Character Required   ✔   3-character code   Unspecified laterality codes were excluded here.   •=New Code   ▲=Revised Code   *Excludes1*—Not coded here, do not use together   *Excludes2*—Not included here

208   PEDIATRIC ICD-10-CM 2022: A MANUAL FOR PROVIDER-BASED CODING

H93.25   **Central auditory processing disorder**
         Congenital auditory imperception
         Word deafness

H93.29   **Other abnormal auditory perceptions**
> **6th**   H93.291   **Other abnormal auditory perceptions, right ear**
>   H93.292   **Other abnormal auditory perceptions, left ear**
>   H93.293   **Other abnormal auditory perceptions, bilateral**

H93.8   **Other specified disorders of ear**
> **5th**   **H93.8X**   **Other specified disorders of ear**
> > **6th**   H93.8X1   **Other specified disorders of right ear**
> >   H93.8X2   **Other specified disorders of left ear**
> >   H93.8X3   **Other specified disorders of ear, bilateral**

(H95) INTRAOPERATIVE AND POSTPROCEDURAL COMPLICATIONS AND DISORDERS OF EAR AND MASTOID PROCESS, NOT ELSEWHERE CLASSIFIED

   4th **5th** **6th** **7th**   Additional Character Required   ✔   3-character code   Unspecified laterality codes were excluded here.   •=New Code   ▲=Revised Code   **Excludes1**—Not coded here, do not use together   **Excludes2**—Not included here

Chapter 9. Diseases of the circulatory system (I00–I99)

GUIDELINES

a. Hypertension

The classification presumes a causal relationship between hypertension and heart involvement and between hypertension and kidney involvement, as the two conditions are linked by the term "with" in the Alphabetic Index. These conditions should be coded as related even in the absence of provider documentation explicitly linking them, unless the documentation clearly states the conditions are unrelated.

For hypertension and conditions not specifically linked by relational terms such as "with," "associated with" or "due to" in the classification, provider documentation must link the conditions in order to code them as related.

1) Hypertension with Heart Disease

Hypertension with heart conditions classified to I50.- or I51.4–I51.7, I51.89, I51.9, are assigned to a code from category I11, Hypertensive heart disease. Use additional code(s) from category I50, Heart failure, to identify the type(s) of heart failure in those patients with heart failure.

The same heart conditions (I50.-, I51.4–I51.7, I51.89, I51.9) with hypertension are coded separately if the provider has documented they are unrelated to the hypertension. Sequence according to the circumstances of the admission/encounter.

Refer to ICD-10-CM Official Guidelines for Coding and Reporting for instructions for reporting atherosclerotic coronary artery disease, cerebrovascular accident, and/or myocardial infarction

Excludes2:
certain conditions originating in the perinatal period (P04–P96)
certain infectious and parasitic diseases (A00–B99)
complications of pregnancy, childbirth and the puerperium (O00–O9A)
congenital malformations, deformations, and chromosomal abnormalities (Q00–Q99)
endocrine, nutritional and metabolic diseases (E00–E88)
injury, poisoning and certain other consequences of external causes (S00–T88)
neoplasms (C00–D49)
symptoms, signs and abnormal clinical and laboratory findings, not elsewhere classified (R00–R94)
systemic connective tissue disorders (M30–M36)
transient cerebral ischemic attacks and related syndromes (G45.-)

(I00–I02) ACUTE RHEUMATIC FEVER

I00 `✓` **RHEUMATIC FEVER WITHOUT HEART INVOLVEMENT**
Includes: arthritis, rheumatic, acute or subacute
Excludes1: rheumatic fever with heart involvement (I01.0–I01.9)

I01 `4th` **RHEUMATIC FEVER WITH HEART INVOLVEMENT**
Excludes1: chronic diseases of rheumatic origin (I05–I09) unless rheumatic fever is also present or there is evidence of reactivation or activity of the rheumatic process.

I01.0 **Acute rheumatic pericarditis**
Any condition in I00 with pericarditis
Rheumatic pericarditis (acute)
Excludes1: acute pericarditis not specified as rheumatic (I30.-)

I01.1 **Acute rheumatic endocarditis**
Any condition in I00 with endocarditis or valvulitis
Acute rheumatic valvulitis

I01.2 **Acute rheumatic myocarditis**
Any condition in I00 with myocarditis

I01.8 **Other acute rheumatic heart disease**
Any condition in I00 with other or multiple types of heart involvement
Acute rheumatic pancarditis

I01.9 **Acute rheumatic heart disease, unspecified**
Any condition in I00 with unspecified type of heart involvement
Rheumatic carditis, acute
Rheumatic heart disease, active or acute

I02 `4th` **RHEUMATIC CHOREA**
Includes: Sydenham's chorea
Excludes1: chorea NOS (G25.5)
Huntington's chorea (G10)

I02.0 **Rheumatic chorea with heart involvement**
Chorea NOS with heart involvement
Rheumatic chorea with heart involvement of any type classifiable under I01.-

I02.9 **Rheumatic chorea without heart involvement**
Rheumatic chorea NOS
Rheumatic heart disease, active or acute

(I05–I09) CHRONIC RHEUMATIC HEART DISEASES

I05 `4th` **RHEUMATIC MITRAL VALVE DISEASES**
Includes: conditions classifiable to both I05.0 and I05.2–I05.9, whether specified as rheumatic or not
Excludes1: mitral valve disease specified as nonrheumatic (I34.-)
mitral valve disease with aortic and/or tricuspid valve involvement (I08.-)

I05.0 **Rheumatic mitral stenosis**
Mitral (valve) obstruction (rheumatic)

I05.1 **Rheumatic mitral insufficiency**
Rheumatic mitral incompetence
Rheumatic mitral regurgitation
Excludes1: mitral insufficiency not specified as rheumatic (I34.0)

I05.2 **Rheumatic mitral stenosis with insufficiency**
Rheumatic mitral stenosis with incompetence or regurgitation

I05.8 **Other rheumatic mitral valve diseases**
Rheumatic mitral (valve) failure

I05.9 **Rheumatic mitral valve disease, unspecified**
Rheumatic mitral (valve) disorder (chronic) NOS

I06 `4th` **RHEUMATIC AORTIC VALVE DISEASES**
Excludes1: aortic valve disease not specified as rheumatic (I35.-)
aortic valve disease with mitral and/or tricuspid valve involvement (I08.-)

I06.0 **Rheumatic aortic stenosis**
Rheumatic aortic (valve) obstruction

I06.1 **Rheumatic aortic insufficiency**
Rheumatic aortic incompetence
Rheumatic aortic regurgitation

I06.2 **Rheumatic aortic stenosis with insufficiency**
Rheumatic aortic stenosis with incompetence or regurgitation

I06.8 **Other rheumatic aortic valve diseases**

I06.9 **Rheumatic aortic valve disease, unspecified**
Rheumatic aortic (valve) disease NOS

I07 `4th` **RHEUMATIC TRICUSPID VALVE DISEASES**
Includes: rheumatic tricuspid valve diseases specified as rheumatic or unspecified
Excludes1: tricuspid valve disease specified as nonrheumatic (I36.-)
tricuspid valve disease with aortic and/or mitral valve involvement (I08.-)

I07.0 **Rheumatic tricuspid stenosis**
Tricuspid (valve) stenosis (rheumatic)

I07.1 **Rheumatic tricuspid insufficiency**
Tricuspid (valve) insufficiency (rheumatic)

I07.2 **Rheumatic tricuspid stenosis and insufficiency**

I07.8 **Other rheumatic tricuspid valve diseases**

I07.9 **Rheumatic tricuspid valve disease, unspecified**
Rheumatic tricuspid valve disorder NOS

I08 `4th` **MULTIPLE VALVE DISEASES**
Includes: multiple valve diseases specified as rheumatic or unspecified
Excludes1: endocarditis, valve unspecified (I38)
multiple valve disease specified a nonrheumatic (I34.-, I35.-, I36.-, I37.-, I38.-, Q22.-, Q23.-, Q24.8-)
rheumatic valve disease NOS (I09.1)

I08.0 **Rheumatic disorders of both mitral and aortic valves**
Involvement of both mitral and aortic valves specified as rheumatic or unspecified

I08.1 **Rheumatic disorders of both mitral and tricuspid valves**

I08.2 **Rheumatic disorders of both aortic and tricuspid valves**

I08.3 **Combined rheumatic disorders of mitral, aortic and tricuspid valves**

I08.8 **Other rheumatic multiple valve diseases**

I08.9 **Rheumatic multiple valve disease, unspecified**

`4th` `5th` `6th` `7th` Additional Character Required `✓` 3-character code

•=New Code
▲=Revised Code

Excludes1—Not coded here, do not use together
Excludes2—Not included here

I09 **OTHER RHEUMATIC HEART DISEASES**
`4th`
   I09.0 **Rheumatic myocarditis**
     Excludes1: myocarditis not specified as rheumatic (I51.4)
   I09.1 **Rheumatic diseases of endocardium, valve unspecified**
     Rheumatic endocarditis (chronic)
     Rheumatic valvulitis (chronic)
     Excludes1: endocarditis, valve unspecified (I38)
   I09.2 **Chronic rheumatic pericarditis**
     Adherent pericardium, rheumatic
     Chronic rheumatic mediastinopericarditis
     Chronic rheumatic myopericarditis
     Excludes1: chronic pericarditis not specified as rheumatic (I31.-)
   I09.8 **Other specified rheumatic heart diseases**
     `5th` **I09.81** **Rheumatic heart failure**
       Use additional code to identify type of heart failure (I50.-)
     I09.89 **Other specified rheumatic heart diseases**
       Rheumatic disease of pulmonary valve
   I09.9 **Rheumatic heart disease, unspecified**
     Rheumatic carditis
     Excludes1: rheumatoid carditis (M05.31)

(I10–I16) HYPERTENSIVE DISEASES

Use additional code to identify: exposure to environmental tobacco smoke (Z77.22)
  history of tobacco dependence (Z87.891)
  occupational exposure to environmental tobacco smoke (Z57.31)
  tobacco dependence (F17.-)
  tobacco use (Z72.0)
Excludes1: neonatal hypertension (P29.2)
  primary pulmonary hypertension (I27.0)
Excludes2: hypertensive disease complicating pregnancy, childbirth and the puerperium (O10–O11, O13–O16)

I10 **ESSENTIAL (PRIMARY) HYPERTENSION**
✔
   Includes: high blood pressure
     hypertension (arterial) (benign) (essential) (malignant) (primary) (systemic)
   Excludes1: hypertensive disease complicating pregnancy, childbirth and the puerperium (O10–O11, O13–O16)
   Excludes2: essential (primary) hypertension involving vessels of brain (I60–I69)
     essential (primary) hypertension involving vessels of eye (H35.0-)

I11 **HYPERTENSIVE HEART DISEASE**
`4th`
   Includes: any condition in I50.-, or I51.4-, I51.7, I51.89, I51.9 due to hypertension
   I11.0 **Hypertensive heart disease with heart failure**
     Hypertensive heart failure
     Use additional code to identify type of heart failure (I50.-)
   I11.9 **Hypertensive heart disease without heart failure**
     Hypertensive heart disease NOS

I12 **HYPERTENSIVE CHRONIC KIDNEY DISEASE**
`4th`
   GUIDELINES

Assign codes from category I12, Hypertensive chronic kidney disease, when both hypertension and a condition classifiable to category N18, Chronic kidney disease (CKD), are present. CKD should not be coded as hypertensive if the provider indicates the CKD is not related to the hypertension.

     The appropriate code from category N18 should be used as a secondary code with a code from category I12 to identify the stage of chronic kidney disease.

     If a patient has hypertensive chronic kidney disease and acute renal failure, an additional code for the acute renal failure is required.
Includes: any condition in N18 and N26 - due to hypertension
  arteriosclerosis of kidney
  arteriosclerotic nephritis (chronic) (interstitial)
  hypertensive nephropathy
  nephrosclerosis
Excludes1: hypertension due to kidney disease (I15.0, I15.1)
  renovascular hypertension (I15.0)
  secondary hypertension (I15.-)
Excludes2: acute kidney failure (N17.-)

   I12.0 **Hypertensive chronic kidney disease with stage 5 chronic kidney disease or end stage renal disease**
     Use additional code to identify the stage of chronic kidney disease (N18.5, N18.6)
   I12.9 **Hypertensive chronic kidney disease with stage 1 through stage 4 chronic kidney disease, or unspecified chronic kidney disease**
     Hypertensive chronic kidney disease NOS
     Hypertensive renal disease NOS
     Use additional code to identify the stage of chronic kidney disease (N18.1-N18.4, N18.9)

I16 **HYPERTENSIVE CRISIS**
`4th`
   GUIDELINES

Assign a code from category I16, Hypertensive crisis, for documented hypertensive urgency, hypertensive emergency or unspecified hypertensive crisis. Code also any identified hypertensive disease (I10-I15). The sequencing is based on the reason for the encounter.
Code also any identified hypertensive disease (I10–I15)
   I16.0 **Hypertensive urgency**
   I16.1 **Hypertensive emergency**
   I16.9 **Hypertensive crisis, unspecified**

(I20–I25) ISCHEMIC HEART DISEASES

Code also the presence of hypertension (I10–I16)
Please see full ICD-10-CM manual for cardiovascular disease with symptoms or infarction.

I20 **ANGINA PECTORIS**
`4th`
   Use additional code to identify:
     exposure to environmental tobacco smoke (Z77.22)
     history of tobacco dependence (Z87.891)
     occupational exposure to environmental tobacco smoke (Z57.31)
     tobacco dependence (F17.-)
     tobacco use (Z72.0)
   Excludes1: angina pectoris with atherosclerotic heart disease of native coronary arteries (I25.1-)
     atherosclerosis of coronary artery bypass graft(s) and coronary artery of transplanted heart with anginapectoris (I25.7-)
     postinfarction angina (I23.7)
   I20.9 **Angina pectoris, unspecified**
     Angina NOS
     Anginal syndrome
     Cardiac angina
     Ischemic chest pain

I23 **CERTAIN CURRENT COMPLICATIONS FOLLOWING ST ELEVATION (STEMI) AND NON-ST ELEVATION (NSTEMI) MYOCARDIALINFARCTION (WITHIN THE 28 DAY PERIOD)**
`4th`
   I23.0 **Hemopericardium as current complication following acute myocardial infarction**
     Excludes1: hemopericardium not specified as current complication following acute myocardial infarction (I31.2)
   I23.3 **Rupture of cardiac wall without hemopericardium as current complication following acute myocardial infarction**

I24 **OTHER ACUTE ISCHEMIC HEART DISEASES**
`4th`
   Excludes1: angina pectoris (I20.-)
     transient myocardial ischemia in newborn (P29.4)
   Excludes2: non-ischemic myocardial injury (I5A)
   I24.1 **Dressler's syndrome**
     Postmyocardial infarction syndrome
     Excludes1: postinfarction angina (I23.7)
   I24.9 **Acute ischemic heart disease, unspecified**
     Excludes1: ischemic heart disease (chronic) NOS (I25.9)

I25 **CHRONIC ISCHEMIC HEART DISEASE**
`4th`
   Use additional history of tobacco dependence (Z87.891)
   Excludes2: non-ischemic myocardial injury (I5A)
   I25.1 **Atherosclerotic cardiovascular disease**
     `5th` Coronary (artery) atheroma
     Coronary (artery) atherosclerosis
     Coronary (artery) disease
     Coronary (artery) sclerosis

`4th` `5th` `6th` `7th` Additional Character Required	✔ 3-character code	•=New Code ▲=Revised Code	*Excludes1*—Not coded here, do not use together *Excludes2*—Not included here

I25.10   **Atherosclerotic heart disease of native coronary artery without angina pectoris**
Atherosclerotic heart disease NOS

(I26–I28) PULMONARY HEART DISEASE AND DISEASES OF PULMONARY CIRCULATION

I27   **OTHER PULMONARY HEART DISEASES**
`4th`

> **GUIDELINES**
>
> Pulmonary hypertension is classified to category I27, Other pulmonary heart diseases. For secondary pulmonary hypertension (I27.1, I27.2-), code also any associated conditions or adverse effects of drugs or toxins. The sequencing is based on the reason for the encounter.

I27.0   **Primary pulmonary hypertension**
Heritable pulmonary arterial hypertension
Idiopathic pulmonary arterial hypertension
Primary group 1 pulmonary hypertension
Primary pulmonary arterial hypertension
Excludes1: persistent pulmonary hypertension of newborn (P29.30)
   pulmonary hypertension NOS (I27.20)
   secondary pulmonary arterial hypertension (I27.21)
   secondary pulmonary hypertension (I27.29)

I27.1   **Kyphoscoliotic heart disease**

I27.2   **Other secondary pulmonary hypertension**
`5th`   **Code also** associated underlying condition
Excludes1: Eisenmenger's syndrome (I27.83)

   I27.20   **Pulmonary hypertension, unspecified**
     Pulmonary hypertension NOS

   I27.21   **Secondary pulmonary arterial hypertension**
     (Associated) (drug-induced) (toxin-induced) pulmonary arterial hypertension NOS
     (Associated) (drug-induced) (toxin-induced) (secondary) group 1 pulmonary hypertension
     Code also associated conditions if applicable, or adverse effects of drugs or toxins, such as:
       adverse effect of appetite depressants (T50.5X5)
       congenital heart disease (Q20-Q28)
       human immunodeficiency virus [HIV] disease (B20)
       polymyositis (M33.2-)
       portal hypertension (K76.6)
       rheumatoid arthritis (M05.-)
       schistosomiasis (B65.-)
       Sjögren syndrome (M35.0-)
       systemic sclerosis (M34.-)

   I27.22   **Pulmonary hypertension due to left heart disease**
     Group 2 pulmonary hypertension
     Code also associated left heart disease, if known, such as:
       multiple valve disease (I08.-)
       rheumatic mitral valve diseases (I05.-)
       rheumatic aortic valve diseases (I06.-)

   I27.23   **Pulmonary hypertension due to lung diseases and hypoxia**
     Group 3 pulmonary hypertension
     Code also associated lung disease, if known, such as:
       bronchiectasis (J47.-)
       cystic fibrosis with pulmonary manifestations (E84.0)
       interstitial lung disease (J84.-)
       pleural effusion (J90)
       sleep apnea (G47.3-)

   I27.24   **Chronic thromboembolic pulmonary hypertension**
     Group 4 pulmonary hypertension
     Code also associated pulmonary embolism, if applicable (I26.-, I27.82)

   I27.29   **Other secondary pulmonary hypertension**
     Group 5 pulmonary hypertension
     Pulmonary hypertension with unclear multifactorial mechanisms
     Pulmonary hypertension due to hematologic disorders
     Pulmonary hypertension due to metabolic disorders
     Pulmonary hypertension due to other systemic disorders

Code also other associated disorders, if known, such as:
   chronic myeloid leukemia (C92.10–C92.22)
   essential thrombocythemia (D47.3)
   Gaucher disease (E75.22)
   hypertensive chronic kidney disease with end stage renal disease (I12.0, I13.11, I13.2)
   hyperthyroidism (E05.-)
   hypothyroidism (E00-E03)
   polycythemia vera (D45)
   sarcoidosis (D86.-)

I27.8   **Other specified pulmonary heart diseases**
`5th`
   I27.81   **Cor pulmonale (chronic)**
     Cor pulmonale NOS
     Excludes1: acute cor pulmonale (I26.0-)

   I27.82   **Chronic pulmonary embolism**
     Use additional code, if applicable, for associated long-term (current) use of anticoagulants (Z79.01)
     Excludes1: personal history of pulmonary embolism (Z86.711)

   I27.83   **Eisenmenger's syndrome**
     Eisenmenger's complex
     (Irreversible) Eisenmenger's disease
     Pulmonary hypertension with right to left shunt related to congenital heart disease
     Code also underlying heart defect, if known, such as:
       atrial septal defect (Q21.1)
       Eisenmenger's defect (Q21.8)
       patent ductus arteriosus (Q25.0)
       ventricular septal defect (Q21.0)

   I27.89   **Other specified pulmonary heart diseases**
     Excludes1: Eisenmenger's defect (Q21.8)

I27.9   **Pulmonary heart disease, unspecified**
Chronic cardiopulmonary disease

I28   **OTHER DISEASES OF PULMONARY VESSELS**
`4th`
I28.0   **Arteriovenous fistula of pulmonary vessels**
Excludes1: congenital arteriovenous fistula (Q25.72)

I28.1   **Aneurysm of pulmonary artery**
Excludes1: congenital aneurysm (Q25.79)
   congenital arteriovenous aneurysm (Q25.72)

I28.8   **Other diseases of pulmonary vessels**
Pulmonary arteritis
Pulmonary endarteritis
Rupture of pulmonary vessels
Stenosis of pulmonary vessels
Stricture of pulmonary vessels

I28.9   **Disease of pulmonary vessels, unspecified**

(I30–I52) OTHER FORMS OF HEART DISEASE

I30   **ACUTE PERICARDITIS**
`4th`
Includes: acute mediastinopericarditis
   acute myopericarditis
   acute pericardial effusion
   acute pleuropericarditis
   acute pneumopericarditis
Excludes1: Dressler's syndrome (I24.1)
   rheumatic pericarditis (acute) (I01.0)
   viral pericarditis due to Coxsakie virus (B33.23)

I30.0   **Acute nonspecific idiopathic pericarditis**

I30.1   **Infective pericarditis**
Pneumococcal pericarditis
Pneumopyopericardium
Purulent pericarditis
Pyopericarditis
Pyopericardium
Pyopneumopericardium
Staphylococcal pericarditis
Streptococcal pericarditis
Suppurative pericarditis
Viral pericarditis
Use additional code (B95–B97) to identify infectious agent

I30.8   **Other forms of acute pericarditis**

I30.9   **Acute pericarditis, unspecified**

CHAPTER 9. DISEASES OF THE CIRCULATORY SYSTEM   (I25.10–I30.9)

`4th` `5th` `6th` `7th`   Additional Character Required   ✔   3-character code   •=New Code   ▲=Revised Code   *Excludes1*—Not coded here, do not use together   *Excludes2*—Not included here

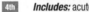

CHAPTER 9. DISEASES OF THE CIRCULATORY SYSTEM   (I31–I43)

I31 `4th` **OTHER DISEASES OF PERICARDIUM**
Excludes1: diseases of pericardium specified as rheumatic (I09.2)
  postcardiotomy syndrome (I97.0)
  traumatic injury to pericardium (S26.-)

I31.0 Chronic adhesive pericarditis
  Accretio cordis
  Adherent pericardium
  Adhesive mediastinopericarditis

I31.1 Chronic constrictive pericarditis
  Concretio cordis
  Pericardial calcification

I31.2 Hemopericardium, not elsewhere classified
  Excludes1: hemopericardium as current complication following
    acute myocardial infarction (I23.0)

I31.3 Pericardial effusion (noninflammatory)
  Chylopericardium
  Excludes1: acute pericardial effusion (I30.9)

I31.4 Cardiac tamponade
  Code first underlying cause

I31.8 Other specified diseases of pericardium
  Epicardial plaques
  Focal pericardial adhesions

I31.9 Disease of pericardium, unspecified
  Pericarditis (chronic) NOS

I33 `4th` **ACUTE AND SUBACUTE ENDOCARDITIS**
Excludes1: acute rheumatic endocarditis (I01.1)
  endocarditis NOS (I38)

I33.0 Acute and subacute infective endocarditis
  Bacterial endocarditis (acute) (subacute)
  Infective endocarditis (acute) (subacute) NOS
  Endocarditis lenta (acute) (subacute)
  Malignant endocarditis (acute) (subacute)
  Purulent endocarditis (acute) (subacute)
  Septic endocarditis (acute) (subacute)
  Ulcerative endocarditis (acute) (subacute)
  Vegetative endocarditis (acute) (subacute)
  Use additional code (B95–B97) to identify infectious agent

I33.9 Acute and subacute endocarditis, unspecified
  Acute endocarditis NOS
  Acute myoendocarditis NOS
  Acute periendocarditis NOS
  Subacute endocarditis NOS
  Subacute myoendocarditis NOS
  Subacute periendocarditis NOS

I34 `4th` **NONRHEUMATIC MITRAL VALVE DISORDERS**
Excludes1: mitral valve disease (I05.9)
  mitral valve failure (I05.8)
  mitral valve stenosis (I05.0)
  mitral valve disorder of unspecified cause with diseases of aortic and/or tricuspid valve(s) (I08.-)
  mitral valve disorder of unspecified cause with mitral stenosis or obstruction (I05.0)
  mitral valve disorder specified as congenital (Q23.2, Q23.9)
  mitral valve disorder specified as rheumatic (I05.-)

I34.0 Nonrheumatic mitral (valve) insufficiency
  Nonrheumatic mitral (valve) incompetence NOS
  Nonrheumatic mitral (valve) regurgitation NOS

I35 `4th` **NONRHEUMATIC AORTIC VALVE DISORDERS**
Excludes1: aortic valve disorder of unspecified cause but with diseases
    of mitral and/or tricuspid valve(s) (I08.-)
  aortic valve disorder specified as congenital (Q23.0, Q23.1)
  aortic valve disorder specified as rheumatic (I06.-)
  hypertrophic subaortic stenosis (I42.1)

I35.0 Nonrheumatic aortic (valve) stenosis
I35.1 Nonrheumatic aortic (valve) insufficiency
  Nonrheumatic aortic (valve) incompetence NOS
  Nonrheumatic aortic (valve) regurgitation NOS
I35.2 Nonrheumatic aortic (valve) stenosis with insufficiency
I35.8 Other nonrheumatic aortic valve disorders
I35.9 Nonrheumatic aortic valve disorder, unspecified

I36 `4th` **NONRHEUMATIC TRICUSPID VALVE DISORDERS**
Excludes1: tricuspid valve disorders of unspecified cause (I07.-)
  tricuspid valve disorders specified as congenital (Q22.4, Q22.8, Q22.9)
  tricuspid valve disorders specified as rheumatic (I07.-)
  tricuspid valve disorders with aortic and/or mitral valve involvement (I08.-)

I36.0 Nonrheumatic tricuspid (valve) stenosis
I36.1 Nonrheumatic tricuspid (valve) insufficiency
  Nonrheumatic tricuspid (valve) incompetence
  Nonrheumatic tricuspid (valve) regurgitation
I36.2 Nonrheumatic tricuspid (valve) stenosis with insufficiency
I36.8 Other nonrheumatic tricuspid valve disorders
I36.9 Nonrheumatic tricuspid valve disorder, unspecified

I37 `4th` **NONRHEUMATIC PULMONARY VALVE DISORDERS**
Excludes1: pulmonary valve disorder specified as congenital (Q22.1, Q22.2, Q22.3)
  pulmonary valve disorder specified as rheumatic (I09.89)

I37.0 Nonrheumatic pulmonary valve stenosis
I37.1 Nonrheumatic pulmonary valve insufficiency
  Nonrheumatic pulmonary valve incompetence
  Nonrheumatic pulmonary valve regurgitation
I37.2 Nonrheumatic pulmonary valve stenosis with insufficiency
I37.8 Other nonrheumatic pulmonary valve disorders
I37.9 Nonrheumatic pulmonary valve disorder, unspecified

I38 `✓` **ENDOCARDITIS, VALVE UNSPECIFIED**
Includes: endocarditis (chronic) NOS
  valvular incompetence NOS
  valvular insufficiency NOS
  valvular regurgitation NOS
  valvular stenosis NOS
  valvulitis (chronic) NOS
Excludes1: congenital insufficiency of cardiac valve NOS (Q24.8)
  congenital stenosis of cardiac valve NOS (Q24.8)
  endocardial fibroelastosis (I42.4)
  endocarditis specified as rheumatic (I09.1)

I40 `4th` **ACUTE MYOCARDITIS**
Includes: subacute myocarditis
Excludes1: acute rheumatic myocarditis (I01.2)

I40.0 Infective myocarditis
  Septic myocarditis
  Use additional code (B95–B97) to identify infectious agent
I40.8 Other acute myocarditis
I40.9 Acute myocarditis, unspecified

I42 `4th` **CARDIOMYOPATHY**
Includes: myocardiopathy
Code first pre-existing cardiomyopathy complicating pregnancy and puerperium (O99.4)
Excludes2: ischemic cardiomyopathy (I25.5)
  peripartum cardiomyopathy (O90.3)
  ventricular hypertrophy (I51.7)

I42.1 Obstructive hypertrophic cardiomyopathy
  Hypertrophic subaortic stenosis (idiopathic)
I42.2 Other hypertrophic cardiomyopathy
  Nonobstructive hypertrophic cardiomyopathy
I42.5 Other restrictive cardiomyopathy
  Constrictive cardiomyopathy NOS
I42.9 Cardiomyopathy, unspecified
  Cardiomyopathy (primary) (secondary) NOS

I43 `✓` **CARDIOMYOPATHY IN DISEASES CLASSIFIED ELSEWHERE**
Code first underlying disease, such as:
  amyloidosis (E85.-)
  glycogen storage disease (E74.0)
  gout (M10.0-)
  thyrotoxicosis (E05.0-E05.9-)
Excludes1: cardiomyopathy (in):
  infectious diseases
  sarcoidosis (D86.85)

`4th` `5th` `6th` `7th` Additional Character Required   `✓` 3-character code

•=New Code
▲=Revised Code

Excludes1—Not coded here, do not use together
Excludes2—Not included here

I44 ATRIOVENTRICULAR AND LEFT BUNDLE-BRANCH BLOCK
4th

I44.0 Atrioventricular block, first degree

I44.1 Atrioventricular block, second degree
Atrioventricular block, type I and II
Möbitz block, type I and II
Second degree block, type I and II
Wenckebach's block

I44.2 Atrioventricular block, complete
Complete heart block NOS
Third degree block

I45 OTHER CONDUCTION DISORDERS
4th

I45.6 Pre-excitation syndrome
Accelerated atrioventricular conduction
Accessory atrioventricular conduction
Anomalous atrioventricular excitation
Lown-Ganong-Levine syndrome
Pre-excitation atrioventricular conduction
Wolff-Parkinson-White syndrome

I45.8 Other specified conduction disorders
5th
 I45.81 Long QT syndrome
 I45.89 Other specified conduction disorders
  Atrioventricular [AV] dissociation
  Interference dissociation
  Isorhythmic dissociation
  Nonparoxysmal AV nodal tachycardia

I45.9 Conduction disorder, unspecified
Heart block NOS
Stokes-Adams syndrome

I46 CARDIAC ARREST
4th

Excludes2: cardiogenic shock (R57.0)

I46.2 Cardiac arrest due to underlying cardiac condition
Code first underlying cardiac condition

I46.8 Cardiac arrest due to other underlying condition
Code first underlying condition

I46.9 Cardiac arrest, cause unspecified

I47 PAROXYSMAL TACHYCARDIA
4th

Code first tachycardia complicating: abortion or ectopic or molar
 pregnancy (O00–O07, O08.8)
 obstetric surgery and procedures (O75.4)

Excludes1: tachycardia NOS (R00.0)
 sinoauricular tachycardia NOS (R00.0)
 sinus [sinusal] tachycardia NOS (R00.0)

I47.1 Supraventricular tachycardia
Atrial (paroxysmal) tachycardia
Atrioventricular [AV] (paroxysmal) tachycardia
Atrioventricular re-entrant (nodal) tachycardia [AVNRT] [AVRT]
Junctional (paroxysmal) tachycardia
Nodal (paroxysmal) tachycardia

I48 ATRIAL FIBRILLATION AND FLUTTER
4th

I48.0 Paroxysmal atrial fibrillation

I48.1 Persistent atrial fibrillation
5th
 Excludes1: Permanent atrial fibrillation (I48.21)
 I48.11 Longstanding persistent atrial fibrillation
 I48.19 Other persistent atrial fibrillation
  Chronic persistent atrial fibrillation
  Persistent atrial fibrillation, NOS

I48.2 Chronic atrial fibrillation
5th
 I48.20 Chronic atrial fibrillation, unspecified
  Excludes1: Chronic persistent atrial fibrillation (I48.19)
 I48.21 Permanent atrial fibrillation

I48.3 Typical atrial flutter
Type I atrial flutter

I48.4 Atypical atrial flutter
Type II atrial flutter

I48.9 Unspecified atrial fibrillation and atrial flutter
5th
 I48.91 Unspecified atrial fibrillation
 I48.92 Unspecified atrial flutter

I49 OTHER CARDIAC ARRHYTHMIAS
4th

Code first cardiac arrhythmia complicating: abortion or ectopic or molar
 pregnancy (O00–O07, O08.8)
 obstetric surgery and procedures (O75.4)

Excludes1: neonatal dysrhythmia (P29.1-)
 sinoatrial bradycardia (R00.1)
 sinus bradycardia (R00.1)
 vagal bradycardia (R00.1)

Excludes2: bradycardia NOS (R00.1)

I49.0 Ventricular fibrillation and flutter
5th
 I49.01 Ventricular fibrillation
 I49.02 Ventricular flutter

I49.1 Atrial premature depolarization
Atrial premature beats

I49.5 Sick sinus syndrome
Tachycardia-bradycardia syndrome

I49.9 Cardiac arrhythmia, unspecified
Arrhythmia (cardiac) NOS

I50 HEART FAILURE
4th

Code first: heart failure complicating abortion or ectopic or molar
 pregnancy (O00–O07, O08.8)
 heart failure due to hypertension (I11.0)
 heart failure due to hypertension with CKD (I13.-)
 heart failure following surgery (I97.13-)
 obstetric surgery and procedures (O75.4)
 rheumatic heart failure (I09.81)

Excludes1: neonatal cardiac failure (P29.0)

Excludes2: cardiac arrest (I46.-)

I50.1 Left ventricular failure, unspecified
Cardiac asthma
Edema of lung with heart disease NOS
Edema of lung with heart failure
Left heart failure
Pulmonary edema with heart disease NOS
Pulmonary edema with heart failure
Excludes1: edema of lung without heart disease or heart failure
 (J81.-)
 pulmonary edema without heart disease or failure (J81.-)

I50.2 Systolic (congestive) heart failure
5th
Heart failure with reduced ejection fraction [HFrEF]
Systolic left ventricular heart failure
Code also end stage heart failure, if applicable (I50.84)
Excludes1: combined systolic (congestive) and diastolic
 (congestive) heart failure (I50.4-)
 I50.20 Unspecified systolic (congestive) heart failure
 I50.21 Acute systolic (congestive) heart failure
 I50.22 Chronic systolic (congestive) heart failure
 I50.23 Acute on chronic systolic (congestive) heart failure

I50.3 Diastolic (congestive) heart failure
5th
Diastolic left ventricular heart failure
Heart failure with normal ejection fraction
Heart failure with preserved ejection fraction [HFpEF]
Code also end stage heart failure, if applicable (I50.84)
Excludes1: combined systolic (congestive) and diastolic
 (congestive) heart failure (I50.4-)
 I50.30 Unspecified diastolic (congestive) heart failure
 I50.31 Acute diastolic (congestive) heart failure
 I50.32 Chronic diastolic (congestive) heart failure
 I50.33 Acute on chronic diastolic (congestive) heart failure

I50.4 Combined systolic (congestive) and diastolic (congestive) heart failure
5th
 I50.40 Unspecified combined systolic (congestive) and diastolic (congestive) heart failure
 I50.41 Acute combined systolic (congestive) and diastolic (congestive) heart failure
 I50.42 Chronic combined systolic (congestive) and diastolic (congestive) heart failure
 I50.43 Acute on chronic combined systolic (congestive) and diastolic (congestive) heart failure

I50.8 Other heart failure
5th
 I50.82 Biventricular heart failure
  Code also the type of left ventricular failure as systolic,
  diastolic, or combined, if known (I50.2-I50.43)

CHAPTER 9. DISEASES OF THE CIRCULATORY SYSTEM (I44–I50.82)

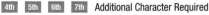 **4th 5th 6th 7th** Additional Character Required   3-character code

•=New Code ***Excludes1***—Not coded here, do not use together
▲=Revised Code ***Excludes2***—Not included here

     I50.83   High output heart failure
     I50.84   End stage heart failure
        Stage D heart failure
        Code also the type of heart failure as systolic, diastolic, or combined, if known (I50.2-I50.43)
     I50.89   Other heart failure
   I50.9   Heart failure, unspecified
       Biventricular (heart) failure NOS
       Cardiac, heart or myocardial failure NOS
       Congestive heart disease
       Congestive heart failure NOS
       Right ventricular failure (secondary to left heart failure)
       Excludes2: fluid overload unrelated to congestive heart failure (E87.70)

I51   **COMPLICATIONS AND ILL-DEFINED DESCRIPTIONS OF HEART DISEASE**
[4th]
   Excludes1: any condition in I51.4–I51.9 due to hypertension (I11.-)
        any condition in I51.4–I51.9 due to hypertension and CKD (I13.-)
        heart disease specified as rheumatic (I00–I09)
   I51.4   Myocarditis, unspecified
       Chronic (interstitial) myocarditis
       Myocardial fibrosis
       Myocarditis NOS
       Excludes1: acute or subacute myocarditis (I40.-)
   I51.5   Myocardial degeneration
       Fatty degeneration of heart or myocardium
       Myocardial disease
       Senile degeneration of heart or myocardium
   I51.7   Cardiomegaly
       Cardiac dilatation
       Cardiac hypertrophy
       Ventricular dilatation
   I51.8   Other ill-defined heart diseases
   [5th]   **I51.81   Takotsubo syndrome**
          Reversible left ventricular dysfunction following sudden emotional stress
          Stress induced cardiomyopathy
          Takotsubo cardiomyopathy
          Transient left ventricular apical ballooning syndrome
      I51.89   Other ill-defined heart diseases
          Carditis (acute)(chronic)
          Pancarditis (acute)(chronic)
   I51.9   Heart disease, unspecified

•**I5A**   **NON-ISCHEMIC MYOCARDIAL INJURY (NON-TRAUMATIC)**
[✓]

I52   **OTHER HEART DISORDERS IN DISEASES CLASSIFIED ELSEWHERE**
[✓]
   Code first underlying disease, such as:
       congenital syphilis (A50.5)
       mucopolysaccharidosis (E76.3)
       schistosomiasis (B65.0-B65.9)
   Excludes1: heart disease (in):
       gonococcal infection (A54.83)
       meningococcal infection (A39.50)
       rheumatoid arthritis (M05.31)
       syphilis (A52.06)

(I60–I69) CEREBROVASCULAR DISEASES

Use additional code to identify presence of:
   alcohol abuse and dependence (F10.-)
   exposure to environmental tobacco smoke (Z77.22)
   history of tobacco dependence (Z87.891)
   hypertension (I10–I16)
   occupational exposure to environmental tobacco smoke (Z57.31)
   tobacco dependence (F17.-)
   tobacco use (Z72.0)
Excludes1: traumatic intracranial hemorrhage (S06.-)

I60   **NONTRAUMATIC SUBARACHNOID HEMORRHAGE**
[4th]   *Excludes1:* syphilitic ruptured cerebral aneurysm (A52.05)
      Excludes2: sequelae of subarachnoid hemorrhage (I69.0-)

I60.0   Nontraumatic subarachnoid hemorrhage from; carotid siphon and bifurcation
[5th]
     I60.00   unspecified carotid siphon and bifurcation
     I60.01   right carotid siphon and bifurcation
     I60.02   left carotid siphon and bifurcation
I60.1   Nontraumatic subarachnoid hemorrhage from; middle cerebral artery
I60.2   Nontraumatic subarachnoid hemorrhage from; anterior communicating artery
I60.3   Nontraumatic subarachnoid hemorrhage from; posterior communicating artery
[5th]
     I60.30   unspecified posterior communicating artery
     I60.31   right posterior communicating artery
     I60.32   left posterior communicating artery
I60.4   Nontraumatic subarachnoid hemorrhage from basilar artery
I60.5   Nontraumatic subarachnoid hemorrhage from; vertebral artery
[5th]
     I60.50   unspecified vertebral artery
     I60.51   from right vertebral artery
     I60.52   from left vertebral artery
I60.6   Nontraumatic subarachnoid hemorrhage from other intracranial arteries
I60.7   Nontraumatic subarachnoid hemorrhage from unspecified intracranial artery
       Ruptured (congenital) berry aneurysm
       Ruptured (congenital) cerebral aneurysm
       Subarachnoid hemorrhage (nontraumatic) from cerebral artery NOS
       Subarachnoid hemorrhage (nontraumatic) from communicating artery NOS
       Excludes1: berry aneurysm, nonruptured (I67.1)
I60.8   Other nontraumatic subarachnoid hemorrhage
       Meningeal hemorrhage
       Rupture of cerebral arteriovenous malformation
I60.9   Nontraumatic subarachnoid hemorrhage, unspecified

I61   **NONTRAUMATIC INTRACEREBRAL HEMORRHAGE**
[4th]   *Excludes2:* sequelae of intracerebral hemorrhage (I69.1-)
I61.0   Nontraumatic intracerebral hemorrhage in hemisphere, subcortical
       Deep intracerebral hemorrhage (nontraumatic)
I61.1   Nontraumatic intracerebral hemorrhage; in hemisphere, cortical
       Cerebral lobe hemorrhage (nontraumatic)
       Superficial intracerebral hemorrhage (nontraumatic)
I61.2   in hemisphere, unspecified
I61.3   in brain stem
I61.4   in cerebellum
I61.5   intraventricular
I61.6   multiple localized
I61.8   Other nontraumatic intracerebral hemorrhage
I61.9   Nontraumatic intracerebral hemorrhage, unspecified

I62   **OTHER AND UNSPECIFIED NONTRAUMATIC INTRACRANIAL HEMORRHAGE**
[4th]   *Excludes2:* sequelae of intracranial hemorrhage (I69.2)
I62.0   Nontraumatic subdural hemorrhage
[5th]
     I62.00   Nontraumatic subdural hemorrhage, unspecified
     I62.01   Nontraumatic acute subdural hemorrhage
     I62.02   Nontraumatic subacute subdural hemorrhage
     I62.03   Nontraumatic chronic subdural hemorrhage
I62.1   Nontraumatic extradural hemorrhage
       Nontraumatic epidural hemorrhage
I62.9   Nontraumatic intracranial hemorrhage, unspecified

I67   **OTHER CEREBROVASCULAR DISEASES**
[4th]   *Excludes2:* sequelae of the listed conditions (I69.8)
I67.1   Cerebral aneurysm, nonruptured
       Cerebral aneurysm NOS
       Cerebral arteriovenous fistula, acquired
       Internal carotid artery aneurysm, intracranial portion
       Internal carotid artery aneurysm, NOS
       Excludes1: congenital cerebral aneurysm, nonruptured (Q28.-)
          ruptured cerebral aneurysm (I60.7)
I67.4   Hypertensive encephalopathy
       Excludes2: insufficiency, NOS, of precerebral arteries (G45.2)

[4th] [5th] [6th] [7th] Additional Character Required   [✓] 3-character code

•=New Code   *Excludes1*—Not coded here, do not use together
▲=Revised Code   *Excludes2*—Not included here

I67.7 Cerebral arteritis, not elsewhere classified
Granulomatous angiitis of the nervous system
Excludes1: allergic granulomatous angiitis (M30.1)

I67.8 Other specified cerebrovascular diseases

`5th` **I67.81 Acute cerebrovascular insufficiency**
Acute cerebrovascular insufficiency unspecified as to location or reversibility

I67.82 Cerebral ischemia
Chronic cerebral ischemia

I67.83 Posterior reversible encephalopathy syndrome
PRES

I67.84 Cerebral vasospasm and vasoconstriction

`6th` **I67.841 Reversible cerebrovascular vasoconstriction syndrome**
Call-Fleming syndrome
Code first underlying condition, if applicable, such as eclampsia (O15.00-O15.9)

I67.848 Other cerebrovascular vasospasm and vasoconstriction

I67.85 Hereditary cerebrovascular diseases

`6th` **I67.850 Cerebral autosomal dominant arteriopathy with subcortical infarcts and leukoencephalopathy CADASIL**
Code also any associated diagnoses, such as:
epilepsy (G40.-)
stroke (I63.-)
vascular dementia (F01.-)

I67.858 Other hereditary cerebrovascular disease

I67.89 Other cerebrovascular disease

I67.9 Cerebrovascular disease, unspecified

(I70–I79) DISEASES OF ARTERIES, ARTERIOLES AND CAPILLARIES

I70 ATHEROSCLEROSIS
`4th` *Includes:* arteriolosclerosis
arterial degeneration
arteriosclerosis
arteriosclerotic vascular disease
arteriovascular degeneration
atheroma
endarteritis deformans or obliterans
senile arteritis
senile endarteritis
vascular degeneration
Use additional code to identify:
exposure to environmental tobacco smoke (Z77.22)
history of tobacco dependence (Z87.891)
occupational exposure to environmental tobacco smoke (Z57.31)
tobacco dependence (F17.-)
tobacco use (Z72.0)
Excludes2: arteriosclerotic cardiovascular disease (I25.1-)
arteriosclerotic heart disease (I25.1-)
atheroembolism (I75.-)
cerebral atherosclerosis (I67.2)
coronary atherosclerosis (I25.1-)
mesenteric atherosclerosis (K55.1)
precerebral atherosclerosis (I67.2)
primary pulmonary atherosclerosis (I27.0)

I70.0 Atherosclerosis of aorta

I70.8 Atherosclerosis of other arteries

I70.9 Other and unspecified atherosclerosis

`5th` **I70.90 Unspecified atherosclerosis**

I70.91 Generalized atherosclerosis

I70.92 Chronic total occlusion of artery of the extremities
Complete occlusion of artery of the extremities
Total occlusion of artery of the extremities
Code first atherosclerosis of arteries of the extremities (I70.2-, I70.3-, I70.4-, I70.5-, I70.6-, I70.7-)

I71 AORTIC ANEURYSM AND DISSECTION
`4th` *Excludes1:* aortic ectasia (I77.81-)
syphilitic aortic aneurysm (A52.01)
traumatic aortic aneurysm (S25.09, S35.09)

I71.8 Aortic aneurysm of unspecified site, ruptured
Rupture of aorta NOS

I71.9 Aortic aneurysm of unspecified site, without rupture
Aneurysm of aorta
Dilatation of aorta
Hyaline necrosis of aorta

I73 OTHER PERIPHERAL VASCULAR DISEASES
`4th` *Excludes2:* chilblains (T69.1)
frostbite (T33–T34)
immersion hand or foot (T69.0-)
spasm of cerebral artery (G45.9)

I73.8 Other specified peripheral vascular diseases
`5th` *Excludes1:* diabetic (peripheral) angiopathy (E08–E13 with .51–.52)

I73.89 Other specified peripheral vascular diseases
Acrocyanosis
Erythrocyanosis
Simple acroparesthesia [Schultze's type]
Vasomotor acroparesthesia [Nothnagel's type]

I73.9 Peripheral vascular disease, unspecified
Intermittent claudication
Peripheral angiopathy NOS
Spasm of artery
Excludes1: atherosclerosis of the extremities (I70.2–I70.7-)

I74 ARTERIAL EMBOLISM AND THROMBOSIS
`4th` *Includes:* embolic infarction
embolic occlusion
thrombotic infarction
thrombotic occlusion
Code first embolism and thrombosis complicating abortion or ectopic or molar pregnancy (O00–O07, O08.2)
embolism and thrombosis complicating pregnancy, childbirth and the puerperium (O88.-)
Excludes2: atheroembolism (I75.-)
basilar embolism and thrombosis (I63.0–I63.2, I65.1)
carotid embolism and thrombosis (I63.0–I63.2, I65.2)
cerebral embolism and thrombosis (I63.3–I63.5, I66.-)
coronary embolism and thrombosis (I21–I25)
mesenteric embolism and thrombosis (K55.0-)
ophthalmic embolism and thrombosis (H34.-)
precerebral embolism and thrombosis NOS (I63.0–I63.2, I65.9)
pulmonary embolism and thrombosis (I26.-)
renal embolism and thrombosis (N28.0)
retinal embolism and thrombosis (H34.-)
septic embolism and thrombosis (I76)
vertebral embolism and thrombosis (I63.0–I63.2, I65.0)

I74.8 Embolism and thrombosis of other arteries

I74.9 Embolism and thrombosis of unspecified artery

I76 SEPTIC ARTERIAL EMBOLISM
`✓` **Code first** underlying infection, such as:
infective endocarditis (I33.0)
lung abscess (J85.-)
Use additional code to identify the site of the embolism (I74.-)
Excludes2: septic pulmonary embolism (I26.01, I26.90)

I77 OTHER DISORDERS OF ARTERIES AND ARTERIOLES
`4th` *Excludes2:* collagen (vascular) diseases (M30–M36)
hypersensitivity angiitis (M31.0)
pulmonary artery (I28.-)

I77.1 Stricture of artery
Narrowing of artery

I77.6 Arteritis, unspecified
Aortitis NOS
Endarteritis NOS
Excludes1: arteritis or endarteritis:
aortic arch (M31.4)
cerebral NEC (I67.7)
coronary (I25.89)
deformans (I70.-)

 `4th` `5th` `6th` `7th` Additional Character Required `✓` 3-character code •=New Code
▲=Revised Code

Excludes1—Not coded here, do not use together
Excludes2—Not included here

giant cell (M31.5, M31.6)
obliterans (I70.-)
senile (I70.-)

I78   DISEASES OF CAPILLARIES
`4th`

I78.0   **Hereditary hemorrhagic telangiectasia**
Rendu-Osler-Weber disease

I78.1   **Nevus, non-neoplastic**
Araneus nevus
Senile nevus
Spider nevus
Stellar nevus
Excludes1: nevus NOS (D22.-)
    vascular NOS (Q82.5)
Excludes2: blue nevus (D22.-)
    flammeus nevus (Q82.5)
    hairy nevus (D22.-)
    melanocytic nevus (D22.-)
    pigmented nevus (D22.-)
    portwine nevus (Q82.5)
    sanguineous nevus (Q82.5)
    strawberry nevus (Q82.5)
    verrucous nevus (Q82.5)

I78.8   **Other diseases of capillaries**

I78.9   **Disease of capillaries, unspecified**

(I80–I89) DISEASES OF VEINS, LYMPHATIC VESSELS AND LYMPH NODES, NOT ELSEWHERE CLASSIFIED

I80   PHLEBITIS AND THROMBOPHLEBITIS
`4th`

Includes: endophlebitis
inflammation, vein
periphlebitis
suppurative phlebitis
Code first phlebitis and thrombophlebitis complicating abortion, ectopic or molar pregnancy (O00–O07, O08.7) phlebitis and thrombophlebitis complicating pregnancy, childbirth and the puerperium (O22.-, O87.-)
Excludes1: venous embolism and thrombosis of lower extremities (I82.4-, I82.5-, I82.81-)

I80.0   **Phlebitis and thrombophlebitis of superficial vessels of; lower extremities**
`5th`
Phlebitis and thrombophlebitis of femoropopliteal vein
   I80.00   **unspecified lower extremity**
   I80.01   **right lower extremity**
   I80.02   **left lower extremity**
   I80.03   **lower extremities, bilateral**

I80.1   **Phlebitis and thrombophlebitis of; femoral vein**
`5th`
Phlebitis and thrombophlebitis of common femoral vein
Phlebitis and thrombophlebitis of deep femoral vein
   I80.10   **unspecified femoral vein**
   I80.11   **right femoral vein**
   I80.12   **left femoral vein**
   I80.13   **femoral vein, bilateral**

I80.2   **Phlebitis and thrombophlebitis of other and unspecified deep vessels of lower extremities**
`5th`
   I80.20   **Phlebitis and thrombophlebitis of unspecified deep vessels of; lower extremities**
   `6th`
     I80.201   **right lower extremity**
     I80.202   **left lower extremity**
     I80.203   **lower extremities, bilateral**
     I80.209   **unspecified lower extremity**
   I80.21   **Phlebitis and thrombophlebitis of; iliac vein**
   `6th`
     Phlebitis and thrombophlebitis of common iliac vein
     Phlebitis and thrombophlebitis of external iliac vein
     Phlebitis and thrombophlebitis of internal iliac vein
     I80.211   **right iliac vein**
     I80.212   **left iliac vein**
     I80.213   **iliac vein, bilateral**
     I80.219   **unspecified iliac vein**
   I80.22   **Phlebitis and thrombophlebitis of; popliteal vein**
   `6th`
     I80.221   **right popliteal vein**
     I80.222   **left popliteal vein**
     I80.223   **popliteal vein, bilateral**
     I80.229   **unspecified popliteal vein**

   I80.23   **Phlebitis and thrombophlebitis of; tibial vein**
   `6th`
     Phlebitis and thrombophlebitis of anterior tibial vein
     Phlebitis and thrombophlebitis of posterior tibial vein
     I80.231   **right tibial vein**
     I80.232   **left tibial vein**
     I80.233   **tibial vein, bilateral**
     I80.239   **unspecified tibial vein**
   I80.24   **Phlebitis and thrombophlebitis of peroneal vein**
   `6th`
     I80.241   **Phlebitis and thrombophlebitis of right peroneal vein**
     I80.242   **Phlebitis and thrombophlebitis of left peroneal vein**
     I80.243   **Phlebitis and thrombophlebitis of peroneal vein, bilateral**
     I80.249   **Phlebitis and thrombophlebitis of unspecified peroneal vein**
   I80.25   **Phlebitis and thrombophlebitis of calf muscular vein**
   `6th`
     Phlebitis and thrombophlebitis of calf muscular vein, NOS
     Phlebitis and thrombophlebitis of gastrocnemial vein
     Phlebitis and thrombophlebitis of soleal vein
     I80.251   **Phlebitis and thrombophlebitis of right calf muscular vein**
     I80.252   **Phlebitis and thrombophlebitis of left calf muscular vein**
     I80.253   **Phlebitis and thrombophlebitis of calf muscular vein, bilateral**
     I80.259   **Phlebitis and thrombophlebitis of unspecified calf muscular vein**
   I80.29   **Phlebitis and thrombophlebitis of other deep vessels of; lower extremities**
   `6th`
     I80.291   **right lower extremity**
     I80.292   **left lower extremity**
     I80.293   **lower extremity, bilateral**
     I80.299   **unspecified lower extremity**

I80.3   **Phlebitis and thrombophlebitis of lower extremities, unspecified**

I80.8   **Phlebitis and thrombophlebitis of other sites**

I80.9   **Phlebitis and thrombophlebitis of unspecified site**

I81   PORTAL VEIN THROMBOSIS
`✓`
Portal (vein) obstruction
Excludes2: hepatic vein thrombosis (I82.0)
    phlebitis of portal vein (K75.1)

I82   OTHER VENOUS EMBOLISM AND THROMBOSIS
`4th`
Code first venous embolism and thrombosis complicating:
   abortion, ectopic or molar pregnancy (O00–O07, O08.7)
   pregnancy, childbirth and the puerperium (O22.-, O87.-)
Excludes2: venous embolism and thrombosis (of):
   cerebral (I63.6, I67.6)
   coronary (I21–I25)
   intracranial and intraspinal, septic or NOS (G08)
   intracranial, nonpyogenic (I67.6)
   intraspinal, nonpyogenic (G95.1)
   mesenteric (K55.0-)
   portal (I81)
   pulmonary (I26.-)

I82.0   **Budd-Chiari syndrome**
Hepatic vein thrombosis

I82.3   **Embolism and thrombosis of renal vein**

I82.9   **Embolism and thrombosis of unspecified vein**
`5th`
   I82.90   **Acute embolism and thrombosis of unspecified vein**
     Embolism of vein NOS
     Thrombosis (vein) NOS

I83   VARICOSE VEINS OF LOWER EXTREMITIES
`4th`
Excludes2: varicose veins complicating pregnancy (O22.0-)
   varicose veins complicating the puerperium (O87.4)

I83.9   **Asymptomatic varicose veins of lower extremities**
`5th`
Phlebectasia of lower extremities
Varicose veins of lower extremities
Varix of lower extremities
   I83.91   **Asymptomatic varicose veins of right lower extremity**

`4th` `5th` `6th` `7th`   Additional Character Required   `✓`   3-character code

• =New Code
▲ =Revised Code

Excludes1—Not coded here, do not use together
Excludes2—Not included here

 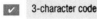

    I83.92 **Asymptomatic varicose veins of left lower extremity**
    I83.93 **Asymptomatic varicose veins of bilateral lower extremities**

I85   ESOPHAGEAL VARICES
`4th`
Use additional code to identify:
alcohol abuse and dependence (F10.-)

I85.0 Esophageal varices
`5th`
Idiopathic esophageal varices
Primary esophageal varices
    I85.00 Esophageal varices without bleeding
        Esophageal varices NOS
    I85.01 Esophageal varices with bleeding

I86   VARICOSE VEINS OF OTHER SITES
`4th`
Excludes1: varicose veins of unspecified site (I83.9-)
Excludes2: retinal varices (H35.0-)

I86.1 Scrotal varices
Varicocele

I88   NONSPECIFIC LYMPHADENITIS
`4th`
Excludes1: acute lymphadenitis, except mesenteric (L04.-)
  enlarged lymph nodes NOS (R59.-)
  HIV disease resulting in generalized lymphadenopathy (B20)

I88.0 Nonspecific mesenteric lymphadenitis
Mesenteric lymphadenitis (acute)(chronic)
I88.1 Chronic lymphadenitis, except mesenteric
Adenitis
Lymphadenitis
I88.8 Other nonspecific lymphadenitis
I88.9 Nonspecific lymphadenitis, unspecified
Lymphadenitis NOS

I89   OTHER NONINFECTIVE DISORDERS OF LYMPHATIC VESSELS AND LYMPH NODES
`4th`
Excludes1: chylocele, tunica vaginalis (nonfilarial) NOS (N50.89)
enlarged lymph nodes NOS (R59.-)
filarial chylocele (B74.-)
hereditary lymphedema (Q82.0)

I89.1 Lymphangitis
Chronic lymphangitis
Lymphangitis NOS
Subacute lymphangitis
Excludes1: acute lymphangitis (L03.-)
I89.8 Other specified noninfective disorders of lymphatic vessels and lymph nodes
Chylocele (nonfilarial)
Chylous ascites
Chylous cyst
Lipomelanotic reticulosis
Lymph node or vessel fistula
Lymph node or vessel infarction
Lymph node or vessel rupture
I89.9 Noninfective disorder of lymphatic vessels and lymph nodes, unspecified
Disease of lymphatic vessels NOS

(I95–I99) OTHER AND UNSPECIFIED DISORDERS OF THE CIRCULATORY SYSTEM

I95   HYPOTENSION
`4th`
Excludes1: cardiovascular collapse (R57.9)
  maternal hypotension syndrome (O26.5-)
  nonspecific low blood pressure reading NOS (R03.1)

I95.1 Orthostatic hypotension
Hypotension, postural
Excludes1: neurogenic orthostatic hypotension [Shy-Drager] (G90.3)
    orthostatic hypotension due to drugs (I95.2)
I95.9 Hypotension, unspecified

I97   INTRAOPERATIVE AND POSTPROCEDURAL COMPLICATIONS AND DISORDERS OF CIRCULATORY SYSTEM, NOT ELSEWHERE CLASSIFIED
`4th`
Excludes2: postprocedural shock (T81.1-)

I97.0 Postcardiotomy syndrome
I97.1 Other postprocedural cardiac functional disturbances
`5th`
Excludes2: acute pulmonary insufficiency following thoracic surgery (J95.1)
intraoperative cardiac functional disturbances (I97.7-)
  I97.11 Postprocedural cardiac insufficiency
  `6th`
    I97.110 Postprocedural cardiac insufficiency following cardiac surgery
    I97.111 Postprocedural cardiac insufficiency following other surgery
  I97.12 Postprocedural cardiac arrest
  `6th`
    I97.120 Postprocedural cardiac arrest following cardiac surgery
    I97.121 Postprocedural cardiac arrest following other surgery
  I97.13 Postprocedural heart failure
  `6th`
  Use additional code to identify the heart failure (I50.-)
    I97.130 Postprocedural heart failure following cardiac surgery
    I97.131 Postprocedural heart failure following other surgery
  I97.19 Other postprocedural cardiac functional disturbances
  `6th`
  Use additional code, if applicable, to further specify disorder
    I97.190 Other postprocedural cardiac functional disturbances following cardiac surgery
    I97.191 Other postprocedural cardiac functional disturbances following other surgery

I97.8 Other intraoperative and postprocedural complications and disorders of the circulatory system, not elsewhere classified
`5th`
Use additional code, if applicable, to further specify disorder
  I97.88 Other intraoperative complications of the circulatory system, NEC
  I97.89 Other postprocedural complications and disorders of the circulatory system, NEC

I99   OTHER AND UNSPECIFIED DISORDERS OF CIRCULATORY SYSTEM
`4th`
I99.8 Other disorder of circulatory system
I99.9 Unspecified disorder of circulatory system

CHAPTER 9. DISEASES OF THE CIRCULATORY SYSTEM   (I83.92–I99.9)

`4th` `5th` `6th` `7th` Additional Character Required   ✔   3-character code   •=New Code   *Excludes1*—Not coded here, do not use together
▲=Revised Code   *Excludes2*—Not included here

Chapter 10. Diseases of the respiratory system (J00–J99)

GUIDELINES

Acute Respiratory Failure

ACUTE RESPIRATORY FAILURE AS PRINCIPAL DIAGNOSIS
Refer to category J96 for guidelines.

ACUTE RESPIRATORY FAILURE AS SECONDARY DIAGNOSIS
Respiratory failure may be listed as a secondary diagnosis if it occurs after admission, or if it is present on admission, but does not meet the definition of principal diagnosis.

SEQUENCING OF ACUTE RESPIRATORY FAILURE AND ANOTHER ACUTE CONDITION
When a patient is admitted with respiratory failure and another acute condition, (e.g., myocardial infarction, cerebrovascular accident, aspiration pneumonia), the principal diagnosis will not be the same in every situation. This applies whether the other acute condition is a respiratory or nonrespiratory condition. Selection of the principal diagnosis will be dependent on the circumstances of admission. If both the respiratory failure and the other acute condition are equally responsible for occasioning the admission to the hospital, and there are no chapter-specific sequencing rules, the guideline regarding two or more diagnoses that equally meet the definition for principal diagnosis may be applied in these situations.

Influenza due to certain identified influenza viruses
See categories J09–J18 for guidelines.

Ventilator associated Pneumonia

DOCUMENTATION OF VENTILATOR ASSOCIATED PNEUMONIA
Refer to category J95 for guidelines.

VENTILATOR ASSOCIATED PNEUMONIA DEVELOPS AFTER ADMISSION
Refer to category J95 for guidelines.

VAPING-RELATED DISORDERS
Refer to code U07.0 for guidelines.

Note: When a respiratory condition is described as occurring in more than one site and is not specifically indexed, it should be classified to the lower anatomic site (e.g. tracheobronchitis to bronchitis in J40).

Use additional code, where applicable, to identify:
    exposure to environmental tobacco smoke (Z77.22)
    exposure to tobacco smoke in the perinatal period (P96.81)
    history of tobacco dependence (Z87.891)
    occupational exposure to environmental tobacco smoke (Z57.31)
    tobacco dependence (F17.-)
    tobacco use (Z72.0)
Excludes2: certain conditions originating in the perinatal period (P04–P96)
    certain infectious and parasitic diseases (A00–B99)
    complications of pregnancy, childbirth and the puerperium (O00–O9A)
    congenital malformations, deformations and chromosomal abnormalities (Q00–Q99)
    endocrine, nutritional and metabolic diseases (E00–E88)
    injury, poisoning and certain other consequences of external causes (S00–T88)
    neoplasms (C00–D49)
    smoke inhalation (T59.81-)
    symptoms, signs and abnormal clinical and laboratory findings, NEC (R00–R94)

(J00–J06) ACUTE UPPER RESPIRATORY INFECTIONS

Excludes1: COPD with acute lower respiratory infection (J44.0)

J00 ✔	**ACUTE NASOPHARYNGITIS [COMMON COLD]**

    Acute rhinitis
    Coryza (acute)
    Infective nasopharyngitis NOS
    Infective rhinitis
    Nasal catarrh, acute
    Nasopharyngitis NOS

Excludes1: acute pharyngitis (J02.-)
    acute sore throat NOS (J02.9)
    influenza virus with other respiratory manifestations (J09.X2, J10.1, J11.1)
    pharyngitis NOS (J02.9)
    rhinitis NOS (J31.0)
    sore throat NOS (J02.9)
Excludes2: allergic rhinitis (J30.1–J30.9)
    chronic pharyngitis (J31.2)
    chronic rhinitis (J31.0)
    chronic sore throat (J31.2)
    nasopharyngitis, chronic (J31.1)
    vasomotor rhinitis (J30.0)

J01 `4th`   **ACUTE SINUSITIS**
Includes: acute abscess of sinus
    acute empyema of sinus
    acute infection of sinus
    acute inflammation of sinus
    acute suppuration of sinus
Use additional code (B95–B97) to identify infectious agent.
Excludes1: sinusitis NOS (J32.9)
Excludes2: chronic sinusitis (J32.0–J32.8)

J01.0   **Acute maxillary sinusitis**
`5th`   Acute antritis
    J01.00   **Acute maxillary sinusitis, unspecified**
    J01.01   **Acute recurrent maxillary sinusitis**
J01.1   **Acute frontal sinusitis**
`5th`   **J01.10**   **Acute frontal sinusitis, unspecified**
    J01.11   **Acute recurrent frontal sinusitis**
J01.2   **Acute ethmoidal sinusitis**
`5th`   **J01.20**   **Acute ethmoidal sinusitis, unspecified**
    J01.21   **Acute recurrent ethmoidal sinusitis**
J01.3   **Acute sphenoidal sinusitis**
`5th`   **J01.30**   **Acute sphenoidal sinusitis, unspecified**
    J01.31   **Acute recurrent sphenoidal sinusitis**
J01.4   **Acute pansinusitis**
`5th`   **J01.40**   **Acute pansinusitis, unspecified**
    J01.41   **Acute recurrent pansinusitis**
J01.8   **Other acute sinusitis**
`5th`   **J01.80**   **Other acute sinusitis**
        Acute sinusitis involving more than one sinus but not pansinusitis
    J01.81   **Other acute recurrent sinusitis**
        Acute recurrent sinusitis involving more than one sinus but not pansinusitis
J01.9   **Acute sinusitis, unspecified**
`5th`   **J01.90**   **Acute sinusitis, unspecified**
    J01.91   **Acute recurrent sinusitis, unspecified**

J02 `4th`   **ACUTE PHARYNGITIS**
Includes: acute sore throat
Excludes1: acute laryngopharyngitis (J06.0)
    peritonsillar abscess (J36)
    pharyngeal abscess (J39.1)
    retropharyngeal abscess (J39.0)
Excludes2: chronic pharyngitis (J31.2)
J02.0   **Streptococcal pharyngitis**
    Septic pharyngitis
    Streptococcal sore throat
    Excludes2: scarlet fever (A38.-)
J02.8   **Acute pharyngitis due to other specified organisms**
    Use additional code (B95–B97) to identify infectious agent
    Excludes1: acute pharyngitis due to coxsackie virus (B08.5)
        acute pharyngitis due to gonococcus (A54.5)
        acute pharyngitis due to herpes [simplex] virus (B00.2)
        acute pharyngitis due to infectious mononucleosis (B27.-)
        enteroviral vesicular pharyngitis (B08.5)

CHAPTER 10. DISEASES OF THE RESPIRATORY SYSTEM (J00–J02.8)

`4th` `5th` `6th` `7th` Additional Character Required	✔ 3-character code	•=New Code ▲=Revised Code	***Excludes1***—Not coded here, do not use together ***Excludes2***—Not included here

J02.9 **Acute pharyngitis, unspecified**
Gangrenous pharyngitis (acute)
Infective pharyngitis (acute) NOS
Pharyngitis (acute) NOS
Sore throat (acute) NOS
Suppurative pharyngitis (acute)
Ulcerative pharyngitis (acute)
Excludes1: influenza virus with other respiratory manifestations (J09.X2, J10.1, J11.1)

J03 **ACUTE TONSILLITIS**
`4th`
Excludes1: acute sore throat (J02.-)
hypertrophy of tonsils (J35.1)
peritonsillar abscess (J36)
sore throat NOS (J02.9)
streptococcal sore throat (J02.0)
Excludes2: chronic tonsillitis (J35.0)
J03.0 **Streptococcal tonsillitis**
`5th` **J03.00** **Acute streptococcal tonsillitis, unspecified**
J03.01 **Acute recurrent streptococcal tonsillitis**
J03.8 **Acute tonsillitis due to other specified organisms**
`5th` **Use additional code** (B95–B97) to identify infectious agent.
Excludes1: diphtheritic tonsillitis (A36.0)
herpesviral pharyngotonsillitis (B00.2)
streptococcal tonsillitis (J03.0)
tuberculous tonsillitis (A15.8)
Vincent's tonsillitis (A69.1)
J03.80 **Acute tonsillitis due to other specified organisms**
J03.81 **Acute recurrent tonsillitis due to other specified organisms**
J03.9 **Acute tonsillitis, unspecified**
`5th` Follicular tonsillitis (acute)
Gangrenous tonsillitis (acute)
Infective tonsillitis (acute)
Tonsillitis (acute) NOS
Ulcerative tonsillitis (acute)
Excludes1: influenza virus with other respiratory manifestations (J09.X2, J10.1, J11.1)
J03.90 **Acute tonsillitis, unspecified**
J03.91 **Acute recurrent tonsillitis, unspecified**

J04 **ACUTE LARYNGITIS AND TRACHEITIS**
`4th`
Use additional code (B95–B97) to identify infectious agent.
Code also influenza, if present, such as:
influenza due to identified novel influenza A virus with other respiratory manifestations (J09.X2)
influenza due to other identified influenza virus with other respiratory manifestations (J10.1)
influenza due to unidentified influenza virus with other respiratory manifestations (J11.1)
Excludes1: acute obstructive laryngitis [croup] and epiglottitis (J05.-)
Excludes2: laryngismus (stridulus) (J38.5)
J04.0 **Acute laryngitis**
Edematous laryngitis (acute)
Laryngitis (acute) NOS
Subglottic laryngitis (acute)
Suppurative laryngitis (acute)
Ulcerative laryngitis (acute)
Excludes1: acute obstructive laryngitis (J05.0)
Excludes2: chronic laryngitis (J37.0)
J04.1 **Acute tracheitis**
`5th` Acute viral tracheitis
Catarrhal tracheitis (acute)
Tracheitis (acute) NOS
Excludes2: chronic tracheitis (J42)
J04.10 **Acute tracheitis without obstruction**
J04.11 **Acute tracheitis with obstruction**
J04.2 **Acute laryngotracheitis**
Laryngotracheitis NOS
Tracheitis (acute) with laryngitis (acute)
Excludes1: acute obstructive laryngotracheitis (J05.0)
Excludes2: chronic laryngotracheitis (J37.1)
J04.3 **Supraglottitis, unspecified**
`5th` **J04.30** **Supraglottitis, unspecified, without obstruction**

J04.31 **Supraglottitis, unspecified, with obstruction**

J05 **ACUTE OBSTRUCTIVE LARYNGITIS [CROUP] AND**
`4th` **EPIGLOTTITIS**
Use additional code (B95–B97) to identify infectious agent.
Code also influenza, if present, such as:
influenza due to identified novel influenza A virus with other respiratory manifestations (J09.X2)
influenza due to other identified influenza virus with other respiratory manifestations (J10.1)
influenza due to unidentified influenza virus with other respiratory manifestations (J11.1)
J05.0 **Acute obstructive laryngitis [croup]**
Obstructive laryngitis (acute) NOS
Obstructive laryngotracheitis NOS
J05.1 **Acute epiglottitis**
`5th` *Excludes2:* epiglottitis, chronic (J37.0)
J05.10 **Acute epiglottitis without obstruction**
Epiglottitis NOS
J05.11 **Acute epiglottitis with obstruction**

J06 **ACUTE UPPER RESPIRATORY INFECTIONS OF MULTIPLE**
`4th` **AND UNSPECIFIED SITES**
Excludes1: acute respiratory infection NOS (J22)
influenza virus with other respiratory manifestations (J09.X2, J10.1, J11.1)
streptococcal pharyngitis (J02.0)
J06.0 **Acute laryngopharyngitis**
J06.9 **Acute upper respiratory infection, unspecified**
Use additional code (B95–B97) to identify infectious agent, if known, such as:
respiratory syncytial virus (RSV) (B97.4)
Upper respiratory disease, acute
Upper respiratory infection NOS

(J09–J18) INFLUENZA AND PNEUMONIA

GUIDELINES

Code only confirmed cases of influenza due to certain identified influenza viruses (category J09), and due to other identified influenza virus (category J10). This is an exception to the hospital inpatient guideline Section II, H. (Uncertain Diagnosis).

In this context, "confirmation" does not require documentation of positive laboratory testing specific for avian or other novel influenza A or other identified influenza virus. However, coding should be based on the provider's diagnostic statement that the patient has avian influenza, or other novel influenza A, for category J09, or has another particular identified strain of influenza, such as H1N1 or H3N2, but not identified as novel or variant, for category J10.

If the provider records "suspected" or "possible" or "probable" avian influenza, or novel influenza, or other identified influenza, then the appropriate influenza code from category J11, Influenza due to unidentified influenza virus, should be assigned. A code from category J09, Influenza due to certain identified influenza viruses, should not be assigned nor should a code from category J10, Influenza due to other identified influenza virus.
Excludes2: allergic or eosinophilic pneumonia (J82)
aspiration pneumonia NOS (J69.0)
meconium pneumonia (P24.01)
neonatal aspiration pneumonia (P24.-)
pneumonia due to solids and liquids (J69.-)
congenital pneumonia (P23.9)
lipid pneumonia (J69.1)
rheumatic pneumonia (I00)
ventilator associated pneumonia (J95.851)

J09 **INFLUENZA DUE TO CERTAIN IDENTIFIED INFLUENZA**
`4th` **VIRUSES**
Excludes1: influenza A/H1N1 (J10.-)
influenza due to other identified influenza virus (J10.-)
influenza due to unidentified influenza virus (J11.-)
seasonal influenza due to other identified influenza virus (J10.-)
seasonal influenza due to unidentified influenza virus (J11.-)

`4th` `5th` `6th` `7th` Additional Character Required | ✓ 3-character code | •=New Code / ▲=Revised Code | *Excludes1*—Not coded here, do not use together / *Excludes2*—Not included here

J09.X **[5th]** **Influenza due to identified novel influenza A virus**
Avian influenza
Bird influenza
Influenza A/H5N1
Influenza of other animal origin, not bird or swine
Swine influenza virus (viruses that normally cause infections in pigs)

J09.X1 **Influenza due to identified novel influenza A virus with pneumonia**
Code also, if applicable, associated: lung abscess (J85.1)
other specified type of pneumonia

J09.X2 **Influenza due to identified novel influenza A virus with other respiratory manifestations**
Influenza due to identified novel influenza A virus NOS
Influenza due to identified novel influenza A virus with laryngitis
Influenza due to identified novel influenza A virus with pharyngitis
Influenza due to identified novel influenza A virus with upper respiratory symptoms
Use additional code, if applicable, for associated: pleural effusion (J91.8) sinusitis (J01.-)

J09.X3 **Influenza due to identified novel influenza A virus with gastrointestinal manifestations**
Influenza due to identified novel influenza A virus gastroenteritis
Excludes1: 'intestinal flu' [viral gastroenteritis] (A08.-)

J09.X9 **Influenza due to identified novel influenza A virus with other manifestations**
Influenza due to identified novel influenza A virus with encephalopathy
Influenza due to identified novel influenza A virus with myocarditis
Influenza due to identified novel influenza A virus with otitis media
Use additional code to identify manifestation

J10 **[4th]** **INFLUENZA DUE TO OTHER IDENTIFIED INFLUENZA VIRUS**
Includes: influenza A (non-novel)
influenza B
influenza C
Excludes1: influenza due to avian influenza virus (J09.X-)
influenza due to swine flu (J09.X-)
influenza due to unidentified influenza virus (J11.-)

J10.0 **[5th]** **Influenza due to other identified influenza virus with pneumonia**
Code also associated lung abscess, if applicable (J85.1)

J10.00 **Influenza due to other identified influenza virus with unspecified type of pneumonia**

J10.01 **Influenza due to other identified influenza virus with the same other identified influenza virus pneumonia**

J10.08 **Influenza due to other identified influenza virus with other specified pneumonia**
Code also other specified type of pneumonia

J10.1 **Influenza due to other identified influenza virus with other respiratory manifestations**
Influenza due to other identified influenza virus NOS
Influenza due to other identified influenza virus with laryngitis
Influenza due to other identified influenza virus with pharyngitis
Influenza due to other identified influenza virus with upper respiratory symptoms
Use additional code for associated pleural effusion, if applicable (J91.8)
Use additional code for associated sinusitis, if applicable (J01.-)

J10.2 **Influenza due to other identified influenza virus with gastrointestinal manifestations**
Influenza due to other identified influenza virus gastroenteritis
Excludes1: 'intestinal flu' [viral gastroenteritis] (A08.-)

J10.8 **[5th]** **Influenza due to other identified influenza virus with other manifestations**

J10.81 **Influenza due to other identified influenza virus with encephalopathy**

J10.82 **Influenza due to other identified influenza virus with myocarditis**

J10.83 **Influenza due to other identified influenza virus with otitis media**
Use additional code for any associated perforated tympanic membrane (H72.-)

J10.89 **Influenza due to other identified influenza virus with other manifestations**
Use additional codes to identify the manifestations

J11 **[4th]** **INFLUENZA DUE TO UNIDENTIFIED INFLUENZA VIRUS**

J11.0 **[5th]** **Influenza due to unidentified influenza virus with pneumonia**
Code also associated lung abscess, if applicable (J85.1)

J11.00 **Influenza due to unidentified influenza virus with unspecified type of pneumonia**
Influenza with pneumonia NOS

J11.08 **Influenza due to unidentified influenza virus with specified pneumonia**
Code also other specified type of pneumonia

J11.1 **Influenza due to unidentified influenza virus with other respiratory manifestations**
Influenza NOS
Influenzal laryngitis NOS
Influenzal pharyngitis NOS
Influenza with upper respiratory symptoms NOS
Use additional code for associated pleural effusion, if applicable (J91.8)
Use additional code for associated sinusitis, if applicable (J01.-)

J11.2 **Influenza due to unidentified influenza virus with gastrointestinal manifestations**
Influenza gastroenteritis NOS
Excludes1: 'intestinal flu' [viral gastroenteritis] (A08.-)

J11.8 **[5th]** **Influenza due to unidentified influenza virus with other manifestations**

J11.81 **Influenza due to unidentified influenza virus with encephalopathy**
Influenzal encephalopathy NOS

J11.82 **Influenza due to unidentified influenza virus with myocarditis**
Influenzal myocarditis NOS

J11.83 **Influenza due to unidentified influenza virus with otitis media**
Influenzal otitis media NOS
Use additional code for any associated perforated tympanic membrane (H72.-)

J11.89 **Influenza due to unidentified influenza virus with other manifestations**
Use additional codes to identify the manifestations

J12 **[4th]** **VIRAL PNEUMONIA, NEC**
Includes: bronchopneumonia due to viruses other than influenza viruses
Code first associated influenza, if applicable (J09.X1, J10.0-, J11.0-)
Code also associated abscess, if applicable (J85.1)
Excludes1: aspiration pneumonia due to solids and liquids (J69.-)
aspiration pneumonia NOS (J69.0)
congenital pneumonia (P23.0)
congenital rubella pneumonitis (P35.0)
interstitial pneumonia NOS (J84.9)
lipid pneumonia (J69.1)
neonatal aspiration pneumonia (P24.-)

J12.0 **Adenoviral pneumonia**

J12.1 **RSV pneumonia**

J12.2 **Parainfluenza virus pneumonia**

J12.3 **Human metapneumovirus pneumonia**

J12.8 **Other viral pneumonia**

[5th] **J12.81** **Pneumonia due to SARS-associated coronavirus**
SARS NOS GUIDELINE
See code U07.1 for further details.

•J12.82 **Pneumonia due to coronavirus disease 2019**

J12.89 **Other viral pneumonia**

J12.9 **Viral pneumonia, unspecified**

[4th] **[5th]** **[6th]** **[7th]** Additional Character Required   [✓]   3-character code

•=New Code   ▲=Revised Code

Excludes1—Not coded here, do not use together
Excludes2—Not included here

CHAPTER 10. DISEASES OF THE RESPIRATORY SYSTEM (J13–J21.8)

J13   PNEUMONIA DUE TO STREPTOCOCCUS PNEUMONIAE
✔
Bronchopneumonia due to S. pneumoniae
Code first associated influenza, if applicable (J09.X1, J10.0-, J11.0-)
Code also associated abscess, if applicable (J85.1)
Excludes1: congenital pneumonia due to S. pneumoniae (P23.6)
     lobar pneumonia, unspecified organism (J18.1)
     pneumonia due to other streptococci (J15.3-J15.4)

J14   PNEUMONIA DUE TO H. INFLUENZAE
✔
Bronchopneumonia due to H. influenzae
Code first associated influenza, if applicable (J09.X1, J10.0-, J11.0-)
Code also associated abscess, if applicable (J85.1)
Excludes1: congenital pneumonia due to H. influenzae (P23.6)

J15   BACTERIAL PNEUMONIA, NEC
4th
Includes: bronchopneumonia due to bacteria other than S. pneumoniae and H. influenzae
Code first associated influenza, if applicable (J09.X1, J10.0-, J11.0-)
Code also associated abscess, if applicable (J85.1)
Excludes1: chlamydial pneumonia (J16.0)
     congenital pneumonia (P23.-)
     Legionnaires' disease (A48.1)
     spirochetal pneumonia (A69.8)

J15.0   Pneumonia due to K. pneumoniae
J15.1   Pneumonia due to Pseudomonas
J15.2   Pneumonia due to staphylococcus
   5th   **J15.20**   Pneumonia due to staphylococcus, unspecified
     J15.21   Pneumonia due to staphylococcus aureus
      6th   **J15.211**   Pneumonia due to MSSA
         MSSA pneumonia
         Pneumonia due to Staphylococcus aureus NOS
         J15.212   Pneumonia due to MRSA
     J15.29   Pneumonia due to other staphylococcus
J15.3   Pneumonia due to streptococcus, group B
J15.4   Pneumonia due to other streptococci
     Excludes1: pneumonia due to streptococcus, group B (J15.3)
       pneumonia due to Streptococcus pneumoniae (J13)
J15.5   Pneumonia due to E. coli
J15.6   Pneumonia due to other (aerobic) Gram-negative bacteria
     Pneumonia due to Serratia marcescens
J15.7   Pneumonia due to M. pneumoniae
J15.8   Pneumonia due to other specified bacteria
J15.9   Unspecified bacterial pneumonia
     Pneumonia due to gram-positive bacteria

J16   PNEUMONIA DUE TO OTHER INFECTIOUS ORGANISMS, NEC
4th
Code first associated influenza, if applicable (J09.X1, J10.0-, J11.0-)
Code also associated abscess, if applicable (J85.1)
Excludes1: congenital pneumonia (P23.-)
     ornithosis (A70)
     pneumocystosis (B59)
     pneumonia NOS (J18.9)
J16.0   Chlamydial pneumonia
J16.8   Pneumonia due to other specified infectious organisms

J17   PNEUMONIA IN DISEASES CLASSIFIED ELSEWHERE
✔
Code first underlying disease, such as:
     Q fever (A78)
     rheumatic fever (I00)
     schistosomiasis (B65.0–B65.9)
Excludes1: candidial pneumonia (B37.1)
     chlamydial pneumonia (J16.0)
     gonorrheal pneumonia (A54.84)
     histoplasmosis pneumonia (B39.0–B39.2)
     measles pneumonia (B05.2)
     nocardiosis pneumonia (A43.0)
     pneumocystosis (B59)
     pneumonia due to Pneumocystis carinii (B59)
     pneumonia due to Pneumocystis jiroveci (B59)
     pneumonia in actinomycosis (A42.0)
     pneumonia in anthrax (A22.1)
     pneumonia in ascariasis (B77.81)

     pneumonia in aspergillosis (B44.0–B44.1)
     pneumonia in coccidioidomycosis (B38.0–B38.2)
     pneumonia in cytomegalovirus disease (B25.0)
     pneumonia in toxoplasmosis (B58.3)
     rubella pneumonia (B06.81)
     salmonella pneumonia (A02.22)
     spirochetal infection NEC with pneumonia (A69.8)
     tularemia pneumonia (A21.2)
     typhoid fever with pneumonia (A01.03)
     varicella pneumonia (B01.2)
     whooping cough with pneumonia (A37 with fifth-character 1)

J18   PNEUMONIA, UNSPECIFIED ORGANISM
4th
Code first associated influenza, if applicable (J09.X1, J10.0-, J11.0-)
Excludes1: abscess of lung with pneumonia (J85.1)
     aspiration pneumonia due to solids and liquids (J69.-)
     aspiration pneumonia NOS (J69.0)
     congenital pneumonia (P23.0)
     drug-induced interstitial lung disorder (J70.2–J70.4)
     interstitial pneumonia NOS (J84.9)
     lipid pneumonia (J69.1)
     neonatal aspiration pneumonia (P24.-)
     pneumonitis due to external agents (J67–J70)
     pneumonitis due to fumes and vapors (J68.0)
     usual interstitial pneumonia (J84.178)
J18.0   Bronchopneumonia, unspecified organism
     Excludes1: hypostatic bronchopneumonia (J18.2)
       lipid pneumonia (J69.1)
     Excludes2: acute bronchiolitis (J21.-)
       chronic bronchiolitis (J44.9)
J18.1   Lobar pneumonia, unspecified organism
J18.8   Other pneumonia, unspecified organism
J18.9   Pneumonia, unspecified organism

(J20–J22) OTHER ACUTE LOWER RESPIRATORY INFECTIONS

Excludes2: COPD with acute lower respiratory infection (J44.0)

J20   ACUTE BRONCHITIS
4th
Includes: acute and subacute bronchitis (with) bronchospasm
     acute and subacute bronchitis (with) tracheitis
     acute and subacute bronchitis (with) tracheobronchitis, acute
     acute and subacute fibrinous bronchitis
     acute and subacute membranous bronchitis
     acute and subacute purulent bronchitis
     acute and subacute septic bronchitis
Excludes1: bronchitis NOS (J40)
     tracheobronchitis NOS
Excludes2: acute bronchitis with bronchiectasis (J47.0)
     acute bronchitis with chronic obstructive asthma (J44.0)
     acute bronchitis with COPD (J44.0)
     allergic bronchitis NOS (J45.909-)
     bronchitis due to chemicals, fumes and vapors (J68.0)
     chronic bronchitis NOS (J42)
     chronic mucopurulent bronchitis (J41.1)
     chronic obstructive bronchitis (J44.-)
     chronic obstructive tracheobronchitis (J44.-)
     chronic simple bronchitis (J41.0)
     chronic tracheobronchitis (J42)
J20.0   Acute bronchitis due to M. pneumoniae
J20.1   Acute bronchitis due to H. influenzae
J20.2   Acute bronchitis due to streptococcus
J20.3   Acute bronchitis due to coxsackievirus
J20.4   Acute bronchitis due to parainfluenza virus
J20.5   Acute bronchitis due to RSV
J20.6   Acute bronchitis due to rhinovirus
J20.7   Acute bronchitis due to echovirus
J20.8   Acute bronchitis due to other specified organisms
J20.9   Acute bronchitis, unspecified

J21   ACUTE BRONCHIOLITIS
4th
Includes: acute bronchiolitis with bronchospasm
Excludes2: respiratory bronchiolitis interstitial lung disease (J84.115)
J21.0   Acute bronchiolitis due to RSV
J21.1   Acute bronchiolitis due to human metapneumovirus
J21.8   Acute bronchiolitis due to other specified organisms

4th **5th** **6th** **7th**   Additional Character Required   ✔   3-character code   •=New Code   *Excludes1*—Not coded here, do not use together
     ▲=Revised Code   *Excludes2*—Not included here

J21.9 Acute bronchiolitis, unspecified
Bronchiolitis (acute)
Excludes1: chronic bronchiolitis (J44.-)

J22 UNSPECIFIED ACUTE LOWER RESPIRATORY INFECTION
☑ Acute (lower) respiratory (tract) infection NOS
Excludes1: upper respiratory infection (acute) (J06.9)

(J30–J39) OTHER DISEASES OF UPPER RESPIRATORY TRACT

J30 VASOMOTOR AND ALLERGIC RHINITIS
[4th] *Includes:* spasmodic rhinorrhea
Excludes1: allergic rhinitis with asthma (bronchial) (J45.909)
    rhinitis NOS (J31.0)
  J30.1 Allergic rhinitis due to pollen
    Allergy NOS due to pollen
    Hay fever
    Pollinosis
  J30.2 Other seasonal allergic rhinitis
  J30.5 Allergic rhinitis due to food
  J30.8 Other allergic rhinitis
    [5th] **J30.81   Allergic rhinitis due to animal (cat) (dog) hair and dander**
      J30.89   Other allergic rhinitis
        Perennial allergic rhinitis
  J30.9 Allergic rhinitis, unspecified

J31 CHRONIC RHINITIS, NASOPHARYNGITIS AND
[4th] **PHARYNGITIS**
Use additional code to identify: (Refer to Chapter 10 guidelines for codes)
  J31.0 Chronic rhinitis
    Atrophic rhinitis (chronic)
    Granulomatous rhinitis (chronic)
    Hypertrophic rhinitis (chronic)
    Obstructive rhinitis (chronic)
    Ozena
    Purulent rhinitis (chronic)
    Rhinitis (chronic) NOS
    Ulcerative rhinitis (chronic)
    Excludes1: allergic rhinitis (J30.1–J30.9)
      vasomotor rhinitis (J30.0)
  J31.1 Chronic nasopharyngitis
    Excludes2: acute nasopharyngitis (J00)
  J31.2 Chronic pharyngitis
    Chronic sore throat
    Atrophic pharyngitis (chronic)
    Granular pharyngitis (chronic)
    Hypertrophic pharyngitis (chronic)
    Excludes2 acute pharyngitis (J02.9)

J32 CHRONIC SINUSITIS
[4th] *Includes:* sinus abscess
    sinus empyema
    sinus infection
    sinus suppuration
Use additional code to identify: (Refer to Chapter 10 guidelines for codes)
Excludes2: acute sinusitis (J01.-)
  J32.0 Chronic maxillary sinusitis
    Antritis (chronic)
    Maxillary sinusitis NOS
  J32.1 Chronic frontal sinusitis
    Frontal sinusitis NOS
  J32.2 Chronic ethmoidal sinusitis
    Ethmoidal sinusitis NOS
    Excludes1: Woakes' ethmoiditis (J33.1)
  J32.3 Chronic sphenoidal sinusitis
    Sphenoidal sinusitis NOS
  J32.4 Chronic pansinusitis
    Pansinusitis NOS
  J32.8 Other chronic sinusitis
    Sinusitis (chronic) involving more than one sinus but not pansinusitis
  J32.9 Chronic sinusitis, unspecified
    Sinusitis (chronic) NOS

J33 NASAL POLYP
[4th] Use additional code to identify: (Refer to Chapter 10 guidelines for codes)
Excludes1: adenomatous polyps (D14.0)
  J33.0 Polyp of nasal cavity
    Choanal polyp
    Nasopharyngeal polyp
  J33.8 Other polyp of sinus
    Accessory polyp of sinus
    Ethmoidal polyp of sinus
    Maxillary polyp of sinus
    Sphenoidal polyp of sinus
  J33.9 Nasal polyp, unspecified

J34 OTHER AND UNSPECIFIED DISORDERS OF NOSE AND
[4th] **NASAL SINUSES**
Excludes2: varicose ulcer of nasal septum (I86.8)
  J34.0 Abscess, furuncle and carbuncle of nose
    Cellulitis of nose
    Necrosis of nose
    Ulceration of nose
  J34.1 Cyst and mucocele of nose and nasal sinus
  J34.2 Deviated nasal septum
    Deflection or deviation of septum (nasal) (acquired)
    Excludes1: congenital deviated nasal septum (Q67.4)
  J34.3 Hypertrophy of nasal turbinates
  J34.8 Other specified disorders of nose and nasal sinuses
    [5th] **J34.81   Nasal mucositis (ulcerative)**
        Code also type of associated therapy, such as:
          antineoplastic and immunosuppressive drugs (T45.1X-)
          radiological procedure and radiotherapy (Y84.2)
        Excludes2: gastrointestinal mucositis (ulcerative) (K92.81)
          mucositis (ulcerative) of vagina and vulva (N76.81)
          oral mucositis (ulcerative) (K12.3-)
      J34.89   Other specified disorders of nose and nasal sinuses
        Perforation of nasal septum NOS
        Rhinolith
  J34.9 Unspecified disorder of nose and nasal sinuses

J35 CHRONIC DISEASES OF TONSILS AND ADENOIDS
[4th] Use additional code to identify: (Refer to Chapter 10 guidelines for codes)
  J35.0 Chronic tonsillitis and adenoiditis
    [5th] *Excludes2:* acute tonsillitis (J03.-)
    J35.01   Chronic tonsillitis
    J35.02   Chronic adenoiditis
    J35.03   Chronic tonsillitis and adenoiditis
  J35.1 Hypertrophy of tonsils
    Enlargement of tonsils
    Excludes1: hypertrophy of tonsils with tonsillitis (J35.0-)
  J35.2 Hypertrophy of adenoids
    Enlargement of adenoids
    Excludes1: hypertrophy of adenoids with adenoiditis (J35.0-)
  J35.3 Hypertrophy of tonsils with hypertrophy of adenoids
    Excludes1: hypertrophy of tonsils and adenoids with tonsillitis and adenoiditis (J35.03)
  J35.8 Other chronic diseases of tonsils and adenoids
    Adenoid vegetations
    Amygdalolith
    Calculus, tonsil
    Cicatrix of tonsil (and adenoid)
    Tonsillar tag
    Ulcer of tonsil
  J35.9 Chronic disease of tonsils and adenoids, unspecified
    Disease (chronic) of tonsils and adenoids NOS

J36 PERITONSILLAR ABSCESS
☑ *Includes:* abscess of tonsil
    peritonsillar cellulitis
    quinsy
Use additional code (B95-B97) to identify infectious agent.
Excludes1: acute tonsillitis (J03.-)
    chronic tonsillitis (J35.0)
    retropharyngeal abscess (J39.0)
    tonsillitis NOS (J03.9-)

[4th] [5th] [6th] [7th] Additional Character Required   ☑ 3-character code

•=New Code   *Excludes1*—Not coded here, do not use together
▲=Revised Code   *Excludes2*—Not included here

J37 **CHRONIC LARYNGITIS AND LARYNGOTRACHEITIS**
[4th]
Use additional code to identify: (Refer to Chapter 10 guidelines for codes)
J37.0 **Chronic laryngitis**
Catarrhal laryngitis
Hypertrophic laryngitis
Sicca laryngitis
Excludes2: acute laryngitis (J04.0)
obstructive (acute) laryngitis (J05.0)
J37.1 **Chronic laryngotracheitis**
Laryngitis, chronic, with tracheitis (chronic)
Tracheitis, chronic, with laryngitis
Excludes1: chronic tracheitis (J42)
Excludes2: acute laryngotracheitis (J04.2)
acute tracheitis (J04.1)

J38 **DISEASES OF VOCAL CORDS AND LARYNX, NEC**
[4th]
Use additional code to identify: (Refer to Chapter 10 guidelines for codes)
Excludes1: congenital laryngeal stridor (P28.89)
obstructive laryngitis (acute) (J05.0)
postprocedural subglottic stenosis (J95.5)
stridor (R06.1)
ulcerative laryngitis (J04.0)
J38.0 **Paralysis of vocal cords and larynx**
[5th]
Laryngoplegia
Paralysis of glottis
J38.00 **Paralysis of vocal cords and larynx, unspecified**
J38.01 **Paralysis of vocal cords and larynx, unilateral**
J38.02 **Paralysis of vocal cords and larynx, bilateral**
J38.4 **Edema of larynx**
Edema (of) glottis
Subglottic edema
Supraglottic edema
Excludes1: acute obstructive laryngitis [croup] (J05.0)
edematous laryngitis (J04.0)
J38.5 **Laryngeal spasm**
Laryngismus (stridulus)

J39 **OTHER DISEASES OF UPPER RESPIRATORY TRACT**
[4th]
Excludes1: acute respiratory infection NOS (J22)
acute upper respiratory infection (J06.9)
upper respiratory inflammation due to chemicals, gases, fumes or vapors (J68.2)
J39.0 **Retropharyngeal and parapharyngeal abscess**
Peripharyngeal abscess
Excludes1: peritonsillar abscess (J36)
J39.2 **Other diseases of pharynx**
Cyst of pharynx
Edema of pharynx
Excludes2: chronic pharyngitis (J31.2)
ulcerative pharyngitis (J02.9)
J39.8 **Other specified diseases of upper respiratory tract**
J39.9 **Disease of upper respiratory tract, unspecified**

(J40–J47) CHRONIC LOWER RESPIRATORY DISEASES

Excludes1: bronchitis due to chemicals, gases, fumes and vapors (J68.0)
Excludes2: cystic fibrosis (E84.-)

J40 **BRONCHITIS, NOT SPECIFIED AS ACUTE OR CHRONIC**
[✔]
Bronchitis NOS
Bronchitis with tracheitis NOS
Catarrhal bronchitis
Tracheobronchitis NOS
Use additional code to identify: (Refer to Chapter 10 guidelines for codes)
Excludes1: acute bronchitis (J20.-)
allergic bronchitis NOS (J45.909-)
asthmatic bronchitis NOS (J45.9-)
bronchitis due to chemicals, gases, fumes and vapors (J68.0)

J42 **UNSPECIFIED CHRONIC BRONCHITIS**
[✔]
Chronic bronchitis NOS
Chronic tracheitis
Chronic tracheobronchitis
Use additional code to identify any associated tobacco use or exposure

Excludes1: chronic asthmatic bronchitis (J44.-)
chronic bronchitis with airway obstruction (J44.-)
chronic emphysematous bronchitis (J44.-)
chronic obstructive pulmonary disease NOS (J44.9)
simple and mucopurulent chronic bronchitis (J41.-)

J45 **ASTHMA**
[4th]
Includes: allergic (predominantly) asthma
allergic bronchitis NOS
allergic rhinitis with asthma
atopic asthma
extrinsic allergic asthma
hay fever with asthma
idiosyncratic asthma
intrinsic nonallergic asthma
nonallergic asthma
Use additional code to identify: (Refer to Chapter 10 guidelines for codes)
eosinophilic asthma (J82.83)
Excludes1: detergent asthma (J69.8)
eosinophilic asthma (J82)
miner's asthma (J60)
wheezing NOS (R06.2)
wood asthma (J67.8)
Excludes2: asthma with COPD (J44.9)
chronic asthmatic (obstructive) bronchitis (J44.9)
chronic obstructive asthma (J44.9)
J45.2 **Mild intermittent asthma**
[5th] **J45.20** **Mild intermittent asthma, uncomplicated**
Mild intermittent asthma NOS
J45.21 **Mild intermittent asthma with (acute) exacerbation**
J45.22 **Mild intermittent asthma with status asthmaticus**
J45.3 **Mild persistent asthma**
[5th] **J45.30** **Mild persistent asthma, uncomplicated**
Mild persistent asthma NOS
J45.31 **Mild persistent asthma with (acute) exacerbation**
J45.32 **Mild persistent asthma with status asthmaticus**
J45.4 **Moderate persistent asthma**
[5th] **J45.40** **Moderate persistent asthma, uncomplicated**
Moderate persistent asthma NOS
J45.41 **Moderate persistent asthma with (acute) exacerbation**
J45.42 **Moderate persistent asthma with status asthmaticus**
J45.5 **Severe persistent asthma**
[5th] **J45.50** **Severe persistent asthma, uncomplicated**
Severe persistent asthma NOS
J45.51 **Severe persistent asthma with (acute) exacerbation**
J45.52 **Severe persistent asthma with status asthmaticus**
J45.9 **Other and unspecified asthma**
[5th] **J45.90** **Unspecified asthma**
[6th] Asthmatic bronchitis NOS
Childhood asthma NOS
Late onset asthma
J45.901 **Unspecified asthma with (acute) exacerbation**
J45.902 **Unspecified asthma with status asthmaticus**
J45.909 **Unspecified asthma, uncomplicated**
Asthma NOS
Excludes2: lung diseases due to external agents (J60–J70)
J45.99 **Other asthma**
[6th] **J45.990** **Exercise induced bronchospasm**
J45.991 **Cough variant asthma**
J45.998 **Other asthma**

(J60–J70) LUNG DISEASES DUE TO EXTERNAL AGENTS

Excludes2: asthma (J45.-)
malignant neoplasm of bronchus and lung (C34.-)

J69 **PNEUMONITIS DUE TO SOLIDS AND LIQUIDS**
[4th]
Excludes1: neonatal aspiration syndromes (P24.-)
postprocedural pneumonitis (J95.4)

J69.0 Pneumonitis due to inhalation of food and vomit
Aspiration pneumonia NOS
Aspiration pneumonia (due to) food (regurgitated)
Aspiration pneumonia (due to) gastric secretions
Aspiration pneumonia (due to) milk
Aspiration pneumonia (due to) vomit
Code also any associated FB in respiratory tract (T17.-)
Excludes1: chemical pneumonitis due to anesthesia (J95.4)

J69.1 Pneumonitis due to inhalation of oils and essences
Exogenous lipoid pneumonia
Lipid pneumonia NOS
Code first (T51–T65) to identify substance
Excludes1: endogenous lipoid pneumonia (J84.89)

J69.8 Pneumonitis due to inhalation of other solids and liquids
Pneumonitis due to aspiration of blood
Pneumonitis due to aspiration of detergent
Code first (T51–T65) to identify substance

J70 RESPIRATORY CONDITIONS DUE TO OTHER EXTERNAL AGENTS `4th`

J70.5 Respiratory conditions due to smoke inhalation
Code first smoke inhalation (T59.81-)
Excludes2: smoke inhalation due to chemicals, gases, fumes and vapors (J68.9)

J70.9 Respiratory conditions due to unspecified external agent
Code first (T51–T65) to identify the external agent

(J80–J84) OTHER RESPIRATORY DISEASES PRINCIPALLY AFFECTING THE INTERSTITIUM

J80 ACUTE RESPIRATORY DISTRESS SYNDROME ✔
Acute respiratory distress syndrome in adult or child
Adult hyaline membrane disease
Excludes1: respiratory distress syndrome in newborn (perinatal) (P22.0)

J81 PULMONARY EDEMA `4th`
Use additional code to identify: (Refer to Chapter 10 guidelines for codes)
Excludes1: chemical (acute) pulmonary edema (J68.1)
hypostatic pneumonia (J18.2)
passive pneumonia (J18.2)
pulmonary edema due to external agents (J60-J70)
pulmonary edema with heart disease NOS (I50.1)
pulmonary edema with heart failure (I50.1)

J81.0 Acute pulmonary edema
Acute edema of lung

J82 PULMONARY EOSINOPHILIA, NOT ELSEWHERE CLASSIFIED `4th`

J82.8 Pulmonary eosinophilia, NEC
`5th` **J82.81 Chronic eosinophilic pneumonia**
Eosinophilic pneumonia, NOS
J82.82 Acute eosinophilic pneumonia
J82.83 Eosinophilic asthma
Code first asthma, by type, such as:
mild intermittent asthma (J45.2-)
mild persistent asthma (J45.3-)
moderate persistent asthma (J45.4-)
severe persistent asthma (J45.5-)
J82.89 Other pulmonary eosinophilia, not elsewhere classified
Allergic pneumonia
Löffler's pneumonia
Tropical (pulmonary) eosinophilia NOS

J84 OTHER INTERSTITIAL PULMONARY DISEASES `4th`
Excludes1: drug-induced interstitial lung disorders (J70.2-J70.4)
interstitial emphysema (J98.2)
Excludes2: lung diseases due to external agents (J60-J70)

J84.0 Alveolar and parieto-alveolar conditions
`5th` **J84.01 Alveolar proteinosis**
J84.02 Pulmonary alveolar microlithiasis
J84.03 Idiopathic pulmonary hemosiderosis
Essential brown induration of lung
Code first underlying disease, such as:
disorders of iron metabolism (E83.1-)

Excludes1: acute idiopathic pulmonary hemorrhage in infants [AIPHI] (R04.81)
J84.09 Other alveolar and parieto-alveolar conditions
J84.8 Other specified interstitial pulmonary diseases
`5th` *Excludes1:* exogenous or unspecified lipoid pneumonia (J69.1)
J84.83 Surfactant mutations of the lung
J84.84 Other interstitial lung diseases of childhood
`6th` **J84.841 Neuroendocrine cell hyperplasia of infancy**
J84.842 Pulmonary interstitial glycogenosis
J84.843 Alveolar capillary dysplasia with vein misalignment
J84.848 Other interstitial lung diseases of childhood
J84.89 Other specified interstitial pulmonary disease
J84.9 Interstitial pulmonary disease, unspecified
Interstitial pneumonia NOS

(J85–J86) SUPPURATIVE AND NECROTIC CONDITIONS OF THE LOWER RESPIRATORY TRACT

J86 PYOTHORAX `4th`
Use additional code (B95–B97) to identify infectious agent.
Excludes1: abscess of lung (J85.-)
pyothorax due to tuberculosis (A15.6)

J86.0 Pyothorax with fistula
Bronchocutaneous fistula
Bronchopleural fistula
Hepatopleural fistula
Mediastinal fistula
Pleural fistula
Thoracic fistula
Any condition classifiable to J86.9 with fistula

J86.9 Pyothorax without fistula
Abscess of pleura
Abscess of thorax
Empyema (chest) (lung) (pleura)
Fibrinopurulent pleurisy
Purulent pleurisy
Pyopneumothorax
Septic pleurisy
Seropurulent pleurisy
Suppurative pleurisy

(J90–J94) OTHER DISEASES OF THE PLEURA

J90 PLEURAL EFFUSION, NEC ✔
Encysted pleurisy
Pleural effusion NOS
Pleurisy with effusion (exudative) (serous)
Excludes1: chylous (pleural) effusion (J94.0)
malignant pleural effusion (J91.0))
pleurisy NOS (R09.1)
tuberculous pleural effusion (A15.6)

J91 PLEURAL EFFUSION IN CONDITIONS CLASSIFIED ELSEWHERE `4th`
Excludes2: pleural effusion in heart failure (I50.-)
pleural effusion in SLE (M32.13)

J91.0 Malignant pleural effusion
Code first underlying neoplasm
J91.8 Pleural effusion in other conditions classified elsewhere
Code first underlying disease, such as:
filariasis (B74.0-B74.9)
influenza (J09.X2, J10.1, J11.1)

J93 PNEUMOTHORAX AND AIR LEAK `4th`
Excludes1: congenital or perinatal pneumothorax (P25.1)
postprocedural air leak (J95.812)
postprocedural pneumothorax (J95.811)
traumatic pneumothorax (S27.0)
tuberculous (current disease) pneumothorax (A15.-)
pyopneumothorax (J86.-)
J93.0 Spontaneous tension pneumothorax

`4th` `5th` `6th` `7th` Additional Character Required   ✔ 3-character code

•=New Code
▲=Revised Code

Excludes1—Not coded here, do not use together
Excludes2—Not included here

J93.1   **Other spontaneous pneumothorax**
> **5th**   **J93.11**   **Primary spontaneous pneumothorax**
>   **J93.12**   **Secondary spontaneous pneumothorax**
>   **Code first** underlying condition, such as:
>   catamenial pneumothorax due to endometriosis (N80.8)
>   cystic fibrosis (E84.-)
>   eosinophilic pneumonia (J82)
>   lymphangioleiomyomatosis (J84.81)
>   malignant neoplasm of bronchus and lung (C34.-)
>   Marfan's syndrome (Q87.4)
>   pneumonia due to Pneumocystis carinii (B59)
>   secondary malignant neoplasm of lung (C78.0-)
>   spontaneous rupture of the esophagus (K22.3)

J93.8   **Other pneumothorax and air leak**
> **5th**   **J93.81**   **Chronic pneumothorax**
>   **J93.82**   **Other air leak**
>   Persistent air leak
>   **J93.83**   **Other pneumothorax**
>   Acute pneumothorax
>   Spontaneous pneumothorax NOS

J93.9   **Pneumothorax, unspecified**
>   Pneumothorax NOS

(J95) INTRAOPERATIVE AND POSTPROCEDURAL COMPLICATIONS AND DISORDERS OF RESPIRATORY SYSTEM, NEC

GUIDELINES

As with all procedural or postprocedural complications, code assignment is based on the provider's documentation of the relationship between the condition and the procedure.

Code J95.851, Ventilator associated pneumonia (VAP), should be assigned only when the provider has documented VAP. An additional code to identify the organism (e.g., Pseudomonas aeruginosa, code B96.5) should also be assigned. Do not assign an additional code from categories J12-J18 to identify the type of pneumonia.

Code J95.851 should not be assigned for cases where the patient has pneumonia and is on a mechanical ventilator and the provider has not specifically stated that the pneumonia is ventilator-associated pneumonia. If the documentation is unclear as to whether the patient has a pneumonia that is a complication attributable to the mechanical ventilator, query the provider.

A patient may be admitted with one type of pneumonia (e.g., code J13, Pneumonia due to Streptococcus pneumonia) and subsequently develop VAP. In this instance, the principal diagnosis would be the appropriate code from categories J12-J18 for the pneumonia diagnosed at the time of admission. Code J95.851, Ventilator associated pneumonia, would be assigned as an additional diagnosis when the provider has also documented the presence of ventilator associated pneumonia.

J95   **INTRAOPERATIVE AND POSTPROCEDURAL**
4th   **COMPLICATIONS AND DISORDERS OF RESPIRATORY SYSTEM, NEC**
> *Excludes2:* aspiration pneumonia (J69.-)
>   emphysema (subcutaneous) resulting from a procedure (T81.82)
>   hypostatic pneumonia (J18.2)
>   pulmonary manifestations due to radiation (J70.0-J70.1)

J95.8   **Other intraoperative and postprocedural complications and**
5th   **disorders of respiratory system, NEC**
> **J95.81**   **Postprocedural pneumothorax and air leak**
> > **6th**   **J95.811**   **Postprocedural pneumothorax**
> >   **J95.812**   **Postprocedural air leak**
> **J95.82**   **Postprocedural respiratory failure**
> > **6th**   *Excludes1:* Respiratory failure in other conditions (J96.-)
> >   **J95.821**   **Acute postprocedural respiratory failure**
> >   Postprocedural respiratory failure NOS
> >   **J95.822**   **Acute and chronic post–procedural respiratory failure**
> **J95.83**   **Postprocedural hemorrhage of a respiratory system**
> > **6th**   **organ or structure; following a procedure**
> >   **J95.830**   **following a respiratory system procedure**
> >   **J95.831**   **following other procedure**
> **J95.84**   **Transfusion-related acute lung injury (TRALI)**

J95.85   **Complication of respirator [ventilator]**
> **6th**   **J95.850**   **Mechanical complication of respirator**
>   *Excludes1:* encounter for respirator [ventilator] dependence during power failure (Z99.12)
>   **J95.851**   **Ventilator associated pneumonia**
>   Ventilator associated pneumonitis
>   **Use additional code** to identify organism, if known (B95.-, B96.-, B97.-)
>   *Excludes1:* ventilator lung in newborn (P27.8)
>   **J95.859**   **Other complication of respirator [ventilator]**

J95.86   **Postprocedural hematoma and seroma of a respiratory**
> **6th**   **system organ or structure following a procedure**
>   **J95.860**   **Postprocedural hematoma of a respiratory system organ or structure following a respiratory system procedure**
>   **J95.861**   **Postprocedural hematoma of a respiratory system organ or structure following other procedure**
>   **J95.862**   **Postprocedural seroma of a respiratory system organ or structure following a respiratory system procedure**
>   **J95.863**   **Postprocedural seroma of a respiratory system organ or structure following other procedure**

J95.88   **Other intraoperative complications of respiratory system, NEC**

J95.89   **Other postprocedural complications and disorders of respiratory system, NEC**
> **Use additional code** to identify disorder, such as:
>   aspiration pneumonia (J69.-)
>   bacterial or viral pneumonia (J12-J18)
> *Excludes2:* acute pulmonary insufficiency following thoracic surgery (J95.1)
>   postprocedural subglottic stenosis (J95.5)

(J96–J99) OTHER DISEASES OF THE RESPIRATORY SYSTEM

J96   **RESPIRATORY FAILURE, NEC**
4th   **GUIDELINES**

Acute Respiratory Failure

AS PRINCIPAL DIAGNOSIS
A code from subcategory J96.0, Acute respiratory failure, or subcategory J96.2, Acute and chronic respiratory failure, may be assigned as a principal diagnosis when it is the condition established after study to be chiefly responsible for occasioning the admission to the hospital, and the selection is supported by the Alphabetic Index and Tabular List. However, chapter-specific coding guidelines (such as obstetrics, poisoning, HIV, newborn) that provide sequencing direction take precedence.

AS SECONDARY DIAGNOSIS
Respiratory failure may be listed as a secondary diagnosis if it occurs after admission, or if it is present on admission, but does not meet the definition of principal diagnosis.

SEQUENCING OF ACUTE RESPIRATORY FAILURE AND ANOTHER ACUTE CONDITION
When a patient is admitted with respiratory failure and another acute condition, (eg, myocardial infarction, cerebrovascular accident, aspiration pneumonia), the principal diagnosis will not be the same in every situation. This applies whether the other acute condition is a respiratory or nonrespiratory condition. Selection of the principal diagnosis will be dependent on the circumstances of admission. If both the respiratory failure and the other acute condition are equally responsible for occasioning the admission to the hospital, and there are no chapter-specific sequencing rules, the guideline regarding two or more diagnoses that equally meet the definition for principal diagnosis may be applied in these situations.

4th   **5th**   **6th**   **7th**   Additional Character Required   ✓   3-character code   •=New Code   ▲=Revised Code   *Excludes1*—Not coded here, do not use together   *Excludes2*—Not included here

Excludes1: acute respiratory distress syndrome (J80)
    cardiorespiratory failure (R09.2)
    newborn respiratory distress syndrome (P22.0)
    postprocedural respiratory failure (J95.82-)
    respiratory arrest (R09.2)
    respiratory arrest of newborn (P28.81)
    respiratory failure of newborn (P28.5)

J96.0 Acute respiratory failure
- `5th` **J96.00 Acute respiratory failure, unspecified whether with hypoxia or hypercapnia**
- **J96.01 Acute respiratory failure with hypoxia**
- **J96.02 Acute respiratory failure with hypercapnia**

J96.1 Chronic respiratory failure
- `5th` **J96.10 Chronic respiratory failure, unspecified whether with hypoxia or hypercapnia**
- **J96.11 Chronic respiratory failure with hypoxia**
- **J96.12 Chronic respiratory failure with hypercapnia**

J96.2 Acute and chronic respiratory failure
- `5th` Acute on chronic respiratory failure
- **J96.20 Acute and chronic respiratory failure, unspecified whether with hypoxia or hypercapnia**
- **J96.21 Acute and chronic respiratory failure with hypoxia**
- **J96.22 Acute and chronic respiratory failure with hypercapnia**

J96.9 Respiratory failure, unspecified
- `5th` **J96.90 Respiratory failure, unspecified, unspecified whether with hypoxia or hypercapnia**
- **J96.91 Respiratory failure, unspecified with hypoxia**
- **J96.92 Respiratory failure, unspecified with hypercapnia**

J98 `4th` OTHER RESPIRATORY DISORDERS

Use additional code to identify (Refer to Chapter 10 guidelines for codes)

Excludes1: newborn apnea (P28.4)
    newborn sleep apnea (P28.3)
Excludes2: apnea NOS (R06.81)
    sleep apnea (G47.3-)

J98.0 Diseases of bronchus, NEC
- `5th` **J98.01 Acute bronchospasm**
  - ***Excludes1:*** acute bronchiolitis with bronchospasm (J21.-)
    - acute bronchitis with bronchospasm (J20.-)
    - asthma (J45.-)
    - exercise induced bronchospasm (J45.990)
- **J98.09 Other diseases of bronchus, not elsewhere classified**
  - Broncholithiasis
  - Calcification of bronchus
  - Stenosis of bronchus
  - Tracheobronchial collapse
  - Tracheobronchial dyskinesia
  - Ulcer of bronchus

J98.1 Pulmonary collapse
- `5th` ***Excludes1:*** therapeutic collapse of lung status (Z98.3)
- **J98.11 Atelectasis**
  - ***Excludes1:*** newborn atelectasis
    - tuberculous atelectasis (current disease) (A15)

J98.2 Interstitial emphysema
    Mediastinal emphysema
    Excludes1: emphysema NOS (J43.9)
      emphysema in newborn (P25.0)
      surgical emphysema (subcutaneous) (T81.82)
      traumatic subcutaneous emphysema (T79.7)

J98.4 Other disorders of lung
    Calcification of lung
    Cystic lung disease (acquired)
    Lung disease NOS
    Pulmolithiasis

J98.6 Disorders of diaphragm
    Diaphragmatitis
    Paralysis of diaphragm
    Relaxation of diaphragm
    Excludes1: congenital malformation of diaphragm NEC (Q79.1)
      congenital diaphragmatic hernia (Q79.0)
    Excludes2: diaphragmatic hernia (K44.-)

J98.8 Other specified respiratory disorders

J98.9 Respiratory disorder, unspecified
    Respiratory disease (chronic) NOS

J99 ✔ RESPIRATORY DISORDERS IN DISEASES CLASSIFIED ELSEWHERE

Code first underlying disease, such as:
    amyloidosis (E85.-)
    ankylosing spondylitis (M45)
    congenital syphilis (A50.5)
    cryoglobulinemia (D89.1)
    early congenital syphilis (A50.0)
    plasminogen deficiency (E88.02)
    schistosomiasis (B65.0-B65.9)
Excludes1: respiratory disorders in:
    amebiasis (A06.5)
    blastomycosis (B40.0-B40.2)
    candidiasis (B37.1)
    coccidioidomycosis (B38.0-B38.2)
    cystic fibrosis with pulmonary manifestations (E84.0)
    dermatomyositis (M33.01, M33.11)
    histoplasmosis (B39.0-B39.2)
    late syphilis (A52.72, A52.73)
    polymyositis (M33.21)
    Sjögren syndrome (M35.02)
    SLE (M32.13)
    systemic sclerosis (M34.81)
    Wegener's granulomatosis (M31.30-M31.31)

CHAPTER 10. DISEASES OF THE RESPIRATORY SYSTEM   (J96.0–J99)

`4th` `5th` `6th` `7th` Additional Character Required   `✔` 3-character code   •=New Code   ▲=Revised Code   ***Excludes1***—Not coded here, do not use together   ***Excludes2***—Not included here

Chapter 11. Diseases of the digestive system (K00–K95)

GUIDELINES

None currently.

Excludes2: certain conditions originating in the perinatal period (P04–P96)
certain infectious and parasitic diseases (A00–B99)
complications of pregnancy, childbirth and the puerperium (O00–O9A)
congenital malformations, deformations and chromosomal abnormalities (Q00–Q99)
endocrine, nutritional and metabolic diseases (E00–E88)
injury, poisoning and certain other consequences of external causes (S00–T88)
neoplasms (C00–D49)
symptoms, signs and abnormal clinical and laboratory findings, NEC (R00–R94)

(K00–K14) DISEASES OF ORAL CAVITY AND SALIVARY GLANDS

K00 **DISORDERS OF TOOTH DEVELOPMENT AND ERUPTION**
`4th` **Excludes2:** embedded and impacted teeth (K01.-)
    K00.0 **Anodontia**
       Hypodontia
       Oligodontia
       Excludes1: acquired absence of teeth (K08.1-)
    K00.1 **Supernumerary teeth**
       Distomolar
       Fourth molar
       Mesiodens
       Paramolar
       Supplementary teeth
       Excludes2: supernumerary roots (K00.2)
    K00.3 **Mottled teeth**
       Dental fluorosis
       Mottling of enamel
       Nonfluoride enamel opacities
       Excludes2: deposits [accretions] on teeth (K03.6)
    K00.6 **Disturbances in tooth eruption**
       Dentia praecox
       Natal tooth
       Neonatal tooth
       Premature eruption of tooth
       Premature shedding of primary [deciduous] tooth
       Prenatal teeth
       Retained [persistent] primary tooth
       Excludes2: embedded and impacted teeth (K01.-)
    K00.7 **Teething syndrome**
    K00.8 **Other disorders of tooth development**
       Color changes during tooth formation
       Intrinsic staining of teeth NOS
       Excludes2: posteruptive color changes (K03.7)
    K00.9 **Disorder of tooth development, unspecified**
       Disorder of odontogenesis NOS

K02 **DENTAL CARIES**
`4th` **Includes:** caries of dentine
       early childhood caries
       pre-eruptive caries
       recurrent caries (dentino enamel junction) (enamel) (to the pulp)
       dental cavities
       tooth decay
    K02.9 **Dental caries, unspecified**

K03 **OTHER DISEASES OF HARD TISSUES OF TEETH**
`4th` **Excludes2:** bruxism (F45.8)
       dental caries (K02.-)
       teeth-grinding NOS (F45.8)
    K03.1 **Abrasion of teeth**
       Dentifrice abrasion of teeth
       Habitual abrasion of teeth
       Occupational abrasion of teeth
       Ritual abrasion of teeth
       Traditional abrasion of teeth
       Wedge defect NOS

    K03.8 **Other specified diseases of hard tissues of teeth**
    `5th` **K03.81** **Cracked tooth**
       Excludes1: broken or fractured tooth due to trauma (S02.5)
    K03.89 **Other specified diseases of hard tissues of teeth**
    K03.9 **Disease of hard tissues of teeth, unspecified**

K04 **DISEASES OF PULP AND PERIAPICAL TISSUES**
`4th` **K04.7** **Periapical abscess without sinus**
       Dental abscess without sinus
       Dentoalveolar abscess without sinus
       Periapical abscess without sinus
    K04.8 **Radicular cyst**
       Apical (periodontal) cyst
       Periapical cyst
       Residual radicular cyst
       Excludes2: lateral periodontal cyst (K09.0)

K05 **GINGIVITIS AND PERIODONTAL DISEASES**
`4th` **Use additional code** to identify:
       alcohol abuse and dependence (F10.-)
       exposure to environmental tobacco smoke (Z77.22)
       exposure to tobacco smoke in the perinatal period (P96.81)
       history of tobacco dependence (Z87.891)
       occupational exposure to environmental tobacco smoke (Z57.31)
       tobacco dependence (F17.-)
       tobacco use (Z72.0)
    K05.0 **Acute gingivitis**
    `5th` **Excludes1:** acute necrotizing ulcerative gingivitis (A69.1)
       herpesviral [herpes simplex] gingivostomatitis (B00.2)
       K05.00 **Acute gingivitis, plaque induced**
          Acute gingivitis NOS
          Plaque-induced gingival disease

K06 **OTHER DISORDERS OF GINGIVA AND EDENTULOUS ALVEOLAR RIDGE**
`4th`
Excludes2: acute gingivitis (K05.0)
       atrophy of edentulous alveolar ridge (K08.2)
       chronic gingivitis (K05.1)
       gingivitis NOS (K05.1)
    K06.1 **Gingival enlargement**
       Gingival fibromatosis

K08 **OTHER DISORDERS OF TEETH AND SUPPORTING STRUCTURES**
`4th`
Excludes2: dentofacial anomalies [including malocclusion] (M26.-)
       disorders of jaw (M27.-)
    K08.1 **Complete loss of teeth**
    `5th` Acquired loss of teeth, complete
       Excludes1: congenital absence of teeth (K00.0)
       exfoliation of teeth due to systemic causes (K08.0)
       partial loss of teeth (K08.4-)
       K08.10 **Complete loss of teeth, unspecified cause**
       `6th` **K08.101** **Complete loss of teeth, unspecified cause; class I**
          K08.102 **class II**
          K08.103 **class III**
          K08.104 **class IV**
          K08.109 **unspecified class**
          Edentulism NOS
       K08.11 **Complete loss of teeth due to trauma**
       `6th` **K08.111** **Complete loss of teeth due to trauma; class I**
          K08.112 **class II**
          K08.113 **class III**
          K08.114 **class IV**
          K08.119 **unspecified class**
       K08.12 **Complete loss of teeth due to periodontal diseases**
       `6th` **K08.121** **Complete loss of teeth due to periodontal diseases, class I**
          K08.122 **class II**
          K08.123 **class III**
          K08.124 **class IV**
          K08.129 **unspecified class**

`4th` `5th` `6th` `7th`   Additional Character Required   ✓   3-character code

•=New Code   **Excludes1**—Not coded here, do not use together
▲=Revised Code   **Excludes2**—Not included here

K08.13 Complete loss of teeth due to caries
- **6th** **K08.131** Complete loss of teeth due to caries; class I
- **K08.132** class II
- **K08.133** class III
- **K08.134** class IV
- **K08.139** unspecified class

K08.19 Complete loss of teeth due to other specified cause
- **6th** **K08.191** Complete loss of teeth due to other specified cause, class I
- **K08.192** class II
- **K08.193** class III
- **K08.194** class IV
- **K08.199** unspecified class

K08.4 **Partial loss of teeth**
5th Acquired loss of teeth, partial
Excludes1: complete loss of teeth (K08.1-)
  congenital absence of teeth (K00.0)
Excludes2: exfoliation of teeth due to systemic causes (K08.0)

K08.40 Partial loss of teeth, unspecified cause
- **6th** **K08.401** Partial loss of teeth, unspecified cause; class I
- **K08.402** class II
- **K08.403** class III
- **K08.404** class IV
- **K08.409** unspecified class
  Tooth extraction status NOS

K08.41 Partial loss of teeth due to trauma
- **6th** **K08.411** Partial loss of teeth due to trauma; class I
- **K08.412** class II
- **K08.413** class III
- **K08.414** class IV
- **K08.419** unspecified class

K08.42 Partial loss of teeth due to periodontal diseases
- **6th** **K08.421** Partial loss of teeth due to periodontal diseases, class I
- **K08.422** class II
- **K08.423** class III
- **K08.424** class IV
- **K08.429** unspecified class

K08.43 Partial loss of teeth due to caries
- **6th** **K08.431** Partial loss of teeth due to caries; class I
- **K08.432** class II
- **K08.433** class III
- **K08.434** class IV
- **K08.439** unspecified class

K08.49 Partial loss of teeth due to other specified cause
- **6th** **K08.491** class I
- **K08.492** class II
- **K08.493** class III
- **K08.494** class IV
- **K08.499** unspecified class

K08.8 **Other specified disorders of teeth and supporting structures**
- **5th** **K08.81** Primary occlusal trauma
- **K08.82** Secondary occlusal trauma
- **K08.89** Other specified disorders of teeth and supporting structures
  Enlargement of alveolar ridge NOS
  Insufficient anatomic crown height
  Insufficient clinical crown length
  Irregular alveolar process
  Toothache NOS

K08.9 **Disorder of teeth and supporting structures, unspecified**

K09 CYSTS OF ORAL REGION, NEC
4th *Includes:* lesions showing histological features both of aneurysmal cyst and of another fibro-osseous lesion
Excludes2: cysts of jaw (M27.0-, M27.4-)
  radicular cyst (K04.8)

K09.0 **Developmental odontogenic cysts**
Dentigerous cyst
Eruption cyst
Follicular cyst
Gingival cyst
Lateral periodontal cyst
Primordial cyst
Excludes2: keratocysts (D16.4, D16.5)
  odontogenic keratocystic tumors (D16.4, D16.5)

K09.1 **Developmental (nonodontogenic) cysts of oral region**
Cyst (of) incisive canal or palatine of papilla
Globulomaxillary cyst
Median palatal cyst
Nasoalveolar cyst
Nasolabial cyst
Nasopalatine duct cyst

K09.8 **Other cysts of oral region, NEC**
Dermoid cyst
Epidermoid cyst
Lymphoepithelial cyst
Epstein's pearl

K09.9 **Cyst of oral region, unspecified**

K11 DISEASES OF SALIVARY GLANDS
4th **Use additional code** to identify:
  alcohol abuse and dependence (F10.-)
  exposure to environmental tobacco smoke (Z77.22)
  exposure to tobacco smoke in the perinatal period (P96.81)
  history of tobacco dependence (Z87.891)
  occupational exposure to environmental tobacco smoke (Z57.31)
  tobacco dependence (F17.-)
  tobacco use (Z72.0)

K11.2 **Sialoadenitis**
5th Parotitis
Excludes1: epidemic parotitis (B26.-)
  mumps (B26.-)
  uveoparotid fever [Heerfordt] (D86.89)
- **K11.20** Sialoadenitis, unspecified
- **K11.21** Acute sialoadenitis
  Excludes1: acute recurrent sialoadenitis (K11.22)
- **K11.22** Acute recurrent sialoadenitis
- **K11.23** Chronic sialoadenitis

K11.3 **Abscess of salivary gland**

K11.4 **Fistula of salivary gland**
Excludes1: congenital fistula of salivary gland (Q38.4)

K11.7 **Disturbances of salivary secretion**
Hypoptyalism
Ptyalism
Xerostomia
Excludes2: dry mouth NOS (R68.2)

K11.8 **Other diseases of salivary glands**
Benign lymphoepithelial lesion of salivary gland
Mikulicz' disease
Necrotizing sialometaplasia
Sialectasia
Stenosis of salivary duct
Stricture of salivary duct
Excludes1: Sjögren syndrome (M35.0-)

K11.9 **Disease of salivary gland, unspecified**
Sialoadenopathy NOS

K12 STOMATITIS AND RELATED LESIONS
4th **Use additional code** to identify: alcohol abuse and dependence (F10.-)
  exposure to environmental tobacco smoke (Z77.22)
  exposure to tobacco smoke in the perinatal period (P96.81)
  history of tobacco dependence (Z87.891)
  occupational exposure to environmental tobacco smoke (Z57.31)
  tobacco dependence (F17.-)
  tobacco use (Z72.0)
Excludes1: cancrum oris (A69.0)
  cheilitis (K13.0)
  gangrenous stomatitis (A69.0)
  herpesviral [herpes simplex] gingivostomatitis (B00.2)
  noma (A69.0)

K12.0   Recurrent oral aphthae
Aphthous stomatitis (major) (minor)
Bednar's aphthae
Periadenitis mucosa necrotica recurrens
Recurrent aphthous ulcer
Stomatitis herpetiformis

K12.1   Other forms of stomatitis
Stomatitis NOS
Denture stomatitis
Ulcerative stomatitis
Vesicular stomatitis
Excludes1: acute necrotizing ulcerative stomatitis (A69.1)

K12.2   Cellulitis and abscess of mouth
Cellulitis of mouth (floor)
Submandibular abscess
Excludes2: abscess of salivary gland (K11.3)
    abscess of tongue (K14.0)
    periapical abscess (K04.6–K04.7)
    periodontal abscess (K05.21)
    peritonsillar abscess (J36)

K12.3   Oral mucositis (ulcerative)
`5th`   Mucositis (oral) (oropharyngeal)
Excludes2: gastrointestinal mucositis (ulcerative) (K92.81)
    mucositis (ulcerative) of vagina and vulva (N76.81)
    nasal mucositis (ulcerative) (J34.81)
    K12.30   Oral mucositis (ulcerative), unspecified

K13   OTHER DISEASES OF LIP AND ORAL MUCOSA
`4th`   *Includes:* epithelial disturbances of tongue
Use additional code to identify:
    alcohol abuse and dependence (F10.-)
    exposure to environmental tobacco smoke (Z77.22)
    exposure to tobacco smoke in the perinatal period (P96.81)
    history of tobacco dependence (Z87.891)
    occupational exposure to environmental tobacco smoke (Z57.31)
    tobacco dependence (F17.-)
    tobacco use (Z72.0)
Excludes2: certain disorders of gingiva and edentulous alveolar ridge
    (K05–K06)
    cysts of oral region (K09.-)
    diseases of tongue (K14.-)
    stomatitis and related lesions (K12.-)

K13.0   Diseases of lips
Abscess of lips
Angular cheilitis
Cellulitis of lips
Cheilitis NOS
Cheilodynia
Cheilosis
Exfoliative cheilitis
Fistula of lips
Glandular cheilitis
Hypertrophy of lips
Perlèche NEC
Excludes1: ariboflavinosis (E53.0)
    cheilitis due to radiation-related disorders (L55–L59)
    congenital fistula of lips (Q38.0)
    congenital hypertrophy of lips (Q18.6)
    Perlèche due to candidiasis (B37.83)
    Perlèche due to riboflavin deficiency (E53.0)

K13.1   Cheek and lip biting
K13.7   Other and unspecified lesions of oral mucosa
`5th`   **K13.70   Unspecified lesions of oral mucosa**
    K13.79   Other lesions of oral mucosa
      Focal oral mucinosis

K14   DISEASES OF TONGUE
`4th`   **Use additional code** to identify: alcohol abuse and dependence (F10.-)
    exposure to environmental tobacco smoke (Z77.22)
    history of tobacco dependence (Z87.891)
    occupational exposure to environmental tobacco smoke (Z57.31)
    tobacco dependence (F17.-)
    tobacco use (Z72.0)

Excludes2: erythroplakia (K13.29)
    focal epithelial hyperplasia (K13.29)
    leukedema of tongue (K13.29)
    leukoplakia of tongue (K13.21)
    hairy leukoplakia (K13.3)
    macroglossia (congenital) (Q38.2)
    submucous fibrosis of tongue (K13.5)

K14.0   Glossitis
Abscess of tongue
Ulceration (traumatic) of tongue
Excludes1: atrophic glossitis (K14.4)

K14.1   Geographic tongue
Benign migratory glossitis
Glossitis areata exfoliativa

K14.3   Hypertrophy of tongue papillae
Black hairy tongue
Coated tongue
Hypertrophy of foliate papillae
Lingua villosa nigra

K14.8   Other diseases of tongue
Atrophy of tongue
Crenated tongue
Enlargement of tongue
Glossocele
Glossoptosis
Hypertrophy of tongue

(K20–K31) DISEASES OF ESOPHAGUS, STOMACH AND DUODENUM

Excludes2: hiatus hernia (K44.-)

K20   ESOPHAGITIS
`4th`   **Use additional code** to identify: alcohol abuse and dependence (F10.-)
Excludes1: erosion of esophagus (K22.1-)
    esophagitis with gastro-esophageal reflux disease (K21.0-)
    reflux esophagitis (K21.0-)
    ulcerative esophagitis (K22.1-)
Excludes2: eosinophilic gastritis or gastroenteritis (K52.81)

K20.0   Eosinophilic esophagitis
K20.8   Other esophagitis
`5th`   **K20.80   Other esophagitis without bleeding**
      Abscess of esophagus
      Other esophagitis NOS
    K20.81   Other esophagitis with bleeding

K20.9   Esophagitis, unspecified
`5th`   **K20.90   Esophagitis, unspecified without bleeding**
      Esophagitis, NOS
    K20.91   Esophagitis, unspecified with bleeding

K21   GASTRO-ESOPHAGEAL REFLUX DISEASE
`4th`   *Excludes1:* newborn esophageal reflux (P78.83)

K21.0   Gastro-esophageal reflux disease (GERD) with esophagitis
`5th`   **K21.00   GERD with esophagitis, without bleeding**
      Reflux esophagitis
    K21.01   GERD with esophagitis, with bleeding

K21.9   GERD without esophagitis
Esophageal reflux NOS

K22   OTHER DISEASES OF ESOPHAGUS
`4th`   *Excludes2:* esophageal varices (I85.-)

K22.0   Achalasia of cardia
Achalasia NOS
Cardiospasm
Excludes1: congenital cardiospasm (Q39.5)

K22.1   Ulcer of esophagus
`5th`   Barrett's ulcer
Erosion of esophagus
Fungal ulcer of esophagus
Peptic ulcer of esophagus
Ulcer of esophagus due to ingestion of chemicals
Ulcer of esophagus due to ingestion of drugs and medicaments
Ulcerative esophagitis
Code first poisoning due to drug or toxin, if applicable (T36-T65
    with fifth or sixth character 1-4 or 6)

`4th` `5th` `6th` `7th`   Additional Character Required   ✔   3-character code   •=New Code   *Excludes1*—Not coded here, do not use together
        ▲=Revised Code   *Excludes2*—Not included here

CHAPTER 11. DISEASES OF THE DIGESTIVE SYSTEM (K22.10–K31.A19)

Use additional code for adverse effect, if applicable, to identify drug (T36-T50 with fifth or sixth character 5)

Excludes1: Barrett's esophagus (K22.7-)

K22.10   Ulcer of esophagus without bleeding
Ulcer of esophagus NOS

K22.11   Ulcer of esophagus with bleeding
Excludes2: bleeding esophageal varices (I85.01, I85.11)

K22.4   Dyskinesia of esophagus
Corkscrew esophagus
Diffuse esophageal spasm
Spasm of esophagus
Excludes1: cardiospasm (K22.0)

▲**K22.8   Other specified diseases of esophagus**
  [5th]   *Excludes2:* esophageal varices (I85.-)
Paterson-Kelly syndrome (D50.1)

•**K22.81   Esophageal polyp**
Excludes1: benign neoplasm of esophagus (D13.0)

•**K22.82   Esophagogastric junction polyp**
Excludes1: benign neoplasm of stomach (D13.1)

•**K22.89   Other specified disease of esophagus**
Hemorrhage of esophagus NOS

K22.9   Disease of esophagus, unspecified

K25   GASTRIC ULCER
 [4th]   *Includes:* erosion (acute) of stomach
pylorus ulcer (peptic)
stomach ulcer (peptic)

Use additional code to identify: alcohol abuse and dependence (F10.-)

Excludes1: acute gastritis (K29.0-)
peptic ulcer NOS (K27.-)

K25.0   Acute gastric ulcer; with hemorrhage
K25.1   with perforation
K25.2   with both hemorrhage and perforation
K25.3   without hemorrhage or perforation
K25.4   Chronic or unspecified gastric ulcer; with hemorrhage
K25.5   with perforation
K25.6   with both hemorrhage and perforation
K25.7   without hemorrhage or perforation
K25.9   Gastric ulcer, unspecified as acute or chronic, without hemorrhage or perforation

K26   DUODENAL ULCER
 [4th]   *Includes:* erosion (acute) of duodenum
duodenum ulcer (peptic)
postpyloric ulcer (peptic)

Use additional code to identify: alcohol abuse and dependence (F10.-)

Excludes1: peptic ulcer NOS (K27.-)

K26.0   Acute duodenal ulcer; with hemorrhage
K26.1   with perforation
K26.2   with both hemorrhage and perforation
K26.3   without hemorrhage or perforation
K26.4   Chronic or unspecified duodenal ulcer; with hemorrhage
K26.5   with perforation
K26.6   with both hemorrhage and perforation
K26.7   without hemorrhage or perforation
K26.9   Duodenal ulcer, unspecified as acute or chronic, without hemorrhage or perforation

K27   PEPTIC ULCER, SITE UNSPECIFIED
 [4th]   *Includes:* gastroduodenal ulcer NOS
peptic ulcer NOS

Use additional code to identify: alcohol abuse and dependence (F10.-)

Excludes1: peptic ulcer of newborn (P78.82)

K27.0   Acute peptic ulcer, site unspecified; with hemorrhage
K27.1   with perforation
K27.2   with both hemorrhage and perforation
K27.3   without hemorrhage or perforation
K27.4   Chronic or unspecified peptic ulcer, site unspecified; with hemorrhage
K27.5   with perforation
K27.6   with both hemorrhage and perforation
K27.7   without hemorrhage or perforation
K27.9   Peptic ulcer, site unspecified, unspecified as acute or chronic, without hemorrhage or perforation

K29   GASTRITIS AND DUODENITIS
 [4th]   *Excludes1:* eosinophilic gastritis or gastroenteritis (K52.81)
Zollinger-Ellison syndrome (E16.4)

K29.0   Acute gastritis
 [5th]   **Use additional code** to identify: alcohol abuse and dependence (F10.-)
Excludes1: erosion (acute) of stomach (K25.-)

K29.00   Acute gastritis without bleeding
K29.01   Acute gastritis with bleeding

K29.7   Gastritis, unspecified
 [5th]   **K29.70   Gastritis, unspecified, without bleeding**
K29.71   Gastritis, unspecified, with bleeding

K29.8   Duodenitis
 [5th]   **K29.80   Duodenitis without bleeding**
K29.81   Duodenitis with bleeding

K29.9   Gastroduodenitis, unspecified
 [5th]   **K29.90   Gastroduodenitis, unspecified, without bleeding**
K29.91   Gastroduodenitis, unspecified, with bleeding

K30   FUNCTIONAL DYSPEPSIA
 [✓]   Indigestion
Excludes1: dyspepsia NOS (R10.13)
heartburn (R12)
nervous dyspepsia (F45.8)
neurotic dyspepsia (F45.8)
psychogenic dyspepsia (F45.8)

K31   OTHER DISEASES OF STOMACH AND DUODENUM
 [4th]   *Includes:* functional disorders of stomach
Excludes2: diabetic gastroparesis (E08.43, E09.43, E10.43, E11.43, E13.43)
diverticulum of duodenum (K57.00–K57.13)

K31.0   Acute dilatation of stomach
Acute distention of stomach

K31.1   Adult hypertrophic pyloric stenosis
Pyloric stenosis NOS
Excludes1: congenital or infantile pyloric stenosis (Q40.0)

K31.3   Pylorospasm, NEC
Excludes1: congenital or infantile pylorospasm (Q40.0)
neurotic pylorospasm (F45.8)
psychogenic pylorospasm (F45.8)

K31.5   Obstruction of duodenum
Constriction of duodenum
Duodenal ileus (chronic)
Stenosis of duodenum
Stricture of duodenum
Volvulus of duodenum
Excludes 1: congenital stenosis of duodenum (Q41.0)

K31.8   Other specified diseases of stomach and duodenum
 [5th]   **K31.83   Achlorhydria**
K31.84   Gastroparesis
Gastroparalysis
Code first underlying disease, if known, such as:
anorexia nervosa (F50.0-)
diabetes mellitus (E08.43, E09.43, E10.43, E11.43, E13.43)
scleroderma (M34.-)

K31.89   Other diseases of stomach and duodenum

K31.9   Disease of stomach and duodenum, unspecified

•**K31.A   Gastric intestinal metaplasia**
 [5th]   •**K31.A0   Gastric intestinal metaplasia, unspecified**
Gastric intestinal metaplasia indefinite for dysplasia
Gastric intestinal metaplasia NOS

•**K31.A1   Gastric intestinal metaplasia without dysplasia**
 [6th]   •**K31.A11   Gastric intestinal metaplasia without dysplasia, involving the antrum**
•**K31.A12   Gastric intestinal metaplasia without dysplasia, involving the body (corpus)**
•**K31.A13   Gastric intestinal metaplasia without dysplasia, involving the fundus**
•**K31.A14   Gastric intestinal metaplasia without dysplasia, involving the cardia**
•**K31.A15   Gastric intestinal metaplasia without dysplasia, involving multiple sites**
•**K31.A19   Gastric intestinal metaplasia without dysplasia, unspecified site**

[4th] [5th] [6th] [7th]   Additional Character Required   [✓]   3-character code

•=New Code
▲=Revised Code

Excludes1—Not coded here, do not use together
Excludes2—Not included here

•K31.A2 **Gastric intestinal metaplasia with dysplasia**
6th •K31.A21 **Gastric intestinal metaplasia with low grade dysplasia**
•K31.A22 **Gastric intestinal metaplasia with high grade dysplasia**
•K31.A29 **Gastric intestinal metaplasia with dysplasia, unspecified**

(K35–K38) DISEASES OF APPENDIX

K35 ACUTE APPENDICITIS
4th **K35.2 Acute appendicitis with generalized peritonitis**
5th K35.20 **Acute appendicitis with generalized peritonitis, without abscess**
(Acute) appendicitis with generalized peritonitis NOS
K35.21 **Acute appendicitis with generalized peritonitis, with abscess**
K35.3 Acute appendicitis with localized peritonitis
5th K35.30 **Acute appendicitis with localized peritonitis, without perforation or gangrene**
Acute appendicitis with localized peritonitis NOS
K35.31 **Acute appendicitis with localized peritonitis and gangrene, without perforation**
K35.32 **Acute appendicitis with perforation and localized peritonitis, without abscess**
(Acute) appendicitis with perforation NOS
Perforated appendix NOS
Ruptured appendix (with localized peritonitis) NOS
K35.33 **Acute appendicitis with perforation and localized peritonitis, with abscess**
(Acute) appendicitis with (peritoneal) abscess NOS
Ruptured appendix with localized peritonitis and abscess
K35.8 Other and unspecified acute appendicitis
5th K35.80 **Unspecified acute appendicitis**
Acute appendicitis NOS
Acute appendicitis without (localized) (generalized) peritonitis
K35.89 **Other acute appendicitis**
6th K35.890 **Other acute appendicitis without perforation or gangrene**
K35.891 **Other acute appendicitis without perforation, with gangrene**

K37 UNSPECIFIED APPENDICITIS
✔ **Excludes1:** unspecified appendicitis with peritonitis (K35.2-, K35.3-)

(K40–K46) HERNIA

Note: Hernia with both gangrene and obstruction is classified to hernia with gangrene.
Includes: acquired hernia
congenital [except diaphragmatic or hiatus] hernia
recurrent hernia

K40 INGUINAL HERNIA
4th **Includes:** bubonocele
direct inguinal hernia
double inguinal hernia
indirect inguinal hernia
inguinal hernia NOS
oblique inguinal hernia
scrotal hernia
K40.0 Bilateral inguinal hernia, with obstruction, without gangrene
5th Inguinal hernia (bilateral) causing obstruction without gangrene
Incarcerated or Irreducible or Strangulated inguinal hernia (bilateral) without gangrene
K40.00 **Bilateral inguinal hernia, with obstruction, without gangrene, not specified as recurrent**
Bilateral inguinal hernia, with obstruction, without gangrene NOS
K40.01 **Bilateral inguinal hernia, with obstruction, without gangrene, recurrent**
K40.1 Bilateral inguinal hernia, with gangrene
5th

K40.10 **Bilateral inguinal hernia, with gangrene, not specified as recurrent**
Bilateral inguinal hernia, with gangrene NOS
K40.11 **Bilateral inguinal hernia, with gangrene, recurrent**
K40.2 Bilateral inguinal hernia, without obstruction or gangrene
5th K40.20 **Bilateral inguinal hernia, without obstruction or gangrene, not specified as recurrent**
Bilateral inguinal hernia NOS
K40.21 **Bilateral inguinal hernia, without obstruction or gangrene, recurrent**
K40.3 Unilateral inguinal hernia, with obstruction, without gangrene
5th Inguinal hernia (unilateral) causing obstruction without gangrene
Incarcerated or Irreducible or Strangulated inguinal hernia (unilateral) without gangrene
K40.30 **Unilateral inguinal hernia, with obstruction, without gangrene, not specified as recurrent**
Inguinal hernia, with obstruction NOS
Unilateral inguinal hernia, with obstruction, without gangrene NOS
K40.31 **Unilateral inguinal hernia, with obstruction, without gangrene, recurrent**
K40.4 Unilateral inguinal hernia, with gangrene
5th K40.40 **Unilateral inguinal hernia, with gangrene, not specified as recurrent**
Inguinal hernia with gangrene NOS
Unilateral inguinal hernia with gangrene NOS
K40.41 **Unilateral inguinal hernia, with gangrene, recurrent**
K40.9 Unilateral inguinal hernia, without obstruction or gangrene
5th K40.90 **Unilateral inguinal hernia, without obstruction or gangrene, not specified as recurrent**
Inguinal hernia NOS
Unilateral inguinal hernia NOS
K40.91 **Unilateral inguinal hernia, without obstruction or gangrene, recurrent**

K42 UMBILICAL HERNIA
4th **Includes:** paraumbilical hernia
Excludes1: omphalocele (Q79.2)
K42.0 Umbilical hernia with obstruction, without gangrene
Umbilical hernia causing obstruction, without gangrene
Incarcerated or Irreducible or Strangulated umbilical hernia, without gangrene
K42.1 Umbilical hernia with gangrene
Gangrenous umbilical hernia
K42.9 Umbilical hernia without obstruction or gangrene
Umbilical hernia NOS

K43 VENTRAL HERNIA
4th **K43.0 Incisional hernia with obstruction, without gangrene**
Incisional hernia causing obstruction, without gangrene
Incarcerated or Irreducible or Strangulated incisional hernia, without gangrene
K43.1 Incisional hernia with gangrene
Gangrenous incisional hernia
K43.2 Incisional hernia without obstruction or gangrene
Incisional hernia NOS
K43.9 Ventral hernia without obstruction or gangrene
Epigastric hernia
Ventral hernia NOS

K44 DIAPHRAGMATIC HERNIA
4th **Includes:** hiatus hernia (esophageal) (sliding)
paraesophageal hernia
Excludes1: congenital diaphragmatic hernia (Q79.0)
congenital hiatus hernia (Q40.1)
K44.0 Diaphragmatic hernia with obstruction, without gangrene
Diaphragmatic hernia causing obstruction
Incarcerated or Irreducible or Strangulated diaphragmatic hernia
K44.1 Diaphragmatic hernia with gangrene
Gangrenous diaphragmatic hernia
K44.9 Diaphragmatic hernia without obstruction or gangrene
Diaphragmatic hernia NOS

4th 5th 6th 7th Additional Character Required ✔ 3-character code •=New Code ▲=Revised Code **Excludes1**—Not coded here, do not use together **Excludes2**—Not included here

K46   UNSPECIFIED ABDOMINAL HERNIA
[4th]

Includes: enterocele
     epiplocele
     hernia NOS
     interstitial hernia
     intestinal hernia
     intra-abdominal hernia
Excludes1: vaginal enterocele (N81.5)

K46.0   Unspecified abdominal hernia with obstruction, without gangrene
     Unspecified abdominal hernia causing obstruction
     Unspecified incarcerated abdominal hernia
     Unspecified irreducible abdominal hernia
     Unspecified strangulated abdominal hernia

K46.1   Unspecified abdominal hernia with gangrene
     Any condition listed under K46 specified as gangrenous

K46.9   Unspecified abdominal hernia without obstruction or gangrene
     Abdominal hernia NOS

(K50–K52) NONINFECTIVE ENTERITIS AND COLITIS

Includes: noninfective inflammatory bowel disease
Excludes1: irritable bowel syndrome (K58.-)
     megacolon (K59.3-)

K50   CROHN'S DISEASE [REGIONAL ENTERITIS]
[4th]

Includes: granulomatous enteritis
Use additional code to identify manifestations, such as: pyoderma gangrenosum (L88)
Excludes1: ulcerative colitis (K51.-)

K50.0   Crohn's disease of small intestine
[5th]   Crohn's disease [regional enteritis] of duodenum or ileum or jejunum
     Regional ileitis
     Terminal ileitis
     Excludes1: Crohn's disease of both small and large intestine (K50.8-)

     K50.00   Crohn's disease of small intestine without complications

     K50.01   Crohn's disease of small intestine with complications
     [6th]
         K50.011   Crohn's disease of small intestine; with rectal bleeding
         K50.012   with intestinal obstruction
         K50.013   with fistula
         K50.014   with abscess
         K50.018   with other complication
         K50.019   with unspecified complications

K50.1   Crohn's disease of large intestine
[5th]   Crohn's disease [regional enteritis] of colon or large bowel or rectum
     Granulomatous colitis
     Regional colitis
     Excludes1: Crohn's disease of both small and large intestine (K50.8)

     K50.10   Crohn's disease of large intestine without complications

     K50.11   Crohn's disease of large intestine with complications
     [6th]
         K50.111   Crohn's disease of large intestine; with rectal bleeding
         K50.112   with intestinal obstruction
         K50.113   with fistula
         K50.114   with abscess
         K50.118   with other complication
         K50.119   with unspecified complications

K50.8   Crohn's disease of both small and large intestine
     [5th]   K50.80   Crohn's disease of both small and large intestine without complications

     K50.81   Crohn's disease of both small and large intestine with complications
     [6th]
         K50.811   Crohn's disease of both small and large intestine; with rectal bleeding
         K50.812   with intestinal obstruction
         K50.813   with fistula

         K50.814   with abscess
         K50.818   with other complication
         K50.819   with unspecified complications

K50.9   Crohn's disease, unspecified
     [5th]   K50.90   Crohn's disease, unspecified, without complications
         Crohn's disease NOS
         Regional enteritis NOS

     K50.91   Crohn's disease, unspecified, with complications
     [6th]   **K50.911   Crohn's disease, unspecified; with rectal bleeding**
         K50.912   with intestinal obstruction
         K50.913   with fistula
         K50.914   with abscess
         K50.918   with other complication
         K50.919   with unspecified complications

K51   ULCERATIVE COLITIS
[4th]

Use additional code to identify manifestations, such as: pyoderma gangrenosum (L88)
Excludes1: Crohn's disease [regional enteritis] (K50.-)

K51.0   Ulcerative (chronic) pancolitis
[5th]   Backwash ileitis

     K51.00   Ulcerative (chronic) pancolitis without complications
         Ulcerative (chronic) pancolitis NOS

     K51.01   Ulcerative (chronic) pancolitis with complications
     [6th]   **K51.011   Ulcerative (chronic) pancolitis; with rectal bleeding**
         K51.012   with intestinal obstruction
         K51.013   with fistula
         K51.014   with abscess
         K51.018   with other complication
         K51.019   with unspecified complications

K51.2   Ulcerative (chronic) proctitis
     [5th]   K51.20   Ulcerative (chronic) proctitis without complications
         Ulcerative (chronic) proctitis NOS

     K51.21   Ulcerative (chronic) proctitis with complications
     [6th]   **K51.211   Ulcerative (chronic) proctitis; with rectal bleeding**
         K51.212   with intestinal obstruction
         K51.213   with fistula
         K51.214   with abscess
         K51.218   with other complication
         K51.219   with unspecified complications

K51.3   Ulcerative (chronic) rectosigmoiditis
     [5th]   K51.30   Ulcerative (chronic) rectosigmoiditis without complications
         Ulcerative (chronic) rectosigmoiditis NOS

     K51.31   Ulcerative (chronic) rectosigmoiditis with complications
     [6th]
         K51.311   Ulcerative (chronic) rectosigmoiditis; with rectal bleeding
         K51.312   with intestinal obstruction
         K51.313   with fistula
         K51.314   with abscess
         K51.318   with other complication
         K51.319   with unspecified complications

K51.4   Inflammatory polyps of colon
[5th]   **Excludes1:** adenomatous polyp of colon (D12.6)
     polyposis of colon (D12.6)
     polyps of colon NOS (K63.5)

     K51.40   Inflammatory polyps of colon without complications
         Inflammatory polyps of colon NOS

     K51.41   Inflammatory polyps of colon with complications
     [6th]   **K51.411   Inflammatory polyps of colon; with rectal bleeding**
         K51.412   with intestinal obstruction
         K51.413   with fistula
         K51.414   with abscess
         K51.418   with other complication
         K51.419   with unspecified complications

K51.5   Left sided colitis
[5th]   Left hemicolitis

     K51.50   Left sided colitis without complications
         Left sided colitis NOS

[4th] [5th] [6th] [7th]   Additional Character Required   **✓**   3-character code   •=New Code   ▲=Revised Code   **Excludes1**—Not coded here, do not use together   **Excludes2**—Not included here

K51.51   **Left sided colitis with complications**
6th   **K51.511**   **Left sided colitis; with rectal bleeding**
     K51.512   **with intestinal obstruction**
     K51.513   **with fistula**
     K51.514   **with abscess**
     K51.518   **with other complication**
     K51.519   **with unspecified complications**

K51.8   **Other ulcerative colitis**
5th   **K51.80**   **Other ulcerative colitis without complications**
     K51.81   **Other ulcerative colitis with complications**
6th   **K51.811**   **Other ulcerative colitis; with rectal bleeding**
       K51.812   **with intestinal obstruction**
       K51.813   **with fistula**
       K51.814   **with abscess**
       K51.818   **with other complication**
       K51.819   **with unspecified complications**

K51.9   **Ulcerative colitis, unspecified**
5th   **K51.90**   **Ulcerative colitis, unspecified, without complications**
     K51.91   **Ulcerative colitis, unspecified, with complications**
6th   **K51.911**   **Ulcerative colitis, unspecified; with rectal bleeding**
       K51.912   **with intestinal obstruction**
       K51.913   **with fistula**
       K51.914   **with abscess**
       K51.918   **with other complication**
       K51.919   **with unspecified complications**

K52   **OTHER AND UNSPECIFIED NONINFECTIVE**
4th   **GASTROENTERITIS AND COLITIS**
K52.2   **Allergic and dietetic gastroenteritis and colitis**
5th   Food hypersensitivity gastroenteritis or colitis
   Use additional code to identify type of food allergy (Z91.01-, Z91.02-)
   Excludes2: allergic eosinophilic colitis (K52.82)
     allergic eosinophilic esophagitis (K20.0)
     allergic eosinophilic gastritis (K52.81)
     allergic eosinophilic gastroenteritis (K52.81)
   K52.21   **Food protein–induced enterocolitis syndrome (FPIES)**
     Use additional code for hypovolemic shock, if present (R57.1)
   K52.22   **Food protein–induced enteropathy**
   K52.29   **Other allergic and dietetic gastroenteritis and colitis**
     Allergic proctocolitis
     Food-induced eosinophilic proctocolitis
     Food protein-induced proctocolitis
     Food hypersensitivity gastroenteritis or colitis
     Immediate gastrointestinal hypersensitivity
     Milk protein-induced proctocolitis

K52.3   **Indeterminate colitis**
   Colonic inflammatory bowel disease unclassified (IBDU)
   Excludes1: unspecified colitis (K52.9)

K52.8   **Other specified noninfective gastroenteritis and colitis**
5th   **K52.81**   **Eosinophilic gastritis or gastroenteritis**
     Eosinophilic enteritis
     Excludes2: eosinophilic esophagitis (K20.0)
   K52.82   **Eosinophilic colitis**
     Excludes2: allergic proctocolitis (K52.29)
     food-induced eosinophilic proctocolitis (K52.29)
     food protein-induced enterocolitis syndrome (FPIES) (K52.21)
     food protein-induced proctocolitis (K52.29)
     milk protein-induced proctocolitis (K52.29)
   K52.83   **Microscopic colitis**
6th   **K52.831**   **Collagenous colitis**
       K52.832   **Lymphocytic colitis**
       K52.838   **Other microscopic colitis**
       K52.839   **Microscopic colitis, unspecified**
   K52.89   **Other specified noninfective gastroenteritis and colitis**

K52.9   **Noninfective gastroenteritis and colitis, unspecified**
   Colitis or Enteritis or Gastroenteritis NOS
   Ileitis or Jejunitis or Sigmoiditis NOS
   Excludes1: diarrhea NOS (R19.7)
     functional diarrhea (K59.1)
     infectious gastroenteritis and colitis NOS (A09)
     neonatal diarrhea (noninfective) (P78.3)
     psychogenic diarrhea (F45.8)

(K55–K64) OTHER DISEASES OF INTESTINES

K55   **VASCULAR DISORDERS OF INTESTINES**
4th   **K55.0**   **Acute vascular disorders of intestine**
5th   Infarction of appendices epiploicae
   Mesenteric (artery) (vein) embolism
   Mesenteric (artery) (vein) infarction
   Mesenteric (artery) (vein) thrombosis
   K55.01   **Ischemia of small intestines**
6th   **K55.011**   **Focal (segmental) acute (reversible) ischemia of small intestine**
       K55.012   **Diffuse acute (reversible) ischemia of small intestine**
       K55.019   **Acute (reversible) ischemia of small intestine, extent unspecified**
   K55.02   **Infarction of small intestines**
6th   Gangrene or necrosis of small intestine
     K55.021   **Focal (segmental) acute infarction of small intestine**
       K55.022   **Diffuse acute infarction of small intestine**
       K55.029   **Acute infarction of small intestine, extent unspecified**
   K55.03   **Ischemia of small intestine**
6th   Acute fulminant ischemic colitis
     Subacute ischemic colitis
     K55.031   **Focal (segmental) acute (reversible) ischemia of large intestine**
       K55.032   **Diffuse acute (reversible) ischemia of large intestine**
       K55.039   **Acute (reversible) ischemia of large intestine, extent unspecified**
   K55.04   **Infarction of intestine, part unspecified**
6th   Gangrene or necrosis of large intestine
     K55.041   **Focal (segmental) acute infarction of large intestine**
       K55.042   **Diffuse acute infarction of large intestine**
       K55.049   **Acute infarction of large intestine, extent unspecified**
   K55.05   **Ischemia of intestine, part unspecified**
6th   **K55.051**   **Focal (segmental) acute (reversible) ischemia of intestine, part unspecified**
       K55.052   **Diffuse acute (reversible) ischemia of intestine, part unspecified**
       K55.059   **Acute (reversible) ischemia of intestine, part and extent unspecified**
   K55.06   **Infarction of intestine, part unspecified**
6th   **K55.061**   **Focal (segmental) acute infarction of intestine, part unspecified**
       K55.062   **Diffuse acute infarction of intestine, part unspecified**
       K55.069   **Acute infarction of intestine, part and extent unspecified**

K55.1   **Chronic vascular disorders of intestine**
   Chronic ischemic colitis
   Chronic ischemic enteritis
   Chronic ischemic enterocolitis
   Ischemic stricture of intestine
   Mesenteric atherosclerosis
   Mesenteric vascular insufficiency

K55.3   **Necrotizing enterocolitis**
5th   *Excludes1:* necrotizing enterocolitis of newborn (P77.-)
   Excludes2: necrotizing enterocolitis due to Clostridium difficile (A04.7-)
   K55.30   **Necrotizing enterocolitis, unspecified**
     Necrotizing enterocolitis, NOS

4th   **5th**   **6th**   **7th**   Additional Character Required   ✓   3-character code

•=New Code   *Excludes1*—Not coded here, do not use together
▲=Revised Code   *Excludes2*—Not included here

CHAPTER 11. DISEASES OF THE DIGESTIVE SYSTEM   (K51.51–K55.30)

CHAPTER 11. DISEASES OF THE DIGESTIVE SYSTEM (K55.31–K61.1)

K55.31 **Stage 1 necrotizing enterocolitis**
Necrotizing enterocolitis without pneumonia or perforation
K55.32 **Stage 2 necrotizing enterocolitis**
Necrotizing enterocolitis with pneumonia, without perforation
K55.33 **Stage 3 necrotizing enterocolitis**
Necrotizing enterocolitis with perforation
Necrotizing enterocolitis with pneumatosis and perforation
K55.9 **Vascular disorder of intestine, unspecified**
Ischemic colitis
Ischemic enteritis
Ischemic enterocolitis

K56 [4th] **PARALYTIC ILEUS AND INTESTINAL OBSTRUCTION WITHOUT HERNIA**
Excludes1: congenital stricture or stenosis of intestine (Q41–Q42)
cystic fibrosis with meconium ileus (E84.11)
ischemic stricture of intestine (K55.1)
meconium ileus NOS (P76.0)
neonatal intestinal obstructions classifiable to P76.-
obstruction of duodenum (K31.5)
postprocedural intestinal obstruction (K91.3-)
Excludes2: stenosis of anus or rectum (K62.4)
K56.0 **Paralytic ileus**
Paralysis of bowel or colon or intestine
Excludes1: gallstone ileus (K56.3)
ileus NOS (K56.7)
obstructive ileus NOS (K56.69-)
K56.1 **Intussusception**
Intussusception or invagination of bowel or colon or intestine or rectum
Excludes2: intussusception of appendix (K38.8)
K56.2 **Volvulus**
Strangulation of colon or intestine
Torsion or Twist of colon or intestine
Excludes2: volvulus of duodenum (K31.5)
K56.4 **Other impaction of intestine**
[5th] K56.41 **Fecal impaction**
Excludes1: constipation (K59.0-)
incomplete defecation (R15.0)
K56.49 **Other impaction of intestine**
K56.6 **Other and unspecified intestinal obstruction**
[5th] K56.60 **Unspecified intestinal obstruction**
[6th] Intestinal obstruction NOS
K56.600 **Partial intestinal obstruction, unspecified as to cause**
Incomplete intestinal obstruction, NOS
K56.601 **Complete intestinal obstruction, unspecified as to cause**
K56.609 **Unspecified intestinal obstruction, unspecified as to partial versus complete obstruction**
Intestinal obstruction NOS
K56.69 **Other intestinal obstruction**
[6th] Enterostenosis NOS
Obstructive ileus NOS
Occlusion or Stenosis or Stricture of colon or intestine NOS
Excludes1: intestinal obstruction due to specified condition-code to condition
K56.690 **Other partial intestinal obstruction**
Other incomplete intestinal obstruction
K56.691 **Other complete intestinal obstruction**
K56.699 **Other intestinal obstruction unspecified as to partial versus complete obstruction**
Other intestinal obstruction, NEC
K56.7 **Ileus, unspecified**
Excludes1: obstructive ileus (K56.69-)
Excludes2: intestinal obstruction with hernia (K40-K46)

K58 [4th] **IRRITABLE BOWEL SYNDROME**
Includes: irritable colon
spastic colon
K58.0 **Irritable bowel syndrome with diarrhea**
K58.1 **Irritable bowel syndrome with constipation**
K58.2 **Mixed irritable bowel syndrome**
K58.8 **Other Irritable bowel syndrome**
K58.9 **Irritable bowel syndrome without diarrhea**
Irritable bowel syndrome NOS

K59 [4th] **OTHER FUNCTIONAL INTESTINAL DISORDERS**
Excludes1: change in bowel habit NOS (R19.4)
intestinal malabsorption (K90.-)
psychogenic intestinal disorders (F45.8)
Excludes2: functional disorders of stomach (K31.-)
K59.0 **Constipation**
[5th] *Excludes1:* fecal impaction (K56.41)
incomplete defecation (R15.0)
K59.00 **Constipation, unspecified**
K59.01 **Slow transit constipation**
K59.02 **Outlet dysfunction constipation**
K59.03 **Drug-induced constipation**
Use additional code for adverse effect, if applicable, to identify drug (T36 –T50) with 5th or 6th character 5
K59.04 **Chronic Idiopathic constipation**
Functional constipation
K59.09 **Other constipation**
Chronic constipation
K59.1 **Functional diarrhea**
Excludes1: diarrhea NOS (R19.7)
irritable bowel syndrome with diarrhea (K58.0)
K59.2 **Neurogenic bowel, not elsewhere classified**
K59.3 **Megacolon, NEC**
[5th] Dilatation of colon
Excludes1: congenital megacolon (aganglionic) (Q43.1)
megacolon (due to) (in) Chagas' disease (B57.32)
megacolon (due to) (in) Clostridium difficile (A04.7-)
megacolon (due to) (in) Hirschsprung's disease (Q43.1)
K59.31 **Toxic megacolon**
Code first (T51–T65) to identify toxic agent, if applicable
K59.39 **Other megacolon**
Megacolon NOS
K59.4 **Anal spasm**
Proctalgia fugax
K59.8 **Other specified functional intestinal disorders**
K59.81 **Ogilvie syndrome**
Acute colonic pseudo-obstruction (ACPO)
K59.89 **Other specified functional intestinal disorders**
Atony of colon
Pseudo-obstruction (acute) (chronic) of intestine
K59.9 **Functional intestinal disorder, unspecified**

K60 [4th] **FISSURE AND FISTULA OF ANAL AND RECTAL REGIONS**
Excludes1: fissure and fistula of anal and rectal regions with abscess or cellulitis (K61.-)
Excludes2: anal sphincter tear (healed) (nontraumatic) (old) (K62.81)
K60.0 **Acute anal fissure**
K60.1 **Chronic anal fissure**
K60.2 **Anal fissure, unspecified**
K60.3 **Anal fistula**
K60.4 **Rectal fistula**
Fistula of rectum to skin
Excludes1: rectovaginal fistula (N82.3)
vesicorectal fistula (N32.1)

K61 [4th] **ABSCESS OF ANAL AND RECTAL REGIONS**
Includes: abscess of anal and rectal regions
cellulitis of anal and rectal regions
K61.0 **Anal abscess**
Perianal abscess
Excludes2: intrasphincteric abscess (K61.4)
K61.1 **Rectal abscess**
Perirectal abscess
Excludes1: ischiorectal abscess (K61.39)

[4th] [5th] [6th] [7th] Additional Character Required   3-character code

•=New Code   *Excludes1*—Not coded here, do not use together
▲=Revised Code   *Excludes2*—Not included here

K61.2 Anorectal abscess
K61.3 Ischiorectal abscess
- **5th** **K61.31 Horseshoe abscess**
- **K61.39 Other ischiorectal abscess**
  Abscess of ischiorectal fossa
  Ischiorectal abscess, NOS
K61.4 Intrasphincteric abscess
  Intersphincteric abscess
K61.5 Supralevator abscess

K62 OTHER DISEASES OF ANUS AND RECTUM
4th
Includes: anal canal
Excludes2: colostomy and enterostomy malfunction (K94.0-, K94.1-)
  fecal incontinence (R15.-)
  hemorrhoids (K64.-)
K62.0 Anal polyp
K62.1 Rectal polyp
  Excludes1: adenomatous polyp (D12.8)
K62.2 Anal prolapse
  Prolapse of anal canal
K62.3 Rectal prolapse
  Prolapse of rectal mucosa
K62.4 Stenosis of anus and rectum
  Stricture of anus (sphincter)
K62.5 Hemorrhage of anus and rectum
  Excludes1: gastrointestinal bleeding NOS (K92.2)
    melena (K92.1)
    neonatal rectal hemorrhage (P54.2)
K62.6 Ulcer of anus and rectum
  Solitary ulcer of anus and rectum
  Stercoral ulcer of anus and rectum
K62.8 Other specified diseases of anus and rectum
  5th *Excludes2:* ulcerative proctitis (K51.2)
- **K62.81 Anal sphincter tear (healed) (nontraumatic) (old)**
  Tear of anus, nontraumatic
  Use additional code for any associated fecal
    incontinence (R15.-)
  Excludes2: anal fissure (K60.-)
    anal sphincter tear (healed) (old) complicating delivery
      (O34.7-)
    traumatic tear of anal sphincter (S31.831)
- **K62.82 Dysplasia of anus**
  Anal intraepithelial neoplasia I and II (AIN I and II)
    (histologically confirmed)
  Dysplasia of anus NOS
  Mild and moderate dysplasia of anus (histologically
    confirmed)
  Excludes1: abnormal results from anal cytologic
    examination without histologic confirmation (R85.61-)
    anal intraepithelial neoplasia III (D01.3)
    carcinoma in situ of anus (D01.3)
    HGSIL of anus (R85.613)
    severe dysplasia of anus (D01.3)
- **K62.89 Other specified diseases of anus and rectum**
  Proctitis NOS
  Use additional code for any associated fecal
    incontinence (R15.-)
K62.9 Disease of anus and rectum, unspecified

K63 OTHER DISEASES OF INTESTINE
4th
- **K63.0 Abscess of intestine**
  Excludes1: abscess of intestine with Crohn's disease (K50.014,
    K50.114, K50.814, K50.914)
    abscess of intestine with diverticular disease (K57.0, K57.2,
    K57.4, K57.8)
    abscess of intestine with ulcerative colitis (K51.014, K51.214,
    K51.314, K51.414, K51.514,K51.814, K51.914)
  Excludes2: abscess of anal and rectal regions (K61.-)
    abscess of appendix (K35.3-)

K63.3 Ulcer of intestine
  Primary ulcer of small intestine
  Excludes1: duodenal ulcer (K26.-)
    gastrointestinal ulcer (K28.-)
    gastrojejunal ulcer (K28.-)
    jejunal ulcer (K28.-)
    peptic ulcer, site unspecified (K27.-)
    ulcer of intestine with perforation (K63.1)
    ulcer of anus or rectum (K62.6)
    ulcerative colitis (K51.-)
K63.5 Polyp of colon
  Excludes1: adenomatous polyp of colon (D12.-)
    inflammatory polyp of colon (K51.4-)
    polyposis of colon (D12.6)
K63.8 Other specified diseases of intestine
  5th **K63.81 Dieulafoy lesion of intestine**
    Excludes2: Dieulafoy lesion of stomach and duodenum
      (K31.82)
  K63.89 Other specified diseases of intestine
K63.9 Disease of intestine, unspecified

K64 HEMORRHOIDS AND PERIANAL VENOUS THROMBOSIS
4th
Includes: piles
Excludes1: hemorrhoids complicating childbirth and the puerperium
  (O87.2)
  hemorrhoids complicating pregnancy (O22.4)
K64.0 First degree hemorrhoids
  Grade/stage I hemorrhoids
  Hemorrhoids (bleeding) without prolapse outside of anal canal
K64.1 Second degree hemorrhoids
  Grade/stage II hemorrhoids
  Hemorrhoids (bleeding) that prolapse with straining, but retract
    spontaneously
K64.2 Third degree hemorrhoids
  Grade/stage III hemorrhoids
  Hemorrhoids (bleeding) that prolapse with straining and require
    manual replacement back inside anal canal
K64.3 Fourth degree hemorrhoids
  Grade/stage IV hemorrhoids
  Hemorrhoids (bleeding) with prolapsed tissue that cannot be
    manually replaced
K64.4 Residual hemorrhoidal skin tags
  External hemorrhoids, NOS
  Skin tags of anus
K64.5 Perianal venous thrombosis
  External hemorrhoids with thrombosis
  Perianal hematoma
  Thrombosed hemorrhoids NOS
K64.8 Other hemorrhoids
  Internal hemorrhoids, without mention of degree
  Prolapsed hemorrhoids, degree not specified
K64.9 Unspecified hemorrhoids
  Hemorrhoids (bleeding) NOS
  Hemorrhoids (bleeding) without mention of degree

(K65–K68) DISEASES OF PERITONEUM AND RETROPERITONEUM

K65 PERITONITIS
4th
Use additional code (B95–B97), to identify infectious agent, if known
Code also if applicable diverticular disease of intestine (K57.-)
Excludes1: acute appendicitis with generalized peritonitis (K35.2-)
  aseptic peritonitis (T81.6)
  benign paroxysmal peritonitis (E85.0)
  chemical peritonitis (T81.6)
  gonococcal peritonitis (A54.85)
  neonatal peritonitis (P78.0–P78.1)
  pelvic peritonitis, female (N73.3–N73.5)
  periodic familial peritonitis (E85.0)
  peritonitis due to talc or other foreign substance (T81.6)
  peritonitis in chlamydia (A74.81) or in diphtheria (A36.89) or syphilis
    (late) (A52.74)

4th **5th** **6th** **7th** Additional Character Required   ✔ 3-character code   •=New Code   ▲=Revised Code   *Excludes1*—Not coded here, do not use together   *Excludes2*—Not included here

peritonitis in tuberculosis (A18.31)
peritonitis with or following appendicitis (K35.-)
retroperitoneal infections (K68.-)

K65.0 Generalized (acute) peritonitis
Pelvic peritonitis (acute), male
Subphrenic peritonitis (acute)
Suppurative peritonitis (acute)

K65.1 Peritoneal abscess
Abdominopelvic abscess
Abscess (of) omentum
Abscess (of) peritoneum
Mesenteric abscess
Retrocecal abscess
Subdiaphragmatic abscess
Subhepatic abscess
Subphrenic abscess

K65.2 Spontaneous bacterial peritonitis
Excludes1: bacterial peritonitis NOS (K65.9)

K65.8 Other peritonitis
Chronic proliferative peritonitis
Peritonitis due to urine

K65.9 Peritonitis, unspecified
Bacterial peritonitis NOS

K68   DISORDERS OF RETROPERITONEUM
`4th`
    K68.1 Retroperitoneal abscess
    `5th`   **K68.19   Other retroperitoneal abscess**

(K70–K77) DISEASES OF LIVER

Excludes1: jaundice NOS (R17)
Excludes2: hemochromatosis (E83.11-)
Reye's syndrome (G93.7)
viral hepatitis (B15–B19)
Wilson's disease (E83.0)

K73   CHRONIC HEPATITIS, NEC
`4th`
    Excludes1: alcoholic hepatitis (chronic) (K70.1-)
    drug-induced hepatitis (chronic) (K71.-)
    granulomatous hepatitis (chronic) NEC (K75.3)
    reactive, nonspecific hepatitis (chronic) (K75.2)
    viral hepatitis (chronic) (B15–B19)

    K73.0 Chronic persistent hepatitis, NEC
    K73.1 Chronic lobular hepatitis, NEC
    K73.2 Chronic active hepatitis, NEC
    K73.8 Other chronic hepatitis, NEC
    K73.9 Chronic hepatitis, unspecified

K74   FIBROSIS AND CIRRHOSIS OF LIVER
`4th`
    Code also, if applicable, viral hepatitis (acute) (chronic) (B15-B19)
    Excludes1: alcoholic cirrhosis (of liver) (K70.3)
    alcoholic fibrosis of liver (K70.2)
    cardiac sclerosis of liver (K76.1)
    cirrhosis (of liver) with toxic liver disease (K71.7)
    congenital cirrhosis (of liver) (P78.81)
    pigmentary cirrhosis (of liver) (E83.110)

    K74.5 Biliary cirrhosis, unspecified
    K74.6 Other and unspecified cirrhosis of liver
    `5th`   **K74.60   Unspecified cirrhosis of liver**
           Cirrhosis (of liver) NOS
        K74.69   Other cirrhosis of liver
           Cryptogenic cirrhosis (of liver)
           Macronodular cirrhosis (of liver)
           Micronodular cirrhosis (of liver)
           Mixed type cirrhosis (of liver)
           Portal cirrhosis (of liver)
           Postnecrotic cirrhosis (of liver)

K75   OTHER INFLAMMATORY LIVER DISEASES
`4th`
    Excludes2: toxic liver disease (K71.-)
    K75.2 Nonspecific reactive hepatitis
        Excludes1: acute or subacute hepatitis (K72.0-)
          chronic hepatitis NEC (K73.-)
          viral hepatitis (B15-B19)

K75.3 Granulomatous hepatitis, not elsewhere classified
Excludes1: acute or subacute hepatitis (K72.0-)
chronic hepatitis NEC (K73.-)
viral hepatitis (B15-B19)

K75.9 Inflammatory liver disease, unspecified
Hepatitis NOS
Excludes1: acute or subacute hepatitis (K72.0-)
chronic hepatitis NEC (K73.-)
viral hepatitis (B15-B19)

K76   OTHER DISEASES OF LIVER
`4th`
    Excludes2: alcoholic liver disease (K70.-)
    amyloid degeneration of liver (E85.-)
    cystic disease of liver (congenital) (Q44.6)
    hepatic vein thrombosis (I82.0)
    hepatomegaly NOS (R16.0)
    pigmentary cirrhosis (of liver) (E83.110)
    portal vein thrombosis (I81)
    toxic liver disease (K71.-)

    K76.0 Fatty (change of) liver, not elsewhere classified
    Nonalcoholic fatty liver disease (NAFLD)
    Excludes1: nonalcoholic steatohepatitis (NASH) (K75.81)

    K76.8 Other specified diseases of liver
    `5th`   **K76.81   Hepatopulmonary syndrome**
          Code first underlying liver disease, such as:
            alcoholic cirrhosis of liver (K70.3-)
            cirrhosis of liver without mention of alcohol (K74.6-)

        K76.89   Other specified diseases of liver
          Cyst (simple) of liver
          Focal nodular hyperplasia of liver
          Hepatoptosis

    K76.9 Liver disease, unspecified

K77   LIVER DISORDERS IN DISEASES CLASSIFIED ELSEWHERE
`✔`
    Code first underlying disease, such as: amyloidosis (E85.-)
    congenital syphilis (A50.0, A50.5)
    congenital toxoplasmosis (P37.1)
    infectious mononucleosis with liver disease (B27.0-B27.9 with .9)
    schistosomiasis (B65.0–B65.9)
    Excludes1: alcoholic hepatitis (K70.1-)
    alcoholic liver disease (K70.-)
    cytomegaloviral hepatitis (B25.1)
    herpesviral [herpes simplex] hepatitis (B00.81)
    mumps hepatitis (B26.81)
    sarcoidosis with liver disease (D86.89)
    secondary syphilis with liver disease (A51.45)
    syphilis (late) with liver disease (A52.74)
    toxoplasmosis (acquired) hepatitis (B58.1)
    tuberculosis with liver disease (A18.83)

(K80–K87) DISORDERS OF GALLBLADDER, BILIARY TRACT AND PANCREAS

K80   CHOLELITHIASIS
`4th`
    Excludes1: retained cholelithiasis following cholecystectomy (K91.86)
    Use additional code if applicable for associated gangrene of gallbladder (K82.A1), or perforation of gallbladder (K82.A2) for sub-categories K80.0-, K80.1-, K80.4-, K80.6-

    K80.0 Calculus of gallbladder with acute cholecystitis
    `5th`   Any condition listed in K80.2 with acute cholecystitis
        K80.00   Calculus of gallbladder with acute cholecystitis without obstruction
        K80.01   Calculus of gallbladder with acute cholecystitis with obstruction

    K80.1 Calculus of gallbladder; with other cholecystitis
    `5th`   **K80.10   with chronic cholecystitis without obstruction**
          Cholelithiasis with cholecystitis NOS
        K80.11   with chronic cholecystitis with obstruction
        K80.12   with acute and chronic cholecystitis without obstruction
        K80.13   with acute and chronic cholecystitis with obstruction
        K80.18   with other cholecystitis without obstruction
        K80.19   with other cholecystitis with obstruction

`4th` `5th` `6th` `7th`   Additional Character Required   `✔`   3-character code

•=New Code   *Excludes1*—Not coded here, do not use together
▲=Revised Code   *Excludes2*—Not included here

K80.2 Calculus of gallbladder without cholecystitis
5th   Cholecystolithiasis with cholecystitis
Cholelithiasis (without cholecystitis)
Colic (recurrent) of gallbladder (without cholecystitis)
Gallstone (impacted) of cystic duct (without cholecystitis)
Gallstone (impacted) of gallbladder (without cholecystitis)
    K80.20 Calculus of gallbladder without cholecystitis without obstruction
    K80.21 Calculus of gallbladder without cholecystitis with obstruction
K80.5 Calculus of bile duct without cholangitis or cholecystitis
5th   Choledocholithiasis (without cholangitis or cholecystitis)
Gallstone (impacted) of bile duct NOS (without cholangitis or cholecystitis)
Gallstone (impacted) of common duct (without cholangitis or cholecystitis)
Gallstone (impacted) of hepatic duct (without cholangitis or cholecystitis)
Hepatic cholelithiasis (without cholangitis or cholecystitis)
Hepatic colic (recurrent) (without cholangitis or cholecystitis)
    K80.50 Calculus of bile duct without cholangitis or cholecystitis without obstruction
    K80.51 Calculus of bile duct without cholangitis or cholecystitis with obstruction
K80.8 Other cholelithiasis
5th   **K80.80 Other cholelithiasis without obstruction**
    K80.81 Other cholelithiasis with obstruction

K81 CHOLECYSTITIS
4th   **Use additional code** if applicable for associated gangrene of gallbladder (K82.A1), or perforation of gallbladder (K82.A2)
Excludes1: cholecystitis with cholelithiasis (K80.-)
K81.0 Acute cholecystitis
Abscess of gallbladder
Angiocholecystitis
Emphysematous (acute) cholecystitis
Empyema of gallbladder
Gangrene of gallbladder
Gangrenous cholecystitis
Suppurative cholecystitis
K81.1 Chronic cholecystitis
K81.2 Acute cholecystitis with chronic cholecystitis
K81.9 Cholecystitis, unspecified

K82 OTHER DISEASES OF GALLBLADDER
4th   *Excludes1:* nonvisualization of gallbladder (R93.2)
postcholecystectomy syndrome (K91.5)
K82.0 Obstruction of gallbladder
Occlusion of cystic duct or gallbladder without cholelithiasis
Stenosis of cystic duct or gallbladder without cholelithiasis
Stricture of cystic duct or gallbladder without cholelithiasis
Excludes1: obstruction of gallbladder with cholelithiasis (K80.-)
K82.8 Other specified diseases of gallbladder
Adhesions of cystic duct or gallbladder
Atrophy of cystic duct or gallbladder
Cyst of cystic duct or gallbladder
Dyskinesia of cystic duct or gallbladder
Hypertrophy of cystic duct or gallbladder
Nonfunctioning of cystic duct or gallbladder
Ulcer of cystic duct or gallbladder
K82.9 Disease of gallbladder, unspecified
K82.A Disorders of gallbladder in diseases classified elsewhere
5th   **Code first** the type of cholecystitis (K81.-), or cholelithiasis with cholecystitis (K80.00-K80.19, K80.40-K80.47,K80.60-K80.67)
    K82.A1 Gangrene of gallbladder in cholecystitis
    K82.A2 Perforation of gallbladder in cholecystitis

K83 OTHER DISEASES OF BILIARY TRACT
4th   *Excludes1:* postcholecystectomy syndrome (K91.5)
Excludes2: conditions involving the gallbladder (K81-K82)
conditions involving the cystic duct (K81-K82)
K83.1 Obstruction of bile duct
Occlusion of bile duct without cholelithiasis
Stenosis of bile duct without cholelithiasis
Stricture of bile duct without cholelithiasis

Excludes1: congenital obstruction of bile duct (Q44.3)
obstruction of bile duct with cholelithiasis (K80.-)
K83.8 Other specified diseases of biliary tract
Adhesions of biliary tract
Atrophy of biliary tract
Hypertrophy of biliary tract
Ulcer of biliary tract
K83.9 Disease of biliary tract, unspecified

K85 ACUTE PANCREATITIS
4th   *Includes:* acute (recurrent) pancreatitis
subacute pancreatitis
K85.0 Idiopathic acute pancreatitis
5th   **K85.00 Idiopathic acute pancreatitis without necrosis or infection**
    K85.01 Idiopathic acute pancreatitis with uninfected necrosis
    K85.02 Idiopathic acute pancreatitis with infected necrosis
K85.8 Other acute pancreatitis
5th   **K85.80 Other acute pancreatitis without necrosis or infection**
    K85.81 Other acute pancreatitis with uninfected necrosis
    K85.82 Other acute pancreatitis with infected necrosis
K85.9 Acute pancreatitis, unspecified
5th   Pancreatitis NOS
    K85.90 Acute pancreatitis without necrosis or infection, unspecified
    K85.91 Acute pancreatitis with uninfected necrosis, unspecified
    K85.92 Acute pancreatitis with infected necrosis, unspecified

K86 OTHER DISEASES OF PANCREAS
4th   *Excludes2:* fibrocystic disease of pancreas (E84.-)
islet cell tumor (of pancreas) (D13.7)
pancreatic steatorrhea (K90.3)
K86.2 Cyst of pancreas
K86.8 Other specified diseases of pancreas
5th   **K86.81 Exocrine pancreatic insufficiency**
    K86.89 Other specified diseases of pancreas
Aseptic pancreatic necrosis, unrelated to acute pancreatitis
Atrophy of pancreas
Calculus of pancreas
Cirrhosis of pancreas
Fibrosis of pancreas
Pancreatic fat necrosis, unrelated to acute pancreatitis
Pancreatic infantilism
Pancreatic necrosis NOS, unrelated to acute pancreatitis
K86.9 Disease of pancreas, unspecified

(K90–K95) OTHER DISEASES OF THE DIGESTIVE SYSTEM

K90 INTESTINAL MALABSORPTION
4th   *Excludes1:* intestinal malabsorption following gastrointestinal surgery (K91.2)
K90.0 Celiac disease
Celiac disease with steatorrhea
Celiac gluten-sensitive enteropathy
Nontropical sprue
Code also exocrine pancreatic insufficiency (K86.81)
Use additional code *for associated disorders including:*
dermatitis herpetiformis (L13.0)
gluten ataxia (G32.81)
K90.1 Tropical sprue
Sprue NOS
Tropical steatorrhea
K90.2 Blind loop syndrome, not elsewhere classified
Blind loop syndrome NOS
Excludes1: congenital blind loop syndrome (Q43.8)
postsurgical blind loop syndrome (K91.2)
K90.3 Pancreatic steatorrhea

K90.4 **Other malabsorption due to intolerance**
[5th] *Excludes2:* celiac gluten-sensitive enteropathy (K90.0)
    lactose intolerance (E73.-)
  K90.41 **Non-celiac gluten sensitivity**
    Gluten sensitivity NOS
    Non-celiac gluten sensitive enteropathy
  K90.49 **Malabsorption due to intolerance, NEC**
    Malabsorption due to intolerance to carbohydrate or fat
    or protein or starch
K90.8 **Other intestinal malabsorption**
[5th]   **K90.81** **Whipple's disease**
  K90.89 **Other intestinal malabsorption**
K90.9 **Intestinal malabsorption, unspecified**

K91 **INTRAOPERATIVE AND POSTPROCEDURAL**
[4th] **COMPLICATIONS AND DISORDERS OF DIGESTIVE**
SYSTEM, NEC
Excludes2: complications of artificial opening of digestive system (K94.-)
  complications of bariatric procedures (K95.-)
  gastrojejunal ulcer (K28.-)
  postprocedural (radiation) retroperitoneal abscess (K68.11)
  radiation colitis (K52.0)
  radiation gastroenteritis (K52.0)
  radiation proctitis (K62.7)
K91.2 **Postsurgical malabsorption, NEC**
  Postsurgical blind loop syndrome
  Excludes1: malabsorption osteomalacia in adults (M83.2)
    malabsorption osteoporosis, postsurgical (M80.8-, M81.8)
K91.3 **Postprocedural intestinal obstruction**
[5th]   **K91.30** **Postprocedural intestinal obstruction, unspecified as**
    to partial versus complete
    Postprocedural intestinal obstruction NOS
  K91.31 **Postprocedural partial intestinal obstruction**
    Postprocedural incomplete intestinal obstruction
  K91.32 **Postprocedural complete intestinal obstruction**
K91.8 **Other intraoperative and postprocedural complications and**
[5th] **disorders of digestive system**
  K91.89 **Other postprocedural complications and disorders of**
    digestive system
    Use additional code, if applicable, to further specify
      disorder
    Excludes2: postprocedural retroperitoneal abscess
      (K68.11)

K92 **OTHER DISEASES OF DIGESTIVE SYSTEM**
[4th] *Excludes1:* neonatal gastrointestinal hemorrhage (P54.0–P54.3)
K92.0 **Hematemesis**
K92.1 **Melena**
  Excludes1: occult blood in feces (R19.5)
K92.2 **Gastrointestinal hemorrhage, unspecified**
  Gastric hemorrhage NOS
  Intestinal hemorrhage NOS
  Excludes1: acute hemorrhagic gastritis (K29.01)
    hemorrhage of anus and rectum (K62.5)
    angiodysplasia of stomach with hemorrhage (K31.811)
    diverticular disease with hemorrhage (K57.-)
    gastritis and duodenitis with hemorrhage (K29.-)
    peptic ulcer with hemorrhage (K25–K28)
K92.8 **Other specified diseases of the digestive system**
[5th]   **K92.81** **Gastrointestinal mucositis (ulcerative)**
    Code also type of associated therapy, such as:
    antineoplastic and immunosuppressive drugs (T45.1X-)
    radiological procedure and radiotherapy (Y84.2)
    Excludes2: mucositis (ulcerative) of vagina and vulva
      (N76.81)
    nasal mucositis (ulcerative) (J34.81)
    oral mucositis (ulcerative) (K12.3-)
  K92.89 **Other specified diseases of the digestive system**
K92.9 **Disease of digestive system, unspecified**

K94 **COMPLICATIONS OF ARTIFICIAL OPENINGS OF THE**
[4th] **DIGESTIVE SYSTEM**
K94.0 **Colostomy complications**
[5th]   **K94.00** **Colostomy complication, unspecified**
  K94.01 **Colostomy hemorrhage**
  K94.02 **Colostomy infection**
    Use additional code to specify type of infection, such as:
      cellulitis of abdominal wall (L03.311)
      sepsis (A40.-, A41.-)
  K94.03 **Colostomy malfunction**
    Mechanical complication of colostomy
  K94.09 **Other complications of colostomy**
K94.2 **Gastrostomy complications**
[5th]   **K94.20** **Gastrostomy complication, unspecified**
  K94.21 **Gastrostomy hemorrhage**
  K94.22 **Gastrostomy infection**
    Use additional code *to specify type of infection,*
      such as: sepsis (A40.-, A41.-)
    cellulitis of abdominal wall (L03.311)
  K94.23 **Gastrostomy malfunction**
    Mechanical complication of gastrostomy
  K94.29 **Other complications of gastrostomy**

 [4th] [5th] [6th] [7th] Additional Character Required   ✔ 3-character code   •=New Code   ▲=Revised Code   *Excludes1*—Not coded here, do not use together   *Excludes2*—Not included here

Chapter 12. Diseases of the skin and subcutaneous tissue (L00–L99)

GUIDELINES

Pressure ulcer stages
Refer to category L89.
Excludes2: certain conditions originating in the perinatal period (P04–P96)
    certain infectious and parasitic diseases (A00–B99)
    complications of pregnancy, childbirth and the puerperium (O00–O9A)
    congenital malformations, deformations, and chromosomal abnormalities
      (Q00–Q99)
    endocrine, nutritional and metabolic diseases (E00–E88)
    lipomelanotic reticulosis (I89.8)
    neoplasms (C00–D49)
    symptoms, signs and abnormal clinical and laboratory findings, NEC (R00–R94)
    systemic connective tissue disorders (M30–M36)
    viral warts (B07.-)

(L00–L08) INFECTIONS OF THE SKIN AND SUBCUTANEOUS TISSUE

Use additional code (B95–B97) to identify infectious agent.
Excludes2: hordeolum (H00.0)
    infective dermatitis (L30.3)
    local infections of skin classified in Chapter 1
    lupus panniculitis (L93.2)
    panniculitis NOS (M79.3)
    panniculitis of neck and back (M54.0-)
    Perlèche NOS (K13.0)
    Perlèche due to candidiasis (B37.0)
    Perlèche due to riboflavin deficiency (E53.0)
    pyogenic granuloma (L98.0)
    relapsing panniculitis [Weber-Christian] (M35.6)
    viral warts (B07.-)
    zoster (B02.-)

L00   **STAPHYLOCOCCAL SCALDED SKIN SYNDROME**
    Ritter's disease
    Use additional code to identify percentage of skin exfoliation (L49.-)
    Excludes1: bullous impetigo (L01.03)
      pemphigus neonatorum (L01.03)
      toxic epidermal necrolysis [Lyell] (L51.2)

L01   **IMPETIGO**
    Excludes1: impetigo herpetiformis (L40.1)
    L01.0   **Impetigo**
      Impetigo contagiosa
      Impetigo vulgaris
      L01.00   **Impetigo, unspecified**
        Impetigo NOS
      L01.01   **Non-bullous impetigo**
      L01.02   **Bockhart's impetigo**
        Impetigo follicularis
        Perifolliculitis NOS
        Superficial pustular perifolliculitis
      L01.03   **Bullous impetigo**
        Impetigo neonatorum
        Pemphigus neonatorum
      L01.09   **Other impetigo**
        Ulcerative impetigo
    L01.1   **Impetiginization of other dermatoses**

L02   **CUTANEOUS ABSCESS, FURUNCLE AND CARBUNCLE**
    Use additional code to identify organism (B95–B96)
    Excludes2: abscess of anus and rectal regions (K61.-)
      abscess of female genital organs (external) (N76.4)
      abscess of male genital organs (external) (N48.2, N49.-)
    L02.0   **Cutaneous abscess, furuncle and carbuncle of face**
      Excludes2: abscess of ear, external (H60.0)
        abscess of eyelid (H00.0)
        abscess of head [any part, except face] (L02.8)
        abscess of lacrimal gland (H04.0)
        abscess of lacrimal passages (H04.3)

        abscess of mouth (K12.2)
        abscess of nose (J34.0)
        abscess of orbit (H05.0)
        submandibular abscess (K12.2)
    L02.01   **Cutaneous abscess of face**
    L02.02   **Furuncle of face**
      Boil of face
      Folliculitis of face
    L02.03   **Carbuncle of face**
  L02.1   **Cutaneous abscess, furuncle and carbuncle of neck**
    L02.11   **Cutaneous abscess of neck**
    L02.12   **Furuncle of neck**
      Boil of neck
      Folliculitis of neck
    L02.13   **Carbuncle of neck**
  L02.2   **Cutaneous abscess, furuncle and carbuncle of trunk**
    Excludes1: non-newborn omphalitis (L08.82)
      omphalitis of newborn (P38.-)
    Excludes2: abscess of breast (N61.1)
      abscess of buttocks (L02.3)
      abscess of female external genital organs (N76.4)
      abscess of male external genital organs (N48.2, N49.-)
      abscess of hip (L02.4)
    L02.21   **Cutaneous abscess of trunk**
      L02.211   **Cutaneous abscess of; abdominal wall**
      L02.212   **back [any part, except buttock]**
      L02.213   **chest wall**
      L02.214   **groin**
      L02.215   **perineum**
      L02.216   **umbilicus**
      L02.219   **trunk, unspecified**
    L02.22   **Furuncle of trunk**
      Boil of trunk
      Folliculitis of trunk
      L02.221   **Furuncle of; abdominal wall**
      L02.222   **back [any part, except buttock]**
      L02.223   **chest wall**
      L02.224   **groin**
      L02.225   **perineum**
      L02.226   **umbilicus**
      L02.229   **trunk, unspecified**
    L02.23   **Carbuncle of trunk**
      L02.231   **Carbuncle of; abdominal wall**
      L02.232   **back [any part, except buttock]**
      L02.233   **chest wall**
      L02.234   **groin**
      L02.235   **perineum**
      L02.236   **umbilicus**
      L02.239   **trunk, unspecified**
  L02.3   **Cutaneous abscess, furuncle and carbuncle of buttock**
    Excludes1: pilonidal cyst with abscess (L05.01)
    L02.31   **Cutaneous abscess of buttock**
      Cutaneous abscess of gluteal region
    L02.32   **Furuncle of buttock**
      Boil of buttock
      Folliculitis of buttock
      Furuncle of gluteal region
    L02.33   **Carbuncle of buttock**
      Carbuncle of gluteal region
  L02.4   **Cutaneous abscess, furuncle and carbuncle of limb**
    Excludes2: Cutaneous abscess, furuncle and carbuncle of groin
      (L02.214, L02.224, L02.234)
      Cutaneous abscess, furuncle and carbuncle of hand (L02.5-)
      Cutaneous abscess, furuncle and carbuncle of foot (L02.6-)
    L02.41   **Cutaneous abscess of; limb**
      L02.411   **right axilla**
      L02.412   **left axilla**
      L02.413   **right upper limb**
      L02.414   **left upper limb**
      L02.415   **right lower limb**
      L02.416   **left lower limb**

4th **5th** **6th** **7th** Additional Character Required   ✔ 3-character code   Unspecified laterality codes were excluded here.   •=New Code ▲=Revised Code   ***Excludes1***—Not coded here, do not use together   ***Excludes2***—Not included here

CHAPTER 12. DISEASES OF THE SKIN AND SUBCUTANEOUS TISSUE   (L02.42–L03.312)

L02.42   **Furuncle of; limb**
    `6th`   Boil of limb
         Folliculitis of limb
         L02.421   **right axilla**
         L02.422   **left axilla**
         L02.423   **right upper limb**
         L02.424   **left upper limb**
         L02.425   **right lower limb**
         L02.426   **left lower limb**

L02.43   **Carbuncle of; limb**
    `6th`   **L02.431**   **right axilla**
         L02.432   **left axilla**
         L02.433   **right upper limb**
         L02.434   **left upper limb**
         L02.435   **right lower limb**
         L02.436   **left lower limb**

L02.5   **Cutaneous abscess, furuncle and carbuncle of hand**
   `5th`   **L02.51**   **Cutaneous abscess of; hand**
       `6th`   **L02.511**   **right hand**
          L02.512   **left hand**
      L02.52   **Furuncle; hand**
       `6th`   Boil of hand
          Folliculitis of hand
          L02.521   **right hand**
          L02.522   **left hand**
      L02.53   **Carbuncle of; hand**
       `6th`   **L02.531**   **right hand**
          L02.532   **left hand**

L02.6   **Cutaneous abscess, furuncle and carbuncle of foot**
   `5th`   **L02.61**   **Cutaneous abscess of; foot**
       `6th`   **L02.611**   **right foot**
          L02.612   **left foot**
      L02.62   **Furuncle of; foot**
       `6th`   Boil of foot
          Folliculitis of foot
          L02.621   **right foot**
          L02.622   **left foot**
      L02.63   **Carbuncle of; foot**
       `6th`   **L02.631**   **right foot**
          L02.632   **left foot**

L02.8   **Cutaneous abscess, furuncle and carbuncle of other sites**
   `5th`   **L02.81**   **Cutaneous abscess of; other sites**
       `6th`   **L02.811**   **head [any part, except face]**
          L02.818   **other sites**
      L02.82   **Furuncle of; other sites**
       `6th`   Boil of other sites
          Folliculitis of other sites
          L02.821   **head [any part, except face]**
          L02.828   **other sites**
      L02.83   **Carbuncle of; other sites**
       `6th`   **L02.831**   **head [any part, except face]**
          L02.838   **other sites**

L02.9   **Cutaneous abscess, furuncle and carbuncle, unspecified**
   `5th`   **L02.91**   **Cutaneous abscess, unspecified**
      L02.92   **Furuncle, unspecified**
         Boil NOS
         Furunculosis NOS
      L02.93   **Carbuncle, unspecified**

L03   **CELLULITIS AND ACUTE LYMPHANGITIS**
  `4th`   ***Excludes2:*** cellulitis of anal and rectal region (K61.-)
       cellulitis of external auditory canal (H60.1)
       cellulitis of eyelid (H00.0)
       cellulitis of female external genital organs (N76.4)
       cellulitis of lacrimal apparatus (H04.3)
       cellulitis of male external genital organs (N48.2, N49.-)
       cellulitis of mouth (K12.2)
       cellulitis of nose (J34.0)
       eosinophilic cellulitis [Wells] (L98.3)
       febrile neutrophilic dermatosis [Sweet] (L98.2)
       lymphangitis (chronic) (subacute) (I89.1)

L03.0   **Cellulitis and acute lymphangitis of finger and toe**
   `5th`   Infection of nail
       Onychia
       Paronychia
       Perionychia
      L03.01   **Cellulitis of; finger**
       `6th`   Felon
          Whitlow
          Excludes1: herpetic whitlow (B00.89)
          L03.011   **right finger**
          L03.012   **left finger**
      L03.02   **Acute lymphangitis of; finger**
       `6th`   Hangnail with lymphangitis of finger
          L03.021   **right finger**
          L03.022   **left finger**
      L03.03   **Cellulitis of; toe**
       `6th`   **L03.031**   **right toe**
          L03.032   **left toe**
      L03.04   **Acute lymphangitis of; toe**
       `6th`   Hangnail with lymphangitis of toe
          L03.041   **right toe**
          L03.042   **left toe**

L03.1   **Cellulitis and acute lymphangitis of other parts of limb**
   `5th`   **L03.11**   **Cellulitis of other parts of limb**
       `6th`   ***Excludes2:*** cellulitis of fingers (L03.01-)
          cellulitis of toes (L03.03-)
          groin (L03.314)
          L03.111   **Cellulitis of; right axilla**
          L03.112   **left axilla**
          L03.113   **right upper limb**
          L03.114   **left upper limb**
          L03.115   **right lower limb**
          L03.116   **left lower limb**
      L03.12   **Acute lymphangitis of other parts of limb**
       `6th`   ***Excludes2:*** acute lymphangitis of fingers (L03.2-)
          acute lymphangitis of toes (L03.04-)
          acute lymphangitis of groin (L03.324)
          L03.121   **Acute lymphangitis of; right axilla**
          L03.122   **left axilla**
          L03.123   **right upper limb**
          L03.124   **left upper limb**
          L03.125   **right lower limb**
          L03.126   **left lower limb**

L03.2   **Cellulitis and acute lymphangitis of face and neck**
   `5th`   **L03.21**   **Cellulitis and acute lymphangitis of face**
       `6th`   **L03.211**   **Cellulitis of face**
          Excludes2: abscess of orbit (H05.01-)
            cellulitis of ear (H60.1-)
            cellulitis of eyelid (H00.0-)
            cellulitis of head or scalp (L03.81-)
            cellulitis of lacrimal apparatus (H04.3)
            cellulitis of lip (K13.0)
            cellulitis of mouth (K12.2)
            cellulitis of nose (internal) (J34.0)
            cellulitis of orbit (H05.01-)
          L03.212   **Acute lymphangitis of face**
          L03.213   **Periorbital cellulitis**
            Preseptal cellulitis
      L03.22   **Cellulitis and acute lymphangitis of neck**
       `6th`   **L03.221**   **Cellulitis of neck**
          L03.222   **Acute lymphangitis of neck**

L03.3   **Cellulitis and acute lymphangitis of trunk**
   `5th`   **L03.31**   **Cellulitis of trunk**
       `6th`   ***Excludes2:*** cellulitis of anal and rectal regions (K61.-)
          cellulitis of breast NOS (N61.0)
          cellulitis of female external genital organs (N76.4)
          cellulitis of male external genital organs (N48.2, N49.-)
          omphalitis of newborn (P38.-)
          puerperal cellulitis of breast (O91.2)
          L03.311   **Cellulitis of; abdominal wall**
            Excludes2: cellulitis of umbilicus (L03.316)
              cellulitis of groin (L03.314)
          L03.312   **back [any part except buttock]**

`4th` `5th` `6th` `7th`   Additional Character Required   ✓   3-character code   Unspecified laterality codes   •=New Code   ***Excludes1***—Not coded here, do not use together
                                                           were excluded here.   ▲=Revised Code   ***Excludes2***—Not included here

L03.313   **chest wall**
L03.314   **groin**
L03.315   **perineum**
L03.316   **umbilicus**
L03.317   **buttock**
L03.319   **trunk, unspecified**

L03.32   **Acute lymphangitis of; trunk**
`6th`
L03.321   **abdominal wall**
L03.322   **back [any part except buttock]**
L03.323   **chest wall**
L03.324   **groin**
L03.325   **perineum**
L03.326   **umbilicus**
L03.327   **buttock**
L03.329   **trunk, unspecified**

L03.8   Cellulitis and acute lymphangitis of other sites
`5th`   **L03.81   Cellulitis of; other sites**
`6th`
     L03.811   head [any part, except face]
        Cellulitis of scalp
        Excludes2: cellulitis of face (L03.211)
     L03.818   other sites

L03.89   Acute lymphangitis of; other sites
`6th`
     L03.891   head [any part, except face]
     L03.898   other sites

L03.9   Cellulitis and acute lymphangitis, unspecified
`5th`   **L03.90   Cellulitis, unspecified**
     L03.91   Acute lymphangitis, unspecified
        Excludes1: lymphangitis NOS (I89.1)

L04   ACUTE LYMPHADENITIS
`4th`
Includes: abscess (acute) of lymph nodes, except mesenteric
     acute lymphadenitis, except mesenteric
Excludes1: chronic or subacute lymphadenitis, except mesenteric (I88.1)
     enlarged lymph nodes (R59.-)
     HIV disease resulting in generalized lymphadenopathy (B20)
     lymphadenitis NOS (I88.9)
     nonspecific mesenteric lymphadenitis (I88.0)

L04.0   Acute lymphadenitis of; face, head and neck
L04.1   trunk
L04.2   upper limb
     Acute lymphadenitis of axilla or shoulder
L04.3   lower limb
     Acute lymphadenitis of hip
     Excludes2: acute lymphadenitis of groin (L04.1)
L04.8   other sites
L04.9   unspecified

L05   PILONIDAL CYST AND SINUS
`4th`
L05.0   Pilonidal cyst and sinus with abscess
`5th`   **L05.01   Pilonidal cyst with abscess**
       Parasacral dimple with abscess
       Excludes 2: congenital sacral dimple (Q82.6)
          parasacral dimple (Q82.6)
     L05.02   Pilonidal sinus with abscess

L05.9   Pilonidal cyst and sinus without abscess
`5th`   **L05.91   Pilonidal cyst without abscess**
       Parasacral or Pilonidal or Postanal dimple
       Pilonidal cyst NOS
       Excludes 2: congenital sacral dimple (Q82.6)
          parasacral dimple (Q82.6)
     L05.92   Pilonidal sinus without abscess
       Coccygeal fistula
       Coccygeal sinus without abscess
       Pilonidal fistula

L08   OTHER LOCAL INFECTIONS OF SKIN AND SUBCUTANEOUS TISSUE
`4th`
L08.0   Pyoderma
     Dermatitis gangrenosa
     Purulent or Septic or Suppurative dermatitis
     Excludes1: pyoderma gangrenosum (L88)
        pyoderma vegetans (L08.81)
L08.9   Local infection of the skin and subcutaneous tissue, unspecified

(L10–L14) BULLOUS DISORDERS

Excludes1: benign familial pemphigus [Hailey-Hailey] (Q82.8)
     staphylococcal scalded skin syndrome (L00)
     toxic epidermal necrolysis [Lyell] (L51.2)

(L20–L30) DERMATITIS AND ECZEMA

Note: In this block the terms dermatitis and eczema are used synonymously and interchangeably.
Excludes2: chronic (childhood) granulomatous disease (D71)
     dermatitis gangrenosa (L08.0)
     dermatitis herpetiformis (L13.0)
     dry skin dermatitis (L85.3)
     factitial dermatitis (L98.1)
     perioral dermatitis (L71.0)
     radiation-related disorders of the skin and subcutaneous tissue (L55–L59)
     stasis dermatitis (I87.2)

L20   ATOPIC DERMATITIS
`4th`
L20.0   Besnier's prurigo
L20.8   Other atopic dermatitis
`5th`   *Excludes2:* circumscribed neurodermatitis (L28.0)
     L20.81   Atopic neurodermatitis
        Diffuse neurodermatitis
     L20.82   Flexural eczema
     L20.83   Infantile (acute) (chronic) eczema
     L20.84   Intrinsic (allergic) eczema
     L20.89   Other atopic dermatitis
L20.9   Atopic dermatitis, unspecified

L21   SEBORRHEIC DERMATITIS
`4th`
Excludes2: infective dermatitis (L30.3)
     seborrheic keratosis (L82.-)
L21.0   Seborrhea capitis
     Cradle cap
L21.1   Seborrheic infantile dermatitis
L21.8   Other seborrheic dermatitis
L21.9   Seborrheic dermatitis, unspecified
     Seborrhea NOS

L22   DIAPER DERMATITIS
`✔`
Diaper erythema
Diaper rash
Psoriasiform diaper rash

L23   ALLERGIC CONTACT DERMATITIS
`4th`
Excludes1: allergy NOS (T78.40)
     contact dermatitis NOS (L25.9)
     dermatitis NOS (L30.9)
Excludes2: dermatitis due to substances taken internally (L27.-)
     dermatitis of eyelid (H01.1-)
     diaper dermatitis (L22)
     eczema of external ear (H60.5-)
     irritant contact dermatitis (L24.-)
     perioral dermatitis (L71.0)
     radiation-related disorders of the skin and subcutaneous tissue (L55–L59)

L23.0   Allergic contact dermatitis due to; metals
     Allergic contact dermatitis due to chromium or nickel
L23.1   adhesives
L23.2   cosmetics
L23.3   drugs in contact with skin
     Use additional code for adverse effect, if applicable, to identify drug (T36–T50 with fifth or sixth character 5)
     Excludes2: dermatitis due to ingested drugs and medicaments (L27.0–L27.1)
L23.4   Allergic contact dermatitis due to; dyes
L23.5   other chemical products
     Allergic contact dermatitis due to cement or to insecticide
L23.6   food in contact with the skin
     Excludes2: dermatitis due to ingested food (L27.2)
L23.7   plants, except food
     Excludes2: allergy NOS due to pollen (J30.1)

CHAPTER 12. DISEASES OF THE SKIN AND SUBCUTANEOUS TISSUE   (L03.313–L23.7)

`4th` `5th` `6th` `7th` Additional Character Required   `✔` 3-character code

Unspecified laterality codes were excluded here.   •=New Code   ▲=Revised Code   *Excludes1*—Not coded here, do not use together   *Excludes2*—Not included here

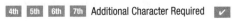

L23.8 Allergic contact dermatitis due to; other agents
5th **L23.81** animal (cat) (dog) dander or hair
L23.89 other agents
L23.9 Allergic contact dermatitis, unspecified cause
Allergic contact eczema NOS

L24 **IRRITANT CONTACT DERMATITIS**
4th ***Excludes1***: allergy NOS (T78.40)
contact dermatitis NOS (L25.9)
dermatitis NOS (L30.9)
Excludes2: allergic contact dermatitis (L23.-)
dermatitis due to substances taken internally (L27.-)
dermatitis of eyelid (H01.1-)
diaper dermatitis (L22)
eczema of external ear (H60.5-)
perioral dermatitis (L71.0)
radiation-related disorders of the skin and subcutaneous tissue
(L55-L59)

L24.0 Irritant contact dermatitis due to detergents
L24.1 Irritant contact dermatitis due to oils and greases
L24.2 Irritant contact dermatitis due to solvents
Irritant contact dermatitis due to chlorocompound or cyclohexane
or glycol or hydrocarbon or ketone
L24.3 Irritant contact dermatitis due to cosmetics
L24.4 Irritant contact dermatitis due to drugs in contact with skin
Use additional code for adverse effect, if applicable, to identify
drug (T36-T50 with fifth or sixth character 5)
L24.5 Irritant contact dermatitis due to other chemical products
Irritant contact dermatitis due to cement
Irritant contact dermatitis due to insecticide
Irritant contact dermatitis due to plastic
Irritant contact dermatitis due to rubber
L24.8 Irritant contact dermatitis due to other agents
5th **L24.81** Irritant contact dermatitis due to metals
Irritant contact dermatitis due to chromium
Irritant contact dermatitis due to nickel
L24.89 Irritant contact dermatitis due to other agents
Irritant contact dermatitis due to dyes
L24.9 Irritant contact dermatitis, unspecified cause
Irritant contact eczema NOS
•**L24.A** Irritant contact dermatitis due to friction or contact with
5th body fluids
Excludes1: irritant contact dermatitis related to stoma or fistula
(L24.B-)
Excludes2: erythema intertrigo (L30.4)
•**L24.A0** Irritant contact dermatitis due to friction or contact
with body fluids, unspecified
•**L24.A1** Irritant contact dermatitis due to saliva
•**L24.A2** Irritant contact dermatitis due to fecal, urinary or
dual incontinence
Excludes1: diaper dermatitis (L22)
•**L24.A9** Irritant contact dermatitis due to friction or contact
with other specified body fluids
Irritant contact dermatitis related to endotracheal tube
Wound fluids, exudate
•**L24.B** Irritant contact dermatitis related to stoma or fistula
5th **Use Additional code** to identify any artificial opening status (Z93.-),
if applicable, for contact dermatitis related to stoma secretions
•**L24.B0** Irritant contact dermatitis related to unspecified
stoma or fistula
Irritant contact dermatitis related to fistula NOS
Irritant contact dermatitis related to stoma NOS
•**L24.B1** Irritant contact dermatitis related to digestive stoma
or fistula
Irritant contact dermatitis related to gastrostomy
Irritant contact dermatitis related to jejunostomy
Irritant contact dermatitis related to saliva or spit fistula
•**L24.B2** Irritant contact dermatitis related to respiratory
stoma or fistula
Irritant contact dermatitis related to tracheostomy

•**L24.B3** Irritant contact dermatitis related to fecal or urinary
stoma or fistula
Irritant contact dermatitis related to colostomy
Irritant contact dermatitis related to enterocutaneous
fistula
Irritant contact dermatitis related to ileostomy

L25 **UNSPECIFIED CONTACT DERMATITIS**
4th ***Excludes1:*** allergic contact dermatitis (L23.-)
allergy NOS (T78.40)
dermatitis NOS (L30.9)
irritant contact dermatitis (L24.-)
Excludes2: dermatitis due to ingested substances (L27.-)
dermatitis of eyelid (H01.1-)
eczema of external ear (H60.5-)
perioral dermatitis (L71.0)
radiation-related disorders of the skin and subcutaneous tissue
(L55–L59)
L25.0 Unspecified contact dermatitis due to cosmetics
L25.1 Unspecified contact dermatitis due to drugs in contact
with skin
Use additional code for adverse effect, if applicable, to identify
drug (T36–T50 with fifth or sixth character 5)
Excludes2: dermatitis due to ingested drugs and medicaments
(L27.0–L27.1)
L25.2 Unspecified contact dermatitis due to dyes
L25.3 Unspecified contact dermatitis due to other chemical products
Unspecified contact dermatitis due to cement
Unspecified contact dermatitis due to insecticide
L25.4 Unspecified contact dermatitis due to food in contact with skin
Excludes2: dermatitis due to ingested food (L27.2)
L25.5 Unspecified contact dermatitis due to plants, except food
Excludes1: nettle rash (L50.9)
Excludes2: allergy NOS due to pollen (J30.1)
L25.8 Unspecified contact dermatitis due to other agents
L25.9 Unspecified contact dermatitis, unspecified cause
Contact dermatitis (occupational) NOS
Contact eczema (occupational) NOS

L26 **EXFOLIATIVE DERMATITIS**
✔ Hebra's pityriasis
Excludes1: Ritter's disease (L00)

L27 **DERMATITIS DUE TO SUBSTANCES TAKEN INTERNALLY**
4th ***Excludes1:*** allergy NOS (T78.40)
Excludes2: adverse food reaction, except dermatitis (T78.0–T78.1)
contact dermatitis (L23–L25)
drug photoallergic response (L56.1)
drug phototoxic response (L56.0)
urticaria (L50.-)
L27.0 Generalized skin eruption due to drugs and medicaments
taken internally
Use additional code for adverse effect, if applicable, to identify
drug (T36–T50 with fifth or sixth character 5)
L27.1 Localized skin eruption due to drugs and medicaments taken
internally
Use additional code for adverse effect, if applicable, to identify
drug (T36–T50 with fifth or sixth character 5)
L27.2 Dermatitis due to ingested food
Excludes2: dermatitis due to food in contact with skin (L23.6,
L24.6, L25.4)
L27.8 Dermatitis due to other substances taken internally
L27.9 Dermatitis due to unspecified substance taken internally

L28 **LICHEN SIMPLEX CHRONICUS AND PRURIGO**
4th **L28.0** Lichen simplex chronicus
Circumscribed neurodermatitis
Lichen NOS
L28.1 Prurigo nodularis
L28.2 Other prurigo
Prurigo NOS
Prurigo Hebra
Prurigo mitis
Urticaria papulosa

4th **5th** **6th** **7th** Additional Character Required　　**✔** 3-character code

Unspecified laterality codes •=New Code ***Excludes1***—Not coded here, do not use together
were excluded here. ▲=Revised Code ***Excludes2***—Not included here

L29 PRURITUS
4th
   Excludes1: neurotic excoriation (L98.1)
      psychogenic pruritus (F45.8)
   L29.0 Pruritus ani
   L29.1 Pruritus scroti
   L29.2 Pruritus vulvae
   L29.3 Anogenital pruritus, unspecified
   L29.8 Other pruritus
   L29.9 Pruritus, unspecified
      Itch NOS

L30 OTHER AND UNSPECIFIED DERMATITIS
4th
   Excludes2: contact dermatitis (L23–L25)
      dry skin dermatitis (L85.3)
      small plaque parapsoriasis (L41.3)
      stasis dermatitis (I83.1–.2)
   L30.1 Dyshidrosis [pompholyx]
   L30.3 Infective dermatitis
      Infectious eczematoid dermatitis
   L30.4 Erythema intertrigo
   L30.5 Pityriasis alba
   L30.8 Other specified dermatitis
   L30.9 Dermatitis, unspecified
      Eczema NOS

(L40–L45) PAPULOSQUAMOUS DISORDERS

L40 PSORIASIS
4th
   L40.5 Arthropathic psoriasis
   5th **L40.54 Psoriatic juvenile arthropathy**
   L40.8 Other psoriasis
      Flexural psoriasis
   L40.9 Psoriasis, unspecified

L42 PITYRIASIS ROSEA
✔

L44 OTHER PAPULOSQUAMOUS DISORDERS
4th
   L44.0 Pityriasis rubra pilaris
   L44.1 Lichen nitidus
   L44.2 Lichen striatus
   L44.3 Lichen ruber moniliformis
   L44.4 Infantile papular acrodermatitis [Gianotti-Crosti]
   L44.8 Other specified papulosquamous disorders
   L44.9 Papulosquamous disorder, unspecified

(L49–L54) URTICARIA AND ERYTHEMA

Excludes1: Lyme disease (A69.2-)
   rosacea (L71.-)

L50 URTICARIA
4th
   Excludes1: allergic contact dermatitis (L23.-)
      angioneurotic edema or giant urticarial or Quincke's edema (T78.3)
      hereditary angio-edema (D84.1)
      serum urticaria (T80.6-)
      solar urticaria (L56.3)
      urticaria neonatorum (P83.8)
      urticaria papulosa (L28.2)
      urticaria pigmentosa (D47.01)
   L50.0 Allergic urticaria
   L50.1 Idiopathic urticaria
   L50.2 Urticaria due to cold and heat
      Excludes2: familial cold urticaria (M04.2)
   L50.3 Dermatographic urticaria
   L50.4 Vibratory urticaria
   L50.5 Cholinergic urticaria
   L50.6 Contact urticaria
   L50.8 Other urticaria
      Chronic urticaria
      Recurrent periodic urticaria
   L50.9 Urticaria, unspecified

L51 ERYTHEMA MULTIFORME
4th
   Use additional code for adverse effect, if applicable, to identify drug (T36–T50 with fifth or sixth character 5)
   Use additional code to identify associated manifestations, such as:
      arthropathy associated with dermatological disorders (M14.8-)
      conjunctival edema (H11.42)
      conjunctivitis (H10.22-)
      corneal scars and opacities (H17.-)
      corneal ulcer (H16.0-)
      edema of eyelid (H02.84-)
      inflammation of eyelid (H01.8)
      keratoconjunctivitis sicca (H16.22-)
      mechanical lagophthalmos (H02.22-)
      stomatitis (K12.-)
      symblepharon (H11.23-)
   Use additional code to identify percentage of skin exfoliation (L49.-)
   Excludes1: staphylococcal scalded skin syndrome (L00)
      Ritter's disease (L00)
   L51.0 Nonbullous erythema multiforme
   L51.1 Stevens-Johnson syndrome
   L51.2 Toxic epidermal necrolysis [Lyell]
   L51.3 Stevens-Johnson syndrome-toxic epidermal necrolysis overlap syndrome
      SJS-TEN overlap syndrome
   L51.8 Other erythema multiforme
   L51.9 Erythema multiforme, unspecified
      Erythema iris
      Erythema multiforme major NOS
      Erythema multiforme minor NOS
      Herpes iris

L52 ERYTHEMA NODOSUM
✔
   Excludes1: tuberculous erythema nodosum (A18.4)

L53 OTHER ERYTHEMATOUS CONDITIONS
4th
   Excludes1: erythema ab igne (L59.0)
      erythema due to external agents in contact with skin (L23-L25)
      erythema intertrigo (L30.4)
   L53.0 Toxic erythema
      Code first poisoning due to drug or toxin, if applicable (T36-T65 with fifth or sixth character 1-4 or 6)
      Use additional code for adverse effect, if applicable, to identify drug (T36-T50 with fifth or sixth character 5)
      Excludes1: neonatal erythema toxicum (P83.1)
   L53.1 Erythema annulare centrifugum
   L53.2 Erythema marginatum
   L53.8 Other specified erythematous conditions
   L53.9 Erythematous condition, unspecified
      Erythema NOS
      Erythroderma NOS

(L55–L59) RADIATION-RELATED DISORDERS OF THE SKIN AND SUBCUTANEOUS TISSUE

L55 SUNBURN
4th
   L55.0 Sunburn of first degree
   L55.1 Sunburn of second degree
   L55.2 Sunburn of third degree
   L55.9 Sunburn, unspecified

L56 OTHER ACUTE SKIN CHANGES DUE TO ULTRAVIOLET RADIATION
4th
   Use additional code to identify the source of the ultraviolet radiation (W89, X32)
   L56.0 Drug phototoxic response
      Use additional code for adverse effect, if applicable, to identify drug (T36-T50 with fifth or sixth character 5)
   L56.1 Drug photoallergic response
      Use additional code for adverse effect, if applicable, to identify drug (T36-T50 with fifth or sixth character 5)
   L56.3 Solar urticaria
   L56.8 Other specified acute skin changes due to ultraviolet radiation
   L56.9 Acute skin change due to ultraviolet radiation, unspecified

CHAPTER 12. DISEASES OF THE SKIN AND SUBCUTANEOUS TISSUE (L29–L56.9)

Unspecified laterality codes • =New Code   *Excludes1*—Not coded here, do not use together
were excluded here. ▲=Revised Code *Excludes2*—Not included here

(L60–L75) DISORDERS OF SKIN APPENDAGES

Excludes1: congenital malformations of integument (Q84.-)

L60   NAIL DISORDERS
`4th`   *Excludes2:* clubbing of nails (R68.3)
        onychia and paronychia (L03.0-)
   L60.0   Ingrowing nail
   L60.1   Onycholysis
   L60.3   Nail dystrophy
   L60.8   Other nail disorders
   L60.9   Nail disorder, unspecified

L65   OTHER NON-SCARRING HAIR LOSS
`4th`   **Use additional code** for adverse effect, if applicable, to identify drug
        (T36–T50 with fifth or sixth character 5)
        Excludes1: trichotillomania (F63.3)
   L65.8   Other specified non-scarring hair loss
   L65.9   Non-scarring hair loss, unspecified
             Alopecia NOS

L68   HYPERTRICHOSIS
`4th`   *Includes:* excess hair
        Excludes1: congenital hypertrichosis (Q84.2)
        persistent lanugo (Q84.2)
   L68.0   Hirsutism

L70   ACNE
`4th`   *Excludes2:* acne keloid (L73.0)
   L70.0   Acne vulgaris
   L70.1   Acne conglobata
   L70.2   Acne varioliformis
             Acne necrotica miliaris
   L70.3   Acne tropica
   L70.4   Infantile acne
   L70.5   Acné excoriée
             Acné excoriée des jeunes filles
             Picker's acne
   L70.8   Other acne
   L70.9   Acne, unspecified

L72   FOLLICULAR CYSTS OF SKIN AND SUBCUTANEOUS
`4th`   **TISSUE**
   L72.0   Epidermal cyst
   L72.1   Pilar and trichodermal cyst
     `5th` **L72.11   Pilar cyst**
            L72.12   Trichodermal cyst
                      Trichilemmal (proliferating) cyst
   L72.3   Sebaceous cyst
             Excludes2: pilar cyst (L72.11)
                       trichilemmal (proliferating) cyst (L72.12)
   L72.8   Other follicular cysts of the skin and subcutaneous tissue
   L72.9   Follicular cyst of the skin and subcutaneous tissue,
             unspecified

L73   OTHER FOLLICULAR DISORDERS
`4th`   **L73.0   Acne keloid**
   L73.1   Pseudofolliculitis barbae
   L73.2   Hidradenitis suppurativa
   L73.8   Other specified follicular disorders
             Sycosis barbae
   L73.9   Follicular disorder, unspecified

L74   ECCRINE SWEAT DISORDERS
`4th`   *Excludes2:* generalized hyperhidrosis (R61)
   L74.0   Miliaria rubra
   L74.1   Miliaria crystallina
   L74.3   Miliaria, unspecified
   L74.5   Focal hyperhidrosis
     `5th` **L74.51   Primary focal hyperhidrosis**
       `6th` **L74.510   Primary focal hyperhidrosis, axilla**
              L74.511   Primary focal hyperhidrosis, face
              L74.512   Primary focal hyperhidrosis, palms
              L74.513   Primary focal hyperhidrosis, soles
              L74.519   Primary focal hyperhidrosis, unspecified
            L74.52   Secondary focal hyperhidrosis
                      Frey's syndrome

(L76) INTRAOPERATIVE AND POSTPROCEDURAL COMPLICATIONS OF SKIN AND SUBCUTANEOUS TISSUE

(L80–L99) OTHER DISORDERS OF THE SKIN AND SUBCUTANEOUS TISSUE

L80   VITILIGO
`✔`   *Excludes2:* vitiligo of eyelids (H02.73-)
        vitiligo of vulva (N90.89)

L81   OTHER DISORDERS OF PIGMENTATION
`4th`   *Excludes1:* birthmark NOS (Q82.5)
        Peutz-Jeghers syndrome (Q85.8)
        Excludes2: nevus — see Alphabetical Index
   L81.2   Freckles
   L81.3   Café au lait spots
   L81.4   Other melanin hyperpigmentation
             Lentigo
   L81.6   Other disorders of diminished melanin formation
   L81.7   Pigmented purpuric dermatosis
             Angioma serpiginosum
   L81.8   Other specified disorders of pigmentation
             Iron pigmentation
             Tattoo pigmentation
   L81.9   Disorder of pigmentation, unspecified

L82   SEBORRHEIC KERATOSIS
`4th`   *Includes:* basal cell papilloma
        dermatosis papulosa nigra
        Leser-Trélat disease
        Excludes2: seborrheic dermatitis (L21.-)
   L82.0   Inflamed seborrheic keratosis
   L82.1   Other seborrheic keratosis
             Seborrheic keratosis NOS

L83   ACANTHOSIS NIGRICANS
`✔`   Confluent and reticulated papillomatosis

L84   CORNS AND CALLOSITIES
`✔`   Callus
      Clavus

L85   OTHER EPIDERMAL THICKENING
`4th`   *Excludes2:* hypertrophic disorders of the skin (L91.-)
   L85.0   Acquired ichthyosis
             Excludes1: congenital ichthyosis (Q80.-)
   L85.1   Acquired keratosis [keratoderma] palmaris et plantaris
             Excludes1: inherited keratosis palmaris et plantaris (Q82.8)
   L85.2   Keratosis punctata (palmaris et plantaris)
   L85.3   Xerosis cutis
             Dry skin dermatitis
   L85.8   Other specified epidermal thickening
             Cutaneous horn
   L85.9   Epidermal thickening, unspecified

L88   PYODERMA GANGRENOSUM
`✔`   Phagedenic pyoderma
      Excludes1: dermatitis gangrenosa (L08.0)

L89   PRESSURE ULCER
`4th`   **GUIDELINES**

Pressure ulcer stages
Codes in category L89, Pressure ulcer, are combination codes that identify the site and stage of the pressure ulcer as well as the stage of the ulcer. The *ICD-10-CM* classifies pressure ulcer stages based on severity, which is designated by stages 1–4, deep tissue pressure injury, unspecified stage and unstageable. Assign as many codes from category L89 as needed to identify all the pressure ulcers the patient has, if applicable. *See Section I.B.14 for pressure ulcer stage documentation by clinicians other than patient's provider.*

`4th` `5th` `6th` `7th` Additional Character Required   `✔` 3-character code

Unspecified laterality codes   •=New Code   *Excludes1*—Not coded here, do not use together
were excluded here.   ▲=Revised Code *Excludes2*—Not included here

Unstageable pressure ulcers

Assignment of the code for unstageable pressure ulcer (L89.--0) should be based on the clinical documentation. These codes are used for pressure ulcers whose stage cannot be clinically determined (e.g., the *ICD-10-CM Official Guidelines for Coding and Reporting* **FY 2022** Page 55 of 115 ulcer is covered by eschar or has been treated with a skin or muscle graft). This code should not be confused with the codes for unspecified stage (L89.--9). When there is no documentation regarding the stage of the pressure ulcer, assign the appropriate code for unspecified stage (L89.--9).

If during an encounter, the stage of an unstageable pressure ulcer is revealed after debridement, assign only the code for the stage revealed following debridement.

Documented pressure ulcer stage

Assignment of the pressure ulcer stage code should be guided by clinical documentation of the stage or documentation of the terms found in the Alphabetic Index. For clinical terms describing the stage that are not found in the Alphabetic Index, and there is no documentation of the stage, the provider should be queried.

Patients admitted with pressure ulcers documented as healed

No code is assigned if the documentation states that the pressure ulcer is completely healed.

Patients admitted with pressure ulcers documented as healing

Refer to the ICD-10-CM manual.

Patient admitted with pressure ulcer evolving into another stage during the admission

Refer to the ICD-10-CM manual.

Pressure-induced deep tissue damage

For pressure-induced deep tissue damage or deep tissue pressure injury, assign only the appropriate code for pressure-induced deep tissue damage (L89.--6).

Includes: bed sore
     decubitus ulcer
     plaster ulcer
     pressure area
     pressure sore
Code first any associated gangrene (I96)
Excludes2: decubitus (trophic) ulcer of
     cervix (uteri) (N86)
     diabetic ulcers (E08.621, E08.622,
       E09.621, E09.622, E10.621, E10.622,
       E11.621, E11.622, E13.621, E13.622)
     non-pressure chronic ulcer of skin
     (L97.-)
     skin infections (L00–L08)
     varicose ulcer (I83.0, I83.2)

> Stage 1 — Pressure pre-ulcer skin changes limited to persistent focal edema
> Stage 2 — Pressure ulcer with abrasion, blister, partial thickness skin loss involving epidermis and/or dermis
> Stage 3 — Pressure ulcer with full thickness skin loss involving damage or necrosis of subcutaneous tissue
> Stage 4 — Pressure ulcer with necrosis of soft tissues through to underlying muscle, tendon, or bone

L89.0 Pressure ulcer of elbow
   `5th` **L89.01 Pressure ulcer of right elbow**
     `6th` Healing pressure ulcer of right elbow
       L89.010 Pressure ulcer of right elbow; unstageable
       L89.011 stage 1
       L89.012 stage 2
       L89.013 stage 3
       L89.014 stage 4
       L89.016 Pressure-induced deep tissue damage of right elbow
       L89.019 unspecified stage
         Healing pressure ulcer right of elbow NOS
   L89.02 Pressure ulcer of left elbow
     `6th` Healing pressure ulcer of left elbow
       L89.020 Pressure ulcer of left elbow; unstageable
       L89.021 stage 1
       L89.022 stage 2
       L89.023 stage 3
       L89.024 stage 4

       L89.026 Pressure-induced deep tissue damage of left elbow
       L89.029 Pressure ulcer of left elbow, unspecified stage
         Healing pressure ulcer of left of elbow NOS

L89.1 Pressure ulcer of back
   `5th` **L89.10 Pressure ulcer of unspecified part of back**
     `6th` Healing pressure ulcer of unspecified part of back
     Pressure pre-ulcer skin changes limited to persistent focal edema, unspecified part of back
       L89.100 Pressure ulcer of unspecified part of back; unstageable
       L89.101 stage 1
       L89.102 stage 2
       L89.103 stage 3
       L89.104 stage 4
       L89.106 Pressure-induced deep tissue damage of unspecified part of back
       L89.109 unspecified stage
         Healing pressure ulcer of unspecified part of back NOS
   L89.11 Pressure ulcer of right upper back
     `6th` Pressure ulcer of right shoulder blade
     Healing pressure ulcer of right upper back
       L89.110 Pressure ulcer of right upper back; unstageable
       L89.111 stage 1
       L89.112 stage 2
       L89.113 stage 3
       L89.114 stage 4
       L89.116 Pressure-induced deep tissue damage of right upper back
       L89.119 unspecified stage
         Healing pressure ulcer of right upper back NOS
   L89.12 Pressure ulcer of left upper back
     `6th` Healing pressure ulcer of left upper back,
     Pressure ulcer of left shoulder blade
       L89.120 Pressure ulcer of left upper back; unstageable
       L89.121 stage 1
       L89.122 stage 2
       L89.123 stage 3
       L89.124 stage 4
       L89.126 Pressure-induced deep tissue damage of left upper back
       L89.129 unspecified stage
         Healing pressure ulcer of left upper back NOS
         Healing pressure ulcer of left upper back, unspecified stage
   L89.13 Pressure ulcer of right lower back
     `6th` Healing pressure ulcer of right lower back
       L89.130 Pressure ulcer of right lower back; unstageable
       L89.131 stage 1
       L89.132 stage 2
       L89.133 stage 3
       L89.134 stage 4
       L89.136 Pressure-induced deep tissue damage of right lower back
       L89.139 unspecified stage
         Healing pressure ulcer of right lower back NOS
   L89.14 Pressure ulcer of left lower back
     `6th` Healing pressure ulcer of left lower back
       L89.140 Pressure ulcer of left lower back; unstageable
       L89.141 stage 1
       L89.142 stage 2
       L89.143 stage 3
       L89.144 stage 4
       L89.146 Pressure-induced deep tissue damage of left lower back

---

`4th` `5th` `6th` `7th` Additional Character Required   ✓   3-character code   Unspecified laterality codes were excluded here.   •=New Code   ▲=Revised Code   ***Excludes1***—Not coded here, do not use together   ***Excludes2***—Not included here

L89.149 **unspecified stage**
Healing pressure ulcer of left lower back NOS

L89.15 **Pressure ulcer of sacral region** [6th]
Healing pressure ulcer of sacral region,
Pressure ulcer of coccyx
Pressure ulcer of tailbone

Stage 1 — Pressure pre-ulcer skin changes limited to persistent focal edema
Stage 2 — Pressure ulcer with abrasion, blister, partial thickness skin loss involving epidermis and/or dermis
Stage 3 — Pressure ulcer with full thickness skin loss involving damage or necrosis of subcutaneous tissue
Stage 4 — Pressure ulcer with necrosis of soft tissues through to underlying muscle, tendon, or bone

L89.150 **Pressure ulcer of sacral region; unstageable**
L89.151 **stage 1**
L89.152 **stage 2**
L89.153 **stage 3**
L89.154 **stage 4**
L89.156 **Pressure-induced deep tissue damage of sacral region**
L89.159 **unspecified stage**
Healing pressure ulcer of sacral region NOS

L89.2 **Pressure ulcer of hip** [5th]
L89.21 **Pressure ulcer of right hip** [6th]
Healing pressure ulcer of right hip
L89.210 **Pressure ulcer of right hip; unstageable**
L89.211 **stage 1**
L89.212 **stage 2**
L89.213 **stage 3**
L89.214 **stage 4**
L89.216 **Pressure-induced deep tissue damage of right hip**
L89.219 **unspecified stage**
Healing pressure ulcer of right hip NOS

L89.22 **Pressure ulcer of left hip** [6th]
Healing pressure ulcer of left hip back
L89.220 **Pressure ulcer of left hip; unstageable**
L89.221 **stage 1**
L89.222 **stage 2**
L89.223 **stage 3**
L89.224 **stage 4**
L89.226 **Pressure-induced deep tissue damage of left hip**
L89.229 **unspecified stage**
Healing pressure ulcer of left hip NOS

L89.3 **Pressure ulcer of buttock** [5th]
L89.31 **Pressure ulcer of right buttock** [6th]
Healing pressure ulcer of right buttock
L89.310 **Pressure ulcer of right buttock; unstageable**
L89.311 **stage 1**
L89.312 **stage 2**
L89.313 **stage 3**
L89.314 **stage 4**
L89.316 **Pressure-induced deep tissue damage of right buttock**
L89.319 **unspecified stage**
Healing pressure ulcer of right buttock NOS

L89.32 **Pressure ulcer of left buttock** [6th]
Healing pressure ulcer of left buttock
L89.320 **Pressure ulcer of left buttock; unstageable**
L89.321 **stage 1**
L89.322 **stage 2**
L89.323 **stage 3**
L89.324 **stage 4**
L89.326 **Pressure-induced deep tissue damage of left buttock**
L89.329 **Pressure ulcer of left buttock, unspecified stage**
Healing pressure ulcer of left buttock NOS

L89.4 **Pressure ulcer of contiguous site of back, buttock and hip** [5th]
Healing pressure ulcer of contiguous site of back, buttock and hip

L89.40 **Pressure ulcer of contiguous site of back, buttock and hip; unspecified stage**
Healing pressure ulcer of contiguous site of back, buttock and hip NOS
L89.41 **stage 1**
L89.42 **stage 2**
L89.43 **stage 3**
L89.44 **stage 4**
L89.45 **unstageable**
L89.46 **Pressure-induced deep tissue damage of contiguous site of back, buttock and hip**

L89.5 **Pressure ulcer of ankle** [5th]
L89.51 **Pressure ulcer of right ankle** [6th]
Healing pressure ulcer of right ankle
L89.510 **Pressure ulcer of right ankle; unstageable**
L89.511 **stage 1**
L89.512 **stage 2**
L89.513 **stage 3**
L89.514 **stage 4**
L89.516 **Pressure-induced deep tissue damage of right ankle**
L89.519 **unspecified stage**
Healing pressure ulcer of right ankle NOS

L89.52 **Pressure ulcer of left ankle** [6th]
Healing pressure ulcer of left ankle
L89.520 **Pressure ulcer of left ankle; unstageable**
L89.521 **stage 1**
Pressure pre-ulcer skin changes limited to persistent focal edema, left ankle
L89.522 **stage 2**
L89.523 **stage 3**
L89.524 **stage 4**
L89.526 **Pressure-induced deep tissue damage of left ankle**
L89.529 **unspecified stage**
Healing pressure ulcer of left ankle NOS

L89.6 **Pressure ulcer of heel** [5th]
L89.61 **Pressure ulcer of right heel** [6th]
Healing pressure ulcer of right heel
L89.610 **Pressure ulcer of right heel; unstageable**
L89.611 **stage 1**
L89.612 **stage 2**
L89.613 **stage 3**
L89.614 **stage 4**
L89.616 **Pressure-induced deep tissue damage of right heel**
L89.619 **unspecified stage**
Healing pressure ulcer of right heel NOS

L89.62 **Pressure ulcer of left heel** [6th]
Healing pressure ulcer of left heel
L89.620 **Pressure ulcer of left heel; unstageable**
L89.621 **stage 1**
L89.622 **stage 2**
L89.623 **stage 3**
L89.624 **stage 4**
L89.626 **Pressure-induced deep tissue damage of left heel**
L89.629 **unspecified stage**
Healing pressure ulcer of left heel NOS

L89.8 **Pressure ulcer of other site** [5th]
L89.81 **Pressure ulcer of head** [6th]
Pressure ulcer of face
Healing pressure ulcer of head
L89.810 **Pressure ulcer of head; unstageable**
L89.811 **stage 1**
L89.812 **stage 2**
L89.813 **stage 3**
L89.814 **stage 4**
L89.816 **Pressure-induced deep tissue damage of head**
L89.819 **unspecified stage**
Healing pressure ulcer of head NOS

[4th] [5th] [6th] [7th] Additional Character Required   [✓] 3-character code

Unspecified laterality codes were excluded here.
•=New Code
▲=Revised Code
Excludes1—Not coded here, do not use together
Excludes2—Not included here

L89.89   **Pressure ulcer of other site**
6th   Healing pressure ulcer of other site

     L89.890   **Pressure ulcer of other site; unstageable**
     L89.891   **stage 1**
     L89.892   **stage 2**
     L89.893   **stage 3**
     L89.894   **stage 4**
     L89.896   **Pressure-induced deep tissue damage of other site**
     L89.899   **unspecified stage**
         Healing pressure ulcer of other site NOS

L89.9   **Pressure ulcer of unspecified site**
5th   Healing pressure ulcer of unspecified site

     L89.90   **Pressure ulcer of unspecified site; unspecified stage**
     L89.91   **stage 1**
     L89.92   **stage 2**
     L89.93   **stage 3**
     L89.94   **stage 4**
     L89.95   **unstageable**
     L89.96   **Pressure-induced deep tissue damage of unspecified site**

L90   **ATROPHIC DISORDERS OF SKIN**
4th
L90.5   **Scar conditions and fibrosis of skin**
   Adherent scar (skin)
   Cicatrix
   Disfigurement of skin due to scar
   Fibrosis of skin NOS

L91   **HYPERTROPHIC DISORDERS OF SKIN**
4th
L91.0   **Hypertrophic scar**
   Keloid
   Keloid scar
   Excludes2: acne keloid (L73.0)
     scar NOS (L90.5)

L91.8   **Other hypertrophic disorders of the skin**
L91.9   **Hypertrophic disorder of the skin, unspecified**

L92   **GRANULOMATOUS DISORDERS OF SKIN AND**
4th   **SUBCUTANEOUS TISSUE**
Excludes2: actinic granuloma (L57.5)

L92.0   **Granuloma annulare**
   Perforating granuloma annulare

L92.3   **FB granuloma of the skin and subcutaneous tissue**
   Use additional code to identify the type of retained FB (Z18.-)

L92.9   **Granulomatous disorder of the skin and subcutaneous tissue, unspecified**
   Excludes2: umbilical granuloma (P83.81)

L94   **OTHER LOCALIZED CONNECTIVE TISSUE DISORDERS**
4th   ***Excludes1:*** systemic connective tissue disorders (M30–M36)
L94.2   **Calcinosis cutis**

L98   **OTHER DISORDERS OF SKIN AND SUBCUTANEOUS**
4th   **TISSUE, NOT ELSEWHERE CLASSIFIED**
L98.0   **Pyogenic granuloma**
   Excludes2: pyogenic granuloma of gingiva (K06.8)
     pyogenic granuloma of maxillary alveolar ridge (K04.5)
     pyogenic granuloma of oral mucosa (K13.4)

L98.1   **Factitial dermatitis**
   Neurotic excoriation
   Excludes1: excoriation (skin-picking) disorder (F42.4)

L98.5   **Mucinosis of the skin**
   Focal mucinosis
   Lichen myxedematosus
   Reticular erythematous mucinosis
   Excludes1: focal oral mucinosis (K13.79)
     myxedema (E03.9)

L98.7   **Excessive and redundant skin and subcutaneous tissue**
   Loose or sagging skin following bariatric surgery weight loss
   Loose or sagging skin following dietary weight loss
   Loose or sagging skin, NOS
   Excludes2: acquired excess or redundant skin of eyelid (H02.3-)
     congenital excess or redundant skin of eyelid (Q10.3)
     skin changes due to chronic exposure to nonionizing radiation   (L57.-)

L98.8   **Other specified disorders of the skin and subcutaneous tissue**
L98.9   **Disorder of the skin and subcutaneous tissue, unspecified**

L99   **OTHER DISORDERS OF SKIN AND SUBCUTANEOUS**
✓   **TISSUE IN DISEASES CLASSIFIED ELSEWHERE**
Code first underlying disease, such as:
   amyloidosis (E85.-)
Excludes1: skin disorders in diabetes (E08–E13 with .62-)
   skin disorders in gonorrhea (A54.89)
   skin disorders in syphilis (A51.31, A52.79)

4th **5th** **6th** **7th** Additional Character Required   **✓**   3-character code   Unspecified laterality codes were excluded here.   •=New Code   ▲=Revised Code   ***Excludes1***—Not coded here, do not use together   ***Excludes2***—Not included here

PEDIATRIC ICD-10-CM 2022: A MANUAL FOR PROVIDER-BASED CODING   251

Chapter 13. Diseases of the musculoskeletal system and connective tissue (M00–M99)

An "X" may be listed at the end of the code to indicate a placeholder digit(s). The X will be required in order to get to the 7th character, which indicates the type of encounter. Be sure to use all indicated placeholder digits prior to the appropriate 7th character digit.

GUIDELINES

Site and laterality

Most of the codes within Chapter 13 have site and laterality designations. The site represents the bone, joint or the muscle involved. For some conditions where more than one bone, joint or muscle is usually involved, such as osteoarthritis, there is a "multiple sites" code available. For categories where no multiple site code is provided and more than one bone, joint or muscle is involved, multiple codes should be used to indicate the different sites involved.

BONE VERSUS JOINT

For certain conditions, the bone may be affected at the upper or lower end. Though the portion of the bone affected may be at the joint, the site designation will be the bone, not the joint.

Acute traumatic versus chronic or recurrent musculoskeletal conditions

Many musculoskeletal conditions are a result of previous injury or trauma to a site, or are recurrent conditions. Bone, joint or muscle conditions that are the result of a healed injury are usually found in Chapter 13. Recurrent bone, joint or muscle conditions are also usually found in Chapter 13. Any current, acute injury should be coded to the appropriate injury code from Chapter 19. Chronic or recurrent conditions should generally be coded with a code from Chapter 13. If it is difficult to determine from the documentation in the record which code is best to describe a condition, query the provider.

Coding of Pathologic Fractures
Refer to category M84.

Note: Use an external cause code following the code for the musculoskeletal condition, if applicable, to identify the cause of the musculoskeletal condition

Excludes2: arthropathic psoriasis (L40.5-)
    certain conditions originating in the perinatal period (P04–P96)
    certain infectious and parasitic diseases (A00–B99)
    compartment syndrome (traumatic) (T79.A-)
    complications of pregnancy, childbirth and the puerperium (O00–O9A)
    congenital malformations, deformations, and chromosomal abnormalities (Q00–Q99)
    endocrine, nutritional and metabolic diseases (E00–E88)
    injury, poisoning and certain other consequences of external causes (S00–T88)
    neoplasms (C00–D49)
    symptoms, signs and abnormal clinical and laboratory findings, NEC (R00–R94)

(M00–M25) ARTHROPATHIES

Includes: disorders affecting predominantly peripheral (limb) joints

(M00–M02) INFECTIOUS ARTHROPATHIES

Note: This block comprises arthropathies due to microbiological agents. Distinction is made between the following types of etiological relationship:
a) direct infection of joint, where organisms invade synovial tissue and microbial antigen is present in the joint;
b) indirect infection, which may be of two types: a reactive arthropathy, where microbial infection of the body is established but neither organisms nor antigens can be identified in the joint, and a postinfective arthropathy, where microbial antigen is present but recovery of an organism is inconstant and evidence of local multiplication is lacking.

M00 PYOGENIC ARTHRITIS
`4th` *Excludes2:* infection and inflammatory reaction due to internal joint prosthesis (T84.5-)
    M00.0 Staphylococcal arthritis and polyarthritis
    `5th` Use additional code (B95.61–B95.8) to identify bacterial agent
        M00.00 Staphylococcal arthritis, unspecified joint
        M00.01 Staphylococcal arthritis, shoulder
        `6th` **M00.011 Staphylococcal arthritis, right shoulder**

M00.012 Staphylococcal arthritis, left shoulder
M00.02 Staphylococcal arthritis, elbow
`6th` **M00.021 Staphylococcal arthritis, right elbow**
M00.022 Staphylococcal arthritis, left elbow
M00.03 Staphylococcal arthritis, wrist
`6th` Staphylococcal arthritis of carpal bones
M00.031 Staphylococcal arthritis, right wrist
M00.032 Staphylococcal arthritis, left wrist
M00.04 Staphylococcal arthritis, hand
`6th` Staphylococcal arthritis of metacarpus and phalanges
M00.041 Staphylococcal arthritis, right hand
M00.042 Staphylococcal arthritis, left hand
M00.05 Staphylococcal arthritis, hip
`6th` **M00.051 Staphylococcal arthritis, right hip**
M00.052 Staphylococcal arthritis, left hip
M00.06 Staphylococcal arthritis, knee
`6th` **M00.061 Staphylococcal arthritis, right knee**
M00.062 Staphylococcal arthritis, left knee
M00.07 Staphylococcal arthritis, ankle and foot
`6th` Staphylococcal arthritis, tarsus, metatarsus and phalanges
M00.071 Staphylococcal arthritis, right ankle and foot
M00.072 Staphylococcal arthritis, left ankle and foot
M00.08 Staphylococcal arthritis, vertebrae
M00.09 Staphylococcal polyarthritis
M00.1 Pneumococcal arthritis and polyarthritis
`5th` **M00.10 Pneumococcal arthritis, unspecified joint**
M00.11 Pneumococcal arthritis, shoulder
`6th` **M00.111 Pneumococcal arthritis, right shoulder**
M00.112 Pneumococcal arthritis, left shoulder
M00.12 Pneumococcal arthritis, elbow
`6th` **M00.121 Pneumococcal arthritis, right elbow**
M00.122 Pneumococcal arthritis, left elbow
M00.13 Pneumococcal arthritis, wrist
`6th` Pneumococcal arthritis of carpal bones
M00.131 Pneumococcal arthritis, right wrist
M00.132 Pneumococcal arthritis, left wrist`
M00.14 Pneumococcal arthritis, hand
`6th` Pneumococcal arthritis of metacarpus and phalanges
M00.141 Pneumococcal arthritis, right hand
M00.142 Pneumococcal arthritis, left hand
M00.15 Pneumococcal arthritis, hip
`6th` **M00.151 Pneumococcal arthritis, right hip**
M00.152 Pneumococcal arthritis, left hip
M00.16 Pneumococcal arthritis, knee
`6th` **M00.161 Pneumococcal arthritis, right knee**
M00.162 Pneumococcal arthritis, left knee
M00.17 Pneumococcal arthritis, ankle and foot
`6th` Pneumococcal arthritis, tarsus, metatarsus and phalanges
M00.171 Pneumococcal arthritis, right ankle and foot
M00.172 Pneumococcal arthritis, left ankle and foot
M00.18 Pneumococcal arthritis, vertebrae
M00.19 Pneumococcal polyarthritis
M00.2 Other streptococcal arthritis and polyarthritis
`5th` Use additional code (B95.0–B95.2, B95.4–B95.5) to identify bacterial agent
M00.20 Other streptococcal arthritis, unspecified joint
M00.21 Other streptococcal arthritis, shoulder
`6th` **M00.211 Other streptococcal arthritis, right shoulder**
M00.212 Other streptococcal arthritis, left shoulder
M00.22 Other streptococcal arthritis, elbow
`6th` **M00.221 Other streptococcal arthritis, right elbow**
M00.222 Other streptococcal arthritis, left elbow
M00.23 Other streptococcal arthritis, wrist
`6th` Other streptococcal arthritis of carpal bones
M00.231 Other streptococcal arthritis, right wrist
M00.232 Other streptococcal arthritis, left wrist

   `4th` `5th` `6th` `7th` Additional Character Required | ✓ 3-character code

Unspecified laterality codes were excluded here. | •=New Code ▲=Revised Code | *Excludes1*—Not coded here, do not use together *Excludes2*—Not included here

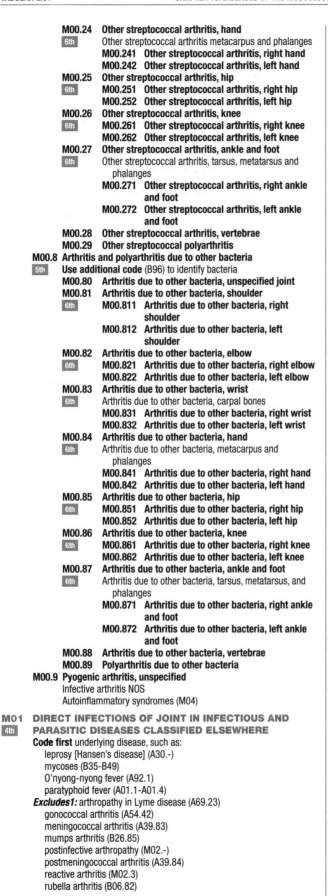

M00.24 Other streptococcal arthritis, hand
6th Other streptococcal arthritis metacarpus and phalanges
    M00.241 Other streptococcal arthritis, right hand
    M00.242 Other streptococcal arthritis, left hand

M00.25 Other streptococcal arthritis, hip
6th **M00.251 Other streptococcal arthritis, right hip**
    M00.252 Other streptococcal arthritis, left hip

M00.26 Other streptococcal arthritis, knee
6th **M00.261 Other streptococcal arthritis, right knee**
    M00.262 Other streptococcal arthritis, left knee

M00.27 Other streptococcal arthritis, ankle and foot
6th Other streptococcal arthritis, tarsus, metatarsus and phalanges
    M00.271 Other streptococcal arthritis, right ankle and foot
    M00.272 Other streptococcal arthritis, left ankle and foot

M00.28 Other streptococcal arthritis, vertebrae
M00.29 Other streptococcal polyarthritis

M00.8 Arthritis and polyarthritis due to other bacteria
5th **Use additional code** (B96) to identify bacteria
M00.80 Arthritis due to other bacteria, unspecified joint
M00.81 Arthritis due to other bacteria, shoulder
6th **M00.811 Arthritis due to other bacteria, right shoulder**
    M00.812 Arthritis due to other bacteria, left shoulder

M00.82 Arthritis due to other bacteria, elbow
6th **M00.821 Arthritis due to other bacteria, right elbow**
    M00.822 Arthritis due to other bacteria, left elbow

M00.83 Arthritis due to other bacteria, wrist
6th Arthritis due to other bacteria, carpal bones
    M00.831 Arthritis due to other bacteria, right wrist
    M00.832 Arthritis due to other bacteria, left wrist

M00.84 Arthritis due to other bacteria, hand
6th Arthritis due to other bacteria, metacarpus and phalanges
    M00.841 Arthritis due to other bacteria, right hand
    M00.842 Arthritis due to other bacteria, left hand

M00.85 Arthritis due to other bacteria, hip
6th **M00.851 Arthritis due to other bacteria, right hip**
    M00.852 Arthritis due to other bacteria, left hip

M00.86 Arthritis due to other bacteria, knee
6th **M00.861 Arthritis due to other bacteria, right knee**
    M00.862 Arthritis due to other bacteria, left knee

M00.87 Arthritis due to other bacteria, ankle and foot
6th Arthritis due to other bacteria, tarsus, metatarsus, and phalanges
    M00.871 Arthritis due to other bacteria, right ankle and foot
    M00.872 Arthritis due to other bacteria, left ankle and foot

M00.88 Arthritis due to other bacteria, vertebrae
M00.89 Polyarthritis due to other bacteria

M00.9 Pyogenic arthritis, unspecified
Infective arthritis NOS
Autoinflammatory syndromes (M04)

M01 DIRECT INFECTIONS OF JOINT IN INFECTIOUS AND
4th **PARASITIC DISEASES CLASSIFIED ELSEWHERE**
Code first underlying disease, such as:
  leprosy [Hansen's disease] (A30.-)
  mycoses (B35-B49)
  O'nyong-nyong fever (A92.1)
  paratyphoid fever (A01.1-A01.4)
Excludes1: arthropathy in Lyme disease (A69.23)
  gonococcal arthritis (A54.42)
  meningococcal arthritis (A39.83)
  mumps arthritis (B26.85)
  postinfective arthropathy (M02.-)
  postmeningococcal arthritis (A39.84)
  reactive arthritis (M02.3)
  rubella arthritis (B06.82)

  sarcoidosis arthritis (D86.86)
  typhoid fever arthritis (A01.04)
  tuberculosis arthritis (A18.01-A18.02)

M01.X Direct infection of joint in infectious and parasitic diseases
5th **classified elsewhere**
M01.X0 Direct infection of unspecified joint in infectious and parasitic diseases classified elsewhere
M01.X1 Direct infection of shoulder joint in infectious and
6th **parasitic diseases classified elsewhere**
    M01.X11 Direct infection of right shoulder in infectious and parasitic diseases classified elsewhere
    M01.X12 Direct infection of left shoulder in infectious and parasitic diseases classified elsewhere

M01.X2 Direct infection of elbow in infectious and parasitic
6th **diseases classified elsewhere**
    M01.X21 Direct infection of right elbow in infectious and parasitic diseases classified elsewhere
    M01.X22 Direct infection of left elbow in infectious and parasitic diseases classified elsewhere

M01.X3 Direct infection of wrist in infectious and parasitic
6th **diseases classified elsewhere**
  Direct infection of carpal bones in infectious and parasitic diseases classified elsewhere
    M01.X31 Direct infection of right wrist in infectious and parasitic diseases classified elsewhere
    M01.X32 Direct infection of left wrist in infectious and parasitic diseases classified elsewhere

M01.X4 Direct infection of hand in infectious and parasitic
6th **diseases classified elsewhere**
  Direct infection of metacarpus and phalanges in infectious and parasitic diseases classified elsewhere
    M01.X41 Direct infection of right hand in infectious and parasitic diseases classified elsewhere
    M01.X42 Direct infection of left hand in infectious and parasitic diseases classified elsewhere

M01.X5 Direct infection of hip in infectious and parasitic
6th **diseases classified elsewhere**
    M01.X51 Direct infection of right hip in infectious and parasitic diseases classified elsewhere
    M01.X52 Direct infection of left hip in infectious and parasitic diseases classified elsewhere

M01.X6 Direct infection of knee in infectious and parasitic
6th **diseases classified elsewhere**
    M01.X61 Direct infection of right knee in infectious and parasitic diseases classified elsewhere
    M01.X62 Direct infection of left knee in infectious and parasitic diseases classified elsewhere

M01.X7 Direct infection of ankle and foot in infectious and
6th **parasitic diseases classified elsewhere**
  Direct infection of tarsus, metatarsus and phalanges in infectious and parasitic diseases classified elsewhere
    M01.X71 Direct infection of right ankle and foot in infectious and parasitic diseases classified elsewhere
    M01.X72 Direct infection of left ankle and foot in infectious and parasitic diseases classified elsewhere

M01.X8 Direct infection of vertebrae in infectious and parasitic diseases classified elsewhere
M01.X9 Direct infection of multiple joints in infectious and parasitic diseases classified elsewhere

---

4th 5th 6th 7th Additional Character Required   ✓ 3-character code

Unspecified laterality codes were excluded here. •=New Code ▲=Revised Code ***Excludes1***—Not coded here, do not use together ***Excludes2***—Not included here

(M04) AUTOINFLAMMATORY SYNDROMES

M04 **AUTOINFLAMMATORY SYNDROMES**
`4th` *Excludes2:* Crohn's disease (K50.-)

M04.1 **Periodic fever syndromes**
Familial Mediterranean fever
Hyperimmunoglobin D syndrome
Mevalonate kinase deficiency
Tumor necrosis factor receptor associated periodic syndrome [TRAPS]

M04.2 **Cryopyrin-associated periodic syndromes**
Chronic infantile neurological, cutaneous and articular syndrome [CINCA]
Familial cold autoinflammatory syndrome
Familial cold urticaria
Muckle-Wells syndrome
Neonatal onset multisystemic inflammatory disorder [NOMID]

M04.8 **Other autoinflammatory syndromes**
Blau syndrome
Deficiency of interleukin 1 receptor antagonist [DIRA]
Majeed syndrome
Periodic fever, aphthous stomatitis, pharyngitis, and adenopathy syndrome [PFAPA]
Pyogenic arthritis, pyoderma gangrenosum, and acne syndrome [PAPA]

M04.9 **Autoinflammatory syndrome, unspecified**

(M05–M14) INFLAMMATORY POLYARTHROPATHIES

M06 **OTHER RHEUMATOID ARTHRITIS**
`4th` **M06.9** **Rheumatoid arthritis, unspecified**

M08 **JUVENILE ARTHRITIS**
`4th` Code also any associated underlying condition, such as: regional enteritis [Crohn's disease] (K50.-)
ulcerative colitis (K51.-)
Excludes1: arthropathy in Whipple's disease (M14.8)
Felty's syndrome (M05.0)
juvenile dermatomyositis (M33.0-)
psoriatic juvenile arthropathy (L40.54)

M08.0 **Unspecified juvenile rheumatoid arthritis**
`5th` Juvenile rheumatoid arthritis with or without rheumatoid factor

  M08.00 **Unspecified juvenile rheumatoid arthritis of unspecified site**

  M08.01 **Unspecified juvenile rheumatoid arthritis, shoulder**
`6th`   M08.011   right shoulder
    M08.012   left shoulder

  M08.02 **Unspecified juvenile rheumatoid arthritis of elbow**
`6th`   M08.021   right elbow
    M08.022   left elbow

  M08.03 **Unspecified juvenile rheumatoid arthritis, wrist**
`6th`   M08.031   right wrist
    M08.032   left wrist

  M08.04 **Unspecified juvenile rheumatoid arthritis, hand**
`6th`   M08.041   right hand
    M08.042   left hand

  M08.05 **Unspecified juvenile rheumatoid arthritis, hip**
`6th`   M08.051   right hip
    M08.052   left hip

  M08.06 **Unspecified juvenile rheumatoid arthritis, knee**
`6th`   M08.061   right knee
    M08.062   left knee

  M08.07 **Unspecified juvenile rheumatoid arthritis, ankle and foot**
`6th`   M08.071   right ankle and foot
    M08.072   left ankle and foot

  M08.08 **Unspecified juvenile rheumatoid arthritis, vertebrae**

  M08.09 **Unspecified juvenile rheumatoid arthritis, multiple sites**

  M08.0A **Unspecified juvenile rheumatoid arthritis, other specified site**

M08.1 **Juvenile ankylosing spondylitis**
Excludes1: ankylosing spondylitis in adults (M45.0-)

M08.2 **Juvenile rheumatoid arthritis with systemic onset**
`5th` Still's disease NOS
Excludes1: adult-onset Still's disease (M06.1-)

  M08.20 **Juvenile rheumatoid arthritis with systemic onset, unspecified site**

  M08.21 **Juvenile rheumatoid arthritis with systemic onset, shoulder**
`6th`   M08.211   right shoulder
    M08.212   left shoulder

  M08.22 **Juvenile rheumatoid arthritis with systemic onset, elbow**
`6th`   M08.221   right elbow
    M08.222   left elbow

  M08.23 **Juvenile rheumatoid arthritis with systemic onset, wrist**
`6th`   M08.231   right wrist
    M08.232   left wrist

  M08.24 **Juvenile rheumatoid arthritis with systemic onset, hand**
`6th`   M08.241   right hand
    M08.242   left hand

  M08.25 **Juvenile rheumatoid arthritis with systemic onset, hip**
`6th`   M08.251   right hip
    M08.252   left hip

  M08.26 **Juvenile rheumatoid arthritis with systemic onset, knee**
`6th`   M08.261   right knee
    M08.262   left knee

  M08.27 **Juvenile rheumatoid arthritis with systemic onset, ankle and foot**
`6th`   M08.271   right ankle and foot
    M08.272   left ankle and foot

  M08.28 **Juvenile rheumatoid arthritis with systemic onset, vertebrae**

  M08.29 **Juvenile rheumatoid arthritis with systemic onset, multiple sites**

  M08.2A **Juvenile rheumatoid arthritis with systemic onset, other specified site**

M08.3 **Juvenile rheumatoid polyarthritis (seronegative)**

M08.4 **Pauciarticular juvenile rheumatoid arthritis**
`5th` **M08.40** **Pauciarticular juvenile rheumatoid arthritis, unspecified site**

  M08.41 **Pauciarticular juvenile rheumatoid arthritis, shoulder**
`6th`   M08.411   right shoulder
    M08.412   left shoulder

  M08.42 **Pauciarticular juvenile rheumatoid arthritis, elbow**
`6th`   M08.421   right elbow
    M08.422   left elbow

  M08.43 **Pauciarticular juvenile rheumatoid arthritis, wrist**
`6th`   M08.431   right wrist
    M08.432   left wrist

  M08.44 **Pauciarticular juvenile rheumatoid arthritis, hand**
`6th`   M08.441   right hand
    M08.442   left hand

  M08.45 **Pauciarticular juvenile rheumatoid arthritis, hip**
`6th`   M08.451   right hip
    M08.452   left hip

  M08.46 **Pauciarticular juvenile rheumatoid arthritis, knee**
`6th`   M08.461   right knee
    M08.462   left knee

  M08.47 **Pauciarticular juvenile rheumatoid arthritis, ankle and foot**
`6th`   M08.471   right ankle and foot
    M08.472   left ankle and foot

  M08.48 **Pauciarticular juvenile rheumatoid arthritis, vertebrae**

  M08.4A **Pauciarticular juvenile rheumatoid arthritis, other specified site**

M08.8 **Other juvenile arthritis**
`5th` **M08.81** **Other juvenile arthritis, shoulder**
`6th`   M08.811   right shoulder
    M08.812   left shoulder

`4th` `5th` `6th` `7th` Additional Character Required ✓ 3-character code

Unspecified laterality codes were excluded here. •=New Code ▲=Revised Code *Excludes1*—Not coded here, do not use together *Excludes2*—Not included here

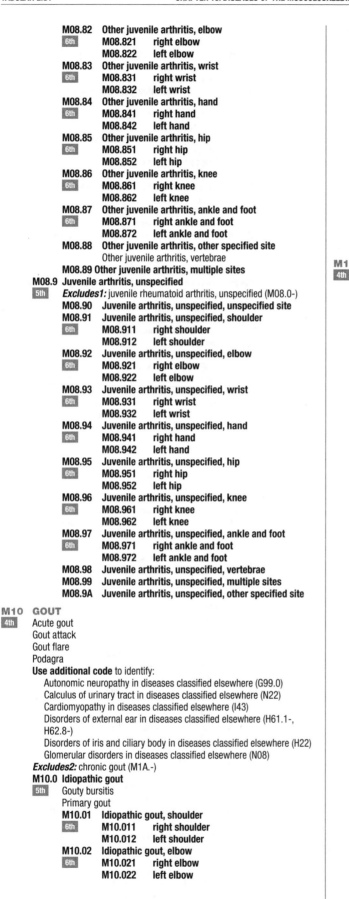

CHAPTER 13. DISEASES OF THE MUSCULOSKELETAL SYSTEM AND CONNECTIVE TISSUE   **(M08.82–M12.562)**

M08.82   Other juvenile arthritis, elbow
- 6th   **M08.821**   right elbow
-       **M08.822**   left elbow

M08.83   Other juvenile arthritis, wrist
- 6th   **M08.831**   right wrist
-       **M08.832**   left wrist

M08.84   Other juvenile arthritis, hand
- 6th   **M08.841**   right hand
-       **M08.842**   left hand

M08.85   Other juvenile arthritis, hip
- 6th   **M08.851**   right hip
-       **M08.852**   left hip

M08.86   Other juvenile arthritis, knee
- 6th   **M08.861**   right knee
-       **M08.862**   left knee

M08.87   Other juvenile arthritis, ankle and foot
- 6th   **M08.871**   right ankle and foot
-       **M08.872**   left ankle and foot

M08.88   Other juvenile arthritis, other specified site
     Other juvenile arthritis, vertebrae

M08.89 Other juvenile arthritis, multiple sites

M08.9 Juvenile arthritis, unspecified
- 5th   *Excludes1:* juvenile rheumatoid arthritis, unspecified (M08.0-)

M08.90   Juvenile arthritis, unspecified, unspecified site

M08.91   Juvenile arthritis, unspecified, shoulder
- 6th   **M08.911**   right shoulder
-       **M08.912**   left shoulder

M08.92   Juvenile arthritis, unspecified, elbow
- 6th   **M08.921**   right elbow
-       **M08.922**   left elbow

M08.93   Juvenile arthritis, unspecified, wrist
- 6th   **M08.931**   right wrist
-       **M08.932**   left wrist

M08.94   Juvenile arthritis, unspecified, hand
- 6th   **M08.941**   right hand
-       **M08.942**   left hand

M08.95   Juvenile arthritis, unspecified, hip
- 6th   **M08.951**   right hip
-       **M08.952**   left hip

M08.96   Juvenile arthritis, unspecified, knee
- 6th   **M08.961**   right knee
-       **M08.962**   left knee

M08.97   Juvenile arthritis, unspecified, ankle and foot
- 6th   **M08.971**   right ankle and foot
-       **M08.972**   left ankle and foot

M08.98   Juvenile arthritis, unspecified, vertebrae

M08.99   Juvenile arthritis, unspecified, multiple sites

M08.9A   Juvenile arthritis, unspecified, other specified site

M10   **GOUT**
- 4th
     Acute gout
     Gout attack
     Gout flare
     Podagra
     Use additional code to identify:
       Autonomic neuropathy in diseases classified elsewhere (G99.0)
       Calculus of urinary tract in diseases classified elsewhere (N22)
       Cardiomyopathy in diseases classified elsewhere (I43)
       Disorders of external ear in diseases classified elsewhere (H61.1-, H62.8-)
       Disorders of iris and ciliary body in diseases classified elsewhere (H22)
       Glomerular disorders in diseases classified elsewhere (N08)
     Excludes2: chronic gout (M1A.-)

M10.0 Idiopathic gout
- 5th
     Gouty bursitis
     Primary gout

M10.01   Idiopathic gout, shoulder
- 6th   **M10.011**   right shoulder
-       **M10.012**   left shoulder

M10.02   Idiopathic gout, elbow
- 6th   **M10.021**   right elbow
-       **M10.022**   left elbow

M10.03   Idiopathic gout, wrist
- 6th   **M10.031**   right wrist
-       **M10.032**   left wrist

M10.04   Idiopathic gout, hand
- 6th   **M10.041**   right hand
-       **M10.042**   left hand

M10.05   Idiopathic gout, hip
- 6th   **M10.051**   right hip
-       **M10.052**   left hip

M10.06   Idiopathic gout, knee
- 6th   **M10.061**   right knee
-       **M10.062**   left knee

M10.07   Idiopathic gout, ankle and foot
- 6th   **M10.071**   right ankle and foot
-       **M10.072**   left ankle and foot

M10.08   Idiopathic gout, vertebrae

M10.09   Idiopathic gout, multiple sites

M10.9 Gout, unspecified
     Gout NOS

M12   **OTHER AND UNSPECIFIED ARTHROPATHY**
- 4th   *Excludes1:* arthrosis (M15-M19)
       cricoarytenoid arthropathy (J38.7)

M12.4 Intermittent hydrarthrosis
- 5th   **M12.41**   Intermittent hydrarthrosis, shoulder
       6th   **M12.411**   right shoulder
            M12.412   left shoulder

     M12.42   Intermittent hydrarthrosis, elbow
       6th   **M12.421**   right elbow
            M12.422   left elbow

     M12.43   Intermittent hydrarthrosis, wrist
       6th   **M12.431**   right wrist
            M12.432   left wrist

     M12.44   Intermittent hydrarthrosis, hand
       6th   **M12.441**   right hand
            M12.442   left hand

     M12.45   Intermittent hydrarthrosis, hip
       6th   **M12.451**   right hip
            M12.452   left hip

     M12.46   Intermittent hydrarthrosis, knee
       6th   **M12.461**   right knee
            M12.462   left knee

     M12.47   Intermittent hydrarthrosis, ankle and foot
       6th   **M12.471**   right ankle and foot
            M12.472   left ankle and foot

     M12.48   Intermittent hydrarthrosis, other site

     M12.49   Intermittent hydrarthrosis, multiple sites

M12.5 Traumatic arthropathy
- 5th   *Excludes1:* current injury — see Alphabetic Index
       post-traumatic osteoarthritis of first carpometacarpal joint (M18.2–M18.3)
       post-traumatic osteoarthritis of hip (M16.4–M16.5)
       post-traumatic osteoarthritis of knee (M17.2–M17.3)
       post-traumatic osteoarthritis NOS (M19.1-)
       post-traumatic osteoarthritis of other single joints (M19.1-)

M12.50   Traumatic arthropathy, unspecified site

M12.51   Traumatic arthropathy, shoulder
- 6th   **M12.511**   right shoulder
-       **M12.512**   left shoulder

M12.52   Traumatic arthropathy, elbow
- 6th   **M12.521**   right elbow
-       **M12.522**   left elbow

M12.53   Traumatic arthropathy, wrist
- 6th   **M12.531**   right wrist
-       **M12.532**   left wrist

M12.54   Traumatic arthropathy, hand
- 6th   **M12.541**   right hand
-       **M12.542**   left hand

M12.55   Traumatic arthropathy, hip
- 6th   **M12.551**   right hip
-       **M12.552**   left hip

M12.56   Traumatic arthropathy, knee
- 6th   **M12.561**   right knee
-       **M12.562**   left knee

 4th   5th   6th   7th   Additional Character Required   ✔   3-character code

Unspecified laterality codes were excluded here.   •=New Code   ▲=Revised Code   *Excludes1*—Not coded here, do not use together   *Excludes2*—Not included here

M12.57   Traumatic arthropathy, ankle and foot
- 6th   **M12.571**   right ankle and foot
- **M12.572**   left ankle and foot

M12.58   Traumatic arthropathy, other specified site
Traumatic arthropathy, vertebrae

M12.59   Traumatic arthropathy, multiple sites

M12.9   Arthropathy, unspecified

M14   **ARTHROPATHIES IN OTHER DISEASES CLASSIFIED ELSEWHERE**
4th

Excludes1: arthropathy in:
DM (E08-E13 with .61-)
hematological disorders (M36.2-M36.3)
hypersensitivity reactions (M36.4)
neoplastic disease (M36.1)
neurosyphillis (A52.16)
sarcoidosis (D86.86)
enteropathic arthropathies (M07.-)
juvenile psoriatic arthropathy (L40.54)
lipoid dermatoarthritis (E78.81)

M14.8   **Arthropathies in other specified diseases classified elsewhere**
5th   **Code first:** underlying disease, such as:
amyloidosis (E85.-)
erythema multiforme (L51.-)
erythema nodosum (L52)
hemochromatosis (E83.11-)
hyperparathyroidism (E21.-)
hypothyroidism (E00–E03)
sickle-cell disorders (D57.-)
thyrotoxicosis [hyperthyroidism] (E05.-)
Whipple's disease (K90.81)

M14.80   Arthropathies in other specified diseases classified elsewhere, unspecified site

M14.81   Arthropathies in other specified diseases classified elsewhere; shoulder
- 6th
- **M14.811**   right shoulder
- **M14.812**   left shoulder

M14.82   Arthropathies in other specified diseases classified elsewhere; elbow
- 6th
- **M14.821**   right elbow
- **M14.822**   left elbow

M14.83   Arthropathies in other specified diseases classified elsewhere; wrist
- 6th
- **M14.831**   right wrist
- **M14.832**   left wrist

M14.84   Arthropathies in other specified diseases classified elsewhere; hand
- 6th
- **M14.841**   right hand
- **M14.842**   left hand

M14.85   Arthropathies in other specified diseases classified elsewhere; hip
- 6th
- **M14.851**   right hip
- **M14.852**   left hip

M14.86   Arthropathies in other specified diseases classified elsewhere; knee
- 6th
- **M14.861**   right knee
- **M14.862**   left knee

M14.87   Arthropathies in other specified diseases classified elsewhere; ankle and foot
- 6th
- **M14.871**   right ankle and foot
- **M14.872**   left ankle and foot

M14.88   Arthropathies in other specified diseases classified elsewhere, vertebrae

M14.89   Arthropathies in other specified diseases classified elsewhere, multiple sites

(M15–M19) OSTEOARTHRITIS

Excludes2: osteoarthritis of spine (M47.-)

(M20–M25) OTHER JOINT DISORDERS

Excludes2: joints of the spine (M40–M54)

M20   **ACQUIRED DEFORMITIES OF FINGERS AND TOES**
4th

Excludes1: acquired absence of fingers and toes (Z89.-)
congenital absence of fingers and toes (Q71.3-, Q72.3-)
congenital deformities and malformations of fingers and toes (Q66.-, Q68–Q70, Q74.-)

M20.0   Deformity of finger(s)
5th   *Excludes1:* clubbing of fingers (R68.3)
palmar fascial fibromatosis [Dupuytren] (M72.0)
trigger finger (M65.3)

M20.00   Unspecified deformity of finger(s)
- 6th
- **M20.001**   Unspecified deformity of right finger(s)
- **M20.002**   Unspecified deformity of left finger(s)

M20.01   Mallet finger
- 6th
- **M20.011**   Mallet finger of right finger(s)
- **M20.012**   Mallet finger of left finger(s)

M20.09   Other deformity of finger(s)
- 6th
- **M20.091**   Other deformity of right finger(s)
- **M20.092**   Other deformity of left finger(s)

M20.1   Hallux valgus (acquired)
5th   *Excludes2:* bunion (M21.6-)
M20.11   Hallux valgus (acquired), right foot
M20.12   Hallux valgus (acquired), left foot

M20.5   Other deformities of toe(s) (acquired)
5th   **M20.5X**   Other deformities of toe(s) (acquired)
- 6th   **M20.5X1**   right foot
- **M20.5X2**   left foot

M20.6   Acquired deformities of toe(s), unspecified
5th   **M20.61**   Acquired deformities of toe(s), unspecified, right foot
M20.62   Acquired deformities of toe(s), unspecified, left foot

M21   **OTHER ACQUIRED DEFORMITIES OF LIMBS**
4th

Excludes1: acquired absence of limb (Z89.-)
congenital absence of limbs (Q71–Q73)
congenital deformities and malformations of limbs (Q65–Q66, Q68–Q74)

Excludes2: acquired deformities of fingers or toes (M20.-)
coxa plana (M91.2)

M21.0   Valgus deformity, NEC
5th   *Excludes1:* metatarsus valgus (Q66.6)
talipes calcaneovalgus (Q66.4-)
M21.06   Valgus deformity, NEC, knee
- 6th   Genu valgum
Knock knee
- **M21.061**   right knee
- **M21.062**   left knee

M21.1   Varus deformity, NEC
5th   *Excludes1:* metatarsus varus (Q66.22-)
tibia vara (M92.51-)
M21.16   Varus deformity, NEC, knee
- 6th   Bow leg
Genu varum
- **M21.161**   right knee
- **M21.162**   left knee

M21.2   Flexion deformity
5th   **M21.21**   Flexion deformity, shoulder
- 6th
- **M21.211**   right shoulder
- **M21.212**   left shoulder

M21.22   Flexion deformity, elbow
- 6th
- **M21.221**   right elbow
- **M21.222**   left elbow

M21.23   Flexion deformity, wrist
- 6th
- **M21.231**   right wrist
- **M21.232**   left wrist

M21.24   Flexion deformity, finger joints
- 6th
- **M21.241**   right finger joints
- **M21.242**   left finger joints

M21.25   Flexion deformity, hip
- 6th
- **M21.251**   right hip
- **M21.252**   left hip

M21.26   Flexion deformity, knee
- 6th
- **M21.261**   right knee
- **M21.262**   left knee

M21.27   Flexion deformity, ankle and toes
- 6th

 4th   5th   6th   7th   Additional Character Required   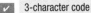 ✓   3-character code

Unspecified laterality codes were excluded here.   •=New Code   ▲=Revised Code   *Excludes1*—Not coded here, do not use together   *Excludes2*—Not included here

M21.271 right ankle and toes
M21.272 left ankle and toes

M21.3 Wrist or foot drop (acquired)
 5th **M21.33** **Wrist drop (acquired)**
  6th M21.331 right wrist
   M21.332 left wrist
  M21.37 **Foot drop (acquired)**
  6th M21.371 right foot
   M21.372 left foot

M21.4 Flat foot [pes planus] (acquired)
 5th *Excludes1:* congenital pes planus (Q66.5-)
  M21.41 right foot
  M21.42 left foot

M21.6 Other acquired deformities of foot
 5th *Excludes2:* deformities of toe (acquired) (M20.1-M20.6-)
  M21.61 **Bunion**
  6th M21.611 right foot
   M21.612 left foot
  M21.62 **Bunionette**
  6th M21.621 right foot
   M21.622 left foot
  M21.6X **Other acquired deformities of foot**
  6th M21.6X1 right foot
   M21.6X2 left foot

M21.8 Other specified acquired deformities of limbs
 5th *Excludes2:* coxa plana (M91.2)
  M21.82 **Other specified acquired deformities of upper arm**
  6th M21.821 right upper arm
   M21.822 left upper arm
  M21.86 **Other specified acquired deformities of lower leg**
  6th M21.861 right lower leg
   M21.862 left lower leg

M22 DISORDER OF PATELLA
 4th *Excludes2:* traumatic dislocation of patella (S83.0-)
 M22.0 Recurrent dislocation of patella
  5th **M22.01** right knee
   M22.02 left knee
 M22.1 Recurrent subluxation of patella
  5th Incomplete dislocation of patella
   M22.11 right knee
   M22.12 left knee
 M22.4 Chondromalacia patellae
  5th **M22.41** right knee
   M22.42 left knee

M23 INTERNAL DERANGEMENT OF KNEE
 4th *Excludes1:* ankylosis (M24.66)
  deformity of knee (M21.-)
  osteochondritis dissecans (M93.2)
 Excludes2: current injury—see injury of knee and lower leg (S80–S89)
  recurrent dislocation or subluxation of joints (M24.4)
  recurrent dislocation or subluxation of patella (M22.0-M22.1)
 M23.5 Chronic instability of knee
  5th **M23.51** **Chronic instability of knee, right knee**
   M23.52 **Chronic instability of knee, left knee**
 M23.8 Other internal derangements of knee
  5th Laxity of ligament of knee
   Snapping knee
  M23.8X **Other internal derangements of knee**
  6th M23.8X1 right knee
   M23.8X2 left knee

M24 OTHER SPECIFIC JOINT DERANGEMENTS
 4th *Excludes1:* current injury — see injury of joint by body region
 Excludes2: ganglion (M67.4)
  snapping knee (M23.8-)
  TMJ disorders (M26.6-)
  M24.51 **Contracture, shoulder**
  6th M24.511 right shoulder
   M24.512 left shoulder
  M24.52 **Contracture, elbow**
  6th M24.521 right elbow
   M24.522 left elbow

M24.53 **Contracture, wrist**
 6th M24.531 right wrist
  M24.532 left wrist
M24.54 **Contracture, hand**
 6th M24.541 right hand
  M24.542 left hand
M24.55 **Contracture, hip**
 6th M24.551 right hip
  M24.552 left hip
M24.56 **Contracture, knee**
 6th M24.561 right knee
  M24.562 left knee
M24.57 **Contracture, ankle and foot**
 6th M24.571 right ankle
  M24.572 left ankle
  M24.574 right foot
  M24.575 left foot
M24.59 **Contracture, other specified joint**

M24.8 Other specific joint derangements, NEC
 5th *Excludes2:* iliotibial band syndrome (M76.3)
  M24.81 **Other specific joint derangements of shoulder, NEC**
  6th M24.811 right shoulder, NEC
   M24.812 left shoulder, NEC
  M24.82 **Other specific joint derangements of elbow, NEC**
  6th M24.821 right elbow, NEC
   M24.822 left elbow, NEC
  M24.83 **Other specific joint derangements of wrist, NEC**
  6th M24.831 right wrist, NEC
   M24.832 left wrist, NEC
  M24.84 **Other specific joint derangements of hand, NEC**
  6th M24.841 right hand, NEC
   M24.842 left hand, NEC
  M24.85 **Other specific joint derangements of hip, NEC**
  6th Irritable hip
   M24.851 right hip, NEC
   M24.852 left hip, NEC
  M24.87 **Other specific joint derangements of ankle and foot, NEC**
  6th M24.871 right ankle, NEC
   M24.872 left ankle, NEC
   M24.874 right foot, NEC
   M24.875 left foot, NEC
  M24.89 **Other specific joint derangement of other specified joint, NEC**

M24.9 Joint derangement, unspecified

M25 OTHER JOINT DISORDER, NEC
 4th *Excludes2:* abnormality of gait and mobility (R26.-)
  acquired deformities of limb (M20–M21)
  calcification of bursa (M71.4-)
  calcification of shoulder (joint) (M75.3)
  calcification of tendon (M65.2-)
  difficulty in walking (R26.2)
  temporomandibular joint disorder (M26.6-)
 M25.0 Hemarthrosis
  5th *Excludes1:* current injury — see injury of joint by body region
   hemophilic arthropathy (M36.2)
  M25.00 **Hemarthrosis, unspecified joint**
  M25.01 **Hemarthrosis, shoulder**
  6th M25.011 right shoulder
   M25.012 left shoulder
  M25.02 **Hemarthrosis, elbow**
  6th M25.021 right elbow
   M25.022 left elbow
  M25.03 **Hemarthrosis, wrist**
  6th M25.031 right wrist
   M25.032 left wrist
  M25.04 **Hemarthrosis, hand**
  6th M25.041 right hand
   M25.042 left hand
  M25.05 **Hemarthrosis, hip**
  6th M25.051 right hip
   M25.052 left hip

4th 5th 6th 7th Additional Character Required ✔ 3-character code Unspecified laterality codes were excluded here. •=New Code ▲=Revised Code *Excludes1*—Not coded here, do not use together *Excludes2*—Not included here

M25.06   **Hemarthrosis, knee**
- 6th   M25.061   right knee
- M25.062   left knee

M25.07   **Hemarthrosis, ankle and foot**
- 6th   M25.071   right ankle
- M25.072   left ankle
- M25.074   right foot
- M25.075   left foot

M25.08   **Hemarthrosis, other specified site**
     Hemarthrosis, vertebrae

M25.2   Flail joint
- 5th   **M25.21   Flail joint, shoulder**
  - 6th   M25.211   right shoulder
  - M25.212   left shoulder
- **M25.22   Flail joint, elbow**
  - 6th   M25.221   right elbow
  - M25.222   left elbow
- **M25.23   Flail joint, wrist**
  - 6th   M25.231   right wrist
  - M25.232   left wrist
- **M25.24   Flail joint, hand**
  - 6th   M25.241   right hand
  - M25.242   left hand
- **M25.25   Flail joint, hip**
  - 6th   M25.251   right hip
  - M25.252   left hip
- **M25.26   Flail joint, knee**
  - 6th   M25.261   right knee
  - M25.262   left knee
- **M25.27   Flail joint, ankle and foot**
  - 6th   M25.271   right ankle and foot
  - M25.272   left ankle and foot
- **M25.28   Flail joint, other site**

M25.3   Other instability of joint
- 5th   ***Excludes1:*** instability of joint secondary to old ligament injury (M24.2-)
  - instability of joint secondary to removal of joint prosthesis (M96.8-)
  - ***Excludes2:*** spinal instabilities (M53.2-)
- **M25.30   Other instability, unspecified joint**
- **M25.31   Other instability, shoulder**
  - 6th   M25.311   right shoulder
  - M25.312   left shoulder
- **M25.32   Other instability, elbow**
  - 6th   M25.321   right elbow
  - M25.322   left elbow
- **M25.33   Other instability, wrist**
  - 6th   M25.331   right wrist
  - M25.332   left wrist
- **M25.34   Other instability, hand**
  - 6th   M25.341   right hand
  - M25.342   left hand
- **M25.35   Other instability, hip**
  - 6th   M25.351   right hip
  - M25.352   left hip
- **M25.36   Other instability, knee**
  - 6th   M25.361   right knee
  - M25.362   left knee
- **M25.37   Other instability, ankle and foot**
  - 6th   M25.371   right ankle
  - M25.372   left ankle
  - M25.374   right foot
  - M25.375   left foot
- **M25.39   Other instability, other specified joint**

M25.4   Effusion of joint
- 5th   ***Excludes1:*** hydrarthrosis in yaws (A66.6)
  - intermittent hydrarthrosis (M12.4-)
  - other infective (teno)synovitis (M65.1-)
- **M25.40   Effusion, unspecified joint**
- **M25.41   Effusion, shoulder**
  - 6th   M25.411   right shoulder
  - M25.412   left shoulder

M25.42   **Effusion, elbow**
- 6th   M25.421   right elbow
- M25.422   left elbow

M25.43   **Effusion, wrist**
- 6th   M25.431   right wrist
- M25.432   left wrist

M25.44   **Effusion, hand**
- 6th   M25.441   right hand
- M25.442   left hand

M25.45   **Effusion, hip**
- 6th   M25.451   right hip
- M25.452   left hip

M25.46   **Effusion, knee**
- 6th   M25.461   right knee
- M25.462   left knee

M25.47   **Effusion, ankle and foot**
- 6th   M25.471   right ankle
- M25.472   left ankle
- M25.474   right foot
- M25.475   left foot

M25.48   **Effusion, other site**

M25.5   Pain in joint
- 5th   ***Excludes2:*** pain in hand (M79.64-)
  - pain in fingers (M79.64-)
  - pain in foot (M79.67-)
  - pain in limb (M79.6-)
  - pain in toes (M79.67-)
- **M25.50   Pain in unspecified joint**
- **M25.51   Pain in shoulder**
  - 6th   M25.511   right shoulder
  - M25.512   left shoulder
- **M25.52   Pain in elbow**
  - 6th   M25.521   right elbow
  - M25.522   left elbow
- **M25.53   Pain in wrist**
  - 6th   M25.531   right wrist
  - M25.532   left wrist
- **M25.54   Pain in hand joints**
  - 6th   M25.541   right hand
  - M25.542   left hand
- **M25.55   Pain in hip**
  - 6th   M25.551   right hip
  - M25.552   left hip
- **M25.56   Pain in knee**
  - 6th   M25.561   right knee
  - M25.562   left knee
- **M25.57   Pain in ankle and joints of foot**
  - 6th   M25.571   Pain in right ankle and joints of right foot
  - M25.572   Pain in left ankle and joints of left foot
- **M25.59   Pain in other specified joint**

M25.6   Stiffness of joint, NEC
- 5th   ***Excludes1:*** ankylosis of joint (M24.6-)
  - contracture of joint (M24.5-)
- **M25.60   Stiffness of unspecified joint, NEC**
- **M25.61   Stiffness of shoulder, NEC**
  - 6th   M25.611   Stiffness of right shoulder, NEC
  - M25.612   Stiffness of left shoulder, NEC
- **M25.62   Stiffness of elbow, NEC**
  - 6th   M25.621   Stiffness of right elbow, NEC
  - M25.622   Stiffness of left elbow, NEC
- **M25.63   Stiffness of wrist, NEC**
  - 6th   M25.631   Stiffness of right wrist, NEC
  - M25.632   Stiffness of left wrist, NEC
- **M25.64   Stiffness of hand, NEC**
  - 6th   M25.641   Stiffness of right hand, NEC
  - M25.642   Stiffness of left hand, NEC
- **M25.65   Stiffness of hip, NEC**
  - 6th   M25.651   Stiffness of right hip, NEC
  - M25.652   Stiffness of left hip, NEC
- **M25.66   Stiffness of knee, NEC**
  - 6th   M25.661   Stiffness of right knee, NEC
  - M25.662   Stiffness of left knee, NEC

| 4th | 5th | 6th | 7th | Additional Character Required | ✓ | 3-character code |

Unspecified laterality codes were excluded here.

•=New Code   ▲=Revised Code

Excludes1—Not coded here, do not use together
Excludes2—Not included here

CHAPTER 13. DISEASES OF THE MUSCULOSKELETAL SYSTEM AND CONNECTIVE TISSUE (M25.67–M31.11)

M25.67 Stiffness of ankle and foot, NEC
- **6th**
  - M25.671   Stiffness of right ankle, NEC
  - M25.672   Stiffness of left ankle, NEC
  - M25.674   Stiffness of right foot, NEC
  - M25.675   Stiffness of left foot, NEC
- **M25.69 Stiffness of other specified joint, NEC**

M25.7 Osteophyte
- **5th**
- **M25.70 Osteophyte, unspecified joint**
- **M25.71 Osteophyte, shoulder**
  - **6th**
    - M25.711   right shoulder
    - M25.712   left shoulder
- **M25.72 Osteophyte, elbow**
  - **6th**
    - M25.721   right elbow
    - M25.722   left elbow
- **M25.73 Osteophyte, wrist**
  - **6th**
    - M25.731   right wrist
    - M25.732   left wrist
- **M25.74 Osteophyte, hand**
  - **6th**
    - M25.741   right hand
    - M25.742   left hand
- **M25.75 Osteophyte, hip**
  - **6th**
    - M25.751   right hip
    - M25.752   left hip
- **M25.76 Osteophyte, knee**
  - **6th**
    - M25.761   right knee
    - M25.762   left knee
- **M25.77 Osteophyte, ankle and foot**
  - **6th**
    - M25.771   right ankle
    - M25.772   left ankle
    - M25.774   right foot
    - M25.775   left foot
- **M25.78 Osteophyte, vertebrae**

M25.9 Joint disorder, unspecified

(M26–M27) DENTOFACIAL ANOMALIES [INCLUDING MALOCCLUSION] AND OTHER DISORDERS OF JAW

Excludes1: hemifacial atrophy or hypertrophy (Q67.4)
   unilateral condylar hyperplasia or hypoplasia (M27.8)

M26 DENTOFACIAL ANOMALIES [INCLUDING MALOCCLUSION]
- **4th**

M26.0 Major anomalies of jaw size
- **5th** *Excludes1:* acromegaly (E22.0)
  -    Robin's syndrome (Q87.0)
- **M26.00 Unspecified anomaly of jaw size**
- **M26.04 Mandibular hypoplasia**
- **M26.09 Other specified anomalies of jaw size**

M26.2 Anomalies of dental arch relationship
- **5th**
- **M26.20 Unspecified anomaly of dental arch relationship**
- **M26.29 Other anomalies of dental arch relationship**
  - Midline deviation of dental arch
  - Overbite (excessive) deep
  - Overbite (excessive) horizontal
  - Overbite (excessive) vertical
  - Posterior lingual occlusion of mandibular teeth

M26.4 Malocclusion, unspecified

M26.6 Temporomandibular joint disorders
- **5th** *Excludes2:* current temporomandibular joint dislocation (S03.0)
  -    current temporomandibular joint sprain (S03.4)
- **M26.60 Temporomandibular joint disorder, unspecified**
  - **6th**
    - M26.601   Right temporomandibular joint disorder
    - M26.602   Left temporomandibular joint disorder
    - M26.603   Bilateral temporomandibular joint disorder
- **M26.61 Adhesions and ankylosis of temporomandibular joint**
  - **6th**
    - M26.611   Adhesions and ankylosis of right temporomandibular joint
    - M26.612   Adhesions and ankylosis of left temporomandibular joint
    - M26.613   Adhesions and ankylosis of bilateral temporomandibular joint
- **M26.62 Arthralgia of temporomandibular joint**
  - **6th**
    - M26.621   Arthralgia of right temporomandibular joint

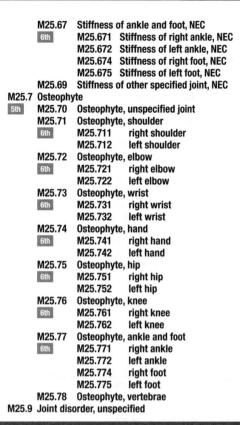

- M26.622   Arthralgia of left temporomandibular joint
- M26.623   Arthralgia of bilateral temporomandibular joint
- **M26.63 Articular disc disorder of temporomandibular joint**
  - **6th**
    - M26.631   Articular disc disorder of right temporomandibular joint
    - M26.632   Articular disc disorder of left temporomandibular joint
    - M26.633   Articular disc disorder of bilateral temporomandibular joint
- **M26.69 Other specified disorders of temporomandibular joint**

M27 OTHER DISEASES OF JAWS
- **4th**
- **M27.0 Developmental disorders of jaws**
  - Latent bone cyst of jaw
  - Stafne's cyst
  - Torus mandibularis
  - Torus palatinus
- **M27.2 Inflammatory conditions of jaws**
  - Osteitis of jaw(s)
  - Osteomyelitis (neonatal) jaw(s)
  - Osteoradionecrosis jaw(s)
  - Periostitis jaw(s)
  - Sequestrum of jaw bone
  - **Use additional code** (W88–W90, X39.0) to identify radiation, if radiation-induced
  - *Excludes2:* osteonecrosis of jaw due to drug (M87.180)
- **M27.4 Other and unspecified cysts of jaw**
  - **5th** *Excludes1:* cysts of oral region (K09.-)
    -    latent bone cyst of jaw (M27.0)
    -    Stafne's cyst (M27.0)
  - **M27.40 Unspecified cyst of jaw**
    - Cyst of jaw NOS
  - **M27.49 Other cysts of jaw**
    - Aneurysmal cyst of jaw
    - Hemorrhagic cyst of jaw
    - Traumatic cyst of jaw
- **M27.8 Other specified diseases of jaws**
  - Cherubism
  - Exostosis
  - Fibrous dysplasia
  - Unilateral condylar hyperplasia
  - Unilateral condylar hypoplasia
  - *Excludes1:* jaw pain (R68.84)

(M30–M36) SYSTEMIC CONNECTIVE TISSUE DISORDERS

Includes: autoimmune disease NOS
   collagen (vascular) disease NOS
   systemic autoimmune disease
   systemic collagen (vascular) disease
Excludes1: autoimmune disease, single organ or single cell type—code to relevant condition category

M30 POLYARTERITIS NODOSA AND RELATED CONDITIONS
- **4th** *Excludes1:* microscopic polyarteritis (M31.7)
- **M30.2 Juvenile polyarteritis**
- **M30.3 Mucocutaneous lymph node syndrome [Kawasaki]**
- **M30.8 Other conditions related to polyarteritis nodosa**
  - Polyangiitis overlap syndrome

M31 OTHER NECROTIZING VASCULOPATHIES
- **4th**
- **M31.0 Hypersensitivity angiitis**
  - Goodpasture's syndrome
- ▲**M31.1 Thrombotic microangiopathy**
  - **5th** •**M31.10 Thrombotic microangiopathy, unspecified**
  - •**M31.11 Hematopoietic stem cell transplantation-associated thrombotic microangiopathy [HSCT-TMA]**
    - Transplant-associated thrombotic microangiopathy [TA-TMA]
    - **Code first** if applicable:
      - complications of bone marrow transplant (T86.0-)
      - complications of stem cell transplant (T86.5)
    - **Use Additional code** to identify specific organ dysfunction, such as:
      - acute kidney failure (N17.-)

4th **5th** **6th** **7th** Additional Character Required   ✔ 3-character code

Unspecified laterality codes were excluded here.   •=New Code   ▲=Revised Code   *Excludes1*—Not coded here, do not use together   *Excludes2*—Not included here

acute respiratory distress syndrome (J80)
capillary leak syndrome (I78.8)
diffuse alveolar hemorrhage (R04.89)
encephalopathy (metabolic) (septic) (G93.41)
fluid overload, unspecified (E87.70)
graft versus host disease (D89.81-)
hemolytic uremic syndrome (D59.3)
hepatic failure (K72.-)
hepatic veno-occlusive disease (K76.5)
idiopathic interstitial pneumonia (J84.11-)
sinusoidal obstruction syndrome (K76.5)
- **M31.19 Other thrombotic microangiopathy**
Thrombotic thrombocytopenic purpura

M31.3 Wegener's granulomatosis
> 5th

Granulomatosis with polyangiitis
Necrotizing respiratory granulomatosis

   M31.30 Wegener's granulomatosis without renal involvement
Wegener's granulomatosis NOS

   M31.31 Wegener's granulomatosis with renal involvement

M31.4 Aortic arch syndrome [Takayasu]

M31.8 Other specified necrotizing vasculopathies
Hypocomplementemic vasculitis
Septic vasculitis

M31.9 Necrotizing vasculopathy, unspecified

M32 SLE
> 4th

Excludes1: lupus erythematosus (discoid) (NOS) (L93.0)

M32.0 Drug-induced systemic lupus erythematosus
Use additional code for adverse effect, if applicable, to identify drug (T36–T50 with fifth or sixth character 5)

M32.1 SLE with organ or system involvement
> 5th

   M32.10 SLE, organ or system involvement unspecified

   M32.11 Endocarditis in SLE
Libman-Sacks disease

   M32.12 Pericarditis in SLE
Lupus pericarditis

   M32.13 Lung involvement in SLE
Pleural effusion due to SLE

   M32.14 Glomerular disease in SLE
Lupus renal disease NOS

   M32.15 Tubulo-interstitial nephropathy in SLE

   M32.19 Other organ or system involvement in SLE

M32.8 Other forms of SLE

M32.9 SLE, unspecified
SLE NOS
SLE NOS
SLE without organ involvement

M33 DERMATOPOLYMYOSITIS
> 4th

M33.0 Juvenile dermatomyositis
> 5th

   M33.00 Juvenile dermatomyositis, organ involvement unspecified

   M33.01 Juvenile dermatomyositis with respiratory involvement

   M33.02 Juvenile dermatomyositis with myopathy

   M33.03 Juvenile dermatomyositis without myopathy

   M33.09 Juvenile dermatomyositis with other organ involvement

M33.1 Other dermatomyositis
> 5th

Adult dermatomyositis

   M33.10 Other dermatomyositis, organ involvement unspecified

   M33.11 Other dermatomyositis with respiratory involvement

   M33.12 Other dermatomyositis with myopathy

   M33.13 Other dermatomyositis without myopathy
Dermatomyositis NOS

   M33.19 Other dermatomyositis with other organ involvement

M33.9 Dermatopolymyositis, unspecified
> 5th

   M33.90 Dermatopolymyositis, unspecified, organ involvement unspecified

   M33.91 Dermatopolymyositis, unspecified with respiratory involvement

   M33.92 Dermatopolymyositis, unspecified with myopathy

   M33.93 Dermatopolymyositis, unspecified without myopathy

   M33.99 Dermatopolymyositis, unspecified with other organ involvement

M35 OTHER SYSTEMIC INVOLVEMENT OF CONNECTIVE TISSUE
> 4th

Excludes1: reactive perforating collagenosis (L87.1)

M35.7 Hypermobility syndrome
Familial ligamentous laxity
Excludes1: Ehlers-Danlos syndromes (Q79.6-)
ligamentous laxity, NOS (M24.2-)

M35.8 Other specified systemic involvement of connective tissue
> 5th

GUIDELINE

See code U07.1 for details.

   M35.81 Multisystem inflammatory syndrome
MIS
MIS-C
Use Additional post COVID-19 condition (U09.9)

-    **M35.89 Other specified systemic involvement of connective tissue**

M35.9 Systemic involvement of connective tissue, unspecified
Autoimmune disease (systemic) NOS
Collagen (vascular) disease NOS

M36 SYSTEMIC DISORDERS OF CONNECTIVE TISSUE IN DISEASES CLASSIFIED ELSEWHERE
> 4th

Excludes2: arthropathies in diseases classified elsewhere (M14.-)

M36.0 Dermato(poly)myositis in neoplastic disease
Code first underlying neoplasm (C00-D49)

M36.1 Arthropathy in neoplastic disease
Code first underlying neoplasm, such as:
leukemia (C91-C95)
malignant histiocytosis (C96.A)
multiple myeloma (C90.0)

M36.2 Hemophilic arthropathy
Hemarthrosis in hemophilic arthropathy
Code first: underlying disease, such as: factor VIII deficiency (D66)
with vascular defect (D68.0)
factor IX deficiency (D67)
hemophilia (classical) (D66)
hemophilia B (D67)
hemophilia C (D68.1)

M36.3 Arthropathy in other blood disorders

M36.4 Arthropathy in hypersensitivity reactions classified elsewhere
Code first underlying disease, such as Henoch (-Schönlein)
purpura (D69.0)
serum sickness (T80.6-)

M36.8 Systemic disorders of connective tissue in other diseases classified elsewhere
Code first underlying disease, such as:
alkaptonuria (E70.2)
hypogammaglobulinemia (D80.-)
ochronosis (E70.2)

(M40–M43) DEFORMING DORSOPATHIES

M40 KYPHOSIS AND LORDOSIS
> 4th

Code first underlying disease
Excludes1: congenital kyphosis and lordosis (Q76.4)
kyphoscoliosis (M41.-)
postprocedural kyphosis and lordosis (M96.-)

M40.2 Other and unspecified kyphosis
> 5th

   M40.20 Unspecified kyphosis
> 6th

	M40.202	cervical region
	M40.203	cervicothoracic region
	M40.204	thoracic region
	M40.205	thoracolumbar region
	M40.209	site unspecified

   M40.29 Other kyphosis
> 6th

	M40.292	cervical region
	M40.293	cervicothoracic region
	M40.294	thoracic region
	M40.295	thoracolumbar region
	M40.299	site unspecified

CHAPTER 13. DISEASES OF THE MUSCULOSKELETAL SYSTEM AND CONNECTIVE TISSUE (M31.19–M40.299)

4th 5th 6th 7th Additional Character Required	✓ 3-character code	Unspecified laterality codes were excluded here.	•=New Code ▲=Revised Code	***Excludes1***—Not coded here, do not use together ***Excludes2***—Not included here

M40.4 Postural lordosis
`5th` Acquired lordosis
- **M40.40**   **site unspecified**
- **M40.45**   **thoracolumbar region**
- **M40.46**   **lumbar region**
- **M40.47**   **lumbosacral region**

M40.5 Lordosis, unspecified
`5th`
- **M40.50**   **site unspecified**
- **M40.55**   **thoracolumbar region**
- **M40.56**   **lumbar region**
- **M40.57**   **lumbosacral region**

M41   SCOLIOSIS
`4th`
Includes: kyphoscoliosis
Excludes1: congenital scoliosis NOS (Q67.5)
     congenital scoliosis due to bony malformation (Q76.3)
     postural congenital scoliosis (Q67.5)
     kyphoscoliotic heart disease (I27.1)
Excludes2: postprocedural scoliosis (M96.-)

M41.0 Infantile idiopathic scoliosis
`5th`
- **M41.00**   **site unspecified**
- **M41.02**   **cervical region**
- **M41.03**   **cervicothoracic region**
- **M41.04**   **thoracic region**
- **M41.05**   **thoracolumbar region**
- **M41.06**   **lumbar region**
- **M41.07**   **lumbosacral region**
- **M41.08**   **sacral and sacrococcygeal region**

M41.1 Juvenile and adolescent idiopathic scoliosis
`5th`
- **M41.11**   **Juvenile idiopathic scoliosis**
  `6th`
  - **M41.112**   **cervical region**
  - **M41.113**   **cervicothoracic region**
  - **M41.114**   **thoracic region**
  - **M41.115**   **thoracolumbar region**
  - **M41.116**   **lumbar region**
  - **M41.117**   **lumbosacral region**
  - **M41.119**   **site unspecified**
- **M41.12**   **Adolescent scoliosis**
  `6th`
  - **M41.122**   **Adolescent idiopathic scoliosis, cervical region**
  - **M41.123**   **Adolescent idiopathic scoliosis, cervicothoracic region**
  - **M41.124**   **Adolescent idiopathic scoliosis, thoracic region**
  - **M41.125**   **Adolescent idiopathic scoliosis, thoracolumbar region**
  - **M41.126**   **Adolescent idiopathic scoliosis, lumbar region**
  - **M41.127**   **Adolescent idiopathic scoliosis, lumbosacral region**
  - **M41.129**   **Adolescent idiopathic scoliosis, site unspecified**

M41.2 Other idiopathic scoliosis
`5th`
- **M41.20**   **Other idiopathic scoliosis, site unspecified**
- **M41.22**   **cervical region**
- **M41.23**   **cervicothoracic region**
- **M41.24**   **thoracic region**
- **M41.25**   **thoracolumbar region**
- **M41.26**   **lumbar region**
- **M41.27**   **lumbosacral region**

M41.9 Scoliosis, unspecified

M43   OTHER DEFORMING DORSOPATHIES
`4th`
Excludes1: congenital spondylolysis and spondylolisthesis (Q76.2)
     hemivertebra (Q76.3–Q76.4)
     Klippel-Feil syndrome (Q76.1)
     lumbarization and sacralization (Q76.4)
     platyspondylisis (Q76.4)
     spina bifida occulta (Q76.0)
     spinal curvature in osteoporosis (M80.-)
     spinal curvature in Paget's disease of bone [osteitis deformans] (M88.-)

M43.0 Spondylolysis
`5th`
Excludes1: congenital spondylolysis (Q76.2)
     spondylolisthesis (M43.1)
- **M43.00**   **Spondylolysis, site unspecified**

- **M43.01**   **occipito-atlanto-axial region**
- **M43.02**   **cervical region**
- **M43.03**   **cervicothoracic region**
- **M43.04**   **thoracic region**
- **M43.05**   **thoracolumbar region**
- **M43.06**   **lumbar region**
- **M43.07**   **lumbosacral region**
- **M43.08**   **sacral and sacrococcygeal region**
- **M43.09**   **multiple sites in spine**

M43.1 Spondylolisthesis
`5th`
Excludes1: acute traumatic of lumbosacral region (S33.1)
     acute traumatic of sites other than lumbosacral- code to
       Fracture, vertebra, by region
     congenital spondylolisthesis (Q76.2)
- **M43.10**   **Spondylolisthesis, site unspecified**
- **M43.11**   **occipito-atlanto-axial region**
- **M43.12**   **cervical region**
- **M43.13**   **cervicothoracic region**
- **M43.14**   **thoracic region**
- **M43.15**   **thoracolumbar region**
- **M43.16**   **lumbar region**
- **M43.17**   **lumbosacral region**
- **M43.18**   **sacral and sacrococcygeal region**
- **M43.19**   **multiple sites in spine**

M43.6 Torticollis
Excludes1: congenital (sternomastoid) torticollis (Q68.0)
     current injury — see Injury, of spine, by body region
     ocular torticollis (R29.891)
     psychogenic torticollis (F45.8)
     spasmodic torticollis (G24.3)
     torticollis due to birth injury (P15.2)

(M45–M49) SPONDYLOPATHIES

M48   OTHER SPONDYLOPATHIES
`4th`
M48.0 Spinal stenosis
`5th` Caudal stenosis
- **M48.00**   **Spinal stenosis, site unspecified**
- **M48.01**   **Spinal stenosis, occipito-atlanto-axial region**
- **M48.02**   **Spinal stenosis, cervical region**
- **M48.03**   **Spinal stenosis, cervicothoracic region**
- **M48.04**   **Spinal stenosis, thoracic region**
- **M48.05**   **Spinal stenosis, thoracolumbar region**
- **M48.06**   **Spinal stenosis, lumbar region**
  `6th`
  - **M48.061**   **Spinal stenosis, lumbar region without neurogenic claudication**
    Spinal stenosis, lumbar region NOS
  - **M48.062**   **Spinal stenosis, lumbar region with neurogenic claudication**
- **M48.07**   **Spinal stenosis, lumbosacral region**
- **M48.08**   **Spinal stenosis, sacral and sacrococcygeal region**

(M50–M54) OTHER DORSOPATHIES

Excludes1: current injury — see injury of spine by body region
     discitis NOS (M46.4-)

M53   OTHER AND UNSPECIFIED DORSOPATHIES, NOT
`4th`   **ELSEWHERE CLASSIFIED**
M53.3 Sacrococcygeal disorders, not elsewhere classified
     Coccygodynia
M53.9 Dorsopathy, unspecified

M54   DORSALGIA
`4th`
Excludes1: psychogenic dorsalgia (F45.41)
M54.2 Cervicalgia
     Excludes1: cervicalgia due to intervertebral cervical disc disorder
       (M50.-)
M54.4 Lumbago with sciatica
`5th`
     Excludes1: lumbago with sciatica due to intervertebral disc
       disorder (M51.1-)
- **M54.40**   **Lumbago with sciatica, unspecified side**
- **M54.41**   **Lumbago with sciatica, right side**
- **M54.42**   **Lumbago with sciatica, left side**

`4th` `5th` `6th` `7th` Additional Character Required   ✓ 3-character code

Unspecified laterality codes were excluded here.   •=New Code   ▲=Revised Code   *Excludes1*—Not coded here, do not use together   *Excludes2*—Not included here

▲**M54.5 Low back pain**
5th ***Excludes1:*** low back strain (S39.012)
  lumbago due to intervertebral disc displacement (M51.2-)
  lumbago with sciatica (M54.4-)
 •**M54.50** **Low back pain, unspecified**
   Loin pain
   Lumbago NOS
 •**M54.51** **Vertebrogenic low back pain**
   Low back vertebral endplate pain
 •**M54.59** **Other low back pain**
M54.9 Dorsalgia, unspecified
 Backache NOS
 Back pain NOS

(M60–M79) SOFT TISSUE DISORDERS

(M60–M63) DISORDERS OF MUSCLES

M60 MYOSITIS
4th ***Excludes2:*** inclusion body myositis [IBM] (G72.41)
 M60.0 Infective myositis
 5th Tropical pyomyositis
  Use additional code (B95–B97) to identify infectious agent
  M60.00 **Infective myositis, unspecified site**
  6th **M60.000** **unspecified right arm**
      Infective myositis, right upper limb NOS
    M60.001 **unspecified left arm**
      Infective myositis, left upper limb NOS
    M60.003 **unspecified right leg**
      Infective myositis, right lower limb NOS
    M60.004 **unspecified left leg**
      Infective myositis, left lower limb NOS
    M60.009 **unspecified site**
  M60.01 **Infective myositis, shoulder**
  6th **M60.011** **right shoulder**
    M60.012 **left shoulder**
  M60.02 **Infective myositis, upper arm**
  6th **M60.021** **right upper arm**
    M60.022 **left upper arm**
  M60.03 **Infective myositis, forearm**
  6th **M60.031** **right forearm**
    M60.032 **left forearm**
  M60.04 **Infective myositis, hand and fingers**
  6th **M60.041** **right hand**
    M60.042 **left hand**
    M60.044 **right finger(s)**
    M60.045 **left finger(s)**
  M60.05 **Infective myositis, thigh**
  6th **M60.051** **right thigh**
    M60.052 **left thigh**
  M60.06 **Infective myositis, lower leg**
  6th **M60.061** **right lower leg**
    M60.062 **left lower leg**
  M60.07 **Infective myositis, ankle, foot and toes**
  6th **M60.070** **right ankle**
    M60.071 **left ankle**
    M60.073 **right foot**
    M60.074 **left foot**
    M60.076 **right toe(s)**
    M60.077 **left toe(s)**
  M60.08 **Infective myositis, other site**
  M60.09 **Infective myositis, multiple sites**
 M60.1 Interstitial myositis
 5th **M60.10** **Interstitial myositis of unspecified site**
  M60.11 **Interstitial myositis, shoulder**
  6th **M60.111** **right shoulder**
    M60.112 **left shoulder**
  M60.12 **Interstitial myositis, upper arm**
  6th **M60.121** **right upper arm**
    M60.122 **left upper arm**
  M60.13 **Interstitial myositis, forearm**
  6th **M60.131** **right forearm**
    M60.132 **left forearm**

  M60.14 **Interstitial myositis, hand**
  6th **M60.141** **right hand**
    M60.142 **left hand**
  M60.15 **Interstitial myositis, thigh**
  6th **M60.151** **right thigh**
    M60.152 **left thigh**
  M60.16 **Interstitial myositis, lower leg**
  6th **M60.161** **right lower leg**
    M60.162 **left lower leg**
 M60.2 Foreign body granuloma of soft tissue, not elsewhere
 5th **classified**
  Use additional code to identify the type of retained foreign body
  (Z18.-)
  Excludes1: foreign body granuloma of skin and subcutaneous
  tissue (L92.3)
  M60.21 **Foreign body granuloma of soft tissue, NEC, shoulder**
  6th **M60.211** **right shoulder**
    M60.212 **left shoulder**
  M60.22 **Foreign body granuloma of soft tissue, NEC, upper**
  6th **arm**
    M60.221 **right upper arm**
    M60.222 **left upper arm**
  M60.23 **Foreign body granuloma of soft tissue, NEC, forearm**
  6th **M60.231** **right forearm**
    M60.232 **left forearm**
  M60.24 **Foreign body granuloma of soft tissue, NEC, hand**
  6th **M60.241** **right hand**
    M60.242 **left hand**
  M60.25 **Foreign body granuloma of soft tissue, NEC, thigh**
  6th **M60.251** **right thigh**
    M60.252 **left thigh**
  M60.26 **Foreign body granuloma of soft tissue, NEC, lower**
  6th **leg**
    M60.261 **right lower leg**
    M60.262 **left lower leg**
  M60.27 **Foreign body granuloma of soft tissue, NEC, ankle**
  6th **and foot**
    M60.271 **right ankle and foot**
    M60.272 **left ankle and foot**
  M60.28 **Foreign body granuloma of soft tissue, NEC, other**
    site
 M60.9 Myositis, unspecified

M62 OTHER DISORDERS OF MUSCLE
4th ***Excludes1:*** alcoholic myopathy (G72.1)
  cramp and spasm (R25.2)
  drug-induced myopathy (G72.0)
  myalgia (M79.1-)
  stiff-man syndrome (G25.82)
 Excludes2: nontraumatic hematoma of muscle (M79.81)
 M62.4 Contracture of muscle
 5th Contracture of tendon (sheath)
  Excludes1: contracture of joint (M24.5-)
  M62.40 **Contracture of muscle, unspecified site**
  M62.41 **Contracture of muscle, shoulder**
  6th **M62.411** **right shoulder**
    M62.412 **left shoulder**
  M62.42 **Contracture of muscle, upper arm**
  6th **M62.421** **right upper arm**
    M62.422 **left upper arm**
  M62.43 **Contracture of muscle, forearm**
  6th **M62.431** **right forearm**
    M62.432 **left forearm**
  M62.44 **Contracture of muscle, hand**
  6th **M62.441** **right hand**
    M62.442 **left hand**
  M62.45 **Contracture of muscle, thigh**
  6th **M62.451** **right thigh**
    M62.452 **left thigh**
  M62.46 **Contracture of muscle, lower leg**
  6th **M62.461** **right lower leg**
    M62.462 **left lower leg**
  M62.47 **Contracture of muscle, ankle and foot**
  6th **M62.471** **right ankle and foot**

4th **5th** **6th** **7th** Additional Character Required ✓ **3-character code**

Unspecified laterality codes •=New Code ***Excludes1***—Not coded here, do not use together
were excluded here. ▲=Revised Code ***Excludes2***—Not included here

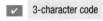

CHAPTER 13. DISEASES OF THE MUSCULOSKELETAL SYSTEM AND CONNECTIVE TISSUE (M62.472–M71.9)

         M62.472   **left ankle and foot**
    M62.48   **Contracture of muscle, other site**
    M62.49   **Contracture of muscle, multiple sites**
M62.8 **Other specified disorders of muscle**
   5th   *Excludes2:* nontraumatic hematoma of muscle (M79.81)
    M62.81   **Muscle weakness (generalized)**
        Excludes1: muscle weakness in sarcopenia (M62.84)
    M62.82   **Rhabdomyolysis**
        Excludes1: traumatic rhabdomyolysis (T79.6)
    M62.83   **Muscle spasm**
     6th   M62.830   **Muscle spasm of back**
        M62.831   **Muscle spasm of calf**
          Charley-horse
        M62.838   **Other muscle spasm**
    M62.89   **Other specified disorders of muscle**
        Muscle (sheath) hernia
M62.9   **Disorder of muscle, unspecified**

(M65–M67) DISORDERS OF SYNOVIUM AND TENDON

M65   **SYNOVITIS AND TENOSYNOVITIS**
4th   *Excludes1:* chronic crepitant synovitis of hand and wrist (M70.0-)
     current injury — see injury of ligament or tendon by body region
     soft tissue disorders related to use, overuse and pressure (M70.-)
M65.4 **Radial styloid tenosynovitis [de Quervain]**
M65.8 **Other synovitis and tenosynovitis**
  5th   M65.80   **Other synovitis and tenosynovitis, unspecified site**
    M65.81   **Other synovitis and tenosynovitis; shoulder**
     6th   M65.811   **right shoulder**
        M65.812   **left shoulder**
    M65.82   **Other synovitis and tenosynovitis; upper arm**
     6th   M65.821   **right upper arm**
        M65.822   **left upper arm**
    M65.83   **Other synovitis and tenosynovitis; forearm**
     6th   M65.831   **right forearm**
        M65.832   **left forearm**
    M65.84   **Other synovitis and tenosynovitis; hand**
     6th   M65.841   **right hand**
        M65.842   **left hand**
    M65.85   **Other synovitis and tenosynovitis; thigh**
     6th   M65.851   **right thigh**
        M65.852   **left thigh**
    M65.86   **Other synovitis and tenosynovitis; lower leg**
     6th   M65.861   **right lower leg**
        M65.862   **left lower leg**
    M65.87   **Other synovitis and tenosynovitis; ankle and foot**
     6th   M65.871   **right ankle and foot**
        M65.872   **left ankle and foot**
    M65.88   **Other synovitis and tenosynovitis, other site**
    M65.89   **Other synovitis and tenosynovitis, multiple sites**
M65.9 **Synovitis and tenosynovitis, unspecified**

M67   **OTHER DISORDERS OF SYNOVIUM AND TENDON**
4th   *Excludes1:* palmar fascial fibromatosis [Dupuytren] (M72.0)
     tendinitis NOS (M77.9-)
     xanthomatosis localized to tendons (E78.2)
M67.0 **Short Achilles tendon (acquired)**
  5th   M67.01   **right ankle**
    M67.02   **left ankle**
M67.4 **Ganglion**
  5th   Ganglion of joint or tendon (sheath)
    Excludes1: ganglion in yaws (A66.6)
    Excludes2: cyst of bursa (M71.2– M71.3)
     cyst of synovium (M71.2–M71.3)
    M67.40   **Ganglion, unspecified site**
    M67.41   **Ganglion, shoulder**
     6th   M67.411   **right shoulder**
        M67.412   **left shoulder**
    M67.42   **Ganglion, elbow**
     6th   M67.421   **right elbow**
        M67.422   **left elbow**
    M67.43   **Ganglion, wrist**
     6th   M67.431   **right wrist**
        M67.432   **left wrist**

    M67.44   **Ganglion, hand**
     6th   M67.441   **right hand**
        M67.442   **left hand**
    M67.45   **Ganglion, hip**
     6th   M67.451   **right hip**
        M67.452   **left hip**
    M67.46   **Ganglion, knee**
     6th   M67.461   **right knee**
        M67.462   **left knee**
    M67.47   **Ganglion, ankle and foot**
     6th   M67.471   **right ankle and foot**
        M67.472   **left ankle and foot**
    M67.48   **Ganglion, other site**
    M67.49   **Ganglion, multiple sites**

(M70–M79) OTHER SOFT TISSUE DISORDERS

M70   **SOFT TISSUE DISORDERS RELATED TO USE, OVERUSE**
4th   **AND PRESSURE**
    Includes: soft tissue disorders of occupational origin
    Use additional external cause code to identify activity causing disorder
     (Y93.-)
    Excludes1: bursitis NOS (M71.9-)
    Excludes2: bursitis of shoulder (M75.5)
     enthesopathies (M76-M77)
     pressure ulcer (pressure area) (L89.-)
M70.3 **Other bursitis of elbow**
  5th   M70.31   **right elbow**
    M70.32   **left elbow**
M70.6 **Trochanteric bursitis**
  5th   Trochanteric tendinitis
    M70.61   **right hip**
    M70.62   **left hip**
M70.7 **Other bursitis of hip**
  5th   Ischial bursitis
    M70.71   **right hip**
    M70.72   **left hip**

M71   **OTHER BURSOPATHIES**
4th   *Excludes1:* bunion (M20.1)
     bursitis related to use, overuse or pressure (M70.-)
     enthesopathies (M76–M77)
M71.2 **Synovial cyst of popliteal space [Baker]**
  5th   *Excludes1:* synovial cyst of popliteal space with rupture (M66.0)
    M71.21   **right knee**
    M71.22   **left knee**
M71.5 **Other bursitis, NEC**
  5th   *Excludes1:* bursitis NOS (M71.9-)
    Excludes2: bursitis of shoulder (M75.5)
     bursitis of tibial collateral [Pellegrini-Stieda] (M76.4-)
    M71.50   **unspecified site**
    M71.52   **elbow**
     6th   M71.521   **right elbow**
        M71.522   **left elbow**
    M71.53   **wrist**
     6th   M71.531   **right wrist**
        M71.532   **left wrist**
    M71.54   **hand**
     6th   M71.541   **right hand**
        M71.542   **left hand**
    M71.55   **hip**
     6th   M71.551   **right hip**
        M71.552   **left hip**
    M71.56   **knee**
     6th   M71.561   **right knee**
        M71.562   **left knee**
    M71.57   **ankle and foot**
     6th   M71.571   **right ankle and foot**
        M71.572   **left ankle and foot**
    M71.58   **other site**
M71.9 **Bursopathy, unspecified**
    Bursitis NOS

 4th **5th** **6th** **7th** Additional Character Required   ✔   3-character code

Unspecified laterality codes   •=New Code   *Excludes1*—Not coded here, do not use together
were excluded here.   ▲=Revised Code   *Excludes2*—Not included here

M72   FIBROBLASTIC DISORDERS
`4th`
  Excludes2: retroperitoneal fibromatosis (D48.3)
  M72.6 Necrotizing fasciitis
      Use additional code (B95.-, B96.-) to identify causative organism
  M72.8 Other fibroblastic disorders
      Abscess of fascia
      Fasciitis NEC
      Other infective fasciitis
      Use additional code to (B95.-, B96.-) identify causative organism
      Excludes1: diffuse (eosinophilic) fasciitis (M35.4)
          necrotizing fasciitis (M72.6)
          nodular fasciitis (M72.4)
          perirenal fasciitis NOS (N13.5)
          perirenal fasciitis with infection (N13.6)
          plantar fasciitis (M72.2)
  M72.9 Fibroblastic disorder, unspecified
      Fasciitis NOS
      Fibromatosis NOS

M75   SHOULDER LESIONS
`4th`
  M75.1 Rotator cuff tear or rupture, not specified as traumatic
    `5th`   Rotator cuff syndrome
            Supraspinatus tear or rupture, not specified as traumatic
            Supraspinatus syndrome
            Excludes1: tear of rotator cuff, traumatic (S46.01-)
            Excludes2: shoulder-hand syndrome (M89.0-)
        M75.10   Unspecified rotator cuff tear or rupture, not specified
        `6th`   **as traumatic**
                **M75.101   Unspecified rotator cuff tear or rupture of
                            right shoulder, not specified as traumatic**
                **M75.102   Unspecified rotator cuff tear or rupture of
                            left shoulder, not specified as traumatic**
        M75.11   Incomplete rotator cuff tear or rupture not specified
        `6th`   **as traumatic**
                **M75.111   Incomplete rotator cuff tear or rupture of
                            right shoulder, not specified as traumatic**
                **M75.112   Incomplete rotator cuff tear or rupture of
                            left shoulder, not specified as traumatic**
        M75.12   Complete rotator cuff tear or rupture not specified as
        `6th`   **traumatic**
                **M75.121   Complete rotator cuff tear or rupture of
                            right shoulder, not specified as traumatic**
                **M75.122   Complete rotator cuff tear or rupture of
                            left shoulder, not specified as traumatic**

M76   ENTHESOPATHIES, LOWER LIMB, EXCLUDING FOOT
`4th`
  Excludes2: bursitis due to use, overuse and pressure (M70.-)
      enthesopathies of ankle and foot (M77.5-)
  M76.0 Gluteal tendinitis
    `5th`   **M76.01   right hip**
            M76.02   left hip
  M76.1 Psoas tendinitis
    `5th`   **M76.11   right hip**
            M76.12   left hip
  M76.2 Iliac crest spur
    `5th`   **M76.21   right hip**
            M76.22   left hip
  M76.3 Iliotibial band syndrome
    `5th`   **M76.31   right leg**
            M76.32   left leg
  M76.4 Tibial collateral bursitis [Pellegrini-Stieda]
    `5th`   **M76.41   right leg**
            M76.42   left leg
  M76.6 Achilles tendinitis
    `5th`   Achilles bursitis
            M76.61   right leg
            M76.62   left leg
  M76.7 Peroneal tendinitis
    `5th`   **M76.71   right leg**
            M76.72   left leg
  M76.8 Other specified enthesopathies of lower limb, excluding foot
    `5th`   **M76.81   Anterior tibial syndrome**
        `6th`   **M76.811   right leg**
                    M76.812   left leg

M76.82   Posterior tibial tendinitis
`6th`   **M76.821   right leg**
           M76.822   left leg
M76.89   Other specified enthesopathies of lower limb,
`6th`   **excluding foot**
               **M76.891   Other specified enthesopathies of right
                           lower limb, excluding foot**
               **M76.892   Other specified enthesopathies of left
                           lower limb, excluding foot**
M76.9 Unspecified enthesopathy, lower limb, excluding foot

M77   OTHER ENTHESOPATHIES
`4th`
  Excludes1: bursitis NOS (M71.9-)
  Excludes2: bursitis due to use, overuse and pressure (M70.-)
      osteophyte (M25.7)
      spinal enthesopathy (M46.0-)
  M77.0 Medial epicondylitis
    `5th`   **M77.01   right elbow**
            M77.02   left elbow
  M77.1 Lateral epicondylitis
    `5th`   Tennis elbow
            M77.11   right elbow
            M77.12   left elbow
  M77.5 Other enthesopathy of foot and ankle
    `5th`   **M77.51   Other enthesopathy of right foot and ankle**
            M77.52   Other enthesopathy of left foot and ankle
  M77.8 Other enthesopathies, NEC
  M77.9 Enthesopathy, unspecified
      Bone spur NOS
      Capsulitis NOS
      Periarthritis NOS
      Tendinitis NOS

M79   OTHER AND UNSPECIFIED SOFT TISSUE DISORDERS,
`4th` **NEC**
  Excludes1: psychogenic rheumatism (F45.8)
      soft tissue pain, psychogenic (F45.41)
  M79.0 Rheumatism, unspecified
      Excludes1: fibromyalgia (M79.7)
          palindromic rheumatism (M12.3-)
  M79.1 Myalgia
    `5th`   Myofascial pain syndrome
            Excludes1: fibromyalgia (M79.7)
                myositis (M60.-)
        M79.10   Myalgia, unspecified site
        M79.11   Myalgia of mastication muscle
        M79.12   Myalgia of auxiliary muscles, head and neck
        M79.18   Myalgia, other site
  M79.2 Neuralgia and neuritis, unspecified
      Excludes1: brachial radiculitis NOS (M54.1)
          lumbosacral radiculitis NOS (M54.1)
          mononeuropathies (G56-G58)
          radiculitis NOS (M54.1)
          sciatica (M54.3-M54.4)
  M79.5 Residual foreign body in soft tissue
      Excludes1: foreign body granuloma of skin and subcutaneous
          tissue (L92.3)
          foreign body granuloma of soft tissue (M60.2-)
  M79.6 Pain in limb, hand, foot, fingers and toes
    `5th`   *Excludes2:* pain in joint (M25.5-)
        M79.60   Pain in limb, unspecified
        `6th`   **M79.601   Pain in right arm**
                            Pain in right upper limb NOS
                    M79.602   Pain in left arm
                            Pain in left upper limb NOS
                    M79.604   Pain in right leg
                            Pain in right lower limb NOS
                    M79.605   Pain in left leg
                            Pain in left lower limb NOS
        M79.62   Pain in upper arm
        `6th`   Pain in axillary region
                    M79.621   Pain in right upper arm
                    M79.622   Pain in left upper arm
        M79.63   Pain in forearm
        `6th`

`4th` `5th` `6th` `7th` Additional Character Required   ✔ 3-character code

Unspecified laterality codes   •=New Code   *Excludes1*—Not coded here, do not use together
were excluded here.   ▲=Revised Code   *Excludes2*—Not included here

CHAPTER 13. DISEASES OF THE MUSCULOSKELETAL SYSTEM AND CONNECTIVE TISSUE   (M79.631–M85.2)

                      M79.631   Pain in right forearm
                      M79.632   Pain in left forearm

M79.64   Pain in hand and fingers
  [6th]
       M79.641   Pain in right hand
       M79.642   Pain in left hand
       M79.644   Pain in right finger(s)
       M79.645   Pain in left finger(s)

M79.65   Pain in thigh
  [6th]
       M79.651   Pain in right thigh
       M79.652   Pain in left thigh

M79.66   Pain in lower leg
  [6th]
       M79.661   Pain in right lower leg
       M79.662   Pain in left lower leg

M79.67   Pain in foot and toes
  [6th]
       M79.671   Pain in right foot
       M79.672   Pain in left foot
       M79.674   Pain in right toe(s)
       M79.675   Pain in left toe(s)

M79.8 Other specified soft tissue disorders
  [5th]   **M79.81**   **Nontraumatic hematoma of soft tissue**
            Nontraumatic hematoma of muscle
            Nontraumatic seroma of muscle and soft tissue

      M79.89   **Other specified soft tissue disorders**
            Polyalgia

M79.9 Soft tissue disorder, unspecified

(M80–M94) OSTEOPATHIES AND CHONDROPATHIES
(M80–M85) DISORDERS OF BONE DENSITY AND STRUCTURE

M84   **DISORDER OF CONTINUITY OF BONE**
[4th]

GUIDELINES

Coding of Pathologic Fractures

7th character A is for use as long as the patient is receiving active treatment for the fracture. Examples of active treatment are: surgical treatment, emergency department encounter, evaluation and continuing treatment by the same or a different physician. While the patient may be seen by a new or different provider over the course of treatment for a pathological fracture, assignment of the 7th character is based on whether the patient is undergoing active treatment and not whether the provider is seeing the patient for the first time. 7th character, D is to be used for encounters after the patient has completed active treatment for the fracture and is receiving routine care for the fracture during the healing or recovery phase. The other 7th characters, listed under each subcategory in the Tabular List, are to be used for subsequent encounters for treatment of problems associated with the healing, such as malunions, nonunions, and sequelae.

Care for complications of surgical treatment for fracture repairs during the healing or recovery phase should be coded with the appropriate complication codes.

Excludes2: traumatic fracture of bone-see fracture, by site

M84.3 Stress fracture
[5th]
    Fatigue fracture
    March fracture
    Stress fracture NOS
    Stress reaction
    Use additional external cause code(s) to identify the cause of the stress fracture

M84 requires 7th character to identify the encounter type
A—initial encounter for fracture care
D—subsequent encounter with routine healing
G—subsequent encounter for fracture with delayed healing
K—subsequent encounter for fracture with nonunion
P—subsequent encounter for fracture with malunion
S—sequela

    Excludes1: pathological fracture NOS (M84.4.-)
        pathological fracture due to osteoporosis (M80.-)
        traumatic fracture (S12.-, S22.-, S32.-, S42.-, S52.-, S62.-, S72.-, S82.-, S92.-)
    Excludes2: personal history of (healed) stress (fatigue) fracture (Z87.312)
        stress fracture of vertebra (M48.4-)
        M84.30X   **Stress fracture, unspecified site**
          [7th]

M84.31   **Stress fracture, shoulder**
  [6th]   **M84.311**   Stress fracture, right shoulder
       [7th]
       M84.312   Stress fracture, left shoulder
       [7th]

M84.32   **Stress fracture, humerus**
  [6th]   **M84.321**   Stress fracture, right humerus
       [7th]
       M84.322   Stress fracture, left humerus
       [7th]

M84.33   **Stress fracture, ulna and radius**
  [6th]   **M84.331**   Stress fracture, right ulna
       [7th]
       M84.332   Stress fracture, left ulna
       [7th]
       M84.333   Stress fracture, right radius
       [7th]
       M84.334   Stress fracture, left radius
       [7th]

M84.34   **Stress fracture, hand and fingers**
  [6th]   **M84.341**   Stress fracture, right hand
       [7th]
       M84.342   Stress fracture, left hand
       [7th]
       M84.344   Stress fracture, right finger(s)
       [7th]
       M84.345   Stress fracture, left finger(s)
       [7th]

M84.35   **Stress fracture, pelvis and femur**
  [6th]   Stress fracture, hip
       M84.350   Stress fracture, pelvis
       [7th]
       M84.351   Stress fracture, right femur
       [7th]
       M84.352   Stress fracture, left femur
       [7th]
       M84.359   Stress fracture, hip, unspecified
       [7th]

M84.36   **Stress fracture, tibia and fibula**
  [6th]   **M84.361**   Stress fracture, right tibia
       [7th]
       M84.362   Stress fracture, left tibia
       [7th]
       M84.363   Stress fracture, right fibula
       [7th]
       M84.364   Stress fracture, left fibula
       [7th]

M84.37   **Stress fracture, ankle, foot and toes**
  [6th]   **M84.371**   Stress fracture, right ankle
       [7th]
       M84.372   Stress fracture, left ankle
       [7th]
       M84.374   Stress fracture, right foot
       [7th]
       M84.375   Stress fracture, left foot
       [7th]
       M84.377   Stress fracture, right toe(s)
       [7th]
       M84.378   Stress fracture, left toe(s)
       [7th]
       M84.38X   Stress fracture, other site
       [7th]   *Excludes2:* stress fracture of vertebra (M48.4-)

      M84.88   **Other disorders of continuity of bone, other site**

M85   **OTHER DISORDERS OF BONE DENSITY AND STRUCTURE**
[4th]   *Excludes1:* osteogenesis imperfecta (Q78.0)
      osteopetrosis (Q78.2)
      osteopoikilosis (Q78.8)
      polyostotic fibrous dysplasia (Q78.1)

M85.2 Hyperostosis of skull

[4th] [5th] [6th] [7th] Additional Character Required   ☑ 3-character code

Unspecified laterality codes were excluded here.   •=New Code   ▲=Revised Code   ***Excludes1***—Not coded here, do not use together   ***Excludes2***—Not included here

M85.6   **Other cyst of bone**
`5th`   ***Excludes1:*** cyst of jaw NEC (M27.4)

osteitis fibrosa cystica generalisata [von Recklinghausen's disease of bone] (E21.0)

M85.60   **Other cyst of bone, unspecified site**
M85.61   **Other cyst of bone, shoulder**
`6th`   **M85.611**   **right shoulder**
     M85.612   **left shoulder**
M85.62   **Other cyst of bone, upper arm**
`6th`   **M85.621**   **right upper arm**
     M85.622   **left upper arm**
M85.63   **Other cyst of bone, forearm**
`6th`   **M85.631**   **right forearm**
     M85.632   **left forearm**
M85.64   **Other cyst of bone, hand**
`6th`   **M85.641**   **right hand**
     M85.642   **left hand**
M85.65   **Other cyst of bone, thigh**
`6th`   **M85.651**   **right thigh**
     M85.652   **left thigh**
M85.66   **Other cyst of bone, lower leg**
`6th`   **M85.661**   **right lower leg**
     M85.662   **left lower leg**
M85.67   **Other cyst of bone, ankle and foot**
`6th`   **M85.671**   **right ankle and foot**
     M85.672   **left ankle and foot**
M85.68   **Other cyst of bone, other site**
M85.69   **Other cyst of bone, multiple sites**

(M86–M90) OTHER OSTEOPATHIES

Excludes1: postprocedural osteopathies (M96.-)

M86   **OSTEOMYELITIS**
`4th`   **Use additional code** (B95–B97) to identify infectious agent
Use additional code to identify major osseous defect, if applicable (M89.7-)
Excludes1: osteomyelitis due to:
Echinococcus (B67.2)
gonococcus (A54.43)
Salmonella (A02.24)
Excludes2: osteomyelitis of:
orbit (H05.0-)
petrous bone (H70.2-)
vertebra (M46.2-)

M86.1   **Other acute osteomyelitis**
`5th`   **M86.10**   **Other acute osteomyelitis, unspecified site**
   M86.11   **Other acute osteomyelitis, shoulder**
`6th`   **M86.111**   **right shoulder**
     M86.112   **left shoulder**
   M86.12   **Other acute osteomyelitis, humerus**
`6th`   **M86.121**   **right humerus**
     M86.122   **left humerus**
   M86.13   **Other acute osteomyelitis, radius and ulna**
`6th`   **M86.131**   **right radius and ulna**
     M86.132   **left radius and ulna**
   M86.14   **Other acute osteomyelitis, hand**
`6th`   **M86.141**   **right hand**
     M86.142   **left hand**
   M86.15   **Other acute osteomyelitis, femur**
`6th`   **M86.151**   **right femur**
     M86.152   **left femur**
   M86.16   **Other acute osteomyelitis, tibia and fibula**
`6th`   **M86.161**   **right tibia and fibula**
     M86.162   **left tibia and fibula**
   M86.17   **Other acute osteomyelitis, ankle and foot**
`6th`   **M86.171**   **right ankle and foot**
     M86.172   **left ankle and foot**
   M86.18   **Other acute osteomyelitis, other site**
   M86.19   **Other acute osteomyelitis, multiple sites**
M86.9   **Osteomyelitis, unspecified**
Infection of bone NOS
Periostitis without osteomyelitis

M88   **OSTEITIS DEFORMANS [PAGET'S DISEASE OF BONE]**
`4th`   ***Excludes1:*** osteitis deformans in neoplastic disease (M90.6)
M88.0   **Osteitis deformans of skull**
M88.1   **Osteitis deformans of vertebrae**
M88.8   **Osteitis deformans of other bones**
`5th`   **M88.81**   **Osteitis deformans of shoulder**
`6th`   **M88.811**   **right shoulder**
     M88.812   **left shoulder**
   M88.82   **Osteitis deformans of upper arm**
`6th`   **M88.821**   **right upper arm**
     M88.822   **left upper arm**
   M88.83   **Osteitis deformans of forearm**
`6th`   **M88.831**   **right forearm**
     M88.832   **left forearm**
   M88.84   **Osteitis deformans of hand**
`6th`   **M88.841**   **right hand**
     M88.842   **left hand**
   M88.85   **Osteitis deformans of thigh**
`6th`   **M88.851**   **right thigh**
     M88.852   **left thigh**
   M88.86   **Osteitis deformans of lower leg**
`6th`   **M88.861**   **right lower leg**
     M88.862   **left lower leg**
   M88.87   **Osteitis deformans of ankle and foot**
`6th`   **M88.871**   **right ankle and foot**
     M88.872   **left ankle and foot**
   M88.88   **Osteitis deformans of other bones**
     Excludes2: osteitis deformans of skull (M88.0)
       osteitis deformans of vertebrae (M88.1)
   M88.89   **Osteitis deformans of multiple sites**
M88.9   **Osteitis deformans of unspecified bone**

M89   **OTHER DISORDERS OF BONE**
`4th`   **M89.1**   **Physeal arrest**
`5th`   Arrest of growth plate
Epiphyseal arrest
Growth plate arrest
   M89.12   **Physeal arrest, humerus**
`6th`   **M89.121**   **Complete physeal arrest, right proximal humerus**
     M89.122   **Complete physeal arrest, left proximal humerus**
     M89.123   **Partial physeal arrest, right proximal humerus**
     M89.124   **Partial physeal arrest, left proximal humerus**
     M89.125   **Complete physeal arrest, right distal humerus**
     M89.126   **Complete physeal arrest, left distal humerus**
     M89.127   **Partial physeal arrest, right distal humerus**
     M89.128   **Partial physeal arrest, left distal humerus**
     M89.129   **Physeal arrest, humerus, unspecified**
   M89.13   **Physeal arrest, forearm**
`6th`   **M89.131**   **Complete physeal arrest, right distal radius**
     M89.132   **Complete physeal arrest, left distal radius**
     M89.133   **Partial physeal arrest, right distal radius**
     M89.134   **Partial physeal arrest, left distal radius**
     M89.138   **Other physeal arrest of forearm**
     M89.139   **Physeal arrest, forearm, unspecified**
   M89.15   **Physeal arrest, femur**
`6th`   **M89.151**   **Complete physeal arrest, right proximal femur**
     M89.152   **Complete physeal arrest, left proximal femur**
     M89.153   **Partial physeal arrest, right proximal femur**
     M89.154   **Partial physeal arrest, left proximal femur**
     M89.155   **Complete physeal arrest, right distal femur**
     M89.156   **Complete physeal arrest, left distal femur**
     M89.157   **Partial physeal arrest, right distal femur**
     M89.158   **Partial physeal arrest, left distal femur**
     M89.159   **Physeal arrest, femur, unspecified**

  `4th` `5th` `6th` `7th`   Additional Character Required   ✔   3-character code

Unspecified laterality codes were excluded here.   •=New Code   ▲=Revised Code   ***Excludes1***—Not coded here, do not use together   ***Excludes2***—Not included here

M89.16 **Physeal arrest, lower leg**
- **6th** **M89.160** Complete physeal arrest, right proximal tibia
- **M89.161** Complete physeal arrest, left proximal tibia
- **M89.162** Partial physeal arrest, right proximal tibia
- **M89.163** Partial physeal arrest, left proximal tibia
- **M89.164** Complete physeal arrest, right distal tibia
- **M89.165** Complete physeal arrest, left distal tibia
- **M89.166** Partial physeal arrest, right distal tibia
- **M89.167** Partial physeal arrest, left distal tibia
- **M89.168** Other physeal arrest of lower leg
- **M89.169** Physeal arrest, lower leg, unspecified
- **M89.18** **Physeal arrest, other site**

M90 OSTEOPATHIES IN DISEASES CLASSIFIED ELSEWHERE
4th
Excludes1: osteochondritis, osteomyelitis, and osteopathy (in):
- cryptococcosis (B45.3)
- DM (E08–E13 with .69-)
- gonococcal (A54.43)
- neurogenic syphilis (A52.11)
- renal osteodystrophy (N25.0)
- salmonellosis (A02.24)
- secondary syphilis (A51.46)
- syphilis (late) (A52.77)

M90.5 **Osteonecrosis in diseases classified elsewhere**
5th
Code first underlying disease, such as: caisson disease (T70.3)
  hemoglobinopathy (D50–D64)
- **M90.50** **Osteonecrosis in diseases classified elsewhere, unspecified site**
- **M90.51** **Osteonecrosis in diseases classified elsewhere; shoulder**
  - **6th**
  - **M90.511** right shoulder
  - **M90.512** left shoulder
- **M90.52** **Osteonecrosis in diseases classified elsewhere; upper arm**
  - **6th**
  - **M90.521** right upper arm
  - **M90.522** left upper arm
- **M90.53** **Osteonecrosis in diseases classified elsewhere; forearm**
  - **6th**
  - **M90.531** right forearm
  - **M90.532** left forearm
- **M90.54** **Osteonecrosis in diseases classified elsewhere; hand**
  - **6th**
  - **M90.541** right hand
  - **M90.542** left hand
- **M90.55** **Osteonecrosis in diseases classified elsewhere; thigh**
  - **6th**
  - **M90.551** right thigh
  - **M90.552** left thigh
- **M90.56** **Osteonecrosis in diseases classified elsewhere; lower leg**
  - **6th**
  - **M90.561** right lower leg
  - **M90.562** left lower leg
- **M90.57** **Osteonecrosis in diseases classified elsewhere; ankle and foot**
  - **6th**
  - **M90.571** right ankle and foot
  - **M90.572** left ankle and foot
- **M90.58** **Osteonecrosis in diseases classified elsewhere, other site**
- **M90.59** **Osteonecrosis in diseases classified elsewhere, multiple sites**

M90.6 **Osteitis deformans in neoplastic diseases**
5th
Osteitis deformans in malignant neoplasm of bone
Code first the neoplasm (C40.-, C41.-)
Excludes1: osteitis deformans [Paget's disease of bone] (M88.-)
Refer to the full *ICD-10-CM* manual for full codes

M90.8 **Osteopathy in diseases classified elsewhere**
5th
Code first underlying disease, such as:
- rickets (E55.0)
- vitamin-D-resistant rickets (E83.3)
- **M90.80** **Osteopathy in diseases classified elsewhere, unspecified site**

(M91–M94) CHONDROPATHIES

Excludes1: postprocedural chondropathies (M96.-)

M91 JUVENILE OSTEOCHONDROSIS OF HIP AND PELVIS
4th
Excludes1: slipped upper femoral epiphysis (nontraumatic) (M93.0)
M91.0 **Juvenile osteochondrosis of pelvis**
- Osteochondrosis (juvenile) of acetabulum
- Osteochondrosis (juvenile) of iliac crest [Buchanan]
- Osteochondrosis (juvenile) of ischiopubic synchondrosis [van Neck]
- Osteochondrosis (juvenile) of symphysis pubis [Pierson]

M91.1 **Juvenile osteochondrosis of head of femur [Legg-Calvé-Perthes]**
5th
- **M91.11** Juvenile osteochondrosis of head of femur [Legg-Calvé-Perthes], right leg
- **M91.12** Juvenile osteochondrosis of head of femur [Legg-Calvé-Perthes], left leg

M91.2 **Coxa plana**
5th
Hip deformity due to previous juvenile osteochondrosis
- **M91.21** Coxa plana, right hip
- **M91.22** Coxa plana, left hip

M91.3 **Pseudocoxalgia**
5th
- **M91.31** Pseudocoxalgia, right hip
- **M91.32** Pseudocoxalgia, left hip

M91.4 **Coxa magna**
5th
- **M91.41** Coxa magna, right hip
- **M91.42** Coxa magna, left hip

M91.8 **Other juvenile osteochondrosis of hip and pelvis**
5th
Juvenile osteochondrosis after reduction of congenital dislocation of hip
- **M91.81** Other juvenile osteochondrosis of hip and pelvis, right leg
- **M91.82** Other juvenile osteochondrosis of hip and pelvis, left leg

M91.9 **Juvenile osteochondrosis of hip and pelvis, unspecified**
5th
- **M91.91** Juvenile osteochondrosis of hip and pelvis, unspecified, right leg
- **M91.92** Juvenile osteochondrosis of hip and pelvis, unspecified, left leg

M92 OTHER JUVENILE OSTEOCHONDROSIS
4th
M92.0 **Juvenile osteochondrosis of humerus**
5th
- Osteochondrosis (juvenile) of capitulum of humerus [Panner]
- Osteochondrosis (juvenile) of head of humerus [Haas]
- **M92.01** right arm
- **M92.02** left arm

M92.1 **Juvenile osteochondrosis of radius and ulna**
5th
- Osteochondrosis (juvenile) of lower ulna [Burns]
- Osteochondrosis (juvenile) of radial head [Brailsford]
- **M92.11** right arm
- **M92.12** left arm

M92.2 **Juvenile osteochondrosis, hand**
5th
- **M92.20** **Unspecified juvenile osteochondrosis; hand**
  - **6th**
  - **M92.201** right hand
  - **M92.202** left hand
- **M92.21** **Osteochondrosis (juvenile) of carpal lunate [Kienböck];**
  - **6th**
  - **M92.211** right hand
  - **M92.212** left hand
- **M92.22** **Osteochondrosis (juvenile) of metacarpal heads [Mauclaire];**
  - **6th**
  - **M92.221** right hand
  - **M92.222** left hand
- **M92.29** **Other juvenile osteochondrosis; hand**
  - **6th**
  - **M92.291** right hand
  - **M92.292** left hand

M92.3 **Other juvenile osteochondrosis; upper limb**
5th
- **M92.31** right upper limb
- **M92.32** left upper limb

M92.4 **Juvenile osteochondrosis of patella;**
5th
- Osteochondrosis (juvenile) of primary patellar center [Köhler]
- Osteochondrosis (juvenile) of secondary patellar centre [Sinding Larsen]
- **M92.41** right knee
- **M92.42** left knee

4th **5th** **6th** **7th** Additional Character Required   ✓ 3-character code

Unspecified laterality codes ●=New Code **Excludes1**—Not coded here, do not use together
were excluded here.   ▲=Revised Code **Excludes2**—Not included here

M92.5 Juvenile osteochondrosis of tibia and fibula;
- `5th` **M92.50 Unspecified juvenile osteochondrosis of tibia and fibula**
  - `6th`
    - M92.501   right leg
    - M92.502   left leg
    - M92.503   bilateral leg
- `5th` **M92.51 Juvenile osteochondrosis of proximal tibia**
  - `6th` Blount disease
    - Tibia vara
    - M92.511   right leg
    - M92.512   left leg
    - M92.513   bilateral
- `5th` **M92.52 Juvenile osteochondrosis of tibia tubercle**
  - `6th` Osgood-Schlatter disease
    - M92.521   right leg
    - M92.522   left leg
    - M92.523   bilateral
- `5th` **M92.59 Other juvenile osteochondrosis of tibia and fibula**
  - `6th`
    - M92.591   right leg
    - M92.592   left leg
    - M92.593   bilateral

M92.6 Juvenile osteochondrosis of tarsus;
- `5th` Osteochondrosis (juvenile) of calcaneum [Sever]
  - Osteochondrosis (juvenile) of os tibiale externum [Haglund]
  - Osteochondrosis (juvenile) of talus [Diaz]
  - Osteochondrosis (juvenile) of tarsal navicular [Köhler]
  - M92.61   right ankle
  - M92.62   left ankle

M92.7 Juvenile osteochondrosis of metatarsus;
- `5th` Osteochondrosis (juvenile) of fifth metatarsus [Iselin]
  - Osteochondrosis (juvenile) of second metatarsus [Freiberg]
  - M92.71   right foot
  - M92.72   left foot

M92.8 Other specified juvenile osteochondrosis
- Calcaneal apophysitis

M92.9 Juvenile osteochondrosis, unspecified
- Juvenile apophysitis NOS
- Juvenile epiphysitis NOS
- Juvenile osteochondritis NOS
- Juvenile osteochondrosis NOS

M93 OTHER OSTEOCHONDROPATHIES
- `4th` *Excludes2:* osteochondrosis of spine (M42.-)

M93.0 Slipped upper femoral epiphysis (nontraumatic)
- `5th` Use additional code for associated chondrolysis (M94.3)
  - **M93.00 Unspecified slipped upper femoral epiphysis**
    - `6th` **(nontraumatic);**
      - M93.001   right hip
      - M93.002   left hip
  - **M93.01 Acute slipped upper femoral epiphysis**
    - `6th` **(nontraumatic);**
      - M93.011   right hip
      - M93.012   left hip
  - **M93.02 Chronic slipped upper femoral epiphysis**
    - `6th` **(nontraumatic);**
      - M93.021   right hip
      - M93.022   left hip

- **M93.03 Acute on chronic slipped upper femoral epiphysis**
  - `6th` **(nontraumatic);**
    - M93.031   right hip
    - M93.032   left hip

M93.9 Osteochondropathy, unspecified
- `5th` Apophysitis NOS
  - Epiphysitis NOS
  - Osteochondritis NOS
  - Osteochondrosis NOS
  - Refer to full *ICD-10-CM* Manual for codes

M94 OTHER DISORDERS OF CARTILAGE
- `4th`

M94.0 Chondrocostal junction syndrome [Tietze]
- Costochondritis

M94.2 Chondromalacia
- `5th` **M94.26 Chondromalacia, knee**
  - `6th`
    - M94.261   Chondromalacia, right knee
    - M94.262   Chondromalacia, left knee

M94.8 Other specified disorders of cartilage
- `5th` **M94.8X Other specified disorders of cartilage**
  - `6th`
    - M94.8X0   multiple sites
    - M94.8X1   shoulder
    - M94.8X2   upper arm
    - M94.8X3   forearm
    - M94.8X4   hand
    - M94.8X5   thigh
    - M94.8X6   lower leg
    - M94.8X7   ankle and foot
    - M94.8X8   other site
    - M94.8X9   unspecified sites

(M95) OTHER DISORDERS OF MUSCULOSKELETAL SYSTEM AND CONNECTIVE TISSUE

M95 OTHER ACQUIRED DEFORMITIES OF
- `4th` **MUSCULOSKELETAL SYSTEM AND CONNECTIVE TISSUE**
  - *Excludes2:* acquired absence of limbs and organs (Z89–Z90)
    - acquired deformities of limbs (M20–M21)
    - congenital malformations and deformations of the musculoskeletal system (Q65–Q79)
    - deforming dorsopathies (M40–M43)
    - dentofacial anomalies [including malocclusion] (M26.-)
    - postprocedural musculoskeletal disorders (M96.-)

M95.0 Acquired deformity of nose
- *Excludes2:* deviated nasal septum (J34.2)

M95.2 Other acquired deformity of head

M95.3 Acquired deformity of neck

M95.4 Acquired deformity of chest and rib

M95.5 Acquired deformity of pelvis

M95.8 Other specified acquired deformities of musculoskeletal system

M95.9 Acquired deformity of musculoskeletal system, unspecified

---

`4th` `5th` `6th` `7th` Additional Character Required   ✓   3-character code   Unspecified laterality codes were excluded here.   •=New Code   ▲=Revised Code   *Excludes1*—Not coded here, do not use together   *Excludes2*—Not included here

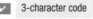

Chapter 14. Diseases of the genitourinary system (N00–N99)

Chronic kidney disease

STAGES OF CKD
Refer to category N18 for guidelines.

CKD AND KIDNEY TRANSPLANT STATUS
Refer to category N18 for guidelines.

CKD WITH OTHER CONDITIONS
Patients with CKD may also suffer from other serious conditions, most commonly DM and hypertension (in adults). The sequencing of the CKD code in relationship to codes for other contributing conditions is based on the conventions in the Tabular List.

   Refer to Chapter 19. CKD and kidney transplant complications.

Excludes2: certain conditions originating in the perinatal period (P04–P96)
   certain infectious and parasitic diseases (A00–B99)
   complications of pregnancy, childbirth and the puerperium (O00–O9A)
   congenital malformations, deformations and chromosomal abnormalities (Q00–Q99)
   endocrine, nutritional and metabolic diseases (E00–E88)
   injury, poisoning and certain other consequences of external causes (S00–T88)
   neoplasms (C00–D49)
   symptoms, signs and abnormal clinical and laboratory findings, NEC (R00–R94)

(N00–N08) GLOMERULAR DISEASES

Code also any associated kidney failure (N17–N19).
Excludes1: hypertensive CKD (I12.-)

N00   **ACUTE NEPHRITIC SYNDROME**
`4th`
   Includes: acute glomerular disease
      acute glomerulonephritis
      acute nephritis
   Excludes1: acute tubulo-interstitial nephritis (N10)
      nephritic syndrome NOS (N05.-)

   N00.0   Acute nephritic syndrome with; minor glomerular abnormality
      Acute nephritic syndrome with minimal change lesion

   N00.1   focal and segmental glomerular lesions
      Acute nephritic syndrome with focal and segmental hyalinosis or with focal and segmental sclerosis or with focal glomerulonephritis

   N00.2   diffuse membranous glomerulonephritis

   N00.3   diffuse mesangial proliferative glomerulonephritis

   N00.4   diffuse endocapillary proliferative glomerulonephritis

   N00.5   diffuse mesangiocapillary glomerulonephritis
      Acute nephritic syndrome with MPGN, types 1 and 3, or NOS
      Excludes1: Acute nephritic syndrome with C3 glomerulonephritis or glomerulopathy (N00.A)

   N00.6   dense deposit disease
      Acute nephritic syndrome with C3 glomerulopathy with dense deposit disease
      Acute nephritic syndrome with MPGN, type 2

   N00.7   diffuse crescentic glomerulonephritis
      Acute nephritic syndrome with extracapillary glomerulonephritis

   N00.8   other morphologic changes
      Acute nephritic syndrome with proliferative glomerulonephritis NOS

   N00.9   unspecified morphologic changes

   N00.A   Acute nephritic syndrome with C3 glomerulonephritis
      Acute nephritic syndrome with C3 glomerulopathy, NOS
      Excludes1: Acute nephritic syndrome (with C3 glomerulopathy) with dense deposit disease(N00.6)

N01   **RAPIDLY PROGRESSIVE NEPHRITIC SYNDROME**
`4th`
   Includes: rapidly progressive glomerular disease
      rapidly progressive glomerulonephritis
      rapidly progressive nephritis
   Excludes1: nephritic syndrome NOS (N05.-)

   N01.0   Rapidly progressive nephritic syndrome with; minor glomerular abnormality
      Rapidly progressive nephritic syndrome with minimal change lesion

   N01.1   focal and segmental glomerular lesions
      Rapidly progressive nephritic syndrome with focal and segmental hyalinosis or with focal and segmental sclerosis or with focal glomerulonephritis

   N01.2   diffuse membranous glomerulonephritis

   N01.3   diffuse mesangial proliferative glomerulonephritis

   N01.4   diffuse endocapillary proliferative glomerulonephritis

   N01.5   diffuse mesangiocapillary glomerulonephritis
      Rapidly progressive nephritic syndrome with MPGN, types 1 and 3, or NOS
      Excludes1: Rapidly progressive nephritic syndrome with C3 glomerulonephritis or glomerulopathy (N01.A)

   N01.6   dense deposit disease
      Rapidly progressive nephritic syndrome with C3 glomerulopathy with dense deposit disease
      Rapidly progressive nephritic syndrome with MPGN, type 2

   N01.7   diffuse crescentic glomerulonephritis
      Rapidly progressive nephritic syndrome with extracapillary glomerulonephritis

   N01.8   other morphologic changes
      Rapidly progressive nephritic syndrome with proliferative glomerulonephritis NOS

   N01.9   unspecified morphologic changes

   N01.A   Rapidly progressive nephritic syndrome with C3 glomerulonephritis
      Rapidly progressive nephritic syndrome with C3 glomerulopathy, NOS
      Excludes1: Rapidly progressive nephritic syndrome (with C3 glomerulopathy) with dense depositdisease (N01.6)

N03   **CHRONIC NEPHRITIC SYNDROME**
`4th`
   Includes: chronic glomerular disease
      chronic glomerulonephritis
      chronic nephritis
   Excludes1: chronic tubulo-interstitial nephritis (N11.-)
      diffuse sclerosing glomerulonephritis (N05.8-)
      nephritic syndrome NOS (N05.-)

   N03.0   Chronic nephritic syndrome with; minor glomerular abnormality
      Chronic nephritic syndrome with minimal change lesion

   N03.1   focal and segmental glomerular lesions
      Chronic nephritic syndrome with focal and segmental hyalinosis or with focal and segmental sclerosis or with focal glomerulonephritis

   N03.2   diffuse membranous glomerulonephritis

   N03.3   diffuse mesangial proliferative glomerulonephritis

   N03.4   diffuse endocapillary proliferative glomerulonephritis

   N03.5   diffuse mesangiocapillary glomerulonephritis
      Chronic nephritic syndrome with MPGN, types 1 and 3, or NOS
      Excludes1: Chronic nephritic syndrome with C3 glomerulonephritis or glomerulopathy (N03.A)

   N03.6   dense deposit disease
      Chronic nephritic syndrome with MPGN, type 2

   N03.7   diffuse crescentic glomerulonephritis
      Chronic nephritic syndrome with C3 glomerulopathy with dense deposit disease
      Chronic nephritic syndrome with extracapillary glomerulonephritis

   N03.8   other morphologic changes
      Chronic nephritic syndrome with proliferative glomerulonephritis NOS

   N03.9   unspecified morphologic changes

   N03.A   Chronic nephritic syndrome with C3 glomerulonephritis
      Chronic nephritic syndrome with C3 glomerulopathy
      Excludes1: Chronic nephritic syndrome (with C3 glomerulopathy) with dense deposit disease (N03.6)

N04   **NEPHROTIC SYNDROME**
`4th`
   Includes: congenital nephrotic syndrome
      lipoid nephrosis

 `4th` `5th` `6th` `7th`   Additional Character Required   3-character code   •=New Code   **_Excludes1_**—Not coded here, do not use together
               ▲=Revised Code   **_Excludes2_**—Not included here

N04.0 Nephrotic syndrome with; minor glomerular abnormality
Nephrotic syndrome with minimal change lesion

N04.1 focal and segmental glomerular lesions
Nephrotic syndrome with focal and segmental hyalinosis or with focal and segmental sclerosis or with focal glomerulonephritis

N04.2 diffuse membranous glomerulonephritis

N04.3 diffuse mesangial proliferative glomerulonephritis

N04.4 diffuse endocapillary proliferative glomerulonephritis

N04.5 diffuse mesangiocapillary glomerulonephritis
Nephrotic syndrome with MPGN, types 1 and 3, or NOS
Excludes1: Nephrotic syndrome with C3 glomerulonephritis or glomerulopathy (N04.A)

N04.6 dense deposit disease
Nephrotic syndrome with C3 glomerulopathy with dense deposit disease
Nephrotic syndrome with MPGN, type 2

N04.7 diffuse crescentic glomerulonephritis
Nephrotic syndrome with extracapillary glomerulonephritis

N04.8 other morphologic changes
Nephrotic syndrome with proliferative glomerulonephritis NOS

N04.9 unspecified morphologic changes

N04.A Nephrotic syndrome with C3 glomerulonephritis
Nephrotic syndrome with C3 glomerulopathy
Excludes1: Nephrotic syndrome (with C3 glomerulopathy) with dense deposit disease (N04.6)

N05 UNSPECIFIED NEPHRITIC SYNDROME
`4th`
Includes: glomerular disease NOS
glomerulonephritis NOS
nephritis NOS
nephropathy NOS and renal disease NOS with morphological lesion specified in .0–.8
Excludes1: nephropathy NOS with no stated morphological lesion (N28.9)
renal disease NOS with no stated morphological lesion (N28.9)
tubulo-interstitial nephritis NOS (N12)

N05.0 Unspecified nephritic syndrome with minor glomerular abnormality
Unspecified nephritic syndrome with minimal change lesion

N05.1 Unspecified nephritic syndrome with focal and segmental glomerular lesions
Unspecified nephritic syndrome with focal and segmental hyalinosis
Unspecified nephritic syndrome with focal and segmental sclerosis
Unspecified nephritic syndrome with focal glomerulonephritis

N05.2 Unspecified nephritic syndrome with diffuse membranous glomerulonephritis

N05.3 Unspecified nephritic syndrome with diffuse mesangial proliferative glomerulonephritis

N05.4 Unspecified nephritic syndrome with diffuse endocapillary proliferative glomerulonephritis

N05.5 Unspecified nephritic syndrome with diffuse mesangiocapillary glomerulonephritis
Unspecified nephritic syndrome with membranoproliferative glomerulonephritis, types 1 and 3, or NOS
Excludes1: Unspecified nephritic syndrome with C3 glomerulonephritis or glomerulopathy (N05.A)

N05.6 Unspecified nephritic syndrome with dense deposit disease
Unspecified nephritic syndrome with membranoproliferative glomerulonephritis, type 2
Unspecified nephritic syndrome with C3 glomerulopathy with dense deposit disease

N05.7 Unspecified nephritic syndrome with diffuse crescentic glomerulonephritis
Unspecified nephritic syndrome with extracapillary glomerulonephritis

N05.8 Unspecified nephritic syndrome with other morphologic changes
Unspecified nephritic syndrome with proliferative glomerulonephritis NOS

N05.9 Unspecified nephritic syndrome with unspecified morphologic changes

N05.A Unspecified nephritic syndrome with C3 glomerulonephritis
Unspecified nephritic syndrome with C3 glomerulopathy
Excludes1: Unspecified nephritic syndrome (with C3 glomerulopathy) with dense deposit disease (N05.6)

N08 GLOMERULAR DISORDERS IN DISEASES CLASSIFIED ELSEWHERE
`✔`
Glomerulonephritis
Nephritis
Nephropathy

Please note the numerous exclusions below.

Code first underlying disease, such as:
amyloidosis (E85.-)
congenital syphilis (A50.5)
cryoglobulinemia (D89.1)
disseminated intravascular coagulation (D65)
gout (M1A.-, M10.-)
microscopic polyangiitis (M31.7)
multiple myeloma (C90.0-)
sepsis (A40.0–A41.9)
sickle-cell disease (D57.0–D57.8)
Excludes1: glomerulonephritis, nephritis and nephropathy (in):
antiglomerular basement membrane disease (M31.0)
diabetes (E08–E13 with .21)
gonococcal (A54.21)
Goodpasture's syndrome (M31.0)
hemolytic-uremic syndrome (D59.3)
lupus (M32.14)
mumps (B26.83)
syphilis (A52.75)
SLE (M32.14)
Wegener's granulomatosis (M31.31)
pyelonephritis in diseases classified elsewhere (N16)
renal tubulo-interstitial disorders classified elsewhere (N16)

(N10–N16) RENAL TUBULO-INTERSTITIAL DISEASES

Includes: pyelonephritis
Excludes1: pyeloureteritis cystica (N28.85)

N10 ACUTE PYELONEPHRITIS
`✔`
Acute infectious interstitial nephritis
Acute pyelitis
Hemoglobin nephrosis
Myoglobin nephrosis
Use additional code (B95–B97), to identify infectious agent.

N11 CHRONIC TUBULO-INTERSTITIAL NEPHRITIS
`4th`
Includes: chronic infectious interstitial nephritis
chronic pyelitis
chronic pyelonephritis
Use additional code (B95–B97), to identify infectious agent

N11.9 Chronic tubulo-interstitial nephritis, unspecified
Chronic interstitial nephritis NOS
Chronic pyelitis NOS
Chronic pyelonephritis NOS

N12 TUBULO-INTERSTITIAL NEPHRITIS, NOT SPECIFIED AS ACUTE OR CHRONIC
`✔`
Interstitial nephritis NOS
Pyelitis NOS
Pyelonephritis NOS
Excludes1: calculous pyelonephritis (N20.9)

N13 OBSTRUCTIVE AND REFLUX UROPATHY
`4th`
Excludes2: calculus of kidney and ureter without hydronephrosis (N20.-)
congenital obstructive defects of renal pelvis and ureter (Q62.0–Q62.3)
hydronephrosis with ureteropelvic junction obstruction (Q62.11)
obstructive pyelonephritis (N11.1)

N13.0 Hydronephrosis with ureteropelvic junction obstruction
Hydronephrosis due to acquired occlusion ureteropelvic junction
Excludes2: hydronephrosis with ureteropelvic junction obstruction due to calculus (N13.2)

N13.1 Hydronephrosis with ureteral stricture, NEC
Excludes1: hydronephrosis with ureteral stricture with infection (N13.6)

`4th` `5th` `6th` `7th` Additional Character Required   `✔` 3-character code

•=New Code
▲=Revised Code

Excludes1—Not coded here, do not use together
Excludes2—Not included here

272   PEDIATRIC ICD-10-CM 2022: A MANUAL FOR PROVIDER-BASED CODING

CHAPTER 14. DISEASES OF THE GENITOURINARY SYSTEM   (N04.0–N13.1)

N13.2 Hydronephrosis with renal and ureteral calculous obstruction
Excludes1: hydronephrosis with renal and ureteral calculous obstruction with infection (N13.6)

N13.3 Other and unspecified hydronephrosis
`5th` *Excludes1:* hydronephrosis with infection (N13.6)
    N13.30 Unspecified hydronephrosis
    N13.39 Other hydronephrosis

N13.5 Crossing vessel and stricture of ureter without hydronephrosis
Kinking and stricture of ureter without hydronephrosis
Excludes1: Crossing vessel and stricture of ureter without hydronephrosis with infection (N13.6)

N13.6 Pyonephrosis
Conditions in N13.0–N13.5 with infection
Obstructive uropathy with infection
Use additional code (B95–B97), to identify infectious agent.

N13.7 Vesicoureteral-reflux
`5th` *Excludes1:* reflux-associated pyelonephritis (N11.0)
    N13.70 Vesicoureteral-reflux, unspecified
    Vesicoureteral-reflux NOS
    N13.71 Vesicoureteral-reflux without reflux nephropathy

N13.8 Other obstructive and reflux uropathy
Urinary tract obstruction due to specified cause
Code first, if applicable, any causal condition, such as:
enlarged prostate (N40.1)

N13.9 Obstructive and reflux uropathy, unspecified
Urinary tract obstruction NOS

N14 **DRUG- AND HEAVY-METAL-INDUCED TUBULO-**
`4th` **INTERSTITIAL AND TUBULAR CONDITIONS**
Code first poisoning due to drug or toxin, if applicable (T36–T65 with fifth or sixth character 1–4 or 6)
Use additional code for adverse effect, if applicable, to identify drug (T36–T50 with fifth or sixth character 5)
N14.0 Analgesic nephropathy

N16 **RENAL TUBULO-INTERSTITIAL DISORDERS**
`✓` **IN DISEASES CLASSIFIED ELSEWHERE**
Pyelonephritis
Tubulo-interstitial nephritis
Code first underlying disease, such as:
brucellosis (A23)
cryoglobulinemia (D89.1)
glycogen storage disease (E74.0)
leukemia (C91-C95)
lymphoma (C81.0-C85.9, C96.0-C96.9)
multiple myeloma (C90.0-)
sepsis (A40.0-A41.9)
Wilson's disease (E83.0)
Excludes1: diphtheritic pyelonephritis and tubulo-interstitial nephritis (A36.84)
pyelonephritis and tubulo-interstitial nephritis in candidiasis (B37.49)
in cystinosis (E72.04)
in Salmonella infection (A02.25)
in sarcoidosis (D86.84)
in Sjögren syndrome (M35.04)
in systemic lupus erythematosus (M32.15)
in toxoplasmosis (B58.83)
renal tubular degeneration in diabetes (E08-E13 with .29)
syphilitic pyelonephritis and tubulo-interstitial nephritis (A52.75)

(N17–N19) ACUTE KIDNEY FAILURE AND CKD

Excludes2: congenital renal failure (P96.0)
drug- and heavy-metal–induced tubulo-interstitial and tubular conditions (N14.-)
extrarenal uremia (R39.2)
hemolytic-uremic syndrome (D59.3)
hepatorenal syndrome (K76.7)
postpartum hepatorenal syndrome (O90.4)
posttraumatic renal failure (T79.5)
prerenal uremia (R39.2)
renal failure complicating abortion or ectopic or molar pregnancy (O00–O07, O08.4)
renal failure following labor and delivery (O90.4)
renal failure postprocedural (N99.0)

N17 **ACUTE KIDNEY FAILURE**
`4th` **Code also associated** underlying condition
Excludes1: posttraumatic renal failure (T79.5)
N17.0 Acute kidney failure with tubular necrosis
Acute tubular necrosis
Renal tubular necrosis
Tubular necrosis NOS

N17.1 Acute kidney failure with acute cortical necrosis
Acute cortical necrosis
Cortical necrosis NOS
Renal cortical necrosis

N17.2 Acute kidney failure with medullary necrosis
Medullary [papillary] necrosis NOS
Acute medullary [papillary] necrosis
Renal medullary [papillary] necrosis

N17.8 Other acute kidney failure
N17.9 Acute kidney failure, unspecified
Acute kidney injury (nontraumatic)
Excludes2: traumatic kidney injury (S37.0-)

N18 **CHRONIC KIDNEY DISEASE (CKD)**
`4th` **GUIDELINES**

Stages of CKD

The *ICD-10-CM* classifies CKD based on severity. The severity of CKD is designated by stages 1–5. Stage 2, code N18.2, equates to mild CKD; stage 3, code N18.3, equates to moderate CKD; and stage 4, code N18.4, equates to severe CKD. Code N18.6, ESRD, is assigned when the provider has documented ESRD.

If both a stage of CKD and ESRD are documented by the provider, only assign code N18.6 for ESRD (CKD requiring dialysis) only.

Patients who have undergone kidney transplant may still have some form of CKD because the kidney transplant may not fully restore kidney function. Therefore, the presence of CKD alone does not constitute a transplant complication. Assign the appropriate N18 code for the patient's stage of CKD and code Z94.0, Kidney transplant status. If a transplant complication such as failure or rejection or other transplant complication is documented, refer to code T86.1 for information on coding complications of a kidney transplant. If the documentation is unclear as to whether the patient has a complication of the transplant, query the provider.
Code first any associated diabetic CKD (E08.22, E09.22, E10.22, E11.22, E13.22)
hypertensive chronic kidney disease (I12.-, I13.-)
Use additional code to identify kidney transplant status, if applicable, (Z94.0)

N18.1 CKD stage 1
N18.2 CKD stage 2 (mild)
N18.3 CKD stage 3 (moderate)
`5th`   **N18.30 CKD, stage 3 unspecified**
    N18.31 CKD, stage 3a
    N18.32 CKD, stage 3b
N18.4 CKD stage 4 (severe)
N18.5 CKD stage 5
Excludes1: CKD, stage 5 requiring chronic dialysis (N18.6)
N18.6 ESRD
CKD requiring chronic dialysis
Use additional code to identify dialysis status (Z99.2)
N18.9 CKD, unspecified
Chronic renal disease
Chronic renal failure NOS
Chronic renal insufficiency
Chronic uremia NOS

N19 **UNSPECIFIED KIDNEY FAILURE**
`✓` Uremia NOS
Excludes1: acute kidney failure (N17.-)
chronic kidney disease (N18.-)
chronic uremia (N18.9)
extrarenal uremia (R39.2)
prerenal uremia (R39.2)
renal insufficiency (acute) (N28.9)
uremia of newborn (P96.0)

CHAPTER 14. DISEASES OF THE GENITOURINARY SYSTEM (N13.2–N19)

 Additional Character Required   `✓` 3-character code

•=New Code   ▲=Revised Code

Excludes1—Not coded here, do not use together
Excludes2—Not included here

CHAPTER 14. DISEASES OF THE GENITOURINARY SYSTEM (N20–N32.2)

(N20–N23) UROLITHIASIS

N20   **CALCULUS OF KIDNEY AND URETER**
`4th`
Calculous pyelonephritis
Excludes1: nephrocalcinosis (E83.5)
that with hydronephrosis (N13.2)

    N20.0   **Calculus of kidney**
      Nephrolithiasis NOS
      Renal calculus
      Renal stone
      Staghorn calculus
      Stone in kidney

    N20.1   **Calculus of ureter**
      Ureteric stone
      Calculus of the ureteropelvic junction

    N20.2   **Calculus of kidney with calculus of ureter**
    N20.9   **Urinary calculus, unspecified**

N21   **CALCULUS OF LOWER URINARY TRACT**
`4th`
Includes: calculus of lower urinary tract with cystitis and urethritis

    N21.0   **Calculus in bladder**
      Calculus in diverticulum of bladder
      Urinary bladder stone
      Excludes2: staghorn calculus (N20.0)

    N21.1   **Calculus in urethra**
      Excludes2: calculus of prostate (N42.0)

N22   **CALCULUS OF URINARY TRACT IN DISEASES**
`✔`   **CLASSIFIED ELSEWHERE**
Code first underlying disease, such as:
   gout (M1A.-, M10.-)
   schistosomiasis (B65.0-B65.9)

N23   **UNSPECIFIED RENAL COLIC**
`✔`

(N25–N29) OTHER DISORDERS OF KIDNEY AND URETER

Excludes2: disorders of kidney and ureter with urolithiasis (N20–N23)

N25   **DISORDERS RESULTING FROM IMPAIRED RENAL**
`4th`   **TUBULAR FUNCTION**
    N25.0   **Renal osteodystrophy**
      Azotemic osteodystrophy
      Phosphate-losing tubular disorders
      Renal rickets
      Renal short stature
      Excludes2: metabolic disorders classifiable to E70–E88

    N25.1   **Nephrogenic diabetes insipidus**
      Excludes1: diabetes insipidus NOS (E23.2)

N27   **SMALL KIDNEY OF UNKNOWN CAUSE**
`4th`
Includes: oligonephronia
    N27.0   **Small kidney, unilateral**
    N27.1   **Small kidney, bilateral**

N28   **OTHER DISORDERS OF KIDNEY AND URETER, NEC**
`4th`
    N28.0   **Ischemia and infarction of kidney**
      Renal artery embolism or obstruction or occlusion or thrombosis
      Renal infarct
      Excludes1: atherosclerosis of renal artery (extrarenal part) (I70.1)
       congenital stenosis of renal artery (Q27.1)
       Goldblatt's kidney (I70.1)

    N28.1   **Cyst of kidney, acquired**
      Cyst (multiple)(solitary) of kidney (acquired)
      Excludes1: cystic kidney disease (congenital) (Q61.-)

    N28.8   **Other specified disorders of kidney and ureter**
     `5th`   ***Excludes1:*** hydroureter (N13.4)
       ureteric stricture with hydronephrosis (N13.1)
       ureteric stricture without hydronephrosis (N13.5)
      N28.85   **Pyeloureteritis cystica**
      N28.89   **Other specified disorders of kidney and ureter**

    N28.9   **Disorder of kidney and ureter, unspecified**
      Nephropathy NOS
      Renal disease (acute) NOS
      Renal insufficiency (acute)
      Excludes1: chronic renal insufficiency (N18.9)
       unspecified nephritic syndrome (N05.-)

N29   **OTHER DISORDERS OF KIDNEY AND URETER IN**
`✔`   **DISEASES CLASSIFIED ELSEWHERE**
Code first underlying disease, such as:
   amyloidosis (E85.-)
   nephrocalcinosis (E83.5)
   schistosomiasis (B65.0-B65.9)
Excludes1: disorders of kidney and ureter in:
   cystinosis (E72.0)
   gonorrhea (A54.21)
   syphilis (A52.75)
   tuberculosis (A18.11)

(N30–N39) OTHER DISEASES OF THE URINARY SYSTEM

Excludes2: urinary infection (complicating): abortion or ectopic or molar pregnancy (O00–O07, O08.8)
pregnancy, childbirth and the puerperium (O23.-, O75.3, O86.2-)

N30   **CYSTITIS**
`4th`
Use additional code to identify infectious agent (B95–B97)
Excludes1: prostatocystitis (N41.3)
    N30.0   **Acute cystitis**
     `5th`   ***Excludes1:*** irradiation cystitis (N30.4-)
       trigonitis (N30.3-)
      N30.00   **Acute cystitis without hematuria**
      N30.01   **Acute cystitis with hematuria**

    N30.3   **Trigonitis**
     `5th`   Urethrotrigonitis
      N30.30   **Trigonitis without hematuria**
      N30.31   **Trigonitis with hematuria**

    N30.4   **Irradiation cystitis**
     `5th`   **N30.40**   **Irradiation cystitis without hematuria**
      N30.41   **Irradiation cystitis with hematuria**

    N30.8   **Other cystitis**
     `5th`   Abscess of bladder
      N30.80   **Other cystitis without hematuria**
      N30.81   **Other cystitis with hematuria**

    N30.9   **Cystitis, unspecified**
     `5th`   **N30.90**   **Cystitis, unspecified without hematuria**
      N30.91   **Cystitis, unspecified with hematuria**

N31   **NEUROMUSCULAR DYSFUNCTION OF BLADDER, NEC**
`4th`
Use additional code to identify any associated urinary incontinence (N39.3–N39.4-)
Excludes1: cord bladder NOS (G95.89)
   neurogenic bladder due to cauda equina syndrome (G83.4)
   neuromuscular dysfunction due to spinal cord lesion (G95.89)
    N31.0   **Uninhibited neuropathic bladder, NEC**
    N31.1   **Reflex neuropathic bladder, NEC**
    N31.2   **Flaccid neuropathic bladder, NEC**
      Atonic (motor) (sensory) neuropathic bladder
      Autonomous neuropathic bladder
      Nonreflex neuropathic bladder
    N31.8   **Other neuromuscular dysfunction of bladder**
    N31.9   **Neuromuscular dysfunction of bladder, unspecified**
      Neurogenic bladder dysfunction NOS

N32   **OTHER DISORDERS OF BLADDER**
`4th`
Excludes2: calculus of bladder (N21.0)
   cystocele (N81.1-)
   hernia or prolapse of bladder, female (N81.1-)
    N32.0   **Bladder-neck obstruction**
      Bladder-neck stenosis (acquired)
      Excludes1: congenital bladder-neck obstruction (Q64.3-)
    N32.1   **Vesicointestinal fistula**
      Vesicorectal fistula
    N32.2   **Vesical fistula, NEC**
      Excludes1: fistula between bladder and female genital tract (N82.0–N82.1)

`4th` `5th` `6th` `7th`   Additional Character Required   `✔`   3-character code

•=New Code   ***Excludes1***—Not coded here, do not use together
▲=Revised Code   ***Excludes2***—Not included here

N32.3 Diverticulum of bladder
Excludes1: congenital diverticulum of bladder (Q64.6)
diverticulitis of bladder (N30.8-)
N32.8 Other specified disorders of bladder
[5th] N32.81 Overactive bladder
Detrusor muscle hyperactivity
Excludes1: frequent urination due to specified bladder
condition — code to condition
N32.89 Other specified disorders of bladder
Bladder hemorrhage
Bladder hypertrophy
Calcified bladder
Contracted bladder
N32.9 Bladder disorder, unspecified

N34 URETHRITIS AND URETHRAL SYNDROME
[4th] Use additional code (B95–B97), to identify infectious agent.
Excludes2: Reiter's disease (M02.3-)
urethritis in diseases with a predominantly sexual mode of transmission
(A50–A64)
urethrotrigonitis (N30.3-)
N34.0 Urethral abscess
Abscess (of) Cowper's gland
Abscess (of) Littré's gland
Abscess (of) urethral (gland)
Periurethral abscess
Excludes1: urethral caruncle (N36.2)
N34.1 Nonspecific urethritis
Nongonococcal urethritis
Nonvenereal urethritis
N34.2 Other urethritis
Meatitis, urethral
Postmenopausal urethritis
Ulcer of urethra (meatus)
Urethritis NOS
N34.3 Urethral syndrome, unspecified

N35 URETHRAL STRICTURE
[4th] *Excludes1:* congenital urethral stricture (Q64.3-)
postprocedural urethral stricture (N99.1-)
N35.0 Post-traumatic urethral stricture
[5th] Urethral stricture due to injury
Excludes1: postprocedural urethral stricture (N99.1-)
N35.01 Post-traumatic urethral stricture, male
**[6th] N35.010 Post-traumatic urethral stricture, male,
meatal**
N35.011 Post-traumatic bulbous urethral stricture
**N35.012 Post-traumatic membranous urethral
stricture**
N35.013 Post-traumatic anterior urethral stricture
**N35.014 Post-traumatic urethral stricture, male,
unspecified**
**N35.016 Post-traumatic urethral stricture, male,
overlapping sites**
N35.02 Post-traumatic urethral stricture, female
[6th] N35.021 Urethral stricture due to childbirth
**N35.028 Other post-traumatic urethral stricture,
female**
N35.1 Postinfective urethral stricture, NEC
[5th] *Excludes1:* urethral stricture associated with schistosomiasis
(B65.-, N29)
gonococcal urethral stricture (A54.01)
syphilitic urethral stricture (A52.76)
N35.11 Postinfective urethral stricture, NEC, male
**[6th] N35.111 Postinfective urethral stricture, NEC, male,
meatal**
**N35.112 Postinfective bulbous urethral stricture,
NEC, male**
**N35.113 Postinfective membranous urethral
stricture, NEC, male**
**N35.114 Postinfective anterior urethral stricture,
NEC, male**
**N35.116 Postinfective urethral stricture, NEC, male,
overlapping sites**

**N35.119 Postinfective urethral stricture, NEC, male,
unspecified**
N35.12 Postinfective urethral stricture, NEC, female
N35.8 Other urethral stricture
[5th] *Excludes1:* postprocedural urethral stricture (N99.1-)
N35.81 Other urethral stricture, male
[6th] N35.811 Other urethral stricture, male, meatal
N35.812 Other urethral bulbous stricture, male
N35.813 Other membranous urethral stricture, male
N35.814 Other anterior urethral stricture, male
**N35.816 Other urethral stricture, male, overlapping
sites**
**N35.819 Other urethral stricture, male, unspecified
site**
N35.82 Other urethral stricture, female
N35.9 Urethral stricture, unspecified
[5th] N35.91 Urethral stricture, unspecified, male
**[6th] N35.911 Unspecified urethral stricture, male,
meatal**
**N35.912 Unspecified bulbous urethral stricture,
male**
**N35.913 Unspecified membranous urethral
stricture, male**
**N35.914 Unspecified anterior urethral stricture,
male**
**N35.916 Unspecified urethral stricture, male,
overlapping sites**
**N35.919 Unspecified urethral stricture, male,
unspecified site**
N35.92 Unspecified urethral stricture, female

N39 OTHER DISORDERS OF URINARY SYSTEM
[4th] *Excludes2:* hematuria NOS (R31.-)
recurrent or persistent hematuria (N02.-)
recurrent or persistent hematuria with specified morphological lesion
(N02.-)
proteinuria NOS (R80.-)
N39.0 Urinary tract infection, site not specified
Use additional code (B95–B97), to identify infectious agent.
Excludes1: candidiasis of urinary tract (B37.4-)
neonatal urinary tract infection (P39.3)
pyuria (R82.81)
urinary tract infection of specified site, such as:
cystitis (N30.-)
urethritis (N34.-)
N39.4 Other specified urinary incontinence
[5th] Code also any associated overactive bladder (N32.81)
Excludes1: enuresis NOS (R32)
functional urinary incontinence (R39.81)
urinary incontinence associated with cognitive impairment
(R39.81)
urinary incontinence NOS (R32)
urinary incontinence of nonorganic origin (F98.0)
N39.44 Nocturnal enuresis
Excludes2: nocturnal polyuria (R35.81)
N39.8 Other specified disorders of urinary system
N39.9 Disorder of urinary system, unspecified

(N40–N53) DISEASES OF MALE GENITAL ORGANS

N41 INFLAMMATORY DISEASES OF PROSTATE
[4th] Use additional code (B95–B97), to identify infectious agent.
N41.0 Acute prostatitis
N41.9 Inflammatory disease of prostate, unspecified
Prostatitis NOS

N43 HYDROCELE AND SPERMATOCELE
[4th] *Includes:* hydrocele of spermatic cord, testis or tunica vaginalis
Excludes1: congenital hydrocele (P83.5)
N43.0 Encysted hydrocele
N43.1 Infected hydrocele
Use additional code (B95–B97), to identify infectious agent
N43.2 Other hydrocele
N43.3 Hydrocele, unspecified

[4th] [5th] [6th] [7th] Additional Character Required **[✓] 3-character code**

•=New Code
▲=Revised Code

Excludes1—Not coded here, do not use together
Excludes2—Not included here

N43.4 Spermatocele of epididymis
5th   Spermatic cyst
     N43.40 Spermatocele of epididymis, unspecified
     N43.41 Spermatocele of epididymis, single
     N43.42 Spermatocele of epididymis, multiple

N44 NONINFLAMMATORY DISORDERS OF TESTIS
4th
   N44.0 Torsion of testis
     5th   **N44.00 Torsion of testis, unspecified**
     N44.01 Extravaginal torsion of spermatic cord
     N44.02 Intravaginal torsion of spermatic cord
       Torsion of spermatic cord NOS
     N44.03 Torsion of appendix testis
     N44.04 Torsion of appendix epididymis
   N44.1 Cyst of tunica albuginea testis
   N44.2 Benign cyst of testis
   N44.8 Other noninflammatory disorders of the testis

N45 ORCHITIS AND EPIDIDYMITIS
4th
   Use additional code (B95–B97), to identify infectious agent.
   N45.1 Epididymitis
   N45.2 Orchitis
   N45.3 Epididymo-orchitis
   N45.4 Abscess of epididymis or testis

N47 DISORDERS OF PREPUCE
4th
   N47.0 Adherent prepuce, newborn
   N47.1 Phimosis
   N47.2 Paraphimosis
   N47.4 Benign cyst of prepuce
   N47.5 Adhesions of prepuce and glans penis
   N47.6 Balanoposthitis
   N47.7 Other inflammatory diseases of prepuce
     Use additional code (B95–B97), to identify infectious agent.
   N47.8 Other disorders of prepuce
     Use additional code (B95–B97), to identify infectious agent.
     Excludes1: balanitis (N48.1)

N48 OTHER DISORDERS OF PENIS
4th
   N48.1 Balanitis
     Use additional code (B95–B97), to identify infectious agent
     Excludes1: amebic balanitis (A06.8)
       balanitis xerotica obliterans (N48.0)
       candidal balanitis (B37.42)
       gonococcal balanitis (A54.23)
       herpesviral [herpes simplex] balanitis (A60.01)
   N48.3 Priapism
     5th   Painful erection
     Code first underlying cause
     N48.30 Priapism, unspecified
     N48.31 Priapism due to trauma
     N48.32 Priapism due to disease classified elsewhere
     N48.33 Priapism, drug-induced
     N48.39 Other priapism
   N48.8 Other specified disorders of penis
     5th   **N48.82 Acquired torsion of penis**
       Acquired torsion of penis NOS
       Excludes1: congenital torsion of penis (Q55.63)
     N48.89 Other specified disorders of penis
   N48.9 Disorder of penis, unspecified

N49 INFLAMMATORY DISORDERS OF MALE GENITAL ORGANS, NOT ELSEWHERE CLASSIFIED
4th
   Use additional code (B95–B97), to identify infectious agent
   Excludes1: inflammation of penis (N48.1, N48.2-)
     orchitis and epididymitis (N45.-)
   N49.0 Inflammatory disorders of seminal vesicle
     Vesiculitis NOS

N50 OTHER AND UNSPECIFIED DISORDERS OF MALE GENITAL ORGANS
4th
   Excludes2: torsion of testis (N44.0-)
   N50.0 Atrophy of testis

N50.8 Other specified disorders of male genital organs
5th   **N50.81 Testicular pain**
     6th   **N50.811 Right testicular pain**
       N50.812 Left testicular pain
   N50.82 Scrotal pain
   N50.89 Other specified disorders of the male genital organs
     Atrophy or edema or hypertrophy or ulcer of scrotum, seminal vesicle, spermatic cord, tunica vaginalis and vas deferens
     Chylocele, tunica vaginalis (nonfilarial) NOS
     Urethroscrotal fistula
     Stricture of spermatic cord, tunica vaginalis, and vas deferens
N50.9 Disorder of male genital organs, unspecified

(N60–N65) DISORDERS OF BREAST

Excludes1: disorders of breast associated with childbirth (O91–O92)

N60 BENIGN MAMMARY DYSPLASIA
4th
   Includes: fibrocystic mastopathy
   N60.0 Solitary cyst of breast
     5th   Cyst of breast
     N60.01 Solitary cyst of right breast
     N60.02 Solitary cyst of left breast
     N60.09 Solitary cyst of unspecified breast

N61 INFLAMMATORY DISORDERS OF BREAST
4th
   Excludes1: inflammatory carcinoma of breast (C50.9)
     inflammatory disorder of breast associated with childbirth (O91.-)
     neonatal infective mastitis (P39.0)
     thrombophlebitis of breast [Mondor's disease] (I80.8)
   N61.0 Mastitis without abscess
     Infective mastitis (acute) (subacute) (nonpuerperal)
     Mastitis (acute) (subacute) (nonpuerperal) NOS
     Cellulitis (acute) (nonpuerperal) (subacute) of breast or nipple NOS
   N61.1 Abscess of the breast and nipple
     Abscess (acute) (chronic) (nonpuerperal) of areola or breast
     Carbuncle of breast
     Mastitis with abscess

N62 HYPERTROPHY OF BREAST
✔
   Gynecomastia
   Hypertrophy of breast NOS
   Massive pubertal hypertrophy of breast
   Excludes1: breast engorgement of newborn (P83.4)
     disproportion of reconstructed breast (N65.1)

N63 UNSPECIFIED LUMP IN BREAST
4th
   Nodule(s) NOS in breast
   N63.0 Unspecified lump in unspecified breast
   N63.1 Unspecified lump in the right breast
     5th   **N63.10 Unspecified lump in the right breast, unspecified quadrant**
     N63.11 upper outer quadrant
     N63.12 upper inner quadrant
     N63.13 lower outer quadrant
     N63.14 lower inner quadrant
     N63.15 overlapping quadrants
   N63.2 Unspecified lump in the left breast
     5th   **N63.20 Unspecified lump in the left breast, unspecified quadrant**
     N63.21 upper outer quadrant
     N63.22 upper inner quadrant
     N63.23 lower outer quadrant
     N63.24 lower inner quadrant
     N63.25 overlapping quadrants
   N63.3 Unspecified lump in axillary tail
     5th   **N63.31 Unspecified lump in axillary tail of the right breast**
     N63.32 Unspecified lump in axillary tail of the left breast
   N63.4 Unspecified lump in breast, subareolar
     5th   **N63.41 Unspecified lump in right breast, subareolar**
     N63.42 Unspecified lump in left breast, subareolar

4th   5th   6th   7th   Additional Character Required   ✔ 3-character code

•=New Code   *Excludes1*—Not coded here, do not use together
▲=Revised Code   *Excludes2*—Not included here

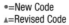

N64 OTHER DISORDERS OF BREAST
`4th`
    Excludes2: mechanical complication of breast prosthesis and implant
(T85.4-)
- **N64.3 Galactorrhea not associated with childbirth**
- **N64.4 Mastodynia**
- **N64.5 Other signs and symptoms in breast**
  `5th`   *Excludes2:* abnormal findings on diagnostic imaging of breast
  (R92.-)
  - **N64.51 Induration of breast**
  - **N64.52 Nipple discharge**
        Excludes1: abnormal findings in nipple discharge
    (R89.-)
  - **N64.53 Retraction of nipple**
  - **N64.59 Other signs and symptoms in breast**
- **N64.8 Other specified disorders of breast**
  `5th` **N64.89 Other specified disorders of breast**
      Galactocele
      Subinvolution of breast (postlactational)

(N70–N77) INFLAMMATORY DISEASES OF FEMALE PELVIC ORGANS

Excludes1: inflammatory diseases of female pelvic organs complicating:
    abortion or ectopic or molar pregnancy (O00–O07, O08.0)
    pregnancy, childbirth and the puerperium (O23.-, O75.3, O85, O86.-)

N70 SALPINGITIS AND OOPHORITIS
`4th`
    Includes: abscess (of) fallopian tube
    abscess (of) ovary
    pyosalpinx
    salpingo-oophoritis
    tubo-ovarian abscess
    tubo-ovarian inflammatory disease
    Use additional code (B95–B97), to identify infectious agent
    Excludes1: gonococcal infection (A54.24)
    tuberculous infection (A18.17)
- **N70.0 Acute salpingitis and oophoritis**
  `5th` **N70.01 Acute salpingitis**
  - **N70.02 Acute oophoritis**
  - **N70.03 Acute salpingitis and oophoritis**
- **N70.1 Chronic salpingitis and oophoritis**
  `5th` Hydrosalpinx
  - **N70.11 Chronic salpingitis**
  - **N70.12 Chronic oophoritis**
  - **N70.13 Chronic salpingitis and oophoritis**
- **N70.9 Salpingitis and oophoritis, unspecified**
  `5th` **N70.91 Salpingitis, unspecified**
  - **N70.92 Oophoritis, unspecified**
  - **N70.93 Salpingitis and oophoritis, unspecified**

N71 INFLAMMATORY DISEASE OF UTERUS, EXCEPT CERVIX
`4th`
    Includes: endo (myo) metritis
    metritis
    myometritis
    pyometra
    uterine abscess
    Use additional code (B95–B97), to identify infectious agent
    Excludes1: hyperplastic endometritis (N85.0-)
    infection of uterus following delivery (O85, O86.-)
- **N71.0 Acute inflammatory disease of uterus**
- **N71.9 Inflammatory disease of uterus, unspecified**

N72 INFLAMMATORY DISEASE OF CERVIX UTERI
`✔`
    Includes: cervicitis or endocervicitis or exocervicitis (all with or without
erosion or ectropion)
    Use additional code (B95–B97), to identify infectious agent
    Excludes1: erosion and ectropion of cervix without cervicitis (N86)

N73 OTHER FEMALE PELVIC INFLAMMATORY DISEASES
`4th`
    Use additional code (B95–B97), to identify infectious agent.
- **N73.0 Acute parametritis and pelvic cellulitis**
      Abscess of broad ligament
      Abscess of parametrium
      Pelvic cellulitis, female
- **N73.1 Chronic parametritis and pelvic cellulitis**
      Any condition in N73.0 specified as chronic

    Excludes1: tuberculous parametritis and pelvic cellulitis (A18.17)
- **N73.3 Female acute pelvic peritonitis**
- **N73.4 Female chronic pelvic peritonitis**
      Excludes1: tuberculous pelvic (female) peritonitis (A18.17)
- **N73.5 Female pelvic peritonitis, unspecified**
- **N73.6 Female pelvic peritoneal adhesions (postinfective)**
      Excludes2: postprocedural pelvic peritoneal adhesions (N99.4)
- **N73.8 Other specified female pelvic inflammatory diseases**
- **N73.9 Female pelvic inflammatory disease, unspecified**
      Female pelvic infection or inflammation NOS

N75 DISEASES OF BARTHOLIN'S GLAND
`4th`
- **N75.0 Cyst of Bartholin's gland**
- **N75.1 Abscess of Bartholin's gland**

N76 OTHER INFLAMMATION OF VAGINA AND VULVA
`4th`
    Use additional code (B95–B97), to identify infectious agent
    Excludes2: vulvar vestibulitis (N94.810)
- **N76.0 Acute vaginitis**
      Acute vulvovaginitis
- **N76.1 Subacute and chronic vaginitis**
      Chronic vulvovaginitis
      Subacute vulvovaginitis
- **N76.2 Acute vulvitis**
      Vulvitis NOS
- **N76.4 Abscess of vulva**
      Furuncle of vulva
- **N76.8 Other specified inflammation of vagina and vulva**
  `5th` **N76.89 Other specified inflammation of vagina and vulva**

N77 VULVOVAGINAL ULCERATION AND INFLAMMATION IN
`4th` **DISEASES CLASSIFIED ELSEWHERE**
- **N77.1 Vaginitis, vulvitis and vulvovaginitis in diseases classified
elsewhere**
      Code first underlying disease, such as:
      pinworm (B80)
      Excludes1: candidal vulvovaginitis (B37.3)
      chlamydial vulvovaginitis (A56.02)
      gonococcal vulvovaginitis (A54.02)
      herpesviral [herpes simplex] vulvovaginitis (A60.04)
      trichomonal vulvovaginitis (A59.01)
      tuberculous vulvovaginitis (A18.18)
      vulvovaginitis in early syphilis (A51.0)
      vulvovaginitis in late syphilis (A52.76)

(N80–N98) NONINFLAMMATORY DISORDERS OF FEMALE GENITAL TRACT

N83 NONINFLAMMATORY DISORDERS OF OVARY, FALLOPIAN
`4th` **TUBE AND BROAD LIGAMENT**
    Excludes2: hydrosalpinx (N70.1-)
- **N83.0 Follicular cyst of ovary**
  `5th` Cyst of graafian follicle
      Hemorrhagic follicular cyst (of ovary)
  - **N83.00 Follicular cyst of ovary, unspecified side**
  - **N83.01 Follicular cyst of right ovary**
  - **N83.02 Follicular cyst of left ovary**
- **N83.1 Corpus luteum cyst**
  `5th` Hemorrhagic corpus luteum cyst
  - **N83.10 Corpus luteum cyst of ovary, unspecified side**
  - **N83.11 Corpus luteum cyst of right ovary**
  - **N83.12 Corpus luteum cyst of left ovary**
- **N83.2 Other and unspecified ovarian cysts**
  `5th` *Excludes1:* developmental ovarian cyst (Q50.1)
      neoplastic ovarian cyst (D27.-)
      polycystic ovarian syndrome (E28.2)
      Stein-Leventhal syndrome (E28.2)
  - **N83.20 Unspecified ovarian cysts**
    `6th` **N83.201 Unspecified ovarian cyst, right side**
        N83.202 Unspecified ovarian cyst, left side
        N83.209 Unspecified ovarian cyst, unspecified side
  - **N83.29 Other ovarian cysts**
    `6th` Retention cyst of ovary
        Simple cyst of ovary

`4th` `5th` `6th` `7th`   Additional Character Required   `✔`   3-character code

•=New Code   *Excludes1*—Not coded here, do not use together
▲=Revised Code   *Excludes2*—Not included here

CHAPTER 14. DISEASES OF THE GENITOURINARY SYSTEM   (N83.291–N92)

         N83.291   **Other ovarian cyst, right side**
         N83.292   **Other ovarian cyst, left side**
         N83.299   **Other ovarian cyst, unspecified side**

N83.4 Prolapse and hernia of ovary and fallopian tube
`5th` **N83.40**   **Prolapse and hernia of ovary and fallopian tube, unspecified side**
         Prolapse and hernia of ovary and fallopian tube, NOS
    N83.41   **Prolapse and hernia of right ovary and fallopian tube**
    N83.42   **Prolapse and hernia of left ovary and fallopian tube**

N83.5 Torsion of ovary, ovarian pedicle and fallopian tube
`5th` Torsion of accessory tube
    N83.51   **Torsion of ovary and ovarian pedicle**
      `6th`   **N83.511**   **Torsion of right ovary and ovarian pedicle**
            N83.512   **Torsion of left ovary and ovarian pedicle**
            N83.519   **Torsion of ovary and ovarian pedicle, unspecified side**
                Torsion of ovary and ovarian pedicle, NOS
    N83.53   **Torsion of ovary, ovarian pedicle and fallopian tube**

N83.8 Other noninflammatory disorders of ovary, fallopian tube and broad ligament
    Broad ligament laceration syndrome [Allen-Masters]

N85 **OTHER NONINFLAMMATORY DISORDERS OF UTERUS, EXCEPT CERVIX**
`4th`
Excludes1: endometriosis (N80.-)
    inflammatory diseases of uterus (N71.-)
    noninflammatory disorders of cervix, except malposition (N86–N88)
    polyp of corpus uteri (N84.0)
    uterine prolapse (N81.-)

N85.0 Endometrial hyperplasia
`5th` **N85.00**   **Endometrial hyperplasia, unspecified**
         Hyperplasia (adenomatous) (cystic) (glandular) of endometrium
         Hyperplastic endometritis

N85.8 Other specified noninflammatory disorders of uterus
    Atrophy of uterus, acquired
    Fibrosis of uterus NOS

N86 **EROSION AND ECTROPION OF CERVIX UTERI**
`✔`
Decubitus (trophic) ulcer of cervix
Eversion of cervix
Excludes1: erosion and ectropion of cervix with cervicitis (N72)

N88 **OTHER NONINFLAMMATORY DISORDERS OF CERVIX UTERI**
`4th`
Excludes2: inflammatory disease of cervix (N72)
    polyp of cervix (N84.1)

N88.1 Old laceration of cervix uteri
    Adhesions of cervix
    Excludes1: current obstetric trauma (O71.3)

N88.2 Stricture and stenosis of cervix uteri
    Excludes1: stricture and stenosis of cervix uteri complicating labor (O65.5)

N89 **OTHER NONINFLAMMATORY DISORDERS OF VAGINA**
`4th`
Excludes1: abnormal results from vaginal cytologic examination without histologic confirmation (R87.62-)
    carcinoma in situ of vagina (D07.2)
    HGSIL of vagina (R87.623)
    inflammation of vagina (N76.-)
    senile (atrophic) vaginitis (N95.2)
    severe dysplasia of vagina (D07.2)
    trichomonal leukorrhea (A59.00)
    vaginal intraepithelial neoplasia [VAIN], grade III (D07.2)

N89.5 Stricture and atresia of vagina
    Vaginal adhesions
    Vaginal stenosis
    Excludes1: congenital atresia or stricture (Q52.4)
         postprocedural adhesions of vagina (N99.2)

N89.6 Tight hymenal ring
    Rigid hymen
    Tight introitus
    Excludes1: imperforate hymen (Q52.3)

N89.7 Hematocolpos
    Hematocolpos with hematometra or hematosalpinx

N89.8 Other specified noninflammatory disorders of vagina
    Leukorrhea NOS
    Old vaginal laceration
    Pessary ulcer of vagina
    Excludes1: current obstetric trauma (O70.-, O71.4, O71.7–O71.8)
         old laceration involving muscles of pelvic floor (N81.8)

N89.9 Noninflammatory disorder of vagina, unspecified

N90 **OTHER NONINFLAMMATORY DISORDERS OF VULVA AND PERINEUM**
`4th`
Excludes1: anogenital (venereal) warts (A63.0)
    carcinoma in situ of vulva (D07.1)
    condyloma acuminatum (A63.0)
    current obstetric trauma (O70.-, O71.7–O71.8)
    inflammation of vulva (N76.-)
    severe dysplasia of vulva (D07.1)
    vulvar intraepithelial neoplasm III [VIN III] (D07.1)

N90.0 Mild vulvar dysplasia
    Vulvar intraepithelial neoplasia [VIN], grade I

N90.1 Moderate vulvar dysplasia
    Vulvar intraepithelial neoplasia [VIN], grade II

N90.3 Dysplasia of vulva, unspecified

N90.4 Leukoplakia of vulva
    Dystrophy of vulva
    Kraurosis of vulva
    Lichen sclerosus of external female genital organs

N90.5 Atrophy of vulva
    Stenosis of vulva

N90.6 Hypertrophy of vulva
`5th` **N90.60**   **Unspecified hypertrophy of vulva**
         Unspecified hypertrophy of labia
    N90.61   **Childhood asymmetric labium majus enlargement CALME**
    N90.69   **Other specified hypertrophy of vulva**
         Other specified hypertrophy of labia

N90.7 Vulvar cyst

N90.8 Other specified noninflammatory disorders of vulva and perineum
`5th`
    N90.81   **Female genital mutilation status**
      `6th`   Female genital cutting status
          N90.810   **Female genital mutilation status, unspecified**
             Female genital cutting status, unspecified
             Female genital mutilation status NOS
          N90.811   **Female genital mutilation Type I status**
             Clitorectomy status
             Female genital cutting Type I status
          N90.812   **Female genital mutilation Type II status**
             Clitorectomy with excision of labia minora status
          N90.813   **Female genital mutilation Type III status**
             Female genital cutting Type III status
             Infibulation status
          N90.818   **Other female genital mutilation status**
             Female genital cutting or mutilation Type IV status
             Other female genital cutting status
    N90.89   **Other specified noninflammatory disorders of vulva and perineum**
         Adhesions of vulva
         Hypertrophy of clitoris

N90.9 Noninflammatory disorder of vulva and perineum, unspecified

N91 **ABSENT, SCANTY AND RARE MENSTRUATION**
`4th`
Excludes1: ovarian dysfunction (E28.-)

N91.0 Primary amenorrhea
N91.1 Secondary amenorrhea
N91.2 Amenorrhea, unspecified

N92 **EXCESSIVE, FREQUENT AND IRREGULAR MENSTRUATION**
`4th`
Excludes1: postmenopausal bleeding (N95.0)
    precocious puberty (menstruation) (E30.1)

 `4th` `5th` `6th` `7th` Additional Character Required   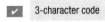 `✔` 3-character code

•=New Code   *Excludes1*—Not coded here, do not use together
▲=Revised Code   *Excludes2*—Not included here

N92.0 Excessive and frequent menstruation with regular cycle
Heavy periods NOS
Menorrhagia NOS
Polymenorrhea

N92.1 Excessive and frequent menstruation with irregular cycle
Irregular intermenstrual bleeding
Irregular, shortened intervals between menstrual bleeding
Menometrorrhagia
Metrorrhagia

N92.2 Excessive menstruation at puberty
Excessive bleeding associated with onset of menstrual periods
Pubertal menorrhagia
Puberty bleeding

N92.3 Ovulation bleeding
Regular intermenstrual bleeding

N92.5 Other specified irregular menstruation

N92.6 Irregular menstruation, unspecified
Irregular bleeding NOS
Irregular periods NOS
Excludes1: irregular menstruation with:
  lengthened intervals or scanty bleeding (N91.3–N91.5)
  shortened intervals or excessive bleeding (N92.1)

N93 OTHER ABNORMAL UTERINE AND VAGINAL BLEEDING
`4th`
Excludes1: neonatal vaginal hemorrhage (P54.6)
  precocious puberty (menstruation) (E30.1)
  pseudomenses (P54.6)

N93.1 Pre-pubertal vaginal bleeding

N93.8 Other specified abnormal uterine and vaginal bleeding
Dysfunctional or functional uterine or vaginal bleeding NOS

N93.9 Abnormal uterine and vaginal bleeding, unspecified

N94 PAIN AND OTHER CONDITIONS ASSOCIATED WITH
`4th` **FEMALE GENITAL ORGANS AND MENSTRUAL CYCLE**

N94.0 Mittelschmerz

N94.1 Dyspareunia
`5th` *Excludes1:* psychogenic dyspareunia (F52.6)
N94.10 Unspecified dyspareunia
N94.11 Superficial (introital) dyspareunia
N94.12 Deep dyspareunia
N94.19 Other specified dyspareunia

N94.2 Vaginismus
Excludes1: psychogenic vaginismus (F52.5)

N94.3 Premenstrual tension syndrome
Excludes 1: premenstrual dysphoric disorder (F32.81)
Code also associated menstrual migraine (G43.82-, G43.83-)

N94.4 Primary dysmenorrhea

N94.5 Secondary dysmenorrhea

N94.6 Dysmenorrhea, unspecified
Excludes1: psychogenic dysmenorrhea (F45.8)

N94.8 Other specified conditions associated with female genital
`5th` **organs and menstrual cycle**
N94.81 Vulvodynia
`6th` **N94.810 Vulvar vestibulitis**
  N94.818 Other vulvodynia
  N94.819 Vulvodynia, unspecified
    Vulvodynia NOS
N94.89 Other specified conditions associated with female
    genital organs and menstrual cycle

N94.9 Unspecified condition associated with female genital organs
and menstrual cycle

N97 FEMALE INFERTILITY
`4th`
Includes: inability to achieve a pregnancy
  sterility, female NOS
Excludes2: female infertility associated with:
  hypopituitarism (E23.0)
  Stein-Leventhal syndrome (E28.2)
  incompetence of cervix uteri (N88.3)

N97.0 Female infertility associated with anovulation

N97.1 Female infertility of tubal origin
Female infertility associated with congenital anomaly of tube
Female infertility due to tubal block
Female infertility due to tubal occlusion
Female infertility due to tubal stenosis

N97.9 Female infertility, unspecified

(N99) INTRAOPERATIVE AND POSTPROCEDURAL COMPLICATIONS AND DISORDERS OF GENITOURINARY SYSTEM, NEC

N99 INTRAOPERATIVE AND POSTPROCEDURAL
`4th` **COMPLICATIONS AND DISORDERS OF GENITOURINARY SYSTEM, NEC**
Excludes2: irradiation cystitis (N30.4-)
  postoophorectomy osteoporosis with current pathological fracture (M80.8-)
  postoophorectomy osteoporosis without current pathological fracture (M81.8)

N99.0 Postprocedural (acute) (chronic) kidney failure
Use additional code to type of kidney disease

N99.1 Postprocedural urethral stricture
`5th` Postcatheterization urethral stricture
N99.11 Postprocedural urethral stricture, male
`6th` **N99.110 Postprocedural urethral stricture, male, meatal**
  N99.111 Postprocedural bulbous urethral stricture, male
  N99.112 Postprocedural membranous urethral stricture, male
  N99.113 Postprocedural anterior bulbous urethral stricture, male
  N99.114 Postprocedural urethral stricture, male, unspecified
  N99.115 Postprocedural fossa navicularis urethral stricture
  N99.116 Postprocedural urethral stricture, male, overlapping sites
N99.12 Postprocedural urethral stricture, female

N99.2 Postprocedural adhesions of vagina

N99.3 Prolapse of vaginal vault after hysterectomy

N99.4 Postprocedural pelvic peritoneal adhesions
Excludes2: pelvic peritoneal adhesions NOS (N73.6)
  postinfective pelvic peritoneal adhesions (N73.6)

N99.5 Complications of stoma of urinary tract
`5th` *Excludes2:* mechanical complication of urinary catheter (T83.0-)
N99.51 Complication of cystostomy
`6th` **N99.510 Cystostomy hemorrhage**
  N99.511 Cystostomy infection
  N99.512 Cystostomy malfunction
  N99.518 Other cystostomy complication
N99.52 Complication of incontinent external stoma of
`6th` **urinary tract**
  N99.520 Hemorrhage of incontinent external stoma of urinary tract
  N99.521 Infection of incontinent external stoma of urinary tract
  N99.522 Malfunction of incontinent external stoma of urinary tract
  N99.523 Herniation of incontinent stoma of urinary tract
  N99.524 Stenosis of incontinent stoma of urinary tract
  N99.528 Other complication of incontinent external stoma of urinary tract
N99.53 Complication of continent stoma of urinary tract
`6th` **N99.530 Hemorrhage of continent stoma of urinary tract**
  N99.531 Infection of continent stoma of urinary tract
  N99.532 Malfunction of continent stoma of urinary tract
  N99.533 Herniation of continent stoma of urinary tract
  N99.534 Stenosis of continent stoma of urinary tract
  N99.538 Other complication of continent stoma of urinary tract

---

`4th` `5th` `6th` `7th` Additional Character Required   3-character code

•=New Code
▲=Revised Code

Excludes1—Not coded here, do not use together
Excludes2—Not included here

N99.8 [5th] **Other intraoperative and postprocedural complications and disorders of GI system**

    N99.81   Other intraoperative complications of GI system

    N99.82 [6th]   Postprocedural hemorrhage of a GI system organ or structure following a procedure

        N99.820   Postprocedural hemorrhage of a GI system organ or structure following a GI system procedure

        N99.821   Postprocedural hemorrhage of a GI system organ or structure following other procedure

    N99.83   Residual ovary syndrome

    N99.84 [6th]   Postprocedural hematoma and seroma of a GI system organ or structure following a procedure

        N99.840   Postprocedural hematoma of a GI system organ or structure following a GI system procedure

        N99.841   Postprocedural hematoma of a GI system organ or structure following other procedure

        N99.842   Postprocedural seroma of a GI system organ or structure following a GI system procedure

        N99.843   Postprocedural seroma of a GI system organ or structure following other procedure

    N99.89   Other postprocedural complications and disorders of GI system

CHAPTER 14. DISEASES OF THE GENITOURINARY SYSTEM   (N99.8–N99.89)

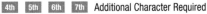

[4th] [5th] [6th] [7th] Additional Character Required   ✔ 3-character code   •=New Code   ▲=Revised Code   ***Excludes1***—Not coded here, do not use together   ***Excludes2***—Not included here

Chapter 15. Pregnancy, childbirth and the puerperium (O00–O9A)

General Rules for Obstetric Cases

CODES FROM CHAPTER 15 AND SEQUENCING PRIORITY
Obstetric cases require codes from Chapter 15, codes in the range O00–O9A, Pregnancy, Childbirth, and the Puerperium. Chapter 15 codes have sequencing priority over codes from other chapters. Additional codes from other chapters may be used in conjunction with Chapter 15 codes to further specify conditions. Should the provider document that the pregnancy is incidental to the encounter, then code Z33.1, Pregnant state, incidental, should be used in place of any Chapter 15 codes. It is the provider's responsibility to state that the condition being treated is not affecting the pregnancy.

CHAPTER 15 CODES USED ONLY ON THE MATERNAL RECORD
Chapter 15 codes are to be used only on the maternal record, never on the record of the newborn.

FINAL CHARACTER FOR TRIMESTER
The majority of codes in Chapter 15 have a final character indicating the trimester of pregnancy. The timeframes for the trimesters are indicated at the beginning of the chapter.

Assignment of the final character for trimester should be based on the provider's documentation of the trimester (or number of weeks) for the current admission/encounter. This applies to the assignment of trimester for pre-existing conditions as well as those that develop during or are due to the pregnancy. The provider's documentation of the number of weeks may be used to assign the appropriate code identifying the trimester.

Whenever delivery occurs during the current admission, and there is an "in childbirth" option for the obstetric complication being coded, the "in childbirth" code should be assigned. **When the classification does not provide an obstetric code with an "in childbirth" option, it is appropriate to assign a code describing the current trimester.**

SELECTION OF TRIMESTER FOR INPATIENT ADMISSIONS THAT ENCOMPASS MORE THAN ONE TRIMESTER
In instances when a patient is admitted to a hospital for complications of pregnancy during one trimester and remains in the hospital into a subsequent trimester, the trimester character for the antepartum complication code should be assigned on the basis of the trimester when the complication developed, not the trimester of the discharge. If the condition developed prior to the current admission/encounter or represents a pre-existing condition, the trimester character for the trimester at the time of the admission/encounter should be assigned.

UNSPECIFIED TRIMESTER
The "unspecified trimester" code should rarely be used, such as when the documentation in the record is insufficient to determine the trimester and it is not possible to obtain clarification.

7TH CHARACTER FOR FETUS IDENTIFICATION
Refer to categories O31, O35, O36, O40, and O41.

Selection of OB Principal or First-listed Diagnosis

ROUTINE OUTPATIENT PRENATAL VISITS
Refer to the *ICD-10-CM* manual for complete guidelines.

PRENATAL OUTPATIENT VISITS FOR HIGH-RISK PATIENTS
For routine prenatal outpatient visits for patients with high-risk pregnancies, a code from category O09, Supervision of high-risk pregnancy, should be used as the first-listed diagnosis. Secondary Chapter 15 codes may be used in conjunction with these codes if appropriate.

EPISODES WHEN NO DELIVERY OCCURS
Refer to the *ICD-10-CM* manual for complete guidelines.

WHEN A DELIVERY OCCURS
Refer to the *ICD-10-CM* manual for complete guidelines.

OUTCOME OF DELIVERY
A code from category Z37, Outcome of delivery, should be included on every maternal record when a delivery has occurred. These codes are not to be used on subsequent records or on the newborn record.

Pre-existing conditions versus conditions due to the pregnancy

Certain categories in Chapter 15 distinguish between conditions of the mother that existed prior to pregnancy (pre-existing) and those that are a direct result of pregnancy. When assigning codes from Chapter 15, it is important to assess if a condition was pre-existing prior to pregnancy or developed during or due to the pregnancy in order to assign the correct code.

Categories that do not distinguish between pre-existing and pregnancy-related conditions may be used for either. It is acceptable to use codes specifically for the puerperium with codes complicating pregnancy and childbirth if a condition arises postpartum during the delivery encounter.

Pre-existing hypertension in pregnancy

Refer to category O10.
Refer to Chapter 9, Hypertension.

Fetal Conditions Affecting the Management of the Mother

CODES FROM CATEGORIES O35 AND O36
Refer to categories O35 and O36.

IN UTERO SURGERY
Refer to category O35.

No code from Chapter 16, the perinatal codes, should be used on the mother's record to identify fetal conditions. Surgery performed in utero on a fetus is still to be coded as an obstetric encounter.

HIV Infection in Pregnancy, Childbirth and the Puerperium

During pregnancy, childbirth or the puerperium, a patient admitted because of an HIV-related illness should receive a principal diagnosis from subcategory O98.7-, HIV disease complicating pregnancy, childbirth and the puerperium, followed by the code(s) for the HIV-related illness(es).

Patients with asymptomatic HIV infection status admitted during pregnancy, childbirth, or the puerperium should receive codes of O98.7- and Z21, Asymptomatic HIV infection status.

DM in pregnancy

Diabetes mellitus is a significant complicating factor in pregnancy. Pregnant women who are diabetic should be assigned a code from category O24, DM in pregnancy, childbirth, and the puerperium, first, followed by the appropriate diabetes code(s) (E08–E13) from Chapter 4.

Long-term use of insulin

Code Z79.4, Long-term (current) use of insulin, should also be assigned if the DM is being treated with insulin.

Gestational (pregnancy induced) diabetes

Gestational (pregnancy induced) diabetes can occur during the second and third trimester of pregnancy in women who were not diabetic prior to pregnancy. Gestational diabetes can cause complications in the pregnancy similar to those of pre-existing DM. It also puts the woman at greater risk of developing diabetes after the pregnancy. Codes for gestational diabetes are in subcategory O24.4, Gestational DM. No other code from category O24, DM in pregnancy, childbirth, and the puerperium, should be used with a code from O24.4

The codes under subcategory O24.4 include diet controlled and insulin controlled. *If a patient with gestational diabetes is treated with both diet and insulin, only the code for insulin-controlled is required.*

Refer to the *ICD-10-CM* manual for complete guidelines.

Refer to the *ICD-10-CM* manual for guidelines for normal delivery (O80); peripartum and postpartum periods; sequela of complication of pregnancy, childbirth, and the puerperium (O94); sepsis and septic shock complicating

---

  4th　5th　6th　7th　Additional Character Required　　　✓　3-character code

•=New Code
▲=Revised Code

Excludes1—Not coded here, do not use together
Excludes2—Not included here

abortion, pregnancy, childbirth and the puerperium; puerperal sepsis; termination of pregnancy and spontaneous abortion and alcohol, tobacco *and drug* use during pregnancy, childbirth and the puerperium.

Abuse in a pregnant patient

Refer to the *ICD-10-CM* manual for complete guidelines.
  Refer to Chapter 19. Adult and child abuse, neglect and other maltreatment.

Note: CODES FROM THIS CHAPTER ARE FOR USE ONLY ON MATERNAL RECORDS, NEVER ON NEWBORN RECORDS.
  Codes from this chapter are for use for conditions related to or aggravated by the pregnancy, childbirth, or by the puerperium (maternal causes or obstetric causes).
  Use additional code from category Z3A, Weeks of gestation, to identify the specific week of the pregnancy, if known
Excludes1: supervision of normal pregnancy (Z34.-)
Excludes2: mental and behavioral disorders associated with the puerperium (F53) obstetrical tetanus (A34) postpartum necrosis of pituitary gland (E23.0) puerperal osteomalacia (M83.0)

> Trimesters are counted from the first day of the last menstrual period. They are defined as follows:
> 1st trimester — less than 14 weeks 0 days
> 2nd trimester — 14 weeks 0 days to less than 28 weeks 0 days
> 3rd trimester — 28 weeks 0 days until delivery

(O00–O08) PREGNANCY WITH ABORTIVE OUTCOME

O00 **ECTOPIC PREGNANCY**
[4th] *Includes:* ruptured ectopic pregnancy
Use additional code from category O08 to identify any associated complication
O00.0 Abdominal pregnancy
[5th] *Excludes1:* maternal care for viable fetus in abdominal pregnancy (O36.7-)
  O00.00   Abdominal pregnancy without intrauterine pregnancy
  O00.01   Abdominal pregnancy with intrauterine pregnancy
O00.1 Tubal pregnancy
[5th] Fallopian pregnancy
  Rupture of (fallopian) tube due to pregnancy
  Tubal abortion
  O00.10   Tubal pregnancy without intrauterine pregnancy
    [6th] **O00.101   Right tubal pregnancy without intrauterine pregnancy**
    O00.102   Left tubal pregnancy without intrauterine pregnancy
    O00.109   Unspecified tubal pregnancy without intrauterine pregnancy
  O00.11   Tubal pregnancy with intrauterine pregnancy
    [6th] **O00.111   Right tubal pregnancy with intrauterine pregnancy**
    O00.112   Left tubal pregnancy with intrauterine pregnancy
    O00.119   Unspecified tubal pregnancy with intrauterine pregnancy
O00.2 Ovarian pregnancy
[5th] **O00.20   Ovarian pregnancy without intrauterine pregnancy**
    [6th] **O00.201   Right ovarian pregnancy without intrauterine pregnancy**
    O00.202   Left ovarian pregnancy without intrauterine pregnancy
    O00.209   Unspecified ovarian pregnancy without intrauterine pregnancy
  O00.21   Ovarian pregnancy with intrauterine pregnancy
    [6th] **O00.211   Right ovarian pregnancy with intrauterine pregnancy**
    O00.212   Left ovarian pregnancy without intrauterine pregnancy
    O00.219   Unspecified ovarian pregnancy with intrauterine pregnancy
O00.8 Other ectopic pregnancy
[5th] Cervical pregnancy
  Cornual pregnancy
  Intraligamentous pregnancy
  Mural pregnancy

  O00.80   Other ectopic pregnancy without intrauterine pregnancy
  O00.81   Other ectopic pregnancy with intrauterine pregnancy
O00.9 Ectopic pregnancy, unspecified
[5th] **O00.90   Unspecified ectopic pregnancy without intrauterine pregnancy**
  O00.91   Unspecified ectopic pregnancy with intrauterine pregnancy

O02 **OTHER ABNORMAL PRODUCTS OF CONCEPTION**
[4th] **Use additional code** from category O08 to identify any associated complication.
Excludes1: papyraceous fetus (O31.0-)
O02.1 Missed abortion
  Early fetal death, before completion of 20 weeks of gestation, with retention of dead fetus
  Excludes1: failed induced abortion (O07.-)
    fetal death (intrauterine) (late) (O36.4)
    missed abortion with blighted ovum (O02.0)
    missed abortion with hydatidiform mole (O01.-)
    missed abortion with nonhydatidiform (O02.0)
    missed abortion with other abnormal products of conception (O02.8-)
    missed delivery (O36.4)
    stillbirth (P95)

O03 **SPONTANEOUS ABORTION**
[4th] **Note:** Incomplete abortion includes retained products of conception following spontaneous abortion
Includes: miscarriage
O03.4 Incomplete spontaneous abortion without complication
O03.9 Complete or unspecified spontaneous abortion without complication
  Miscarriage NOS
  Spontaneous abortion NOS

(O09) SUPERVISION OF HIGH RISK PREGNANCY

O09 **SUPERVISION OF HIGH RISK PREGNANCY**
[4th] **O09.6 Supervision of young primigravida and multigravida**
  [5th] Supervision of pregnancy for a female <16 years old at expected date of delivery
    O09.61   Supervision of young
    [6th]   **primigravida**
    O09.62   Supervision of young
    [6th]   **multigravida**

> Requires 6th character to identify trimester
> 1 first trimester
> 2 second trimester
> 3 third trimester
> 9 unspecified trimester

(O10–O16) EDEMA, PROTEINURIA AND HYPERTENSIVE DISORDERS IN PREGNANCY, CHILDBIRTH AND THE PUERPERIUM

Category O10, Pre-existing hypertension complicating pregnancy, childbirth and the puerperium, includes codes for hypertensive heart and hypertensive CKD. When assigning one of the O10 codes that includes hypertensive heart disease or hypertensive CKD, it is necessary to add a secondary code from the appropriate hypertension category to specify the type of heart failure or CKD.

O10 **PRE-EXISTING HYPERTENSION COMPLICATING**
[4th] **PREGNANCY, CHILDBIRTH AND THE PUERPERIUM**
Includes: pre-existing hypertension with pre-existing proteinuria complicating pregnancy, childbirth and the puerperium
Excludes2: pre-existing hypertension with superimposed pre-eclampsia complicating pregnancy, childbirth and the puerperium (O11.-)
O10.0   Pre-existing essential hypertension complicating pregnancy, childbirth and the puerperium
[5th] Any condition in I10 specified as a reason for obstetric care during pregnancy, childbirth or the puerperium
  O10.01   Pre-existing essential hypertension complicating
  [6th]   **pregnancy**
  O10.02   Pre-existing essential hypertension complicating
  [6th]   **childbirth**
  O10.03   Pre-existing essential hypertension complicating the puerperium

---

[4th] [5th] [6th] [7th] Additional Character Required   ✔ 3-character code

•=New Code   *Excludes1*—Not coded here, do not use together
▲=Revised Code   *Excludes2*—Not included here

O10.1 `5th` **Pre-existing hypertensive heart disease complicating pregnancy, childbirth and the puerperium**

> Requires 6th character to identify trimester
> 1 first trimester
> 2 second trimester
> 3 third trimester
> 9 unspecified trimester

Any condition in I11 specified as a reason for obstetric care during pregnancy, childbirth or the puerperium

Use additional code from I11 to identify the type of hypertensive heart disease

O10.11 `6th` **Pre-existing hypertensive heart disease complicating pregnancy**

O10.4 `5th` **Pre-existing secondary hypertension complicating pregnancy, childbirth and the puerperium**

Any condition in I15 specified as a reason for obstetric care during pregnancy, childbirth or the puerperium

Use additional code from I15 to identify the type of secondary hypertension

O10.41 `6th` **Pre-existing secondary hypertension complicating pregnancy**

O11 `4th` **PRE-EXISTING HYPERTENSION WITH PRE-ECLAMPSIA**

Includes: conditions in OI0 complicated by pre-eclampsia
pre-eclampsia superimposed pre-existing hypertension

Use additional code from O10 to identify the type of hypertension

O11.1 Pre-existing hypertension with pre-eclampsia, first trimester

O11.2 Pre-existing hypertension with pre-eclampsia, second trimester

O11.3 Pre-existing hypertension with pre-eclampsia, third trimester

O14 `4th` **PRE-ECLAMPSIA**

Excludes1: pre-existing hypertension with pre-eclampsia (O11)

O14.0 `5th` **Mild to moderate pre-eclampsia**

O14.1 `5th` **Severe pre-eclampsia**

> O14 requires 5th character
> 4 complicating childbirth
> 5 complicating the puerperium

Excludes1: HELLP syndrome (O14.2-)

O14.2 `5th` **HELLP syndrome**

Severe pre-eclampsia with hemolysis, elevated liver enzymes and low platelet count (HELLP)

O14.9 `5th` **Unspecified pre-eclampsia**

(O20–O29) OTHER MATERNAL DISORDERS PREDOMINANTLY RELATED TO PREGNANCY

Excludes2: maternal care related to the fetus and amniotic cavity and possible delivery problems (O30–O48)
maternal diseases classifiable elsewhere but complicating pregnancy, labor and delivery, and the puerperium (O98–O99)

O20 `4th` **HEMORRHAGE IN EARLY PREGNANCY**

Includes: hemorrhage before completion of 20 weeks gestation
Excludes1: pregnancy with abortive outcome (O00–O08)

O20.0 **Threatened abortion**

Hemorrhage specified as due to threatened abortion

O20.8 **Other hemorrhage in early pregnancy**

O20.9 **Hemorrhage in early pregnancy, unspecified**

O24 `4th` **DM IN PREGNANCY, CHILDBIRTH, AND THE PUERPERIUM**

O24.0 `5th` **Pre-existing type 1 DM**

Juvenile onset DM, in pregnancy, childbirth and the puerperium
Ketosis-prone DM in pregnancy, childbirth and the puerperium

Use additional code from category E10 to further identify any manifestations

O24.01 `6th` **Pre-existing type 1 DM, in pregnancy**

> O24.01 and O24.11 require 6th character to identify trimester
> 1 first trimester
> 2 second trimester
> 3 third trimester
> 9 unspecified trimester

O24.1 `5th` **Pre-existing type 2 DM**

Insulin-resistant DM

Use additional code (for): from category E11 to further identify any manifestations long-term (current) use of insulin (Z79.4)

O24.11 `6th` **Pre-existing type 2 DM, in pregnancy**

O24.4 `5th` **Gestational DM**

DM arising in pregnancy
Gestational diabetes mellitus NOS

O24.41 `6th` **Gestational DM in pregnancy**

O24.410 **Gestational DM in pregnancy, diet controlled**

O24.414 **Gestational DM in pregnancy, insulin controlled**

O24.415 **Gestational DM in pregnancy, controlled by oral hypoglycemic drugs**

Gestational diabetes mellitus in pregnancy, controlled by oral antidiabetic drugs

O28 `4th` **ABNORMAL FINDINGS ON ANTENATAL SCREENING OF MOTHER**

Excludes1: diagnostic findings classified elsewhere—**see Alphabetical Index**

O28.0 Abnormal hematological finding on antenatal screening of mother

O28.1 Abnormal biochemical finding on antenatal screening of mother

O28.2 Abnormal cytological finding on antenatal screening of mother

O28.3 Abnormal ultrasonic finding on antenatal screening of mother

O28.4 Abnormal radiological finding on antenatal screening of mother

O28.5 Abnormal chromosomal and genetic finding on antenatal screening of mother

O28.8 Other abnormal findings on antenatal screening of mother

O28.9 Unspecified abnormal findings on antenatal screening of mother

(O30–O48) MATERNAL CARE RELATED TO THE FETUS AND AMNIOTIC CAVITY AND POSSIBLE DELIVERY PROBLEMS

O30 `4th` **MULTIPLE GESTATION**

Code also any complications specific to multiple gestation

O30.0 `5th` **Twin pregnancy**

O30.00 `6th` **Twin pregnancy, unspecified number of placenta and unspecified number of amniotic sacs**

O30.01 `6th` **Twin pregnancy, monochorionic/monoamniotic**

Twin pregnancy, one placenta, one amniotic sac

Excludes1: conjoined twins (O30.02-)

O30.02 `6th` **Conjoined twin pregnancy**

O30.03 `6th` **Twin pregnancy, monochorionic/diamniotic**

Twin pregnancy, one placenta, two amniotic sacs

O30.04 `6th` **Twin pregnancy, dichorionic/diamniotic**

Twin pregnancy, two placentae, two amniotic sacs

O30.09 `6th` **Twin pregnancy, unable to determine number of placenta and number of amniotic sacs**

O30.1 `5th` **Triplet pregnancy**

O30.10 `6th` **Triplet pregnancy, unspecified number of placenta and unspecified number of amniotic sacs**

O30.11 `6th` **Triplet pregnancy with two or more monochorionic fetuses**

O30.12 `6th` **Triplet pregnancy with two or more monoamniotic fetuses**

> O30 requires 6th character to identify trimester
> 1 first trimester
> 2 second trimester
> 3 third trimester
> 9 unspecified trimester

O30.13 `6th` **Triplet pregnancy, trichorionic/triamniotic**

O30.19 `6th` **Triplet pregnancy, unable to determine number of placenta and number of amniotic sacs**

O30.2 `5th` **Quadruplet pregnancy**

O30.20 `6th` **Quadruplet pregnancy, unspecified number of placenta**

O30.21 `6th` **Quadruplet pregnancy with two or more monochorionic fetuses**

O30.22 `6th` **Quadruplet pregnancy with two or more monoamniotic fetuses**

O30.23 `6th` **Quadruplet pregnancy, quadrachorionic/quadra-amniotic**

`4th` `5th` `6th` `7th` Additional Character Required   ✓ 3-character code

•=New Code
▲=Revised Code

Excludes1—Not coded here, do not use together
Excludes2—Not included here

 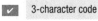

O30.29 `6th` Quadruplet pregnancy, unable to determine number of placenta and number of amniotic sacs

O30.8 Other specified multiple gestation
`5th` Multiple gestation pregnancy greater then quadruplets

  O30.80 `6th` Other specified multiple gestation, unspecified number of placenta and unspecified number of amniotic sacs

  O30.81 `6th` Other specified multiple gestation with two or more monochorionic fetuses

  O30.82 `6th` Other specified multiple gestation with two or more monoamniotic fetuses

> O30 requires 6th character to identify trimester
> 1 first trimester
> 2 second trimester
> 3 third trimester
> 9 unspecified trimester

  O30.83 `6th` Other specified multiple gestation, number of chorions and amnions are both equal to the number of fetuses
Pentachorionic, penta-amniotic pregnancy (quintuplets)
Hexachorionic, hexa-amniotic pregnancy (sextuplets)
Heptachorionic, hepta-amniotic pregnancy (septuplets)

  O30.89 `6th` Other specified multiple gestation, unable to determine number of placenta and number ofamniotic sacs

O31 `4th` **COMPLICATIONS SPECIFIC TO MULTIPLE GESTATION**
Assign a 7th character to identify the fetus for which the complication code applies.
Assign 7th character "0" for either a single gestation or when the documentation is insufficient to determine the fetus affected and it is not possible to obtain clarification or when it is not possible to clinically determine which fetus is affected.

> Requires 7th character to identify affected fetus
> 0 not applicable (ie, only one fetus) or unspecified
> 1 fetus 1
> 2 fetus 2
> 3 fetus 3
> 4 fetus 4
> 5 fetus 5
> 9 other fetus

Excludes2: delayed delivery of second twin, triplet, etc. (O63.2)
malpresentation of one fetus or more (O32.9)
placental transfusion syndromes (O43.0-)
Code also the appropriate code from category O30, Multiple gestation, when assigning a code from category O31 that has a 7th character of 1 through 9.

O31.1 `5th` Continuing pregnancy after spontaneous abortion of one fetus or more

  O31.10 Continuing pregnancy after spontaneous abortion of one fetus or more, unspecified trimester

  O31.11 Continuing pregnancy after spontaneous abortion of one fetus or more, first trimester

  O31.12 Continuing pregnancy after spontaneous abortion of one fetus or more, second trimester

  O31.13 Continuing pregnancy after spontaneous abortion of one fetus or more, third trimester

O31.2 `5th` Continuing pregnancy after intrauterine death of one fetus or more

  O31.20 Continuing pregnancy after intrauterine death of one fetus or more, unspecified trimester

  O31.21 Continuing pregnancy after intrauterine death of one fetus or more, first trimester

  O31.22 Continuing pregnancy after intrauterine death of one fetus or more, second trimester

  O31.23 Continuing pregnancy after intrauterine death of one fetus or more, third trimester

O31.8 Other complications specific to multiple gestation
`5th` **O31.8X** `6th` Other complications specific to multiple gestation

    O31.8X1 `7th` Other complications specific to multiple gestation, first trimester

    O31.8X2 `7th` Other complications specific to multiple gestation, second trimester

    O31.8X3 `7th` Other complications specific to multiple gestation, third trimester

O35 `4th` **MATERNAL CARE FOR KNOWN OR SUSPECTED FETAL ABNORMALITY AND DAMAGE**
Assign only when the fetal condition is actually responsible for modifying the management of the mother, ie, by requiring diagnostic studies, additional observation, special care, or termination of pregnancy. The fact that the fetal condition exists does not justify assigning a code from this series to the mother's record.
In cases when surgery is performed on the fetus, a diagnosis code from category O35, Maternal care for known or suspected fetal abnormality and damage, should be assigned identifying the fetal condition. Assign the appropriate procedure code for the procedure performed.
No code from Chapter 16, the perinatal codes, should be used on the mother's record to identify fetal conditions. Surgery performed in utero on a fetus is still to be coded as an obstetric encounter.
Assign a 7th character to identify the fetus for which the complication code applies.
Assign 7th character "0" for either a single gestation or when the documentation is insufficient to determine the fetus affected and it is not possible to obtain clarification or when it is not possible to clinically determine which fetus is affected.
Includes: the listed conditions in the fetus as a reason for hospitalization or other obstetric care to the mother, or
for termination of pregnancy
Code also any associated maternal condition
Excludes1: encounter for suspected maternal and fetal conditions ruled out (Z03.7-)
Code also the appropriate code from category O30, Multiple gestation, when assigning a code from category O35 that has a 7th character of 1 through 9.
Use placeholder X to complete the full code

  O35.0XX `7th` Maternal care for (suspected) central nervous system malformation in fetus
Maternal care for fetal anencephaly
Maternal care for fetal hydrocephalus
Maternal care for fetal spina bifida
Excludes2: chromosomal abnormality in fetus (O35.1)

  O35.1XX `7th` Maternal care for (suspected) chromosomal abnormality in fetus

  O35.2XX `7th` Maternal care for (suspected) hereditary disease in fetus
Excludes2: chromosomal abnormality in fetus (O35.1)

  O35.3XX `7th` Maternal care for (suspected) damage to fetus from viral disease in mother
Maternal care for damage to fetus from maternal cytomegalovirus infection
Maternal care for damage to fetus from maternal rubella

  O35.4XX `7th` Maternal care for (suspected) damage to fetus from alcohol

  O35.5XX `7th` Maternal care for (suspected) damage to fetus by drugs
Maternal care for damage to fetus from drug addiction

  O35.6XX `7th` Maternal care for (suspected) damage to fetus by radiation

  O35.7XX `7th` Maternal care for (suspected) damage to fetus by other medical procedures
Maternal care for damage to fetus by amniocentesis
Maternal care for damage to fetus by biopsy procedures
Maternal care for damage to fetus by hematological investigation
Maternal care for damage to fetus by intrauterine contraceptive device
Maternal care for damage to fetus by intrauterine surgery

  O35.8XX `7th` Maternal care for other (suspected) fetal abnormality and damage
Maternal care for other (suspected) fetal abnormality and damage
Maternal care for damage to fetus from maternal listeriosis
Maternal care for damage to fetus from maternal toxoplasmosis

---

`4th` `5th` `6th` `7th` Additional Character Required   3-character code

●=New Code
▲=Revised Code

Excludes1—Not coded here, do not use together
Excludes2—Not included here

O35.9XX `7th` **Maternal care for (suspected) fetal abnormality and damage, unspecified**

Requires 7th character to identify affected fetus
0 not applicable (ie, only one fetus) or unspecified
1 fetus 1
2 fetus 2
3 fetus 3
4 fetus 4
5 fetus 5
9 other fetus

O36 `4th` **MATERNAL CARE FOR OTHER FETAL PROBLEMS**

Assign only when the fetal condition is actually responsible for modifying the management of the mother, ie, by requiring diagnostic studies, additional observation, special care, or termination of pregnancy. The fact that the fetal condition exists does not justify assigning a code from this series to the mother's record.

No code from Chapter 16, the perinatal codes, should be used on the mother's record to identify fetal conditions. Surgery performed in utero on a fetus is still to be coded as an obstetric encounter.

Assign a 7th character to identify the fetus for which the complication code applies.

Assign 7th character "0" for either a single gestation or when the documentation is insufficient to determine the fetus affected and it is not possible to obtain clarification or when it is not possible to clinically determine which fetus is affected.

Includes: the listed conditions in the fetus as a reason for hospitalization or other obstetric care of the mother, or for termination of pregnancy

Excludes1: encounter for suspected maternal and fetal conditions ruled out (Z03.7-)
placental transfusion syndromes (O43.0-)

Excludes2: labor and delivery complicated by fetal stress (O77.-)

Code also the appropriate code from category O30, Multiple gestation, when assigning a code from category O36 that has a 7th character of 1 through 9.

O36.0 `5th` **Maternal care for rhesus isoimmunization**
Maternal care for Rh incompatibility (with hydrops fetalis)

    O36.01 `6th` **Maternal care for anti-D [Rh] antibodies**

        O36.011 `7th` **Maternal care for anti-D [Rh] antibodies, first trimester**

        O36.012 `7th` **Maternal care for anti-D [Rh] antibodies, second trimester**

        O36.013 `7th` **Maternal care for anti-D [Rh] antibodies, third trimester**

    O36.09 `6th` **Maternal care for other rhesus isoimmunization**

        O36.091 `7th` **Maternal care for other rhesus isoimmunization, first trimester**

        O36.092 `7th` **Maternal care for other rhesus isoimmunization, second trimester**

        O36.093 `7th` **Maternal care for other rhesus isoimmunization, third trimester**

O36.1 `5th` **Maternal care for other isoimmunization**
Maternal care for ABO isoimmunization

    O36.11 `6th` **Maternal care for Anti-A sensitization**
Maternal care for isoimmunization NOS (with hydrops fetalis)

        O36.111 `7th` **Maternal care for Anti-A sensitization, first trimester**

        O36.112 `7th` **Maternal care for Anti-A sensitization, second trimester**

        O36.113 `7th` **Maternal care for Anti-A sensitization, third trimester**

    O36.19 `6th` **Maternal care for other isoimmunization**
Maternal care for Anti-B sensitization

        O36.191 `7th` **Maternal care for other isoimmunization, first trimester**

        O36.192 `7th` **Maternal care for other isoimmunization, second trimester**

        O36.193 `7th` **Maternal care for other isoimmunization, third trimester**

O36.2 `5th` **Maternal care for hydrops fetalis**
Maternal care for hydrops fetalis NOS
Maternal care for hydrops fetalis not associated with isoimmunization

Excludes1: hydrops fetalis associated with ABO isoimmunization (O36.1-)
hydrops fetalis associated with rhesus isoimmunization (O36.0-)

    O36.21X `7th` **Maternal care for hydrops fetalis, first trimester**

    O36.22X `7th` **Maternal care for hydrops fetalis, second trimester**

    O36.23X `7th` **Maternal care for hydrops fetalis, third trimester**

O36.4XX `7th` **Maternal care for intrauterine death**
Maternal care for intrauterine fetal death NOS
Maternal care for intrauterine fetal death after completion of 20 weeks of gestation
Maternal care for late fetal death
Maternal care for missed delivery

Excludes1: missed abortion (O02.1)
stillbirth (P95)

O36.5 `5th` **Maternal care for known or suspected poor fetal growth**

    O36.51 `6th` **Maternal care for known or suspected placental insufficiency**

        O36.511 `7th` **Maternal care for known or suspected placental insufficiency, first trimester**

        O36.512 `7th` **Maternal care for known or suspected placental insufficiency, second trimester**

        O36.513 `7th` **Maternal care for known or suspected placental insufficiency, third trimester**

    O36.59 `6th` **Maternal care for other known or suspected poor fetal growth**
Maternal care for known or suspected light-for-dates NOS
Maternal care for known or suspected small-for-dates NOS

        O36.591 `7th` **Maternal care for other known or suspected poor fetal growth, first trimester**

        O36.592 `7th` **Maternal care for other known or suspected poor fetal growth, second trimester**

        O36.593 `7th` **Maternal care for other known or suspected poor fetal growth, third trimester**

O36.6 `5th` **Maternal care for excessive fetal growth**
Maternal care for known or suspected large-for-dates

    O36.61X `7th` **Maternal care for excessive fetal growth, first trimester**

    O36.62X `7th` **Maternal care for excessive fetal growth, second trimester**

    O36.63X `7th` **Maternal care for excessive fetal growth, third trimester**

O36.7 `5th` **Maternal care for viable fetus in abdominal pregnancy**

    O36.71X `7th` **Maternal care for viable fetus in abdominal pregnancy, first trimester**

    O36.72X `7th` **Maternal care for viable fetus in abdominal pregnancy, second trimester**

    O36.73X `7th` **Maternal care for viable fetus in abdominal pregnancy, third trimester**

O36.8 `5th` **Maternal care for other specified fetal problems**

    O36.80 **Pregnancy with inconclusive fetal viability**
Encounter to determine fetal viability of pregnancy

    O36.81 `6th` **Decreased fetal movements**

        O36.812 **Decreased fetal movements, second trimester**

        O36.813 `7th` **Decreased fetal movements, third trimester**

    O36.82 `6th` **Fetal anemia and thrombocytopenia**

        O36.821 `7th` **Fetal anemia and thrombocytopenia, first trimester**

        O36.822 `7th` **Fetal anemia and thrombocytopenia, second trimester**

`4th` `5th` `6th` `7th` Additional Character Required   ✔ 3-character code

•=New Code
▲=Revised Code

Excludes1—Not coded here, do not use together
Excludes2—Not included here

O36.823 **Fetal anemia and thrombo-cytopenia, third trimester**
`7th`

Requires 7th character to identify affected fetus
0 not applicable (ie, only one fetus) or unspecified
1 fetus 1
2 fetus 2
3 fetus 3
4 fetus 4
5 fetus 5
9 other fetus

O36.83 **Maternal care for abnormalities of the fetal heart rate or rhythm**
`6th`

Maternal care for depressed fetal heart rate tones
Maternal care for fetal bradycardia
Maternal care for fetal heart rate abnormal variability
Maternal care for fetal heart rate decelerations
Maternal care for fetal heart rate irregularity
Maternal care for fetal tachycardia
Maternal care for non-reassuring fetal heart rate or rhythm

O36.831 **Maternal care for abnormalities of the fetal heart rate or rhythm, first trimester**
`7th`

O36.832 **Maternal care for abnormalities of the fetal heart rate or rhythm, second trimester**
`7th`

O36.833 **Maternal care for abnormalities of the fetal heart rate or rhythm, third trimester**
`7th`

O36.839 **Maternal care for abnormalities of the fetal heart rate or rhythm, unspecified trimester**
`7th`

O36.89 **Maternal care for other specified fetal problems**
`6th`

O36.891 **Maternal care for other specified fetal problems, first trimester**
`7th`

O36.892 **Maternal care for other specified fetal problems, second trimester**
`7th`

O36.893 **Maternal care for other specified fetal problems, third trimester**
`7th`

O40 POLYHYDRAMNIOS
`4th`

Assign a 7th character to identify the fetus for which the complication code applies.
Assign 7th character "0" for either a single
  gestation or when the documentation is insufficient to determine the fetus affected and it is not possible to obtain clarification or when it is not possible to clinically determine which fetus is affected.
Includes: hydramnios
Excludes1: encounter for suspected maternal and fetal conditions ruled out (Z03.7-)

O40.1XX Polyhydramnios, first trimester
`7th`

O40.2XX Polyhydramnios, second trimester
`7th`

O40.3XX Polyhydramnios, third trimester
`7th`

O40.9XX Polyhydramnios, unspecified trimester
`7th`

O41 OTHER DISORDERS OF AMNIOTIC FLUID AND MEMBRANES
`4th`

Assign a 7th character to identify the fetus
  for which the complication code applies.
Assign 7th character "0" for either a single gestation or when the documentation is insufficient to determine the fetus affected and it is not possible to obtain clarification or when it is not possible to clinically determine which fetus is affected.
Excludes1: encounter for suspected maternal and fetal conditions ruled out (Z03.7-)
Code also the appropriate code from category O30, Multiple gestation, when assigning a code from category O41 that has a 7th character of 1 through 9.

O41.01X Oligohydramnios, first trimester, not applicable or unspecified
`7th`

O41.02X Oligohydramnios, second trimester, not applicable or unspecified
`7th`

O41.03X Oligohydramnios, third trimester, not applicable or unspecified
`7th`

O42 PREMATURE RUPTURE OF MEMBRANES
`4th`

O42.00 **Premature rupture of membranes, onset of labor within 24 hours of rupture, unspecified weeks of gestation**

O42.01 **Preterm premature rupture of membranes, onset of labor within 24 hours of rupture**
`6th`
Premature rupture of membranes before 37 completed weeks of gestation

O42.011 **Preterm premature rupture of membranes, onset of labor within 24 hours of rupture, first trimester**

O42.012 **second trimester**

O42.013 **third trimester**

O42.019 **unspecified trimester**

O42.02 **Full-term premature rupture of membranes, onset of labor within 24 hours of rupture**
Premature rupture of membranes at or after 37 completed weeks of gestation, onset of labor within 24hours of rupture

O42.1 Premature rupture of membranes, onset of labor more than 24 hours following rupture
`5th`

O42.10 **Premature rupture of membranes, onset of labor more than 24 hours following rupture, unspecified weeks of gestation**

O42.11 **Preterm premature rupture of membranes, onset of labor more than 24 hours following rupture**
`6th`
Premature rupture of membranes before 37 completed weeks of gestation

O42.111 **Preterm premature rupture of membranes, onset of labor more than 24 hours following rupture, first trimester**

O42.112 **second trimester**

O42.113 **third trimester**

O42.119 **unspecified trimester**

O42.12 **Full-term premature rupture of membranes, onset of labor more than 24 hours following rupture**
Premature rupture of membranes at or after 37 completed weeks of gestation, onset of labor more than 24 hours following rupture

O42.9 Premature rupture of membranes, unspecified as to length of time between rupture and onset of labor

O42.90 **Premature rupture of membranes, unspecified as to length of time between rupture and onset of labor, unspecified weeks of gestation**

O42.91 **Preterm premature rupture of membranes, unspecified as to length of time between rupture and onset of labor**
`6th`
Premature rupture of membranes before 37 completed weeks of gestation

O42.911 **Preterm premature rupture of membranes, unspecified as to length of time between rupture and onset of labor; first trimester**

O42.912 **second trimester**

O42.913 **third trimester**

O42.92 **Full-term premature rupture of membranes, unspecified as to length of time between rupture and onset of labor**
Premature rupture of membranes at or after 37 completed weeks of gestation, unspecified as to length of time between rupture and onset of labor

O43 PLACENTAL DISORDERS
`4th`
Excludes2: maternal care for poor fetal growth due to placental insufficiency (O36.5-)
placenta previa (O44.-)
placental polyp (O90.89)
placentitis (O41.14-)
premature separation of placenta [abruptio placentae] (O45.-)

O43.0 Placental transfusion syndromes
`5th`

O43.01 **Fetomaternal placental transfusion syndrome**
`6th`
Maternofetal placental transfusion syndrome

O43.011 **Fetomaternal placental transfusion syndrome; first trimester**

O43.012 **second trimester**

`4th` `5th` `6th` `7th` Additional Character Required   ✓ 3-character code   •=New Code   ▲=Revised Code   *Excludes1*—Not coded here, do not use together   *Excludes2*—Not included here

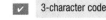

	O43.013	third trimester	Requires 7th character to identify affected fetus

O43.02 **Fetus-to-fetus placental transfusion syndrome**
[6th]

> Requires 7th character to identify affected fetus
> 0 not applicable (ie, only one fetus) or unspecified
> 1 fetus 1
> 2 fetus 2
> 3 fetus 3
> 4 fetus 4
> 5 fetus 5
> 9 other fetus

O43.021 **Fetus-to-fetus placental transfusion syndrome; first trimester**

O43.022 **second trimester**

O43.023 **third trimester**

(O60–O77) COMPLICATIONS OF LABOR AND DELIVERY

O60 PRETERM LABOR
[4th]
Includes: onset (spontaneous) of labor before 37 completed weeks of gestation
Excludes1: false labor (O47.0-)
threatened labor NOS (O47.0-)

O60.0 Preterm labor without delivery
[5th]　**O60.02 Preterm labor without delivery, second trimester**
　O60.03 Preterm labor without delivery, third trimester

O75 OTHER COMPLICATIONS OF LABOR AND DELIVERY, NOT ELSEWHERE CLASSIFIED
[4th]
Excludes2: puerperal (postpartum) infection (O86.-)
puerperal (postpartum) sepsis (O85)

O75.0 Maternal distress during labor and delivery

O75.1 Shock during or following labor and delivery
Obstetric shock following labor and delivery

O75.2 Pyrexia during labor, not elsewhere classified

O75.3 Other infection during labor
Sepsis during labor
Use additional code (B95–B97), to identify infectious agent

O75.4 Other complications of obstetric surgery and procedures
Cardiac arrest following obstetric surgery or procedures
Cardiac failure following obstetric surgery or procedures
Cerebral anoxia following obstetric surgery or procedures
Pulmonary edema following obstetric surgery or procedures
Use additional code to identify specific complication
Excludes2: complications of anesthesia during labor and delivery (O74.-)
disruption of obstetrical (surgical) wound (O90.0–O90.1)
hematoma of obstetrical (surgical) wound (O90.2)
infection of obstetrical (surgical) wound (O86.0-)

O75.5 Delayed delivery after artificial rupture of membranes

O75.8 Other specified complications of labor and delivery
[5th]　**O75.81 Maternal exhaustion complicating labor and delivery**
　O75.82 Onset (spontaneous) of labor after 37 completed weeks of gestation but before 39 completed weeks gestation, with delivery by (planned) cesarean section
Delivery by (planned) cesarean section occurring after 37 completed weeks of gestation but before 39 completed weeks gestation due to (spontaneous) onset of labor
Code first to specify reason for planned cesarean section such as:
cephalopelvic disproportion (normally formed fetus) (O33.9)
previous cesarean delivery (O34.21)
　O75.89 Other specified complications of labor and delivery

O75.9 Complication of labor and delivery, unspecified

(O80–O82) ENCOUNTER FOR DELIVERY

(O85–O92) COMPLICATIONS PREDOMINANTLY RELATED TO THE PUERPERIUM

O92 OTHER DISORDERS OF BREAST AND DISORDERS OF LACTATION ASSOCIATED WITH PREGNANCY AND THE PUERPERIUM
[4th]

O92.0 Retracted nipple associated with pregnancy, the puerperium, and lactation
[5th]
　O92.02 Retracted nipple associated with the puerperium
　O92.03 Retracted nipple associated with lactation

O92.1 Cracked nipple associated with pregnancy, the puerperium, and lactation
[5th]
Fissure of nipple, gestational or puerperal
　O92.12 Cracked nipple associated with the puerperium
　O92.13 Cracked nipple associated with lactation

O92.2 Other and unspecified disorders of breast associated with pregnancy and the puerperium
[5th]
　O92.20 Unspecified disorder of breast associated with pregnancy and the puerperium
　O92.29 Other disorders of breast associated with pregnancy and the puerperium

O92.3 Agalactia
Primary agalactia
Excludes1: Elective agalactia (O92.5)
Secondary agalactia (O92.5)
Therapeutic agalactia (O92.5)

O92.4 Hypogalactia

O92.5 Suppressed lactation
Elective agalactia
Secondary agalactia
Therapeutic agalactia
Excludes1: primary agalactia (O92.3)

O92.6 Galactorrhea

O92.7 Other and unspecified disorders of lactation
[5th]　**O92.70 Unspecified disorders of lactation**
　O92.79 Other disorders of lactation
Puerperal galactocele

(O94–O9A) OTHER OBSTETRIC CONDITIONS, NOT ELSEWHERE CLASSIFIED

[4th] [5th] [6th] [7th] Additional Character Required　　[✓] 3-character code　　•=New Code　▲=Revised Code　*Excludes1*—Not coded here, do not use together　*Excludes2*—Not included here

Chapter 16. Certain conditions originating in the perinatal period (P00–P96)

GUIDELINES

For coding and reporting purposes the perinatal period is defined as before birth through the 28th day following birth. The following guidelines are provided for reporting purposes

General Perinatal Rules

Codes in this chapter are <u>never</u> for use on the maternal record. Codes from Chapter 15, the obstetric chapter, are never permitted on the newborn record. Chapter 16 codes may be used throughout the life of the patient if the condition is still present.

PRINCIPAL DIAGNOSIS FOR BIRTH RECORD

When coding the birth episode in a newborn record, assign a code from category Z38, Liveborn infants according to place of birth and type of delivery, as the principal diagnosis. Refer to code Z38 for further guidelines.

    A code from category Z38 is used only on the newborn record, not on the mother's record.

USE OF CODES FROM OTHER CHAPTERS WITH CODES FROM CHAPTER 16

Codes from other chapters may be used with codes from Chapter 16 if the codes from the other chapters provide more specific detail. Codes for signs and symptoms may be assigned when a definitive diagnosis has not been established. If the reason for the encounter is a perinatal condition, the code from Chapter 16 should be sequenced first.

USE OF CHAPTER 16 CODES AFTER THE PERINATAL PERIOD

Should a condition originate in the perinatal period, and continue throughout the life of the patient, the perinatal code should continue to be used regardless of the patient's age.

BIRTH PROCESS OR COMMUNITY ACQUIRED CONDITIONS

If a newborn has a condition that may be either due to the birth process or community acquired and the documentation does not indicate which it is, the default is due to the birth process and the code from Chapter 16 should be used. If the condition is community-acquired, a code from Chapter 16 should not be assigned.

CODE ALL CLINICALLY SIGNIFICANT CONDITIONS

All clinically significant conditions noted on routine newborn examination should be coded. A condition is clinically significant if it requires:

- clinical evaluation; or
- therapeutic treatment; or
- diagnostic procedures; or
- extended length of hospital stay; or
- increased nursing care and/or monitoring; or
- has implications for future health care needs

Note: The perinatal guidelines listed above are the same as the general coding guidelines for "additional diagnoses," except for the final point regarding implications for future health care needs. Codes should be assigned for conditions that have been specified by the provider as having implications for future health care needs.

Observation and Evaluation of Newborns for Suspected Condition not Found

See category Z05.

Coding Additional Perinatal Diagnoses

ASSIGNING CODES FOR CONDITIONS THAT REQUIRE TREATMENT

Assign codes for conditions that require treatment or further investigation, prolong the length of stay, or require resource utilization.

CODES FOR CONDITIONS SPECIFIED AS HAVING IMPLICATIONS FOR FUTURE HEALTH CARE NEEDS

Assign codes for conditions that have been specified by the provider as having implications for future health care needs.

Prematurity and Fetal Growth Retardation

Refer to categories P05–P07 for guidelines for prematurity and fetal growth retardation.

LBW and immaturity status

Refer to category P07, Disorders of newborn related to short gestation and LBW, not elsewhere classified, for associated guidelines.

Bacterial Sepsis of Newborn

Refer to category P36, Bacterial sepsis of newborn for guidelines for reporting newborn bacterial sepsis.

Stillbirth

Refer to code P95 for guidelines.

COVID-19 Infection in Newborn

For a newborn that tests positive for COVID-19, assign code U07.1, COVID-19, and the appropriate codes for associated manifestation(s) in neonates/newborns in the absence of documentation indicating a specific type of transmission. For a newborn that tests positive for COVID-19 and the provider documents the condition was contracted in utero or during the birth process, assign codes P35.8, Other congenital viral diseases, and U07.1, COVID-19. When coding the birth episode in a newborn record, the appropriate code from category Z38, Liveborn infants according to place of birth and type of delivery, should be assigned as the principal diagnosis.

Note: Codes from this chapter are for use on newborn records only, never on maternal records

Includes: conditions that have their origin in the fetal or perinatal period (before birth through the first 28 days after birth) even if morbidity occurs later

Excludes2: congenital malformations, deformations and chromosomal abnormalities (Q00–Q99)
endocrine, nutritional and metabolic diseases (E00–E88)
injury, poisoning and certain other consequences of external causes (S00–T88)
neoplasms (C00–D49)
tetanus neonatorum (A33)

(P00–P04) NEWBORN AFFECTED BY MATERNAL FACTORS AND BY COMPLICATIONS OF PREGNANCY, LABOR, AND DELIVERY

Note: These codes are for use when the listed maternal conditions are specified as the cause of confirmed morbidity or potential morbidity which have their origin in the perinatal period (before birth through the first 28 days after birth). Codes from these categories are also for use for newborns who are suspected of having an abnormal condition resulting from exposure from the mother or the birth process.

P00 **NEWBORN AFFECTED BY MATERNAL CONDITIONS THAT**
[4th] **MAY BE UNRELATED TO PRESENT PREGNANCY**
    Code first any current condition in newborn
    Excludes2: encounter for observation and evaluation of newborn for suspected diseases and conditions ruled out (Z05.-)
       newborn affected by maternal complications of pregnancy (P01.-)
       newborn affected by maternal endocrine and metabolic disorders (P70–P74)
       newborn affected by noxious substances transmitted via placenta or breast milk (P04.-)
    P00.0 **Newborn affected by maternal hypertensive disorders**
       Newborn affected by maternal conditions classifiable to O10–O11, O13–O16
    P00.1 **Newborn affected by maternal renal and urinary tract diseases**
       Newborn affected by maternal conditions classifiable to N00–N39
    P00.2 **Newborn affected by maternal infectious and parasitic diseases**
       Newborn affected by maternal infectious disease classifiable to A00–B99, J09 and J10
       Excludes2: infections specific to the perinatal period (P35–P39)
          maternal genital tract or other localized infections (P00.8-)

    Additional Character Required   ✔ 3-character code   •=New Code   ***Excludes1***—Not coded here, do not use together
    ▲=Revised Code   ***Excludes2***—Not included here

CHAPTER 16. CERTAIN CONDITIONS ORIGINATING IN THE PERINATAL PERIOD   (P00.3–P03.81)

P00.3 Newborn affected by other maternal circulatory and respiratory diseases
Newborn affected by maternal conditions classifiable to I00–I99, J00–J99, Q20–Q34 and not included in P00.0, P00.2

P00.4 Newborn affected by maternal nutritional disorders
Newborn affected by maternal disorders classifiable to E40–E64
Maternal malnutrition NOS

P00.5 Newborn affected by maternal injury
Newborn affected by maternal conditions classifiable to O9A.2-

P00.6 Newborn affected by surgical procedure on mother
Newborn affected by amniocentesis
Excludes1: cesarean delivery for present delivery (P03.4)
damage to placenta from amniocentesis, cesarean delivery or surgical induction (P02.1)
previous surgery to uterus or pelvic organs (P03.89)
Excludes2: newborn affected by complication of (fetal) intrauterine procedure (P96.5)

P00.7 Newborn affected by other medical procedures on mother, NEC
Newborn affected by radiation to mother
Excludes1: damage to placenta from amniocentesis, cesarean delivery or surgical induction (P02.1)
newborn affected by other complications of labor and delivery (P03.-)

P00.8 Newborn affected by other maternal conditions
  `5th`   **P00.81 Newborn affected by periodontal disease in mother**
     •**P00.82 Newborn affected by (positive) maternal group B streptococcus (GBS) colonization**
Contact with positive maternal group B streptococcus
     P00.89 Newborn affected by other maternal conditions
Newborn affected by conditions classifiable to T80–T88
Newborn affected by maternal genital tract or other localized infections
Newborn affected by maternal SLE
Use additional code to identify infectious agent, if known
Excludes 2: newborn affected by positive maternal group B streptococcus(GBS) colonization (P00.82)

P00.9 Newborn affected by unspecified maternal condition

P01   **NEWBORN AFFECTED BY MATERNAL COMPLICATIONS**
`4th`   **OF PREGNANCY**
Code first any current condition in newborn
Excludes2: encounter for observation of newborn for suspected diseases and conditions ruled out (Z05.-)

P01.0 Newborn affected by incompetent cervix

P01.1 Newborn affected by premature rupture of membranes

P01.2 Newborn affected by oligohydramnios
Excludes1: oligohydramnios due to premature rupture of membranes (P01.1)

P01.3 Newborn affected by polyhydramnios
Newborn affected by hydramnios

P01.4 Newborn affected by ectopic pregnancy
Newborn affected by abdominal pregnancy

P01.5 Newborn affected by multiple pregnancy
Newborn affected by triplet (pregnancy)
Newborn affected by twin (pregnancy)

P01.6 Newborn affected by maternal death

P01.7 Newborn affected by malpresentation before labor
Newborn affected by breech presentation before labor
Newborn affected by external version before labor
Newborn affected by face presentation before labor
Newborn affected by transverse lie before labor
Newborn affected by unstable lie before labor

P01.8 Newborn affected by other maternal complications of pregnancy

P01.9 Newborn affected by maternal complication of pregnancy, unspecified

P02   **NEWBORN AFFECTED BY COMPLICATIONS OF**
`4th`   **PLACENTA, CORD AND MEMBRANES**
Code first any current condition in newborn
Excludes2: encounter for observation of newborn for suspected diseases and conditions ruled out (Z05.-)

P02.0 Newborn affected by placenta previa

P02.1 Newborn affected by other forms of placental separation and hemorrhage
Newborn affected by abruptio placenta
Newborn affected by accidental hemorrhage
Newborn affected by antepartum hemorrhage
Newborn affected by damage to placenta from amniocentesis, cesarean delivery or surgical induction
Newborn affected by maternal blood loss
Newborn affected by premature separation of placenta

P02.2 Newborn affected by other and unspecified morphological and
`5th`   **functional abnormalities of placenta**
     P02.20 Newborn affected by unspecified morphological and functional abnormalities of placenta
     P02.29 Newborn affected by other morphological and functional abnormalities of placenta
Newborn affected by placental dysfunction
Newborn affected by placental infarction
Newborn affected by placental insufficiency

P02.3 Newborn affected by placental transfusion syndromes
Newborn affected by placental and cord abnormalities resulting in twin-to-twin or other transplacental transfusion

P02.4 Newborn affected by prolapsed cord

P02.5 Newborn affected by other compression of umbilical cord
Newborn affected by umbilical cord (tightly) around neck
Newborn affected by entanglement of umbilical cord
Newborn affected by knot in umbilical cord

P02.6 Newborn affected by other and unspecified conditions of
`5th`   **umbilical cord**
     P02.60 Newborn affected by unspecified conditions of umbilical cord
     P02.69 Newborn affected by other conditions of umbilical cord
Newborn affected by short umbilical cord
Newborn affected by vasa previa
Excludes1: newborn affected by single umbilical artery (Q27.0)

P02.7 Newborn affected by chorioamnionitis
`5th`   **P02.70 Newborn affected by fetal inflammatory response syndrome**
     P02.78 Newborn affected by other conditions from chorioamnionitis
Newborn affected by amnionitis
Newborn affected by membranitis
Newborn affected by placentitis

P02.8 Newborn affected by other abnormalities of membranes

P02.9 Newborn affected by abnormality of membranes, unspecified

P03   **NEWBORN AFFECTED BY OTHER COMPLICATIONS OF**
`4th`   **LABOR AND DELIVERY**
Code first any current condition in newborn
Excludes2: encounter for observation of newborn for suspected diseases and conditions ruled out (Z05.-)

P03.0 Newborn affected by breech delivery and extraction

P03.1 Newborn affected by other malpresentation, malposition and disproportion during labor and delivery
Newborn affected by contracted pelvis
Newborn affected by conditions classifiable to O64–O66
Newborn affected by persistent occipitoposterior
Newborn affected by transverse lie

P03.2 Newborn affected by forceps delivery

P03.3 Newborn affected by delivery by vacuum extractor [ventouse]

P03.4 Newborn affected by cesarean delivery

P03.5 Newborn affected by precipitate delivery
Newborn affected by rapid second stage

P03.6 Newborn affected by abnormal uterine contractions
Newborn affected by conditions classifiable to O62.-, except O62.3
Newborn affected by hypertonic labor
Newborn affected by uterine inertia

P03.8 Newborn affected by other specified complications of labor
`5th`   **and delivery**
     P03.81 Newborn affected by abnormality in fetal
     `6th`   **(intrauterine) heart rate or rhythm**
Excludes1: neonatal cardiac dysrhythmia (P29.1-)

   Additional Character Required   ✔ 3-character code

•=New Code   *Excludes1*—Not coded here, do not use together
▲=Revised Code   *Excludes2*—Not included here

P03.810 Newborn affected by abnormality in fetal (intrauterine) heart rate or rhythm before the onset of labor

P03.811 Newborn affected by abnormality in fetal (intrauterine) heart rate or rhythm during labor

P03.819 Newborn affected by abnormality in fetal (intrauterine) heart rate or rhythm, unspecified as to time of onset

P03.82 Meconium passage during delivery
Excludes1: meconium aspiration (P24.00, P24.01)
meconium staining (P96.83)

P03.89 Newborn affected by other specified complications of labor and delivery
Newborn affected by abnormality of maternal soft tissues
Newborn affected by conditions classifiable to O60–O75 and by procedures used in labor and delivery not included in P02.- and P03.0–P03.6
Newborn affected by induction of labor

P03.9 Newborn affected by complication of labor and delivery, unspecified

P04 NEWBORN AFFECTED BY NOXIOUS SUBSTANCES
[4th] TRANSMITTED VIA PLACENTA OR BREAST MILK
Includes: nonteratogenic effects of substances transmitted via placenta
Code first any current condition in newborn, if applicable
Excludes2: congenital malformations (Q00–Q99)
encounter for observation of newborn for suspected diseases and conditions ruled out (Z05.-)
neonatal jaundice from excessive hemolysis due to drugs or toxins transmitted from mother (P58.4)
newborn in contact with and (suspected) exposures hazardous to health not transmitted via placenta or breast milk (Z77.-)

P04.0 Newborn affected by maternal anesthesia and analgesia in pregnancy, labor and delivery
Newborn affected by reactions and intoxications from maternal opiates and tranquilizers administered for procedures during pregnancy or labor and delivery
Excludes2: newborn affected by other maternal medication (P04.1-)

P04.1 Newborn affected by other maternal medication
[5th] **Code first** withdrawal symptoms from maternal use of drugs of addiction, if applicable (P96.1)
Excludes1: dysmorphism due to warfarin (Q86.2)
fetal hydantoin syndrome (Q86.1)
Excludes2: maternal anesthesia and analgesia in pregnancy, labor and delivery (P04.0)
maternal use of drugs of addiction (P04.4-)

P04.11 Newborn affected by maternal antineoplastic chemotherapy

P04.12 Newborn affected by maternal cytotoxic drugs

P04.13 Newborn affected by maternal use of anticonvulsants

P04.14 Newborn affected by maternal use of opiates

P04.15 Newborn affected by maternal use of antidepressants

P04.16 Newborn affected by maternal use of amphetamines

P04.17 Newborn affected by maternal use of sedative-hypnotics

P04.18 Newborn affected by other maternal medication

P04.19 Newborn affected by maternal use of unspecified medication

P04.1A Newborn affected by maternal use of anxiolytics

P04.2 Newborn affected by maternal use of tobacco
Newborn affected by exposure in utero to tobacco smoke
Excludes2: newborn exposure to environmental tobacco smoke (P96.81)

P04.3 Newborn affected by maternal use of alcohol
Excludes1: fetal alcohol syndrome (Q86.0)

P04.4 Newborn affected by maternal use of drugs of addiction
[5th] **P04.40** Newborn affected by maternal use of unspecified drugs of addiction

P04.41 Newborn affected by maternal use of cocaine

P04.42 Newborn affected by maternal use of hallucinogens
Excludes2: newborn affected by other maternal medication (P04.1-)

P04.49 Newborn affected by maternal use of other drugs of addiction
Excludes2: newborn affected by maternal anesthesia and analgesia (P04.0)
withdrawal symptoms from maternal use of drugs of addiction (P96.1)

P04.5 Newborn affected by maternal use of nutritional chemical substances

P04.6 Newborn affected by maternal exposure to environmental chemical substances

P04.8 Newborn affected by other maternal noxious substances
[5th] **P04.81** Newborn affected by maternal use of cannabis
P04.89 Newborn affected by other maternal noxious substances

P04.9 Newborn affected by maternal noxious substance, unspecified

(P05–P08) DISORDERS OF NEWBORN RELATED TO LENGTH OF GESTATION AND FETAL GROWTH

Providers utilize different criteria in determining prematurity. A code for prematurity should not be assigned unless it is documented. Assignment of codes in categories P05, Disorders of newborn related to slow fetal growth and fetal malnutrition, and P07, Disorders of newborn related to short gestation and LBW, not elsewhere classified, should be based on the recorded birth weight and estimated gestational age. Codes from category P05 should not be assigned with codes from category P07.

P05 DISORDERS OF NEWBORN RELATED TO SLOW FETAL
[4th] GROWTH AND FETAL MALNUTRITION

P05.0 Newborn light for gestational age
[5th] *Light-for-dates newborns are those who are smaller in size than normal for the gestational age, most commonly defined as weight below the 10th percentile but length above the 10th percentile for gestational age.*
Newborn light-for-dates

P05.00 Newborn light for gestational age, unspecified weight

P05.01 Newborn light for gestational age, less than 500 g

P05.02 Newborn light for gestational age, 500–749 g

P05.03 Newborn light for gestational age, 750–999 g

P05.04 Newborn light for gestational age, 1000–1249 g

P05.05 Newborn light for gestational age, 1250–1499 g

P05.06 Newborn light for gestational age, 1500–1749 g

P05.07 Newborn light for gestational age, 1750–1999 g

P05.08 Newborn light for gestational age, 2000–2499 g

P05.09 Newborn light for gestational age, 2500 g and over

P05.1 Newborn small for gestational age
[5th] *Small for gestational age newborns are those who are smaller in size than normal for the gestational age, most commonly defined as weight below the 10th percentile and length below 10th percentile for the gestational age.*
Newborn small-and-light-for-dates
Newborn small-for-dates

P05.10 Newborn small for gestational age, unspecified weight

P05.11 Newborn small for gestational age, less than 500 g

P05.12 Newborn small for gestational age, 500–749 g

P05.13 Newborn small for gestational age, 750–999 g

P05.14 Newborn small for gestational age, 1000–1249 g

P05.15 Newborn small for gestational age, 1250–1499 g

P05.16 Newborn small for gestational age, 1500–1749 g

P05.17 Newborn small for gestational age, 1750–1999 g

P05.18 Newborn small for gestational age, 2000–2499 g

P05.19 Newborn small for gestational age, other
Newborn small for gestational age, 2500 g and over

 [4th] [5th] [6th] [7th] Additional Character Required   ✔ 3-character code

•=New Code
▲=Revised Code

Excludes1—Not coded here, do not use together
Excludes2—Not included here

CHAPTER 16. CERTAIN CONDITIONS ORIGINATING IN THE PERINATAL PERIOD   (P05.2–P09.4)

P05.2 **Newborn affected by fetal (intrauterine) malnutrition not light or small for gestational age**
Infant, not light or small for gestational age, showing signs of fetal malnutrition, such as dry, peeling skin and loss of subcutaneous tissue
  Excludes1: newborn affected by fetal malnutrition with light for gestational age (P05.0-)
    newborn affected by fetal malnutrition with small for gestational age (P05.1-)

P05.9 **Newborn affected by slow intrauterine growth, unspecified**
Newborn affected by fetal growth retardation NOS

P07 **DISORDERS OF NEWBORN RELATED TO SHORT**
[4th] **GESTATION AND LBW, NEC**
Note: When both birth weight and gestational age of the newborn are available, both should be coded with birth weight sequenced before gestational age
Includes: the listed conditions, without further specification, as the cause of morbidity or additional care, in newborn

P07.0 **Extremely LBW newborn**
[5th] Newborn birth weight 999 g or less
  Excludes1: LBW due to slow fetal growth and fetal malnutrition (P05.-)
    P07.00 **Extremely LBW newborn, unspecified weight**
    P07.01 **Extremely LBW newborn, less than 500 g**
    P07.02 **Extremely LBW newborn, 500–749 g**
    P07.03 **Extremely LBW newborn, 750–999 g**

P07.1 **Other LBW newborn**
[5th] Newborn birth weight 1000–2499 g.
  Excludes1: LBW due to slow fetal growth and fetal malnutrition (P05.-)
    P07.10 **Other LBW newborn, unspecified weight**
    P07.14 **Other LBW newborn, 1000–1249 g**
    P07.15 **Other LBW newborn, 1250–1499 g**
    P07.16 **Other LBW newborn, 1500–1749 g**
    P07.17 **Other LBW newborn, 1750–1999 g**
    P07.18 **Other LBW newborn, 2000–2499 g**

P07.2 **Extreme immaturity of newborn**
[5th] Less than 28 completed weeks (less than 196 completed days) of gestation.
    P07.20 **Extreme immaturity of newborn; unspecified weeks of gestation**
    Gestational age less than 28 completed weeks NOS
    P07.21 **gestational age less than 23 completed weeks**
    gestational age less than 23 weeks, 0 days
    P07.22 **gestational age 23 completed weeks**
    gestational age 23 weeks, 0 days through 23 weeks, 6 days
    P07.23 **gestational age 24 completed weeks**
    gestational age 24 weeks, 0 days through 24 weeks, 6 days
    P07.24 **gestational age 25 completed weeks**
    gestational age 25 weeks, 0 days through 25 weeks, 6 days
    P07.25 **gestational age 26 completed weeks**
    gestational age 26 weeks, 0 days through 26 weeks, 6 days
    P07.26 **gestational age 27 completed weeks**
    gestational age 27 weeks, 0 days through 27 weeks, 6 days

P07.3 **Preterm [premature] newborn [other]**
[5th] 28 completed weeks or more but less than 37 completed weeks (196 completed days but less than 259 completed days) of gestation.
Prematurity NOS
    P07.30 **Preterm newborn, unspecified weeks of gestation**
    P07.31 **Preterm newborn, gestational age 28 completed weeks**
    Preterm newborn, gestational age 28 weeks, 0 days through 28 weeks, 6 days
    P07.32 **Preterm newborn, gestational age 29 completed weeks**
    Preterm newborn, gestational age 29 weeks, 0 days through 29 weeks, 6 days

P07.33 **Preterm newborn, gestational age 30 completed weeks**
Preterm newborn, gestational age 30 weeks, 0 days through 30 weeks, 6 days

P07.34 **Preterm newborn, gestational age 31 completed weeks**
Preterm newborn, gestational age 31 weeks, 0 days through 31 weeks, 6 days

P07.35 **Preterm newborn, gestational age 32 completed weeks**
Preterm newborn, gestational age 32 weeks, 0 days through 32 weeks, 6 days

P07.36 **Preterm newborn, gestational age 33 completed weeks**
Preterm newborn, gestational age 33 weeks, 0 days through 33 weeks, 6 days

P07.37 **Preterm newborn, gestational age 34 completed weeks**
Preterm newborn, gestational age 34 weeks, 0 days through 34 weeks, 6 days

P07.38 **Preterm newborn, gestational age 35 completed weeks**
Preterm newborn, gestational age 35 weeks, 0 days through 35 weeks, 6 days

P07.39 **Preterm newborn, gestational age 36 completed weeks**
Preterm newborn, gestational age 36 weeks, 0 days through 36 weeks, 6 days

P08 **DISORDERS OF NEWBORN RELATED TO LONG**
[4th] **GESTATION AND HIGH BIRTH WEIGHT**
Note: When both birth weight and gestational age of the newborn are available, priority of assignment should be given to birth weight
Includes: the listed conditions, without further specification, as causes of morbidity or additional care, in newborn

P08.0 **Exceptionally large newborn baby**
Usually implies a birth weight of 4500 g. or more
  Excludes1: syndrome of infant of diabetic mother (P70.1)
    syndrome of infant of mother with gestational diabetes (P70.0)

P08.1 **Other heavy for gestational age newborn**
Other newborn heavy- or large-for-dates regardless of period of gestation
Usually implies a birth weight of 4000 g. to 4499 g.
  Excludes1: newborn with a birth weight of 4500 or more (P08.0)
    syndrome of infant of diabetic mother (P70.1)
    syndrome of infant of mother with gestational diabetes (P70.0).

P08.2 **Late newborn, not heavy for gestational age**
[5th]   **P08.21** **Post-term newborn**
    Newborn with gestation period over 40 completed weeks to 42 completed weeks
  P08.22 **Prolonged gestation of newborn**
    Newborn with gestation period over 42 completed weeks (294 days or more), not heavy- or large-for-dates.
    Postmaturity NOS

(P09) ABNORMAL FINDINGS ON NEONATAL SCREENING

▲**P09** **ABNORMAL FINDINGS ON NEONATAL SCREENING**
[4th] *Includes:* Abnormal findings on state mandated newborn screens
Failed newborn screening
•**P09.1** **Abnormal findings on neonatal screening for inborn errors of metabolism**
Abnormal findings on neonatal screening for congenital adrenal hyperplasia
Abnormal findings on neonatal screening for hypothyroidism screen
•**P09.2** **Abnormal findings on neonatal screening for congenital endocrine disease**
•**P09.3** **Abnormal findings on neonatal screening for congenital hematologic disorders**
Abnormal findings for hemoglobinothies screen
Abnormal findings on red cell membrane defects screen
Abnormal findings on sickle cell screen
•**P09.4** **Abnormal findings on neonatal screening for cystic fibrosis**

[4th] [5th] [6th] [7th]   Additional Character Required   ✔   3-character code   •=New Code   *Excludes1*—Not coded here, do not use together
▲=Revised Code   *Excludes2*—Not included here

- **P09.5 Abnormal findings on neonatal screening for critical congenital heart disease**
  Neonatal congenital heart disease screening failure
- **P09.6 Abnormal findings on neonatal screening for neonatal hearing loss**
  Excludes2: Encounter for hearing examination following failed hearing screening (Z01.110)
- **P09.8 Other abnormal findings on neonatal screening**
- **P09.9 Abnormal findings on neonatal screening, unspecified**

(P10–P15) BIRTH TRAUMA

P10 **INTRACRANIAL LACERATION AND HEMORRHAGE DUE TO BIRTH INJURY**
`4th`
Excludes1: intracranial hemorrhage of newborn NOS (P52.9)
    intracranial hemorrhage of newborn due to anoxia or hypoxia (P52.-)
    nontraumatic intracranial hemorrhage of newborn (P52.-)

- **P10.0 Subdural hemorrhage due to birth injury**
  Subdural hematoma (localized) due to birth injury
- **P10.1 Cerebral hemorrhage due to birth injury**
- **P10.2 Intraventricular hemorrhage due to birth injury**
- **P10.3 Subarachnoid hemorrhage due to birth injury**
- **P10.4 Tentorial tear due to birth injury**
- **P10.8 Other intracranial lacerations and hemorrhages due to birth injury**
- **P10.9 Unspecified intracranial laceration and hemorrhage due to birth injury**
  Excludes1: subdural hemorrhage accompanying tentorial tear (P10.4)

P11 **OTHER BIRTH INJURIES TO CENTRAL NERVOUS SYSTEM**
`4th`
- **P11.0 Cerebral edema due to birth injury**
- **P11.1 Other specified brain damage due to birth injury**
- **P11.2 Unspecified brain damage due to birth injury**
- **P11.3 Birth injury to facial nerve**
  Facial palsy due to birth injury
- **P11.4 Birth injury to other cranial nerves**
- **P11.5 Birth injury to spine and spinal cord**
  Fracture of spine due to birth injury
- **P11.9 Birth injury to central nervous system, unspecified**

P12 **BIRTH INJURY TO SCALP**
`4th`
- **P12.0 Cephalhematoma due to birth injury**
- **P12.1 Chignon (from vacuum extraction) due to birth injury**
- **P12.2 Epicranial subaponeurotic hemorrhage due to birth injury**
  Subgaleal hemorrhage
- **P12.3 Bruising of scalp due to birth injury**
- **P12.4 Injury of scalp of newborn due to monitoring equipment**
  Sampling incision of scalp of newborn
  Scalp clip (electrode) injury of newborn
- **P12.8 Other birth injuries to scalp**
  - `5th` **P12.81 Caput succedaneum**
  - **P12.89 Other birth injuries to scalp**
- **P12.9 Birth injury to scalp, unspecified**

P13 **BIRTH INJURY TO SKELETON**
`4th`
Excludes2: birth injury to spine (P11.5)
- **P13.0 Fracture of skull due to birth injury**
- **P13.1 Other birth injuries to skull**
  Excludes1: cephalhematoma (P12.0)
- **P13.2 Birth injury to femur**
- **P13.3 Birth injury to other long bones**
- **P13.4 Fracture of clavicle due to birth injury**
- **P13.8 Birth injuries to other parts of skeleton**
- **P13.9 Birth injury to skeleton, unspecified**

P14 **BIRTH INJURY TO PERIPHERAL NERVOUS SYSTEM**
`4th`
- **P14.0 Erb's paralysis due to birth injury**
- **P14.1 Klumpke's paralysis due to birth injury**
- **P14.2 Phrenic nerve paralysis due to birth injury**
- **P14.3 Other brachial plexus birth injuries**
- **P14.8 Birth injuries to other parts of peripheral nervous system**
- **P14.9 Birth injury to peripheral nervous system, unspecified**

P15 **OTHER BIRTH INJURIES**
`4th`
- **P15.0 Birth injury to liver**
  Rupture of liver due to birth injury
- **P15.1 Birth injury to spleen**
  Rupture of spleen due to birth injury
- **P15.2 Sternomastoid injury due to birth injury**
- **P15.3 Birth injury to eye**
  Subconjunctival hemorrhage due to birth injury
  Traumatic glaucoma due to birth injury
- **P15.4 Birth injury to face**
  Facial congestion due to birth injury
- **P15.5 Birth injury to external genitalia**
- **P15.6 Subcutaneous fat necrosis due to birth injury**
- **P15.8 Other specified birth injuries**
- **P15.9 Birth injury, unspecified**

(P19–P29) RESPIRATORY AND CARDIOVASCULAR DISORDERS SPECIFIC TO THE PERINATAL PERIOD

P19 **METABOLIC ACIDEMIA IN NEWBORN**
`4th`
Includes: metabolic acidemia in newborn
- **P19.0 Metabolic acidemia in newborn first noted before onset of labor**
- **P19.1 Metabolic acidemia in newborn first noted during labor**
- **P19.2 Metabolic acidemia noted at birth**
- **P19.9 Metabolic acidemia, unspecified**

P22 **RESPIRATORY DISTRESS OF NEWBORN**
`4th`
- **P22.0 Respiratory distress syndrome of newborn**
  Cardiorespiratory distress syndrome of newborn
  Hyaline membrane disease
  Idiopathic respiratory distress syndrome [IRDS or RDS] of newborn
  Pulmonary hypoperfusion syndrome
  Respiratory distress syndrome, type I
  Excludes2: respiratory arrest of newborn (P28.81)
      respiratory failure of newborn NOS (P28.5)
- **P22.1 Transient tachypnea of newborn**
  Idiopathic tachypnea of newborn
  Respiratory distress syndrome, type II
  Wet lung syndrome
- **P22.8 Other respiratory distress of newborn**
  Excludes1: respiratory arrest of newborn (P28.81)
      respiratory failure of newborn NOS (P28.5)
- **P22.9 Respiratory distress of newborn, unspecified**
  Excludes1: respiratory arrest of newborn (P28.81)
      respiratory failure of newborn NOS (P28.5)

P23 **CONGENITAL PNEUMONIA**
`4th`
Includes: infective pneumonia acquired in utero or during birth
Excludes1: neonatal pneumonia resulting from aspiration (P24.-)
- **P23.0 Congenital pneumonia; due to viral agent**
  Use additional code (B97) to identify organism
  Excludes1: congenital rubella pneumonitis (P35.0)
- **P23.1 due to Chlamydia**
- **P23.2 due to Staphylococcus**
- **P23.3 due to Streptococcus, group B**
- **P23.4 due to E. coli**
- **P23.5 due to Pseudomonas**
- **P23.6 due to other bacterial agents**
  due to H. influenzae
  due to K. pneumoniae
  due to Mycoplasma
  due to Streptococcus, except group B
  Use additional code (B95–B96) to identify organism
- **P23.8 due to other organisms**
- **P23.9 unspecified**

P24 **NEONATAL ASPIRATION**
`4th`
Includes: aspiration in utero and during delivery
- **P24.0 Meconium aspiration**
  `5th` *Excludes1:* meconium passage (without aspiration) during delivery (P03.82)
      meconium staining (P96.83)
  - **P24.00 Meconium aspiration without respiratory symptoms**
    Meconium aspiration NOS

   6th **7th** Additional Character Required   3-character code

•=New Code
▲=Revised Code

Excludes1—Not coded here, do not use together
Excludes2—Not included here

CHAPTER 16. CERTAIN CONDITIONS ORIGINATING IN THE PERINATAL PERIOD   (P24.01–P35)

P24.01 Meconium aspiration with respiratory symptoms
Meconium aspiration pneumonia
Meconium aspiration pneumonitis
Meconium aspiration syndrome NOS
Use additional code to identify any secondary pulmonary hypertension, if applicable (I27.2-)

P24.1 Neonatal aspiration of (clear) amniotic fluid and mucus
`5th` Neonatal aspiration of liquor (amnii)

  P24.10 Neonatal aspiration of (clear) amniotic fluid and mucus; without respiratory symptoms
Neonatal aspiration of amniotic fluid and mucus NOS

  P24.11 with respiratory symptoms
with pneumonia
with pneumonitis
Use additional code to identify any secondary pulmonary hypertension, if applicable (I27.2-)

P24.2 Neonatal aspiration of blood;
`5th`
  P24.20 without respiratory symptoms
Neonatal aspiration of blood NOS

  P24.21 with respiratory symptoms
with pneumonia
with pneumonitis
Use additional code to identify any secondary pulmonary hypertension, if applicable (I27.2-)

P24.3 Neonatal aspiration of milk and regurgitated food
`5th` Neonatal aspiration of stomach contents

  P24.30 Neonatal aspiration of milk and regurgitated food; without respiratory symptoms
Neonatal aspiration of milk and regurgitated food NOS

  P24.31 with respiratory symptoms
Use additional code to identify any secondary pulmonary hypertension, if applicable (I27.2-)

P24.8 Other neonatal aspiration;
`5th`
  P24.80 without respiratory symptoms
Neonatal aspiration NEC

  P24.81 with respiratory symptoms
Neonatal aspiration pneumonia NEC
Neonatal aspiration with pneumonitis NEC
Neonatal aspiration with pneumonia NOS
Neonatal aspiration with pneumonitis NOS
Use additional code to identify any secondary pulmonary hypertension, if applicable (I27.2-)

P24.9 Neonatal aspiration, unspecified

P25 INTERSTITIAL EMPHYSEMA AND RELATED CONDITIONS ORIGINATING IN THE PERINATAL PERIOD
`4th`
Do not report codes from P25 that do not originate in the perinatal period.

P25.0 Interstitial emphysema originating in the perinatal period
P25.1 Pneumothorax originating in the perinatal period
P25.2 Pneumomediastinum originating in the perinatal period
P25.3 Pneumopericardium originating in the perinatal period
P25.8 Other conditions related to interstitial emphysema originating in the perinatal period

P26 PULMONARY HEMORRHAGE ORIGINATING IN THE PERINATAL PERIOD
`4th`
Do not report codes from P26 that do not originate in the perinatal period
Excludes1: acute idiopathic hemorrhage in infants over 28 days old (R04.81)

P26.0 Tracheobronchial hemorrhage
P26.1 Massive pulmonary hemorrhage
P26.8 Other pulmonary hemorrhages
P26.9 Unspecified pulmonary hemorrhage

P27 CHRONIC RESPIRATORY DISEASE ORIGINATING IN THE PERINATAL PERIOD
`4th`
Do not report codes from P27 that do not originate in the perinatal period
Excludes2: respiratory distress of newborn (P22.0–P22.9)

P27.0 Wilson-Mikity syndrome
Pulmonary dysmaturity
P27.1 Bronchopulmonary dysplasia
P27.8 Other chronic respiratory diseases
Congenital pulmonary fibrosis
Ventilator lung in newborn
P27.9 Unspecified chronic respiratory disease

P28 OTHER RESPIRATORY CONDITIONS ORIGINATING IN THE PERINATAL PERIOD
`4th`
Excludes1: congenital malformations of the respiratory system (Q30–Q34)

P28.0 Primary atelectasis of newborn
Primary failure to expand terminal respiratory units
Pulmonary hypoplasia associated with short gestation
Pulmonary immaturity NOS

P28.1 Other and unspecified atelectasis of newborn
`5th`
  P28.10 Unspecified atelectasis of newborn
Atelectasis of newborn NOS

  P28.11 Resorption atelectasis without respiratory distress syndrome
Excludes1: resorption atelectasis with respiratory distress syndrome (P22.0)

  P28.19 Other atelectasis of newborn
Partial atelectasis of newborn
Secondary atelectasis of newborn

P28.2 Cyanotic attacks of newborn
Excludes1: apnea of newborn (P28.3–P28.4)

P28.3 Primary sleep apnea of newborn
Central sleep apnea of newborn
Obstructive sleep apnea of newborn
Sleep apnea of newborn NOS

P28.4 Other apnea of newborn
Apnea of prematurity
Obstructive apnea of newborn
Excludes1: obstructive sleep apnea of newborn (P28.3)

P28.5 Respiratory failure of newborn
Excludes1: respiratory arrest of newborn (P28.81) respiratory distress of newborn (P22.0-)

P28.8 Other specified respiratory conditions of newborn
`5th`
  P28.81 Respiratory arrest of newborn
  P28.89 Other specified respiratory conditions of newborn
Congenital laryngeal stridor
Sniffles in newborn
Snuffles in newborn
Excludes1: early congenital syphilitic rhinitis (A50.05)

P28.9 Respiratory condition of newborn, unspecified
Respiratory depression in newborn

P29 CARDIOVASCULAR DISORDERS ORIGINATING IN THE PERINATAL PERIOD
`4th`
Excludes2: congenital malformations of the circulatory system (Q20–Q28)

P29.0 Neonatal cardiac failure
P29.1 Neonatal cardiac dysrhythmia
`5th`
  P29.11 Neonatal tachycardia
  P29.12 Neonatal bradycardia
P29.2 Neonatal hypertension
P29.3 Persistent fetal circulation
`5th`
  P29.30 Pulmonary hypertension of newborn
Persistent pulmonary hypertension of newborn
  P29.38 Other persistent fetal circulation
Delayed closure of ductus arteriosus
P29.4 Transient myocardial ischemia in newborn
P29.8 Other cardiovascular disorders originating in the perinatal period
`5th`
  P29.81 Cardiac arrest of newborn
  P29.89 Other cardiovascular disorders originating in the perinatal period
P29.9 Cardiovascular disorder originating in the perinatal period, unspecified

(P35–P39) INFECTIONS SPECIFIC TO THE PERINATAL PERIOD

Infections acquired in utero, during birth via the umbilicus, or during the first 28 days after birth
Excludes2: asymptomatic HIV infection status (Z21)
congenital gonococcal infection (A54.-)
congenital pneumonia (P23.-)
congenital syphilis (A50.-)
HIV disease (B20)
infant botulism (A48.51)
infectious diseases not specific to the perinatal period (A00–B99, J09, J10.-)
intestinal infectious disease (A00–A09)
laboratory evidence of HIV (R75)
tetanus neonatorum (A33)

`4th` `5th` `6th` `7th` Additional Character Required   ✔ 3-character code

•=New Code
▲=Revised Code

Excludes1—Not coded here, do not use together
Excludes2—Not included here

P35 CONGENITAL VIRAL DISEASES
4th

Includes: infections acquired in utero or during birth

P35.0 Congenital rubella syndrome
Congenital rubella pneumonitis

P35.1 Congenital cytomegalovirus infection

P35.2 Congenital herpesviral [herpes simplex] infection

P35.3 Congenital viral hepatitis

P35.4 Congenital Zika virus disease
Use additional code to identify manifestations of congenital Zika virus disease

P35.8 Other congenital viral diseases
Congenital varicella [chickenpox]

P35.9 Congenital viral disease, unspecified

P36 BACTERIAL SEPSIS OF NEWBORN
4th

> **GUIDELINES**
>
> Category P36, Bacterial sepsis of newborn, includes congenital sepsis. If a perinate is documented as having sepsis without documentation of congenital or community acquired, the default is congenital and a code from category P36 should be assigned. If the P36 code includes the causal organism, an additional code from category B95, Streptococcus, Staphylococcus, and Enterococcus as the cause of diseases classified elsewhere, or B96, Other bacterial agents as the cause of diseases classified elsewhere, should not be assigned. If the P36 code does not include the causal organism, assign an additional code from category B96. If applicable, use additional codes to identify severe sepsis (R65.2-) and any associated acute organ dysfunction.

Includes: congenital sepsis

Use additional code(s), if applicable, to identify severe sepsis (R65.2-) and associated acute organ dysfunction(s)

P36.0 Sepsis of newborn due to Streptococcus, group B

P36.1 Sepsis of newborn due to other and unspecified streptococci
5th **P36.10 Sepsis of newborn due to unspecified streptococci**
P36.19 Sepsis of newborn due to other streptococci

P36.2 Sepsis of newborn due to Staphylococcus aureus

P36.3 Sepsis of newborn due to other and unspecified staphylococci
5th **P36.30 Sepsis of newborn due to unspecified staphylococci**
P36.39 Sepsis of newborn due to other staphylococci

P36.4 Sepsis of newborn due to E. coli

P36.5 Sepsis of newborn due to anaerobes

P36.8 Other bacterial sepsis of newborn
Use additional code from category B96 to identify organism

P36.9 Bacterial sepsis of newborn, unspecified

P37 OTHER CONGENITAL INFECTIOUS AND PARASITIC DISEASES
4th

Excludes2: congenital syphilis (A50.-)
infectious neonatal diarrhea (A00–A09)
necrotizing enterocolitis in newborn (P77.-)
noninfectious neonatal diarrhea (P78.3)
ophthalmia neonatorum due to gonococcus (A54.31)
tetanus neonatorum (A33)

P37.0 Congenital tuberculosis

P37.1 Congenital toxoplasmosis
Hydrocephalus due to congenital toxoplasmosis

P37.2 Neonatal (disseminated) listeriosis

P37.3 Congenital falciparum malaria

P37.4 Other congenital malaria

P37.5 Neonatal candidiasis

P37.8 Other specified congenital infectious and parasitic diseases

P37.9 Congenital infectious or parasitic disease, unspecified

P38 OMPHALITIS OF NEWBORN
4th

Excludes1: omphalitis not of newborn (L08.82)
tetanus omphalitis (A33)
umbilical hemorrhage of newborn (P51.-)

P38.1 Omphalitis with mild hemorrhage

P38.9 Omphalitis without hemorrhage
Omphalitis of newborn NOS

P39 OTHER INFECTIONS SPECIFIC TO THE PERINATAL PERIOD
4th

Use additional code to identify organism or specific infection

P39.0 Neonatal infective mastitis
Excludes1: breast engorgement of newborn (P83.4)
noninfective mastitis of newborn (P83.4)

P39.1 Neonatal conjunctivitis and dacryocystitis
Neonatal chlamydial conjunctivitis
Ophthalmia neonatorum NOS
Excludes1: gonococcal conjunctivitis (A54.31)

P39.2 Intra-amniotic infection affecting newborn, NEC

P39.3 Neonatal urinary tract infection

P39.4 Neonatal skin infection
Neonatal pyoderma
Excludes1: pemphigus neonatorum (L00)
staphylococcal scalded skin syndrome (L00)

P39.8 Other specified infections specific to the perinatal period

P39.9 Infection specific to the perinatal period, unspecified

(P50–P61) HEMORRHAGIC AND HEMATOLOGICAL DISORDERS OF NEWBORN

Excludes1: congenital stenosis and stricture of bile ducts (Q44.3)
Crigler-Najjar syndrome (E80.5)
Dubin-Johnson syndrome (E80.6)
Gilbert syndrome (E80.4)
hereditary hemolytic anemias (D55–D58)

P50 NEWBORN AFFECTED BY INTRAUTERINE (FETAL) BLOOD LOSS
4th

Excludes1: congenital anemia from intrauterine (fetal) blood loss (P61.3)

P50.0 Newborn affected by intrauterine (fetal) blood loss from vasa previa

P50.1 Newborn affected by intrauterine (fetal) blood loss from ruptured cord

P50.2 Newborn affected by intrauterine (fetal) blood loss from placenta

P50.3 Newborn affected by hemorrhage into co-twin

P50.4 Newborn affected by hemorrhage into maternal circulation

P50.5 Newborn affected by intrauterine (fetal) blood loss from cut end of co-twin's cord

P50.8 Newborn affected by other intrauterine (fetal) blood loss

P50.9 Newborn affected by intrauterine (fetal) blood loss, unspecified
Newborn affected by fetal hemorrhage NOS

P51 UMBILICAL HEMORRHAGE OF NEWBORN
4th

Excludes1: omphalitis with mild hemorrhage (P38.1)
umbilical hemorrhage from cut end of co-twins cord (P50.5)

P51.0 Massive umbilical hemorrhage of newborn

P51.8 Other umbilical hemorrhages of newborn
Slipped umbilical ligature NOS

P51.9 Umbilical hemorrhage of newborn, unspecified

P52 INTRACRANIAL NONTRAUMATIC HEMORRHAGE OF NEWBORN
4th

Includes: intracranial hemorrhage due to anoxia or hypoxia
Excludes1: intracranial hemorrhage due to birth injury (P10.-)
intracranial hemorrhage due to other injury (S06.-)

P52.0 Intraventricular (nontraumatic) hemorrhage, grade 1, of newborn
Subependymal hemorrhage (without intraventricular extension)
Bleeding into germinal matrix

P52.1 Intraventricular (nontraumatic) hemorrhage, grade 2, of newborn
Subependymal hemorrhage with intraventricular extension
Bleeding into ventricle

P52.2 Intraventricular (nontraumatic) hemorrhage, grade 3 and grade 4, of newborn
5th
P52.21 Intraventricular (nontraumatic) hemorrhage, grade 3, of newborn
Subependymal hemorrhage with intraventricular extension with enlargement of ventricle
P52.22 Intraventricular (nontraumatic) hemorrhage, grade 4, of newborn
Bleeding into cerebral cortex
Subependymal hemorrhage with intracerebral extension

P52.3 Unspecified intraventricular (nontraumatic) hemorrhage of newborn

P52.4 Intracerebral (nontraumatic) hemorrhage of newborn

P52.5 Subarachnoid (nontraumatic) hemorrhage of newborn

4th **5th** **6th** **7th** Additional Character Required   ✔ 3-character code

•=New Code   *Excludes1*—Not coded here, do not use together
▲=Revised Code   *Excludes2*—Not included here

P52.6 Cerebellar (nontraumatic) and posterior fossa hemorrhage of newborn

P52.8 Other intracranial (nontraumatic) hemorrhages of newborn

P52.9 Intracranial (nontraumatic) hemorrhage of newborn, unspecified

P53 HEMORRHAGIC DISEASE OF NEWBORN
☑
Vitamin K deficiency of newborn

P54 OTHER NEONATAL HEMORRHAGES
4th
Excludes1: newborn affected by (intrauterine) blood loss (P50.-)
pulmonary hemorrhage originating in the perinatal period (P26.-)

P54.0 Neonatal hematemesis
Excludes1: neonatal hematemesis due to swallowed maternal blood (P78.2)

P54.1 Neonatal melena
Excludes1: neonatal melena due to swallowed maternal blood (P78.2)

P54.2 Neonatal rectal hemorrhage

P54.3 Other neonatal gastrointestinal hemorrhage

P54.4 Neonatal adrenal hemorrhage

P54.5 Neonatal cutaneous hemorrhage
Neonatal bruising
Neonatal ecchymoses
Neonatal petechiae
Neonatal superficial hematomata
Excludes2: bruising of scalp due to birth injury (P12.3)
cephalhematoma due to birth injury (P12.0)

P54.6 Neonatal vaginal hemorrhage
Neonatal pseudomenses

P54.8 Other specified neonatal hemorrhages

P54.9 Neonatal hemorrhage, unspecified

P55 HEMOLYTIC DISEASE OF NEWBORN
4th
P55.0 Rh isoimmunization of newborn

P55.1 ABO isoimmunization of newborn

P55.8 Other hemolytic diseases of newborn

P55.9 Hemolytic disease of newborn, unspecified

P56 HYDROPS FETALIS DUE TO HEMOLYTIC DISEASE
4th
Excludes1: hydrops fetalis NOS (P83.2)

P56.0 Hydrops fetalis due to isoimmunization

P56.9 Hydrops fetalis due to other and unspecified hemolytic disease
5th **P56.90 Hydrops fetalis due to unspecified hemolytic disease**
P56.99 Hydrops fetalis due to other hemolytic disease

P57 KERNICTERUS
4th
P57.0 Kernicterus due to isoimmunization

P57.8 Other specified kernicterus
Excludes1: Crigler-Najjar syndrome (E80.5)

P57.9 Kernicterus, unspecified

P59 NEONATAL JAUNDICE FROM OTHER AND UNSPECIFIED CAUSES
4th
Excludes1: jaundice due to inborn errors of metabolism (E70–E88)
kernicterus (P57.-)

P59.0 Neonatal jaundice associated with preterm delivery
Hyperbilirubinemia of prematurity
Jaundice due to delayed conjugation associated with preterm delivery

P59.1 Inspissated bile syndrome

P59.2 Neonatal jaundice from other and unspecified hepatocellular
5th **damage**
Excludes1: congenital viral hepatitis (P35.3)
P59.20 Neonatal jaundice from unspecified hepatocellular damage
P59.29 Neonatal jaundice from other hepatocellular damage
Neonatal giant cell hepatitis
Neonatal (idiopathic) hepatitis

P59.3 Neonatal jaundice from breast milk inhibitor

P59.8 Neonatal jaundice from other specified causes

P59.9 Neonatal jaundice, unspecified
Neonatal physiological jaundice (intense)(prolonged) NOS

P60 DISSEMINATED INTRAVASCULAR COAGULATION
☑ **OF NEWBORN**
Defibrination syndrome of newborn

P61 OTHER PERINATAL HEMATOLOGICAL DISORDERS
4th
Excludes1: transient hypogammaglobulinemia of infancy (D80.7)

P61.0 Transient neonatal thrombocytopenia
Neonatal thrombocytopenia due to exchange transfusion
Neonatal thrombocytopenia due to idiopathic maternal thrombocytopenia
Neonatal thrombocytopenia due to isoimmunization

P61.1 Polycythemia neonatorum

P61.2 Anemia of prematurity

P61.3 Congenital anemia from fetal blood loss

P61.4 Other congenital anemias, NEC
Congenital anemia NOS

P61.5 Transient neonatal neutropenia
Excludes1: congenital neutropenia (nontransient) (D70.0)

P61.6 Other transient neonatal disorders of coagulation

P61.8 Other specified perinatal hematological disorders

P61.9 Perinatal hematological disorder, unspecified

(P70–P74) TRANSITORY ENDOCRINE AND METABOLIC DISORDERS SPECIFIC TO NEWBORN

Includes: transitory endocrine and metabolic disturbances caused by the infant's response to maternal endocrine and metabolic factors, or its adjustment to extrauterine environment

P70 TRANSITORY DISORDERS OF CARBOHYDRATE
4th **METABOLISM SPECIFIC TO NEWBORN**

P70.0 Syndrome of infant of mother with gestational diabetes
Newborn (with hypoglycemia) affected by maternal gestational diabetes
Excludes1: newborn (with hypoglycemia) affected by maternal (pre-existing) DM (P70.1)
syndrome of infant of a diabetic mother (P70.1)

P70.1 Syndrome of infant of a diabetic mother
Newborn (with hypoglycemia) affected by maternal (pre-existing) DM
Excludes1: newborn (with hypoglycemia) affected by maternal gestational diabetes (P70.0)
syndrome of infant of mother with gestational diabetes (P70.0)

P70.2 Neonatal DM

P70.3 Iatrogenic neonatal hypoglycemia

P70.4 Other neonatal hypoglycemia
Transitory neonatal hypoglycemia

P70.8 Other transitory disorders of carbohydrate metabolism of newborn

P71 TRANSITORY NEONATAL DISORDERS OF CALCIUM AND
4th **MAGNESIUM METABOLISM**

P71.0 Cow's milk hypocalcemia in newborn

P71.1 Other neonatal hypocalcemia
Excludes1: neonatal hypoparathyroidism (P71.4)

P71.3 Neonatal tetany without calcium or magnesium deficiency
Neonatal tetany NOS

P71.4 Transitory neonatal hypoparathyroidism

P71.8 Other transitory neonatal disorders of calcium and magnesium metabolism

P71.9 Transitory neonatal disorder of calcium and magnesium metabolism, unspecified

P72 OTHER TRANSITORY NEONATAL ENDOCRINE
4th **DISORDERS**
Excludes1: congenital hypothyroidism with or without goiter (E03.0-E03.1)
dyshormogenetic goiter (E07.1)
Pendred's syndrome (E07.1)

P72.0 Neonatal goiter, not elsewhere classified
Transitory congenital goiter with normal functioning

P72.1 Transitory neonatal hyperthyroidism
Neonatal thyrotoxicosis

P72.2 Other transitory neonatal disorders of thyroid function, not elsewhere classified
Transitory neonatal hypothyroidism

P72.8 Other specified transitory neonatal endocrine disorders

P72.9 Transitory neonatal endocrine disorder, unspecified

4th 5th 6th 7th Additional Character Required   ☑ 3-character code

•=New Code   *Excludes1*—Not coded here, do not use together
▲=Revised Code   *Excludes2*—Not included here

P74 **OTHER TRANSITORY NEONATAL ELECTROLYTE AND**
`4th` **METABOLIC DISTURBANCES**
   P74.0 **Late metabolic acidosis of newborn**
      Excludes1: (fetal) metabolic acidosis of newborn (P19)
   P74.1 **Dehydration of newborn**
   P74.2 **Disturbances of sodium balance of newborn**
     `5th` **P74.21** **Hypernatremia of newborn**
          P74.22 **Hyponatremia of newborn**
   P74.3 **Disturbances of potassium balance of newborn**
     `5th` **P74.31** **Hyperkalemia of newborn**
          P74.32 **Hypokalemia of newborn**
   P74.4 **Other transitory electrolyte disturbances of newborn**
     `5th` **P74.41** **Alkalosis of newborn**
          P74.42 **Disturbances of chlorine balance of newborn**
        `6th` **P74.421** **Hyperchloremia of newborn**
                Hyperchloremic metabolic acidosis
                Excludes2: late metabolic acidosis of the
                    newborn (P47.0)
          P74.422 **Hypochloremia of newborn**
        P74.49 **Other transitory electrolyte disturbance of newborn**
   P74.5 **Transitory tyrosinemia of newborn**
   P74.6 **Transitory hyperammonemia of newborn**
   P74.8 **Other transitory metabolic disturbances of newborn**
      Amino-acid metabolic disorders described as transitory
   P74.9 **Transitory metabolic disturbance of newborn, unspecified**

(P76–P78) DIGESTIVE SYSTEM DISORDERS OF NEWBORN

P76 **OTHER INTESTINAL OBSTRUCTION OF NEWBORN**
`4th` **P76.0** **Meconium plug syndrome**
      Meconium ileus NOS
      Excludes1: meconium ileus in cystic fibrosis (E84.11)
   P76.1 **Transitory ileus of newborn**
      Excludes1: Hirschsprung's disease (Q43.1)
   P76.2 **Intestinal obstruction due to inspissated milk**
   P76.8 **Other specified intestinal obstruction of newborn**
      Excludes1: intestinal obstruction classifiable to K56.-
   P76.9 **Intestinal obstruction of newborn, unspecified**

P77 **NECROTIZING ENTEROCOLITIS OF NEWBORN**
`4th` **P77.1** **Stage 1 necrotizing enterocolitis in newborn**
      Necrotizing enterocolitis without
        pneumatosis, without perforation
   P77.2 **Stage 2 necrotizing enterocolitis**
      in newborn
      Necrotizing enterocolitis with
        pneumatosis, without perforation
   P77.3 **Stage 3 necrotizing enterocolitis**
      in newborn
      Necrotizing enterocolitis with perforation
      Necrotizing enterocolitis with pneumatosis and perforation
   P77.9 **Necrotizing enterocolitis in newborn, unspecified**
      Necrotizing enterocolitis in newborn, NOS

> For necrotizing enterocolitis that begins after the 28th day, see the alphabetic index for the appropriate reference (eg, necrotizing enterocolitis due to C. difficile A04.7).

P78 **OTHER PERINATAL DIGESTIVE SYSTEM DISORDERS**
`4th` *Excludes1:* cystic fibrosis (E84.0–E84.9)
      neonatal gastrointestinal hemorrhages (P54.0–P54.3)
   P78.0 **Perinatal intestinal perforation**
      Meconium peritonitis
   P78.1 **Other neonatal peritonitis**
      Neonatal peritonitis NOS
   P78.2 **Neonatal hematemesis and melena due to swallowed maternal blood**
   P78.3 **Noninfective neonatal diarrhea**
      Neonatal diarrhea NOS
   P78.8 **Other specified perinatal digestive system disorders**
     `5th` **P78.81** **Congenital cirrhosis (of liver)**
          P78.82 **Peptic ulcer of newborn**
          P78.83 **Newborn esophageal reflux**
               Neonatal esophageal reflux
          P78.84 **Gestational alloimmune liver disease**
               GALD
               Neonatal hemochromatosis
               Excludes 1: hemochromatosis (E83.11-)

   P78.89 **Other specified perinatal digestive system disorders**
   P78.9 **Perinatal digestive system disorder, unspecified**

(P80–P83) CONDITIONS INVOLVING THE INTEGUMENT AND TEMPERATURE REGULATION OF NEWBORN

P80 **HYPOTHERMIA OF NEWBORN**
`4th` **P80.0** **Cold injury syndrome**
      Severe and usually chronic hypothermia associated with a pink
        flushed appearance, edema and neurological and biochemical
        abnormalities.
      Excludes1: mild hypothermia of newborn (P80.8)
   P80.8 **Other hypothermia of newborn**
      Mild hypothermia of newborn
   P80.9 **Hypothermia of newborn, unspecified**

P81 **OTHER DISTURBANCES OF TEMPERATURE REGULATION**
`4th` **OF NEWBORN**
   P81.0 **Environmental hyperthermia of newborn**
   P81.8 **Other specified disturbances of temperature regulation of newborn**
   P81.9 **Disturbance of temperature regulation of newborn, unspecified**
      Fever of newborn NOS

P83 **OTHER CONDITIONS OF INTEGUMENT SPECIFIC TO**
`4th` **NEWBORN**
   Excludes1: congenital malformations of skin and integument (Q80–Q84)
      hydrops fetalis due to hemolytic disease (P56.-)
      neonatal skin infection (P39.4)
      staphylococcal scalded skin syndrome (L00)
   Excludes2: cradle cap (L21.0)
      diaper [napkin] dermatitis (L22)
   P83.0 **Sclerema neonatorum**
   P83.1 **Neonatal erythema toxicum**
   P83.2 **Hydrops fetalis not due to hemolytic disease**
      Hydrops fetalis NOS
   P83.3 **Other and unspecified edema specific to newborn**
          P83.30 **Unspecified edema specific to newborn**
          P83.39 **Other edema specific to newborn**
   P83.4 **Breast engorgement of newborn**
      Noninfective mastitis of newborn
   P83.5 **Congenital hydrocele**
   P83.6 **Umbilical polyp of newborn**
   P83.8 **Other specified conditions of integument specific to newborn**
     `5th` **P83.81** **Umbilical granuloma**
               Excludes2: Granulomatous disorder of the skin and
                  subcutaneous tissue, unspecified (L92.9)
          P83.88 **Other specified conditions of integument specific to newborn**
               Bronze baby syndrome
               Neonatal scleroderma
               Urticaria neonatorum
   P83.9 **Condition of the integument specific to newborn, unspecified**

(P84) OTHER PROBLEMS WITH NEWBORN

P84 **OTHER PROBLEMS WITH NEWBORN**
`✔` Acidemia of newborn
      Acidosis of newborn
      Anoxia of newborn NOS
      Asphyxia of newborn NOS
      Hypercapnia of newborn
      Hypoxemia of newborn
      Hypoxia of newborn NOS
      Mixed metabolic and respiratory acidosis of newborn
      Excludes1: intracranial hemorrhage due to anoxia or hypoxia (P52.-)
      hypoxic ischemic encephalopathy [HIE] (P91.6-)
      late metabolic acidosis of newborn (P74.0)

CHAPTER 16. CERTAIN CONDITIONS ORIGINATING IN THE PERINATAL PERIOD (P74–P84)

| `4th` `5th` `6th` `7th` Additional Character Required | `✔` 3-character code | •=New Code ▲=Revised Code | *Excludes1*—Not coded here, do not use together *Excludes2*—Not included here |

CHAPTER 16. CERTAIN CONDITIONS ORIGINATING IN THE PERINATAL PERIOD (P90–P96.9)

(P90–P96) OTHER DISORDERS ORIGINATING IN THE PERINATAL PERIOD

P90 CONVULSIONS OF NEWBORN
☑ ***Excludes1:*** benign myoclonic epilepsy in infancy (G40.3-)
    benign neonatal convulsions (familial) (G40.3-)

P91 OTHER DISTURBANCES OF CEREBRAL STATUS OF
`4th` **NEWBORN**
  P91.0 Neonatal cerebral ischemia
    Excludes1: Neonatal cerebral infarction (P91.82-)
  P91.1 Acquired periventricular cysts of newborn
  P91.2 Neonatal cerebral leukomalacia
    Periventricular leukomalacia
  P91.3 Neonatal cerebral irritability
  P91.4 Neonatal cerebral depression
  P91.5 Neonatal coma
  P91.6 Hypoxic ischemic encephalopathy [HIE]
   `5th` ***Excludes1:*** Neonatal cerebral depression (P91.4)
    Neonatal cerebral irritability (P91.3)
    Neonatal coma (P91.5)
    P91.60 HIE, unspecified
    P91.61 Mild HIE
    P91.62 Moderate HIE
    P91.63 Severe HIE
  P91.8 Other specified disturbances of cerebral status of newborn
  `5th` **P91.81 Neonatal encephalopathy**
    `6th` **P91.811 Neonatal encephalopathy in diseases classified elsewhere**
      Code first underlying condition, if known, such as:
      congenital cirrhosis (of liver) (P78.81)
      intracranial nontraumatic hemorrhage of newborn (P52.-)
      kernicterus (P57.-)
      P91.819 Neonatal encephalopathy, unspecified
    P91.82 Neonatal cerebral infarction
    `6th` Neonatal stroke
      Perinatal arterial ischemic stroke
      Perinatal cerebral infarction
      Excludes1: cerebral infarction (I63.-)
      Excludes2: intracranial hemorrhage of newborn (P52.-)
      P91.821 Neonatal cerebral infarction, right side of brain
      P91.822 Neonatal cerebral infarction, left side of brain
      P91.823 Neonatal cerebral infarction, bilateral
      P91.829 Neonatal cerebral infarction, unspecified side
    P91.88 Other specified disturbances of cerebral status of newborn
  P91.9 Disturbance of cerebral status of newborn, unspecified

P92 FEEDING PROBLEMS OF NEWBORN
`4th` ***Excludes1:*** eating disorders (F50.-)
Excludes2: feeding problems in child over 28 days old (R63.3)

> Note: Report a code from P92 after 28 days of life if the feeding problem began within the first 28 days of life

  P92.0 Vomiting of newborn
  `5th` ***Excludes1:*** vomiting of child over 28 days old (R11.-)
    P92.01 Bilious vomiting of newborn
      Excludes1: bilious vomiting in child over 28 days old (R11.14)
    P92.09 Other vomiting of newborn
      Excludes1: regurgitation of food in newborn (P92.1)
  P92.1 Regurgitation and rumination of newborn
  P92.2 Slow feeding of newborn
  P92.3 Underfeeding of newborn
  P92.4 Overfeeding of newborn
  P92.5 Neonatal difficulty in feeding at breast

  P92.6 Failure to thrive in newborn
    Excludes1: failure to thrive in child over 28 days old (R62.51)
  P92.8 Other feeding problems of newborn
  P92.9 Feeding problem of newborn, unspecified

P93 REACTIONS AND INTOXICATIONS DUE TO DRUGS
`4th` **ADMINISTERED TO NEWBORN**
Includes: reactions and intoxications due to drugs administered to fetus affecting newborn
Excludes1: jaundice due to drugs or toxins transmitted from mother or given to newborn (P58.4-)
reactions and intoxications from maternal opiates, tranquilizers and other medication (P04.0-P04.1, P04.4-)
withdrawal symptoms from maternal use of drugs of addiction (P96.1)
withdrawal symptoms from therapeutic use of drugs in newborn (P96.2)
  P93.0 Grey baby syndrome
  P93.8 Other reactions and intoxications due to drugs administered to newborn
    Use additional code for adverse effect, if applicable, to identify drug (T36-T50 with fifth or sixth character 5)

P94 DISORDERS OF MUSCLE TONE OF NEWBORN
`4th`   **P94.0 Transient neonatal myasthenia gravis**
    myasthenia gravis (G70.0)
  P94.1 Congenital hypertonia
  P94.2 Congenital hypotonia
    Floppy baby syndrome, unspecified
  P94.8 Other disorders of muscle tone of newborn
  P94.9 Disorder of muscle tone of newborn, unspecified

P95 STILLBIRTH
☑ Deadborn fetus NOS
Fetal death of unspecified cause
Stillbirth NOS
Excludes1: maternal care for intrauterine death (O36.4)
  missed abortion (O02.1)
  outcome of delivery, stillbirth (Z37.1, Z37.3, Z37.4, Z37.7)
Code P95, Stillbirth, is only for use in institutions that maintain separate records for stillbirths. No other code should be used with P95. Code P95 should not be used on the mother's record.

P96 OTHER CONDITIONS ORIGINATING IN THE PERINATAL
`4th` **PERIOD**
  P96.0 Congenital renal failure
    Uremia of newborn
  P96.1 Neonatal withdrawal symptoms from maternal use of drugs of addiction
    Drug withdrawal syndrome in infant of dependent mother
    Neonatal abstinence syndrome
    Excludes1: reactions and intoxications from maternal opiates and tranquilizers administered during labor and delivery (P04.0)
  P96.2 Withdrawal symptoms from therapeutic use of drugs in newborn
  P96.3 Wide cranial sutures of newborn
    Neonatal craniotabes
  P96.5 Complication to newborn due to (fetal) intrauterine procedure
    newborn affected by amniocentesis (P00.6)
  P96.8 Other specified conditions originating in the perinatal period
  `5th` **P96.81 Exposure to (parental) (environmental) tobacco smoke in the perinatal period**
      Excludes2: newborn affected by in utero exposure to tobacco (P04.2)
      exposure to environmental tobacco smoke after the perinatal period (Z77.22)
    P96.82 Delayed separation of umbilical cord
    P96.83 Meconium staining
      Excludes1: meconium aspiration (P24.00, P24.01)
      meconium passage during delivery (P03.82)
    P96.89 Other specified conditions originating in the perinatal period
      Use additional code to specify condition
  P96.9 Condition originating in the perinatal period, unspecified
    Congenital debility NOS

  Additional Character Required   ☑ 3-character code

•=New Code   ***Excludes1***—Not coded here, do not use together
▲=Revised Code   ***Excludes2***—Not included here

Chapter 17. Congenital malformations, deformations and chromosomal abnormalities (Q00–Q99)

GUIDELINES

Assign an appropriate code(s) from categories Q00–Q99, Congenital malformations, deformations, and chromosomal abnormalities when a malformation/deformation or chromosomal abnormality is documented. A malformation/deformation or chromosomal abnormality may be the principal/first-listed diagnosis on a record or a secondary diagnosis.

When a malformation/deformation or chromosomal abnormality does not have a unique code assignment, assign additional code(s) for any manifestations that may be present.

When the code assignment specifically identifies the malformation/deformation or chromosomal abnormality, manifestations that are an inherent component of the anomaly should not be coded separately. Additional codes should be assigned for manifestations that are not an inherent component.

Codes from Chapter 17 may be used throughout the life of the patient. If a congenital malformation or deformity has been corrected, a personal history code should be used to identify the history of the malformation or deformity. Although present at birth, a malformation/deformation or chromosomal abnormality may not be identified until later in life. Whenever the condition is diagnosed by the provider, it is appropriate to assign a code from codes Q00–Q99.For the birth admission, the appropriate code from category Z38, Liveborn infants, according to place of birth and type of delivery, should be sequenced as the principal diagnosis, followed by any congenital anomaly codes, Q00–Q99.
Note: Codes from this chapter are not for use on maternal records
Excludes2: inborn errors of metabolism (E70–E88)

(Q00–Q07) CONGENITAL MALFORMATIONS OF THE NERVOUS SYSTEM

Q00   ANENCEPHALY AND SIMILAR MALFORMATIONS
`4th`
    Q00.0   Anencephaly
            Acephaly
            Acrania
            Amyelencephaly
            Hemianencephaly
            Hemicephaly
    Q00.1   Craniorachischisis
    Q00.2   Iniencephaly

Q01   ENCEPHALOCELE
`4th`
    Includes: Arnold-Chiari syndrome, type III
            encephalocystocele
            encephalomyelocele
            hydroencephalocele
            hydromeningocele, cranial
            meningocele, cerebral
            meningoencephalocele
    Excludes1: Meckel-Gruber syndrome (Q61.9)
    Q01.0   Frontal encephalocele
    Q01.1   Nasofrontal encephalocele
    Q01.2   Occipital encephalocele
    Q01.8   Encephalocele of other sites
    Q01.9   Encephalocele, unspecified

Q02   MICROCEPHALY
`✔`
    Includes: hydromicrocephaly
            micrencephalon
    Code first, if applicable, to identify congenital Zika virus disease
    Excludes1: Meckel-Gruber syndrome (Q61.9)

Q03   CONGENITAL HYDROCEPHALUS
`4th`
    Includes: hydrocephalus in newborn
    Excludes1: Arnold-Chiari syndrome, type II (Q07.0-)
            acquired hydrocephalus (G91.-)
            hydrocephalus due to congenital toxoplasmosis (P37.1)
            hydrocephalus with spina bifida (Q05.0–Q05.4)
    Q03.0   Malformations of aqueduct of Sylvius
            Anomaly of aqueduct of Sylvius
            Obstruction of aqueduct of Sylvius, congenital
            Stenosis of aqueduct of Sylvius
    Q03.1   Atresia of foramina of Magendie and Luschka
            Dandy-Walker syndrome
    Q03.8   Other congenital hydrocephalus

    Q03.9   Congenital hydrocephalus, unspecified

Q04   OTHER CONGENITAL MALFORMATIONS OF BRAIN
`4th`
    Excludes1: cyclopia (Q87.0)
            macrocephaly (Q75.3)
    Q04.0   Congenital malformations of corpus callosum
            Agenesis of corpus callosum
    Q04.3   Other reduction deformities of brain
            Absence of part of brain
            Agenesis of part of brain
            Agyria
            Aplasia of part of brain
            Hydranencephaly
            Hypoplasia of part of brain
            Lissencephaly
            Microgyria
            Pachygyria
            Excludes1: congenital malformations of corpus callosum (Q04.0)
    Q04.6   Congenital cerebral cysts
            Porencephaly
            Schizencephaly
            Excludes1: acquired porencephalic cyst (G93.0)
    Q04.8   Other specified congenital malformations of brain
            Arnold-Chiari syndrome, type IV
            Macrogyria
    Q04.9   Congenital malformation of brain, unspecified
            Congenital anomaly NOS of brain
            Congenital deformity NOS of brain
            Congenital disease or lesion NOS of brain
            Multiple anomalies NOS of brain, congenital

Q05   SPINA BIFIDA
`4th`
    Includes: hydromeningocele (spinal)
            meningocele (spinal)
            meningomyelocele
            myelocele
            myelomeningocele
            rachischisis
            spina bifida (aperta) (cystica)
            syringomyelocele

> Lipomeningocele in spina bifida is also included in category Q05.

    Use additional code for any associated paraplegia (paraparesis) (G82.2-)
    Excludes1: Arnold-Chiari syndrome, type II (Q07.0-)
            spina bifida occulta (Q76.0)
    Q05.0   Cervical spina bifida with hydrocephalus
    Q05.1   Thoracic spina bifida with hydrocephalus
            Dorsal spina bifida with hydrocephalus
            Thoracolumbar spina bifida with hydrocephalus
    Q05.2   Lumbar spina bifida with hydrocephalus
            Lumbosacral spina bifida with hydrocephalus
    Q05.3   Sacral spina bifida with hydrocephalus
    Q05.4   Unspecified spina bifida with hydrocephalus
    Q05.5   Cervical spina bifida without hydrocephalus
    Q05.6   Thoracic spina bifida without hydrocephalus
            Dorsal spina bifida NOS
            Thoracolumbar spina bifida NOS
    Q05.7   Lumbar spina bifida without hydrocephalus
            Lumbosacral spina bifida NOS
    Q05.8   Sacral spina bifida without hydrocephalus
    Q05.9   Spina bifida, unspecified

Q06   OTHER CONGENITAL MALFORMATIONS OF SPINAL CORD
`4th`
    Q06.0   Amyelia
    Q06.1   Hypoplasia and dysplasia of spinal cord
            Atelomyelia
            Myelatelia
            Myelodysplasia of spinal cord
    Q06.2   Diastematomyelia
    Q06.3   Other congenital cauda equina malformations
    Q06.4   Hydromyelia
            Hydrorachis
    Q06.8   Other specified congenital malformations of spinal cord

---

`4th` `5th` `6th` `7th`   Additional Character Required   `✔`   3-character code

•=New Code   **Excludes1**—Not coded here, do not use together
▲=Revised Code   **Excludes2**—Not included here

CHAPTER 17. CONGENITAL MALFORMATIONS, DEFORMATIONS AND CHROMOSOMAL ABNORMALITIES (Q06.9–Q15.9)

Q06.9 Congenital malformation of spinal cord, unspecified
Congenital anomaly NOS of spinal cord
Congenital deformity NOS of spinal cord
Congenital disease or lesion NOS of spinal cord

Q07 OTHER CONGENITAL MALFORMATIONS OF NERVOUS SYSTEM `4th`
Excludes2: congenital central alveolar hypoventilation syndrome (G47.35)
familial dysautonomia [Riley-Day] (G90.1)
neurofibromatosis (nonmalignant) (Q85.0-)

Q07.0 Arnold-Chiari syndrome `5th`
Arnold-Chiari syndrome, type II
Excludes1: Arnold-Chiari syndrome, type III (Q01.-)
Arnold-Chiari syndrome, type IV (Q04.8)
Q07.00 without spina bifida or hydrocephalus
Q07.01 with spina bifida
Q07.02 with hydrocephalus
Q07.03 with spina bifida and hydrocephalus

Q07.8 Other specified congenital malformations of nervous system
Agenesis of nerve
Displacement of brachial plexus
Jaw-winking syndrome
Marcus Gunn's syndrome

Q07.9 Congenital malformation of nervous system, unspecified
Congenital anomaly NOS of nervous system
Congenital deformity NOS of nervous system
Congenital disease or lesion NOS of nervous system

(Q10–Q18) CONGENITAL MALFORMATIONS OF EYE, EAR, FACE AND NECK

Excludes2: cleft lip and cleft palate (Q35–Q37)
congenital malformation of cervical spine (Q05.0, Q05.5, Q67.5, Q76.0–Q76.4)
congenital malformation of larynx (Q31.-)
congenital malformation of lip NEC (Q38.0)
congenital malformation of nose (Q30.-)
congenital malformation of parathyroid gland (Q89.2)
congenital malformation of thyroid gland (Q89.2)

Q10 CONGENITAL MALFORMATIONS OF EYELID, LACRIMAL APPARATUS AND ORBIT `4th`
Excludes1: cryptophthalmos NOS (Q11.2)
cryptophthalmos syndrome (Q87.0)

Q10.0 Congenital ptosis
Q10.1 Congenital ectropion
Q10.2 Congenital entropion
Q10.3 Other congenital malformations of eyelid
Ablepharon
Blepharophimosis, congenital
Coloboma of eyelid
Congenital absence or agenesis of cilia
Congenital absence or agenesis of eyelid
Congenital accessory eyelid
Congenital accessory eye muscle
Congenital malformation of eyelid NOS
Q10.4 Absence and agenesis of lacrimal apparatus
Congenital absence of punctum lacrimale
Q10.5 Congenital stenosis and stricture of lacrimal duct
Q10.6 Other congenital malformations of lacrimal apparatus
Congenital malformation of lacrimal apparatus NOS
Q10.7 Congenital malformation of orbit

Q11 ANOPHTHALMOS, MICROPHTHALMOS AND MACROPHTHALMOS `4th`
Q11.0 Cystic eyeball
Q11.1 Other anophthalmos
Anophthalmos NOS
Agenesis of eye
Aplasia of eye
Q11.2 Microphthalmos
Cryptophthalmos NOS
Dysplasia of eye
Hypoplasia of eye
Rudimentary eye
Excludes1: cryptophthalmos syndrome (Q87.0)

Q11.3 Macrophthalmos
Excludes1: macrophthalmos in congenital glaucoma (Q15.0)

Q12 CONGENITAL LENS MALFORMATIONS `4th`
Q12.0 Congenital cataract
Q12.1 Congenital displaced lens
Q12.2 Coloboma of lens
Q12.3 Congenital aphakia
Q12.4 Spherophakia
Q12.8 Other congenital lens malformations
Microphakia
Q12.9 Congenital lens malformation, unspecified

Q13 CONGENITAL MALFORMATIONS OF ANTERIOR SEGMENT OF EYE `4th`
Q13.0 Coloboma of iris
Coloboma NOS
Q13.1 Absence of iris
Aniridia
Use additional code for associated glaucoma (H42)
Q13.2 Other congenital malformations of iris
Anisocoria, congenital
Atresia of pupil
Congenital malformation of iris NOS
Corectopia
Q13.3 Congenital corneal opacity
Q13.4 Other congenital corneal malformations
Congenital malformation of cornea NOS
Microcornea
Peter's anomaly
Q13.5 Blue sclera
Q13.8 Other congenital malformations of anterior segment of eye
`5th` **Q13.81 Rieger's anomaly**
Use additional code for associated glaucoma (H42)
Q13.89 Other congenital malformations of anterior segment of eye
Q13.9 Congenital malformation of anterior segment of eye, unspecified

Q14 CONGENITAL MALFORMATIONS OF POSTERIOR SEGMENT OF EYE `4th`
Excludes2: optic nerve hypoplasia (H47.03-)
Q14.0 Congenital malformation of vitreous humor
Congenital vitreous opacity
Q14.1 Congenital malformation of retina
Congenital retinal aneurysm
Q14.2 Congenital malformation of optic disc
Coloboma of optic disc
Q14.3 Congenital malformation of choroid
Q14.8 Other congenital malformations of posterior segment of eye
Coloboma of the fundus
Q14.9 Congenital malformation of posterior segment of eye, unspecified

Q15 OTHER CONGENITAL MALFORMATIONS OF EYE `4th`
Excludes1: congenital nystagmus (H55.01)
ocular albinism (E70.31-)
optic nerve hypoplasia (H47.03-)
retinitis pigmentosa (H35.52)
Q15.0 Congenital glaucoma
Axenfeld's anomaly
Buphthalmos
Glaucoma of childhood
Glaucoma of newborn
Hydrophthalmos
Keratoglobus, congenital, with glaucoma
Macrocornea with glaucoma
Macrophthalmos in congenital glaucoma
Megalocornea with glaucoma
Q15.8 Other specified congenital malformations of eye
Q15.9 Congenital malformation of eye, unspecified
Congenital anomaly of eye
Congenital deformity of eye

  `4th` `5th` `6th` `7th` Additional Character Required   ✔ 3-character code   •=New Code   *Excludes1*—Not coded here, do not use together
▲=Revised Code   *Excludes2*—Not included here

Q16   CONGENITAL MALFORMATIONS OF EAR CAUSING IMPAIRMENT OF HEARING
`4th`

Excludes1: congenital deafness (H90.-)

Q16.0   Congenital absence of (ear) auricle

Q16.1   Congenital absence, atresia and stricture of auditory canal (external)
Congenital atresia or stricture of osseous meatus

Q16.2   Absence of eustachian tube

Q16.3   Congenital malformation of ear ossicles
Congenital fusion of ear ossicles

Q16.4   Other congenital malformations of middle ear
Congenital malformation of middle ear NOS

Q16.5   Congenital malformation of inner ear
Congenital anomaly of membranous labyrinth
Congenital anomaly of organ of Corti

Q16.9   Congenital malformation of ear causing impairment of hearing, unspecified
Congenital absence of ear NOS

Q17   OTHER CONGENITAL MALFORMATIONS OF EAR
`4th`

*Excludes*1: congenital malformations of ear with impairment of hearing (Q16.0–Q16.9)
preauricular sinus (Q18.1)

Q17.0   Accessory auricle
Accessory tragus
Polyotia
Preauricular appendage or tag
Supernumerary ear
Supernumerary lobule

Q17.1   Macrotia

Q17.2   Microtia

Q17.3   Other misshapen ear
Pointed ear

Q17.4   Misplaced ear
Low-set ears
Excludes1: cervical auricle (Q18.2)

Q17.5   Prominent ear
Bat ear

Q17.8   Other specified congenital malformations of ear
Congenital absence of lobe of ear

Q17.9   Congenital malformation of ear, unspecified
Congenital anomaly of ear NOS

Q18   OTHER CONGENITAL MALFORMATIONS OF FACE AND NECK
`4th`

Excludes1: cleft lip and cleft palate (Q35-Q37)
conditions classified to Q67.0-Q67.4
congenital malformations of skull and face bones (Q75.-)
cyclopia (Q87.0)
dentofacial anomalies [including malocclusion] (M26.-)
malformation syndromes affecting facial appearance (Q87.0)
persistent thyroglossal duct (Q89.2)

Q18.0   Sinus, fistula and cyst of branchial cleft
Branchial vestige

Q18.1   Preauricular sinus and cyst
Fistula of auricle, congenital
Cervicoaural fistula

Q18.2   Other branchial cleft malformations
Branchial cleft malformation NOS
Cervical auricle
Otocephaly

Q18.6   Macrocheilia
Hypertrophy of lip, congenital

Q18.8   Other specified congenital malformations of face and neck
Medial cyst of face and neck
Medial fistula of face and neck
Medial sinus of face and neck

Q18.9   Congenital malformation of face and neck, unspecified
Congenital anomaly NOS of face and neck

(Q20–Q28) CONGENITAL MALFORMATIONS OF THE CIRCULATORY SYSTEM

Q20   CONGENITAL MALFORMATIONS OF CARDIAC CHAMBERS AND CONNECTIONS
`4th`

Excludes1: dextrocardia with situs inversus (Q89.3)
mirror-image atrial arrangement with situs inversus (Q89.3)

Q20.0   Common arterial trunk
Persistent truncus arteriosus
Excludes1: aortic septal defect (Q21.4)

Q20.3   Discordant ventriculoarterial connection
Dextrotransposition of aorta
Transposition of great vessels (complete)

Q20.8   Other congenital malformations of cardiac chambers and connections
Cor binoculare

Q21   CONGENITAL MALFORMATIONS OF CARDIAC SEPTA
`4th`

Excludes1: acquired cardiac septal defect (I51.0)

Q21.0   Ventricular septal defect
Roger's disease

Q21.1   Atrial septal defect
Coronary sinus defect
Patent or persistent foramen ovale
Patent or persistent ostium secundum defect (type II)
Patent or persistent sinus venosus defect

Q21.2   Atrioventricular septal defect
Common atrioventricular canal
Endocardial cushion defect
Ostium primum atrial septal defect (type I)

Q21.3   Tetralogy of Fallot
Ventricular septal defect with pulmonary stenosis or atresia, dextroposition of aorta and hypertrophy of right ventricle

Q21.8   Other congenital malformations of cardiac septa
Eisenmenger's defect
Pentalogy of Fallot
Code also Eisenmenger's complex or syndrome (I27.83)

Q21.9   Congenital malformation of cardiac septum, unspecified
Septal (heart) defect NOS

Q22   CONGENITAL MALFORMATIONS OF PULMONARY AND TRICUSPID VALVES
`4th`

Q22.0   Pulmonary valve atresia

Q22.1   Congenital pulmonary valve stenosis

Q22.2   Congenital pulmonary valve insufficiency
Congenital pulmonary valve regurgitation

Q22.3   Other congenital malformations of pulmonary valve
Congenital malformation of pulmonary valve NOS
Supernumerary cusps of pulmonary valve

Q22.4   Congenital tricuspid stenosis
Congenital tricuspid atresia

Q22.5   Ebstein's anomaly

Q22.6   Hypoplastic right heart syndrome

Q22.8   Other congenital malformations of tricuspid valve

Q22.9   Congenital malformation of tricuspid valve, unspecified

Q23   CONGENITAL MALFORMATIONS OF AORTIC AND MITRAL VALVES
`4th`

Q23.0   Congenital stenosis of aortic valve
Congenital aortic atresia
Congenital aortic stenosis NOS
Excludes1: congenital stenosis of aortic valve in hypoplastic left heart syndrome (Q23.4)
congenital subaortic stenosis (Q24.4)
supravalvular aortic stenosis (congenital) (Q25.3)

Q23.1   Congenital insufficiency of aortic valve
Bicuspid aortic valve
Congenital aortic insufficiency

Q23.2   Congenital mitral stenosis
Congenital mitral atresia

Q23.3   Congenital mitral insufficiency

Q23.4   Hypoplastic left heart syndrome

Q23.8   Other congenital malformations of aortic and mitral valves

CHAPTER 17. CONGENITAL MALFORMATIONS, DEFORMATIONS AND CHROMOSOMAL ABNORMALITIES   (Q16–Q23.8)

`4th` `5th` `6th` `7th` Additional Character Required	`✓` 3-character code	•=New Code ▲=Revised Code	*Excludes1*—Not coded here, do not use together *Excludes2*—Not included here

CHAPTER 17. CONGENITAL MALFORMATIONS, DEFORMATIONS AND CHROMOSOMAL ABNORMALITIES (Q23.9–Q28.8)

Q23.9 Congenital malformation of aortic and mitral valves, unspecified

Q24 OTHER CONGENITAL MALFORMATIONS OF HEART
4th *Excludes1:* endocardial fibroelastosis (I42.4)

Q24.0 Dextrocardia
Excludes1: dextrocardia with situs inversus (Q89.3)
   isomerism of atrial appendages (with asplenia or polysplenia) (Q20.6)
   mirror-image atrial arrangement with situs inversus (Q89.3)

Q24.1 Levocardia

Q24.3 Pulmonary infundibular stenosis
Subvalvular pulmonic stenosis

Q24.4 Congenital subaortic stenosis

Q24.6 Congenital heart block

Q24.8 Other specified congenital malformations of heart
Congenital diverticulum of left ventricle
Congenital malformation of myocardium
Congenital malformation of pericardium
Malposition of heart
Uhl's disease

Q24.9 Congenital malformation of heart, unspecified
Congenital anomaly of heart
Congenital disease of heart

Q25 CONGENITAL MALFORMATIONS OF GREAT ARTERIES
4th **Q25.0 Patent ductus arteriosus**
Patent ductus Botallo
Persistent ductus arteriosus

Q25.1 Coarctation of aorta
Coarctation of aorta (preductal) (postductal)
Stenosis of aorta

Q25.2 Atresia of aorta
5th **Q25.21 Interruption of aortic arch**
   Atresia of aortic arch
Q25.29 Other atresia of aorta
   Atresia of aorta

Q25.3 Supravalvular aortic stenosis
Excludes1: congenital aortic stenosis NOS (Q23.0)
   congenital stenosis of aortic valve (Q23.0)

Q25.4 Other congenital malformations of aorta
5th **Q25.40 Congenital malformation of aorta unspecified**
Q25.41 Absence and aplasia of aorta
Q25.42 Hypoplasia of aorta
Q25.43 Congenital aneurysm of aorta
   Congenital aneurysm of aortic root
   Congenital aneurysm of aortic sinus
Q25.44 Congenital dilation of aorta
Q25.45 Double aortic arch
   Vascular ring of aorta
Q25.46 Tortuous aortic arch
   Persistent convolutions of aortic arch
Q25.47 Right aortic arch
   Persistent right aortic arch
Q25.48 Anomalous origin of subclavian artery
Q25.49 Other congenital malformations of aorta
   Aortic arch
   Bovine arch

Q25.5 Atresia of pulmonary artery

Q25.6 Stenosis of pulmonary artery
Supravalvular pulmonary stenosis

Q25.7 Other congenital malformations of pulmonary artery
5th **Q25.71 Coarctation of pulmonary artery**
Q25.72 Congenital pulmonary arteriovenous malformation
   Congenital pulmonary arteriovenous aneurysm
Q25.79 Other congenital malformations of pulmonary artery
   Aberrant pulmonary artery
   Agenesis of pulmonary artery
   Congenital aneurysm of pulmonary artery
   Congenital anomaly of pulmonary artery
   Hypoplasia of pulmonary artery

Q25.9 Congenital malformation of great arteries, unspecified

Q26 CONGENITAL MALFORMATIONS OF GREAT VEINS
4th **Q26.2 Total anomalous pulmonary venous connection**
TAPVR, subdiaphragmatic
TAPVR, supradiaphragmatic

Q26.3 Partial anomalous pulmonary venous connection
Partial anomalous pulmonary venous return

Q26.4 Anomalous pulmonary venous connection, unspecified

Q26.8 Other congenital malformations of great veins
Absence of vena cava (inferior) (superior)
Azygos continuation of inferior vena cava
Persistent left posterior cardinal vein
Scimitar syndrome

Q26.9 Congenital malformation of great vein, unspecified
Congenital anomaly of vena cava (inferior) (superior) NOS

Q27 OTHER CONGENITAL MALFORMATIONS OF PERIPHERAL VASCULAR SYSTEM
4th *Excludes2:* anomalies of cerebral and precerebral vessels (Q28.0–Q28.3)
   anomalies of coronary vessels (Q24.5)
   anomalies of pulmonary artery (Q25.5–Q25.7)
   congenital retinal aneurysm (Q14.1)
   hemangioma and lymphangioma (D18.-)

Q27.0 Congenital absence and hypoplasia of umbilical artery
Single umbilical artery

Q27.3 Arteriovenous malformation (peripheral)
5th Arteriovenous aneurysm
Excludes1: acquired arteriovenous aneurysm (I77.0)
Excludes2: arteriovenous malformation of cerebral vessels (Q28.2)
   arteriovenous malformation of precerebral vessels (Q28.0)
Q27.30 Arteriovenous malformation, site unspecified
Q27.31 Arteriovenous malformation of vessel of upper limb
Q27.32 Arteriovenous malformation of vessel of lower limb
Q27.33 Arteriovenous malformation of digestive system vessel
Q27.34 Arteriovenous malformation of renal vessel
Q27.39 Arteriovenous malformation, other site

Q27.8 Other specified congenital malformations of peripheral vascular system
Absence of peripheral vascular system
Atresia of peripheral vascular system
Congenital aneurysm (peripheral)
Congenital stricture, artery
Congenital varix
Excludes 1: arteriovenous malformation (Q27.3-)

Q27.9 Congenital malformation of peripheral vascular system, unspecified
Anomaly of artery or vein NOS

Q28 OTHER CONGENITAL MALFORMATIONS OF CIRCULATORY SYSTEM
4th *Excludes1:* congenital aneurysm NOS (Q27.8)
   congenital coronary aneurysm (Q24.5)
   ruptured cerebral arteriovenous malformation (I60.8)
   ruptured malformation of precerebral vessels (I72.0)
Excludes2: congenital peripheral aneurysm (Q27.8)
   congenital pulmonary aneurysm (Q25.79)
   congenital retinal aneurysm (Q14.1)

Q28.2 Arteriovenous malformation of cerebral vessels
Arteriovenous malformation of brain NOS
Congenital arteriovenous cerebral aneurysm (nonruptured)

Q28.3 Other malformations of cerebral vessels
Congenital cerebral aneurysm (nonruptured)
Congenital malformation of cerebral vessels NOS
Developmental venous anomaly

Q28.8 Other specified congenital malformations of circulatory system
Congenital aneurysm, specified site NEC
Spinal vessel anomaly

   4th **5th** **6th** **7th** Additional Character Required   ✓ 3-character code   •=New Code ▲=Revised Code   *Excludes1*—Not coded here, do not use together   *Excludes2*—Not included here

(Q30–Q34) CONGENITAL MALFORMATIONS OF THE RESPIRATORY SYSTEM

Q30 **CONGENITAL MALFORMATIONS OF NOSE**
[4th] *Excludes1:* congenital deviation of nasal septum (Q67.4)
- **Q30.0** **Choanal atresia**
  Atresia of nares (anterior) (posterior)
  Congenital stenosis of nares (anterior) (posterior)
- **Q30.3** **Congenital perforated nasal septum**
- **Q30.8** **Other congenital malformations of nose**
  Accessory nose
  Congenital anomaly of nasal sinus wall
- **Q30.9** **Congenital malformation of nose, unspecified**

Q31 **CONGENITAL MALFORMATIONS OF LARYNX**
[4th] *Excludes1:* congenital laryngeal stridor NOS (P28.89)
- **Q31.2** **Laryngeal hypoplasia**
- **Q31.5** **Congenital laryngomalacia**
- **Q31.8** **Other congenital malformations of larynx**
  Absence of larynx
  Agenesis of larynx
  Atresia of larynx
  Congenital cleft thyroid cartilage
  Congenital fissure of epiglottis
  Congenital stenosis of larynx NEC
  Posterior cleft of cricoid cartilage

Q32 **CONGENITAL MALFORMATIONS OF TRACHEA AND**
[4th] **BRONCHUS**
Excludes1: congenital bronchiectasis (Q33.4)

> For congenital tracheoesophageal fistula, see category Q39.

- **Q32.0** **Congenital tracheomalacia**
- **Q32.4** **Other congenital malformations of bronchus**
  Absence of bronchus
  Agenesis of bronchus
  Atresia of bronchus
  Congenital diverticulum of bronchus
  Congenital malformation of bronchus NOS

Q33 **CONGENITAL MALFORMATIONS OF LUNG**
[4th] *Excludes1:* pulmonary hypoplasia associated with short gestation (P28.0)
- **Q33.6** **Congenital hypoplasia and dysplasia of lung**
- **Q33.9** **Congenital malformation of lung, unspecified**

Q34 **OTHER CONGENITAL MALFORMATIONS OF**
[4th] **RESPIRATORY SYSTEM**
Excludes2: congenital central alveolar hypoventilation syndrome (G47.35)
- **Q34.8** **Other specified congenital malformations of respiratory system**
  Atresia of nasopharynx
- **Q34.9** **Congenital malformation of respiratory system, unspecified**
  Congenital absence of respiratory system
  Congenital anomaly of respiratory system NOS

(Q35–Q37) CLEFT LIP AND CLEFT PALATE

Use additional code to identify associated malformation of the nose (Q30.2)
Excludes2: Robin's syndrome (Q87.0)

Q35 **CLEFT PALATE**
[4th] *Includes:* fissure of palate
  palatoschisis
Excludes1: cleft palate with cleft lip (Q37.-)
- **Q35.1** **Cleft hard palate**
- **Q35.3** **Cleft soft palate**
- **Q35.5** **Cleft hard palate with cleft soft palate**
- **Q35.7** **Cleft uvula**
- **Q35.9** **Cleft palate, unspecified**
  Cleft palate NOS

Q36 **CLEFT LIP**
[4th] *Includes:* cheiloschisis
  congenital fissure of lip
  harelip
  labium leporinum
Excludes1: cleft lip with cleft palate (Q37.-)

- **Q36.0** **Cleft lip, bilateral**
- **Q36.1** **Cleft lip, median**
- **Q36.9** **Cleft lip, unilateral**
  Cleft lip NOS

Q37 **CLEFT PALATE WITH CLEFT LIP**
[4th] *Includes:* cheilopalatoschisis
- **Q37.0** **Cleft hard palate with bilateral cleft lip**
- **Q37.1** **Cleft hard palate with unilateral cleft lip**
  Cleft hard palate with cleft lip NOS
- **Q37.2** **Cleft soft palate with bilateral cleft lip**
- **Q37.3** **Cleft soft palate with unilateral cleft lip**
  Cleft soft palate with cleft lip NOS
- **Q37.4** **Cleft hard and soft palate with bilateral cleft lip**
- **Q37.5** **Cleft hard and soft palate with unilateral cleft lip**
  Cleft hard and soft palate with cleft lip NOS
- **Q37.8** **Unspecified cleft palate with bilateral cleft lip**
- **Q37.9** **Unspecified cleft palate with unilateral cleft lip**

(Q38–Q45) OTHER CONGENITAL MALFORMATIONS OF THE DIGESTIVE SYSTEM

Q38 **OTHER CONGENITAL MALFORMATIONS OF TONGUE,**
[4th] **MOUTH AND PHARYNX**
Excludes1: dentofacial anomalies (M26.-)
  macrostomia (Q18.4)
  microstomia (Q18.5)
- **Q38.0** **Congenital malformations of lips, not elsewhere classified**
  Congenital fistula of lip
  Congenital malformation of lip NOS
  Van der Woude's syndrome
  Excludes1: cleft lip (Q36.-)
    cleft lip with cleft palate (Q37.-)
    macrocheilia (Q18.6)
    microcheilia (Q18.7)
- **Q38.1** **Ankyloglossia**
  Tongue tie
- **Q38.2** **Macroglossia**
  Congenital hypertrophy of tongue
- **Q38.3** **Other congenital malformations of tongue**
  Aglossia
  Bifid tongue
  Congenital adhesion of tongue
  Congenital fissure of tongue
  Congenital malformation of tongue NOS
  Double tongue
  Hypoglossia
  Hypoplasia of tongue
  Microglossia
- **Q38.5** **Congenital malformations of palate, not elsewhere classified**
  Congenital absence of uvula
  Congenital malformation of palate NOS
  Congenital high arched palate
  Excludes1: cleft palate (Q35.-)
    cleft palate with cleft lip (Q37.-)
- **Q38.6** **Other congenital malformations of mouth**
  Congenital malformation of mouth NOS
- **Q38.8** **Other congenital malformations of pharynx**
  Congenital malformation of pharynx NOS
  Imperforate pharynx

Q39 **CONGENITAL MALFORMATIONS OF ESOPHAGUS**
[4th]
- **Q39.0** **Atresia of esophagus without fistula**
  Atresia of esophagus NOS

  > Code Q39.1 may be used to report congenital tracheo-esophageal fistula with atresia of esophagus.

- **Q39.1** **Atresia of esophagus with tracheo-esophageal fistula**
  Atresia of esophagus with broncho-esophageal fistula
- **Q39.2** **Congenital tracheo-esophageal fistula without atresia**
  Congenital tracheo-esophageal fistula NOS
- **Q39.5** **Congenital dilatation of esophagus**
  Congenital cardiospasm

[4th] [5th] [6th] [7th] Additional Character Required | ✓ 3-character code | •=New Code ▲=Revised Code | *Excludes1*—Not coded here, do not use together *Excludes2*—Not included here

Q40 OTHER CONGENITAL MALFORMATIONS OF UPPER ALIMENTARY TRACT
4th

Q40.0 Congenital hypertrophic pyloric stenosis
Congenital or infantile constriction or hypertrophy or spasm
Congenital or infantile stenosis
Congenital or infantile stricture or stricture

Q40.1 Congenital hiatus hernia
Congenital displacement of cardia through esophageal hiatus
Excludes1: congenital diaphragmatic hernia (Q79.0)

Q40.2 Other specified congenital malformations of stomach
Congenital displacement of stomach
Congenital diverticulum of stomach
Congenital hourglass stomach
Congenital duplication of stomach
Megalogastria
Microgastria

Q40.8 Other specified congenital malformations of upper alimentary tract

Q40.9 Congenital malformation of upper alimentary tract, unspecified
Congenital anomaly of upper alimentary tract
Congenital deformity of upper alimentary tract

Q41 CONGENITAL ABSENCE, ATRESIA AND STENOSIS OF SMALL INTESTINE
4th

Includes: congenital obstruction, occlusion or stricture of small intestine or intestine NOS
Excludes1: cystic fibrosis with intestinal manifestation (E84.11)
meconium ileus NOS (without cystic fibrosis) (P76.0)

Q41.0 Congenital absence, atresia and stenosis of duodenum

Q41.1 Congenital absence, atresia and stenosis of jejunum
Apple peel syndrome
Imperforate jejunum

Q41.2 Congenital absence, atresia and stenosis of ileum

Q41.8 Congenital absence, atresia and stenosis of other specified parts of small intestine

Q41.9 Congenital absence, atresia and stenosis of small intestine, part unspecified
Congenital absence, atresia and stenosis of intestine NOS

Q42 CONGENITAL ABSENCE, ATRESIA AND STENOSIS OF LARGE INTESTINE
4th

Includes: congenital obstruction, occlusion and stricture of large intestine

Q42.0 Congenital absence, atresia and stenosis of rectum with fistula

Q42.1 Congenital absence, atresia and stenosis of rectum without fistula
Imperforate rectum

Q42.2 Congenital absence, atresia and stenosis of anus with fistula

Q42.3 Congenital absence, atresia and stenosis of anus without fistula
Imperforate anus

Q42.8 Congenital absence, atresia and stenosis of other parts of large intestine

Q42.9 Congenital absence, atresia and stenosis of large intestine, part unspecified

Q43 OTHER CONGENITAL MALFORMATIONS OF INTESTINE
4th

Q43.0 Meckel's diverticulum (displaced) (hypertrophic)
Persistent omphalomesenteric duct
Persistent vitelline duct

Q43.1 Hirschsprung's disease
Aganglionosis
Congenital (aganglionic) megacolon

Q43.2 Other congenital functional disorders of colon
Congenital dilatation of colon

Q43.3 Congenital malformations of intestinal fixation
Congenital omental, anomalous adhesions [bands]
Congenital peritoneal adhesions [bands]
Incomplete rotation of cecum and colon
Insufficient rotation of cecum and colon
Jackson's membrane
Malrotation of colon
Rotation failure of cecum and colon
Universal mesentery

Q43.6 Congenital fistula of rectum and anus
Excludes1: congenital fistula of anus with absence, atresia and stenosis (Q42.2)
congenital fistula of rectum with absence, atresia and stenosis (Q42.0)
congenital rectovaginal fistula (Q52.2)
congenital urethrorectal fistula (Q64.73)
pilonidal fistula or sinus (L05.-)

Q43.8 Other specified congenital malformations of intestine
Congenital blind loop syndrome
Congenital diverticulitis, colon
Congenital diverticulum, intestine
Dolichocolon
Megaloappendix
Megaloduodenum
Microcolon
Transposition of appendix
Transposition of colon
Transposition of intestine

Q43.9 Congenital malformation of intestine, unspecified

Q44 CONGENITAL MALFORMATIONS OF GALLBLADDER, BILE DUCTS AND LIVER
4th

Q44.0 Agenesis, aplasia and hypoplasia of gallbladder
Congenital absence of gallbladder

Q44.1 Other congenital malformations of gallbladder
Congenital malformation of gallbladder NOS
Intrahepatic gallbladder

Q44.2 Atresia of bile ducts

Q44.3 Congenital stenosis and stricture of bile ducts

Q44.4 Choledochal cyst

Q44.5 Other congenital malformations of bile ducts
Accessory hepatic duct
Biliary duct duplication
Congenital malformation of bile duct NOS
Cystic duct duplication

Q44.7 Other congenital malformations of liver
Accessory liver
Alagille's syndrome
Congenital absence of liver
Congenital hepatomegaly
Congenital malformation of liver NOS

Q45 OTHER CONGENITAL MALFORMATIONS OF DIGESTIVE SYSTEM
4th

Excludes2: congenital diaphragmatic hernia (Q79.0)
congenital hiatus hernia (Q40.1)

Q45.8 Other specified congenital malformations of digestive system
Absence (complete) (partial) of alimentary tract NOS
Duplication of digestive system
Malposition, congenital of digestive system

Q45.9 Congenital malformation of digestive system, unspecified
Congenital anomaly of digestive system
Congenital deformity of digestive system

(Q50–Q56) CONGENITAL MALFORMATIONS OF GENITAL ORGANS

Excludes1: androgen insensitivity syndrome (E34.5-)
syndromes associated with anomalies in the number and form of chromosomes (Q90–Q99)

Q50 CONGENITAL MALFORMATIONS OF OVARIES, FALLOPIAN TUBES AND BROAD LIGAMENTS
4th

Q50.0 Congenital absence of ovary
5th *Excludes1:* Turner's syndrome (Q96.-)
Q50.01 Congenital absence of ovary, unilateral
Q50.02 Congenital absence of ovary, bilateral

Q50.1 Developmental ovarian cyst

Q50.2 Congenital torsion of ovary

Q50.3 Other congenital malformations of ovary
5th **Q50.31 Accessory ovary**
Q50.32 Ovarian streak
46, XX with streak gonads

| 4th | 5th | 6th | 7th | Additional Character Required | ✔ 3-character code |

•=New Code   *Excludes1*—Not coded here, do not use together
▲=Revised Code   *Excludes2*—Not included here

Q50.39 Other congenital malformation of ovary
Congenital malformation of ovary NOS

Q50.4 Embryonic cyst of fallopian tube
Fimbrial cyst

Q50.5 Embryonic cyst of broad ligament
Epoophoron cyst
Parovarian cyst

Q50.6 Other congenital malformations of fallopian tube and broad ligament
Absence of fallopian tube and broad ligament
Accessory fallopian tube and broad ligament
Atresia of fallopian tube and broad ligament
Congenital malformation of fallopian tube or broad ligament NOS

Q51 CONGENITAL MALFORMATIONS OF UTERUS AND CERVIX
`4th`

Q51.0 Agenesis and aplasia of uterus
Congenital absence of uterus

Q51.1 Doubling of uterus with doubling of cervix and vagina
`5th` **Q51.10 Doubling of uterus with doubling of cervix and vagina without obstruction**
Doubling of uterus with doubling of cervix and vagina NOS

Q51.11 Doubling of uterus with doubling of cervix and vagina with obstruction

Q51.2 Other doubling of uterus
`5th` Doubling of uterus NOS
Septate uterus

Q51.21 Complete doubling of uterus
Complete septate uterus

Q51.22 Partial doubling of uterus
Partial septate uterus

Q51.28 Other and unspecified doubling of uterus
Septate uterus NOS

Q51.3 Bicornate uterus
Bicornate uterus, complete or partial

Q51.4 Unicornate uterus
Unicornate uterus with or without a separate uterine horn
Uterus with only one functioning horn

Q51.5 Agenesis and aplasia of cervix
Congenital absence of cervix

Q51.6 Embryonic cyst of cervix

Q51.7 Congenital fistulae between uterus and digestive and urinary tracts

Q51.8 Other congenital malformations of uterus and cervix
`5th` **Q51.81 Other congenital malformations of uterus**
`6th` **Q51.810 Arcuate uterus**
Arcuatus uterus
Q51.811 Hypoplasia of uterus
Q51.818 Other congenital malformations of uterus
Müllerian anomaly of uterus NEC

Q51.82 Other congenital malformations of cervix
`6th` **Q51.820 Cervical duplication**
Q51.821 Hypoplasia of cervix
Q51.828 Other congenital malformations of cervix

Q51.9 Congenital malformation of uterus and cervix, unspecified

Q52 OTHER CONGENITAL MALFORMATIONS OF FEMALE GENITALIA
`4th`

Q52.0 Congenital absence of vagina
Vaginal agenesis, total or partial

Q52.1 Doubling of vagina
`5th` *Excludes1:* doubling of vagina with doubling of uterus and cervix (Q51.1-)

Q52.10 Doubling of vagina, unspecified
Septate vagina NOS
Q52.11 Transverse vaginal septum
Q52.12 Longitudinal vaginal septum
`6th` **Q52.120 Longitudinal vaginal septum, nonobstructing**
Q52.121 Longitudinal vaginal septum, obstructing, right side
Q52.122 Longitudinal vaginal septum, obstructing, left side

Q52.123 Longitudinal vaginal septum, microperforate, right side
Q52.124 Longitudinal vaginal septum, microperforate, left side
Q52.129 Other and unspecified longitudinal vaginal septum

Q52.2 Congenital rectovaginal fistula
Excludes1: cloaca (Q43.7)

Q52.4 Other congenital malformations of vagina
Canal of Nuck cyst, congenital
Congenital malformation of vagina NOS
Embryonic vaginal cyst
Gartner's duct cyst

Q52.5 Fusion of labia

Q52.6 Congenital malformation of clitoris

Q52.7 Other and unspecified congenital malformations of vulva
`5th` **Q52.70 Unspecified congenital malformations of vulva**
Congenital malformation of vulva NOS
Q52.71 Congenital absence of vulva
Q52.79 Other congenital malformations of vulva
Congenital cyst of vulva

Q52.3 Imperforate hymen

Q52.8 Other specified congenital malformations of female genitalia

Q52.9 Congenital malformation of female genitalia, unspecified

Q53 UNDESCENDED AND ECTOPIC TESTICLE
`4th`

Q53.0 Ectopic testis
`5th` **Q53.00 Ectopic testis, unspecified**
Q53.01 Ectopic testis, unilateral
Q53.02 Ectopic testes, bilateral

Q53.1 Undescended testicle, unilateral
`5th` **Q53.10 Unspecified undescended testicle, unilateral**
Q53.11 Abdominal testis, unilateral
`6th` **Q53.111 Unilateral intraabdominal testis**
Q53.112 Unilateral inguinal testis
Q53.12 Ectopic perineal testis, unilateral
Q53.13 Unilateral high scrotal testis

Q53.2 Undescended testicle, bilateral
`5th` **Q53.20 Undescended testicle, unspecified, bilateral**
Q53.21 Abdominal testis, bilateral
`6th` **Q53.211 Bilateral intraabdominal testes**
Q53.212 Bilateral inguinal testes
Q53.22 Ectopic perineal testis, bilateral
Q53.23 Bilateral high scrotal testes

Q53.9 Undescended testicle, unspecified
Cryptorchism NOS

Q54 HYPOSPADIAS
`4th` *Excludes1:* epispadias (Q64.0)

Q54.0 Hypospadias, balanic
Hypospadias, coronal
Hypospadias, glandular

Q54.1 Hypospadias, penile

Q54.2 Hypospadias, penoscrotal

Q54.3 Hypospadias, perineal

Q54.4 Congenital chordee
Chordee without hypospadias

Q54.8 Other hypospadias
Hypospadias with intersex state

Q54.9 Hypospadias, unspecified

Q55 OTHER CONGENITAL MALFORMATIONS OF MALE GENITAL ORGANS
`4th` *Excludes1:* congenital hydrocele (P83.5)
hypospadias (Q54.-)

Q55.0 Absence and aplasia of testis
Monorchism

Q55.1 Hypoplasia of testis and scrotum
Fusion of testes

Q55.2 Other and unspecified congenital malformations of testis and scrotum
`5th` **Q55.20 Unspecified congenital malformations of testis and scrotum**
Congenital malformation of testis or scrotum NOS

`4th` `5th` `6th` `7th` Additional Character Required   `✓` 3-character code   •=New Code   *Excludes1*—Not coded here, do not use together
▲=Revised Code   *Excludes2*—Not included here

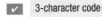

CHAPTER 17. CONGENITAL MALFORMATIONS, DEFORMATIONS AND CHROMOSOMAL ABNORMALITIES   (Q55.21–Q64.6)

Q55.21 **Polyorchism**
Q55.22 **Retractile testis**
Q55.23 **Scrotal transposition**
Q55.29 **Other congenital malformations of testis and scrotum**
Q55.4 **Other congenital malformations of vas deferens, epididymis, seminal vesicles and prostate**
Absence or aplasia of prostate
Absence or aplasia of spermatic cord
Congenital malformation of vas deferens, epididymis, seminal vesicles or prostate NOS
Q55.5 **Congenital absence and aplasia of penis**
Q55.6 **Other congenital malformations of penis**
[5th] Q55.61 **Curvature of penis (lateral)**
Q55.62 **Hypoplasia of penis**
Micropenis
Q55.63 **Congenital torsion of penis**
Excludes1: acquired torsion of penis (N48.82)
Q55.64 **Hidden penis**
Buried penis
Concealed penis
Excludes1: acquired buried penis (N48.83)
Q55.69 **Other congenital malformation of penis**
Congenital malformation of penis NOS
Q55.8 **Other specified congenital malformations of male genital organs**
Q55.9 **Congenital malformation of male genital organ, unspecified**
Congenital anomaly of male genital organ
Congenital deformity of male genital organ

Q56 **INDETERMINATE SEX AND PSEUDOHERMAPHRODITISM**
[4th] *Excludes1:* 46, XX true hermaphrodite (Q99.1)
androgen insensitivity syndrome (E34.5-)
chimera 46, XX/46, XY true hermaphrodite (Q99.0)
female pseudohermaphroditism with adrenocortical disorder (E25.-)
pseudohermaphroditism with specified chromosomal anomaly (Q96–Q99)
pure gonadal dysgenesis (Q99.1)
Q56.1 **Male pseudohermaphroditism, not elsewhere classified**
46, XY with streak gonads
Male pseudohermaphroditism NOS
Q56.2 **Female pseudohermaphroditism, not elsewhere classified**
Female pseudohermaphroditism NOS
Q56.3 **Pseudohermaphroditism, unspecified**
Q56.4 **Indeterminate sex, unspecified**
Ambiguous genitalia

(Q60–Q64) CONGENITAL MALFORMATIONS OF THE URINARY SYSTEM

Q60 **RENAL AGENESIS AND OTHER REDUCTION DEFECTS OF KIDNEY**
[4th]
Includes: congenital absence of kidney
congenital atrophy of kidney
infantile atrophy of kidney
Q60.0 **Renal agenesis, unilateral**
Q60.1 **Renal agenesis, bilateral**
Q60.3 **Renal hypoplasia, unilateral**
Q60.4 **Renal hypoplasia, bilateral**
Q60.6 **Potter's syndrome**

Q61 **CYSTIC KIDNEY DISEASE**
[4th] *Excludes1:* acquired cyst of kidney (N28.1)
Potter's syndrome (Q60.6)
Q61.0 **Congenital renal cyst**
[5th] Q61.00 **Congenital renal cyst, unspecified**
Cyst of kidney NOS (congenital)
Q61.01 **Congenital single renal cyst**
Q61.02 **Congenital multiple renal cysts**
Q61.1 **Polycystic kidney, infantile type**
[5th] Polycystic kidney, autosomal recessive
Q61.11 **Cystic dilatation of collecting ducts**
Q61.19 **Other polycystic kidney, infantile type**

Q61.2 **Polycystic kidney, adult type**
Polycystic kidney, autosomal dominant
Q61.3 **Polycystic kidney, unspecified**
Q61.4 **Renal dysplasia**
Multicystic dysplastic kidney
Multicystic kidney (development)
Multicystic kidney disease
Multicystic renal dysplasia
Excludes1: polycystic kidney disease (Q61.11–Q61.3)
Q61.5 **Medullary cystic kidney**
Nephronopthisis
Sponge kidney NOS
Q61.8 **Other cystic kidney diseases**
Fibrocystic kidney
Fibrocystic renal degeneration or disease
Q61.9 **Cystic kidney disease, unspecified**
Meckel-Gruber syndrome

Q62 **CONGENITAL OBSTRUCTIVE DEFECTS OF RENAL PELVIS**
[4th] **AND CONGENITAL MALFORMATIONS OF URETER**
Q62.0 **Congenital hydronephrosis**
Q62.1 **Congenital occlusion of ureter**
[5th] Atresia and stenosis of ureter
Q62.10 **Congenital occlusion of ureter, unspecified**
Q62.11 **Congenital occlusion of ureteropelvic junction**
Q62.12 **Congenital occlusion of ureterovesical orifice**
Q62.3 **Other obstructive defects of renal pelvis and ureter**
[5th] Q62.31 **Congenital ureterocele, orthotopic**
Q62.32 **Cecoureterocele**
Ectopic ureterocele
Q62.39 **Other obstructive defects of renal pelvis and ureter**
Ureteropelvic junction obstruction NOS
Q62.8 **Other congenital malformations of ureter**
Anomaly of ureter NOS

Q63 **OTHER CONGENITAL MALFORMATIONS OF KIDNEY**
[4th] *Excludes1:* congenital nephrotic syndrome (N04.-)
Q63.0 **Accessory kidney**
Q63.1 **Lobulated, fused and horseshoe kidney**
Q63.2 **Ectopic kidney**
Congenital displaced kidney
Malrotation of kidney
Q63.3 **Hyperplastic and giant kidney**
Compensatory hypertrophy of kidney
Q63.8 **Other specified congenital malformations of kidney**
Congenital renal calculi
Q63.9 **Congenital malformation of kidney, unspecified**

Q64 **OTHER CONGENITAL MALFORMATIONS OF**
[4th] **URINARY SYSTEM**
Q64.0 **Epispadias**
Excludes1: hypospadias (Q54.-)
Q64.1 **Exstrophy of urinary bladder**
[5th] Q64.10 **Exstrophy of urinary bladder, unspecified**
Ectopia vesicae
Q64.11 **Supravesical fissure of urinary bladder**
Q64.12 **Cloacal exstrophy of urinary bladder**
Q64.19 **Other exstrophy of urinary bladder**
Extroversion of bladder
Q64.2 **Congenital posterior urethral valves**
Q64.3 **Other atresia and stenosis of urethra and bladder neck**
[5th] Q64.31 **Congenital bladder neck obstruction**
Congenital obstruction of vesicourethral orifice
Q64.39 **Other atresia and stenosis of urethra and bladder neck**
Atresia and stenosis of urethra and bladder neck NOS
Q64.4 **Malformation of urachus**
Cyst of urachus
Patent urachus
Prolapse of urachus
Q64.5 **Congenital absence of bladder and urethra**
Q64.6 **Congenital diverticulum of bladder**

   [4th] [5th] [6th] [7th] Additional Character Required   ✔ 3-character code

•=New Code   *Excludes1*—Not coded here, do not use together
▲=Revised Code   *Excludes2*—Not included here

Q64.7 **Other and unspecified congenital malformations of bladder and urethra**
> 5th

> ***Excludes1:*** congenital prolapse of bladder (mucosa) (Q79.4)

    Q64.70 **Unspecified congenital malformation of bladder and urethra**
         Malformation of bladder or urethra NOS

    Q64.79 **Other congenital malformations of bladder and urethra**

Q64.9 **Congenital malformation of urinary system, unspecified**
     Congenital anomaly NOS of urinary system
     Congenital deformity NOS of urinary system

(Q65–Q79) CONGENITAL MALFORMATIONS AND DEFORMATIONS OF THE MUSCULOSKELETAL SYSTEM

Q65 **CONGENITAL DEFORMITIES OF HIP**
> 4th

> ***Excludes1:*** clicking hip (R29.4)

Q65.0 **Congenital dislocation of hip, unilateral**
> 5th

    Q65.00 **Congenital dislocation of unspecified hip, unilateral**
    Q65.01 **Congenital dislocation of right hip, unilateral**
    Q65.02 **Congenital dislocation of left hip, unilateral**

Q65.1 **Congenital dislocation of hip, bilateral**

Q65.2 **Congenital dislocation of hip, unspecified**

Q65.3 **Congenital partial dislocation of hip, unilateral**
> 5th

    Q65.30 **Congenital partial dislocation of unspecified hip, unilateral**
    Q65.31 **Congenital partial dislocation of right hip, unilateral**
    Q65.32 **Congenital partial dislocation of left hip, unilateral**

Q65.4 **Congenital partial dislocation of hip, bilateral**

Q65.5 **Congenital partial dislocation of hip, unspecified**

Q65.6 **Congenital unstable hip**
     Congenital dislocatable hip

Q65.8 **Other congenital deformities of hip**
> 5th

    Q65.81 **Congenital coxa valga**
    Q65.82 **Congenital coxa vara**
    Q65.89 **Other specified congenital deformities of hip**
         Anteversion of femoral neck
         Congenital acetabular dysplasia

Q66 **CONGENITAL DEFORMITIES OF FEET**
> 4th

> ***Excludes1:*** reduction defects of feet (Q72.-)
>   valgus deformities (acquired) (M21.0-)
>   varus deformities (acquired) (M21.1-)

Q66.0 **Congenital talipes equinovarus**
> 5th

    Q66.01 **Congenital talipes equinovarus, right foot**
    Q66.02 **Congenital talipes equinovarus, left foot**

Q66.1 **Congenital talipes calcaneovarus**
> 5th

    Q66.11 **Congenital talipes calcaneovarus, right foot**
    Q66.12 **Congenital talipes calcaneovarus, left foot**

Q66.2 **Congenital metatarsus deformities**
> 5th

    Q66.21 **Congenital metatarsus primus varus**
>   6th

        Q66.211 **Congenital metatarsus primus varus, right foot**
        Q66.212 **Congenital metatarsus primus varus, left foot**

    Q66.22 **Congenital metatarsus adductus**
>   6th

         Congenital metatarsus varus
        Q66.221 **Congenital metatarsus adductus, right foot**
        Q66.222 **Congenital metatarsus adductus, left foot**

Q66.3 **Other congenital varus deformities of feet**
> 5th

     Hallux varus, congenital
    Q66.31 **Other congenital varus deformities of feet, right foot**
    Q66.32 **Other congenital varus deformities of feet, left foot**

Q66.4 **Congenital talipes calcaneovalgus**
> 5th

    Q66.41 **Congenital talipes calcaneovalgus, right foot**
    Q66.42 **Congenital talipes calcaneovalgus, left foot**

Q66.5 **Congenital pes planus**
> 5th

     Congenital flat foot
     Congenital rigid flat foot
     Congenital spastic (everted) flat foot

> ***Excludes1:*** pes planus, acquired (M21.4)

    Q66.50 **Congenital pes planus, unspecified foot**
    Q66.51 **Congenital pes planus, right foot**

    Q66.52 **Congenital pes planus, left foot**

Q66.6 **Other congenital valgus deformities of feet**
     Congenital metatarsus valgus

Q66.7 **Congenital pes cavus**
> 5th

    Q66.71 **Congenital pes cavus, right foot**
    Q66.72 **Congenital pes cavus, left foot**

Q66.8 **Other congenital deformities of feet**
> 5th

    Q66.80 **Congenital vertical talus deformity, unspecified foot**
    Q66.81 **Congenital vertical talus deformity, right foot**
    Q66.82 **Congenital vertical talus deformity, left foot**
    Q66.89 **Other specified congenital deformities of feet**
         Congenital asymmetric talipes
         Congenital clubfoot NOS
         Congenital talipes NOS
         Congenital tarsal coalition
         Hammer toe, congenital

Q66.9 **Congenital deformity of feet, unspecified**
> 5th

    Q66.91 **Congenital deformity of feet, unspecified, right foot**
    Q66.92 **Congenital deformity of feet, unspecified, left foot**

Q67 **CONGENITAL MUSCULOSKELETAL DEFORMITIES OF HEAD, FACE, SPINE AND CHEST**
> 4th

> ***Excludes1:*** congenital malformation syndromes classified to Q87.-
>   Potter's syndrome (Q60.6)

Q67.0 **Congenital facial asymmetry**

Q67.1 **Congenital compression facies**

Q67.2 **Dolichocephaly**

Q67.3 **Plagiocephaly**

Q67.4 **Other congenital deformities of skull, face and jaw**
     Congenital depressions in skull
     Congenital hemifacial atrophy or hypertrophy
     Deviation of nasal septum, congenital
     Squashed or bent nose, congenital

> ***Excludes1:*** dentofacial anomalies [including malocclusion] (M26.-)
>   syphilitic saddle nose (A50.5)

Q67.5 **Congenital deformity of spine**
     Congenital postural scoliosis
     Congenital scoliosis NOS

> ***Excludes1:*** infantile idiopathic scoliosis (M41.0)
>   scoliosis due to congenital bony malformation (Q76.3)

Q67.6 **Pectus excavatum**
     Congenital funnel chest

Q67.7 **Pectus carinatum**
     Congenital pigeon chest

Q67.8 **Other congenital deformities of chest**
     Congenital deformity of chest wall NOS

Q68 **OTHER CONGENITAL MUSCULOSKELETAL DEFORMITIES**
> 4th

> ***Excludes1:*** reduction defects of limb(s) (Q71-Q73)
> ***Excludes2:*** congenital myotonic chondrodystrophy (G71.13)

Q68.0 **Congenital deformity of sternocleidomastoid muscle**
     Congenital contracture of sternocleidomastoid (muscle)
     Congenital (sternomastoid) torticollis
     Sternomastoid tumor (congenital)

Q68.1 **Congenital deformity of finger(s) and hand**
     Congenital clubfinger
     Spade-like hand (congenital)

Q68.2 **Congenital deformity of knee**
     Congenital dislocation of knee
     Congenital genu recurvatum

Q68.5 **Congenital bowing of long bones of leg, unspecified**

Q68.8 **Other specified congenital musculoskeletal deformities**
     Congenital deformity of clavicle or scapula
     Congenital deformity of elbow or forearm or wrist
     Congenital dislocation of elbow or shoulder or wrist

Q69 **POLYDACTYLY**
> 4th

Q69.0 **Accessory finger(s)**

Q69.1 **Accessory thumb(s)**

Q69.2 **Accessory toe(s)**
     Accessory hallux

Q69.9 **Polydactyly, unspecified**
     Supernumerary digit(s) NOS

> 4th   5th   6th   7th   Additional Character Required   ✔   3-character code

●=New Code   ***Excludes1***—Not coded here, do not use together
▲=Revised Code   ***Excludes2***—Not included here

CHAPTER 17. CONGENITAL MALFORMATIONS, DEFORMATIONS AND CHROMOSOMAL ABNORMALITIES   (Q70–Q75.3)

Q70   SYNDACTYLY
`4th`

Q70.0 Fused fingers
`5th`   Complex syndactyly of fingers with synostosis
- **Q70.00 Fused fingers, unspecified hand**
- **Q70.01 Fused fingers, right hand**
- **Q70.02 Fused fingers, left hand**
- **Q70.03 Fused fingers, bilateral**

Q70.1 Webbed fingers
`5th`   Simple syndactyly of fingers without synostosis
- **Q70.10 Webbed fingers, unspecified hand**
- **Q70.11 Webbed fingers, right hand**
- **Q70.12 Webbed fingers, left hand**
- **Q70.13 Webbed fingers, bilateral**

Q70.2 Fused toes
`5th`   Complex syndactyly of toes with synostosis
- **Q70.20 Fused toes, unspecified foot**
- **Q70.21 Fused toes, right foot**
- **Q70.22 Fused toes, left foot**
- **Q70.23 Fused toes, bilateral**

Q70.3 Webbed toes
`5th`   Simple syndactyly of toes without synostosis
- **Q70.30 Webbed toes, unspecified foot**
- **Q70.31 Webbed toes, right foot**
- **Q70.32 Webbed toes, left foot**
- **Q70.33 Webbed toes, bilateral**

Q70.4 Polysyndactyly, unspecified
Excludes1: specified syndactyly of hand and feet—code to specified conditions (Q70.0–Q70.3-)

Q70.9 Syndactyly, unspecified
Symphalangy NOS

Q71   REDUCTION DEFECTS OF UPPER LIMB
`4th`

Q71.4 Longitudinal reduction defect of radius
`5th`   Clubhand (congenital)
Radial clubhand
- **Q71.41 Longitudinal reduction defect of right radius**
- **Q71.42 Longitudinal reduction defect of left radius**
- **Q71.43 Longitudinal reduction defect of radius, bilateral**

Q71.5 Longitudinal reduction defect of ulna
`5th`
- **Q71.51 Longitudinal reduction defect of right ulna**
- **Q71.52 Longitudinal reduction defect of left ulna**
- **Q71.53 Longitudinal reduction defect of ulna, bilateral**

Q71.6 Lobster-claw hand
`5th`
- **Q71.61 Lobster-claw right hand**
- **Q71.62 Lobster-claw left hand**
- **Q71.63 Lobster-claw hand, bilateral**

Q71.8 Other reduction defects of upper limb
`5th`   **Q71.81 Congenital shortening of upper limb**
   `6th`   **Q71.811 Congenital shortening of right upper limb**
     Q71.812 Congenital shortening of left upper limb
     Q71.813 Congenital shortening of upper limb, bilateral
  Q71.89 Other reduction defects of upper limb
   `6th`   **Q71.891 Other reduction defects of right upper limb**
     Q71.892 Other reduction defects of left upper limb
     Q71.893 Other reduction defects of upper limb, bilateral

Q71.9 Unspecified reduction defect of upper limb
`5th`
- **Q71.91 Unspecified reduction defect of right upper limb**
- **Q71.92 Unspecified reduction defect of left upper limb**
- **Q71.93 Unspecified reduction defect of upper limb, bilateral**

Q72   REDUCTION DEFECTS OF LOWER LIMB
`4th`

Q72.4 Longitudinal reduction defect of femur
`5th`   Proximal femoral focal deficiency
- **Q72.41 Longitudinal reduction defect of right femur**
- **Q72.42 Longitudinal reduction defect of left femur**
- **Q72.43 Longitudinal reduction defect of femur, bilateral**

Q72.5 Longitudinal reduction defect of tibia
`5th`
- **Q72.51 Longitudinal reduction defect of right tibia**
- **Q72.52 Longitudinal reduction defect of left tibia**
- **Q72.53 Longitudinal reduction defect of tibia, bilateral**

Q72.6 Longitudinal reduction defect of fibula
`5th`
- **Q72.61 Longitudinal reduction defect of right fibula**
- **Q72.62 Longitudinal reduction defect of left fibula**
- **Q72.63 Longitudinal reduction defect of fibula, bilateral**

Q72.7 Split foot
`5th`
- **Q72.71 Split foot, right lower limb**
- **Q72.72 Split foot, left lower limb**
- **Q72.73 Split foot, bilateral**

Q72.8 Other reduction defects of lower limb
`5th`   **Q72.81 Congenital shortening of lower limb**
   `6th`   **Q72.811 Congenital shortening of right lower limb**
     Q72.812 Congenital shortening of left lower limb
     Q72.813 Congenital shortening of lower limb, bilateral
  Q72.89 Other reduction defects of lower limb
   `6th`   **Q72.891 Other reduction defects of right lower limb**
     Q72.892 Other reduction defects of left lower limb
     Q72.893 Other reduction defects of lower limb, bilateral

Q72.9 Unspecified reduction defect of lower limb
`5th`
- **Q72.91 Unspecified reduction defect of right lower limb**
- **Q72.92 Unspecified reduction defect of left lower limb**
- **Q72.93 Unspecified reduction defect of lower limb, bilateral**

Q74   OTHER CONGENITAL MALFORMATIONS OF LIMB(S)
`4th`
Excludes1: polydactyly (Q69.-)
reduction defect of limb (Q71–Q73)
syndactyly (Q70.-)

Q74.0 Other congenital malformations of upper limb(s), including shoulder girdle
Accessory carpal bones
Cleidocranial dysostosis
Congenital pseudarthrosis of clavicle
Macrodactylia (fingers)
Madelung's deformity
Radioulnar synostosis
Sprengel's deformity
Triphalangeal thumb

Q74.1 Congenital malformation of knee
Congenital absence of patella
Congenital dislocation of patella
Congenital genu valgum
Congenital genu varum
Rudimentary patella
Excludes1: congenital dislocation of knee (Q68.2)
congenital genu recurvatum (Q68.2)
nail patella syndrome (Q87.2)

Q74.2 Other congenital malformations of lower limb(s), including pelvic girdle
Congenital fusion of sacroiliac joint
Congenital malformation of ankle joint
Congenital malformation of sacroiliac joint
Excludes1: anteversion of femur (neck) (Q65.89)

Q74.3 Arthrogryposis multiplex congenita
Q74.8 Other specified congenital malformations of limb(s)
Q74.9 Unspecified congenital malformation of limb(s)
Congenital anomaly of limb(s) NOS

Q75   OTHER CONGENITAL MALFORMATIONS OF SKULL AND FACE BONES
`4th`
Excludes1: congenital malformation of face NOS (Q18.-)
congenital malformation syndromes classified to Q87.-
dentofacial anomalies [including malocclusion] (M26.-)
musculoskeletal deformities of head and face (Q67.0–Q67.4)
skull defects associated with congenital anomalies of brain such as:
anencephaly (Q00.0)
encephalocele (Q01.-)
hydrocephalus (Q03.-)
microcephaly (Q02)

Q75.0 Craniosynostosis
Acrocephaly
Imperfect fusion of skull
Oxycephaly
Trigonocephaly

Q75.1 Craniofacial dysostosis
Crouzon's disease

Q75.2 Hypertelorism

Q75.3 Macrocephaly

`4th` `5th` `6th` `7th` Additional Character Required   ✔ 3-character code

•=New Code   *Excludes1*—Not coded here, do not use together
▲=Revised Code   *Excludes2*—Not included here

Q75.4　Mandibulofacial dysostosis
Franceschetti syndrome
Treacher Collins syndrome

Q75.5　Oculomandibular dysostosis

Q75.8　Other specified congenital malformations of skull and face bones
Absence of skull bone, congenital
Congenital deformity of forehead
Platybasia

Q75.9　Congenital malformation of skull and face bones, unspecified
Congenital anomaly of face bones NOS
Congenital anomaly of skull NOS

Q76　CONGENITAL MALFORMATIONS OF SPINE AND
`4th`　**BONY THORAX**
Excludes1: congenital musculoskeletal deformities of spine and chest (Q67.5–Q67.8)

Q76.0　Spina bifida occulta
Excludes1: meningocele (spinal) (Q05.-)
spina bifida (aperta) (cystica) (Q05.-)

Q76.2　Congenital spondylolisthesis
Congenital spondylolysis
Excludes1: spondylolisthesis (acquired) (M43.1-)
spondylolysis (acquired) (M43.0-)

Q76.3　Congenital scoliosis due to congenital bony malformation
Hemivertebra fusion or failure of segmentation with scoliosis

Q76.4　Other congenital malformations of spine, not associated with
`5th`　scoliosis

　　Q76.42　Congenital lordosis
　　`6th`　**Q76.425　Congenital lordosis, thoracolumbar region**
　　　　　　　Q76.426　Congenital lordosis, lumbar region
　　　　　　　Q76.427　Congenital lordosis, lumbosacral region
　　　　　　　Q76.428　Congenital lordosis, sacral and sacrococcygeal region
　　　　　　　Q76.429　Congenital lordosis, unspecified region
　　Q76.49　Other congenital malformations of spine, not associated with scoliosis
　　　　Congenital absence of vertebra NOS
　　　　Congenital fusion of spine NOS
　　　　Congenital malformation of lumbosacral (joint) (region) NOS
　　　　Congenital malformation of spine NOS
　　　　Hemivertebra NOS
　　　　Malformation of spine NOS
　　　　Platyspondylisis NOS
　　　　Supernumerary vertebra NOS

Q77　OSTEOCHONDRODYSPLASIA WITH DEFECTS OF
`4th`　**GROWTH OF TUBULAR BONES AND SPINE**
Excludes1: mucopolysaccharidosis (E76.0-E76.3)
Excludes2: congenital myotonic chondrodystrophy (G71.13)

Q77.0　Achondrogenesis
Hypochondrogenesis

Q77.1　Thanatophoric short stature

Q77.2　Short rib syndrome
Asphyxiating thoracic dysplasia [Jeune]

Q77.3　Chondrodysplasia punctata
Excludes1: Rhizomelic chondrodysplasia punctata (E71.43)

Q77.4　Achondroplasia
Hypochondroplasia
Osteosclerosis congenita

Q77.5　Diastrophic dysplasia

Q77.6　Chondroectodermal dysplasia
Ellis-van Creveld syndrome

Q77.7　Spondyloepiphyseal dysplasia

Q77.8　Other osteochondrodysplasia with defects of growth of tubular bones and spine

Q77.9　Osteochondrodysplasia with defects of growth of tubular bones and spine, unspecified

Q78　OTHER OSTEOCHONDRODYSPLASIAS
`4th`　*Excludes2:* congenital myotonic chondrodystrophy (G71.13)

Q78.0　Osteogenesis imperfecta
Fragilitas ossium
Osteopsathyrosis

Q78.2　Osteopetrosis
Albers-Schönberg syndrome
Osteosclerosis NOS

Q78.4　Enchondromatosis
Maffucci's syndrome
Ollier's disease

Q78.8　Other specified osteochondrodysplasias
Osteopoikilosis

Q78.9　Osteochondrodysplasia, unspecified
Chondrodystrophy NOS
Osteodystrophy NOS

Q79　CONGENITAL MALFORMATIONS OF MUSCULOSKELETAL
`4th`　**SYSTEM, NEC**
Excludes2: congenital (sternomastoid) torticollis (Q68.0)

Q79.0　Congenital diaphragmatic hernia
Excludes1: congenital hiatus hernia (Q40.1)

Q79.1　Other congenital malformations of diaphragm
Absence of diaphragm
Congenital malformation of diaphragm NOS
Eventration of diaphragm

Q79.2　Exomphalos
Omphalocele
Excludes1: umbilical hernia (K42.-)

Q79.3　Gastroschisis

Q79.4　Prune belly syndrome
Congenital prolapse of bladder mucosa
Eagle-Barrett syndrome

Q79.5　Other congenital malformations of abdominal wall
`5th`　*Excludes1:* umbilical hernia (K42.-)
　　Q79.51　Congenital hernia of bladder
　　Q79.59　Other congenital malformations of abdominal wall

Q79.6　Ehlers-Danlos syndromes
`5th`　**Q79.60　Ehlers-Danlos syndrome, unspecified**
　　Q79.61　Classical Ehlers-Danlos syndrome
　　　　Classical EDS (cEDS)
　　Q79.62　Hypermobile Ehlers-Danlos syndrome
　　　　Hypermobile EDS (hEDS)
　　Q79.63　Vascular Ehlers-Danlos syndrome
　　　　Vascular EDS (vEDS)
　　Q79.69　Other Ehlers-Danlos syndromes

Q79.8　Other congenital malformations of musculoskeletal system
Absence of muscle
Absence of tendon
Accessory muscle
Amyotrophia congenita
Congenital constricting bands
Congenital shortening of tendon
Poland syndrome

Q79.9　Congenital malformation of musculoskeletal system, unspecified
Congenital anomaly of musculoskeletal system NOS
Congenital deformity of musculoskeletal system NOS

(Q80–Q89) OTHER CONGENITAL MALFORMATIONS

Q80　CONGENITAL ICHTHYOSIS
`4th`　*Excludes1:* Refsum's disease (G60.1)

Q80.0　Ichthyosis vulgaris

Q80.1　X-linked ichthyosis

Q80.2　Lamellar ichthyosis
Collodion baby

Q80.3　Congenital bullous ichthyosiform erythroderma

Q80.4　Harlequin fetus

Q80.8　Other congenital ichthyosis

Q80.9　Congenital ichthyosis, unspecified

Q81　EPIDERMOLYSIS BULLOSA
`4th`　**Q81.0　Epidermolysis bullosa simplex**
　　Excludes1: Cockayne's syndrome (Q87.19)

Q81.1　Epidermolysis bullosa letalis
Herlitz' syndrome

Q81.2　Epidermolysis bullosa dystrophica

Q81.8　Other epidermolysis bullosa

Q81.9　Epidermolysis bullosa, unspecified

`4th`　`5th`　`6th`　`7th`　Additional Character Required　　　✔　3-character code

•=New Code　　　*Excludes1*—Not coded here, do not use together
▲=Revised Code　　　*Excludes2*—Not included here

CHAPTER 17. CONGENITAL MALFORMATIONS, DEFORMATIONS AND CHROMOSOMAL ABNORMALITIES   (Q82–Q87.2)

Q82   **OTHER CONGENITAL MALFORMATIONS OF SKIN**
`4th`   *Excludes1:* acrodermatitis enteropathica (E83.2)
     congenital erythropoietic porphyria (E80.0)
     pilonidal cyst or sinus (L05.-)
     Sturge-Weber (-Dimitri) syndrome (Q85.8)

Q82.0   **Hereditary lymphedema**

Q82.1   **Xeroderma pigmentosum**

Q82.2   **Congenital cutaneous mastocytosis**
     Congenital diffuse cutaneous mastocytosis
     Congenital maculopapular cutaneous mastocytosis
     Congenital urticaria pigmentosa
     Excludes1: cutaneous mastocytosis NOS (D47.01)
       diffuse cutaneous mastocytosis (with onset after newborn
       period) (D47.01)
       malignant mastocytosis (C96.2-)
       systemic mastocytosis (D47.02)
       urticaria pigmentosa (non-congenital) (with onset after newborn
       period) (D47.01)

Q82.3   **Incontinentia pigmenti**

Q82.4   **Ectodermal dysplasia (anhidrotic)**
     Excludes1: Ellis-van Creveld syndrome (Q77.6)

Q82.5   **Congenital non-neoplastic nevus**
     Birthmark NOS
     Flammeus nevus
     Portwine nevus
     Sanguineous nevus
     Strawberry nevus
     Vascular nevus NOS
     Verrucous nevus
     Excludes2: Café au lait spots (L81.3)
       lentigo (L81.4)
       nevus NOS (D22.-)
       araneus nevus (I78.1)
       melanocytic nevus (D22.-)
       pigmented nevus (D22.-)
       spider nevus (I78.1)
       stellar nevus (I78.1)

Q82.6   **Congenital sacral dimple**
     Parasacral dimple
     Excludes2: pilonidal cyst with abscess (L05.01)
     pilonidal cyst without abscess (L05.91)

Q82.8   **Other specified congenital malformations of skin**
     Abnormal palmar creases
     Accessory skin tags
     Benign familial pemphigus [Hailey-Hailey]
     Congenital poikiloderma
     Cutis laxa (hyperelastica)
     Dermatoglyphic anomalies
     Inherited keratosis palmaris et plantaris
     Keratosis follicularis *[Darier-White]*
     Excludes1: Ehlers-Danlos syndromes (Q79.6-).

Q82.9   **Congenital malformation of skin, unspecified**

Q83   **CONGENITAL MALFORMATIONS OF BREAST**
`4th`   *Excludes2:* absence of pectoral muscle (Q79.8)
     hypoplasia of breast (N64.82)
     micromastia (N64.82)

Q83.0   **Congenital absence of breast with absent nipple**

Q83.3   **Accessory nipple**
     Supernumerary nipple

Q83.8   **Other congenital malformations of breast**

Q84   **OTHER CONGENITAL MALFORMATIONS OF INTEGUMENT**
`4th`   **Q84.2**   **Other congenital malformations of hair**
     Congenital hypertrichosis
     Congenital malformation of hair NOS
     Persistent lanugo

Q84.3   **Anonychia**
     Excludes1: nail patella syndrome (Q87.2)

Q84.4   **Congenital leukonychia**

Q84.6   **Other congenital malformations of nails**
     Congenital clubnail
     Congenital koilonychia
     Congenital malformation of nail NOS

Q84.8   **Other specified congenital malformations of integument**
     Aplasia cutis congenita

Q84.9   **Congenital malformation of integument, unspecified**
     Congenital anomaly of integument NOS
     Congenital deformity of integument NOS

Q85   **PHAKOMATOSES, NES**
`4th`   *Excludes1:* ataxia telangiectasia [Louis-Bar] (G11.3)
     familial dysautonomia [Riley-Day] (G90.1)

Q85.0   **Neurofibromatosis (nonmalignant)**
`5th`   **Q85.00**   **Neurofibromatosis, unspecified**
     Q85.01   **Neurofibromatosis, type 1**
       Von Recklinghausen disease
     Q85.02   **Neurofibromatosis, type 2**
       Acoustic neurofibromatosis
     Q85.03   **Schwannomatosis**
     Q85.09   **Other neurofibromatosis**

Q85.1   **Tuberous sclerosis**
     Bourneville's disease
     Epiloia

Q85.8   **Other phakomatoses, NEC**
     Peutz-Jeghers syndrome
     Sturge-Weber (-Dimitri) syndrome
     von Hippel-Lindau syndrome
     Excludes1: Meckel-Gruber syndrome (Q61.9)

Q85.9   **Phakomatosis, unspecified**
     Hamartosis NOS

Q86   **CONGENITAL MALFORMATION SYNDROMES DUE TO**
`4th`   **KNOWN EXOGENOUS CAUSES, NEC**
     Excludes2: iodine-deficiency-related hypothyroidism (E00–E02)
     nonteratogenic effects of substances transmitted via placenta or
     breast milk (P04.-)

Q86.0   **Fetal alcohol syndrome (dysmorphic)**

Q87   **OTHER SPECIFIED CONGENITAL MALFORMATION**
`4th`   **SYNDROMES AFFECTING MULTIPLE SYSTEMS**
     Use additional code(s) to identify all associated manifestations

Q87.0   **Congenital malformation syndromes predominantly affecting**
     facial appearance
     Acrocephalopolysyndactyly
     Acrocephalosyndactyly [Apert]
     Cryptophthalmos syndrome
     Cyclopia
     Goldenhar syndrome
     Moebius syndrome
     Oro-facial-digital syndrome
     Robin syndrome
     Whistling face
     Production note-replace text with Insert 17E:

Q87.1   **Congenital malformation syndromes predominantly associated**
`5th`   **with short stature**
     Excludes1: Ellis-van Creveld syndrome (Q77.6)
     Smith-Lemli-Opitz syndrome (E78.72)
     Q87.11   **Prader-Willi syndrome**
     Q87.19   **Other congenital malformation syndromes**
       predominantly associated with short stature
       Aarskog syndrome
       Cockayne syndrome
       De Lange syndrome
       Dubowitz syndrome
       Noonan syndrome
       Robinow-Silverman-Smith syndrome
       Russell-Silver syndrome
       Seckel syndrome

Q87.2   **Congenital malformation syndromes predominantly involving**
     limbs
     Holt-Oram syndrome
     Klippel-Trenaunay-Weber syndrome
     Nail patella syndrome
     Rubinstein-Taybi syndrome
     Sirenomelia syndrome
     TAR syndrome
     VATER syndrome

`4th` `5th` `6th` `7th`   Additional Character Required   ✓   3-character code

•=New Code   *Excludes1*—Not coded here, do not use together
▲=Revised Code   *Excludes2*—Not included here

Q87.3 Congenital malformation syndromes involving early overgrowth
Beckwith-Wiedemann syndrome
Sotos syndrome
Weaver syndrome

Q87.4 Marfan's syndrome `5th`
    Q87.40 Marfan's syndrome, unspecified
    Q87.41 Marfan's syndrome with cardiovascular manifestations `6th`
        Q87.410 Marfan's syndrome with aortic dilation
        Q87.418 Marfan's syndrome with other cardiovascular manifestations
    Q87.42 Marfan's syndrome with ocular manifestations
    Q87.43 Marfan's syndrome with skeletal manifestation

Q87.8 Other specified congenital malformation syndromes, NEC `5th`
    Excludes1: Zellweger syndrome (E71.510)
    Q87.81 Alport syndrome
        Use additional code to identify stage of CKD (N18.1–N18.6)
    Q87.82 Arterial tortuosity syndrome
    Q87.89 Other specified congenital malformation syndromes, NEC
        Laurence-Moon (-Bardet)-Biedl syndrome

Q89 OTHER CONGENITAL MALFORMATIONS, NEC `4th`
Q89.0 Congenital absence and malformations of spleen `5th`
    Excludes1: isomerism of atrial appendages (with asplenia or polysplenia) (Q20.6)
    Q89.01 Asplenia (congenital)
    Q89.09 Congenital malformations of spleen
        Congenital splenomegaly

Q89.1 Congenital malformations of adrenal gland
    Excludes1: adrenogenital disorders (E25.-)
        congenital adrenal hyperplasia (E25.0)

Q89.2 Congenital malformations of other endocrine glands
Congenital malformation of parathyroid or thyroid gland
Persistent thyroglossal duct
Thyroglossal cyst
    Excludes1: congenital goiter (E03.0)
        congenital hypothyroidism (E03.1)

Q89.3 Situs inversus
Dextrocardia with situs inversus
Mirror-image atrial arrangement with situs inversus
Situs inversus or transversus abdominalis
Situs inversus or transversus thoracis
Transposition of abdominal viscera
Transposition of thoracic viscera
    Excludes1: dextrocardia NOS (Q24.0)

Q89.7 Multiple congenital malformations, NEC
Multiple congenital anomalies NOS
Multiple congenital deformities NOS
    Excludes1: congenital malformation syndromes affecting multiple systems (Q87.-)

Q89.8 Other specified congenital malformations
    Use additional code(s) to identify all associated manifestations

Q89.9 Congenital malformation, unspecified
Congenital anomaly NOS
Congenital deformity NOS

(Q90–Q99) CHROMOSOMAL ABNORMALITIES, NEC

Excludes2: mitochondrial metabolic disorders (E88.4-)

Q90 DOWN SYNDROME `4th`
Use additional code(s) to identify any associated physical conditions and degree of intellectual disabilities (F70–F79)
Q90.0 Trisomy 21, nonmosaicism (meiotic nondisjunction)
Q90.1 Trisomy 21, mosaicism (mitotic nondisjunction)
Q90.2 Trisomy 21, translocation
Q90.9 Down syndrome, unspecified
Trisomy 21 NOS

Q91 TRISOMY 18 AND TRISOMY 13 `4th`
Q91.0 Trisomy 18, nonmosaicism (meiotic nondisjunction)
Q91.1 Trisomy 18, mosaicism (mitotic nondisjunction)
Q91.2 Trisomy 18, translocation

Q91.3 Trisomy 18, unspecified
Q91.4 Trisomy 13, nonmosaicism (meiotic nondisjunction)
Q91.5 Trisomy 13, mosaicism (mitotic nondisjunction)
Q91.6 Trisomy 13, translocation
Q91.7 Trisomy 13, unspecified

Q92 OTHER TRISOMIES AND PARTIAL TRISOMIES OF THE AUTOSOMES, NOT ELSEWHERE CLASSIFIED `4th`
Includes: unbalanced translocations and insertions
Excludes1: trisomies of chromosomes 13, 18, 21 (Q90-Q91)
Q92.9 Trisomy and partial trisomy of autosomes, unspecified

Q93 MONOSOMIES AND DELETIONS FROM THE AUTOSOMES, NEC `4th`
Q93.0 Whole chromosome monosomy, nonmosaicism (meiotic nondisjunction)
Q93.1 Whole chromosome monosomy, mosaicism (mitotic nondisjunction)
Q93.2 Chromosome replaced with ring, dicentric or isochromosome
Q93.3 Deletion of short arm of chromosome 4
Wolff-Hirschorn syndrome
Q93.4 Deletion of short arm of chromosome 5
Cri-du-chat syndrome
Q93.5 Other deletions of part of a chromosome `5th`
    Q93.51 Angelman syndrome
    Q93.59 Other deletions of part of a chromosome
Q93.7 Deletions with other complex rearrangements
Deletions due to unbalanced translocations, inversions and insertions
Code also any associated duplications due to unbalanced translocations, inversions and insertions (Q92.5)
Q93.8 Other deletions from the autosomes `5th`
    Q93.81 Velo-cardio-facial syndrome
        Deletion 22q11.2
    Q93.82 Williams syndrome
    Q93.88 Other microdeletions
        Miller-Dieker syndrome
        Smith-Magenis syndrome
    Q93.89 Other deletions from the autosomes
        Deletions identified by fluorescence in situ hybridization (FISH)
        Deletions identified by in situ hybridization (ISH)
        Deletions seen only at prometaphase
Q93.9 Deletion from autosomes, unspecified

Q95 BALANCED REARRANGEMENTS AND STRUCTURAL MARKERS, NOT ELSEWHERE CLASSIFIED `4th`
Includes: Robertsonian and balanced reciprocal translocations and insertions
Q95.0 Balanced translocation and insertion in normal individual
Q95.9 Balanced rearrangement and structural marker, unspecified

Q96 TURNER'S SYNDROME `4th`
Excludes1: Noonan syndrome (Q87.19)
Q96.0 Karyotype 45, X
Q96.1 Karyotype 46, X iso (Xq)
Karyotype 46, isochromosome Xq
Q96.2 Karyotype 46, X with abnormal sex chromosome, except iso (Xq)
Karyotype 46, X with abnormal sex chromosome, except isochromosome Xq
Q96.3 Mosaicism, 45, X/46, XX or XY
Q96.4 Mosaicism, 45, X/other cell line(s) with abnormal sex chromosome
Q96.8 Other variants of Turner's syndrome
Q96.9 Turner's syndrome, unspecified

Q97 OTHER SEX CHROMOSOME ABNORMALITIES, FEMALE PHENOTYPE, NEC `4th`
Excludes1: Turner's syndrome (Q96.-)
Q97.0 Karyotype 47, XXX
Q97.2 Mosaicism, lines with various numbers of X chromosomes
Q97.8 Other specified sex chromosome abnormalities, female phenotype
Q97.9 Sex chromosome abnormality, female phenotype, unspecified

---

`4th` `5th` `6th` `7th` Additional Character Required   ✔ 3-character code

•=New Code   *Excludes1*—Not coded here, do not use together
▲=Revised Code   *Excludes2*—Not included here

CHAPTER 17. CONGENITAL MALFORMATIONS, DEFORMATIONS AND CHROMOSOMAL ABNORMALITIES   (Q98–Q99.9)

Q98   **OTHER SEX CHROMOSOME ABNORMALITIES, MALE**
`4th`   **PHENOTYPE, NEC**

     Q98.3   **Other male with 46, XX karyotype**

     Q98.4   **Klinefelter syndrome, unspecified**

     Q98.5   **Karyotype 47, XYY**

     Q98.7   **Male with sex chromosome mosaicism**

     Q98.9   **Sex chromosome abnormality, male phenotype, unspecified**

Q99   **OTHER CHROMOSOME ABNORMALITIES, NEC**
`4th`   **Q99.1**   **46, XX true hermaphrodite**

           46, XX with streak gonads

           46, XY with streak gonads

           Pure gonadal dysgenesis

     Q99.2   **Fragile X chromosome**

           Fragile X syndrome

     Q99.8   **Other specified chromosome abnormalities**

     Q99.9   **Chromosomal abnormality, unspecified**

   `4th` `5th` `6th` `7th`   Additional Character Required   3-character code   •=New Code   ▲=Revised Code   *Excludes1*—Not coded here, do not use together   *Excludes2*—Not included here

312   **PEDIATRIC ICD-10-CM 2022: A MANUAL FOR PROVIDER-BASED CODING**

Chapter 18. Symptoms, signs, and abnormal clinical and laboratory findings, not elsewhere classified (R00–R99)

GUIDELINES

Chapter 18 includes symptoms, signs, abnormal results of clinical or other investigative procedures, and ill-defined conditions regarding which no diagnosis classifiable elsewhere is recorded. Signs and symptoms that point to a specific diagnosis have been assigned to a category in other chapters of the classification.

Use of symptom codes

Codes that describe symptoms and signs are acceptable for reporting purposes when a related definitive diagnosis has not been established (confirmed) by the provider.

Use of a symptom code with a definitive diagnosis code

Codes for signs and symptoms may be reported in addition to a related definitive diagnosis when the sign or symptom is not routinely associated with that diagnosis, such as the various signs and symptoms associated with complex syndromes. The definitive diagnosis code should be sequenced before the symptom code.

Signs or symptoms that are associated routinely with a disease process should not be assigned as additional codes, unless otherwise instructed by the classification.

Combination codes that include symptoms

ICD-10-CM contains a number of combination codes that identify both the definitive diagnosis and common symptoms of that diagnosis. When using one of these combination codes, an additional code should not be assigned for the symptom.

Repeated falls

Refer to the ICD-10-CM manual.

Coma

Refer to subcategory R40.2 for guidelines.

SIRS due to Non-Infectious Process

Refer to codes R65.10-R65.11.

Death NOS

Refer to code R99.

Note: This chapter includes symptoms, signs, abnormal results of clinical or other investigative procedures, and ill-defined conditions regarding which no diagnosis classifiable elsewhere is recorded.

Signs and symptoms that point rather definitely to a given diagnosis have been assigned to a category in other chapters of the classification. In general, categories in this chapter include the less well-defined conditions and symptoms that, without the necessary study of the case to establish a final diagnosis, point perhaps equally to two or more diseases or to two or more systems of the body. Practically all categories in the chapter could be designated 'not otherwise specified,' 'unknown etiology' or 'transient'. The Alphabetical Index should be consulted to determine which symptoms and signs are to be allocated here and which to other chapters. The residual subcategories, numbered .8, are generally provided for other relevant symptoms that cannot be allocated elsewhere in the classification.

The conditions and signs or symptoms included in categories R00–R94 consist of:
a) cases for which no more specific diagnosis can be made even after all the facts bearing on the case have been investigated;
b) signs or symptoms existing at the time of initial encounter that proved to be transient and whose causes could not be determined;
c) provisional diagnosis in a patient who failed to return for further investigation or care;
d) cases referred elsewhere for investigation or treatment before the diagnosis was made;
e) cases in which a more precise diagnosis was not available for any other reason;
f) certain symptoms, for which supplementary information is provided, that represent important problems in medical care in their own right.

Excludes2: abnormal findings on antenatal screening of mother (O28.-)
certain conditions originating in the perinatal period (P04–P96)
signs and symptoms classified in the body system chapters signs and symptoms of breast (N63, N64.5)

(R00–R09) SYMPTOMS AND SIGNS INVOLVING THE CIRCULATORY AND RESPIRATORY SYSTEMS

R00 **ABNORMALITIES OF HEART BEAT**
`4th` **Excludes1:** abnormalities originating in the perinatal period (P29.1-)
Excludes 2: specified arrhythmias (I47–I49)
  R00.0 **Tachycardia, unspecified**
    Rapid heart beat
    Sinoauricular tachycardia NOS
    Sinus [sinusal] tachycardia NOS
    Excludes1: neonatal tachycardia (P29.11)
      paroxysmal tachycardia (I47.-)
  R00.1 **Bradycardia, unspecified**
    Sinoatrial bradycardia
    Sinus bradycardia
    Slow heart beat
    Vagal bradycardia
    Use additional code for adverse effect, if applicable, to identify drug (T36–T50 with fifth or sixth character 5)
    Excludes1: neonatal bradycardia (P29.12)
  R00.2 **Palpitations**
    Awareness of heart beat
  R00.8 **Other abnormalities of heart beat**
  R00.9 **Unspecified abnormalities of heart beat**

R01 **CARDIAC MURMURS AND OTHER CARDIAC SOUNDS**
`4th` **Excludes1:** cardiac murmurs and sounds originating in the perinatal period (P29.8)
  R01.0 **Benign and innocent cardiac murmurs**
    Functional cardiac murmur
  R01.1 **Cardiac murmur, unspecified**
    Cardiac bruit NOS
    Heart murmur NOS
    Systolic murmur NOS
  R01.2 **Other cardiac sounds**
    Cardiac dullness, increased or decreased
    Precordial friction

R03 **ABNORMAL BLOOD-PRESSURE READING, WITHOUT**
`4th` **DIAGNOSIS**
  R03.0 **Elevated blood-pressure reading, without diagnosis of hypertension**
    Note: This category is to be used to record an episode of elevated blood pressure in a patient in whom no formal diagnosis of hypertension has been made, or as an isolated incidental finding.
  R03.1 **Nonspecific low blood-pressure reading**
    Excludes1: hypotension (I95.-)
      maternal hypotension syndrome (O26.5-)
      neurogenic orthostatic hypotension (G90.3)

R04 **HEMORRHAGE FROM RESPIRATORY PASSAGES**
`4th` **R04.0** **Epistaxis**
    Hemorrhage from nose
    Nosebleed
  R04.2 **Hemoptysis**
    Blood-stained sputum
    Cough with hemorrhage
  R04.8 **Hemorrhage from other sites in respiratory passages**
   `5th` **R04.81** **Acute idiopathic pulmonary hemorrhage in infants**
      AIPHI
      Acute idiopathic hemorrhage in infants over 28 days old
      Excludes1: perinatal pulmonary hemorrhage (P26.-)
        von Willebrand's disease (D68.0)
   R04.89 **Hemorrhage from other sites in respiratory passages**
      Pulmonary hemorrhage NOS
  R04.9 **Hemorrhage from respiratory passages, unspecified**

`4th` `5th` `6th` `7th`   Additional Character Required   ✓   3-character code

•=New Code
▲=Revised Code

Excludes1—Not coded here, do not use together
Excludes2—Not included here

▲R05 **COUGH**
`4th`
> **Excludes1:** paroxysmal cough due to Bordetella pertussis (A37.0-)
>   smoker's cough (J41.0)
>
> **Excludes2:** cough with hemorrhage (R04.2)

- **•R05.1** **Acute cough**
- **•R05.2** **Subacute cough**
- **•R05.3** **Chronic cough**
  > Persistent cough
  > Refractory cough
  > Unexplained cough
- **•R05.4** **Cough syncope**
  > **Code first** syncope and collapse (R55)
- **•R05.8** **Other specified cough**
- **•R05.9** **Cough, unspecified**

R06 **ABNORMALITIES OF BREATHING**
`4th`
> **Excludes1:** acute respiratory distress syndrome (J80)
>   respiratory arrest (R09.2)
>   respiratory arrest of newborn (P28.81)
>   respiratory distress syndrome of newborn (P22.-)
>   respiratory failure (J96.-)
>   respiratory failure of newborn (P28.5)

R06.0 **Dyspnea**
`5th`
> **Excludes1:** tachypnea NOS (R06.82)
>   transient tachypnea of newborn (P22.1)

    R06.00 **Dyspnea, unspecified**
    R06.01 **Orthopnea**
    R06.02 **Shortness of breath**
    R06.03 **Acute respiratory distress**

R06.1 **Stridor**
> **Excludes1:** congenital laryngeal stridor (P28.89)
>   laryngismus (stridulus) (J38.5)

R06.2 **Wheezing**
> **Excludes1:** Asthma (J45.-)

R06.3 **Periodic breathing**
> Cheyne-Stokes breathing

R06.4 **Hyperventilation**
> **Excludes1:** psychogenic hyperventilation (F45.8)

R06.5 **Mouth breathing**
> **Excludes2:** dry mouth NOS (R68.2)

R06.6 **Hiccough**
> **Excludes1:** psychogenic hiccough (F45.8)

R06.7 **Sneezing**

R06.8 **Other abnormalities of breathing**
`5th`
    R06.81 **Apnea, NEC**
        Apnea NOS
        > **Excludes1:** apnea (of) newborn (P28.4)
        >   sleep apnea (G47.3-)
        >   sleep apnea of newborn (primary) (P28.3)

    R06.82 **Tachypnea, NEC**
        Tachypnea NOS
        > **Excludes1:** transitory tachypnea of newborn (P22.1)

    R06.83 **Snoring**
    R06.89 **Other abnormalities of breathing**
        Breath-holding (spells)
        Sighing
        Hypercapnia

R07 **PAIN IN THROAT AND CHEST**
`4th`
> **Excludes1:** epidemic myalgia (B33.0)
>
> **Excludes2:** jaw pain R68.84
>   pain in breast (N64.4)

R07.0 **Pain in throat**
> **Excludes1:** chronic sore throat (J31.2)
>   sore throat (acute) NOS (J02.9)
>
> **Excludes2:** dysphagia (R13.1-)
>   pain in neck (M54.2)

R07.1 **Chest pain on breathing**
> Painful respiration

R07.8 **Other chest pain**
`5th`
    R07.81 **Pleurodynia**
        Pleurodynia NOS
        > **Excludes1:** epidemic pleurodynia (B33.0)

    R07.82 **Intercostal pain**

    R07.89 **Other chest pain**
        Anterior chest-wall pain NOS

R07.9 **Chest pain, unspecified**

R09 **OTHER SYMPTOMS AND SIGNS INVOLVING THE**
`4th` **CIRCULATORY AND RESPIRATORY SYSTEM**
> **Excludes1:** acute respiratory distress syndrome (J80)
>   respiratory arrest of newborn (P28.81)
>   respiratory distress syndrome of newborn (P22.0)
>   respiratory failure (J96.-)
>   respiratory failure of newborn (P28.5)

R09.0 **Asphyxia and hypoxemia**
`5th`
> **Excludes1:** asphyxia due to carbon monoxide (T58.-)
>   asphyxia due to FB in respiratory tract (T17.-)
>   birth (intrauterine) asphyxia (P84)
>   hyperventilation (R06.4)
>   traumatic asphyxia (T71.-)
>
> **Excludes 2:** hypercapnia (R06.89)

    R09.01 **Asphyxia**
    R09.02 **Hypoxemia**

R09.1 **Pleurisy**
> **Excludes1:** pleurisy with effusion (J90)

R09.2 **Respiratory arrest**
> Cardiorespiratory failure
> **Excludes1:** cardiac arrest (I46.-)
>   respiratory arrest of newborn (P28.81)
>   respiratory distress of newborn (P22.0)
>   respiratory failure (J96.-)
>   respiratory failure of newborn (P28.5)
>   respiratory insufficiency (R06.89)
>   respiratory insufficiency of newborn (P28.5)

R09.3 **Abnormal sputum**
> Abnormal amount of sputum
> Abnormal color of sputum
> Abnormal odor of sputum
> Excessive sputum
> **Excludes1:** blood-stained sputum (R04.2)

R09.8 **Other specified symptoms and signs involving the circulatory**
`5th` **and respiratory systems**
    R09.81 **Nasal congestion**
    R09.82 **Postnasal drip**
    R09.89 **Other specified symptoms and signs involving the circulatory and respiratory systems**
        Bruit (arterial)
        Abnormal chest percussion
        Feeling of FB in throat
        Friction sounds in chest
        Chest tympany
        Choking sensation
        Rales
        Weak pulse
        > **Excludes2:** FB in throat (T17.2-)
        >   wheezing (R06.2)

(R10–R19) SYMPTOMS AND SIGNS INVOLVING THE DIGESTIVE SYSTEM AND ABDOMEN

Excludes2: congenital or infantile pylorospasm (Q40.0)
  gastrointestinal hemorrhage (K92.0–K92.2)
  intestinal obstruction (K56.-)
  newborn gastrointestinal hemorrhage (P54.0–P54.3)
  newborn intestinal obstruction (P76.-)
  pylorospasm (K31.3)
  signs and symptoms involving the urinary system (R30–R39)
  symptoms referable to female genital organs (N94.-)
  symptoms referable to male genital organs male (N48–N50)

R10 **ABDOMINAL AND PELVIC PAIN**
`4th`
> **Excludes1:** renal colic (N23)
>
> **Excludes2:** dorsalgia (M54.-)
>   flatulence and related conditions (R14.-)

`4th` `5th` `6th` `7th` Additional Character Required   3-character code

    •=New Code   **Excludes1**—Not coded here, do not use together
    ▲=Revised Code   **Excludes2**—Not included here

R10.0 Acute abdomen
Severe abdominal pain (generalized) (with abdominal rigidity)
Excludes1: abdominal rigidity NOS (R19.3)
  generalized abdominal pain NOS (R10.84)
  localized abdominal pain (R10.1-R10.3-)
R10.1 Pain localized to upper abdomen
`5th`   **R10.10 Upper abdominal pain, unspecified**
  R10.11 RUQ pain
  R10.12 LUQ pain
  R10.13 Epigastric pain
    Dyspepsia
    Excludes1: functional dyspepsia (K30)
R10.2 Pelvic and perineal pain
  Excludes1: vulvodynia (N94.81)
R10.3 Pain localized to other parts of lower abdomen
`5th`   **R10.30 Lower abdominal pain, unspecified**
  R10.31 RLQ pain
  R10.32 LLQ pain
  R10.33 Periumbilical pain
R10.8 Other abdominal pain
`5th`   **R10.81 Abdominal tenderness**
    Abdominal tenderness NOS
  `6th`
    R10.811 RUQ abdominal tenderness
    R10.812 LUQ abdominal tenderness
    R10.813 RLQ abdominal tenderness
    R10.814 LLQ abdominal tenderness
    R10.815 Periumbilic abdominal tenderness
    R10.816 Epigastric abdominal tenderness
    R10.817 Generalized abdominal tenderness
    R10.819 Abdominal tenderness, unspecified site
  R10.82 Rebound abdominal tenderness
  `6th`
    R10.821 RUQ rebound abdominal tenderness
    R10.822 LUQ rebound abdominal tenderness
    R10.823 RLQ rebound abdominal tenderness
    R10.824 LLQ rebound abdominal tenderness
    R10.825 Periumbilic rebound abdominal tenderness
    R10.826 Epigastric rebound abdominal tenderness
    R10.827 Generalized rebound abdominal tenderness
    R10.829 Rebound abdominal tenderness, unspecified site
  R10.83 Colic
    Colic NOS
    Infantile colic
    Excludes1: colic in adult and child over 12 months old (R10.84)
  R10.84 Generalized abdominal pain
    Excludes1: generalized abdominal pain associated with acute abdomen (R10.0)
R10.9 Unspecified abdominal pain

R11 NAUSEA AND VOMITING
`4th` *Excludes1:* cyclical vomiting associated with migraine (G43.A-)
  excessive vomiting in pregnancy (O21.-)
  hematemesis (K92.0)
  neonatal hematemesis (P54.0)
  newborn vomiting (P92.0-)
  psychogenic vomiting (F50.89)
  vomiting associated with bulimia nervosa (F50.2)
  vomiting following gastrointestinal surgery (K91.0)
R11.0 Nausea
  Nausea NOS
  Nausea without vomiting
R11.1 Vomiting
`5th`   **R11.10 Vomiting, unspecified**
    Vomiting NOS
  R11.11 Vomiting without nausea
  R11.12 Projectile vomiting
  R11.13 Vomiting of fecal matter
  R11.14 Bilious vomiting
    Bilious emesis

R11.15 Cyclical vomiting syndrome unrelated to migraine
  Cyclic vomiting syndrome NOS
  Persistent vomiting
  Excludes1: cyclical vomiting in migraine (G43.A-)
  Excludes2: bulimia nervosa (F50.2)
    diabetes mellitus due to underlying condition (E08.-)
R11.2 Nausea with vomiting, unspecified
  Persistent nausea with vomiting NOS

R12 HEARTBURN
✔ *Excludes1:* dyspepsia NOS (R10.13)
  functional dyspepsia (K30)

R13 APHAGIA AND DYSPHAGIA
`4th` **R13.0 Aphagia**
  Inability to swallow
  Excludes1: psychogenic aphagia (F50.9)
R13.1 Dysphagia
`5th` **Code first**, if applicable, dysphagia following cerebrovascular disease (I69. with final characters -91)
  Excludes1: psychogenic dysphagia (F45.8)
  R13.10 Dysphagia, unspecified
    Difficulty in swallowing NOS
  R13.11 Dysphagia, oral phase
  R13.12 Dysphagia, oropharyngeal phase
  R13.13 Dysphagia, pharyngeal phase
  R13.14 Dysphagia, pharyngoesophageal phase
  R13.19 Other dysphagia
    Cervical dysphagia
    Neurogenic dysphagia

R14 FLATULENCE AND RELATED CONDITIONS
`4th` *Excludes1:* psychogenic aerophagy (F45.8)
R14.0 Abdominal distension (gaseous)
  Bloating
  Tympanites (abdominal) (intestinal)
R14.1 Gas pain
R14.2 Eructation
R14.3 Flatulence

R15 FECAL INCONTINENCE
`4th` *Includes:* encopresis NOS
Excludes1: fecal incontinence of nonorganic origin (F98.1)
R15.0 Incomplete defecation
  Excludes1: constipation (K59.0-)
    fecal impaction (K56.41)
R15.1 Fecal smearing
  Fecal soiling
R15.2 Fecal urgency
R15.9 Full incontinence of feces
  Fecal incontinence NOS

R16 HEPATOMEGALY AND SPLENOMEGALY, NEC
`4th` **R16.0 Hepatomegaly, NEC**
  Hepatomegaly NOS
R16.1 Splenomegaly, NEC
  Splenomegaly NOS
R16.2 Hepatomegaly with splenomegaly, NEC
  Hepatosplenomegaly NOS

R17 UNSPECIFIED JAUNDICE
✔ *Excludes1:* neonatal jaundice (P55, P57–P59)

R18 ASCITES
`4th` *Includes:* fluid in peritoneal cavity
Excludes1: ascites in alcoholic cirrhosis (K70.31)
  ascites in alcoholic hepatitis (K70.11)
  ascites in toxic liver disease with chronic active hepatitis (K71.51)
R18.0 Malignant ascites
  Code first malignancy, such as: malignant neoplasm of ovary (C56.-)
    secondary malignant neoplasm of retroperitoneum and peritoneum (C78.6)
R18.8 Other ascites
  Ascites NOS
  Peritoneal effusion (chronic)

`4th` `5th` `6th` `7th` Additional Character Required   ✔ 3-character code

•=New Code   *Excludes1*—Not coded here, do not use together
▲=Revised Code   *Excludes2*—Not included here

CHAPTER 18. SYMPTOMS, SIGNS, AND ABNORMAL CLINICAL AND LABORATORY FINDINGS, NOT ELSEWHERE CLASSIFIED (R19–R25.9)

R19 **OTHER SYMPTOMS AND SIGNS INVOLVING THE DIGESTIVE SYSTEM AND ABDOMEN**
`4th`
Excludes1: acute abdomen (R10.0)

R19.0 **Intra-abdominal and pelvic swelling, mass and lump**
`5th` *Excludes1:* abdominal distension (gaseous) (R14.-)
ascites (R18.-)

R19.00 **Intra-abdominal and pelvic swelling, mass and lump, unspecified site**

R19.01 **RUQ abdominal swelling, mass and lump**

R19.02 **LUQ abdominal swelling, mass and lump**

R19.03 **RLQ abdominal swelling, mass and lump**

R19.04 **LLQ abdominal swelling, mass and lump**

R19.05 **Periumbilic swelling, mass or lump**
Diffuse or generalized umbilical swelling or mass

R19.06 **Epigastric swelling, mass or lump**

R19.07 **Generalized intra-abdominal and pelvic swelling, mass and lump**
Diffuse or generalized intra-abdominal swelling or mass NOS
Diffuse or generalized pelvic swelling or mass NOS

R19.09 **Other intra-abdominal and pelvic swelling, mass and lump**

R19.1 **Abnormal bowel sounds**
`5th` **R19.11** **Absent bowel sounds**

R19.12 **Hyperactive bowel sounds**

R19.15 **Other abnormal bowel sounds**
Abnormal bowel sounds NOS

R19.2 **Visible peristalsis**
Hyperperistalsis

R19.3 **Abdominal rigidity**
`5th` *Excludes1:* abdominal rigidity with severe abdominal pain (R10.0)

R19.30 **Abdominal rigidity, unspecified site**

R19.31 **RUQ abdominal rigidity**

R19.32 **LUQ abdominal rigidity**

R19.33 **RLQ abdominal rigidity**

R19.34 **LLQ abdominal rigidity**

R19.35 **Periumbilic abdominal rigidity**

R19.36 **Epigastric abdominal rigidity**

R19.37 **Generalized abdominal rigidity**

R19.4 **Change in bowel habit**
Excludes1: constipation (K59.0-)
functional diarrhea (K59.1)

R19.5 **Other fecal abnormalities**
Abnormal stool color
Bulky stools
Mucus in stools
Occult blood in feces
Occult blood in stools
Excludes1: melena (K92.1)
neonatal melena (P54.1)

R19.6 **Halitosis**

R19.7 **Diarrhea, unspecified**
Diarrhea NOS
Excludes1: functional diarrhea (K59.1)
neonatal diarrhea (P78.3)
psychogenic diarrhea (F45.8)

R19.8 **Other specified symptoms and signs involving the digestive system and abdomen**

(R20–R23) SYMPTOMS AND SIGNS INVOLVING THE SKIN AND SUBCUTANEOUS TISSUE

Excludes2: symptoms relating to breast (N64.4–N64.5)

R20 **DISTURBANCES OF SKIN SENSATION**
`4th` *Excludes1:* dissociative anesthesia and sensory loss (F44.6)
psychogenic disturbances (F45.8)

R20.0 **Anesthesia of skin**

R20.1 **Hypoesthesia of skin**

R20.2 **Paresthesia of skin**
Formication
Pins and needles
Tingling skin
Excludes1: acroparesthesia (I73.8)

R20.3 **Hyperesthesia**

R20.8 **Other disturbances of skin sensation**

R20.9 **Unspecified disturbances of skin sensation**

R21 **RASH AND OTHER NONSPECIFIC SKIN ERUPTION**
`✔`
Includes: rash NOS
Excludes1: specified type of rash — code to condition
vesicular eruption (R23.8)

R22 **LOCALIZED SWELLING, MASS AND LUMP OF SKIN AND SUBCUTANEOUS TISSUE**
`4th`
Includes: subcutaneous nodules (localized)(superficial)
Excludes1: abnormal findings on diagnostic imaging (R90–R93)
edema (R60.-)
enlarged lymph nodes (R59.-)
localized adiposity (E65)
swelling of joint (M25.4-)

R22.0 **Localized swelling, mass and lump; head**

R22.1   **neck**

R22.2   **trunk**
Excludes1: intra-abdominal or pelvic mass and lump (R19.0-)
intra-abdominal or pelvic swelling (R19.0-)
Excludes2: breast mass and lump (N63)

R22.3 **Localized swelling, mass and lump, upper limb**
`5th` **R22.31** **Localized swelling, mass and lump; right upper limb**

R22.32   **left upper limb**

R22.33   **upper limb, bilateral**

R22.4 **Localized swelling, mass and lump, lower limb**
`5th` **R22.41** **Localized swelling, mass and lump; right lower limb**

R22.42   **left lower limb**

R22.43   **lower limb, bilateral**

R22.9 **Localized swelling, mass and lump, unspecified**

R23 **OTHER SKIN CHANGES**
`4th` **R23.0** **Cyanosis**
Excludes1: acrocyanosis (I73.8)
cyanotic attacks of newborn (P28.2)

R23.1 **Pallor**
Clammy skin

R23.2 **Flushing**
Excessive blushing
Code first, if applicable, menopausal and female climacteric states (N95.1)

R23.3 **Spontaneous ecchymoses**
Petechiae
Excludes1: ecchymoses of newborn (P54.5)
purpura (D69.-)

R23.8 **Other skin changes**

R23.9 **Unspecified skin changes**

(R25–R29) SYMPTOMS AND SIGNS INVOLVING THE NERVOUS AND MUSCULOSKELETAL SYSTEMS

R25 **ABNORMAL INVOLUNTARY MOVEMENTS**
`4th` *Excludes1:* specific movement disorders (G20–G26)
stereotyped movement disorders (F98.4)
tic disorders (F95.-)

R25.0 **Abnormal head movements**

R25.1 **Tremor, unspecified**
Excludes1: chorea NOS (G25.5)
essential tremor (G25.0)
hysterical tremor (F44.4)
intention tremor (G25.2)

R25.2 **Cramp and spasm**
Excludes2: carpopedal spasm (R29.0)
charley-horse (M62.831)
infantile spasms (G40.4-)
muscle spasm of back (M62.830)
muscle spasm of calf (M62.831)

R25.8 **Other abnormal involuntary movements**

R25.9 **Unspecified abnormal involuntary movements**

`4th` `5th` `6th` `7th` Additional Character Required	`✔` 3-character code	•=New Code ▲=Revised Code	*Excludes1*—Not coded here, do not use together *Excludes2*—Not included here

R26 ABNORMALITIES OF GAIT AND MOBILITY
4th

Excludes1: ataxia NOS (R27.0)
 hereditary ataxia (G11.-)
 locomotor (syphilitic) ataxia (A52.11)
 immobility syndrome (paraplegic) (M62.3)

R26.0 Ataxic gait
 Staggering gait

R26.1 Paralytic gait
 Spastic gait

R26.2 Difficulty in walking, NEC
 Excludes1: falling (R29.6)
  unsteadiness on feet (R26.81)

R26.8 Other abnormalities of gait and mobility
 5th **R26.81 Unsteadiness on feet**
 R26.89 Other abnormalities of gait and mobility

R26.9 Unspecified abnormalities of gait and mobility

R27 OTHER LACK OF COORDINATION
4th

Excludes1: ataxic gait (R26.0)
 hereditary ataxia (G11.-)
 vertigo NOS (R42)

R27.0 Ataxia, unspecified
 Excludes1: ataxia following cerebrovascular disease (I69. with final characters -93)

R27.8 Other lack of coordination

R27.9 Unspecified lack of coordination

R29 OTHER SYMPTOMS AND SIGNS INVOLVING THE NERVOUS AND MUSCULOSKELETAL SYSTEMS
4th

R29.0 Tetany
 Carpopedal spasm
 Excludes1: hysterical tetany (F44.5)
  neonatal tetany (P71.3)
  parathyroid tetany (E20.9)
  post-thyroidectomy tetany (E89.2)

R29.1 Meningismus

R29.2 Abnormal reflex
 Excludes2: abnormal pupillary reflex (H57.0)
  hyperactive gag reflex (J39.2)
  vasovagal reaction or syncope (R55)

R29.3 Abnormal posture

R29.4 Clicking hip
 Excludes1: congenital deformities of hip (Q65.-)

R29.8 Other symptoms and signs involving the nervous and musculoskeletal systems
 5th
 R29.81 Other symptoms and signs involving the nervous system
  6th
  R29.810 Facial weakness
   Facial droop
  R29.818 Other symptoms and signs involving the nervous system
 R29.89 Other symptoms and signs involving the musculoskeletal system
  6th
  Excludes2: pain in limb (M79.6-)
  R29.891 Ocular torticollis
   Excludes1: congenital (sternomastoid) torticollis Q68.0
    psychogenic torticollis (F45.8)
    spasmodic torticollis (G24.3)
    torticollis due to birth injury (P15.8)
    torticollis NOS M43.6
  R29.898 Other symptoms and signs involving the musculoskeletal system

R29.9 Unspecified symptoms and signs involving the; nervous and musculoskeletal systems
 5th
 R29.90 Nervous system
 R29.91 Musculoskeletal system

(R30–R39) SYMPTOMS AND SIGNS INVOLVING THE GENITOURINARY SYSTEM

R30 PAIN ASSOCIATED WITH MICTURITION
4th

Excludes1: psychogenic pain associated with micturition (F45.8)

R30.0 Dysuria
 Strangury

R30.9 Painful micturition, unspecified
 Painful urination NOS

R31 HEMATURIA
4th

Excludes1: hematuria included with underlying conditions, such as:
 acute cystitis with hematuria (N30.01)
 recurrent and persistent hematuria in glomerular diseases (N02.-)

R31.0 Gross hematuria

R31.1 Benign essential microscopic hematuria

R31.2 Other microscopic hematuria
 5th **R31.21 Asymptomatic microscopic hematuria**
 R31.29 Other microscopic hematuria

R31.9 Hematuria, unspecified

R32 UNSPECIFIED URINARY INCONTINENCE
✔

Enuresis NOS

Excludes1: functional urinary incontinence (R39.81)
 nonorganic enuresis (F98.0)
 stress incontinence and other specified urinary incontinence (N39.3–N39.4-)
 urinary incontinence associated with cognitive impairment (R39.81)

R33 RETENTION OF URINE
4th

Excludes1: psychogenic retention of urine (F45.8)

R33.8 Other retention of urine
 Code first, if applicable, any causal condition, such as: enlarged prostate (N40.1)

R33.9 Retention of urine, unspecified

R34 ANURIA AND OLIGURIA
✔

Excludes1: anuria and oliguria complicating abortion or ectopic or molar pregnancy (O00–O07, O08.4)
 anuria and oliguria complicating pregnancy (O26.83–)

R35 POLYURIA
4th

Code first, if applicable, any causal condition, such as: enlarged prostate (N40.1)

Excludes1: psychogenic polyuria (F45.8)

R35.0 Frequency of micturition

R35.1 Nocturia

▲**R35.8 Other polyuria**
 5th •**R35.81 Nocturnal polyuria**
  Excludes2: nocturnal enuresis (N39.44)
 •**R35.89 Other polyuria**
  Polyuria NOS

R36 URETHRAL DISCHARGE
4th

R36.0 Urethral discharge without blood

R36.1 Hematospermia

R36.9 Urethral discharge, unspecified
 Penile discharge NOS
 Urethrorrhea

R37 SEXUAL DYSFUNCTION, UNSPECIFIED
✔

R39 OTHER AND UNSPECIFIED SYMPTOMS AND SIGNS INVOLVING THE GENITOURINARY SYSTEM
4th

R39.0 Extravasation of urine

R39.1 Other difficulties with micturition
 5th
 Code first, if applicable, any causal condition, such as: enlarged prostate (N40.1)
 R39.11 Hesitancy of micturition
 R39.12 Poor urinary stream
  Weak urinary steam
 R39.13 Splitting of urinary stream
 R39.14 Feeling of incomplete bladder emptying
 R39.15 Urgency of urination
  Excludes1: urge incontinence (N39.41, N39.46)

 4th **5th** **6th** **7th** Additional Character Required **✔** 3-character code

•=New Code
▲=Revised Code

Excludes1—Not coded here, do not use together
Excludes2—Not included here

R39.16   Straining to void
R39.19   Other difficulties with micturition
  6th   R39.191   Need to immediately re-void
          R39.192   Position dependent micturition
          R39.198   Other difficulties with micturition
R39.8 Other symptoms and signs involving the genitourinary system
  5th   R39.81   Functional urinary incontinence
          R39.82   Chronic bladder pain
          R39.83   Unilateral non-palpable testicle
          R39.84   Bilateral non-palpable testicles
          R39.89   Other symptoms and signs involving the genitourinary system
R39.9 Unspecified symptoms and signs involving the genitourinary system

(R40–R46) SYMPTOMS AND SIGNS INVOLVING COGNITION, PERCEPTION, EMOTIONAL STATE AND BEHAVIOR

Excludes2: symptoms and signs constituting part of a pattern of mental disorder (F01–F99)

R40 SOMNOLENCE, STUPOR AND COMA
4th
  Excludes1: neonatal coma (P91.5)
      somnolence, stupor and coma in diabetes (E08–E13)
      somnolence, stupor and coma in hepatic failure (K72.-)
      somnolence, stupor and coma in hypoglycemia (nondiabetic) (E15)
  R40.0 Somnolence
      Drowsiness
      Excludes1: coma (R40.2-)
  R40.1 Stupor
      Catatonic stupor
      Semicoma
      Excludes1: catatonic schizophrenia (F20.2)
          coma (R40.2-)
          depressive stupor (F31–F33)
          dissociative stupor (F44.2)
          manic stupor (F30.2)
  R40.2 Coma
  5th
GUIDELINES

  Code R40.20, Unspecified coma, may be assigned in conjunction with codes for any medical condition.
       Do not report codes for unspecified coma, individual or total Glasgow coma scale scores for a patient with a medically induced coma or a sedated patient.
       The coma scale codes **R40.21- to R40.24-** can be used in conjunction with traumatic brain injury codes, acute cerebrovascular disease or sequelae of cerebrovascular disease codes. These codes are primarily for use by trauma registries, but they may be used in any setting where this information is collected. The coma scale codes should be sequenced after the diagnosis code(s).
       These codes, one from each subcategory, are needed to complete the scale. The 7th character indicates when the scale was recorded. The 7th character should match for all three codes.
       At a minimum, report the initial score documented on presentation at your facility. This may be a score from the emergency medicine technician (EMT) or in the emergency department. If desired, a facility may choose to capture multiple coma scale scores.
       Assign code R40.24, Glasgow coma scale, total score, when only the total score is documented in the medical record and not the individual score(s). **If multiple coma scores are captured within the first 24 hours after hospital admission, assign only the code for the score at the time of admission. ICD-10-CM does not classify coma scores that are reported after admission but less than 24 hours later.**
       See Section I.B.14 for coma scale documentation by clinicians other than patient's provider.
  Code first any associated: fracture of skull (S02.-)
      intracranial injury (S06.-)
  Note: One code from each subcategory R40.21–R40.23 is required to complete the coma scale

R40.20 Unspecified coma
      Coma NOS
      Unconsciousness NOS
R40.21 Coma scale, eyes open
  6th   R40.211   Coma scale, eyes open, never
      7th   Coma scale eye opening score of 1

7th character is to be added to subcategory R40.21- or R40.22-
0–unspecified time
1–in the field [EMT/ambulance]
2–at arrival to ED
3–at hospital admission
4–24 hours or more after hospital admission

      R40.212   Coma scale, eyes open, to pain
      7th   Coma scale eye opening score of 2
      R40.213   Coma scale, eyes open, to sound
      7th   Coma scale eye opening score of 3
      R40.214   Coma scale, eyes open, spontaneous
      7th   Coma scale eye opening score of 4
R40.22 Coma scale, best verbal response
  6th   R40.221   Coma scale, best verbal response, none
      7th   Coma scale verbal score of 1
      R40.222   Coma scale, best verbal response, incomprehensible words
      7th   Coma scale verbal score of 2
          Incomprehensible sounds (2–5 years of age)
          Moans/grunts to pain; restless (<2 years old)
      R40.223   Coma scale, best verbal response, inappropriate words
      7th   Coma scale verbal score of 3
          Inappropriate crying or screaming (< 2 years of age)
          Screaming (2–5 years of age)
      R40.224   Coma scale, best verbal response, confused conversation
      7th   Coma scale verbal score of 4
          Inappropriate words (2–5 years of age)
          Irritable cries (< 2 years of age)
      R40.225   Coma scale, best verbal response, oriented
      7th   Coma scale verbal score of 5
          Cooing or babbling or crying appropriately (< 2 years of age)
          Uses appropriate words (2–5 years of age)
R40.23 Coma scale, best motor response
  6th   R40.231   Coma scale, best motor response, none
      7th   Coma scale motor score of 1

7th character is to be added to subcategory R40.23- or R40.24-
0–unspecified time
1–in the field [EMT/ambulance]
2–at arrival to ED
3–at hospital admission
4–24 hours or more after hospital admission

      R40.232   Coma scale, best motor response, extension
      7th   Coma scale motor score of 2
          Abnormal extensor posturing to pain or noxious stimuli (< 2 years of age)
          Extensor posturing to pain or noxious stimuli (2–5 years of age)
      R40.233   Coma scale, best motor response, abnormal
      7th   Coma scale motor score of 3
          Abnormal flexure posturing to pain or noxious stimuli (0–5 years of age)
          Flexion/decorticate posturing (< 2 years of age)
      R40.234   Coma scale, best motor response, flexion withdrawal
      7th   Coma scale motor score of 4
          Withdraws from pain or noxious stimuli (0–5 years of age)

 | **4th** **5th** **6th** **7th** Additional Character Required | ✓ 3-character code | •=New Code
▲=Revised Code | ***Excludes1***—Not coded here, do not use together
Excludes2—Not included here |

R40.235 **Coma scale, best motor response, localizes pain**
[7th]
Coma scale motor score of 5
Localizes pain (2-5 years of age)
Withdraws to touch (< 2 years of age)

R40.236 **Coma scale, best motor response, obeys commands**
[7th]
Coma scale motor score of 6
Normal or spontaneous movement (< 2 years of age)
Obeys commands (2-5 years of age)

R40.24 **Glasgow coma scale, total score**
[6th]
Note: Assign a code from subcategory R40.24, when only the total coma score is documented

R40.241 **Glasgow coma scale score 13–15**
[7th]

R40.242 **Glasgow coma scale score 9–12**
[7th]

R40.243 **Glasgow coma scale score 3–8**
[7th]

R40.244 **Other coma, without documented Glasgow coma scale score, or with partial score reported**
[7th]

R40.3 **Persistent vegetative state**

R41 **OTHER SYMPTOMS AND SIGNS INVOLVING COGNITIVE FUNCTIONS AND AWARENESS**
[4th]
Excludes1: dissociative [conversion] disorders (F44.-)
mild cognitive impairment, so stated (G31.84)

R41.0 **Disorientation, unspecified**
Confusion NOS
Delirium NOS

R41.8 **Other symptoms and signs involving cognitive functions and awareness**
[5th]

R41.82 **Altered mental status, unspecified**
Change in mental status NOS
Excludes1: altered level of consciousness (R40.-)
altered mental status due to known condition—code to condition
delirium NOS (R41.0)

R41.83 **Borderline intellectual functioning**
IQ level 71 to 84
Excludes1: intellectual disabilities (F70–F79)

R41.84 **Other specified cognitive deficit**
[6th]
Excludes1: cognitive deficits as sequelae of cerebrovascular disease (I69.01-, I69.11-, I69.21-, I69.31-, I69.81-, I69.91-)

R41.840 **Attention and concentration deficit**
Excludes1: attention-deficit hyperactivity disorders (F90.-)

R41.841 **Cognitive communication deficit**
R41.842 **Visuospatial deficit**
R41.843 **Psychomotor deficit**
R41.844 **Frontal lobe and executive function deficit**

R41.89 **Other symptoms and signs involving cognitive functions and awareness**
Anosognosia

R41.9 **Unspecified symptoms and signs involving cognitive functions and awareness**
Unspecified neurocognitive disorder

R42 **DIZZINESS AND GIDDINESS**
[✓]
Light-headedness
Vertigo NOS
Excludes1: vertiginous syndromes (H81.-)
vertigo from infrasound (T75.23)

R43 **DISTURBANCES OF SMELL AND TASTE**
[4th]
R43.0 **Anosmia**
R43.1 **Parosmia**
R43.2 **Parageusia**
R43.8 **Other disturbances of smell and taste**
Mixed disturbance of smell and taste
R43.9 **Unspecified disturbances of smell and taste**

R44 **OTHER SYMPTOMS AND SIGNS INVOLVING GENERAL SENSATIONS AND PERCEPTIONS**
[4th]
Excludes1: alcoholic hallucinations (F10.151, F10.251, F10.951)
hallucinations in drug psychosis (F11-F19 with fifth to sixth characters 51)
hallucinations in mood disorders with psychotic symptoms (F30.2, F31.5, F32.3, F33.3)
hallucinations in schizophrenia, schizotypal and delusional disorders (F20–F29)
Excludes2: disturbances of skin sensation (R20.-)

R44.0 **Auditory hallucinations**
R44.1 **Visual hallucinations**
R44.2 **Other hallucinations**
R44.3 **Hallucinations, unspecified**
R44.8 **Other symptoms and signs involving general sensations and perceptions**
R44.9 **Unspecified symptoms and signs involving general sensations and perceptions**

R45 **SYMPTOMS AND SIGNS INVOLVING EMOTIONAL STATE**
[4th]
R45.0 **Nervousness**
Nervous tension
R45.1 **Restlessness and agitation**
R45.2 **Unhappiness**
R45.3 **Demoralization and apathy**
Excludes1: anhedonia (R45.84)
R45.4 **Irritability and anger**
R45.5 **Hostility**
R45.6 **Violent behavior**
R45.7 **State of emotional shock and stress, unspecified**
R45.8 **Other symptoms and signs involving emotional state**
[5th]
R45.81 **Low self-esteem**
R45.82 **Worries**
R45.83 **Excessive crying of child, adolescent or adult**
Excludes1: excessive crying of infant (baby) R68.11
R45.84 **Anhedonia**
R45.85 **Homicidal and suicidal ideations**
[6th]
Excludes1: suicide attempt (T14.91)
R45.850 **Homicidal ideations**
R45.851 **Suicidal ideations**
R45.86 **Emotional lability**
R45.87 **Impulsiveness**
•**R45.88** **Nonsuicidal self-harm**
Nonsuicidal self-injury
Nonsuicidal self-mutilation
Self-inflicted injury without suicidal intent
Code also injury, if known
R45.89 **Other symptoms and signs involving emotional state**

R46 **SYMPTOMS AND SIGNS INVOLVING APPEARANCE AND BEHAVIOR**
[4th]
Excludes1: appearance and behavior in schizophrenia, schizotypal and delusional disorders (F20–F29)
mental and behavioral disorders (F01– F99)
R46.0 **Very low level of personal hygiene**
R46.1 **Bizarre personal appearance**
R46.2 **Strange and inexplicable behavior**
R46.3 **Overactivity**
R46.4 **Slowness and poor responsiveness**
Excludes 1: stupor (R40.1)
R46.5 **Suspiciousness and marked evasiveness**
R46.6 **Undue concern and preoccupation with stressful events**
R46.7 **Verbosity and circumstantial detail obscuring reason for contact**
R46.8 **Other symptoms and signs involving appearance and behavior**
[5th]
R46.81 **Obsessive-compulsive behavior**
obsessive-compulsive disorder (F42.-)
R46.89 **Other symptoms and signs involving appearance and behavior**

[4th] [5th] [6th] [7th] Additional Character Required   [✓] 3-character code   •=New Code   ▲=Revised Code   *Excludes1*—Not coded here, do not use together   *Excludes2*—Not included here

(R47–R49) SYMPTOMS AND SIGNS INVOLVING SPEECH AND VOICE

R47 **SPEECH DISTURBANCES, NEC**
`4th`
Excludes1: autism (F84.0)
cluttering (F80.81)
specific developmental disorders of speech and language (F80.-)
stuttering (F80.81)

R47.1 **Dysarthria and anarthria**
Excludes1: dysarthria following cerebrovascular disease (I69. with final characters -22)

R47.8 **Other speech disturbances**
`5th`
Excludes1: dysarthria following cerebrovascular disease (I69. with final characters -28)

R47.81 **Slurred speech**

R47.82 **Fluency disorder in conditions classified elsewhere**
Stuttering in conditions classified elsewhere
Code first underlying disease or condition, such as:
Parkinson's disease (G20)
Excludes1: adult onset fluency disorder (F98.5)
childhood onset fluency disorder (F80.81)
fluency disorder (stuttering) following cerebrovascular disease (I69. with final characters -23)

R47.89 **Other speech disturbances**

R47.9 **Unspecified speech disturbances**

R48 **DYSLEXIA AND OTHER SYMBOLIC DYSFUNCTIONS, NEC**
`4th`
Excludes1: specific developmental disorders of scholastic skills (F81.-)

R48.0 **Dyslexia and alexia**

R48.1 **Agnosia**
Astereognosia (astereognosis)
Autotopagnosia
Excludes1: visual object agnosia (R48.3)

R48.8 **Other symbolic dysfunctions**
Acalculia
Agraphia

R48.9 **Unspecified symbolic dysfunctions**

R49 **VOICE AND RESONANCE DISORDERS**
`4th`
Excludes1: psychogenic voice and resonance disorders (F44.4)

R49.0 **Dysphonia**
Hoarseness

R49.1 **Aphonia**
Loss of voice

R49.2 **Hypernasality and hyponasality**
`5th`
R49.21 **Hypernasality**
R49.22 **Hyponasality**

R49.8 **Other voice and resonance disorders**

R49.9 **Unspecified voice and resonance disorder**
Change in voice NOS
Resonance disorder NOS

(R50–R69) GENERAL SYMPTOMS AND SIGNS

R50 **FEVER OF OTHER AND UNKNOWN ORIGIN**
`4th`
Excludes1: chills without fever (R68.83)
febrile convulsions (R56.0-)
fever of unknown origin during labor (O75.2)
fever of unknown origin in newborn (P81.9)
hypothermia due to illness (R68.0)
malignant hyperthermia due to anesthesia (T88.3)
puerperal pyrexia NOS (O86.4)

R50.2 **Drug-induced fever**
Use additional code for adverse effect, if applicable, to identify drug (T36–T50 with fifth or sixth character 5)
Excludes1: postvaccination (postimmunization) fever (R50.83)

R50.8 **Other specified fever**
`5th`
R50.81 **Fever presenting with conditions classified elsewhere**
Code first underlying condition when associated fever is present, such as with: leukemia (C91–C95)
neutropenia (D70.-)
sickle-cell disease (D57.-)

> Do not use R50.81 with acute conditions

R50.82 **Postprocedural fever**
Excludes1: postprocedural infection (T81.4-)
posttransfusion fever (R50.84)
postvaccination (postimmunization) fever (R50.83)

R50.83 **Postvaccination fever**
Postimmunization fever

R50.84 **Febrile nonhemolytic transfusion reaction**
FNHTR
Posttransfusion fever

R50.9 **Fever, unspecified**
Fever NOS
Fever of unknown origin [FUO]
Fever with chills
Fever with rigors
Hyperpyrexia NOS
Persistent fever

R51 **HEADACHE**
`4th`
Excludes2: atypical face pain (G50.1)
migraine and other headache syndromes (G43–G44)
trigeminal neuralgia (G50.0)

R51.0 **Headache with orthostatic component, NEC**
Headache with positional component, NEC

R51.9 **Headache, unspecified**
Facial pain NOS

R52 **PAIN, UNSPECIFIED**
`✔`
Acute pain NOS
Generalized pain NOS
Pain NOS
Excludes1: acute and chronic pain, NEC (G89.-)
localized pain, unspecified type — code to pain by site, such as:
abdomen pain (R10.-)
back pain (M54.9)
breast pain (N64.4)
chest pain (R07.1–R07.9)
ear pain (H92.0-)
eye pain (H57.1)
headache (R51.9)
joint pain (M25.5-)
limb pain (M79.6-)
lumbar region pain (M54.5-)
pelvic and perineal pain (R10.2)
shoulder pain (M25.51-)
spine pain (M54.-)
throat pain (R07.0)
tongue pain (K14.6)
tooth pain (K08.8)
renal colic (N23)
pain disorders exclusively related to psychological factors (F45.41)

R53 **MALAISE AND FATIGUE**
`4th`
R53.1 **Weakness**
Asthenia NOS
Excludes1: muscle weakness (M62.81)
sarcopenia (M62.84)

R53.8 **Other malaise and fatigue**
`5th`
Excludes1: combat exhaustion and fatigue (F43.0)
congenital debility (P96.9)
exhaustion and fatigue due to excessive exertion (T73.3)
exhaustion and fatigue due to exposure (T73.2)
exhaustion and fatigue due to heat (T67.-)
exhaustion and fatigue due to recurrent depressive episode (F33)

R53.81 **Other malaise**
Chronic debility
Debility NOS
General physical deterioration
Malaise NOS
Nervous debility
Excludes1: age-related physical debility (R54)

R53.82 **Chronic fatigue, unspecified**
Chronic fatigue syndrome NOS
Excludes1: postviral fatigue syndrome (G93.3)

`4th` `5th` `6th` `7th` Additional Character Required   3-character code

•=New Code
▲=Revised Code

Excludes1—Not coded here, do not use together
Excludes2—Not included here

R53.83   **Other fatigue**
Fatigue NOS
Lack of energy
Lethargy
Tiredness
Excludes 2: exhaustion and fatigue due to depressive episode (F32.-)

R55   SYNCOPE AND COLLAPSE
☑
Blackout
Fainting
Vasovagal attack
Excludes1: cardiogenic shock (R57.0)
carotid sinus syncope (G90.01)
heat syncope (T67.1)
neurocirculatory asthenia (F45.8)
neurogenic orthostatic hypotension (G90.3)
orthostatic hypotension (I95.1)
postprocedural shock (T81.1-)
psychogenic syncope (F48.8)
shock NOS (R57.9)
shock complicating or following abortion or ectopic or molar pregnancy (O00–O07, O08.3)
Stokes-Adams attack (I45.9)
unconsciousness NOS (R40.2-)

R56   CONVULSIONS, NEC
`4th`
Excludes1: dissociative convulsions and seizures (F44.5)
epileptic convulsions and seizures (G40.-)
newborn convulsions and seizures (P90)

R56.0   **Febrile convulsions**
  `5th`   **R56.00**   **Simple febrile convulsions**
Febrile convulsion NOS
Febrile seizure NOS
      R56.01   **Complex febrile convulsions**
Atypical febrile seizure
Complex febrile seizure
Complicated febrile seizure
Excludes1: status epilepticus (G40.901)

R56.1   **Post traumatic seizures**
Excludes1: post traumatic epilepsy (G40.-)

R56.9   **Unspecified convulsions**
Convulsion disorder
Fit NOS
Recurrent convulsions
Seizure(s) (convulsive) NOS

R57   SHOCK, NEC
`4th`
Excludes1: anaphylactic shock NOS (T78.2)
anaphylactic reaction or shock due to adverse food reaction (T78.0-)
anaphylactic shock due to adverse effect of correct drug or medicament properly administered (T88.6)
anaphylactic shock due to serum (T80.5-)
shock due to anesthetic (T88.3)
electric shock (T75.4)
obstetric shock (O75.1)
postprocedural shock (T81.1-)
psychic shock (F43.0)
shock complicating or following ectopic or molar pregnancy (O00–O07, O08.3)
shock due to anesthesia (T88.2)
shock due to lightning (T75.01)
traumatic shock (T79.4)
toxic shock syndrome (A48.3)

R57.0   **Cardiogenic shock**
Excludes 2: septic shock (R65.21)
R57.1   **Hypovolemic shock**
R57.8   **Other shock**
R57.9   **Shock, unspecified**
Failure of peripheral circulation NOS

R58   HEMORRHAGE, NEC
☑
Hemorrhage NOS
Excludes1: hemorrhage included with underlying conditions, such as:
acute duodenal ulcer with hemorrhage (K26.0)
acute gastritis with bleeding (K29.01)
ulcerative enterocolitis with rectal bleeding (K51.01)

R59   ENLARGED LYMPH NODES
`4th`
Includes: swollen glands
Excludes1: lymphadenitis NOS (I88.9)
acute lymphadenitis (L04.-)
chronic lymphadenitis (I88.1)
mesenteric (acute) (chronic) lymphadenitis (I88.0)

R59.0   **Localized enlarged lymph nodes**
R59.1   **Generalized enlarged lymph nodes**
Lymphadenopathy NOS
R59.9   **Enlarged lymph nodes, unspecified**

R60   EDEMA, NEC
`4th`
Excludes1: angioneurotic edema (T78.3)
ascites (R18.-)
cerebral edema (G93.6)
cerebral edema due to birth injury (P11.0)
edema of larynx (J38.4)
edema of nasopharynx (J39.2)
edema of pharynx (J39.2)
gestational edema (O12.0-)
hereditary edema (Q82.0)
hydrops fetalis NOS (P83.2)
hydrothorax (J94.8)
hydrops fetalis NOS (P83.2)
newborn edema (P83.3)
pulmonary edema (J81.-)

R60.0   **Localized edema**
R60.1   **Generalized edema**
Excludes 2: nutritional edema (E40–E46)
R60.9   **Edema, unspecified**
Fluid retention NOS

R61   GENERALIZED HYPERHIDROSIS
☑
Excessive sweating
Night sweats
Secondary hyperhidrosis
Code first, if applicable, menopausal and female climacteric states (N95.1)
Excludes1: focal (primary) (secondary) hyperhidrosis (L74.5-)
Frey's syndrome (L74.52)
localized (primary) (secondary) hyperhidrosis (L74.5-)

R62   LACK OF EXPECTED NORMAL PHYSIOLOGICAL DEVELOPMENT IN CHILDHOOD AND ADULTS
`4th`
Excludes1: delayed puberty (E30.0)
gonadal dysgenesis (Q99.1)
hypopituitarism (E23.0)

R62.0   **Delayed milestone in childhood**
Delayed attainment of expected physiological developmental stage
Late talker
Late walker
R62.5   **Other and unspecified lack of expected normal physiological development in childhood**
  `5th`
Excludes1: HIV disease resulting in failure to thrive (B20)
physical retardation due to malnutrition (E45)
      R62.50   **Unspecified lack of expected normal physiological development in childhood**
Infantilism NOS
      R62.51   **Failure to thrive (child)**
Failure to gain weight
Excludes1: failure to thrive in child under 28 days old (P92.6)
      R62.52   **Short stature (child)**
Lack of growth
Physical retardation
Short stature NOS
Excludes1: short stature due to endocrine disorder (E34.3)
      R62.59   **Other lack of expected normal physiological development in childhood**

  `4th` `5th` `6th` `7th` Additional Character Required   ☑ 3-character code   •=New Code   ▲=Revised Code   ***Excludes1***—Not coded here, do not use together   ***Excludes2***—Not included here

R63 **SYMPTOMS AND SIGNS CONCERNING FOOD AND**
4th **FLUID INTAKE**
Excludes1: bulimia NOS (F50.2)
R63.0 Anorexia
Loss of appetite
Excludes1: anorexia nervosa (F50.0-)
loss of appetite of nonorganic origin (F50.89)
R63.1 Polydipsia
Excessive thirst
R63.2 Polyphagia
Excessive eating
Hyperalimentation NOS
▲**R63.3 Feeding difficulties**
5th *Excludes2:* eating disorders (F50.-)
feeding problems of newborn (P92.-)
infant feeding disorder of nonorganic origin (F98.2-)
•**R63.30 Feeding difficulties, unspecified**
•**R63.31 Pediatric feeding disorder, acute**
Pediatric feeding dysfunction, acute
Code also, if applicable, associated conditions such as:
aspiration pneumonia (J69.0)
dysphagia (R13.1-)
gastro-esophageal reflux disease (K21.-)
malnutrition (E40-E46)
•**R63.32 Pediatric feeding disorder, chronic**
Pediatric feeding dysfunction, chronic
Code also, if applicable, associated conditions such as:
aspiration pneumonia (J69.0)
dysphagia (R13.1-)
gastro-esophageal reflux disease (K21.-)
malnutrition (E40-E46)
•**R63.39 Other feeding difficulties**
Feeding problem (elderly) (infant) NOS
Picky eater
R63.4 Abnormal weight loss
R63.5 Abnormal weight gain
Excludes1: excessive weight gain in pregnancy (O26.0-)
obesity (E66.-)
R63.6 Underweight
Use additional code to identify body mass index (BMI), if known (Z68.-)
Excludes1: abnormal weight loss (R63.4)
anorexia nervosa (F50.0-)
malnutrition (E40–E46)
R63.8 Other symptoms and signs concerning food and fluid intake

R64 **CACHEXIA**
✔ Wasting syndrome
Code first underlying condition, if known
Excludes1: abnormal weight loss (R63.4)
nutritional marasmus (E41)

R65 **SYMPTOMS AND SIGNS SPECIFICALLY ASSOCIATED**
4th **WITH SYSTEMIC INFLAMMATION AND INFECTION**
R65.1 SIRS of non-infectious origin
5th

GUIDELINE

The SIRS can develop as a result of certain non-infectious disease processes, such as trauma, malignant neoplasm, or pancreatitis. When SIRS is documented with a noninfectious condition, and no subsequent infection is documented, the code for the underlying condition, such as an injury, should be assigned, followed by code R65.10 or code R65.11. If an associated acute organ dysfunction is documented, the appropriate code(s) for the specific type of organ dysfunction(s) should be assigned in addition to code R65.11. If acute organ dysfunction is documented, but it cannot be determined if the acute organ dysfunction is associated with SIRS or due to another condition (e.g., directly due to the trauma), the provider should be queried.
Code first underlying condition, such as: heatstroke (T67.0-)
injury and trauma (S00–T88)
Excludes1: sepsis- code to infection
severe sepsis (R65.2)
R65.10 SIRS of non-infectious origin without acute organ
dysfunction
SIRS NOS

R65.11 SIRS of non-infectious origin with acute organ
dysfunction
Use additional code to identify specific acute organ dysfunction, such as:
acute kidney failure (N17.-)
cute respiratory failure (J96.0-)
critical illness myopathy (G72.81)
critical illness polyneuropathy (G62.81)
disseminated intravascular coagulopathy [DIC] (D65)
encephalopathy (metabolic) (septic) (G93.41)
hepatic failure (K72.0-)
R65.2 Severe sepsis
5th Infection with associated acute organ dysfunction
Sepsis with acute organ dysfunction
Sepsis with multiple organ dysfunction
SIRS due to infectious process with acute organ dysfunction
Code first underlying infection, such as: infection following a procedure (T81.4-)
infections following infusion, transfusion and therapeutic injection (T80.2-)
puerperal sepsis (O85)
sepsis following complete or unspecified spontaneous abortion (O03.87)
sepsis following ectopic and molar pregnancy (O08.82)
sepsis following incomplete spontaneous abortion (O03.37)
sepsis following (induced) termination of pregnancy (O04.87)
sepsis NOS (A41.9)
Use additional code to identify specific acute organ dysfunction, such as:
acute kidney failure (N17.-)
acute respiratory failure (J96.0-)
critical illness myopathy (G72.81)
critical illness polyneuropathy (G62.81)
disseminated intravascular coagulopathy [DIC] (D65)
encephalopathy (metabolic) (septic) (G93.41)
hepatic failure (K72.0-)
R65.20 Severe sepsis without septic shock
Severe sepsis NOS
R65.21 Severe sepsis with septic shock

R68 **OTHER GENERAL SYMPTOMS AND SIGNS**
4th **R68.0 Hypothermia, not associated with low environmental**
temperature
Excludes1: hypothermia NOS (accidental) (T68)
hypothermia due to anesthesia (T88.51)
hypothermia due to low environmental temperature (T68)
newborn hypothermia (P80.-)
R68.1 Nonspecific symptoms peculiar to infancy
5th *Excludes1:* colic, infantile (R10.83)
neonatal cerebral irritability (P91.3)
teething syndrome (K00.7)
R68.11 Excessive crying of infant (baby)
Excludes1: excessive crying of child, adolescent, or adult (R45.83)
R68.12 Fussy infant (baby)
Irritable infant
R68.13 Apparent life threatening event in infant (ALTE)
Apparent life threatening event in newborn
Brief resolved unexplained event (BRUE)
Code first confirmed diagnosis, if known
Use additional code(s) for associated signs and symptoms if no confirmed diagnosis established, or if signs and symptoms are not associated routinely with confirmed diagnosis, or provide additional information for cause of ALTE
R68.19 Other nonspecific symptoms peculiar to infancy
R68.2 Dry mouth, unspecified
Excludes1: dry mouth due to dehydration (E86.0)
dry mouth due to Sjögren syndrome (M35.0-)
salivary gland hyposecretion (K11.7)
R68.3 Clubbing of fingers
Clubbing of nails
Excludes1: congenital club finger (Q68.1)

4th 5th 6th 7th Additional Character Required ✔ 3-character code

•=New Code *Excludes1*—Not coded here, do not use together
▲=Revised Code *Excludes2*—Not included here

R68.8 Other general symptoms and signs
- **5th**   **R68.81 Early satiety**
- **R68.83 Chills (without fever)**
  Chills NOS
  Excludes1: chills with fever (R50.9)
- **R68.84 Jaw pain**
  Mandibular pain
  Maxilla pain
  Excludes1: temporomandibular joint arthralgia (M26.62-)
- **R68.89 Other general symptoms and signs**

R69   ILLNESS, UNSPECIFIED
✔
Unknown and unspecified cases of morbidity

(R70–R79) ABNORMAL FINDINGS ON EXAMINATION OF BLOOD, WITHOUT DIAGNOSIS

Excludes2: abnormalities (of) (on):
    abnormal findings on antenatal screening of mother (O28.-)
    coagulation hemorrhagic disorders (D65–D68)
    lipids (E78.-)
    platelets and thrombocytes (D69.-)
    white blood cells classified elsewhere (D70–D72)
    diagnostic abnormal findings classified elsewhere—see Alphabetical Index
    hemorrhagic and hematological disorders of newborn (P50–P61)

R70   ELEVATED ERYTHROCYTE SEDIMENTATION RATE AND ABNORMALITY OF PLASMA VISCOSITY
4th
- **R70.0 Elevated erythrocyte sedimentation rate**
- **R70.1 Abnormal plasma viscosity**

R71   ABNORMALITY OF RED BLOOD CELLS
4th
Excludes1: anemias (D50–D64)
    anemia of premature infant (P61.2)
    benign (familial) polycythemia (D75.0)
    congenital anemias (P61.2–P61.4)
    newborn anemia due to isoimmunization (P55.-)
    polycythemia neonatorum (P61.1)
    polycythemia NOS (D75.1)
    polycythemia vera (D45)
    secondary polycythemia (D75.1)
- **R71.0 Precipitous drop in hematocrit**
  Drop (precipitous) in hemoglobin
  Drop in hematocrit
- **R71.8 Other abnormality of red blood cells**
  Abnormal red-cell morphology NOS
  Abnormal red-cell volume NOS
  Anisocytosis
  Poikilocytosis

R73   ELEVATED BLOOD GLUCOSE LEVEL
4th
Excludes1: DM (E08–E13)
    DM in pregnancy, childbirth and the puerperium (O24.-)
    neonatal disorders (P70.0–P70.2)
    postsurgical hypoinsulinemia (E89.1)
- **R73.0 Abnormal glucose**
  - **5th**   *Excludes1:* abnormal glucose in pregnancy (O99.81-)
        DM (E08–E13)
        dysmetabolic syndrome X (E88.81)
        gestational diabetes (O24.4-)
        glycosuria (R81)
        hypoglycemia (E16.2)
  - **R73.01 Impaired fasting glucose**
    Elevated fasting glucose
  - **R73.02 Impaired glucose tolerance (oral)**
    Elevated glucose tolerance
  - **R73.03 Prediabetes**
    Latent diabetes
  - **R73.09 Other abnormal glucose**
    Abnormal glucose NOS
    Abnormal non-fasting glucose tolerance

    > Do not report for hyperglycemia caused by DM
- **R73.9 Hyperglycemia, unspecified**

R74   ABNORMAL SERUM ENZYME LEVELS
4th
- **R74.0 Nonspecific elevation of levels of transaminase and lactic acid dehydrogenase [LDH]**
  - **5th**   **R74.01 Elevation of levels of liver transaminase levels**
    Elevation of levels of alanine transaminase (ALT)
    Elevation of levels of aspartate transaminase (AST)
  - **R74.02 Elevation of levels of lactic acid dehydrogenase [LDH]**
- **R74.8 Abnormal levels of other serum enzymes**
  Abnormal level of acid phosphatase
  Abnormal level of alkaline phosphatase
  Abnormal level of amylase
  Abnormal level of lipase [triacylglycerol lipase]
- **R74.9 Abnormal serum enzyme level, unspecified**

R75   INCONCLUSIVE LABORATORY EVIDENCE OF HIV
✔

GUIDELINES

Patients with inconclusive HIV serology, but no definitive diagnosis or manifestations of the illness, may be assigned code R75, Inconclusive laboratory evidence of HIV.
Nonconclusive HIV-test finding in infants
Excludes1: asymptomatic HIV infection status (Z21)
    HIV disease (B20)

R76   OTHER ABNORMAL IMMUNOLOGICAL FINDINGS IN SERUM
4th
- **R76.0 Raised antibody titer**
  Excludes1: isoimmunization in pregnancy (O36.0–O36.1)
      isoimmunization affecting newborn (P55.-)
- **R76.1 Nonspecific reaction to test for tuberculosis**
  - **5th**   **R76.11 Nonspecific reaction to tuberculin skin test without active tuberculosis**
    Abnormal result of Mantoux test
    PPD positive
    Tuberculin (skin test) positive
    Tuberculin (skin test) reactor
    Excludes1: nonspecific reaction to cell mediated immunity measurement of gamma interferon antigen response without active tuberculosis (R76.12)
  - **R76.12 Nonspecific reaction to cell mediated immunity measurement of gamma interferon antigen response without active tuberculosis**
    Nonspecific reaction to QFT without active tuberculosis
    Excludes1: nonspecific reaction to tuberculin skin test without active tuberculosis (R76.11)
        positive tuberculin skin test (R76.11)
- **R76.8 Other specified abnormal immunological findings in serum**
  Raised level of immunoglobulins NOS
- **R76.9 Abnormal immunological finding in serum, unspecified**

R77   OTHER ABNORMALITIES OF PLASMA PROTEINS
4th
Excludes1: disorders of plasma-protein metabolism (E88.0-)
- **R77.1 Abnormality of globulin**
  Hyperglobulinemia NOS
- **R77.8 Other specified abnormalities of plasma proteins**
- **R77.9 Abnormality of plasma protein, unspecified**

R78   FINDINGS OF DRUGS AND OTHER SUBSTANCES, NOT NORMALLY FOUND IN BLOOD
4th
Use additional code to identify the any retained FB, if applicable (Z18.-)
Excludes1: mental or behavioral disorders due to psychoactive substance use (F10–F19)
- **R78.0 Finding of alcohol in blood**
  Use additional external cause code (Y90.-), for detail regarding alcohol level
- **R78.1 Finding of opiate drug in blood**
- **R78.2 Finding of cocaine in blood**
- **R78.3 Finding of hallucinogen in blood**
- **R78.4 Finding of other drugs of addictive potential in blood**
- **R78.5 Finding of other psychotropic drug in blood**
- **R78.6 Finding of steroid agent in blood**
- **R78.7 Finding of abnormal level of heavy metals in blood**
  - **5th**   **R78.71 Abnormal lead level in blood**
    Excludes1: lead poisoning (T56.0-)
  - **R78.79 Finding of abnormal level of heavy metals in blood**

4th   **5th**   **6th**   **7th**   Additional Character Required   **✔**   3-character code

•=New Code   *Excludes1*—Not coded here, do not use together
▲=Revised Code   *Excludes2*—Not included here

CHAPTER 18. SYMPTOMS, SIGNS, AND ABNORMAL CLINICAL AND LABORATORY FINDINGS, NOT ELSEWHERE CLASSIFIED   (R78.8–R84.4)

R78.8 **5th** **Finding of other specified substances, not normally found in blood**

    R78.81 **Bacteremia**

        Excludes1: sepsis-code to specified infection

    R78.89 **Finding of other specified substances, not normally found in blood**

        Finding of abnormal level of lithium in blood

  R78.9 **Finding of unspecified substance, not normally found in blood**

R79 **4th** **OTHER ABNORMAL FINDINGS OF BLOOD CHEMISTRY**

Use additional code to identify any retained FB, if applicable (Z18.-)

Excludes1: asymptomatic hyperuricemia (E79.0)

  hyperglycemia NOS (R73.9)

  hypoglycemia NOS (E16.2)

  neonatal hypoglycemia (P70.3–P70.4)

  specific findings indicating disorder of amino-acid metabolism (E70–E72)

  specific findings indicating disorder of carbohydrate metabolism (E73–E74)

  specific findings indicating disorder of lipid metabolism (E75.-)

R79.1 **Abnormal coagulation profile**

  Abnormal or prolonged bleeding time

  Abnormal or prolonged coagulation time

  Abnormal or prolonged partial thromboplastin time [PTT]

  Abnormal or prolonged prothrombin time [PT]

  Excludes1: coagulation defects (D68.-)

  Excludes2: abnormality of fluid, electrolyte or acid-base balance (E86–E87)

R79.8 **5th** **Other specified abnormal findings of blood chemistry**

  R79.81 **Abnormal blood-gas level**

  R79.82 **Elevated C-reactive protein (CRP)**

  •**R79.83** **Abnormal findings of blood amino-acid level**

    Homocysteinemia

    Excludes1: disorders of amino-acid metabolism (E70–E72)

  R79.89 **Other specified abnormal findings of blood chemistry**

R79.9 **Abnormal finding of blood chemistry, unspecified**

(R80–R82) ABNORMAL FINDINGS ON EXAMINATION OF URINE, WITHOUT DIAGNOSIS

Excludes1: abnormal findings on antenatal screening of mother (O28.-)

  diagnostic abnormal findings classified elsewhere—see Alphabetical Index

  specific findings indicating disorder of amino-acid metabolism (E70–E72)

  specific findings indicating disorder of carbohydrate metabolism (E73–E74)

R80 **4th** **PROTEINURIA**

Excludes1: gestational proteinuria (O12.1-)

R80.0 **Isolated proteinuria**

  Idiopathic proteinuria

  Excludes1: isolated proteinuria with specific morphological lesion (N06.-)

R80.1 **Persistent proteinuria, unspecified**

R80.2 **Orthostatic proteinuria, unspecified**

  Postural proteinuria

R80.3 **Bence Jones proteinuria**

R80.8 **Other proteinuria**

R80.9 **Proteinuria, unspecified**

  Albuminuria NOS

R81 **✓** **GLYCOSURIA**

Excludes1: renal glycosuria (E74.818)

R82 **4th** **OTHER AND UNSPECIFIED ABNORMAL FINDINGS IN URINE**

Includes: chromoabnormalities in urine

Use additional code to identify any retained FB, if applicable (Z18.-)

Excludes2: hematuria (R31.-)

R82.0 **Chyluria**

  Excludes1: filarial chyluria (B74.-)

R82.1 **Myoglobinuria**

R82.2 **Biliuria**

R82.3 **Hemoglobinuria**

  Excludes1: hemoglobinuria due to hemolysis from external causes NEC (D59.6)

    hemoglobinuria due to paroxysmal nocturnal [Marchiafava-Micheli] (D59.5)

R82.7 **5th** **Abnormal findings on microbiological examination of urine**

Excludes1: colonization status (Z22.-)

  R82.71 **Bacteriuria**

  R82.79 **Other abnormal findings on microbiological examination of urine**

R82.8 **5th** **Abnormal findings on cytological and histological examination of urine**

  R82.81 **Pyuria**

    sterile pyuria

  R82.89 **Other abnormal findings on cytological and histological examination of urine**

R82.9 **5th** **Other and unspecified abnormal findings in urine**

  R82.90 **Unspecified abnormal findings in urine**

  R82.91 **Other chromoabnormalities of urine**

    Chromoconversion (dipstick)

    Idiopathic dipstick converts positive for blood with no cellular forms in sediment

    Excludes1: hemoglobinuria (R82.3)

    myoglobinuria (R82.1)

  R82.99 **6th** **Other abnormal findings in urine**

    R82.991 **Hypocitraturia**

    R82.992 **Hyperoxaluria**

      Excludes1: primary hyperoxaluria (E72.53)

    R82.993 **Hyperuricosuria**

    R82.994 **Hypercalciuria**

      Idiopathic hypercalciuria

    R82.998 **Other abnormal findings in urine**

      Cells and casts in urine

      Crystalluria

      Melanuria

(R83–R89) ABNORMAL FINDINGS ON EXAMINATION OF OTHER BODY FLUIDS, SUBSTANCES AND TISSUES, WITHOUT DIAGNOSIS

Excludes1: abnormal findings on antenatal screening of mother (O28.-)

  diagnostic abnormal findings classified elsewhere — see Alphabetical Index

Excludes2: abnormal findings on examination of blood, without diagnosis (R70–R79)

  abnormal findings on examination of urine, without diagnosis (R80–R82)

  abnormal tumor markers (R97.-)

R83 **4th** **ABNORMAL FINDINGS IN CEREBROSPINAL FLUID**

R83.3 **Abnormal level of substances chiefly nonmedicinal as to source in cerebrospinal fluid**

R83.4 **Abnormal immunological findings in cerebrospinal fluid**

R83.5 **Abnormal microbiological findings in cerebrospinal fluid**

  Positive culture findings in cerebrospinal fluid

  Excludes1: colonization status (Z22.-)

R83.6 **Abnormal cytological findings in cerebrospinal fluid**

R83.8 **Other abnormal findings in cerebrospinal fluid**

  Abnormal chromosomal findings in cerebrospinal fluid

R83.9 **Unspecified abnormal finding in cerebrospinal fluid**

R84 **4th** **ABNORMAL FINDINGS IN SPECIMENS FROM RESPIRATORY ORGANS AND THORAX**

Includes: abnormal findings in bronchial washings

  abnormal findings in nasal secretions

  abnormal findings in pleural fluid

  abnormal findings in sputum

  abnormal findings in throat scrapings

Excludes1: blood-stained sputum (R04.2)

R84.3 **Abnormal level of substances chiefly nonmedicinal as to source in specimens from respiratory organs and thorax**

R84.4 **Abnormal immunological findings in specimens from respiratory organs and thorax**

4th **5th** **6th** **7th** Additional Character Required   3-character code

•=New Code   *Excludes1*—Not coded here, do not use together

▲=Revised Code   *Excludes2*—Not included here

R84.5 Abnormal microbiological findings in specimens from respiratory organs and thorax
Positive culture findings in specimens from respiratory organs and thorax
Excludes1: colonization status (Z22.-)

R84.6 Abnormal cytological findings in specimens from respiratory organs and thorax

R89 ABNORMAL FINDINGS IN SPECIMENS FROM OTHER ORGANS, SYSTEMS AND TISSUES
Includes: abnormal findings in nipple discharge
abnormal findings in synovial fluid
abnormal findings in wound secretions

R89.0 Abnormal level of enzymes in specimens from other organs, systems and tissues

R89.1 Abnormal level of hormones in specimens from other organs, systems and tissues

R89.2 Abnormal level of other drugs, medicaments and biological substances in specimens from other organs, systems and tissues

R89.3 Abnormal level of substances chiefly nonmedicinal as to source in specimens from other organs, systems and tissues

R89.4 Abnormal immunological findings in specimens from other organs, systems and tissues

R89.5 Abnormal microbiological findings in specimens from other organs, systems and tissues
Positive culture findings in specimens from other organs, systems and tissues
Excludes1: colonization status (Z22.-)

R89.6 Abnormal cytological findings in specimens from other organs, systems and tissues

R89.7 Abnormal histological findings in specimens from other organs, systems and tissues

R89.8 Other abnormal findings in specimens from other organs, systems and tissues
Abnormal chromosomal findings in specimens from other organs, systems and tissues

R89.9 Unspecified abnormal finding in specimens from other organs, systems and tissues

(R90–R94) ABNORMAL FINDINGS ON DIAGNOSTIC IMAGING AND IN FUNCTION STUDIES, WITHOUT DIAGNOSIS

Includes: nonspecific abnormal findings on diagnostic imaging by CAT scan
nonspecific abnormal findings on diagnostic imaging by MRI [NMR] or PET scan
nonspecific abnormal findings on diagnostic imaging by thermography
nonspecific abnormal findings on diagnostic imaging by ultrasound [echogram]
nonspecific abnormal findings on diagnostic imaging by X-ray examination
Excludes1: abnormal findings on antenatal screening of mother (O28.-)
diagnostic abnormal findings classified elsewhere — **see Alphabetical Index**

R91 ABNORMAL FINDINGS ON DIAGNOSTIC IMAGING OF LUNG

R91.1 Solitary pulmonary nodule
Coin lesion lung
Solitary pulmonary nodule, subsegmental branch of the bronchial tree

R91.8 Other nonspecific abnormal finding of lung field
Lung mass NOS found on diagnostic imaging of lung
Pulmonary infiltrate NOS
Shadow, lung

R93 ABNORMAL FINDINGS ON DIAGNOSTIC IMAGING OF OTHER BODY STRUCTURES

R93.0 Abnormal findings on diagnostic imaging of skull and head, NEC
Excludes1: intracranial space-occupying lesion found on diagnostic imaging (R90.0)

R93.1 Abnormal findings on diagnostic imaging of heart and coronary circulation
Abnormal echocardiogram NOS
Abnormal heart shadow

R93.2 Abnormal findings on diagnostic imaging of liver and biliary tract
Nonvisualization of gallbladder

R93.3 Abnormal findings on diagnostic imaging of other parts of digestive tract

R93.4 Abnormal findings on diagnostic imaging of urinary organs
Excludes2: hypertrophy of kidney (N28.81)

R93.41 Abnormal radiologic findings on diagnostic imaging of renal pelvis, ureter, or bladder
Filling defect of bladder found on diagnostic imaging
Filling defect of renal pelvis found on diagnostic imaging
Filling defect of ureter found on diagnostic imaging

R93.42 Abnormal radiologic findings on diagnostic imaging of kidney
    R93.421 right kidney
    R93.422 left kidney
    R93.429 unspecified kidney

R93.49 Abnormal radiologic findings on diagnostic imaging of other urinary organs

R93.5 Abnormal findings on diagnostic imaging of other abdominal regions, including retroperitoneum

R93.6 Abnormal findings on diagnostic imaging of limbs
Excludes2: abnormal finding in skin and subcutaneous tissue (R93.8-)

R93.7 Abnormal findings on diagnostic imaging of other parts of musculoskeletal system
Excludes2: abnormal findings on diagnostic imaging of skull (R93.0)

R93.8 Abnormal findings on diagnostic imaging of other specified body structures

R93.81 Abnormal radiologic findings on diagnostic imaging of testicles
    R93.811 Abnormal radiologic findings on diagnostic imaging of right testicle
    R93.812 Abnormal radiologic findings on diagnostic imaging of left testicle
    R93.813 Abnormal radiologic findings on diagnostic imaging of testicles, bilateral
    R93.819 Abnormal radiologic findings on diagnostic imaging of unspecified testicle

R93.89 Abnormal findings on diagnostic imaging of other specified body structures
Abnormal finding by radioisotope localization of placenta
Abnormal radiological finding in skin and subcutaneous tissue
Mediastinal shift

R94 ABNORMAL RESULTS OF FUNCTION STUDIES
Includes: abnormal results of radionuclide [radioisotope] uptake studies
abnormal results of scintigraphy

R94.0 Abnormal results of function studies of central nervous system
    R94.01 Abnormal electroencephalogram [EEG]
    R94.02 Abnormal brain scan
    R94.09 Abnormal results of other function studies of central nervous system

R94.1 Abnormal results of function studies of peripheral nervous system and special senses
    R94.11 Abnormal results of function studies of eye
        R94.110 Abnormal electro-oculogram [EOG]
        R94.111 Abnormal electroretinogram[ERG]
        Abnormal retinal function study
        R94.112 Abnormal visually evoked potential [VEP]
        R94.113 Abnormal oculomotor study
        R94.118 Abnormal results of other function studies of eye
    R94.12 Abnormal results of function studies of ear and other special senses
        R94.120 Abnormal auditory function study
        R94.121 Abnormal vestibular function study
        R94.128 Abnormal results of other function studies of ear and other special senses
    R94.13 Abnormal results of function studies of peripheral nervous system
        R94.130 Abnormal response to nerve stimulation, unspecified
        R94.131 Abnormal electromyogram [EMG]
        Excludes1: electromyogram of eye (R94.113)

4th   5th   6th   7th   Additional Character Required   ✓   3-character code

•=New Code
▲=Revised Code

Excludes1—Not coded here, do not use together
Excludes2—Not included here

R94.138 **Abnormal results of other function studies of peripheral nervous system**

R94.2 **Abnormal results of pulmonary function studies**
Reduced ventilatory capacity
Reduced vital capacity

R94.3 **Abnormal results of cardiovascular function studies**

5th R94.30 **Abnormal result of cardiovascular function study, unspecified**

R94.31 **Abnormal electrocardiogram [ECG] [EKG]**
Excludes1: long QT syndrome (I45.81)

R94.39 **Abnormal result of other cardiovascular function study**
Abnormal electrophysiological intracardiac studies
Abnormal phonocardiogram
Abnormal vectorcardiogram

R94.4 **Abnormal results of kidney function studies**
Abnormal renal function test

R94.5 **Abnormal results of liver function studies**

R94.6 **Abnormal results of thyroid function studies**

R94.7 **Abnormal results of other endocrine function studies**
Excludes2: abnormal glucose (R73.0-)

R94.8 **Abnormal results of function studies of other organs and systems**
Abnormal basal metabolic rate [BMR]
Abnormal bladder function test
Abnormal splenic function test

(R97) ABNORMAL TUMOR MARKERS

R97 **ABNORMAL TUMOR MARKERS**
4th Elevated tumor associated antigens [TAA]
Elevated tumor specific antigens [TSA]
R97.0 **Elevated carcinoembryonic antigen [CEA]**
R97.1 **Elevated cancer antigen 125 [CA 125]**
R97.8 **Other abnormal tumor markers**

(R99) ILL-DEFINED AND UNKNOWN CAUSE OF MORTALITY

R99 **ILL-DEFINED AND UNKNOWN CAUSE OF MORTALITY**
✔ Code R99, Ill-defined and unknown cause of mortality, is only for use in the very limited circumstance when a patient who has already died is brought into an emergency department or other healthcare facility and is pronounced dead upon arrival. It does not represent the discharge disposition of death.
Death (unexplained) NOS
Unspecified cause of mortality

   Additional Character Required 3-character code

•=New Code
▲=Revised Code

Excludes1—Not coded here, do not use together
Excludes2—Not included here

326 PEDIATRIC ICD-10-CM 2022: A MANUAL FOR PROVIDER-BASED CODING

Chapter 19. Injury, poisoning and certain other consequences of external causes (S00–T88)

Application of 7th Characters in Chapter 19

Most categories in Chapter 19 have a 7th character requirement for each applicable code. Most categories in this chapter have three 7th character values (with the exception of fractures): A, initial encounter, D, subsequent encounter and S, sequela. Categories for traumatic fractures have additional 7th character values. While the patient may be seen by a new or different provider over the course of treatment for an injury, assignment of the 7th character is based on whether the patient is undergoing active treatment and not whether the provider is seeing the patient for the first time.

For complication codes, active treatment refers to treatment for the condition described by the code, even though it may be related to an earlier precipitating problem. For example, code T84.50XA, Infection and inflammatory reaction due to unspecified internal joint prosthesis, initial encounter, is used when active treatment is provided for the infection, even though the condition relates to the prosthetic device, implant or graft that was placed at a previous encounter.

7th character "A," initial encounter, is used while the patient is receiving active treatment for the condition. Examples of active treatment are: surgical treatment, emergency department encounter, and evaluation and continuing treatment by the same or a different physician.

7th character "D," subsequent encounter, is used for encounters after the patient has received active treatment of the condition and is receiving routine care for the condition during the healing or recovery phase. Examples of subsequent care are: cast change or removal, an x-ray to check healing status of fracture, removal of external or internal fixation device, medication adjustment, other aftercare and follow up visits following treatment of the injury or condition.

The aftercare Z codes should not be used for aftercare for conditions such as injuries or poisonings, where 7th characters are provided to identify subsequent care. For example, for aftercare of an injury, assign the acute injury code with the 7th character "D" (subsequent encounter).

7th character "S," sequela, is for use for complications or conditions that arise as a direct result of a condition, such as scar formation after a burn. The scars are sequelae of the burn. When using 7th character "S," it is necessary to use both the injury code that precipitated the sequela and the code for the sequela itself. The "S" is added only to the injury code, not the sequela code. The 7th character "S" identifies the injury responsible for the sequela. The specific type of sequela (eg, scar) is sequenced first, followed by the injury code.

An "X" may be listed at the end of the code to indicate a placeholder digit(s). The X will be required in order to get to the 7th character, which indicates the type of encounter. Be sure to use all indicated placeholder digits prior to the appropriate 7th character digit.

Coding of Injuries

When coding injuries, assign separate codes for each injury unless a combination code is provided, in which case the combination code is assigned. Codes from category T07, Unspecified multiple injuries should not be assigned in the inpatient setting unless information for a more specific code is not available. Traumatic injury codes (S00–T14.9) are not to be used for normal, healing surgical wounds or to identify complications of surgical wounds.

The code for the most serious injury, as determined by the provider and the focus of treatment, is sequenced first.

SUPERFICIAL INJURIES
Superficial injuries such as abrasions or contusions are not coded when associated with more severe injuries of the same site.

PRIMARY INJURY WITH DAMAGE TO NERVES/BLOOD VESSELS
When a primary injury results in minor damage to peripheral nerves or blood vessels, the primary injury is sequenced first with additional code(s) for injuries to nerves and spinal cord (such as category S04), and/or injury to blood vessels (such as category S15). When the primary injury is to the blood vessels or nerves, that injury should be sequenced first.

IATROGENIC INJURIES
Injury codes from Chapter 19 should not be assigned for injuries that occur during, or as a result of, a medical intervention. Assign the appropriate complication code(s).

Coding of Traumatic Fractures
The principles of multiple coding of injuries should be followed in coding fractures. Fractures of specified sites are coded individually by site in accordance with both

the provisions within categories S02, S12, S22, S32, S42, S49, S52, S59, S62, S72, S79, S82, S89, S92 and the level of detail furnished by medical record content.

A fracture not indicated as open or closed should be coded to closed. A fracture not indicated whether displaced or not displaced should be coded to displaced.

More specific guidelines are as follows:

INITIAL VS. SUBSEQUENT ENCOUNTER FOR FRACTURES
Traumatic fractures are coded using the appropriate 7th character for initial encounter (A, B, C) while the patient is receiving active treatment for the fracture. Examples of active treatment are: surgical treatment, emergency department encounter, and evaluation and continuing (ongoing) treatment by the same or different physician. The appropriate 7th character for initial encounter should also be assigned for a patient who delayed seeking treatment for the fracture or nonunion. Fractures are coded using the appropriate 7th character for subsequent care for encounters after the patient has completed active treatment of the fracture and is receiving routine care for the fracture during the healing or recovery phase. Examples of fracture aftercare are: cast change or removal, an x-ray to check healing status of fracture, removal of external or internal fixation device, medication adjustment, and follow-up visits following fracture treatment.

Care for complications of surgical treatment for fracture repairs during the healing or recovery phase should be coded with the appropriate complication codes.

Care of complications of fractures, such as malunion and nonunion, should be reported with the appropriate 7th character for subsequent care with nonunion (K, M, N,) or subsequent care with malunion (P, Q, R).

Malunion/nonunion: The appropriate 7th character for initial encounter should also be assigned for a patient who delayed seeking treatment for the fracture or nonunion.

A code from category M80, not a traumatic fracture code, should be used for any patient with known osteoporosis who suffers a fracture, even if the patient had a minor fall or trauma, if that fall or trauma would not usually break a normal, healthy bone.

The aftercare Z codes should not be used for aftercare for traumatic fractures. For aftercare of a traumatic fracture, assign the acute fracture code with the appropriate 7th character.

MULTIPLE FRACTURES SEQUENCING
Multiple fractures are sequenced in accordance with the severity of the fracture.

PHYSEAL FRACTURES
For physeal fractures, assign only the code identifying the type of physeal fracture. Do not assign a separate code to identify the specific bone that is fractured.

Coding of Burns and Corrosions
Refer to category T20 for guidelines.

Adverse Effects, Poisoning, Underdosing and Toxic Effects
Refer to category T36 for guidelines.

Adult and Child Abuse, Neglect and Other Maltreatment
Refer to category T74 for guidelines.

Complications of care

GENERAL GUIDELINES FOR COMPLICATIONS OF CARE
See Section I.B.16 (page XVIII) for information on documentation of complications of care.

PAIN DUE TO MEDICAL DEVICES
Pain associated with devices, implants or grafts left in a surgical site (for example painful hip prosthesis) is assigned to the appropriate code(s) found in Chapter 19, Injury, poisoning, and certain other consequences of external causes. Specific codes for pain due to medical devices are found in the T code section of the *ICD-10-CM*. **Use additional code(s)** from category G89 to identify acute or chronic pain due to presence of the device, implant or graft (G89.18 or G89.28).

TRANSPLANT COMPLICATIONS
Transplant complications other than kidney

Please see category T86 for guidelines for complications of transplanted organs and tissue other than kidney.

Kidney transplant complications
Refer to code T86.1 for guidelines for complications of kidney transplant.

COMPLICATION CODES THAT INCLUDE THE EXTERNAL CAUSE
As with certain other T codes, some of the complications of care codes have the external cause included in the code. The code includes the nature of the complication as well as the type of procedure that caused the complication. No external cause code indicating the type of procedure is necessary for these codes.

COMPLICATIONS OF CARE CODES WITHIN THE BODY SYSTEM CHAPTERS
Intraoperative and postprocedural complication codes are found within the body system chapters with codes specific to the organs and structures of that body system. These codes should be sequenced first, followed by a code(s) for the specific complication, if applicable.

Note: Use secondary code(s) from Chapter 20, External causes of morbidity, to indicate cause of injury. Codes within the T-section that include the external cause do not require an additional external cause code

Use additional code to identify any retained FB, if applicable (Z18.-)

Excludes1: birth trauma (P10–P15)
obstetric trauma (O70–O71)

Note: The chapter uses the S-section for coding different types of injuries related to single body regions and the T-section to cover injuries to unspecified body regions as well as poisoning and certain other consequences of external causes.

Most codes in Chapter 19 require the addition of 7th characters to form complete codes. Descriptors for 7th characters are provided in text boxes throughout the chapter.

(S00–S09) INJURIES TO THE HEAD

Includes: Injuries of ear
injuries of eye
injuries of face [any part]
injuries of gum
injuries of jaw
injuries of oral cavity
injuries of palate
injuries of periocular area
injuries of scalp
injuries of temporomandibular joint area
injuries of tongue
injuries of tooth

7th characters for category S00
A—initial encounter
D—subsequent encounter
S—sequela

Code also for any associated infection
Excludes2: burns and corrosions (T20–T32)
effects of FB in ear (T16)
effects of FB in larynx (T17.3)
effects of FB in mouth NOS (T18.0)
effects of FB in nose (T17.0–T17.1)
effects of FB in pharynx (T17.2)
effects of FB on external eye (T15.-)
frostbite (T33–T34)
insect bite or sting, venomous (T63.4)

S00 `4th` **SUPERFICIAL INJURY OF HEAD**
Excludes1: diffuse cerebral contusion (S06.2-)
focal cerebral contusion (S06.3-)
injury of eye and orbit (S05.-)
open wound of head (S01.-)

S00.0 **Superficial injury of scalp**
`5th` **S00.00X** **Unspecified superficial injury of scalp**
`7th`

S00.01X **Abrasion of scalp**
`7th`

S00.02X **Blister (nonthermal) of scalp**
`7th`

S00.03X **Contusion of scalp**
`7th` Bruise of scalp
Hematoma of scalp

S00.04X **External constriction of part of scalp**
`7th`

S00.05X **Superficial FB of scalp**
`7th` Splinter in the scalp

S00.06X **Insect bite (nonvenomous) of scalp**
`7th`

S00.07X **Other superficial bite of scalp**
`7th` ***Excludes1:*** open bite of scalp (S01.05)

S00.1 **Contusion of eyelid and periocular area**
`5th` Black eye
Excludes2: contusion of eyeball and orbital tissues (S05.1-)

S00.10X **Contusion of unspecified eyelid and periocular area**
`7th`

S00.11X **Contusion of right eyelid and periocular area**
`7th`

S00.12X **Contusion of left eyelid and periocular area**
`7th`

S00.2 **Other and unspecified superficial injuries of eyelid and**
`5th` **periocular area**
Excludes2: superficial injury of conjunctiva and cornea (S05.0-)

S00.20 **Unspecified superficial injury of eyelid and**
`6th` **periocular area**
S00.201 **Unspecified superficial injury of right**
`7th` **eyelid and periocular area**
S00.202 **Unspecified superficial injury of left eyelid**
`7th` **and periocular area**

S00.21 **Abrasion of eyelid and periocular area**
`6th` **S00.211** **Abrasion of right eyelid and periocular**
`7th` **area**
S00.212 **Abrasion of left eyelid and periocular area**
`7th`

S00.22 **Blister (nonthermal) of eyelid and periocular area**
`6th` **S00.221** **Blister (nonthermal) of right eyelid and**
`7th` **periocular area**
S00.222 **Blister (nonthermal) of left eyelid and**
`7th` **periocular area**

S00.24 **External constriction of eyelid and periocular area**
`6th` **S00.241** **External constriction of right eyelid and**
`7th` **periocular area**
S00.242 **External constriction of left eyelid and**
`7th` **periocular area**

S00.25 **Superficial FB of eyelid and periocular area**
`6th` Splinter of eyelid and periocular area
Excludes2: retained FB in eyelid (H02.81-)
S00.251 **Superficial FB of right eyelid and**
`7th` **periocular area**
S00.252 **Superficial FB of left eyelid and periocular**
`7th` **area**

S00.26 **Insect bite (nonvenomous) of eyelid and periocular**
`6th` **area**
S00.261 **Insect bite (nonvenomous) of right eyelid**
`7th` **and periocular area**
S00.262 **Insect bite (nonvenomous) of left eyelid**
`7th` **and periocular area**

S00.27 **Other superficial bite of eyelid and periocular area**
`6th` ***Excludes1:*** open bite of eyelid and periocular area
(S01.15)
S00.271 **Other superficial bite of right eyelid and**
`7th` **periocular area**
S00.272 **Other superficial bite of left eyelid and**
`7th` **periocular area**

S00.3 **Superficial injury of nose**
`5th` **S00.30X** **Unspecified superficial injury of nose**
S00.31X **Abrasion of nose**
`7th`

S00.32X **Blister (nonthermal) of nose**
`7th`

S00.33X **Contusion of nose**
`7th` Bruise of nose
Hematoma of nose

S00.34X **External constriction of nose**
`7th`

S00.35X **Superficial FB of nose**
`7th` Splinter in the nose

S00.36X **Insect bite (nonvenomous) of nose**
`7th`

S00.37X **Other superficial bite of nose**
`7th` ***Excludes1:*** open bite of nose (S01.25)

| `4th` `5th` `6th` `7th` Additional Character Required | ✓ 3-character code | Unspecified laterality codes were excluded here. | • =New Code
▲ =Revised Code
◘ =Social determinants of health | ***Excludes1***—Not coded here, do not use together
Excludes2—Not included here |

S00.4 Superficial injury of ear

5th	

S00.40 Unspecified superficial injury of ear

6th

7th characters for category S00
A—initial encounter
D—subsequent encounter
S—sequela

S00.401 Unspecified superficial injury of right ear
7th

S00.402 Unspecified superficial injury of left ear
7th

S00.41 Abrasion of ear
6th

S00.411 Abrasion of right ear
7th

S00.412 Abrasion of left ear
7th

S00.42 Blister (nonthermal) of ear
6th

S00.421 Blister (nonthermal) of right ear
7th

S00.422 Blister (nonthermal) of left ear
7th

S00.43 Contusion of ear
6th
Bruise of ear
Hematoma of ear

S00.431 Contusion of right ear
7th

S00.432 Contusion of left ear
7th

S00.44 External constriction of ear
6th

S00.441 External constriction of right ear
7th

S00.442 External constriction of left ear
7th

S00.45 Superficial FB of ear
6th
Splinter in the ear

S00.451 Superficial FB of right ear
7th

S00.452 Superficial FB of left ear
7th

S00.46 Insect bite (nonvenomous) of ear
6th

S00.461 Insect bite (nonvenomous) of right ear
7th

S00.462 Insect bite (nonvenomous) of left ear
7th

S00.47 Other superficial bite of ear
6th
Excludes1: open bite of ear (S01.35)

S00.471 Other superficial bite of right ear
7th

S00.472 Other superficial bite of left ear
7th

S00.5 Superficial injury of lip and oral cavity
5th

S00.50 Unspecified superficial injury of lip and oral cavity
6th

S00.501 Unspecified superficial injury of lip
7th

S00.502 Unspecified superficial injury of oral cavity
7th

S00.51 Abrasion of lip and oral cavity
6th

S00.511 Abrasion of lip
7th

S00.512 Abrasion of oral cavity
7th

S00.52 Blister (nonthermal) of lip and oral cavity
6th

S00.521 Blister (nonthermal) of lip
7th

S00.522 Blister (nonthermal) of oral cavity
7th

S00.53 Contusion of lip and oral cavity
6th

S00.531 Contusion of lip
7th
Bruise of lip
Hematoma of lip

S00.532 Contusion of oral cavity
7th
Bruise of oral cavity
Hematoma of oral cavity

S00.54 External constriction of lip and oral cavity
6th

S00.541 External constriction of lip
7th

S00.542 External constriction of oral cavity
7th

S00.55 Superficial FB of lip and oral cavity
6th

S00.551 Superficial FB of lip
7th
Splinter of lip and oral cavity

S00.552 Superficial FB of oral cavity
7th
Splinter of lip and oral cavity

S00.56 Insect bite (nonvenomous) of lip and oral cavity
6th

S00.561 Insect bite (nonvenomous) of lip
7th

S00.562 Insect bite (nonvenomous) of oral cavity
7th

S00.57 Other superficial bite of lip and oral cavity
6th

S00.571 Other superficial bite of lip
7th
Excludes1: open bite of lip (S01.551)

S00.572 Other superficial bite of oral cavity
7th
Excludes1: open bite of oral cavity (S01.552)

S00.8 Superficial injury of other parts of head
5th
Superficial injuries of face [any part]

S00.80X Unspecified superficial injury of other part of head
7th

S00.81X Abrasion of other part of head
7th

S00.82X Blister (nonthermal) of other part of head
7th

S00.83X Contusion of other part of head
7th
Bruise of other part of head
Hematoma of other part of head

S00.84X External constriction of other part of head
7th

S00.85X Superficial FB of other part of head
7th
Splinter in other part of head

S00.86X Insect bite (nonvenomous) of other part of head
7th

S00.87X Other superficial bite of other part of head
7th
Excludes1: open bite of other part of head (S01.85)

S00.9 Superficial injury of unspecified part of head
5th

S00.90X Unspecified superficial injury of unspecified part of head
7th

S00.91X Abrasion of unspecified part of head
7th

S00.92X Blister (nonthermal) of unspecified part of head
7th

S00.93X Contusion of unspecified part of head
7th
Bruise of head
Hematoma of head

S00.94X External constriction of unspecified part of head
7th

S00.95X Superficial FB of unspecified part of head
7th
Splinter of head

S00.96X Insect bite (nonvenomous) of unspecified part of head
7th

S00.97X Other superficial bite of unspecified part of head
7th
Excludes1: open bite of head (S01.95)

S01 OPEN WOUND OF HEAD
4th
Code also any associated:
  injury of cranial nerve (S04.-)
  injury of muscle and tendon of head (S09.1-)
  intracranial injury (S06.-)
  wound infection

7th characters for category S01
A—initial encounter
D—subsequent encounter
S—sequela

Excludes1: open skull fracture (S02.- with 7th character)
Excludes2: injury of eye and orbit (S05.-)
  traumatic amputation of part of head (S08.-)

S01.0 Open wound of scalp
5th
Excludes1: avulsion of scalp (S08.0-)

S01.01X Laceration without FB of scalp
7th

S01.02X Laceration with FB of scalp
7th

S01.03X Puncture wound without FB of scalp
7th

| **4th** | **5th** | **6th** | **7th** | Additional Character Required | ✓ | 3-character code | Unspecified laterality codes were excluded here. | ● =New Code
▲ =Revised Code
◻ =Social determinants of health | *Excludes1*—Not coded here, do not use together
Excludes2—Not included here |

CHAPTER 19. INJURY, POISONING AND CERTAIN OTHER CONSEQUENCES OF EXTERNAL CAUSES   (S01.04X–S01.81X)

S01.04X [7th] **Puncture wound with FB of scalp**

S01.05X [7th] **Open bite of scalp**
Bite of scalp NOS
Excludes1: superficial bite of scalp (S00.06, S00.07-)

7th characters for category S01
A—initial encounter
D—subsequent encounter
S—sequela

S01.1 [5th] **Open wound of eyelid and periocular area**
Open wound of eyelid and periocular area with or without involvement of lacrimal passages

S01.11 [6th] **Laceration without FB of eyelid and periocular area**
    S01.111 [7th] **Laceration without FB of right eyelid and periocular area**
    S01.112 [7th] **Laceration without FB of left eyelid and periocular area**

S01.12 [6th] **Laceration with FB of eyelid and periocular area**
    S01.121 [7th] **Laceration with FB of right eyelid and periocular area**
    S01.122 [7th] **Laceration with FB of left eyelid and periocular area**

S01.13 [6th] **Puncture wound without FB of eyelid and periocular area**
    S01.131 [7th] **Puncture wound without FB of right eyelid and periocular area**
    S01.132 [7th] **Puncture wound without FB of left eyelid and periocular area**

S01.14 [6th] **Puncture wound with FB of eyelid and periocular area**
    S01.141 [7th] **Puncture wound with FB of right eyelid and periocular area**
    S01.142 [7th] **Puncture wound with FB of left eyelid and periocular area**

S01.15 [6th] **Open bite of eyelid and periocular area**
Bite of eyelid and periocular area NOS
Excludes1: superficial bite of eyelid and periocular area (S00.26, S00.27)
    S01.151 [7th] **Open bite of right eyelid and periocular area**
    S01.152 [7th] **Open bite of left eyelid and periocular area**

S01.2 [5th] **Open wound of nose**

S01.21X [7th] **Laceration without FB of nose**

S01.22X [7th] **Laceration with FB of nose**

S01.23X [7th] **Puncture wound without FB of nose**

S01.24X [7th] **Puncture wound with FB of nose**

S01.25X [7th] **Open bite of nose**
Bite of nose NOS
Excludes1: superficial bite of nose (S00.36, S00.37)

S01.3 [5th] **Open wound of ear**

S01.31 [6th] **Laceration without FB of ear**
    S01.311 [7th] **Laceration without FB of right ear**
    S01.312 [7th] **Laceration without FB of left ear**

S01.32 [6th] **Laceration with FB of ear**
    S01.321 [7th] **Laceration with FB of right ear**
    S01.322 [7th] **Laceration with FB of left ear**

S01.33 [6th] **Puncture wound without FB of ear**
    S01.331 [7th] **Puncture wound without FB of right ear**
    S01.332 [7th] **Puncture wound without FB of left ear**

S01.34 [6th] **Puncture wound with FB of ear**
    S01.341 [7th] **Puncture wound with FB of right ear**
    S01.342 [7th] **Puncture wound with FB of left ear**

S01.35 [6th] **Open bite of ear**
Bite of ear NOS
Excludes1: superficial bite of ear (S00.46, S00.47)
    S01.351 [7th] **Open bite of right ear**
    S01.352 [7th] **Open bite of left ear**

S01.4 [5th] **Open wound of cheek and temporomandibular area**

S01.41 [6th] **Laceration without FB of cheek and temporomandibular area**
    S01.411 [7th] **Laceration without FB of right cheek and temporomandibular area**
    S01.412 [7th] **Laceration without FB of left cheek and temporomandibular area**

S01.42 [6th] **Laceration with FB of cheek and temporomandibular area**
    S01.421 [7th] **Laceration with FB of right cheek and temporomandibular area**
    S01.422 [7th] **Laceration with FB of left cheek and temporomandibular area**

S01.43 [6th] **Puncture wound without FB of cheek and temporomandibular area**
    S01.431 [7th] **Puncture wound without FB of right cheek and temporomandibular area**
    S01.432 [7th] **Puncture wound without FB of left cheek and temporomandibular area**

S01.44 [6th] **Puncture wound with FB of cheek and temporomandibular area**
    S01.441 [7th] **Puncture wound with FB of right cheek and temporomandibular area**
    S01.442 [7th] **Puncture wound with FB of left cheek and temporomandibular area**

S01.45 [6th] **Open bite of cheek and temporomandibular area**
Bite of cheek and temporomandibular area NOS
Excludes2: superficial bite of cheek and temporomandibular area (S00.86, S00.87)
    S01.451 [7th] **Open bite of right cheek and temporomandibular area**
    S01.452 [7th] **Open bite of left cheek and temporomandibular area**

S01.5 [5th] **Open wound of lip and oral cavity**
Excludes2: tooth dislocation (S03.2)
tooth fracture (S02.5)

S01.51 [6th] **Laceration of lip and oral cavity without FB**
    S01.511 [7th] **Laceration without FB of lip**
    S01.512 [7th] **Laceration without FB of oral cavity**

S01.52 [6th] **Laceration of lip and oral cavity with FB**
    S01.521 [7th] **Laceration with FB of lip**
    S01.522 [7th] **Laceration with FB of oral cavity**

S01.53 [6th] **Puncture wound of lip and oral cavity without FB**
    S01.531 [7th] **Puncture wound without FB of lip**
    S01.532 [7th] **Puncture wound without FB of oral cavity**

S01.54 [6th] **Puncture wound of lip and oral cavity with FB**
    S01.541 [7th] **Puncture wound with FB of lip**
    S01.542 [7th] **Puncture wound with FB of oral cavity**

S01.55 [6th] **Open bite of lip and oral cavity**
    S01.551 [7th] **Open bite of lip**
    Bite of lip NOS
    Excludes1: superficial bite of lip (S00.571)
    S01.552 [7th] **Open bite of oral cavity**
    Bite of oral cavity NOS
    Excludes1: superficial bite of oral cavity (S00.572)

S01.8 [5th] **Open wound of other parts of head**

S01.81X [7th] **Laceration without FB of other part of head**

[4th] [5th] [6th] [7th] Additional Character Required   ✔ 3-character code

Unspecified laterality codes were excluded here.

• =New Code
▲ =Revised Code
◘ =Social determinants of health

Excludes1—Not coded here, do not use together
Excludes2—Not included here

330   **PEDIATRIC ICD-10-CM 2022: A MANUAL FOR PROVIDER-BASED CODING**

S01.82X `7th` **Laceration with FB of other part of head**

S01.83X `7th` **Puncture wound without FB of other part of head**

S01.84X `7th` **Puncture wound with FB of other part of head**

S01.85X `7th` **Open bite of other part of head**
Bite of other part of head NOS
Excludes1: superficial bite of other part of head (S00.87)

S01.9 **Open wound of unspecified part of head**
`5th`
  S01.90X `7th` **Unspecified open wound of unspecified part of head**

  S01.91X `7th` **Laceration without FB of unspecified part of head**

  S01.92X `7th` **Laceration with FB of unspecified part of head**

  S01.93X `7th` **Puncture wound without FB of unspecified part of head**

  S01.94X `7th` **Puncture wound with FB of unspecified part of head**

  S01.95X `7th` **Open bite of unspecified part of head**
Bite of head NOS
Excludes1: superficial bite of head NOS (S00.97)

S02 **FRACTURE OF SKULL AND FACIAL BONES**
`4th`
Note: A fracture not indicated as open or closed should be coded to closed
Code also any associated intracranial injury (S06.-)

S02.0 **Fracture of vault of skull**
Fracture of frontal bone
Fracture of parietal bone

S02.1 **Fracture of base of skull**
`5th`
Excludes2: lateral orbital wall (S02.84-)
  medial orbital wall (S02.83-)
  orbital floor (S02.3-)

  S02.101 `7th` **Fracture of base of skull, right side**

  S02.102 `7th` **Fracture of base of skull, left side**

  S02.109 `7th` **Fracture of base of skull, unspecified side**

  S02.11 `6th` **Fracture of occiput**
    S02.111 `7th` **Type II occipital condyle fracture, unspecified side**
    S02.112 `7th` **Type III occipital condyle fracture, unspecified side**
    S02.113 `7th` **Unspecified occipital condyle fracture**
    S02.118 `7th` **Other fracture of occiput, unspecified side**
    S02.119 `7th` **Unspecified fracture of occiput**
    S02.11A `7th` **Type I occipital condyle fracture, right side**
    S02.11B `7th` **Type I occipital condyle fracture, left side**
    S02.11C `7th` **Type II occipital condyle fracture, right side**
    S02.11D `7th` **Type II occipital condyle fracture, left side**
    S02.11E `7th` **Type III occipital condyle fracture, right side**
    S02.11F `7th` **Type III occipital condyle fracture, left side**
    S02.11G `7th` **Other fracture of occiput, right side**
    S02.11H `7th` **Other fracture of occiput, left side**

  S02.12 `6th` **Fracture of orbital roof**
    S02.121 `7th` **Fracture of orbital roof, right side, closed fracture**
    S02.122 `7th` **Fracture of orbital roof, left side, closed fracture**

7th characters for category S01
A—initial encounter
D—subsequent encounter
S—sequela

    S02.129 `7th` **Fracture of orbital roof, unspecified side, closed fracture**

S02.19X `7th` **Other fracture of base of skull**
Fracture of anterior fossa of base of skull
Fracture of ethmoid or frontal sinus
Fracture of middle fossa of base of skull
Fracture of orbital roof
Fracture of posterior fossa of base of skull
Fracture of sphenoid
Fracture of temporal bone

S02.2XX `7th` **Fracture of nasal bones**

S02.3 **Fracture of orbital floor**
`5th`
Fracture of inferior orbital wall
Excludes1: orbit NOS (S02.85)
Excludes2: lateral orbital wall (S02.84-)
  medial orbital wall (S02.83-)
  orbital roof (S02.1-)

  S02.30X `7th` **Fracture of orbital floor, unspecified side**
    Excludes1: orbit NOS (S02.85)
    Excludes2: orbital roof (S02.1-)

  S02.31X `7th` **Fracture of orbital floor, right side**
    Excludes1: orbit NOS (S02.8)
    Excludes2: orbital roof (S02.1-)

  S02.32X `7th` **Fracture of orbital floor, left side**
    Excludes1: orbit NOS (S02.8)
    Excludes2: orbital roof (S02.1-)

S02.4 **Fracture of malar, maxillary and zygoma bones**
`5th`
Fracture of superior maxilla
Fracture of upper jaw (bone)
Fracture of zygomatic process of temporal bone

  S02.40 `6th` **Fracture of malar, maxillary and zygoma bones, unspecified**
    S02.400 `7th` **Malar fracture, unspecified side**
    S02.401 `7th` **Maxillary fracture, unspecified side**
    S02.402 `7th` **Zygomatic fracture, unspecified side**
    S02.40A `7th` **Malar fracture, right side**
    S02.40B `7th` **Malar fracture, left side**
    S02.40C `7th` **Maxillary fracture, right side**
    S02.40D `7th` **Maxillary fracture, left side**
    S02.40E `7th` **Zygomatic fracture, right side**
    S02.40F `7th` **Zygomatic fracture, left side**

S02.5XX `7th` **Fracture of tooth (traumatic)**
Broken tooth
Excludes1: cracked tooth (nontraumatic) (K03.81)

S02.6 **Fracture of mandible**
`5th`
Fracture of lower jaw (bone)

  S02.60 `6th` **Fracture of mandible, unspecified**
    S02.600 `7th` **Fracture of unspecified part of body of mandible, unspecified side**
    S02.601 `7th` **Fracture of unspecified part of body of right mandible**
    S02.602 `7th` **Fracture of unspecified part of body of left mandible**
    S02.609 `7th` **Fracture of mandible, unspecified**

  S02.61 `6th` **Fracture of condylar process of mandible**
    S02.610 `7th` **Fracture of condylar process of mandible, unspecified side**
    S02.611 `7th` **Fracture of condylar process of right mandible**
    S02.612 `7th` **Fracture of condylar process of left mandible**

  S02.62 `6th` **Fracture of subcondylar process of mandible**

7th characters for category S02
A—initial encounter for closed fracture
B—initial encounter for open fracture
D—subsequent encounter for fracture with routine healing
G—subsequent encounter for fracture with delayed healing
K—subsequent encounter for fracture with nonunion
S—sequela

`4th` `5th` `6th` `7th` Additional Character Required   ✓   3-character code   Unspecified laterality codes were excluded here.

• =New Code
▲ =Revised Code
⌑ =Social determinants of health

Excludes1—Not coded here, do not use together
Excludes2—Not included here

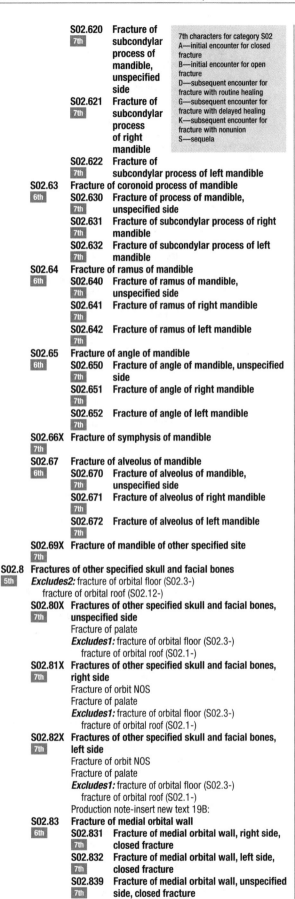

S02.620 **Fracture of subcondylar process of mandible, unspecified side**
[7th]

S02.621 **Fracture of subcondylar process of right mandible**
[7th]

7th characters for category S02
A—initial encounter for closed fracture
B—initial encounter for open fracture
D—subsequent encounter for fracture with routine healing
G—subsequent encounter for fracture with delayed healing
K—subsequent encounter for fracture with nonunion
S—sequela

S02.622 **Fracture of subcondylar process of left mandible**
[7th]

S02.63 **Fracture of coronoid process of mandible**
[6th]
    S02.630 **Fracture of process of mandible, unspecified side**
    [7th]
    S02.631 **Fracture of subcondylar process of right mandible**
    [7th]
    S02.632 **Fracture of subcondylar process of left mandible**
    [7th]

S02.64 **Fracture of ramus of mandible**
[6th]
    S02.640 **Fracture of ramus of mandible, unspecified side**
    [7th]
    S02.641 **Fracture of ramus of right mandible**
    [7th]
    S02.642 **Fracture of ramus of left mandible**
    [7th]

S02.65 **Fracture of angle of mandible**
[6th]
    S02.650 **Fracture of angle of mandible, unspecified side**
    [7th]
    S02.651 **Fracture of angle of right mandible**
    [7th]
    S02.652 **Fracture of angle of left mandible**
    [7th]

S02.66X **Fracture of symphysis of mandible**
[7th]

S02.67 **Fracture of alveolus of mandible**
[6th]
    S02.670 **Fracture of alveolus of mandible, unspecified side**
    [7th]
    S02.671 **Fracture of alveolus of right mandible**
    [7th]
    S02.672 **Fracture of alveolus of left mandible**
    [7th]

S02.69X **Fracture of mandible of other specified site**
[7th]

S02.8 **Fractures of other specified skull and facial bones**
[5th]
Excludes2: fracture of orbital floor (S02.3-)
    fracture of orbital roof (S02.12-)

S02.80X **Fractures of other specified skull and facial bones, unspecified side**
[7th]
Fracture of palate
Excludes1: fracture of orbital floor (S02.3-)
    fracture of orbital roof (S02.1-)

S02.81X **Fractures of other specified skull and facial bones, right side**
[7th]
Fracture of orbit NOS
Fracture of palate
Excludes1: fracture of orbital floor (S02.3-)
    fracture of orbital roof (S02.1-)

S02.82X **Fractures of other specified skull and facial bones, left side**
[7th]
Fracture of orbit NOS
Fracture of palate
Excludes1: fracture of orbital floor (S02.3-)
    fracture of orbital roof (S02.1-)
Production note-insert new text 19B:

S02.83 **Fracture of medial orbital wall**
[6th]
    S02.831 **Fracture of medial orbital wall, right side, closed fracture**
    [7th]
    S02.832 **Fracture of medial orbital wall, left side, closed fracture**
    [7th]
    S02.839 **Fracture of medial orbital wall, unspecified side, closed fracture**
    [7th]

S02.84 **Fracture of lateral orbital wall**
[6th]
    S02.841 **Fracture of lateral orbital wall, right side, closed fracture**
    [7th]
    S02.842 **Fracture of lateral orbital wall, left side, closed fracture**
    [7th]
    S02.849 **Fracture of lateral orbital wall, unspecified side, closed fracture**
    [7th]

S02.85 **Fracture of orbit, unspecified**
[7th]
Fracture of orbit NOS
Fracture of orbit wall NOS
Excludes1: lateral orbital wall (S02.84-)
    medial orbital wall (S02.83-)
    orbital floor (S02.3-)
    orbital roof (S02.12-)

S02.9 **Fracture of unspecified skull and facial bones**
[5th]
    S02.91X **Unspecified fracture of skull**
    [7th]

    S02.92X **Unspecified fracture of facial bones**
    [7th]

S03 **DISLOCATION AND SPRAIN OF JOINTS AND LIGAMENTS OF HEAD**
[4th]
Includes: avulsion of joint (capsule) or ligament of head
    laceration of cartilage, joint (capsule) or ligament of head
    sprain of cartilage, joint (capsule) or ligament of head
    traumatic hemarthrosis of joint or ligament of head
    traumatic rupture of joint or ligament of head
    traumatic subluxation of joint or ligament of head
    traumatic tear of joint or ligament of head
Code also any associated open wound
Excludes2: Strain of muscle or tendon of head (S09.1)

S03.0 **Dislocation of jaw**
[5th]
Dislocation of jaw (cartilage) (meniscus)
Dislocation of mandible or of temporomandibular (joint)
    S03.00X **Dislocation of jaw, unspecified side**
    [7th]

    S03.01X **Dislocation of jaw, right side**
    [7th]

    S03.02X **Dislocation of jaw, left side**
    [7th]

    S03.03X **Dislocation of jaw, bilateral**
    [7th]

S03.1XX **Dislocation of septal cartilage of nose**
[7th]

S03.2XX **Dislocation of tooth**
[7th]

S03.4 **Sprain of jaw**
[5th]
Sprain of temporomandibular (joint) (ligament)
    S03.40X **Sprain of jaw, unspecified side**
    [7th]

    S03.41X **Sprain of jaw, right side**
    [7th]

    S03.42X **Sprain of jaw, left side**
    [7th]

    S03.43X **Sprain of jaw, bilateral**
    [7th]

S04 **INJURY OF CRANIAL NERVE**
[4th]
The selection of side should be based on the side of the body being affected
Code first any associated intracranial injury (S06.-)
Code also any associated:
    open wound of head (S01.-)
    skull fracture (S02.-)

S04.5 **Injury of facial nerve**
[5th]
Injury of 7th cranial nerve
    S04.51X **Injury of facial nerve, right side**
    [7th]

    S04.52X **Injury of facial nerve, left side**
    [7th]

[4th] [5th] [6th] [7th] Additional Character Required   ✓   3-character code   Unspecified laterality codes were excluded here.

• =New Code
▲ =Revised Code
▫ =Social determinants of health

Excludes1—Not coded here, do not use together
Excludes2—Not included here

CHAPTER 19. INJURY, POISONING AND CERTAIN OTHER CONSEQUENCES OF EXTERNAL CAUSES   (S02.620–S04.52X)

S05 INJURY OF EYE AND ORBIT
`4th`

Includes: open wound of eye and orbit
Excludes2: 2nd cranial [optic] nerve injury (S04.0-)
3rd cranial [oculomotor] nerve injury (S04.1-)
open wound of eyelid and periocular area (S01.1-)
orbital bone fracture (S02.1-, S02.3-, S02.8-)
superficial injury of eyelid (S00.1–S00.2)

> 7th characters for categories
> S05 & S06
> A—initial encounter
> D—subsequent encounter
> S—sequela

S05.0 Injury of conjunctiva and corneal abrasion without FB
`5th`

Excludes1: FB in conjunctival sac (T15.1)
FB in cornea (T15.0)

S05.01X Injury of conjunctiva and corneal abrasion without FB, right eye
`7th`

S05.02X Injury of conjunctiva and corneal abrasion without FB, left eye
`7th`

S05.1 Contusion of eyeball and orbital tissues
`5th`

Traumatic hyphema
Excludes2: black eye NOS (S00.1)
contusion of eyelid and periocular area (S00.1)

S05.11X Contusion of eyeball and orbital tissues, right eye
`7th`

S05.12X Contusion of eyeball and orbital tissues, left eye
`7th`

S05.8 Other injuries of eye and orbit
`5th`

Lacrimal duct injury

S05.8X Other injuries of eye and orbit
`6th`

   S05.8X1 Other injuries of right eye and orbit
`7th`

   S05.8X2 Other injuries of left eye and orbit
`7th`

S05.9 Unspecified injury of eye and orbit
`5th`

Injury of eye NOS

S05.91X Unspecified injury of right eye and orbit
`7th`

S05.92X Unspecified injury of left eye and orbit
`7th`

S06 INTRACRANIAL INJURY
`4th`

Includes: traumatic brain injury
Code also any associated:
open wound of head (S01.-)
skull fracture (S02.-)
Excludes1: head injury NOS (S09.90)

> 7th characters for categories
> S05 & S06
> A—initial encounter
> D—subsequent encounter
> S—sequela

S06.0 Concussion
`5th`

Commotio cerebri
Excludes1: concussion with other intracranial injuries classified in subcategories S06.1- to S06.6-, S06.81- and S06.82- code to specified intracranial injury

S06.0X Concussion
`6th`

   S06.0X0 Concussion without LOC
`7th`

   S06.0X1 Concussion with LOC of 30 min or less
`7th`

   S06.0X9 Concussion with LOC unspecified duration
`7th`   Concussion NOS

S06.3 Focal traumatic brain injury
`5th`

Use additional code, if applicable, for traumatic brain compression or herniation (S06.A-)
Excludes1: any condition classifiable to S06.4–S06.6
Excludes2: focal cerebral edema (S06.1)

S06.30 Unspecified focal traumatic brain injury

   S06.300 Unspecified focal traumatic brain injury without LOC
`7th`

   S06.301 Unspecified focal traumatic brain injury with LOC of; 30 min or less
`7th`

   S06.302 31 min to 59 min
`7th`

   S06.303 1 hour to 5 h 59 min
`7th`

   S06.304 6 h to 24 h
`7th`

   S06.305 greater than 24 h with return to pre-existing conscious level
`7th`

   S06.306 greater than 24 h without return to pre-existing conscious level with patient surviving
`7th`

   S06.307A any duration with death due to brain injury prior to regaining consciousness

   S06.308A any duration with death due to other cause prior to regaining consciousness

   S06.309 unspecified duration
`7th`   Unspecified focal traumatic brain injury NOS

S06.31 Contusion and laceration of right cerebrum
`6th`

   S06.310 Contusion and laceration of right cerebrum without loss of consciousness
`7th`

   S06.311 Contusion and laceration of right cerebrum with LOC of; 30 min or less
`7th`

   S06.312 31 min to 59 min
`7th`

   S06.313 1 hour to 5 h 59 min
`7th`

   S06.314 6 h to 24 h
`7th`

   S06.315 greater than 24 h with return to pre-existing conscious level
`7th`

   S06.316 greater than 24 h without return to pre-existing conscious level with patient surviving
`7th`

   S06.317A any duration with death due to brain injury prior to regaining consciousness

   S06.318A any duration with death due to other cause prior to regaining consciousness

   S06.319 unspecified duration
`7th`   Contusion and laceration of right cerebrum NOS

S06.32 Contusion and laceration of left cerebrum
`6th`

   S06.320 Contusion and laceration of left cerebrum without loss of consciousness
`7th`

   S06.321 Contusion and laceration of left cerebrum with LOC of; 30 min or less
`7th`

   S06.322 31 min to 59 min
`7th`

   S06.323 1 hour to 5 h 59 min
`7th`

   S06.324 6 h to 24 h
`7th`

   S06.325 greater than 24 h with return to pre-existing conscious level
`7th`

   S06.326 greater than 24 h without return to pre-existing conscious level with patient surviving
`7th`

   S06.327A any duration with death due to brain injury prior to regaining consciousness

   S06.328A any duration with death due to other cause prior to regaining consciousness

   S06.329 unspecified duration
`7th`   Contusion and laceration of left cerebrum NOS

S06.34 Traumatic hemorrhage of right cerebrum
`6th`

Traumatic intracerebral hemorrhage and hematoma of right cerebrum

   S06.340 Traumatic hemorrhage of right cerebrum without LOC
`7th`

   S06.341 Traumatic hemorrhage of right cerebrum with LOC of; 30 min or less
`7th`

   S06.342 31 min to 59 min
`7th`

   S06.343 1 h to 5 h 59 min
`7th`

   S06.344 6 h to 24 h
`7th`

   S06.345 greater than 24 h with return to pre-existing conscious level
`7th`

   S06.346 greater than 24 h without return to pre-existing conscious level with patient surviving
`7th`

     Additional Character Required ✔ 3-character code   Unspecified laterality codes were excluded here.   • =New Code   ▲ =Revised Code   ◘ =Social determinants of health   ***Excludes1***—Not coded here, do not use together   ***Excludes2***—Not included here

S06.347A any dura-tion with death due to brain injury prior to regaining consciousness

> 7th characters for categories S06
> A—initial encounter
> D—subsequent encounter
> S—sequela

S06.348A any duration with death due to other cause prior to regaining consciousness

S06.349 unspecified duration
> 7th   Traumatic hemorrhage of right cerebrum NOS

S06.35 Traumatic hemorrhage of left cerebrum
> 6th
Traumatic intracerebral hemorrhage and hematoma of left cerebrum

S06.350 Traumatic hemorrhage of left cerebrum
> 7th   without LOC

S06.351 Traumatic hemorrhage of left cerebrum
> 7th   with LOC of; 30 min or less

S06.352 31 min to 59 min
> 7th

S06.353 1 h to 5 h 59 min
> 7th

S06.354 6 h to 24 h
> 7th

S06.355 greater than 24 h with return to pre-existing conscious level
> 7th

S06.356 greater than 24 h without return to pre-existing conscious level with patient surviving
> 7th

S06.357A any duration with death due to brain injury prior to regaining consciousness

S06.358A any duration with death due to other cause prior to regaining consciousness

S06.359 unspecified duration
> 7th   Traumatic hemorrhage of left cerebrum NOS

S06.37 Contusion, laceration, and hemorrhage of cerebellum
> 6th

S06.370 Contusion, laceration, and hemorrhage of cerebellum without LOC
> 7th

S06.371 Contusion, laceration, and hemorrhage of cerebellum with LOC of; 30 min or less
> 7th

S06.372 31 min to 59 min
> 7th

S06.373 1 hour to 5 h 59 min
> 7th

S06.374 6 h to 24 h
> 7th

S06.375 greater than 24 h with return to pre-existing conscious level
> 7th

S06.376 greater than 24 h without return to pre-existing conscious level with patient surviving
> 7th

S06.377A any duration with death due to brain injury prior to regaining consciousness

S06.378A any duration with death due to other cause prior to regaining consciousness

S06.379 unspecified duration
> 7th   Contusion, laceration, and hemorrhage of cerebellum NOS

S06.38 Contusion, laceration, and hemorrhage of brainstem
> 6th

S06.380 Contusion, laceration, and hemorrhage of brainstem without LOC
> 7th

S06.381 Contusion, laceration, and hemorrhage of brainstem with LOC of; 30 min or less
> 7th

S06.382 31 min to 59 min
> 7th

S06.383 1 hour to 5 h 59 min
> 7th

S06.384 6 h to 24 h
> 7th

S06.385 greater than 24 h with return to pre-existing conscious level
> 7th

S06.386 greater than 24 h without return to pre-existing conscious level with patient surviving
> 7th

S06.387A any duration with death due to brain injury prior to regaining consciousness

S06.388A any duration with death due to other cause prior to regaining consciousness

S06.389 unspecified duration
> 7th   Contusion, laceration, and hemorrhage of brainstem NOS

S06.4 Epidural hemorrhage
> 5th
Extradural hemorrhage NOS
Extradural hemorrhage (traumatic)

S06.4X Epidural hemorrhage
> 6th

S06.4X0 Epidural hemorrhage without loss of
> 7th   consciousness

S06.4X1 Epidural hemorrhage with loss of
> 7th   consciousness of 30 minutes or less

S06.4X2 Epidural hemorrhage with loss of
> 7th   consciousness of 31 minutes to 59 minutes

S06.4X3 Epidural hemorrhage with loss of
> 7th   consciousness of 1 hour to 5 hours 59 minutes

S06.4X4 Epidural hemorrhage with loss of
> 7th   consciousness of 6 hours to 24 hours

S06.4X5 Epidural hemorrhage with loss of
> 7th   consciousness greater than 24 hours with return to pre-existing conscious level

S06.4X6 Epidural hemorrhage with loss of
> 7th   consciousness greater than 24 hours without return to pre-existing conscious level with patient surviving

S06.4X7A Epidural hemorrhage with loss of consciousness of any duration with death due to brain injury prior to regaining consciousness

S06.4X8A Epidural hemorrhage with loss of consciousness of any duration with death due to other causes prior to regaining consciousness

S06.4X9 Epidural hemorrhage with loss of
> 7th   consciousness of unspecified duration
Epidural hemorrhage NOS

S06.5 Traumatic subdural hemorrhage
> 5th
Use additional code, if applicable, for traumatic brain compression or herniation (S06.A-)

S06.5X Traumatic subdural hemorrhage
> 6th

S06.5X0 Traumatic subdural hemorrhage without
> 7th   LOC

S06.5X1 Traumatic subdural hemorrhage with LOC
> 7th   of; 30 min or less

S06.5X2 31 min to 59 min
> 7th

S06.5X3 1 hour to 5 h 59 min
> 7th

S06.5X4 6 h to 24 h
> 7th

S06.5X5 greater than 24 h with return to pre-existing conscious level
> 7th

S06.5X6 greater than 24 h without return to pre-existing conscious level with patient surviving
> 7th

S06.5X7A any duration with death due to brain injury before regaining consciousness

S06.5X8A any duration with death due to other cause before regaining consciousness

S06.5X9 unspecified duration
> 7th   Traumatic subdural hemorrhage NOS

S06.6 Traumatic subarachnoid hemorrhage
> 5th
Use additional code, if applicable, for traumatic brain compression or herniation (S06.A-)

S06.6X Traumatic subarachnoid hemorrhage
> 6th

S06.6X0 Traumatic subarachnoid hemorrhage
> 7th   without LOC

S06.6X1 Traumatic subarachnoid hemorrhage with
> 7th   LOC of; 30 min or less

4th 5th 6th 7th Additional Character Required   ✓   3-character code   Unspecified laterality codes were excluded here.   • =New Code   ▲ =Revised Code   ▢ =Social determinants of health   **Excludes1**—Not coded here, do not use together   **Excludes2**—Not included here

S06.6X2 `7th` **31 min to 59 min**

S06.6X3 `7th` **1 hour to 5 h 59 min**

S06.6X4 `7th` **6 h to 24 h**

S06.6X5 `7th` **greater than 24 h with return to pre-existing conscious level**

S06.6X6 `7th` **greater than 24 h without return to pre-existing conscious level with patient surviving**

S06.6X7A **any duration with death due to brain injury prior to regaining consciousness**

S06.6X8A **any duration with death due to other cause prior to regaining consciousness**

S06.6X9 `7th` **unspecified duration**
Traumatic subarachnoid hemorrhage NOS

> 7th characters for categories S06
> A—initial encounter
> D—subsequent encounter
> S—sequela

S06.8 `5th` **Other specified intracranial injuries**

   S06.89 `6th` **Other specified intracranial injury**
      Excludes1: concussion (S06.0X-)

      S06.890 `7th` **Other specified intracranial injury without LOC**

      S06.891 `7th` **Other specified intracranial injury with LOC of 30 min or less**

      S06.892 `7th` **Other specified intracranial injury with LOC of; 31 min to 59 min**

      S06.893 `7th` **1 hour to 5 h 59 min**

      S06.894 `7th` **6 h to 24 h**

      S06.895 `7th` **greater than 24 h with return to pre-existing conscious level**

      S06.896 `7th` **greater than 24 h without return to pre-existing conscious level with patient surviving**

      S06.897A **any duration with death due to brain injury prior to regaining consciousness**

      S06.898A **any duration with death due to other cause prior to regaining consciousness**

      S06.899 `7th` **unspecified duration**

S06.9 `5th` **Unspecified intracranial injury**
Brain injury NOS
Head injury NOS with LOC
Traumatic brain injury NOS
Excludes1: conditions classifiable to S06.0- to S06.8- code to specified intracranial injury
head injury NOS (S09.90)

   S06.9X `6th` **Unspecified intracranial injury**

      S06.9X0 `7th` **Unspecified intracranial injury without LOC**

      S06.9X1 `7th` **Unspecified intracranial injury with LOC of; 30 min or less**

      S06.9X2 `7th` **31 min to 59 min**

      S06.9X3 `7th` **1 hour to 5 h 59 min**

      S06.9X4 `7th` **6 h to 24 h**

      S06.9X5 `7th` **greater than 24 h with return to pre-existing conscious level**

      S06.9X6 `7th` **greater than 24 h without return to pre-existing conscious level with patient surviving**

      S06.9X7A **any duration with death due to brain injury prior to regaining consciousness**

      S06.9X8A **any duration with death due to other cause prior to regaining consciousness**

      S06.9X9 `7th` **unspecified duration**

• **S06.A** `5th` **Traumatic brain compression**
Traumatic cerebral compression
Code first the underlying traumatic brain injury, such as:
diffuse traumatic brain injury (S06.2-)
focal traumatic brain injury (S06.3-)
traumatic subdural hemorrhage (S06.5-)
traumatic subarachnoid hemorrhage (S06.6-)

   • **S06.A0X** `7th` **Traumatic brain compression without herniation**
Traumatic brain or cerebral compression NOS

   • **S06.A1X** `7th` **Traumatic brain compression with herniation**
Traumatic brain herniation
Traumatic brainstem or cerebellar or cerebral compression with herniation

S09 `4th` **OTHER AND UNSPECIFIED INJURIES OF HEAD**

S09.0 **Injury of blood vessels of head, NEC**
Excludes1: injury of cerebral blood vessels (S06.-)
injury of precerebral blood vessels (S15.-)

> 7th characters for categories S09
> A—initial encounter
> D—subsequent encounter
> S—sequela

S09.1 `5th` **Injury of muscle and tendon of head**
Code also any associated open wound (S01.-)
Excludes2: sprain to joints and ligament of head (S03.9)

   S09.10X `7th` **Unspecified injury of muscle and tendon of head**
Injury of muscle and tendon of head NOS

   S09.11X `7th` **Strain of muscle and tendon of head**

   S09.12X `7th` **Laceration of muscle and tendon of head**

   S09.19X **Other specified injury of muscle and tendon of head**

S09.2 `5th` **Traumatic rupture of ear drum**
Excludes1: traumatic rupture of ear drum due to blast injury (S09.31-)

   S09.21X `7th` **Traumatic rupture of right ear drum**

   S09.22X `7th` **Traumatic rupture of left ear drum**

S09.8 `5th` **Other specified injuries of head**

S09.9 `5th` **Unspecified injury of face and head**

   S09.90X `7th` **Unspecified injury of head**
Head injury NOS
Excludes1: brain injury NOS (S06.9-)
head injury NOS with LOC (S06.9-)
intracranial injury NOS (S06.9-)

   S09.91X `7th` **Unspecified injury of ear**
Injury of ear NOS

   S09.92X `7th` **Unspecified injury of nose**
Injury of nose NOS

   S09.93X `7th` **Unspecified injury of face**
Injury of face NOS
Injuries to the neck (S10–S19)
Includes: injuries of nape
injuries of supraclavicular region
injuries of throat
Excludes2: burns and corrosions (T20–T32)
effects of FB in esophagus (T18.1)
effects of FB in larynx (T17.3)
effects of FB in pharynx (T17.2)
effects of FB in trachea (T17.4)
frostbite (T33–T34)
insect bite or sting, venomous (T63.4)

(S10–S19) INJURIES TO THE NECK

Includes: injuries of nape
injuries of supraclavicular region
injuries of throat
Excludes2: burns and corrosions (T20–T32)
effects of FB in esophagus (T18.1)
effects of FB in larynx (T17.3)
effects of FB in pharynx (T17.2)
effects of FB in trachea (T17.4)

`4th` `5th` `6th` `7th` Additional Character Required   ✓ 3-character code   Unspecified laterality codes were excluded here.   • =New Code   ▲ =Revised Code   ◘ =Social determinants of health   *Excludes1*—Not coded here, do not use together   *Excludes2*—Not included here

CHAPTER 19. INJURY, POISONING AND CERTAIN OTHER CONSEQUENCES OF EXTERNAL CAUSES   (S10–S12.400)

frostbite (T33–T34)
insect bite or sting, venomous (T63.4)

S10 **SUPERFICIAL INJURY OF NECK**
[4th]

S10.0XX **Contusion of throat**
[7th]
     Contusion of cervical esophagus
     Contusion of larynx
     Contusion of pharynx
     Contusion of trachea

> 7th characters for category S10 & S11
> A—initial encounter
> D—subsequent encounter
> S—sequela

S10.1 **Other and unspecified superficial injuries of throat**
[5th]

S10.10X **Unspecified superficial injuries of throat**
[7th]

S10.11X **Abrasion of throat**
[7th]

> 7th characters for category S10 & S11
> A—initial encounter
> D—subsequent encounter
> S—sequela

S10.12X **Blister (nonthermal) of throat**
[7th]

S10.14X **External constriction of part of throat**
[7th]

S10.15X **Superficial FB of throat**
[7th]
     Splinter in the throat

S10.16X **Insect bite (nonvenomous) of throat**
[7th]

S10.17X **Other superficial bite of throat**
[7th]
     Excludes1: open bite of throat (S11.85)

S10.8 **Superficial injury of other specified parts of neck**
[5th]

S10.80X **Unspecified superficial injury of other specified part of neck**
[7th]

S10.81X **Abrasion of other specified part of neck**
[7th]

S10.82X **Blister (nonthermal) of other specified part of neck**
[7th]

S10.83X **Contusion of other specified part of neck**
[7th]

S10.84X **External constriction of other specified part of neck**
[7th]

S10.85X **Superficial FB of other specified part of neck**
[7th]
     Splinter in other specified part of neck

S10.86X **Insect bite of other specified part of neck**
[7th]

S10.87X **Other superficial bite of other specified part of neck**
[7th]
     Excludes1: open bite of other specified parts of neck (S11.85)

S10.9 **Superficial injury of unspecified part of neck**
[5th]

S10.90X **Unspecified superficial injury of unspecified part of neck**
[7th]

S10.91X **Abrasion of unspecified part of neck**
[7th]

S10.92X **Blister (nonthermal) of unspecified part of neck**
[7th]

S10.93X **Contusion of unspecified part of neck**
[7th]

S10.94X **External constriction of unspecified part of neck**
[7th]

S10.95X **Superficial FB of unspecified part of neck**
[7th]

S10.96X **Insect bite of unspecified part of neck**
[7th]

S10.97X **Other superficial bite of unspecified part of neck**
[7th]

S11 **OPEN WOUND OF NECK**
[4th]
Code also any associated:
     spinal cord injury (S14.0, S14.1-)
     wound infection
Excludes2: open fracture of vertebra (S12.- with 7th character B)

S11.8 **Open wound of other specified parts of neck**
[5th]

S11.80X **Unspecified open wound of other specified part of neck**
[7th]

S11.81X **Laceration without foreign body of other specified part of neck**
[7th]

S11.82X **Laceration with foreign body of other specified part of neck**
[7th]

S11.83X **Puncture wound without foreign body of other specified part of neck**
[7th]

S11.84X **Puncture wound with foreign body of other specified part of neck**
[7th]

S11.85X **Open bite of other specified part of neck**
[7th]
     Bite of other specified part of neck NOS
     Excludes1: superficial bite of other specified part of neck (S10.87)

S11.9 **Open wound of unspecified part of neck**

S11.91X **Laceration without FB of unspecified part of neck**
[5th]
[7th]

S11.92X **Laceration with FB of unspecified part of neck**
[7th]

S11.93X **Puncture wound without FB of unspecified part of neck**
[7th]

S11.94X **Puncture wound with FB of unspecified part of neck**
[7th]

S11.95X **Open bite of unspecified part of neck**
[7th]
     Bite of neck NOS
     Excludes1: superficial bite of neck (S10.97)

S12 **FRACTURE OF CERVICAL VERTEBRA AND OTHER PARTS OF NECK**
[4th]
Note: A fracture not indicated as displaced or nondisplaced should be coded to displaced
A fracture not indicated as open or closed should be coded to closed
Includes: fracture of cervical neural arch
     fracture of cervical spine
     fracture of cervical spinous process
     fracture of cervical transverse process
     fracture of cervical vertebral arch
     fracture of neck
Code first any associated cervical spinal cord injury (S14.0, S14.1-)

S12.0 **Fracture of first cervical vertebra**
[5th]
     Atlas

S12.00 **Unspecified fracture of first cervical vertebra**
[6th]

> 7th characters for category S12.0–S12.6
> A—initial encounter for closed fracture
> B—initial encounter for open fracture
> D—subsequent encounter for fracture with routine healing
> G—subsequent encounter for fracture with delayed healing
> K—subsequent encounter for fracture with nonunion
> S—sequela

     S12.000 **Unspecified displaced fracture of first cervical vertebra**
     [7th]

     S12.001 **Unspecified nondisplaced fracture of first cervical vertebra**
     [7th]

S12.03 **Posterior arch fracture of first cervical vertebra**
[6th]
     S12.030 **Displaced posterior arch fracture of first cervical vertebra**
     [7th]
     S12.031 **Nondisplaced posterior arch fracture of first cervical vertebra**
     [7th]

S12.1 **Fracture of second cervical vertebra**
[5th]
     Axis

S12.10 **Unspecified fracture of second cervical vertebra**
[6th]
     S12.100 **Unspecified displaced fracture of second cervical vertebra**
     [7th]
     S12.101 **Unspecified nondisplaced fracture of second cervical vertebra**
     [7th]

S12.2 **Fracture of third cervical vertebra**
[5th]
S12.20 **Unspecified fracture of third cervical vertebra**
[6th]
     S12.200 **Unspecified displaced fracture of third cervical vertebra**
     [7th]
     S12.201 **Unspecified nondisplaced fracture of third cervical vertebra**
     [7th]

S12.3 **Fracture of fourth cervical vertebra**
[5th]
S12.30 **Unspecified fracture of fourth cervical vertebra**
[6th]
     S12.300 **Unspecified displaced fracture of fourth cervical vertebra**
     [7th]
     S12.301 **Unspecified nondisplaced fracture of fourth cervical vertebra**
     [7th]

S12.4 **Fracture of fifth cervical vertebra**
[5th]
S12.40 **Unspecified fracture of fifth cervical vertebra**
[6th]
     S12.400 **Unspecified displaced fracture of fifth cervical vertebra**
     [7th]

[4th] [5th] [6th] [7th] Additional Character Required   ✓   3-character code   Unspecified laterality codes were excluded here.

• =New Code
▲ =Revised Code
¤ =Social determinants of health

Excludes1—Not coded here, do not use together
Excludes2—Not included here

S12.401 **Unspecified nondisplaced fracture of fifth**
7th cervical vertebra

S12.5 Fracture of sixth cervical vertebra
5th **S12.50** **Unspecified fracture of sixth cervical vertebra**
6th **S12.500** **Unspecified displaced fracture of sixth**
7th cervical vertebra
S12.501 **Unspecified nondisplaced fracture of sixth**
7th cervical vertebra

S12.6 Fracture of seventh cervical vertebra
5th **S12.60** **Unspecified fracture of seventh cervical vertebra**
6th **S12.600** **Unspecified displaced fracture of seventh**
7th cervical vertebra
S12.601 **Unspecified nondisplaced fracture of**
7th seventh cervical vertebra

S12.8XX **Fracture of other parts of neck**
7th Hyoid bone
Larynx
Thyroid cartilage
Trachea

> 7th characters for category S12.8 & S12.9
> A—initial encounter
> D—subsequent encounter
> S—sequela

S12.9XX **Fracture of neck, unspecified**
7th Fracture of neck NOS
Fracture of cervical spine NOS
Fracture of cervical vertebra NOS

S13 **DISLOCATION AND SPRAIN OF JOINTS AND LIGAMENTS**
4th **AT NECK LEVEL**
Includes: avulsion of joint or ligament at
neck level
laceration of cartilage, joint or ligament
at neck level
sprain of cartilage, joint or ligament at
neck level
traumatic hemarthrosis of joint or ligament at neck level
traumatic rupture of joint or ligament at neck level
traumatic subluxation of joint or ligament at neck level
traumatic tear of joint or ligament at neck level

> 7th characters for category S13
> A—initial encounter
> D—subsequent encounter
> S—sequela

Code also any associated open wound
Excludes2: strain of muscle or tendon at neck level (S16.1)
S13.4XX **Sprain of ligaments of cervical spine**
7th Sprain of anterior longitudinal (ligament), cervical
Sprain of atlanto-axial (joints)
Sprain of atlanto-occipital (joints)
Whiplash injury of cervical spine
S13.8XX **Sprain of joints and ligaments of other parts of neck**
7th
S13.9XX **Sprain of joints and ligaments of unspecified parts of neck**
7th

S14 **INJURY OF NERVES AND SPINAL CORD AT NECK LEVEL**
4th **Note:** Code to highest level of cervical cord injury
Code also any associated:
fracture of cervical vertebra
(S12.0–S12.6.-)
open wound of neck (S11.-)
transient paralysis (R29.5)

> 7th characters for category S14
> A—initial encounter
> D—subsequent encounter
> S—sequela

S14.0XX **Concussion and edema of**
7th cervical spinal cord
S14.1 **Other and unspecified injuries of cervical spinal cord**
5th **S14.10** **Unspecified injury of cervical spinal cord**
6th **S14.101** **Unspecified injury at; C1 level of cervical**
7th spinal cord
S14.102 **C2 level of cervical spinal cord**
7th
S14.103 **C3 level of cervical spinal cord**
7th
S14.104 **C4 level of cervical spinal cord**
7th
S14.105 **C5 level of cervical spinal cord**
7th
S14.106 **C6 level of cervical spinal cord**
7th
S14.107 **C7 level of cervical spinal cord**
7th
S14.108 **C8 level of cervical spinal cord**
7th

S14.109 **unspecified level of cervical spinal cord**
7th Injury of cervical spinal cord NOS
S14.2XX **Injury of nerve root of cervical spine**
7th
S14.3XX **Injury of brachial plexus**
7th
S14.4XX **Injury of peripheral nerves of neck**
7th
S14.5XX **Injury of cervical sympathetic nerves**
7th
S14.8XX **Injury of other specified nerves of neck**
7th
S14.9XX **Injury of unspecified nerves of neck**
7th

S15 **INJURY OF BLOOD VESSELS AT NECK LEVEL**
4th **Code also** any associated open wound (S11.-)
S15.8XX **Injury of other specified**
7th **blood vessels at neck level**
S15.9XX **Injury of unspecified blood vessel at neck level**
7th

S16 **INJURY OF MUSCLE, FASCIA AND TENDON AT**
4th **NECK LEVEL**
Code also any associated open wound (S11.-)
Excludes2: sprain of joint or ligament at neck level (S13.9)
S16.1XX **Strain of muscle, fascia and tendon at neck level**
7th
S16.2XX **Laceration of muscle, fascia and tendon at neck level**
7th
S16.8XX **Other specified injury of muscle, fascia and tendon at neck**
7th **level**
S16.9XX **Unspecified injury of muscle, fascia and tendon at neck**
7th **level**
Injuries to the thorax (S20–S29)
Includes: injuries of breast
injuries of chest (wall)
injuries of interscapular area
Excludes2: burns and corrosions (T20–T32)
effects of FB in bronchus (T17.5)
effects of FB in esophagus (T18.1)
effects of FB in lung (T17.8)
effects of FB in trachea (T17.4)
frostbite (T33–T34)
injuries of axilla
injuries of clavicle
injuries of scapular region
injuries of shoulder
insect bite or sting, venomous (T63.4)

(S20–S29) INJURIES TO THE THORAX

Includes: injuries of breast
injuries of chest (wall)
injuries of interscapular area
Excludes2: burns and corrosions (T20–T32)
effects of FB in bronchus (T17.5)
effects of FB in esophagus (T18.1)
effects of FB in lung (T17.8)
effects of FB in trachea (T17.4)
frostbite (T33–T34)
injuries of axilla
injuries of clavicle
injuries of scapular region
injuries of shoulder
insect bite or sting, venomous (T63.4)

> 7th characters for category S20
> A—initial encounter
> D—subsequent encounter
> S—sequela

S20 **SUPERFICIAL INJURY OF THORAX**
4th **S20.0** **Contusion of breast**
5th **S20.00X** **Contusion of breast, unspecified breast**
7th
S20.01X **Contusion of right breast**
7th
S20.02X **Contusion of left breast**
7th

4th **5th** **6th** **7th** Additional Character Required	✓ 3-character code	Unspecified laterality codes were excluded here.	• =New Code ▲ =Revised Code ¤ =Social determinants of health	*Excludes1*—Not coded here, do not use together *Excludes2*—Not included here

S20.1 **Other and unspecified superficial injuries of breas**

S20.11 **Abrasion of breast**

S20.111 Abrasion of breast, right breast

S20.112 Abrasion of breast, left breast

S20.119 Abrasion of breast, unspecified breast

S20.12 **Blister (nonthermal) of breast**

S20.121 Blister (nonthermal) of breast, right breast

S20.122 Blister (nonthermal) of breast, left breast

7th characters for category S20
A—initial encounter
D—subsequent encounter
S—sequela

S20.129 Blister (nonthermal) of breast, unspecified breast

S20.14 **External constriction of part of breast**

S20.141 External constriction of part of breast, right breast

S20.142 External constriction of part of breast, left breast

S20.15 **Superficial FB of breast**

Splinter in the breast

S20.151 Superficial FB of breast, right breast

S20.152 Superficial FB of breast, left breast

S20.16 **Insect bite (nonvenomous) of breast**

S20.161 Insect bite (nonvenomous) of breast, right breast

S20.162 Insect bite (nonvenomous) of breast, left breast

S20.17 **Other superficial bite of breast**

Excludes1: open bite of breast (S21.05-)

S20.171 Other superficial bite of breast, right breast

S20.172 Other superficial bite of breast, left breast

S20.2 **Contusion of thorax**

S20.20X Contusion of thorax, unspecified

S20.21 **Contusion of front wall of thorax**

S20.211 Contusion of right front wall of thorax

S20.212 Contusion of left front wall of thorax

S20.213 Contusion of bilateral front wall of thorax

S20.214 Contusion of middle front wall of thorax

S20.219 Contusion of unspecified front wall of thorax

S20.22 **Contusion of back wall of thorax**

S20.221 Contusion of right back wall of thorax

S20.222 Contusion of left back wall of thorax

S20.223 Contusion of bilateral back wall of thorax

S20.224 Contusion of middle back wall of thorax

S20.229 Contusion of unspecified back wall of thorax

Interscapular contusion

S20.3 **Other and unspecified superficial injuries of front wall of thorax**

S20.30 **Unspecified superficial injuries of front wall of thorax**

S20.301 Unspecified superficial injuries of right front wall of thorax

S20.302 Unspecified superficial injuries of left front wall of thorax

S20.303 Unspecified superficial injuries of bilateral front wall of thorax

S20.304 Unspecified superficial injuries of middle front wall of thorax

S20.309 Unspecified superficial injuries of unspecified front wall of thorax

S20.31 **Abrasion of front wall of thorax**

S20.311 Abrasion of right front wall of thorax

S20.312 Abrasion of left front wall of thorax

S20.313 Abrasion of bilateral front wall of thorax

S20.314 Abrasion of middle front wall of thorax

S20.319 Abrasion of unspecified front wall of thorax

S20.32 **Blister (nonthermal) of front wall of thorax**

S20.321 Blister (nonthermal) of right front wall of thorax

S20.322 Blister (nonthermal) of left front wall of thorax

S20.323 Blister (nonthermal) of bilateral front wall of thorax

S20.324 Blister (nonthermal) of middle front wall of thorax

S20.329 Blister (nonthermal) of unspecified front wall of thorax

S20.34 **External constriction of front wall of thorax**

S20.341 External constriction of right front wall of thorax

S20.342 External constriction of left front wall of thorax

S20.343 External constriction of bilateral front wall of thorax

S20.344 External constriction of middle front wall of thorax

S20.349 External constriction of unspecified front wall of thorax

S20.35 **Superficial foreign body of front wall of thorax**

Splinter in front wall of thorax

S20.351 Superficial foreign body of right front wall of thorax

S20.352 Superficial foreign body of left front wall of thorax

S20.353 Superficial foreign body of bilateral front wall of thorax

S20.354 Superficial foreign body of middle front wall of thorax

S20.359 Superficial foreign body of unspecified front wall of thorax

S20.36 **Insect bite (nonvenomous) of front wall of thorax**

S20.361 Insect bite (nonvenomous) of right front wall of thorax

S20.362 Insect bite (nonvenomous) of left front wall of thorax

S20.363 Insect bite (nonvenomous) of bilateral front wall of thorax

S20.364 Insect bite (nonvenomous) of middle front wall of thorax

S20.369 Insect bite (nonvenomous) of unspecified front wall of thorax

S20.37 **Other superficial bite of front wall of thorax**

Excludes1: open bite of front wall of thorax (S21.14)

S20.371 Other superficial bite of right front wall of thorax

S20.372 Other superficial bite of left front wall of thorax

S20.373 Other superficial bite of bilateral front wall of thorax

S20.374 Other superficial bite of middle front wall of thorax

S20.379 Other superficial bite of unspecified front wall of thorax

4th 5th 6th 7th	Additional Character Required	✔ 3-character code

Unspecified laterality codes were excluded here.

• =New Code
▲ =Revised Code
☐ =Social determinants of health

Excludes1—Not coded here, do not use together
Excludes2—Not included here

S20.4 [5th] Other and unspecified superficial injuries of back wall of thorax

    S20.40 [6th] Unspecified superficial injuries of back wall of thorax

        S20.401 [7th] Unspecified superficial injuries of right back wall of thorax

        S20.402 [7th] Unspecified superficial injuries of left back wall of thorax

        S20.409 [7th] Unspecified superficial injuries of unspecified back wall of thorax

    S20.41 [6th] Abrasion of back wall of thorax

7th characters for category S20
A—initial encounter
D—subsequent encounter
S—sequela

        S20.411 [7th] Abrasion of right back wall of thorax

        S20.412 [7th] Abrasion of left back wall of thorax

        S20.419 [7th] Abrasion of unspecified back wall of thorax

    S20.42 [6th] Blister (nonthermal) of back wall of thorax

        S20.421 [7th] Blister (nonthermal) of right back wall of thorax

        S20.422 [7th] Blister (nonthermal) of left back wall of thorax

        S20.429 [7th] Blister (nonthermal) of unspecified back wall of thorax

    S20.44 [6th] External constriction of back wall of thorax

        S20.441 [7th] External constriction of right back wall of thorax

        S20.442 [7th] External constriction of left back wall of thorax

        S20.449 [7th] External constriction of unspecified back wall of thorax

    S20.46 [6th] Insect bite (nonvenomous) of back wall of thorax

        S20.461 [7th] Insect bite (nonvenomous) of right back wall of thorax

        S20.462 [7th] Insect bite (nonvenomous) of left back wall of thorax

        S20.469 [7th] Insect bite (nonvenomous) of unspecified back wall of thorax

    S20.47 [6th] Other superficial bite of back wall of thorax

    Excludes1: open bite of back wall of thorax (S21.24)

        S20.471 [7th] Other superficial bite of right back wall of thorax

        S20.472 [7th] Other superficial bite of left back wall of thorax

        S20.479 [7th] Other superficial bite of unspecified back wall of thorax

S20.9 [5th] Superficial injury of unspecified parts of thorax

    Excludes1: contusion of thorax NOS (S20.20)

    S20.90X [7th] Unspecified superficial injury of unspecified parts of thorax

    Superficial injury of thoracic wall NOS

    S20.91X [7th] Abrasion of unspecified parts of thorax

    S20.92X [7th] Blister (nonthermal) of unspecified parts of thorax

    S20.94X [7th] External constriction of unspecified parts of thorax

    S20.95X [7th] Superficial FB of unspecified parts of thorax

    Splinter in thorax NOS

    S20.96X [7th] Insect bite (nonvenomous) of unspecified parts of thorax

    S20.97X [7th] Other superficial bite of unspecified parts of thorax

    Excludes1: open bite of thorax NOS (S21.95)

S21 [4th] **OPEN WOUND OF THORAX**

Code also any associated injury, such as:
    rib fracture (S22.3-, S22.4-)
    wound infection

Excludes1: traumatic amputation (partial) of thorax (S28.1)

7th characters for category S21
A—initial encounter
D—subsequent encounter
S—sequela

S21.1 [5th] Open wound of front wall of thorax without penetration into thoracic cavity

    S21.11 [6th] Laceration without FB of front wall of thorax without penetration into thoracic cavity

        S21.111 [7th] Laceration without FB of; right front wall of thorax without penetration into thoracic cavity

        S21.112 [7th] of left front wall of thorax without penetration into thoracic cavity

        S21.119 [7th] unspecified front wall of thorax without penetration into thoracic cavity

    S21.12 [6th] Laceration with FB of; front wall of thorax without penetration into thoracic cavity

        S21.121 [7th] right front wall of thorax without penetration into thoracic cavity

        S21.122 [7th] left front wall of thorax without penetration into thoracic cavity

        S21.129 [7th] unspecified front wall of thorax without penetration into thoracic cavity

    S21.13 [6th] Puncture wound without FB of; front wall of thorax without penetration into thoracic cavity

        S21.131 [7th] right front wall of thorax without penetration into thoracic cavity

        S21.132 [7th] left front wall of thorax without penetration into thoracic cavity

        S21.139 [7th] unspecified front wall of thorax without penetration into thoracic cavity

    S21.14 [6th] Puncture wound with FB of; front wall of thorax without penetration into thoracic cavity

        S21.141 [7th] right front wall of thorax without penetration into thoracic cavity

        S21.142 [7th] left front wall of thorax without penetration into thoracic cavity

        S21.149 [7th] unspecified front wall of thorax without penetration into thoracic cavity

S21.2 [5th] Open wound of back wall of thorax without penetration into thoracic cavity

    S21.21 [6th] Laceration without FB of; back wall of thorax without penetration into thoracic cavity

        S21.211 [7th] right back wall of thorax without penetration into thoracic cavity

        S21.212 [7th] left back wall of thorax without penetration into thoracic cavity

        S21.219 [7th] unspecified back wall of thorax without penetration into thoracic cavity

    S21.22 [6th] Laceration with FB of; back wall of thorax without penetration into thoracic cavity

        S21.221 [7th] right back wall of thorax without penetration into thoracic cavity

        S21.222 [7th] left back wall of thorax without penetration into thoracic cavity

        S21.229 [7th] unspecified back wall of thorax without penetration into thoracic cavity

    S21.23 [6th] Puncture wound without FB of; back wall of thorax without penetration into thoracic cavity

        S21.231 [7th] right back wall of thorax without penetration into thoracic cavity

        S21.232 [7th] left back wall of thorax without penetration into thoracic cavity

        S21.239 [7th] unspecified back wall of thorax without penetration into thoracic cavity

    S21.24 [6th] Puncture wound with FB of; back wall of thorax without penetration into thoracic cavity

        S21.241 [7th] right back wall of thorax without penetration into thoracic cavity

        S21.242 [7th] left back wall of thorax without penetration into thoracic cavity

        S21.249 [7th] unspecified back wall of thorax without penetration into thoracic cavity

S21.9 [5th] Open wound of unspecified part of thorax

    Open wound of thoracic wall NOS

    S21.91X [7th] Laceration without FB of unspecified part of thorax

---

| [4th] | [5th] | [6th] | [7th] | Additional Character Required | ✔ | 3-character code | Unspecified laterality codes were excluded here. | • =New Code ▲ =Revised Code ▫ =Social determinants of health | *Excludes1*—Not coded here, do not use together *Excludes2*—Not included here |

S21.92X Laceration with FB of unspecified part of thorax
`7th`

S21.93X Puncture wound without FB of unspecified part of thorax
`7th`

S21.94X Puncture wound with FB of unspecified part of thorax
`7th`

S21.95X Open bite of unspecified part of thorax
`7th`
> *Excludes1:* superficial bite of thorax (S20.97)

S22 `4th` **FRACTURE OF RIB(S), STERNUM AND THORACIC SPINE**

Note: A fracture not indicated as displaced or nondisplaced should be coded to displaced
A fracture not indicated as open or closed should be coded to closed

Includes: fracture of thoracic neural arch
fracture of thoracic spinous process
fracture of thoracic transverse process
fracture of thoracic vertebra or of thoracic vertebral arch

Code first any associated:
injury of intrathoracic organ (S27.-)
spinal cord injury (S24.0-, S24.1-)

Excludes1: transection of thorax (S28.1)

Excludes2: fracture of clavicle (S42.0-)
fracture of scapula (S42.1-)

> 7th characters for category S22
> A—initial encounter for closed fracture
> B —initial encounter for open fracture
> D—subsequent encounter for fracture with routine healing
> G —subsequent encounter for fracture with delayed healing
> K—subsequent encounter for fracture with nonunion
> S—sequela

S22.2 **Fracture of sternum**

`5th` **S22.20X** Unspecified fracture of sternum
`7th`

S22.21X Fracture of manubrium
`7th`

S22.22X Fracture of body of sternum
`7th`

S22.23X Sternal manubrial dissociation
`7th`

S22.24X Fracture of xiphoid process
`7th`

S22.3 **Fracture of one rib**

`5th` **S22.31X** Fracture of one rib, right side
`7th`

S22.32X Fracture of one rib, left side
`7th`

S22.39X Fracture of one rib, unspecified side
`7th`

S22.4 **Multiple fractures of ribs**

`5th` Fractures of two or more ribs
Excludes1: flail chest (S22.5-)

S22.41X Multiple fractures of ribs, right side
`7th`

S22.42X Multiple fractures of ribs, left side
`7th`

S22.43X Multiple fractures of ribs, bilateral
`7th`

S22.49X Multiple fractures of ribs, unspecified side
`7th`

S22.5XX **Flail chest**
`7th`

S22.9XX **Fracture of bony thorax, part unspecified**
`7th`

S24 `4th` **INJURY OF NERVES AND SPINAL CORD AT THORAX LEVEL**

Note: Code to highest level of thoracic spinal cord injury
Injuries to the spinal cord (S24.0 and S24.1) refer to the cord level and not bone level injury, and can affect nerve roots at and below the level given.

Code also any associated:
fracture of thoracic vertebra (S22.0-)
open wound of thorax (S21.-)
transient paralysis (R29.5)

> 7th characters for category S24
> A—initial encounter
> D—subsequent encounter
> S—sequela

Excludes2: injury of brachial plexus (S14.3)

S24.0XX **Concussion and edema of thoracic spinal cord**
`7th`

S24.1 **Other and unspecified injuries of thoracic spinal cord**

`5th` **S24.10** Unspecified injury of thoracic spinal cord

`6th` **S24.101** Unspecified injury at; T1 level of thoracic spinal cord
`7th`

S24.102 T2–T6 level of thoracic spinal cord
`7th`

S24.103 T7–T10 level of thoracic spinal cord
`7th`

S24.104 T11–T12 level of thoracic spinal cord
`7th`

S24.109 unspecified level of thoracic spinal cord
`7th` Injury of thoracic spinal cord NOS

S27 `4th` **INJURY OF OTHER AND UNSPECIFIED INTRATHORACIC ORGANS**

Code also any associated open wound of thorax (S21.-)

Excludes2: injury of cervical esophagus (S10–S19)
injury of trachea (cervical) (S10–S19)

> 7th characters for category S27
> A—initial encounter
> D—subsequent encounter
> S—sequela

S27.0XX **Traumatic pneumothorax**
`7th` *Excludes1:* spontaneous pneumothorax (J93.-)

S27.3 **Other and unspecified injuries of lung**

`5th` **S27.30** Unspecified injury of lung

`6th` **S27.301** Unspecified injury of lung, unilateral
`7th`

S27.302 Unspecified injury of lung, bilateral
`7th`

S27.32 Contusion of lung

`6th` **S27.321** Contusion of lung, unilateral
`7th`

S27.322 Contusion of lung, bilateral
`7th`

S27.329 Contusion of lung, unspecified
`7th`

(S30–S39) INJURIES TO THE ABDOMEN, LOWER BACK, LUMBAR SPINE, PELVIS AND EXTERNAL GENITALS

Includes: injuries to the abdominal wall
injuries to the anus
injuries to the buttock
injuries to the external genitalia
injuries to the flank
injuries to the groin

Excludes2: burns and corrosions (T20–T32)
effects of FB in anus and rectum (T18.5)
effects of FB in genitourinary tract (T19.-)
effects of FB in stomach, small intestine and colon (T18.2–T18.4)
frostbite (T33–T34)
insect bite or sting, venomous (T63.4)

S30 `4th` **SUPERFICIAL INJURY OF ABDOMEN, LOWER BACK, PELVIS AND EXTERNAL GENITALS**

Excludes2: superficial injury of hip (S70.-)

S30.0XX **Contusion of lower back and pelvis**
`7th` Contusion of buttock

> 7th characters for category S30
> A—initial encounter
> D—subsequent encounter
> S—sequela

S30.1XX **Contusion of abdominal wall**
`7th` Contusion of flank
Contusion of groin

S30.2 **Contusion of external genital organs**

`5th` **S30.20** Contusion of unspecified external genital organ

`6th` **S30.201** Contusion of unspecified external genital organ, male
`7th`

S30.202 Contusion of unspecified external genital organ, female
`7th`

S30.21X Contusion of penis
`7th`

S30.22X Contusion of scrotum and testes
`7th`

S30.23X Contusion of vagina and vulva
`7th`

S30.3XX **Contusion of anus**
`7th`

• =New Code
▲ =Revised Code
▣ =Social determinants of health

Excludes1—Not coded here, do not use together
Excludes2—Not included here

S30.8 `5th` **Other superficial injuries of abdomen, lower back, pelvis and external genitals**

   S30.81 `6th` **Abrasion of abdomen, lower back, pelvis and external genitals**

      S30.810 `7th` **Abrasion of lower back and pelvis**

      S30.811 `7th` **Abrasion of abdominal wall**

      S30.812 `7th` **Abrasion of penis**

      S30.813 `7th` **Abrasion of scrotum and testes**

> 7th characters for category S30
> A—initial encounter
> D—subsequent encounter
> S—sequela

      S30.814 `7th` **Abrasion of vagina and vulva**

      S30.815 `7th` **Abrasion of unspecified external genital organs, male**

      S30.816 `7th` **Abrasion of unspecified external genital organs, female**

      S30.817 `7th` **Abrasion of anus**

   S30.82 `6th` **Blister (nonthermal) of abdomen, lower back, pelvis and external genitals**

      S30.820 `7th` **Blister (non-thermal) of lower back and pelvis**

      S30.821 `7th` **Blister (nonthermal) of abdominal wall**

      S30.822 `7th` **Blister (nonthermal) of penis**

      S30.823 `7th` **Blister (nonthermal) of scrotum and testes**

      S30.824 `7th` **Blister (nonthermal) of vagina and vulva**

      S30.825 `7th` **Blister (nonthermal) of unspecified external genital organs, male**

      S30.826 `7th` **Blister (nonthermal) of unspecified external genital organs, female**

      S30.827 `7th` **Blister (nonthermal) of anus**

   S30.84 `6th` **External constriction of abdomen, lower back, pelvis and external genitals**

      S30.840 `7th` **External constriction of lower back and pelvis**

      S30.841 `7th` **External constriction of abdominal wall**

      S30.842 `7th` **External constriction of penis**
        Hair tourniquet syndrome of penis
        Use additional cause code to identify the constricting item (W49.0-)

      S30.843 `7th` **External constriction of scrotum and testes**

      S30.844 `7th` **External constriction of vagina and vulva**

      S30.845 `7th` **External constriction of unspecified external genital organs, male**

      S30.846 `7th` **External constriction of unspecified external genital organs, female**

   S30.85 `6th` **Superficial FB of abdomen, lower back, pelvis and external genitals**
     Splinter in the abdomen, lower back, pelvis and external genitals

      S30.850 `7th` **Superficial FB of; lower back and pelvis**

      S30.851 `7th` **abdominal wall**

      S30.852 `7th` **penis**

      S30.853 `7th` **scrotum and testes**

      S30.854 `7th` **vagina and vulva**

      S30.855 `7th` **unspecified external genital organs, male**

      S30.856 `7th` **unspecified external genital organs, female**

      S30.857 `7th` **anus**

   S30.86 `6th` **Insect bite (nonvenomous) of abdomen, lower back, pelvis and external genitals**

      S30.860 `7th` **Insect bite (nonvenomous) of; lower back and pelvis**

      S30.861 `7th` **abdominal wall**

      S30.862 `7th` **penis**

      S30.863 `7th` **scrotum and testes**

      S30.864 `7th` **vagina and vulva**

      S30.865 `7th` **unspecified external genital organs, male**

      S30.866 `7th` **unspecified external genital organs, female**

      S30.867 `7th` **anus**

   S30.87 `6th` **Other superficial bite of abdomen, lower back, pelvis and external genitals**
     Excludes1: open bite of abdomen, lower back, pelvis and external genitals (S31.05, S31.15, S31.25, S31.35, S31.45, S31.55)

      S30.870 `7th` **Other superficial bite of; lower back and pelvis**

      S30.871 `7th` **abdominal wall**

      S30.872 `7th` **penis**

      S30.873 `7th` **scrotum and testes**

      S30.874 `7th` **vagina and vulva**

      S30.875 `7th` **unspecified external genital organs, male**

      S30.876 `7th` **unspecified external genital organs, female**

      S30.877 `7th` **anus**

S30.9 `5th` **Unspecified superficial injury of abdomen, lower back, pelvis and external genitals**

   S30.91X `7th` **Unspecified superficial injury of; lower back and pelvis**

   S30.92X `7th` **abdominal wall**

   S30.93X `7th` **penis**

   S30.94X `7th` **scrotum and testes**

   S30.95X `7th` **vagina and vulva**

   S30.96X `7th` **unspecified external genital organs, male**

   S30.97X `7th` **unspecified external genital organs, female**

   S30.98X `7th` **anus**

S31 `4th` **OPEN WOUND OF ABDOMEN, LOWER BACK, PELVIS AND EXTERNAL GENITALS**
Code also any associated:
  spinal cord injury (S24.0, S24.1-, S34.0-, S34.1-)
  wound infection
Excludes1: traumatic amputation of part of abdomen, lower back and pelvis (S38.2-, S38.3)
Excludes2: open wound of hip (S71.00–S71.02)
  open fracture of pelvis (S32.1–S32.9 with 7th character B)

> 7th characters for categories S31
> A—initial encounter
> D—subsequent encounter
> S—sequela

`4th` `5th` `6th` `7th` Additional Character Required   ✔   3-character code   Unspecified laterality codes were excluded here.

• =New Code
▲ =Revised Code
◻ =Social determinants of health

Excludes1—Not coded here, do not use together
Excludes2—Not included here

 PEDIATRIC ICD-10-CM 2022: A MANUAL FOR PROVIDER-BASED CODING   341

S31.0 **Open wound of lower back and**
5th **pelvis**

    S31.01 **Laceration without**
    6th **FB of lower back and**
    pelvis;

        S31.010 **without**
        7th **penetration into retroperitoneum**
        Laceration without FB of lower back and pelvis NOS

> For subcategory S31.0, use 6th character of 1 for penetration into the retroperitoneum, along with the appropriate 7th character.

    S31.02 **Laceration with FB of**
    6th **lower back and pelvis;**

        S31.020 **without**
        7th **penetration into retroperitoneum**
        Laceration with FB of lower back and pelvis NOS

> 7th characters for category S31
> A—initial encounter
> D—subsequent encounter
> S—sequela

    S31.03 **Puncture wound without FB of lower back and pelvis**
    6th
        S31.030 **Puncture wound without FB of lower**
        7th **back and pelvis without penetration into retroperitoneum**
        Puncture wound without FB of lower back and pelvis NOS

    S31.04 **Puncture wound with FB of lower back and pelvis**
    6th
        S31.040 **Puncture wound with FB of lower back**
        7th **and pelvis; without penetration into retroperitoneum**
        Puncture wound with FB of lower back and pelvis NOS

    S31.05 **Open bite of lower back and pelvis**
    6th Bite of lower back and pelvis NOS
    Excludes1: superficial bite of lower back and pelvis (S30.860, S30.870)

        S31.050 **Open bite of lower back and pelvis without**
        7th **penetration into retroperitoneum**
        Open bite of lower back and pelvis NOS

S31.1 **Open wound of abdominal wall without penetration into**
5th **peritoneal cavity**
Open wound of abdominal wall NOS
Excludes2: open wound of abdominal wall with penetration into peritoneal cavity (S31.6-)

    S31.11 **Laceration without FB of abdominal wall without**
    6th **penetration into peritoneal cavity**

        S31.110 **Laceration without FB of abdominal wall;**
        7th **RUQ without penetration into peritoneal cavity**
        S31.111 **LUQ without penetration into peritoneal**
        7th **cavity**
        S31.112 **epigastric region without penetration**
        7th **into peritoneal cavity**
        S31.113 **RLQ without penetration into peritoneal**
        7th **cavity**
        S31.114 **LLQ without penetration into peritoneal**
        7th **cavity**
        S31.115 **periumbilic region without penetration**
        7th **into peritoneal cavity**
        S31.119 **unspecified quadrant without**
        7th **penetration into peritoneal cavity**

    S31.12 **Laceration with FB of abdominal wall without**
    6th **penetration into peritoneal cavity**

        S31.120 **Laceration of abdominal wall with FB; RUQ**
        7th **without penetration into peritoneal cavity**
        S31.121 **LUQ without penetration into peritoneal**
        7th **cavity**
        S31.122 **epigastric region without penetration**
        7th **into peritoneal cavity**
        S31.123 **RLQ without penetration into peritoneal**
        7th **cavity**
        S31.124 **LLQ without penetration into peritoneal**
        7th **cavity**
        S31.125 **periumbilic region without penetration**
        7th **into peritoneal cavity**
        S31.129 **unspecified quadrant without**
        7th **penetration into peritoneal cavity**

S31.13 **Puncture wound of abdominal wall without FB**
6th **without penetration into peritoneal cavity**

    S31.130 **Puncture wound of abdominal wall**
    7th **without FB; RUQ without penetration into peritoneal cavity**
    S31.131 **LUQ without penetration into peritoneal**
    7th **cavity**
    S31.132 **epigastric region without penetration into peritoneal cavity**
    7th
    S31.133 **RLQ without penetration into peritoneal**
    7th **cavity**
    S31.134 **LLQ without penetration into peritoneal**
    7th **cavity**
    S31.135 **periumbilic region without penetration into peritoneal cavity**
    7th
    S31.139 **unspecified quadrant without penetration into peritoneal cavity**
    7th

S31.14 **Puncture wound of abdominal wall with FB without**
6th **penetration into peritoneal cavity**

    S31.140 **Puncture wound of abdominal wall**
    7th **with FB; RUQ without penetration into peritoneal cavity**
    S31.141 **LUQ without penetration into peritoneal**
    7th **cavity**
    S31.142 **epigastric region without penetration into peritoneal cavity**
    7th
    S31.143 **RLQ without penetration into peritoneal**
    7th **cavity**
    S31.144 **LLQ without penetration into peritoneal**
    7th **cavity**
    S31.145 **periumbilic region without penetration into peritoneal cavity**
    7th
    S31.149 **unspecified quadrant without penetration into peritoneal cavity**
    7th

S31.15 **Open bite of abdominal wall without penetration into**
6th **peritoneal cavity**
Bite of abdominal wall NOS
Excludes1: superficial bite of abdominal wall (S30.871)

    S31.150 **Open bite of abdominal wall; RUQ without**
    7th **penetration into peritoneal cavity**
    S31.151 **LUQ without penetration into peritoneal**
    7th **cavity**
    S31.152 **epigastric region without penetration into peritoneal cavity**
    7th
    S31.153 **RLQ without penetration into peritoneal cavity**
    7th
    S31.154 **LLQ without penetration into peritoneal**
    7th **cavity**
    S31.155 **periumbilic region without penetration into peritoneal cavity**
    7th
    S31.159 **unspecified quadrant without penetration into peritoneal cavity**
    7th

S31.2 **Open wound of penis**
5th **S31.21X** **Laceration without FB of penis**
    7th
    S31.23X **Puncture wound without foreign body of penis**
    7th
    S31.24X **Puncture wound with foreign body of penis**
    7th
    S31.25X **Open bite of penis**
    7th Bite of penis NOS
    Excludes1: superficial bite of penis (S30.862, S30.872)

S31.3 **Open wound of scrotum and testes**
5th **S31.31X** **Laceration without FB of scrotum and testes**
    7th
    S31.33X **Puncture wound without foreign body of scrotum**
    7th **and testes**
    S31.34X **Puncture wound with foreign body of scrotum and**
    7th **testes**
    S31.35X **Open bite of scrotum and testes**
    7th Bite of scrotum and testes NOS
    Excludes1: superficial bite of scrotum and testes (S30.863, S30.873)

4th	5th	6th	7th	Additional Character Required	✓	3-character code

Unspecified laterality codes were excluded here.

• =New Code
▲ =Revised Code
¤ =Social determinants of health

Excludes1—Not coded here, do not use together
Excludes2—Not included here

S31.4   **Open wound of vagina and vulva**
`5th`   *Excludes1:* injury to vagina and vulva during delivery (O70.-, O71.4)

    S31.41X   **Laceration without FB of vagina and vulva**
    `7th`

    S31.42X   **Laceration with FB of vagina and vulva**
    `7th`

    S31.43X   **Puncture wound without FB of vagina and vulva**
    `7th`

    S31.44X   **Puncture wound with FB of vagina and vulva**
    `7th`

    S31.45X   **Open bite of vagina and vulva**
    `7th`   Bite of vagina and vulva NOS

    Excludes1: superficial bite of vagina and vulva (S30.864, S30.874)

> **7th characters for category S31**
> A—initial encounter
> D—subsequent encounter
> S—sequela

S31.8   **Open wound of other parts of abdomen, lower back and pelvis**
`5th`

    S31.81   **Open wound of right buttock**
    `6th`
       S31.811   **Laceration without FB of right buttock**
       `7th`

       S31.812   **Laceration with FB of right buttock**
       `7th`

       S31.813   **Puncture wound without FB of right buttock**
       `7th`

       S31.814   **Puncture wound with FB of right buttock**
       `7th`

       S31.815   **Open bite of right buttock**
       `7th`   Bite of right buttock NOS
       Excludes1: superficial bite of buttock (S30.870)

    S31.82   **Open wound of left buttock**
    `6th`
       S31.821   **Laceration without FB of left buttock**
       `7th`

       S31.822   **Laceration with FB of left buttock**
       `7th`

       S31.823   **Puncture wound without FB of left buttock**
       `7th`

       S31.824   **Puncture wound with FB of left buttock**
       `7th`

       S31.825   **Open bite of left buttock**
       `7th`   Bite of left buttock NOS
       Excludes1: superficial bite of buttock (S30.870)

    S31.83   **Open wound of anus**
    `6th`
       S31.831   **Laceration without FB of anus**
       `7th`

       S31.832   **Laceration with FB of anus**
       `7th`

       S31.833   **Puncture wound without FB of anus**
       `7th`

       S31.834   **Puncture wound with FB of anus**
       `7th`

       S31.835   **Open bite of anus**
       `7th`   Bite of anus NOS
       Excludes1: superficial bite of anus (S30.877)

S32   **FRACTURE OF LUMBAR SPINE AND PELVIS**
`4th`   **Note:** A fracture not indicated as displaced or nondisplaced should be coded to displaced
A fracture not indicated as opened or closed should be coded to closed
Includes: fracture of lumbosacral neural arch
    fracture of lumbosacral spinous process
    fracture of lumbosacral transverse process
    fracture of lumbosacral vertebra or of lumbosacral vertebral arch
Code first any associated spinal cord and spinal nerve injury (S34.-)
Excludes1: transection of abdomen (S38.3)
Excludes2: fracture of hip NOS (S72.0-)

> **7th characters for category S32**
> A—initial encounter for closed fracture
> B—initial encounter for open fracture
> D—subsequent encounter for fracture with routine healing
> G—subsequent encounter for fracture with delayed healing
> K—subsequent encounter for fracture with nonunion
> S—sequela

S32.1   **Fracture of sacrum**
`5th`   For vertical fractures, code to most medial fracture extension
Use two codes if both a vertical and transverse fracture are present
Code also any associated fracture of pelvic ring (S32.8-)

    S32.10X   **Unspecified fracture of sacrum**
    `7th`

    S32.11   **Zone I fracture of sacrum**
    `6th`   **Vertical sacral ala fracture of sacrum**
       S32.110   **Nondisplaced Zone I fracture of sacrum**
       `7th`

       S32.111   **Minimally displaced Zone I fracture of sacrum**
       `7th`
       S32.112   **Severely displaced Zone I fracture of sacrum**
       `7th`
       S32.119   **Unspecified Zone I fracture of sacrum**

    S32.12   **Zone II fracture of sacrum**
    `6th`   Vertical foraminal region fracture of sacrum
       S32.120   **Nondisplaced Zone II fracture of sacrum**
       `7th`

       S32.121   **Minimally displaced Zone II fracture of sacrum**
       `7th`
       S32.122   **Severely displaced Zone II fracture of sacrum**
       `7th`
       S32.129   **Unspecified Zone II fracture of sacrum**
       `7th`

    S32.13   **Zone III fracture of sacrum**
    `6th`   Vertical fracture into spinal canal region of sacrum
       S32.130   **Nondisplaced Zone III fracture of sacrum**
       `7th`

       S32.131   **Minimally displaced Zone III fracture of sacrum**
       `7th`
       S32.132   **Severely displaced Zone III fracture of sacrum**
       `7th`
       S32.139   **Unspecified Zone III fracture of sacrum**
       `7th`

    S32.14X   **Type 1 fracture of sacrum**
    `7th`   Transverse flexion fracture of sacrum without displacement

    S32.15X   **Type 2 fracture of sacrum**
    `7th`   Transverse flexion fracture of sacrum with posterior displacement

    S32.16X   **Type 3 fracture of sacrum**
    `7th`   Transverse extension fracture of sacrum with anterior displacement

    S32.17X   **Type 4 fracture of sacrum**
    `7th`   Transverse segmental comminution of upper sacrum

    S32.19X   **Other fracture of sacrum**

S32.2XX   **Fracture of coccyx**
`7th`

S32.3   **Fracture of ilium**
`5th`   *Excludes1:* fracture of ilium with associated disruption of pelvic ring (S32.8-)

    S32.30   **Unspecified fracture of ilium**
    `6th`
       S32.301   **Unspecified fracture of right ilium**
       `7th`

       S32.302   **Unspecified fracture of left ilium**
       `7th`

       S32.309   **Unspecified fracture of unspecified ilium**
       `7th`

    S32.31   **Avulsion fracture of ilium**
    `6th`
       S32.311   **Displaced avulsion fracture of right ilium**
       `7th`

       S32.312   **Displaced avulsion fracture of left ilium**
       `7th`

       S32.313   **Displaced avulsion fracture of unspecified ilium**
       `7th`
       S32.314   **Nondisplaced avulsion fracture of right ilium**
       `7th`
       S32.315   **Nondisplaced avulsion fracture of left ilium**
       `7th`
       S32.316   **Nondisplaced avulsion fracture of unspecified ilium**
       `7th`

`4th` `5th` `6th` `7th`   Additional Character Required   ✓   3-character code   Unspecified laterality codes were excluded here.

• =New Code
▲ =Revised Code
☐ =Social determinants of health

Excludes1—Not coded here, do not use together
Excludes2—Not included here

CHAPTER 19. INJURY, POISONING AND CERTAIN OTHER CONSEQUENCES OF EXTERNAL CAUSES   (S32.39–S32.81)

S32.39 Other fracture of ilium

    6th **S32.391** Other fracture of right ilium
        7th

    S32.392 Other fracture of left ilium
        7th

    S32.399 Other fracture of unspecified ilium
        7th

S32.4 Fracture of acetabulum
  5th **Code also** any associated fracture of pelvic ring (S32.8-)

    S32.40 Unspecified fracture of acetabulum
    6th

        S32.401 Unspecified fracture of right acetabulum
        7th

        S32.402 Unspecified fracture of left acetabulum
        7th

> 7th characters for category S32
> A—initial encounter for closed fracture
> B—initial encounter for open fracture
> D—subsequent encounter for fracture with routine healing
> G—subsequent encounter for fracture with delayed healing
> K—subsequent encounter for fracture with nonunion
> S—sequela

    S32.41 Fracture of anterior wall of acetabulum
    6th

        S32.411 Displaced fracture of anterior wall of right acetabulum
        7th

        S32.412 Displaced fracture of anterior wall of left acetabulum
        7th

        S32.414 Nondisplaced fracture of anterior wall of right acetabulum
        7th

        S32.415 Nondisplaced fracture of anterior wall of left acetabulum
        7th

    S32.42 Fracture of posterior wall of acetabulum
    6th

        S32.421 Displaced fracture of posterior wall of right acetabulum
        7th

        S32.422 Displaced fracture of posterior wall of left acetabulum
        7th

        S32.424 Nondisplaced fracture of posterior wall of right acetabulum
        7th

        S32.425 Nondisplaced fracture of posterior wall of left acetabulum
        7th

    S32.43 Fracture of anterior column [iliopubic] of acetabulum
    6th

        S32.431 Displaced fracture of anterior column [iliopubic] of right acetabulum
        7th

        S32.432 Displaced fracture of anterior column [iliopubic] of left acetabulum
        7th

        S32.434 Nondisplaced fracture of anterior column [iliopubic] of right aceta-bulum
        7th

        S32.435 Nondisplaced fracture of anterior column [iliopubic] of left aceta-bulum
        7th

    S32.44 Fracture of posterior column [ilioischial] of acetabulum
    6th

        S32.441 Displaced fracture of posterior column [ilioischial] of right acetabulum
        7th

        S32.442 Displaced fracture of posterior column [ilioischial] of left acetabulum
        7th

        S32.444 Nondisplaced fracture of posterior column [ilioischial] of right acetabulum
        7th

        S32.445 Nondisplaced fracture of posterior column [ilioischial] of left acetabulum
        7th

    S32.45 Transverse fracture of acetabulum
    6th

        S32.451 Displaced transverse fracture of right acetabulum
        7th

        S32.452 Displaced transverse fracture of left acetabulum
        7th

        S32.454 Nondisplaced transverse fracture of right acetabulum
        7th

        S32.455 Nondisplaced transverse fracture of left acetabulum
        7th

        S32.456 Nondisplaced transverse fracture of unspecified acetabulum
        7th

    S32.46 Associated transverse-posterior fracture of acetabulum
    6th

        S32.461 Displaced associated transverse-posterior fracture of right acetabulum
        7th

        S32.462 Displaced associated transverse-posterior fracture of left acetabulum
        7th

        S32.464 Nondisplaced associated transverse-posterior fracture of right acetabulum
        7th

        S32.465 Nondisplaced associated transverse-posterior fracture of left acetabulum
        7th

    S32.47 Fracture of medial wall of acetabulum
    6th

        S32.471 Displaced fracture of medial wall of right acetabulum
        7th

        S32.472 Displaced fracture of medial wall of left acetabulum
        7th

        S32.474 Nondisplaced fracture of medial wall of right acetabulum
        7th

        S32.475 Nondisplaced fracture of medial wall of left acetabulum
        7th

    S32.48 Dome fracture of acetabulum
    6th

        S32.481 Displaced dome fracture of right acetabulum
        7th

        S32.482 Displaced dome fracture of left acetabulum
        7th

        S32.484 Nondisplaced dome fracture of right acetabulum
        7th

        S32.485 Nondisplaced dome fracture of left acetabulum
        7th

    S32.49 Other specified fracture of acetabulum
    6th

        S32.491 Other specified fracture of right acetabulum
        7th

        S32.492 Other specified fracture of left acetabulum
        7th

S32.5 Fracture of pubis
  5th ***Excludes1:*** fracture of pubis with associated disruption of pelvic ring (S32.8-)

    S32.50 Unspecified fracture of pubis
    6th

        S32.501 Unspecified fracture of right pubis
        7th

        S32.502 Unspecified fracture of left pubis
        7th

    S32.51 Fracture of superior rim of pubis
    6th

        S32.511 Fracture of superior rim of right pubis
        7th

        S32.512 Fracture of superior rim of left pubis
        7th

    S32.59 Other specified fracture of pubis
    6th

        S32.591 Other specified fracture of right pubis
        7th

        S32.592 Other specified fracture of left pubis
        7th

S32.6 Fracture of ischium
  5th ***Excludes1:*** fracture of ischium with associated disruption of pelvic ring (S32.8-)

    S32.60 Unspecified fracture of ischium
    6th

        S32.601 Unspecified fracture of right ischium
        7th

        S32.602 Unspecified fracture of left ischium
        7th

    S32.61 Avulsion fracture of ischium
    6th

        S32.611 Displaced avulsion fracture of right ischium
        7th

        S32.612 Displaced avulsion fracture of left ischium
        7th

        S32.614 Nondisplaced avulsion fracture of right ischium
        7th

        S32.615 Nondisplaced avulsion fracture of left ischium
        7th

    S32.69 Other specified fracture of ischium
    6th

        S32.691 Other specified fracture of right ischium
        7th

        S32.692 Other specified fracture of left ischium
        7th

S32.8 Fracture of other parts of pelvis
  5th **Code also** any associated: fracture of acetabulum (S32.4-)
                          sacral fracture (S32.1-)

    S32.81 Multiple fractures of pelvis with disruption of pelvic ring
    6th
        Multiple pelvic fractures with disruption of pelvic circle

4th 5th 6th 7th Additional Character Required ✓ 3-character code   Unspecified laterality codes were excluded here.   • =New Code ▲ =Revised Code ¤ =Social determinants of health   ***Excludes1***—Not coded here, do not use together ***Excludes***—Not included here

344   PEDIATRIC ICD-10-CM 2022: A MANUAL FOR PROVIDER-BASED CODING

S32.810 **Multiple fractures of pelvis with stable disruption of pelvic ring**
7th

S32.811 **Multiple fractures of pelvis with unstable disruption of pelvic ring**
7th

S32.82X **Multiple fractures of pelvis without disruption of pelvic ring**
7th
Multiple pelvic fractures without disruption of pelvic circle

S32.89X **Fracture of other parts of pelvis**
7th

S32.9XX **Fracture of unspecified parts of lumbosacral spine and pelvis**
7th
Fracture of lumbosacral spine NOS
Fracture of pelvis NOS

S33 **DISLOCATION AND SPRAIN OF JOINTS AND LIGAMENTS OF LUMBAR SPINE AND PELVIS**
4th
Includes: avulsion of joint or ligament of lumbar spine and pelvis
laceration of cartilage, joint or ligament of lumbar spine and pelvis
sprain of cartilage, joint or ligament of lumbar spine and pelvis
traumatic hemarthrosis of joint or ligament of lumbar spine and pelvis
traumatic rupture of joint or ligament of lumbar spine and pelvis
traumatic subluxation of joint or ligament of lumbar spine and pelvis
traumatic tear of joint or ligament of lumbar spine and pelvis

7th characters for category S33
A—initial encounter
D—subsequent encounter
S—sequela

Code also any associated open wound
Excludes1: nontraumatic rupture or displacement of lumbar intervertebral disc NOS (M51.-)
obstetric damage to pelvic joints and ligaments (O71.6)
Excludes2: dislocation and sprain of joints and ligaments of hip (S73.-)
strain of muscle of lower back and pelvis (S39.01-)

S33.2XX **Dislocation of sacroiliac and sacrococcygeal joint**
7th

S33.5XX **Sprain of ligaments of lumbar spine**
7th

S33.6XX **Sprain of sacroiliac joint**
7th

S33.8XX **Sprain of other parts of lumbar spine and pelvis**
7th

S33.9XX **Sprain of unspecified parts of lumbar spine and pelvis**
7th

S34 **INJURY OF LUMBAR AND SACRAL SPINAL CORD AND NERVES AT ABDOMEN, LOWER BACK AND PELVIS LEVEL**
4th
Note: Code to highest level of lumbar cord injury
Injuries to the spinal cord (S34.0 and S34.1) refer to the cord level and not bone level injury, and can affect nerve roots at and below the level given.

7th characters for category S34
A—initial encounter
D—subsequent encounter
S—sequela

Code also any associated: fracture of vertebra (S22.0-, S32.0-)
open wound of abdomen, lower back and pelvis (S31.-)
transient paralysis (R29.5)

S34.0 **Concussion and edema of lumbar and sacral spinal cord**
5th
S34.01X **Concussion and edema of lumbar spinal cord**
7th

S34.02X **Concussion and edema of sacral spinal cord**
7th
Concussion and edema of conus medullaris

S34.1 **Other and unspecified injury of lumbar and sacral spinal cord**
5th
S34.10 **Unspecified injury to lumbar spinal cord (level)**
6th
S34.101 **Unspecified injury to; L1 level of lumbar spinal cord**
7th
S34.102 **L2 level of lumbar spinal cord**
7th
S34.103 **L3 level of lumbar spinal cord**
7th
S34.104 **L4 level of lumbar spinal cord**
7th
S34.105 **L5 level of lumbar spinal cord**
7th
S34.109 **unspecified level of lumbar spinal cord**
7th

S34.12 **Incomplete lesion of lumbar spinal cord (level)**
6th
S34.121 **Incomplete lesion of; L1 level of lumbar spinal cord**
7th
S34.123 **L3 level of lumbar spinal cord**
7th
S34.124 **L4 level of lumbar spinal cord**
7th
S34.125 **L5 level of lumbar spinal cord**
7th
S34.129 **unspecified level of lumbar spinal cord**
7th

S34.13 **Other and unspecified injury to sacral spinal cord**
6th
Other injury to conus medullaris
S34.131 **Complete lesion of sacral spinal cord**
7th
Complete lesion of conus medullaris
S34.132 **Incomplete lesion of sacral spinal cord**
7th
Incomplete lesion of conus medullaris
S34.139 **Unspecified injury to sacral spinal cord**
7th
Unspecified injury of conus medullaris

S34.2 **Injury of nerve root of lumbar and sacral spine**
5th
S34.21X **Injury of nerve root of lumbar spine**
7th

S34.22X **Injury of nerve root of sacral spine**
7th

S34.3XX **Injury of cauda equina**
7th

S34.4XX **Injury of lumbosacral plexus**
7th

S34.5XX **Injury of lumbar, sacral and pelvic sympathetic nerves**
7th
Injury of celiac ganglion or plexus
Injury of hypogastric plexus
Injury of mesenteric plexus (inferior) (superior)
Injury of splanchnic nerve

S34.6XX **Injury of peripheral nerve(s) at abdomen, lower back and pelvis level**
7th

S34.8XX **Injury of other nerves at abdomen, lower back and pelvis level**
7th

S34.9XX **Injury of unspecified nerves at abdomen, lower back and pelvis level**
7th

S36 **INJURY OF INTRA-ABDOMINAL ORGANS**
4th
Code also any associated open wound (S31.-)
S36.0 **Injury of spleen**
5th
S36.02 **Contusion of spleen**
6th
S36.020 **Minor contusion of spleen**
7th
Contusion of spleen less than 2 cm
S36.021 **Major contusion of spleen**
7th
Contusion of spleen greater than 2 cm
S36.03 **Laceration of spleen**
6th
S36.030 **Superficial (capsular) laceration of spleen**
7th

7th characters for category S36
A—initial encounter
D—subsequent encounter
S—sequela

Laceration of spleen less than 1 cm
Minor laceration of spleen
S36.032 **Major laceration of spleen**
7th
Avulsion of spleen
Laceration of spleen greater than 3 cm
Massive laceration of spleen
Multiple moderate lacerations of spleen
Stellate laceration of spleen

S36.3 **Injury of stomach**
5th
S36.30 **Unspecified injury of stomach**
S36.32 **Contusion of stomach**
S36.6 **Injury of rectum**
5th
S36.60X **Unspecified injury of rectum**
7th
S36.62X **Contusion of rectum**
7th
S36.63X **Laceration of rectum**
7th

CHAPTER 19. INJURY, POISONING AND CERTAIN OTHER CONSEQUENCES OF EXTERNAL CAUSES (S32.810–S36.63X)

4th 5th 6th 7th Additional Character Required ✓ 3-character code Unspecified laterality codes were excluded here.

• =New Code
▲ =Revised Code
▱ =Social determinants of health

Excludes1—Not coded here, do not use together
Excludes2—Not included here

CHAPTER 19. INJURY, POISONING AND CERTAIN OTHER CONSEQUENCES OF EXTERNAL CAUSES   (S36.9–S40.861)

S36.9   Injury of unspecified intra-abdominal organ

5th   **S36.90X**   Unspecified injury of unspecified intra-abdominal organ

7th

     S36.92X   Contusion of unspecified intra-abdominal organ

7th

     S36.93X   Laceration of unspecified intra-abdominal organ

7th

     S36.99X   Other injury of unspecified intra-abdominal organ

7th

S37   **INJURY OF URINARY AND PELVIC ORGANS**

4th

Code also any associated open wound (S31.-)

Excludes1: obstetric trauma to pelvic organs (O71.-)

Excludes2: injury of peritoneum (S36.81)

    injury of retroperitoneum (S36.89-)

S37.0   Injury of kidney

5th   *Excludes2:* acute kidney injury (nontraumatic) (N17.9)

> 7th characters for category S37
> A—initial encounter
> D—subsequent encounter
> S—sequela

    S37.01   Minor contusion of kidney

6th   Contusion of kidney less than 2 cm

    Contusion of kidney NOS

     S37.011   Minor contusion of right kidney

7th

     S37.012   Minor contusion of left kidney

7th

    S37.02   Major contusion of kidney

6th   Contusion of kidney greater than 2 cm

     S37.021   Major contusion of right kidney

7th

     S37.022   Major contusion of left kidney

7th

S39   **OTHER AND UNSPECIFIED INJURIES OF ABDOMEN, LOWER BACK, PELVIS AND EXTERNAL GENITALS**

4th

Code also any associated open wound (S31.-)

Excludes2: sprain of joints and ligaments of lumbar spine and pelvis (S33.-)

S39.0   Injury of muscle, fascia and tendon of abdomen, lower back and pelvis

5th

    S39.01   Strain of muscle, fascia and tendon of abdomen, lower back and pelvis

6th

> 7th characters for category S39
> A—initial encounter
> D—subsequent encounter
> S—sequela

     S39.011   Strain of muscle, fascia and tendon of abdomen

7th

     S39.012   Strain of muscle, fascia and tendon of lower back

7th

S39.8   Other specified injuries of abdomen, lower back, pelvis and external genitals

5th

    S39.83X   Other specified injuries of pelvis

7th

    S39.84   Other specified injuries of external genitals

6th   **S39.848**   Other specified injuries of external genitals

7th

S39.9   Unspecified injury of abdomen, lower back, pelvis and external genitals

5th

    S39.91X   Unspecified injury of abdomen

7th

    S39.92X   Unspecified injury of lower back

7th

    S39.93X   Unspecified injury of pelvis

7th

    S39.94X   Unspecified injury of external genitals

7th

(S40–S49) INJURIES TO THE SHOULDER AND UPPER ARM

Includes: injuries of axilla

    injuries of scapular region

Excludes2: burns and corrosions (T20–T32)

    frostbite (T33–T34)

    injuries of elbow (S50–S59)

    insect bite or sting, venomous (T63.4)

S40   **SUPERFICIAL INJURY OF SHOULDER AND UPPER ARM**

4th

S40.0   Contusion of shoulder and upper arm

5th

    S40.01   Contusion of shoulder

6th   **S40.011**   Contusion of right shoulder

7th

     S40.012   Contusion of left shoulder

7th

> 7th characters for category S40
> A—initial encounter
> D—subsequent encounter
> S—sequela

    S40.02   Contusion of upper arm

6th   **S40.021**   Contusion of right upper arm

7th

     S40.022   Contusion of left upper arm

7th

S40.2   Other superficial injuries of shoulder

5th

    S40.21   Abrasion of shoulder

6th   **S40.211**   Abrasion of right shoulder

7th

     S40.212   Abrasion of left shoulder

7th

    S40.22   Blister (nonthermal) of shoulder

6th   **S40.221**   Blister (nonthermal) of right shoulder

7th

     S40.222   Blister (nonthermal) of left shoulder

7th

    S40.24   External constriction of shoulder

6th   **S40.241**   External constriction of right shoulder

7th

     S40.242   External constriction of left shoulder

7th

    S40.25   Superficial FB of shoulder

6th   Splinter in the shoulder

     S40.251   Superficial FB of right shoulder

7th

     S40.252   Superficial FB of left shoulder

7th

    S40.26   Insect bite (nonvenomous) of shoulder

6th   **S40.261**   Insect bite (nonvenomous) of right shoulder

7th

     S40.262   Insect bite (nonvenomous) of left shoulder

7th

    S40.27   Other superficial bite of shoulder

6th   *Excludes1:* open bite of shoulder (S41.05)

     S40.271   Other superficial bite of right shoulder

7th

     S40.272   Other superficial bite of left shoulder

7th

S40.8   Other superficial injuries of upper arm

5th

    S40.81   Abrasion of upper arm

6th   **S40.811**   Abrasion of right upper arm

7th

     S40.812   Abrasion of left upper arm

7th

    S40.82   Blister (nonthermal) of upper arm

6th   **S40.821**   Blister (nonthermal) of right upper arm

7th

     S40.822   Blister (nonthermal) of left upper arm

7th

    S40.84   External constriction of upper arm

6th   **S40.841**   External constriction of right upper arm

7th

     S40.842   External constriction of left upper arm

7th

    S40.85   Superficial FB of upper arm

6th   Splinter in the upper arm

     S40.851   Superficial FB of right upper arm

7th

     S40.852   Superficial FB of left upper arm

7th

    S40.86   Insect bite (nonvenomous) of upper arm

6th   **S40.861**   Insect bite (nonvenomous) of right upper arm

7th

4th   **5th**   **6th**   **7th**   Additional Character Required   ✓   3-character code

Unspecified laterality codes were excluded here.

• =New Code
▲ =Revised Code
▫ =Social determinants of health

Excludes1—Not coded here, do not use together
Excludes2—Not included here

S40.862 `7th` Insect bite (nonvenomous) of left upper arm

S40.87 `6th` Other superficial bite of upper arm
Excludes1: open bite of upper arm (S41.14)
Excludes2: other superficial bite of shoulder (S40.27-)

   S40.871 `7th` Other superficial bite of right upper arm

   S40.872 `7th` Other superficial bite of left upper arm

S40.9 `5th` Unspecified superficial injury of shoulder and upper arm

   S40.91 `6th` Unspecified superficial injury of shoulder

      S40.911 `7th` Unspecified superficial injury of right shoulder

      S40.912 `7th` Unspecified superficial injury of left shoulder

   S40.92 `6th` Unspecified superficial injury of upper arm

      S40.921 `7th` Unspecified superficial injury of right upper arm

      S40.922 `7th` Unspecified superficial injury of left upper arm

> 7th characters for categories S40 & S41
> A—initial encounter
> D—subsequent encounter
> S—sequela

S41 `4th` OPEN WOUND OF SHOULDER AND UPPER ARM

Code also any associated wound infection
Excludes1: traumatic amputation of shoulder and upper arm (S48.-)
Excludes2: open fracture of shoulder and upper arm (S42.- with 7th character B or C)

S41.0 `5th` Open wound of shoulder

   S41.01 `6th` Laceration without FB of shoulder

      S41.011 `7th` Laceration without FB of right shoulder

      S41.012 `7th` Laceration without FB of left shoulder

   S41.02 `6th` Laceration with FB of shoulder

      S41.021 `7th` Laceration with FB of right shoulder

      S41.022 `7th` Laceration with FB of left shoulder

   S41.03 `6th` Puncture wound without FB of shoulder

      S41.031 `7th` Puncture wound without FB of right shoulder

      S41.032 `7th` Puncture wound without FB of left shoulder

   S41.04 `6th` Puncture wound with FB of shoulder

      S41.041 `7th` Puncture wound with FB of right shoulder

      S41.042 `7th` Puncture wound with FB of left shoulder

   S41.05 `6th` Open bite of shoulder
Bite of shoulder NOS
Excludes1: superficial bite of shoulder (S40.27)

      S41.051 `7th` Open bite of right shoulder

      S41.052 `7th` Open bite of left shoulder

S41.1 `5th` Open wound of upper arm

   S41.11 `6th` Laceration without FB of upper arm

      S41.111 `7th` Laceration without FB of right upper arm

      S41.112 `7th` Laceration without FB of left upper arm

   S41.12 `6th` Laceration with FB of upper arm

      S41.121 `7th` Laceration with FB of right upper arm

      S41.122 `7th` Laceration with FB of left upper arm

   S41.13 `6th` Puncture wound without FB of upper arm

      S41.131 `7th` Puncture wound without FB of right upper arm

      S41.132 `7th` Puncture wound without FB of left upper arm

   S41.14 Puncture wound with FB of upper arm

      S41.141 `6th` Puncture wound with FB of right upper arm

      S41.142 `7th` Puncture wound with FB of left upper arm

   S41.15 `6th` Open bite of upper arm
Bite of upper arm NOS
Excludes1: superficial bite of upper arm (S40.87)

      S41.151 `7th` Open bite of right upper arm

      S41.152 `7th` Open bite of left upper arm

S42 `4th` FRACTURE OF SHOULDER AND UPPER ARM

Note: A fracture not indicated as displaced or nondisplaced should be coded to displaced
A fracture not indicated as open or closed should be coded to closed
Excludes1: traumatic amputation of shoulder and upper arm (S48.-)

S42.0 `5th` Fracture of clavicle

   S42.00 `6th` Fracture of unspecified part of clavicle

      S42.001 `7th` Fracture of unspecified part of right clavicle

      S42.002 `7th` Fracture of unspecified part of left clavicle

> 7th characters for category S42
> A—initial encounter for closed fracture
> B—initial encounter for open fracture
> D—subsequent encounter for fracture with routine healing
> G—subsequent encounter for fracture with delayed healing
> K—subsequent encounter for fracture with nonunion
> P—subsequent encounter for fracture with malunion
> S—sequela

   S42.01 `6th` Fracture of sternal end of clavicle

      S42.011 `7th` Anterior displaced fracture of sternal end of right clavicle

      S42.012 `7th` Anterior displaced fracture of sternal end of left clavicle

      S42.014 `7th` Posterior displaced fracture of sternal end of right clavicle

      S42.015 `7th` Posterior displaced fracture of sternal end of left clavicle

      S42.017 `7th` Nondisplaced fracture of sternal end of right clavicle

      S42.018 `7th` Nondisplaced fracture of sternal end of left clavicle

   S42.02 `6th` Fracture of shaft of clavicle

      S42.021 `7th` Displaced fracture of shaft of right clavicle

      S42.022 `7th` Displaced fracture of shaft of left clavicle

      S42.024 `7th` Nondisplaced fracture of shaft of right clavicle

      S42.025 `7th` Nondisplaced fracture of shaft of left clavicle

   S42.03 `6th` Fracture of lateral end of clavicle
Fracture of acromial end of clavicle

      S42.031 `7th` Displaced fracture of lateral end of right clavicle

      S42.032 `7th` Displaced fracture of lateral end of left clavicle

      S42.034 `7th` Nondisplaced fracture of lateral end of right clavicle

      S42.035 `7th` Nondisplaced fracture of lateral end of left clavicle

S42.2 `5th` Fracture of upper end of humerus
Fracture of proximal end of humerus
Excludes2: fracture of shaft of humerus (S42.3-)
physeal fracture of upper end of humerus (S49.0-)

   S42.20 `6th` Unspecified fracture of upper end of; humerus

      S42.201 `7th` right humerus

      S42.202 `7th` left humerus

   S42.21 `6th` Unspecified fracture of surgical neck of humerus
Fracture of neck of humerus NOS

`4th` `5th` `6th` `7th` Additional Character Required ✓ 3-character code Unspecified laterality codes were excluded here. • =New Code ▲ =Revised Code ◨ =Social determinants of health *Excludes1*—Not coded here, do not use together *Excludes2*—Not included here

CHAPTER 19. INJURY, POISONING AND CERTAIN OTHER CONSEQUENCES OF EXTERNAL CAUSES   (S42.211–S42.40)

S42.211 **7th** Unspecified displaced fracture of surgical neck of right humerus

S42.212 **7th** Unspecified displaced fracture of surgical neck of left humerus

S42.214 **7th** Unspecified nondisplaced fracture of surgical neck of right humerus

S42.215 **7th** Unspecified nondisplaced fracture of surgical neck of left humerus

S42.22 **6th** 2-part fracture of surgical neck of humerus

S42.221 **7th** 2-part displaced fracture of surgical neck of right humerus

S42.222 **7th** 2-part displaced fracture of surgical neck of left humerus

> 7th characters for category S42
> A—initial encounter for closed fracture
> B—initial encounter for open fracture
> D—subsequent encounter for fracture with routine healing
> G—subsequent encounter for fracture with delayed healing
> K—subsequent encounter for fracture with nonunion
> P—subsequent encounter for fracture with malunion
> S—sequela

S42.224 **7th** 2-part nondisplaced fracture of surgical neck of right humerus

S42.225 **7th** 2-part nondisplaced fracture of surgical neck of left humerus

S42.23 **6th** 3-part fracture of surgical neck of humerus

S42.231 **7th** 3-part fracture of surgical neck of right humerus

S42.232 **7th** 3-part fracture of surgical neck of left humerus

S42.24 **6th** 4-part fracture of surgical neck of humerus

S42.241 **7th** 4-part fracture of surgical neck of right humerus

S42.242 **7th** 4-part fracture of surgical neck of left humerus

S42.25 **6th** Fracture of greater tuberosity of humerus

S42.251 **7th** Displaced fracture of greater tuberosity of right humerus

S42.252 **7th** Displaced fracture of greater tuberosity of left humerus

S42.254 **7th** Nondisplaced fracture of greater tuberosity of right humerus

S42.255 **7th** Nondisplaced fracture of greater tuberosity of left humerus

S42.26 **6th** Fracture of lesser tuberosity of humerus

S42.261 **7th** Displaced fracture of lesser tuberosity of right humerus

S42.262 **7th** Displaced fracture of lesser tuberosity of left humerus

S42.264 **7th** Nondisplaced fracture of lesser tuberosity of right humerus

S42.265 **7th** Nondisplaced fracture of lesser tuberosity of left humerus

S42.27 **6th** Torus fracture of upper end of humerus

S42.271 **7th** Torus fracture of upper end of right humerus

S42.272 **7th** Torus fracture of upper end of left humerus

S42.29 **6th** Other fracture of upper end of humerus
Fracture of anatomical neck of humerus
Fracture of articular head of humerus

S42.291 **7th** Other displaced fracture of upper end of right humerus

S42.292 **7th** Other displaced fracture of upper end of left humerus

S42.293 **7th** Other displaced fracture of upper end of unspecified humerus

S42.294 **7th** Other nondisplaced fracture of upper end of right humerus

S42.295 **7th** Other nondisplaced fracture of upper end of left humerus

S42.3 **5th** **Fracture of shaft of humerus**
Fracture of humerus NOS
Fracture of upper arm NOS
Excludes2: physeal fractures of upper end of humerus (S49.0-)
physeal fractures of lower end of humerus (S49.1-)

S42.30 **6th** Unspecified fracture of shaft of humerus

S42.301 **7th** Unspecified fracture of shaft of humerus, right arm

S42.302 **7th** Unspecified fracture of shaft of humerus, left arm

S42.31 **6th** Greenstick fracture of shaft of humerus

S42.311 **7th** Greenstick fracture of shaft of humerus, right arm

S42.312 **7th** Greenstick fracture of shaft of humerus, left arm

S42.32 **6th** Transverse fracture of shaft of humerus

S42.321 **7th** Displaced transverse fracture of shaft of humerus, right arm

S42.322 **7th** Displaced transverse fracture of shaft of humerus, left arm

S42.324 **7th** Nondisplaced transverse fracture of shaft of humerus, right arm

S42.325 **7th** Nondisplaced transverse fracture of shaft of humerus, left arm

S42.33 **6th** Oblique fracture of shaft of humerus

S42.331 **7th** Displaced oblique fracture of shaft of humerus, right arm

S42.332 **7th** Displaced oblique fracture of shaft of humerus, left arm

S42.334 **7th** Nondisplaced oblique fracture of shaft of humerus, right arm

S42.335 **7th** Nondisplaced oblique fracture of shaft of humerus, left arm

S42.34 **6th** Spiral fracture of shaft of humerus

S42.341 **7th** Displaced spiral fracture of shaft of humerus, right arm

S42.342 **7th** Displaced spiral fracture of shaft of humerus, left arm

S42.343 **7th** Displaced spiral fracture of shaft of humerus, unspecified arm

S42.344 **7th** Nondisplaced spiral fracture of shaft of humerus, right arm

S42.345 **7th** Nondisplaced spiral fracture of shaft of humerus, left arm

S42.35 **6th** Comminuted fracture of shaft of humerus

S42.351 **7th** Displaced comminuted fracture of shaft of humerus, right arm

S42.352 **7th** Displaced comminuted fracture of shaft of humerus, left arm

S42.354 **7th** Nondisplaced comminuted fracture of shaft of humerus, right arm

S42.355 **7th** Nondisplaced comminuted fracture of shaft of humerus, left arm

S42.36 **6th** Segmental fracture of shaft of humerus

S42.361 **7th** Displaced segmental fracture of shaft of humerus, right arm

S42.362 **7th** Displaced segmental fracture of shaft of humerus, left arm

S42.364 **7th** Nondisplaced segmental fracture of shaft of humerus, right arm

S42.365 **7th** Nondisplaced segmental fracture of shaft of humerus, left arm

S42.39 **6th** Other fracture of shaft of humerus

S42.391 **7th** Other fracture of shaft of right humerus

S42.392 **7th** Other fracture of shaft of left humerus

S42.4 **5th** **Fracture of lower end of humerus**
Fracture of distal end of humerus
Excludes2: fracture of shaft of humerus (S42.3-)
physeal fracture of lower end of humerus (S49.1-)

S42.40 **6th** Unspecified fracture of lower end of humerus
Fracture of elbow NOS

 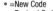

4th **5th** **6th** **7th** Additional Character Required   ✓   3-character code   Unspecified laterality codes were excluded here.   • =New Code ▲ =Revised Code ▫ =Social determinants of health   *Excludes1*—Not coded here, do not use together   *Excludes2*—Not included here

S42.401 `7th` Unspecified fracture of lower end of right humerus

S42.402 `7th` Unspecified fracture of lower end of left humerus

S42.41 `6th` Simple supracondylar fracture without intercondylar fracture of humerus

S42.411 `7th` Displaced simple supracondylar fracture without intercondylar fracture of right humerus

S42.412 `7th` Displaced simple supracondylar fracture without intercondylar fracture of left humerus

S42.414 `7th` Nondisplaced simple supracondylar fracture without intercondylar fracture of right humerus

7th characters for category S42
A—initial encounter for closed fracture
B—initial encounter for open fracture
D—subsequent encounter for fracture with routine healing
G—subsequent encounter for fracture with delayed healing
K—subsequent encounter for fracture with nonunion
P—subsequent encounter for fracture with malunion
S—sequela

S42.415 `7th` Nondisplaced simple supracondylar fracture without intercondylar fracture of left humerus

S42.42 `6th` Comminuted supracondylar fracture without intercondylar fracture of humerus

S42.421 `7th` Displaced comminuted supracondylar fracture without intercondylar fracture of right humerus

S42.422 `7th` Displaced comminuted supracondylar fracture without intercondylar fracture of left humerus

S42.424 `7th` Nondisplaced comminuted supracondylar fracture without intercondylar fracture of right humerus

S42.425 `7th` Nondisplaced comminuted supracondylar fracture without intercondylar fracture of left humerus

S42.43 `6th` Fracture (avulsion) of lateral epicondyle of humerus

S42.431 `7th` Displaced fracture (avulsion) of lateral epicondyle of right humerus

S42.432 `7th` Displaced fracture (avulsion) of lateral epicondyle of left humerus

S42.434 `7th` Nondisplaced fracture (avulsion) of lateral epicondyle of right humerus

S42.435 `7th` Nondisplaced fracture (avulsion) of lateral epicondyle of left humerus

S42.44 `6th` Fracture (avulsion) of medial epicondyle of humerus

S42.441 `7th` Displaced fracture (avulsion) of medial epicondyle of right humerus

S42.442 `7th` Displaced fracture (avulsion) of medial epicondyle of left humerus

S42.444 `7th` Nondisplaced fracture (avulsion) of medial epicondyle of right humerus

S42.445 `7th` Nondisplaced fracture (avulsion) of medial epicondyle of left humerus

S42.447 `7th` Incarcerated fracture (avulsion) of medial epicondyle of right humerus

S42.448 `7th` Incarcerated fracture (avulsion) of medial epicondyle of left humerus

S42.45 `6th` Fracture of lateral condyle of humerus
Fracture of capitellum of humerus

S42.451 `7th` Displaced fracture of lateral condyle of right humerus

S42.452 `7th` Displaced fracture of lateral condyle of left humerus

S42.454 `7th` Nondisplaced fracture of lateral condyle of right humerus

S42.455 `7th` Nondisplaced fracture of lateral condyle of left humerus

S42.46 `6th` Fracture of medial condyle of humerus
Trochlea fracture of humerus

S42.461 `7th` Displaced fracture of medial condyle of right humerus

S42.462 `7th` Displaced fracture of medial condyle of left humerus

S42.464 `7th` Nondisplaced fracture of medial condyle of right humerus

S42.465 `7th` Nondisplaced fracture of medial condyle of left humerus

S42.47 `6th` Transcondylar fracture of humerus

S42.471 `7th` Displaced transcondylar fracture of right humerus

S42.472 `7th` Displaced transcondylar fracture of left humerus

S42.474 `7th` Nondisplaced transcondylar fracture of right humerus

S42.475 `7th` Nondisplaced transcondylar fracture of left humerus

S42.48 `6th` Torus fracture of lower end of humerus

S42.481 `7th` Torus fracture of lower end of right humerus

S42.482 `7th` Torus fracture of lower end of left humerus

S42.49 `6th` Other fracture of lower end of humerus

S42.491 `7th` Other displaced fracture of lower end of right humerus

S42.492 `7th` Other displaced fracture of lower end of left humerus

S42.494 `7th` Other nondisplaced fracture of lower end of right humerus

S42.495 `7th` Other nondisplaced fracture of lower end of left humerus

S42.9 `5th` Fracture of shoulder girdle, part unspecified
Fracture of shoulder NOS

S42.91X `7th` Fracture of right shoulder girdle, part unspecified

S42.92X `7th` Fracture of left shoulder girdle, part unspecified

S43 `4th` **DISLOCATION AND SPRAIN OF JOINTS AND LIGAMENTS OF SHOULDER GIRDLE**

Includes: avulsion of joint or ligament of shoulder girdle
laceration of cartilage, joint or ligament of shoulder girdle
sprain of cartilage, joint or ligament of shoulder girdle
traumatic hemarthrosis of joint or ligament of shoulder girdle
traumatic rupture of joint or ligament of shoulder girdle
traumatic subluxation of joint or ligament of shoulder girdle
traumatic tear of joint or ligament of shoulder girdle

7th characters for category S43
A—initial encounter
D—subsequent encounter
S—sequela

Code also any associated open wound
Excludes2: strain of muscle, fascia and tendon of shoulder and upper arm (S46.-)

S43.0 `5th` Subluxation and dislocation of shoulder joint
Dislocation of glenohumeral joint
Subluxation of glenohumeral joint

S43.00 `6th` Unspecified subluxation and dislocation of shoulder joint
Dislocation of humerus NOS
Subluxation of humerus NOS

S43.001 `7th` Unspecified subluxation of right shoulder joint

S43.002 `7th` Unspecified subluxation of left shoulder joint

S43.004 `7th` Unspecified dislocation of right shoulder joint

S43.005 `7th` Unspecified dislocation of left shoulder joint

S43.01 `6th` Anterior subluxation and dislocation of humerus

S43.011 `7th` Anterior subluxation of right humerus

`4th` `5th` `6th` `7th`   Additional Character Required   ✔   `3-character code`   Unspecified laterality codes were excluded here.   • =New Code   ▲ =Revised Code   ▫ =Social determinants of health   *Excludes1*—Not coded here, do not use together   *Excludes2*—Not included here

S43.012 **7th** Anterior subluxation of left humerus

S43.014 **7th** Anterior dislocation of right humerus

S43.015 **7th** Anterior dislocation of left humerus

S43.02 **6th** Posterior subluxation and dislocation of humerus

S43.021 **7th** Posterior subluxation of right humerus

S43.022 **7th** Posterior subluxation of left humerus

S43.024 **7th** Posterior dislocation of right humerus

S43.025 **7th** Posterior dislocation of left humerus

> 7th characters for category S43
> A—initial encounter
> D—subsequent encounter
> S—sequela

S43.03 **6th** Inferior subluxation and dislocation of humerus

S43.031 **7th** Inferior subluxation of right humerus

S43.032 **7th** Inferior subluxation of left humerus

S43.034 **7th** Inferior dislocation of right humerus

S43.035 **7th** Inferior dislocation of left humerus

S43.08 **6th** Other subluxation and dislocation of shoulder joint

S43.081 **7th** Other subluxation of right shoulder joint

S43.082 **7th** Other subluxation of left shoulder joint

S43.084 **7th** Other dislocation of right shoulder joint

S43.085 **7th** Other dislocation of left shoulder joint

S43.1 **5th** Subluxation and dislocation of acromioclavicular joint

S43.10 **6th** Unspecified dislocation of acromioclavicular joint

S43.101 **7th** Unspecified dislocation of right acromioclavicular joint

S43.102 **7th** Unspecified dislocation of left acromioclavicular joint

S43.11 **6th** Subluxation of acromioclavicular joint

S43.111 **7th** Subluxation of right acromioclavicular joint

S43.112 **7th** Subluxation of left acromioclavicular joint

S43.12 **6th** Dislocation of acromioclavicular joint, 100%–200% displacement

S43.121 **7th** Dislocation of right acromioclavicular joint, 100%–200% displacement

S43.122 **7th** Dislocation of left acromioclavicular joint, 100%–200% displacement

S43.13 **6th** Dislocation of acromioclavicular joint, greater than 200% displacement

S43.131 **7th** Dislocation of right acromioclavicular joint, greater than 200% displacement

S43.132 **7th** Dislocation of left acromioclavicular joint, greater than 200% displacement

S43.14 **6th** Inferior dislocation of acromioclavicular joint

S43.141 **7th** Inferior dislocation of right acromioclavicular joint

S43.142 **7th** Inferior dislocation of left acromioclavicular joint

S43.15 **6th** Posterior dislocation of acromioclavicular joint

S43.151 **7th** Posterior dislocation of right acromioclavicular joint

S43.152 **7th** Posterior dislocation of left acromioclavicular joint

S43.2 **5th** Subluxation and dislocation of sternoclavicular joint

S43.20 **6th** Unspecified subluxation and dislocation of sternoclavicular joint

S43.201 **7th** Unspecified subluxation of right sternoclavicular joint

S43.202 **7th** Unspecified subluxation of left sternoclavicular joint

S43.204 **7th** Unspecified dislocation of right sternoclavicular joint

S43.205 **7th** Unspecified dislocation of left sternoclavicular joint

S43.21 **6th** Anterior subluxation and dislocation of sternoclavicular joint

S43.211 **7th** Anterior subluxation of right sternoclavicular joint

S43.212 **7th** Anterior subluxation of left sternoclavicular joint

S43.214 **7th** Anterior dislocation of right sternoclavicular joint

S43.215 **7th** Anterior dislocation of left sternoclavicular joint

S43.22 **6th** Posterior subluxation and dislocation of sternoclavicular joint

S43.221 **7th** Posterior subluxation of right sternoclavicular joint

S43.222 **7th** Posterior subluxation of left sternoclavicular joint

S43.224 **7th** Posterior dislocation of right sternoclavicular joint

S43.225 **7th** Posterior dislocation of left sternoclavicular joint

S43.3 **5th** Subluxation and dislocation of other and unspecified parts of shoulder girdle

S43.30 **6th** Subluxation and dislocation of unspecified parts of shoulder girdle
Dislocation/subluxation of shoulder girdle NOS

S43.301 **7th** Subluxation of unspecified parts of right shoulder girdle

S43.302 **7th** Subluxation of unspecified parts of left shoulder girdle

S43.304 **7th** Dislocation of unspecified parts of right shoulder girdle

S43.305 **7th** Dislocation of unspecified parts of left shoulder girdle

S43.31 **6th** Subluxation and dislocation of scapula

S43.311 **7th** Subluxation of right scapula

S43.312 **7th** Subluxation of left scapula

S43.314 **7th** Dislocation of right scapula

S43.315 **7th** Dislocation of left scapula

S43.39 **6th** Subluxation and dislocation of other parts of shoulder girdle

S43.391 **7th** Subluxation of other parts of right shoulder girdle

S43.392 **7th** Subluxation of other parts of left shoulder girdle

S43.394 **7th** Dislocation of other parts of right shoulder girdle

S43.395 **7th** Dislocation of other parts of left shoulder girdle

S43.4 **5th** Sprain of shoulder joint

S43.40 **6th** Unspecified sprain of shoulder joint

S43.401 **7th** Unspecified sprain of right shoulder joint

S43.402 **7th** Unspecified sprain of left shoulder joint

S43.41 **6th** Sprain of coracohumeral (ligament)

S43.411 **7th** Sprain of right coracohumeral (ligament)

S43.412 **7th** Sprain of left coracohumeral (ligament)

S43.42 **6th** Sprain of rotator cuff capsule
Excludes1: rotator cuff syndrome (complete) (incomplete), not specified as traumatic (M75.1-)
Excludes2: injury of tendon of rotator cuff (S46.0-)

4th **5th** **6th** **7th** Additional Character Required ✔ 3-character code Unspecified laterality codes were excluded here.

• =New Code
▲ =Revised Code
¤ =Social determinants of health

Excludes1—Not coded here, do not use together
Excludes2—Not included here

S43.421   Sprain of right rotator cuff capsule
`7th`

S43.422   Sprain of left rotator cuff capsule
`7th`

S43.43   Superior glenoid labrum lesion
`6th`
     SLAP lesion

S43.431   Superior glenoid labrum lesion of right
`7th`   shoulder

S43.432   Superior glenoid labrum lesion of left
`7th`   shoulder

S43.49   Other sprain of shoulder joint
`6th`

S43.491   Other sprain of right shoulder joint
`7th`

S43.492   Other sprain of left shoulder joint
`7th`

S43.5   Sprain of acromioclavicular joint
`5th`
     Sprain of acromioclavicular ligament

S43.51X   Sprain of right acromioclavicular joint
`7th`

S43.52X   Sprain of left acromioclavicular joint
`7th`

S43.6   Sprain of sternoclavicular joint
`5th`

S43.61X   Sprain of right sternoclavicular joint
`7th`

S43.62X   Sprain of left sternoclavicular joint
`7th`

S43.8   Sprain of other specified parts of shoulder girdle
`5th`

S43.81X   Sprain of other specified parts of right shoulder
`7th`   girdle

S43.82X   Sprain of other
`7th`   specified parts of left
     shoulder girdle

> 7th characters for categories
> S43 & S46
> A—initial encounter
> D—subsequent encounter
> S—sequela

S46   INJURY OF MUSCLE, FASCIA AND TENDON AT SHOULDER AND UPPER ARM LEVEL
`4th`

Code also any associated open wound (S41.-)

Excludes2: injury of muscle, fascia and tendon at elbow (S56.-)
     sprain of joints and ligaments of shoulder girdle (S43.9)

S46.0   Injury of muscle(s) and tendon(s) of the rotator cuff of shoulder
`5th`

S46.00   Unspecified injury of muscle(s) and tendon(s) of the
`6th`   rotator cuff of shoulder

S46.001   Unspecified injury of muscle(s) and ten-
`7th`   don(s) of the rotator cuff of right shoulder

S46.002   Unspecified injury of muscle(s) and
`7th`   tendon(s) of the rotator cuff of left
     shoulder

S46.01   Strain of muscle(s) and tendon(s) of the rotator cuff
`6th`   of shoulder

S46.011   Strain of muscle(s) and tendon(s) of the
`7th`   rotator cuff of right shoulder

S46.012   Strain of muscle(s) and tendon(s) of the
`7th`   rotator cuff of left shoulder

S46.02   Laceration of muscle(s) and tendon(s) of the rotator
`6th`   cuff of shoulder

S46.021   Laceration of muscle(s) and tendon(s) of
`7th`   the rotator cuff of right shoulder

S46.022   Laceration of muscle(s) and tendon(s) of
`7th`   the rotator cuff of left shoulder

S46.09   Other injury of muscle(s) and tendon(s) of the rotator
`6th`   cuff of shoulder

S46.091   Other injury of muscle(s) and tendon(s) of
`7th`   the rotator cuff of right shoulder

S46.092   Other injury of muscle(s) and tendon(s) of
`7th`   the rotator cuff of left shoulder

S46.91   Strain of unspecified muscle, fascia and tendon at
`6th`   shoulder and upper arm level

S46.911   Strain of unspecified muscle, fascia and
`7th`   tendon at shoulder and upper arm level,
     right arm

S46.912   Strain of unspecified muscle, fascia and
`7th`   tendon at shoulder and upper arm level,
     left arm

S46.92   Laceration of unspecified muscle, fascia and tendon
`6th`   at shoulder and upper arm level

S46.921   Laceration of unspecified muscle, fascia
`7th`   and tendon at shoulder and upper arm
     level, right arm

S46.922   Laceration of unspecified muscle, fascia
`7th`   and tendon at shoulder and upper arm
     level, left arm

S46.99   Other injury of unspecified muscle, fascia and tendon
`6th`   at shoulder and upper arm level

S46.991   Other injury of unspecified muscle, fascia
`7th`   and tendon at shoulder and upper arm
     level, right arm

S46.992   Other injury of unspecified muscle, fascia
`7th`   and tendon at shoulder and upper arm
     level, left arm

S49   OTHER AND UNSPECIFIED INJURIES OF SHOULDER AND UPPER ARM
`4th`

S49.0   Physeal fracture of upper end
`5th`   of humerus

S49.00   Unspecified physeal
`6th`   fracture of upper end
     of humerus

> 7th characters for category S49
> A—initial encounter for closed fracture
> D—subsequent encounter for fracture with routine healing
> G—subsequent encounter for fracture with delayed healing
> K—subsequent encounter for fracture with nonunion
> P—subsequent encounter for fracture with malunion
> S—sequela

S49.001   Unspecified
`7th`   physeal
     fracture of
     upper end
     of humerus,
     right arm

S49.002   Unspecified
`7th`   physeal fracture of upper end of humerus,
     left arm

S49.01   Salter-Harris Type I physeal fracture of upper end of
`6th`   humerus

S49.011   Salter-Harris Type I physeal fractureof
`7th`   upper end of humerus, right arm

S49.012   Salter-Harris Type I physeal fracture of
`7th`   upper end of humerus, left arm

S49.02   Salter-Harris Type II physeal fracture of upper end of
`6th`   humerus

S49.021   Salter-Harris Type II physeal fracture of
`7th`   upper end of humerus, right arm

S49.022   Salter-Harris Type II physeal fracture of
`7th`   upper end of humerus, left arm

S49.03   Salter-Harris Type III physeal fracture of upper end of
`6th`   humerus

S49.031   Salter-Harris Type III physeal fracture of
`7th`   upper end of humerus, right arm

S49.032   Salter-Harris Type III physeal fracture of
`7th`   upper end of humerus, left arm

S49.04   Salter-Harris Type IV physeal fracture of upper end of
`6th`   humerus

S49.041   Salter-Harris Type IV physeal fracture of
`7th`   upper end of humerus, right arm

S49.042   Salter-Harris Type IV physeal fracture of
`7th`   upper end of humerus, left arm

S49.09   Other physeal fracture of upper end of humerus
`6th`

S49.091   Other physeal fracture of upper end of
`7th`   humerus, right arm

S49.092   Other physeal fracture of upper end of
`7th`   humerus, left arm

S49.1   Physeal fracture of lower end of humerus
`5th`

S49.10   Unspecified physeal fracture of lower end of
`6th`   humerus

S49.101   Unspecified physeal fracture of lower end
`7th`   of humerus, right arm

S49.102   Unspecified physeal fracture of lower end
`7th`   of humerus, left arm

S49.11   Salter-Harris Type I physeal fracture of lower end of
`6th`   humerus

S49.111   Salter-Harris Type I physeal fracture of
`7th`   lower end of humerus, right arm

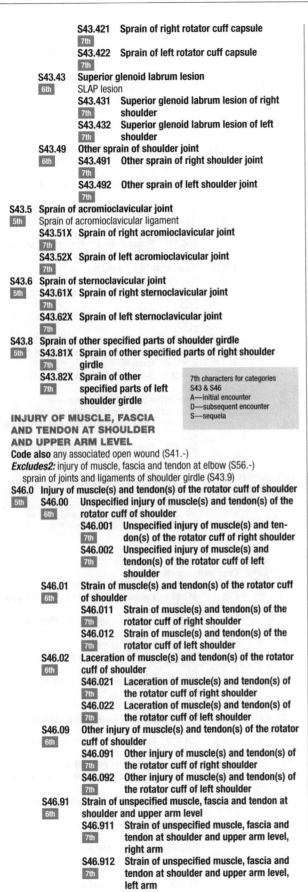

`4th` `5th` `6th` `7th`   Additional Character Required   ✓   3-character code   Unspecified laterality codes were excluded here.

• =New Code
▲ =Revised Code
◘ =Social determinants of health

Excludes1—Not coded here, do not use together
Excludes2—Not included here

S49.112 **7th** Salter-Harris Type I physeal fracture of lower end of humerus, left arm

S49.12 **6th** Salter-Harris Type II physeal fracture of lower end of humerus

S49.121 **7th** Salter-Harris Type II physeal fracture of lower end of humerus, right arm

S49.122 **7th** Salter-Harris Type II physeal fracture of lower end of humerus, left arm

S49.13 **6th** Salter-Harris Type III physeal fracture of lower end of humerus

S49.131 **7th** Salter-Harris Type III physeal fracture of lower end of humerus, right arm

S49.132 **7th** Salter-Harris Type III physeal fracture of lower end of humerus, left arm

S49.14 **6th** Salter-Harris Type IV physeal fracture of lower end of humerus

S49.141 **7th** Salter-Harris Type IV physeal fracture of lower end of humerus, right arm

S49.142 **7th** Salter-Harris Type IV physeal fracture of lower end of humerus, left arm

S49.19 **6th** Other physeal fracture of lower end of humerus

S49.191 **7th** Other physeal fracture of lower end of humerus, right arm

S49.192 **7th** Other physeal fracture of lower end of humerus, left arm

(S50–S59) INJURIES TO THE ELBOW AND FOREARM

Excludes2: burns and corrosions (T20–T32)
frostbite (T33–T34)
injuries of wrist and hand (S60–S69)
insect bite or sting, venomous (T63.4)

> 7th characters for category S50
> A—initial encounter
> D—subsequent encounter
> S—sequela

S50 **4th** **SUPERFICIAL INJURY OF ELBOW AND FOREARM**

Excludes2: superficial injury of wrist and hand (S60.-)

S50.0 Contusion of elbow
5th **S50.01X** **7th** Contusion of right elbow

S50.02X **7th** Contusion of left elbow

S50.1 Contusion of forearm
5th **S50.11X** **7th** Contusion of right forearm

S50.12X **7th** Contusion of left forearm

S50.3 Other superficial injuries of elbow
5th **S50.31** **6th** Abrasion of elbow
     S50.311 **7th** Abrasion of right elbow

     S50.312 **7th** Abrasion of left elbow

S50.32 **6th** Blister (nonthermal) of elbow
     S50.321 **7th** Blister (nonthermal) of right elbow

     S50.322 **7th** Blister (nonthermal) of left elbow

S50.34 **6th** External constriction of elbow
     S50.341 **7th** External constriction of right elbow

     S50.342 **7th** External constriction of left elbow

S50.35 **6th** Superficial FB of elbow
Splinter in the elbow
     S50.351 **7th** Superficial FB of right elbow

     S50.352 **7th** Superficial FB of left elbow

S50.36 **6th** Insect bite (nonvenomous) of elbow
     S50.361 **7th** Insect bite (nonvenomous) of right elbow

     S50.362 **7th** Insect bite (nonvenomous) of left elbow

S50.37 **6th** Other superficial bite of elbow
Excludes1: open bite of elbow (S51.04)

S50.371 **7th** Other superficial bite of right elbow

S50.372 **7th** Other superficial bite of left elbow

S50.8 Other superficial injuries of forearm
5th **S50.81** **6th** Abrasion of forearm
     S50.811 **7th** Abrasion of right forearm

     S50.812 **7th** Abrasion of left forearm

S50.82 **6th** Blister (nonthermal) of forearm
     S50.821 **7th** Blister (nonthermal) of right forearm

     S50.822 **7th** Blister (nonthermal) of left forearm

S50.84 **6th** External constriction of forearm
     S50.841 **7th** External constriction of right forearm

     S50.842 **7th** External constriction of left forearm

S50.85 **6th** Superficial FB of forearm
Splinter in the forearm
     S50.851 **7th** Superficial FB of right forearm

     S50.852 **7th** Superficial FB of left forearm

S50.86 **6th** Insect bite (nonvenomous) of forearm
     S50.861 **7th** Insect bite (nonvenomous) of right forearm

     S50.862 **7th** Insect bite (nonvenomous) of left forearm

S50.87 **6th** Other superficial bite of forearm
Excludes1: open bite of forearm (S51.84)

     S50.871 **7th** Other superficial bite of right forearm

     S50.872 **7th** Other superficial bite of left forearm

S51 **4th** **OPEN WOUND OF ELBOW AND FOREARM**

Code also any associated wound infection

Excludes1: open fracture of elbow and forearm (S52.- with open fracture 7th character)
traumatic amputation of elbow and forearm (S58.-)

> 7th characters for category S51
> A—initial encounter
> D—subsequent encounter
> S—sequela

Excludes2: open wound of wrist and hand (S61.-)

S51.0 Open wound of elbow
5th **S51.01** **6th** Laceration without FB of elbow
     S51.011 **7th** Laceration without FB of right elbow

     S51.012 **7th** Laceration without FB of left elbow

S51.02 **6th** Laceration with FB of elbow
     S51.021 **7th** Laceration with FB of right elbow

     S51.022 **7th** Laceration with FB of left elbow

S51.03 **6th** Puncture wound without FB of elbow
     S51.031 **7th** Puncture wound without FB of right elbow

     S51.032 **7th** Puncture wound without FB of left elbow

S51.04 **6th** Puncture wound with FB of elbow
     S51.041 **7th** Puncture wound with FB of right elbow

     S51.042 **7th** Puncture wound with FB of left elbow

S51.05 **6th** Open bite of elbow
Bite of elbow NOS
Excludes1: superficial bite of elbow (S50.36, S50.37)
     S51.051 **7th** Open bite, right elbow

     S51.052 **7th** Open bite, left elbow

4th **5th** **6th** **7th** Additional Character Required   ✔   3-character code   Unspecified laterality codes were excluded here.   • =New Code   ▲ =Revised Code   ▫ =Social determinants of health   *Excludes1*—Not coded here, do not use together   *Excludes2*—Not included here

S51.8 `5th` **Open wound of forearm**
    Excludes2: open wound of elbow (S51.0-)

    S51.81 `6th` **Laceration without FB of forearm**
        S51.811 `7th` **Laceration without FB of right forearm**
        S51.812 `7th` **Laceration without FB of left forearm**

    S51.82 `6th` **Laceration with FB of forearm**
        S51.821 `7th` **Laceration with FB of right forearm**
        S51.822 `7th` **Laceration with FB of left forearm**

    S51.83 `6th` **Puncture wound without FB of forearm**
        S51.831 `7th` **Puncture wound without FB of right forearm**
        S51.832 `7th` **Puncture wound without FB of left forearm**

    S51.84 `6th` **Puncture wound with FB of forearm**
        S51.841 `7th` **Puncture wound with FB of right forearm**
        S51.842 `7th` **Puncture wound with FB of left forearm**

    S51.85 `6th` **Open bite of forearm**
    Bite of forearm NOS
    Excludes1: superficial bite of forearm (S50.86, S50.87)
        S51.851 `7th` **Open bite of right forearm**
        S51.852 `7th` **Open bite of left forearm**

S52 `4th` **FRACTURE OF FOREARM**
    Note: A fracture not indicated as displaced or nondisplaced should be coded to displaced
    A fracture not indicated as open or closed should be coded to closed
    The open fracture designations are based on the Gustilo open fracture classification
    Excludes1: traumatic amputation of forearm (S58.-)
    Excludes2: fracture at wrist and hand level (S62.-)

S52.0 `5th` **Fracture of upper end of ulna**
    Fracture of proximal end of ulna
    Excludes2: fracture of elbow NOS (S42.40-)
    fractures of shaft of ulna (S52.2-)

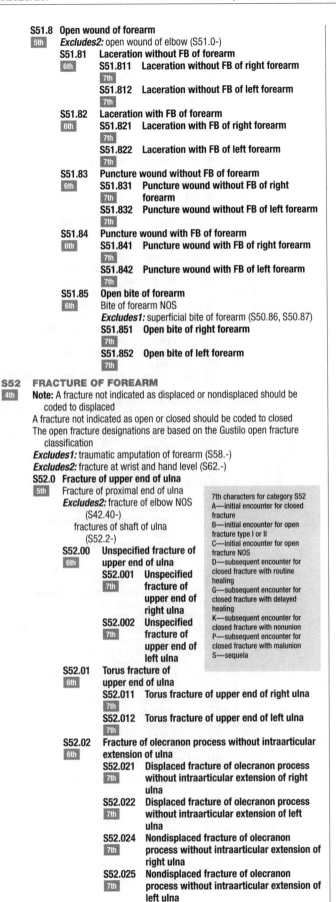

7th characters for category S52
A—initial encounter for closed fracture
B—initial encounter for open fracture type I or II
C—initial encounter for open fracture NOS
D—subsequent encounter for closed fracture with routine healing
G—subsequent encounter for closed fracture with delayed healing
K—subsequent encounter for closed fracture with nonunion
P—subsequent encounter for closed fracture with malunion
S—sequela

    S52.00 `6th` **Unspecified fracture of upper end of ulna**
        S52.001 `7th` **Unspecified fracture of upper end of right ulna**
        S52.002 `7th` **Unspecified fracture of upper end of left ulna**

    S52.01 `6th` **Torus fracture of upper end of ulna**
        S52.011 `7th` **Torus fracture of upper end of right ulna**
        S52.012 `7th` **Torus fracture of upper end of left ulna**

    S52.02 `6th` **Fracture of olecranon process without intraarticular extension of ulna**
        S52.021 `7th` **Displaced fracture of olecranon process without intraarticular extension of right ulna**
        S52.022 `7th` **Displaced fracture of olecranon process without intraarticular extension of left ulna**
        S52.024 `7th` **Nondisplaced fracture of olecranon process without intraarticular extension of right ulna**
        S52.025 `7th` **Nondisplaced fracture of olecranon process without intraarticular extension of left ulna**

S52.03 `6th` **Fracture of olecranon process with intraarticular extension of ulna**
    S52.031 `7th` **Displaced fracture of olecranon process with intraarticular extension of right ulna**
    S52.032 `7th` **Displaced fracture of olecranon process with intraarticular extension of left ulna**
    S52.034 `7th` **Nondisplaced fracture of olecranon process with intraarticular extension of right ulna**
    S52.035 `7th` **Nondisplaced fracture of olecranon process with intraarticular extension of left ulna**

S52.04 `6th` **Fracture of coronoid process of ulna**
    S52.041 `7th` **Displaced fracture of coronoid process of right ulna**
    S52.042 `7th` **Displaced fracture of coronoid process of left ulna**
    S52.044 `7th` **Nondisplaced fracture of coronoid process of right ulna**
    S52.045 `7th` **Nondisplaced fracture of coronoid process of left ulna**

S52.09 `6th` **Other fracture of upper end of ulna**
    S52.091 `7th` **Other fracture of upper end of right ulna**
    S52.092 `7th` **Other fracture of upper end of left ulna**

S52.1 `5th` **Fracture of upper end of radius**
    Fracture of proximal end of radius
    Excludes2: physeal fractures of upper end of radius (S59.2-)
    fracture of shaft of radius (S52.3-)

    S52.10 `6th` **Unspecified fracture of upper end of radius**
        S52.101 `7th` **Unspecified fracture of upper end of right radius**
        S52.102 `7th` **Unspecified fracture of upper end of left radius**

    S52.11 `6th` **Torus fracture of upper end of radius**
        S52.111 `7th` **Torus fracture of upper end of right radius**
        S52.112 `7th` **Torus fracture of upper end of left radius**

    S52.12 `6th` **Fracture of head of radius**
        S52.121 `7th` **Displaced fracture of head of right radius**
        S52.122 `7th` **Displaced fracture of head of left radius**
        S52.124 `7th` **Nondis-placed fracture of head of right radius**
        S52.125 `7th` **Nondisplaced fracture of head of left radius**

    S52.13 `6th` **Fracture of neck of radius**
        S52.131 `7th` **Displaced fracture of neck of right radius**
        S52.132 `7th` **Displaced fracture of neck of eft radius**
        S52.134 `7th` **Nondisplaced fracture of neck of right radius**
        S52.135 `7th` **Nondisplaced fracture of neck of left radius**

    S52.18 `6th` **Other fracture of upper end of radius**
        S52.181 `7th` **Other fracture of upper end of right radius**
        S52.182 `7th` **Other fracture of upper end of left radius**

S52.2 `5th` **Fracture of shaft of ulna**
    S52.20 `6th` **Unspecified fracture of shaft of ulna**
    Fracture of ulna NOS
        S52.201 `7th` **Unspecified fracture of shaft of right ulna**
        S52.202 `7th` **Unspecified fracture of shaft of left ulna**

    S52.21 `6th` **Greenstick fracture of shaft of ulna**
        S52.211 `7th` **Greenstick fracture of shaft of right ulna**

`4th` `5th` `6th` `7th` Additional Character Required   ✓ **3-character code**   Unspecified laterality codes were excluded here.

• =New Code
▲ =Revised Code
▣ =Social determinants of health

Excludes1—Not coded here, do not use together
Excludes2—Not included here

S52.212   Greenstick fracture of shaft of left ulna
`7th`

S52.22 `6th`   Transverse fracture of shaft of ulna
    S52.221   Displaced transverse fracture of shaft of right ulna `7th`
    S52.222   Displaced transverse fracture of shaft of left ulna `7th`
    S52.224   Nondisplaced transverse fracture of shaft of right ulna `7th`
    S52.225   Nondisplaced transverse fracture of shaft of left ulna `7th`

S52.23 `6th`   Oblique fracture of shaft of ulna
    S52.231   Displaced oblique fracture of shaft of right ulna `7th`
    S52.232   Displaced oblique fracture of shaft of left ulna `7th`
    S52.234   Nondisplaced oblique fracture of shaft of right ulna `7th`
    S52.235   Nondisplaced oblique fracture of shaft of left ulna `7th`

S52.24 `6th`   Spiral fracture of shaft of ulna
    S52.241   Displaced spiral fracture of shaft of ulna, right arm `7th`
    S52.242   Displaced spiral fracture of shaft of ulna, left arm `7th`
    S52.244   Nondisplaced spiral fracture of shaft of ulna, right arm `7th`
    S52.245   Nondisplaced spiral fracture of shaft of ulna, left arm `7th`

> 7th characters for category S52
> A—initial encounter for closed fracture
> B—initial encounter for open fracture type I or II
> C—initial encounter for open fracture NOS
> D—subsequent encounter for closed fracture with routine healing
> G—subsequent encounter for closed fracture with delayed healing
> K—subsequent encounter for closed fracture with nonunion
> P—subsequent encounter for closed fracture with malunion
> S—sequela

S52.25 `6th`   Comminuted fracture of shaft of ulna
    S52.251   Displaced comminuted fracture of shaft of ulna, right arm `7th`
    S52.252   Displaced comminuted fracture of shaft of ulna, left arm `7th`
    S52.254   Nondisplaced comminuted fracture of shaft of ulna, right arm `7th`
    S52.255   Nondisplaced comminuted fracture of shaft of ulna, left arm `7th`

S52.26 `6th`   Segmental fracture of shaft of ulna
    S52.261   Displaced segmental fracture of shaft of ulna, right arm `7th`
    S52.262   Displaced segmental fracture of shaft of ulna, left arm `7th`
    S52.264   Nondisplaced segmental fracture of shaft of ulna, right arm `7th`
    S52.265   Nondisplaced segmental fracture of shaft of ulna, left arm `7th`

S52.27 `6th`   Monteggia's fracture of ulna
    Fracture of upper shaft of ulna with dislocation of radial head
    S52.271   Monteggia's fracture of right ulna `7th`
    S52.272   Monteggia's fracture of left ulna `7th`

S52.28 `6th`   Bent bone of ulna
    S52.281   Bent bone of right ulna `7th`
    S52.282   Bent bone of left ulna `7th`

S52.29 `6th`   Other fracture of shaft of ulna
    S52.291   Other fracture of shaft of right ulna `7th`

S52.292   Other fracture of shaft of left ulna `7th`

S52.3 `5th`   Fracture of shaft of radius
  S52.30 `6th`   Unspecified fracture of shaft of radius
    S52.301   Unspecified fracture of shaft of right radius `7th`
    S52.302   Unspecified fracture of shaft of left radius `7th`

  S52.31 `6th`   Greenstick fracture of shaft of radius
    S52.311   Greenstick fracture of shaft of radius, right arm `7th`
    S52.312   Greenstick fracture of shaft of radius, left arm `7th`

  S52.32 `6th`   Transverse fracture of shaft of radius
    S52.321   Displaced transverse fracture of shaft of right radius `7th`
    S52.322   Displaced transverse fracture of shaft of left radius `7th`
    S52.324   Nondisplaced transverse fracture of shaft of right radius `7th`
    S52.325   Nondisplaced transverse fracture of shaft of left radius `7th`

  S52.33 `6th`   Oblique fracture of shaft of radius
    S52.331   Displaced oblique fracture of shaft of right radius `7th`
    S52.332   Displaced oblique fracture of shaft of left radius `7th`
    S52.334   Nondisplaced oblique fracture of shaft of right radius `7th`
    S52.335   Nondisplaced oblique fracture of shaft of left radius `7th`

  S52.34 `6th`   Spiral fracture of shaft of radius
    S52.341   Displaced spiral fracture of shaft of radius, right arm `7th`
    S52.342   Displaced spiral fracture of shaft of radius, left arm `7th`
    S52.344   Nondisplaced spiral fracture of shaft of radius, right arm `7th`
    S52.345   Nondisplaced spiral fracture of shaft of radius, left arm `7th`

  S52.35 `6th`   Comminuted fracture of shaft of radius
    S52.351   Displaced comminuted fracture of shaft of radius, right arm `7th`
    S52.352   Displaced comminuted fracture of shaft of radius, left arm `7th`
    S52.354   Nondisplaced comminuted fracture of shaft of radius, right arm `7th`
    S52.355   Nondisplaced comminuted fracture of shaft of radius, left arm `7th`

  S52.36 `6th`   Segmental fracture of shaft of radius
    S52.361   Displaced segmental fracture of shaft of radius, right arm `7th`
    S52.362   Displaced segmental fracture of shaft of radius, left arm `7th`
    S52.364   Nondisplaced segmental fracture of shaft of radius, right arm `7th`
    S52.365   Nondisplaced segmental fracture of shaft of radius, left arm `7th`

  S52.37 `6th`   Galeazzi's fracture
    Fracture of lower shaft of radius with radioulnar joint dislocation
    S52.371   Galeazzi's fracture of right radius `7th`
    S52.372   Galeazzi's fracture of left radius `7th`

  S52.38 `6th`   Bent bone of radius
    S52.381   Bent bone of right radius `7th`
    S52.382   Bent bone of left radius `7th`

  S52.39 `6th`   Other fracture of shaft of radius
    S52.391   Other fracture of shaft of radius, right arm `7th`

`4th` `5th` `6th` `7th`   Additional Character Required   ✔   3-character code   Unspecified laterality codes were excluded here.

• =New Code
▲ =Revised Code
¤ =Social determinants of health

Excludes1—Not coded here, do not use together
Excludes2—Not included here

S52.392 Other fracture of shaft of radius, left arm
`7th`

S52.5 Fracture of lower end of radius
`5th`
Fracture of distal end of radius
Excludes: physeal fractures of lower end of radius (S59.2-)

S52.50 Unspecified fracture of the lower end of radius
`6th`
    S52.501 Unspecified fracture of the lower end of right radius `7th`
    S52.502 Unspecified fracture of the lower end of left radius `7th`

S52.51 Fracture of radial styloid process
`6th`
    S52.511 Displaced fracture of right radial styloid process `7th`
    S52.512 Displaced fracture of left radial styloid process `7th`
    S52.514 Nondisplaced fracture of right radial styloid process `7th`
    S52.515 Nondisplaced fracture of left radial styloid process `7th`

S52.52 Torus fracture of lower end of radius
`6th`
    S52.521 Torus fracture of lower end of right radius `7th`
    S52.522 Torus fracture of lower end of left radius `7th`

S52.53 Colles' fracture
`6th`
    S52.531 Colles' fracture of right radius `7th`
    S52.532 Colles' fracture of left radius `7th`

S52.54 Smith's fracture
`6th`
    S52.541 Smith's fracture of right radius `7th`
    S52.542 Smith's fracture of left radius `7th`

S52.55 Other extraarticular fracture of lower end of radius
`6th`
    S52.551 Other extra-articular fracture of lower end of right radius `7th`
    S52.552 Other extra-articular fracture of lower end of left radius `7th`

S52.56 Barton's fracture
`6th`
    S52.561 Barton's fracture of right radius `7th`
    S52.562 Barton's fracture of left radius `7th`

S52.57 Other intraarticular fracture of lower end of radius
`6th`
    S52.571 Other intraarticular fracture of lower end of right radius `7th`
    S52.572 Other intraarticular fracture of lower end of left radius `7th`

S52.59 Other fractures of lower end of radius
`6th`
    S52.591 Other fractures of lower end of right radius `7th`
    S52.592 Other fractures of lower end of left radius `7th`

S52.6 Fracture of lower end of ulna
`5th`
S52.60 Unspecified fracture of lower end of ulna
`6th`
    S52.601 Unspecified fracture of lower end of right ulna `7th`
    S52.602 Unspecified fracture of lower end of left ulna `7th`

S52.61 Fracture of ulna styloid process
`6th`
    S52.611 Displaced fracture of right ulna styloid process `7th`
    S52.612 Displaced fracture of left ulna styloid process `7th`

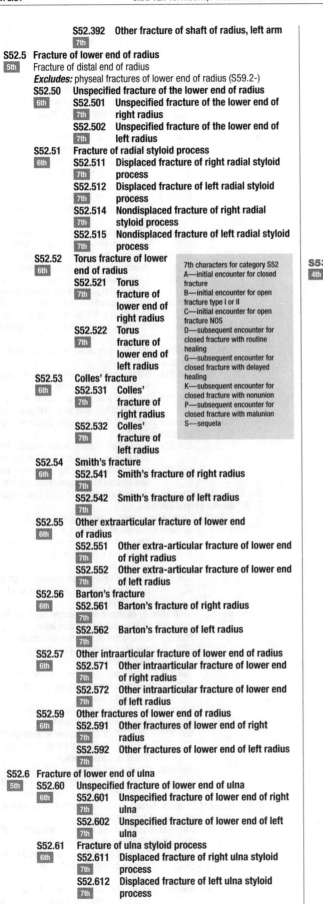

7th characters for category S52
A—initial encounter for closed fracture
B—initial encounter for open fracture type I or II
C—initial encounter for open fracture NOS
D—subsequent encounter for closed fracture with routine healing
G—subsequent encounter for closed fracture with delayed healing
K—subsequent encounter for closed fracture with nonunion
P—subsequent encounter for closed fracture with malunion
S—sequela

    S52.614 Nondisplaced fracture of right ulna styloid process `7th`
    S52.615 Nondisplaced fracture of left ulna styloid process `7th`

S52.62 Torus fracture of lower end of ulna
`6th`
    S52.621 Torus fracture of lower end of right ulna `7th`
    S52.622 Torus fracture of lower end of left ulna `7th`

S52.69 Other fracture of lower end of ulna
`6th`
    S52.691 Other fracture of lower end of right ulna `7th`
    S52.692 Other fracture of lower end of left ulna `7th`

S52.9 Unspecified fracture of forearm
`5th`
S52.91X Unspecified fracture of right forearm `7th`
S52.92X Unspecified fracture of left forearm `7th`

S53 DISLOCATION AND SPRAIN OF JOINTS AND LIGAMENTS OF ELBOW
`4th`
Includes: avulsion of joint or ligament of elbow
laceration of cartilage, joint or ligament of elbow
sprain of cartilage, joint or ligament of elbow
traumatic hemarthrosis of joint or ligament of elbow
traumatic rupture of joint or ligament of elbow
traumatic subluxation of joint or ligament of elbow
traumatic tear of joint or ligament of elbow
Code also any associated open wound
Excludes2: strain of muscle, fascia and tendon at forearm level (S56.-)

7th characters for category S53
A—initial encounter
D—subsequent encounter
S—sequela

S53.0 Subluxation and dislocation of radial head
`5th`
Dislocation of radiohumeral joint
Subluxation of radiohumeral joint
Excludes1: Monteggia's fracture-dislocation (S52.27-)

S53.00 Unspecified subluxation and dislocation of radial head
`6th`
    S53.001 Unspecified subluxation of right radial head `7th`
    S53.002 Unspecified subluxation of left radial head `7th`
    S53.004 Unspecified dislocation of right radial head `7th`
    S53.005 Unspecified dislocation of left radial head `7th`

S53.02 Posterior subluxation and dislocation of radial head
`6th`
Posteriolateral subluxation and dislocation of radial head
    S53.021 Posterior subluxation of right radial head `7th`
    S53.022 Posterior subluxation of left radial head `7th`
    S53.024 Posterior dislocation of right radial head `7th`
    S53.025 Posterior dislocation of left radial head `7th`

S53.03 Nursemaid's elbow
`6th`
    S53.031 Nursemaid's elbow, right elbow `7th`
    S53.032 Nursemaid's elbow, left elbow `7th`

S53.09 Other subluxation and dislocation of radial head
`6th`
    S53.091 Other subluxation of right radial head `7th`
    S53.092 Other subluxation of left radial head `7th`
    S53.094 Other dislocation of right radial head `7th`
    S53.095 Other dislocation of left radial head `7th`

S53.4 Sprain of elbow
`5th`
Excludes2: traumatic rupture of radial collateral ligament (S53.2-)
traumatic rupture of ulnar collateral ligament (S53.3-)

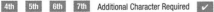

`4th` `5th` `6th` `7th` Additional Character Required   ✓   3-character code   Unspecified laterality codes were excluded here.

• =New Code
▲ =Revised Code
◘ =Social determinants of health

Excludes1—Not coded here, do not use together
Excludes2—Not included here

CHAPTER 19. INJURY, POISONING AND CERTAIN OTHER CONSEQUENCES OF EXTERNAL CAUSES   (S53.40–S56.412)

S53.40 Unspecified sprain of elbow
6th
    S53.401 Unspecified sprain of right elbow
    7th
    S53.402 Unspecified sprain of left elbow
    7th

S53.41 Radiohumeral (joint) sprain
6th
    S53.411 Radiohumeral (joint) sprain of right elbow
    7th
    S53.412 Radiohumeral (joint) sprain of left elbow
    7th

S53.42 Ulnohumeral (joint) sprain
6th
    S53.421 Ulnohumeral (joint) sprain of right elbow
    7th
    S53.422 Ulnohumeral (joint) sprain of left elbow
    7th

S53.43 Radial collateral ligament sprain
6th
    S53.431 Radial collateral ligament sprain of right elbow
    7th
    S53.432 Radial collateral ligament sprain of left elbow
    7th

S53.44 Ulnar collateral ligament sprain
6th

> 7th characters for category S53
> A—initial encounter
> D—subsequent encounter
> S—sequela

    S53.441 Ulnar collateral ligament sprain of right elbow
    7th
    S53.442 Ulnar collateral ligament sprain of left elbow
    7th

S53.49 Other sprain of elbow
6th
    S53.491 Other sprain of right elbow
    7th
    S53.492 Other sprain of left elbow
    7th

S56 INJURY OF MUSCLE, FASCIA AND TENDON AT FOREARM LEVEL
4th

Code also any associated open wound (S51.-)

Excludes2: injury of muscle, fascia and tendon at or below wrist (S66.-)
sprain of joints and ligaments of elbow (S53.4-)

> 7th characters for category S56
> A—initial encounter
> D—subsequent encounter
> S—sequela

S56.0 Injury of flexor muscle, fascia and tendon of thumb at forearm level
5th
  S56.01 Strain of flexor muscle, fascia and tendon of thumb at forearm level
  6th
    S56.011 Strain of flexor muscle, fascia and tendon of right thumb at forearm level
    7th
    S56.012 Strain of flexor muscle, fascia and tendon of left thumb at forearm level
    7th
  S56.02 Laceration of flexor muscle, fascia and tendon of thumb at forearm level
  6th
    S56.021 Laceration of flexor muscle, fascia and tendon of right thumb at forearm level
    7th
    S56.022 Laceration of flexor muscle, fascia and tendon of left thumb at forearm level
    7th

S56.1 Injury of flexor muscle, fascia and tendon of other and unspecified finger at forearm level
5th
  S56.11 Strain of flexor muscle, fascia and tendon of other and unspecified finger at forearm level
  6th
    S56.111 Strain of flexor muscle, fascia and tendon of right index finger at forearm level
    7th
    S56.112 Strain of flexor muscle, fascia and tendon of left index finger at forearm level
    7th
    S56.113 Strain of flexor muscle, fascia and tendon of right middle finger at forearm level
    7th
    S56.114 Strain of flexor muscle, fascia and tendon of left middle finger at forearm level
    7th
    S56.115 Strain of flexor muscle, fascia and tendon of right ring finger at forearm level
    7th
    S56.116 Strain of flexor muscle, fascia and tendon of left ring finger at forearm level
    7th
    S56.117 Strain of flexor muscle, fascia and tendon of right little finger at forearm level
    7th
    S56.118 Strain of flexor muscle, fascia and tendon of left little finger at forearm level
    7th
  S56.12 Laceration of flexor muscle, fascia and tendon of other and unspecified finger at forearm level
  6th
    S56.121 Laceration of flexor muscle, fascia and tendon of right index finger at forearm level
    7th
    S56.122 Laceration of flexor muscle, fascia and tendon of left index finger at forearm level
    7th
    S56.123 Laceration of flexor muscle, fascia and tendon of right middle finger at forearm level
    7th
    S56.124 Laceration of flexor muscle, fascia and tendon of left middle finger at forearm level
    7th
    S56.125 Laceration of flexor muscle, fascia and tendon of right ring finger at forearm level
    7th
    S56.126 Laceration of flexor muscle, fascia and tendon of left ring finger at forearm level
    7th
    S56.127 Laceration of flexor muscle, fascia and tendon of right little finger at forearm level
    7th
    S56.128 Laceration of flexor muscle, fascia and tendon of left little finger at forearm level
    7th

S56.2 Injury of other flexor muscle, fascia and tendon at forearm level
5th
  S56.21 Strain of other flexor muscle, fascia and tendon at forearm level
  6th
    S56.211 Strain of other flexor muscle, fascia and tendon at forearm level, right arm
    7th
    S56.212 Strain of other flexor muscle, fascia and tendon at forearm level, left arm
    7th
  S56.22 Laceration of other flexor muscle, fascia and tendon at forearm level
  6th
    S56.221 Laceration of other flexor muscle, fascia and tendon at forearm level, right arm
    7th
    S56.222 Laceration of other flexor muscle, fascia and tendon at forearm level, left arm
    7th

S56.3 Injury of extensor or abductor muscles, fascia and tendons of thumb at forearm level
5th
  S56.31 Strain of extensor or abductor muscles, fascia and tendons of thumb at forearm level
  6th
    S56.311 Strain of extensor or abductor muscles, fascia and tendons of right thumb at forearm level
    7th
    S56.312 Strain of extensor or abductor muscles, fascia and tendons of left thumb at forearm level
    7th
  S56.32 Laceration of extensor or abductor muscles, fascia and tendons of thumb at forearm level
  6th
    S56.321 Laceration of extensor or abductor muscles, fascia and tendons of right thumb at forearm level
    7th
    S56.322 Laceration of extensor or abductor muscles, fascia and tendons of left thumb at forearm level
    7th
  S56.39 Other injury of extensor or abductor muscles, fascia and tendons of thumb at forearm level
  6th
    S56.391 Other injury of extensor or abductor muscles, fascia and tendons of right thumb at forearm level
    7th
    S56.392 Other injury of extensor or abductor muscles, fascia and tendons of left thumb at forearm level
    7th

S56.4 Injury of extensor muscle, fascia and tendon of other and unspecified finger at forearm level
5th
  S56.41 Strain of extensor muscle, fascia and tendon of other and unspecified finger at forearm level
  6th
    S56.411 Strain of extensor muscle, fascia and tendon of right index finger at forearm level
    7th
    S56.412 Strain of extensor muscle, fascia and tendon of left index finger at forearm level
    7th

4th **5th** **6th** **7th** Additional Character Required   ✔   3-character code   Unspecified laterality codes were excluded here.

• =New Code
▲ =Revised Code
▫ =Social determinants of health

Excludes1—Not coded here, do not use together
Excludes2—Not included here

S56.413 **Strain of extensor muscle, fascia and tendon of right middle finger at forearm level** [7th]

S56.414 **Strain of extensor muscle, fascia and tendon of left middle finger at forearm level** [7th]

S56.415 **Strain of extensor muscle, fascia and tendon of right ring finger at forearm level** [7th]

S56.416 **Strain of extensor muscle, fascia and tendon of left ring finger at forearm level** [7th]

S56.417 **Strain of extensor muscle, fascia and tendon of right little finger at forearm level** [7th]

S56.418 **Strain of extensor muscle, fascia and tendon of left little finger at forearm level** [7th]

S56.42 **Laceration of extensor muscle, fascia and tendon of other and unspecified finger at forearm level** [6th]

> 7th characters for category S56
> A—initial encounter
> D—subsequent encounter
> S—sequela

S56.421 **Laceration of extensor muscle, fascia and tendon of right index finger at forearm level** [7th]

S56.422 **Laceration of extensor muscle, fascia and tendon of left index finger at forearm level** [7th]

S56.423 **Laceration of extensor muscle, fascia and tendon of right middle finger at forearm level** [7th]

S56.424 **Laceration of extensor muscle, fascia and tendon of left middle finger at forearm level** [7th]

S56.425 **Laceration of extensor muscle, fascia and tendon of right ring finger at forearm level** [7th]

S56.426 **Laceration of extensor muscle, fascia and tendon of left ring finger at forearm level** [7th]

S56.427 **Laceration of extensor muscle, fascia and tendon of right little finger at forearm level** [7th]

S56.428 **Laceration of extensor muscle, fascia and tendon of left little finger at forearm level** [7th]

S56.5 **Injury of other extensor muscle, fascia and tendon at forearm level** [5th]

S56.51 **Strain of other extensor muscle, fascia and tendon at forearm level** [6th]

S56.511 **Strain of other extensor muscle, fascia and tendon at forearm level, right arm** [7th]

S56.512 **Strain of other extensor muscle, fascia and tendon at forearm level, left arm** [7th]

S56.52 **Laceration of other extensor muscle, fascia and tendon at forearm level** [6th]

S56.521 **Laceration of other extensor muscle, fascia and tendon at forearm level, right arm** [7th]

S56.522 **Laceration of other extensor muscle, fascia and tendon at forearm level, left arm** [7th]

S56.8 **Injury of other muscles, fascia and tendons at forearm level** [5th]

S56.81 **Strain of other muscles, fascia and tendons at forearm level** [6th]

S56.811 **Strain of other muscles, fascia and tendons at forearm level, right arm** [7th]

S56.812 **Strain of other muscles, fascia and tendons at forearm level, left arm** [7th]

S56.82 **Laceration of other muscles, fascia and tendons at forearm level** [6th]

S56.821 **Laceration of other muscles, fascia and tendons at forearm level, right arm** [7th]

S56.822 **Laceration of other muscles, fascia and tendons at forearm level, left arm** [7th]

S56.9 **Injury of unspecified muscles, fascia and tendons at forearm level** [5th]

S56.90 **Unspecified injury of unspecified muscles, fascia and tendons at forearm level** [6th]

S56.901 **Unspecified injury of unspecified muscles, fascia and tendons at forearm level, right arm** [7th]

S56.902 **Unspecified injury of unspecified muscles, fascia and tendons at forearm level, left arm** [7th]

S56.91 **Strain of unspecified muscles, fascia and tendons at forearm level** [6th]

S56.911 **Strain of unspecified muscles, fascia and tendons at forearm level, right arm** [7th]

S56.912 **Strain of unspecified muscles, fascia and tendons at forearm level, left arm** [7th]

S56.92 **Laceration of unspecified muscles, fascia and tendons at forearm level** [6th]

S56.921 **Laceration of unspecified muscles, fascia and tendons at forearm level, right arm** [7th]

S56.922 **Laceration of unspecified muscles, fascia and tendons at forearm level, left arm** [7th]

S59 **OTHER AND UNSPECIFIED INJURIES OF ELBOW AND FOREARM** [4th]

Excludes2: other and unspecified injuries of wrist and hand (S69.-)

S59.0 **Physeal fracture of lower end of ulna** [5th]

> 7th characters for category S59
> A—initial encounter for closed fracture
> D—subsequent encounter for fracture with routine healing
> G—subsequent encounter for fracture with delayed healing
> K—subsequent encounter for fracture with nonunion
> P—subsequent encounter for fracture with malunion
> S—sequela

S59.00 **Unspecified physeal fracture of lower end of ulna** [6th]

S59.001 **Unspecified physeal fracture of lower end of ulna, right arm** [7th]

S59.002 **Unspecified physeal fracture of lower end of ulna, left arm** [7th]

S59.01 **Salter-Harris Type I physeal fracture of lower end of ulna** [6th]

S59.011 **Salter-Harris Type I physeal fracture of lower end of ulna, right arm** [7th]

S59.012 **Salter-Harris Type I physeal fracture of lower end of ulna, left arm** [7th]

S59.02 **Salter-Harris Type II physeal fracture of lower end of ulna** [6th]

S59.021 **Salter-Harris Type II physeal fracture of lower end of ulna, right arm** [7th]

S59.022 **Salter-Harris Type II physeal fracture of lower end of ulna, left arm** [7th]

S59.03 **Salter-Harris Type III physeal fracture of lower end of ulna** [6th]

S59.031 **Salter-Harris Type III physeal fracture of lower end of ulna, right arm** [7th]

S59.032 **Salter-Harris Type III physeal fracture of lower end of ulna, left arm** [7th]

S59.04 **Salter-Harris Type IV physeal fracture of lower end of ulna** [6th]

S59.041 **Salter-Harris Type IV physeal fracture of lower end of ulna, right arm** [7th]

S59.042 **Salter-Harris Type IV physeal fracture of lower end of ulna, left arm** [7th]

S59.09 **Other physeal fracture of lower end of ulna** [6th]

S59.091 **Other physeal fracture of lower end of ulna, right arm** [7th]

S59.092 **Other physeal fracture of lower end of ulna, left arm** [7th]

S59.1 **Physeal fracture of upper end of radius** [5th]

S59.10 **Unspecified physeal fracture of upper end of radius** [6th]

S59.101 **Unspecified physeal fracture of upper end of radius, right arm** [7th]

S59.102 **Unspecified physeal fracture of upper end of radius, left arm** [7th]

S59.11 **Salter-Harris Type I physeal fracture of upper end of radius** [6th]

S59.111 **Salter-Harris Type I physeal fracture of upper end of radius, right arm** [7th]

S59.112 **Salter-Harris Type I physeal fracture of upper end of radius, left arm** [7th]

[4th] [5th] [6th] [7th] Additional Character Required ✓ 3-character code | Unspecified laterality codes were excluded here. | • =New Code ▲ =Revised Code ¤ =Social determinants of health | *Excludes1*—Not coded here, do not use together *Excludes2*—Not included here

S59.12 `6th` Salter-Harris Type II physeal fracture of upper end of radius

    S59.121 `7th` Salter-Harris Type II physeal fracture of upper end of radius, right arm

    S59.122 `7th` Salter-Harris Type II physeal fracture of upper end of radius, left arm

S59.13 `6th` Salter-Harris Type III physeal fracture of upper end of radius

    S59.131 `7th` Salter-Harris Type III physeal fracture of upper end of radius, right arm

    S59.132 `7th` Salter-Harris Type III physeal fracture of upper end of radius, left arm

S59.14 `6th` Salter-Harris Type IV physeal fracture of upper end of radius

    S59.141 `7th` Salter-Harris Type IV physeal fracture of upper end of radius, right arm

    S59.142 `7th` Salter-Harris Type IV physeal fracture of upper end of radius, left arm

> **7th characters for category S59**
> A—initial encounter for closed fracture
> D—subsequent encounter for fracture with routine healing
> G—subsequent encounter for fracture with delayed healing
> K—subsequent encounter for fracture with nonunion
> P—subsequent encounter for fracture with malunion
> S—sequela

S59.19 `6th` Other physeal fracture of upper end of radius

    S59.191 `7th` Other physeal fracture of upper end of radius, right arm

    S59.192 `7th` Other physeal fracture of upper end of radius, left arm

S59.2 Physeal fracture of lower end of radius

`5th` **S59.20** `6th` Unspecified physeal fracture of lower end of radius

    S59.201 `7th` Unspecified physeal fracture of lower end of radius, right arm

    S59.202 `7th` Unspecified physeal fracture of lower end of radius, left arm

S59.21 `6th` Salter-Harris Type I physeal fracture of lower end of radius

    S59.211 `7th` Salter-Harris Type I physeal fracture of lower end of radius, right arm

    S59.212 `7th` Salter-Harris Type I physeal fracture of lower end of radius, left arm

S59.22 `6th` Salter-Harris Type II physeal fracture of lower end of radius

    S59.221 `7th` Salter-Harris Type II physeal fracture of lower end of radius, right arm

    S59.222 `7th` Salter-Harris Type II physeal fracture of lower end of radius, left arm

S59.23 `6th` Salter-Harris Type III physeal fracture of lower end of radius

    S59.231 `7th` Salter-Harris Type III physeal fracture of lower end of radius, right arm

    S59.232 `7th` Salter-Harris Type III physeal fracture of lower end of radius, left arm

S59.24 `6th` Salter-Harris Type IV physeal fracture of lower end of radius

    S59.241 `7th` Salter-Harris Type IV physeal fracture of lower end of radius, right arm

    S59.242 `7th` Salter-Harris Type IV physeal fracture of lower end of radius, left arm

S59.29 `6th` Other physeal fracture of lower end of radius

    S59.291 `7th` Other physeal fracture of lower end of radius, right arm

    S59.292 `7th` Other physeal fracture of lower end of radius, left arm

S59.8 Other specified injuries of elbow and forearm

`5th` **S59.80** `6th` Other specified injuries of elbow

    S59.801 `7th` Other specified injuries of right elbow

> **7th characters for subcategory S59.8**
> A—initial encounter
> D—subsequent encounter
> S—sequela

    S59.802 Other specified injuries of left elbow

S59.81 `7th` Other specified injuries of forearm

`6th`   **S59.811** `7th` Other specified injuries right forearm

    S59.812 `7th` Other specified injuries left forearm

(S60–S69) INJURIES TO THE WRIST, HAND AND FINGERS

Excludes2: burns and corrosions (T20–T32)
    frostbite (T33–T34)
    insect bite or sting, venomous (T63.4)

S60 `4th` **SUPERFICIAL INJURY OF WRIST, HAND AND FINGERS**

S60.0 `5th` Contusion of finger without damage to nail

    Excludes1: contusion involving nail (matrix) (S60.1)

> **7th characters for category S60**
> A—initial encounter
> D—subsequent encounter
> S—sequela

    S60.00X `7th` Contusion of unspecified finger without damage to nail

    Contusion of finger(s) NOS

S60.01 Contusion of thumb without damage to nail

`6th`   **S60.011** `7th` Contusion of right thumb without damage to nail

S60.02 Contusion of index finger without damage to nail

`6th`   **S60.021** `7th` Contusion of right index finger without damage to nail

    S60.022 `7th` Contusion of left index finger without damage to nail

S60.03 Contusion of middle finger without damage to nail

`6th`   **S60.031** `7th` Contusion of right middle finger without damage to nail

    S60.032 `7th` Contusion of left middle finger without damage to nail

S60.04 Contusion of ring finger without damage to nail

`6th`   **S60.041** `7th` Contusion of right ring finger without damage to nail

    S60.042 `7th` Contusion of left ring finger without damage to nail

S60.05 Contusion of little finger without damage to nail

`6th`   **S60.051** `7th` Contusion of right little finger without damage to nail

    S60.052 `7th` Contusion of left little finger without damage to nail

S60.1 Contusion of finger with damage to nail

`5th` **S60.11** Contusion of thumb with damage to nail

`6th`   **S60.111** `7th` Contusion of right thumb with damage to nail

    S60.112 `7th` Contusion of left thumb with damage to nail

S60.12 Contusion of index finger with damage to nail

`6th`   **S60.121** `7th` Contusion of right index finger with damage to nail

    S60.122 `7th` Contusion of left index finger with damage to nail

S60.13 Contusion of middle finger with damage to nail

`6th`   **S60.131** `7th` Contusion of right middle finger with damage to nail

    S60.132 `7th` Contusion of left middle finger with damage to nail

S60.14 Contusion of ring finger with damage to nail

`6th`   **S60.141** `7th` Contusion of right ring finger with damage to nail

    S60.142 `7th` Contusion of left ring finger with damage to nail

S60.15 Contusion of little finger with damage to nail

`6th`   **S60.151** `7th` Contusion of right little finger with damage to nail

    S60.152 `7th` Contusion of left little finger with damage to nail

S60.2 Contusion of wrist and hand

`5th`   ***Excludes2:*** contusion of fingers (S60.0-, S60.1-)

`4th` `5th` `6th` `7th` Additional Character Required ✓ 3-character code

Unspecified laterality codes were excluded here.

• =New Code
▲ =Revised Code
◘ =Social determinants of health

Excludes1—Not coded here, do not use together
Excludes2—Not included here

S60.21 **Contusion of wrist**
6th
    S60.211 **Contusion of right wrist**
    7th
    S60.212 **Contusion of left wrist**
    7th

S60.22 **Contusion of hand**
6th
    S60.221 **Contusion of right hand**
    7th
    S60.222 **Contusion**
    7th   **of left hand**

S60.3 **Other superficial injuries of thumb**
5th
S60.31 **Abrasion of thumb**
6th
    S60.311 **Abrasion of right thumb**
    7th
    S60.312 **Abrasion of**
    7th   **left thumb**

> 7th characters for category S60
> A—initial encounter
> D—subsequent encounter
> S—sequela

S60.32 **Blister (nonthermal)**
6th **of thumb**
    S60.321 **Blister**
    7th   **(nonthermal) of right thumb**
    S60.322 **Blister (nonthermal) of left thumb**
    7th

S60.34 **External constriction of thumb**
6th
Hair tourniquet syndrome of thumb
Use additional cause code to identify the constricting item (W49.0-)
    S60.341 **External constriction of right thumb**
    7th
    S60.342 **External constriction of left thumb**
    7th

S60.35 **Superficial FB of thumb**
6th
Splinter in the thumb
    S60.351 **Superficial FB of right thumb**
    7th
    S60.352 **Superficial FB of left thumb**
    7th

S60.36 **Insect bite (nonvenomous) of thumb**
6th
    S60.361 **Insect bite (nonvenomous) of right thumb**
    7th
    S60.362 **Insect bite (nonvenomous) of left thumb**
    7th

S60.37 **Other superficial bite of thumb**
6th
Excludes1: open bite of thumb (S61.05-, S61.15-)
    S60.371 **Other superficial bite of right thumb**
    7th
    S60.372 **Other superficial bite of left thumb**
    7th

S60.4 **Other superficial injuries of other fingers**
5th
S60.41 **Abrasion of fingers**
6th
    S60.410 **Abrasion of right index finger**
    7th
    S60.411 **Abrasion of left index finger**
    7th
    S60.412 **Abrasion of right middle finger**
    7th
    S60.413 **Abrasion of left middle finger**
    7th
    S60.414 **Abrasion of right ring finger**
    7th
    S60.415 **Abrasion of left ring finger**
    7th
    S60.416 **Abrasion of right little finger**
    7th
    S60.417 **Abrasion of left little finger**
    7th

S60.42 **Blister (nonthermal) of fingers**
6th
    S60.420 **Blister (nonthermal) of right index finger**
    7th
    S60.421 **Blister (nonthermal) of left index finger**
    7th
    S60.422 **Blister (nonthermal) of right middle finger**
    7th
    S60.423 **Blister (nonthermal) of left middle finger**
    7th

    S60.424 **Blister (nonthermal) of right ring finger**
    7th
    S60.425 **Blister (nonthermal) of left ring finger**
    7th
    S60.426 **Blister (nonthermal) of right little finger**
    7th
    S60.427 **Blister (nonthermal) of left little finger**
    7th

S60.44 **External constriction of fingers**
6th
Hair tourniquet syndrome of finger
Use additional cause code to identify the constricting item (W49.0-)
    S60.440 **External constriction of right index finger**
    7th
    S60.441 **External constriction of left index finger**
    7th
    S60.442 **External constriction of right middle finger**
    7th
    S60.443 **External constriction of left middle finger**
    7th
    S60.444 **External constriction of right ring finger**
    7th
    S60.445 **External constriction of left ring finger**
    7th
    S60.446 **External constriction of right little finger**
    7th
    S60.447 **External constriction of left little finger**
    7th

S60.45 **Superficial FB of fingers**
6th
Splinter in the finger(s)
    S60.450 **Superficial FB of right index finger**
    7th
    S60.451 **Superficial FB of left index finger**
    7th
    S60.452 **Superficial FB of right middle finger**
    7th
    S60.453 **Superficial FB of left middle finger**
    7th
    S60.454 **Superficial FB of right ring finger**
    7th
    S60.455 **Superficial FB of left ring finger**
    7th
    S60.456 **Superficial FB of right little finger**
    7th
    S60.457 **Superficial FB of left little finger**
    7th

S60.46 **Insect bite (nonvenomous) of fingers**
6th
    S60.460 **Insect bite (nonvenomous) of right index finger**
    7th
    S60.461 **Insect bite (nonvenomous) of left index finger**
    7th
    S60.462 **Insect bite (nonvenomous) of right middle finger**
    7th
    S60.463 **Insect bite (nonvenomous) of left middle finger**
    7th
    S60.464 **Insect bite (nonvenomous) of right ring finger**
    7th
    S60.465 **Insect bite (nonveno-mous) of left ring finger**
    7th
    S60.466 **Insect bite (nonvenomous) of right little finger**
    7th
    S60.467 **Insect bite (nonvenomous) of left little finger**
    7th

S60.47 **Other superficial bite of fingers**
6th
Excludes1: open bite of fingers (S61.25-, S61.35-)
    S60.470 **Other superficial bite of right index finger**
    7th
    S60.471 **Other superficial bite of left index finger**
    7th
    S60.472 **Other superficial bite of right middle finger**
    7th
    S60.473 **Other superficial bite of left middle finger**
    7th

CHAPTER 19. INJURY, POISONING AND CERTAIN OTHER CONSEQUENCES OF EXTERNAL CAUSES (S60.21–S60.473)

4th 5th 6th 7th Additional Character Required ✓ 3-character code | Unspecified laterality codes were excluded here. | • =New Code / ▲ =Revised Code / ⊡ =Social determinants of health | *Excludes1*—Not coded here, do not use together / *Excludes2*—Not included here

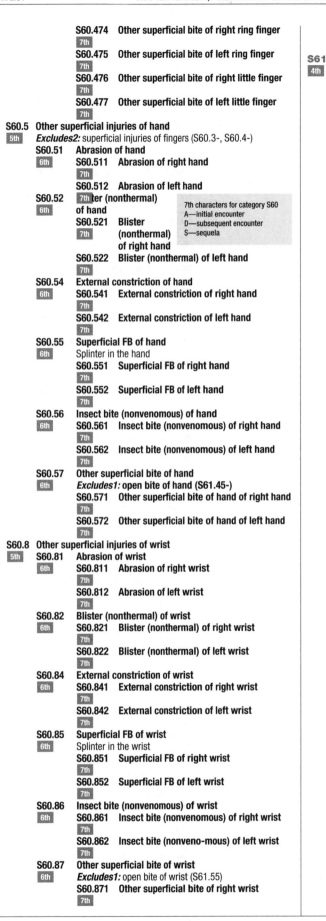

S60.474   Other superficial bite of right ring finger
`7th`

S60.475   Other superficial bite of left ring finger
`7th`

S60.476   Other superficial bite of right little finger
`7th`

S60.477   Other superficial bite of left little finger
`7th`

S60.5   **Other superficial injuries of hand**
`5th`   *Excludes2:* superficial injuries of fingers (S60.3-, S60.4-)

   S60.51   **Abrasion of hand**
   `6th`   **S60.511**   Abrasion of right hand
     `7th`
     S60.512   Abrasion of left hand
     `7th`

   S60.52   Blister (nonthermal)
   `6th`   of hand

> 7th characters for category S60
> A—initial encounter
> D—subsequent encounter
> S—sequela

     S60.521   Blister (nonthermal) of right hand
     `7th`
     S60.522   Blister (nonthermal) of left hand
     `7th`

   S60.54   **External constriction of hand**
   `6th`   **S60.541**   External constriction of right hand
     `7th`
     S60.542   External constriction of left hand
     `7th`

   S60.55   **Superficial FB of hand**
   `6th`   Splinter in the hand
     S60.551   Superficial FB of right hand
     `7th`
     S60.552   Superficial FB of left hand
     `7th`

   S60.56   **Insect bite (nonvenomous) of hand**
   `6th`   **S60.561**   Insect bite (nonvenomous) of right hand
     `7th`
     S60.562   Insect bite (nonvenomous) of left hand
     `7th`

   S60.57   **Other superficial bite of hand**
   `6th`   *Excludes1:* open bite of hand (S61.45-)
     S60.571   Other superficial bite of hand of right hand
     `7th`
     S60.572   Other superficial bite of hand of left hand
     `7th`

S60.8   **Other superficial injuries of wrist**
`5th`   **S60.81**   **Abrasion of wrist**
   `6th`   **S60.811**   Abrasion of right wrist
     `7th`
     S60.812   Abrasion of left wrist
     `7th`

   S60.82   **Blister (nonthermal) of wrist**
   `6th`   **S60.821**   Blister (nonthermal) of right wrist
     `7th`
     S60.822   Blister (nonthermal) of left wrist
     `7th`

   S60.84   **External constriction of wrist**
   `6th`   **S60.841**   External constriction of right wrist
     `7th`
     S60.842   External constriction of left wrist
     `7th`

   S60.85   **Superficial FB of wrist**
   `6th`   Splinter in the wrist
     S60.851   Superficial FB of right wrist
     `7th`
     S60.852   Superficial FB of left wrist
     `7th`

   S60.86   **Insect bite (nonvenomous) of wrist**
   `6th`   **S60.861**   Insect bite (nonvenomous) of right wrist
     `7th`
     S60.862   Insect bite (nonveno-mous) of left wrist
     `7th`

   S60.87   **Other superficial bite of wrist**
   `6th`   *Excludes1:* open bite of wrist (S61.55)
     S60.871   Other superficial bite of right wrist
     `7th`

S60.872   Other superficial bite of left wrist
`7th`

S61   **OPEN WOUND OF WRIST, HAND AND FINGERS**
`4th`   **Code also** any associated wound infection
   Excludes1: open fracture of wrist, hand and finger (S62.- with
     7th character B)
   traumatic amputation of wrist and hand (S68.-)

S61.0   **Open wound of thumb without damage to nail**
`5th`   *Excludes1:* open wound of thumb
     with damage to nail (S61.1-)

> 7th characters for category S61
> A—initial encounter
> D—subsequent encounter
> S—sequela

   S61.01   **Laceration without**
   `6th`   **FB of thumb without**
     damage to nail
     S61.011   Laceration without FB of right thumb without damage to nail
     `7th`
     S61.012   Laceration without FB of left thumb without damage to nail
     `7th`

   S61.02   **Laceration with FB of thumb without damage to nail**
   `6th`   **S61.021**   Laceration with FB of right thumb without damage to nail
     `7th`
     S61.022   Laceration with FB of left thumb without damage to nail
     `7th`

   S61.03   **Puncture wound without FB of thumb without damage to nail**
   `6th`   **S61.031**   Puncture wound without FB of right thumb without damage to nail
     `7th`
     S61.032   Puncture wound without FB of left thumb without damage to nail
     `7th`

   S61.04   **Puncture wound with FB of thumb without damage to nail**
   `6th`   **S61.041**   Puncture wound with FB of right thumb without damage to nail
     `7th`
     S61.042   Puncture wound with FB of left thumb without damage to nail
     `7th`

   S61.05   **Open bite of thumb without damage to nail**
   `6th`   Bite of thumb NOS
     Excludes1: superficial bite of thumb (S60.36-, S60.37-)
     S61.051   Open bite of right thumb without damage to nail
     `7th`
     S61.052   Open bite of left thumb without damage to nail
     `7th`

S61.1   **Open wound of thumb with damage to nail**
`5th`   **S61.11**   **Laceration without FB of thumb with damage to nail**
   `6th`   **S61.111**   Laceration without FB of right thumb with damage to nail
     `7th`
     S61.112   Laceration without FB of left thumb with damage to nail
     `7th`

   S61.12   **Laceration with FB of thumb with damage to nail**
   `6th`   **S61.121**   Laceration with FB of right thumb with damage to nail
     `7th`
     S61.122   Laceration with FB of left thumb with damage to nail
     `7th`

   S61.13   **Puncture wound without FB of thumb with damage to nail**
   `6th`   **S61.131**   Puncture wound without FB of right thumb with damage to nail
     `7th`
     S61.132   Puncture wound without FB of left thumb with damage to nail
     `7th`

   S61.14   **Puncture wound with FB of thumb with damage to nail**
   `6th`   **S61.141**   Puncture wound with FB of right thumb with damage to nail
     `7th`
     S61.142   Puncture wound with FB of left thumb with damage to nail
     `7th`

   S61.15   **Open bite of thumb with damage to nail**
   `6th`   Bite of thumb with damage to nail NOS
     Excludes1: superficial bite of thumb (S60.36-, S60.37-)
     S61.151   Open bite of right thumb with damage to nail
     `7th`
     S61.152   Open bite of left thumb with damage to nail
     `7th`

`4th` `5th` `6th` `7th`   Additional Character Required   ✓   3-character code   Unspecified laterality codes were excluded here.   • =New Code   ▲ =Revised Code   ▫ =Social determinants of health   *Excludes1*—Not coded here, do not use together   *Excludes2*—Not included here

S61.2 **Open wound of other finger without damage to nail**
`5th` *Excludes1:* open wound of finger involving nail (matrix) (S61.3-)
Excludes2: open wound of thumb without damage to nail (S61.0-)

S61.21 **Laceration without FB of finger without damage to nail**
`6th`

S61.210 Laceration without FB of right index finger without damage to nail
`7th`

S61.211 Laceration without FB of left index finger without damage to nail
`7th`

S61.212 Laceration without FB of right middle finger without damage to nail
`7th`

S61.213 Laceration without FB of left middle finger without damage to nail
`7th`

S61.214 Laceration without FB of right ring finger without damage to nail
`7th`

S61.215 Laceration without FB of left ring finger without damage to nail
`7th`

> 7th characters for category S61
> A—initial encounter
> D—subsequent encounter
> S—sequela

S61.216 Laceration without FB of right little finger without damage to nail
`7th`

S61.217 Laceration without FB of left little finger without damage to nail
`7th`

S61.22 **Laceration with FB of finger without damage to nail**
`6th`

S61.220 Laceration with FB of right index finger without damage to nail
`7th`

S61.221 Laceration with FB of left index finger without damage to nail
`7th`

S61.222 Laceration with FB of right middle finger without damage to nail
`7th`

S61.223 Laceration with FB of left middle finger without damage to nail
`7th`

S61.224 Laceration with FB of right ring finger without damage to nail
`7th`

S61.225 Laceration with FB of left ring finger without damage to nail
`7th`

S61.226 Laceration with FB of right little finger without damage to nail
`7th`

S61.227 Laceration with FB of left little finger without damage to nail
`7th`

S61.23 **Puncture wound without FB of finger without damage to nail**
`6th`

S61.230 Puncture wound without FB of right index finger without damage to nail
`7th`

S61.231 Puncture wound without FB of left index finger without damage to nail
`7th`

S61.232 Puncture wound without FB of right middle finger without damage to nail
`7th`

S61.233 Puncture wound without FB of left middle finger without damage to nail
`7th`

S61.234 Puncture wound without FB of right ring finger without damage to nail
`7th`

S61.235 Puncture wound without FB of left ring finger without damage to nail
`7th`

S61.236 Puncture wound without FB of right little finger without damage to nail
`7th`

S61.237 Puncture wound without FB of left little finger without damage to nail
`7th`

S61.24 **Puncture wound with FB of finger without damage to nail**
`6th`

S61.240 Puncture wound with FB of right index finger with-out damage to nail
`7th`

S61.241 Puncture wound with FB of left index finger without damage to nail
`7th`

S61.242 Puncture wound with FB of right middle finger without damage to nail
`7th`

S61.243 Puncture wound with FB of left middle finger without damage to nail
`7th`

S61.244 Puncture wound with FB of right ring finger without damage to nail
`7th`

S61.245 Puncture wound with FB of left ring finger without damage to nail
`7th`

S61.246 Puncture wound with FB of right little finger without damage to nail
`7th`

S61.247 Puncture wound with FB of left little finger without damage to nail
`7th`

S61.25 **Open bite of finger without damage to nail**
`6th` Bite of finger without damage to nail NOS
Excludes1: superficial bite of finger (S60.46-, S60.47-)

S61.250 Open bite of right index finger without damage to nail
`7th`

S61.251 Open bite of left index finger without damage to nail
`7th`

S61.252 Open bite of right middle finger without damage to nail
`7th`

S61.253 Open bite of left middle finger without damage to nail
`7th`

S61.254 Open bite of right ring finger without damage to nail
`7th`

S61.255 Open bite of left ring finger without damage to nail
`7th`

S61.256 Open bite of right little finger without damage to nail
`7th`

S61.257 Open bite of left little finger without damage to nail
`7th`

S61.3 **Open wound of other finger with damage to nail**
`5th`

S61.31 **Laceration without FB of finger with damage to nail**
`6th`

S61.310 Laceration without FB of right index finger with damage to nail
`7th`

S61.311 Laceration without FB of left index finger with damage to nail
`7th`

S61.312 Laceration without FB of right middle finger with damage to nail
`7th`

S61.313 Laceration without FB of left middle finger with damage to nail
`7th`

S61.314 Laceration without FB of right ring finger with damage to nail
`7th`

S61.315 Laceration without FB of left ring finger with damage to nail
`7th`

S61.316 Laceration without FB of right little finger with damage to nail
`7th`

S61.317 Laceration without FB of left little finger with damage to nail
`7th`

S61.32 **Laceration with FB of finger with damage to nail**
`6th`

S61.320 Laceration with FB of right index finger with damage to nail
`7th`

S61.321 Laceration with FB of left index finger with damage to nail
`7th`

S61.322 Laceration with FB of right middle finger with damage to nail
`7th`

S61.323 Laceration with FB of left middle finger with damage to nail
`7th`

S61.324 Laceration with FB of right ring finger with damage to nail
`7th`

S61.325 Laceration with FB of left ring finger with damage to nail
`7th`

S61.326 Laceration with FB of right little finger with damage to nail
`7th`

S61.327 Laceration with FB of left little finger with damage to nail
`7th`

S61.33 **Puncture wound without FB of finger with damage to nail**
`6th`

S61.330 Puncture wound without FB of right index finger with damage to nail
`7th`

S61.331 Puncture wound without FB of left index finger with damage to nail
`7th`

S61.332 Puncture wound without FB of right middle finger with damage to nail
`7th`

S61.333 Puncture wound without FB of left middle finger with damage to nail
`7th`

S61.334 Puncture wound without FB of right ring finger with damage to nail
`7th`

S61.335 Puncture wound without FB of left ring finger with damage to nail
`7th`

S61.336 Puncture wound without FB of right little finger with damage to nail
`7th`

`4th` `5th` `6th` `7th` Additional Character Required   ✔ 3-character code   Unspecified laterality codes were excluded here.

• =New Code
▲ =Revised Code
� =Social determinants of health

Excludes1—Not coded here, do not use together
Excludes2—Not included here

S61.337 `7th` Puncture wound without FB of left little finger with damage to nail

S61.34 `6th` Puncture wound with FB of finger with damage to nail

S61.340 `7th` Puncture wound with FB of right index finger with damage to nail

S61.341 `7th` Puncture wound with FB of left index finger with damage to nail

S61.342 `7th` Puncture wound with FB of right middle finger with damage to nail

S61.343 `7th` Puncture wound with FB of left middle finger with damage to nail

S61.344 `7th` Puncture wound with FB of right ring finger with damage to nail

S61.345 `7th` Puncture wound with FB of left ring finger with damage to nail

> 7th characters for category S61
> A—initial encounter
> D—subsequent encounter
> S—sequela

S61.346 `7th` Puncture wound with FB of right little finger with damage to nail

S61.347 `7th` Puncture wound with FB of left little finger with damage to nail

S61.35 `6th` Open bite of finger with damage to nail
Bite of finger with damage to nail NOS
Excludes1: superficial bite of finger (S60.46-, S60.47-)

S61.350 `7th` Open bite of right index finger with damage to nail

S61.351 `7th` Open bite of left index finger with damage to nail

S61.352 `7th` Open bite of right middle finger with damage to nail

S61.353 `7th` Open bite of left middle finger with damage to nail

S61.354 `7th` Open bite of right ring finger with damage to nail

S61.355 `7th` Open bite of left ring finger with damage to nail

S61.356 `7th` Open bite of right little finger with damage to nail

S61.357 `7th` Open bite of left little finger with damage to nail

S61.4 `5th` Open wound of hand

S61.41 `6th` Laceration without FB of hand

S61.411 `7th` Laceration without FB of right hand

S61.412 `7th` Laceration without FB of left hand

S61.42 `6th` Laceration with FB of hand

S61.421 `7th` Laceration with FB of right hand

S61.422 `7th` Laceration with FB of left hand

S61.43 `6th` Puncture wound without FB of hand

S61.431 `7th` Puncture wound without FB of right hand

S61.432 `7th` Puncture wound without FB of left hand

S61.44 `6th` Puncture wound with FB of hand

S61.441 `7th` Puncture wound with FB of right hand

S61.442 `7th` Puncture wound with FB of left hand

S61.45 `6th` Open bite of hand
Bite of hand NOS
Excludes1: superficial bite of hand (S60.56-, S60.57-)

S61.451 `7th` Open bite of right hand

S61.452 `7th` Open bite of left hand

S61.5 `5th` Open wound of wrist

S61.51 `6th` Laceration without FB of wrist

S61.511 `7th` Laceration without FB of right wrist

S61.512 `7th` Laceration without FB of left wrist

S61.52 `6th` Laceration with FB of wrist

S61.521 `7th` Laceration with FB of right wrist

S61.522 `7th` Laceration with FB of left wrist

S61.53 `6th` Puncture wound without FB of wrist

S61.531 `7th` Puncture wound without FB of right wrist

S61.532 `7th` Puncture wound without FB of left wrist

S61.54 `6th` Puncture wound with FB of wrist

S61.541 `7th` Puncture wound with FB of right wrist

S61.542 `7th` Puncture wound with FB of left wrist

S61.55 `6th` Open bite of wrist
Bite of wrist NOS
Excludes1: superficial bite of wrist (S60.86-, S60.87-)

S61.551 `7th` Open bite of right wrist

S61.552 `7th` Open bite of left wrist

S62 FRACTURE AT WRIST AND HAND LEVEL
`4th` **Note:** A fracture not indicated as displaced or nondisplaced should be coded to displaced
A fracture not indicated as open or closed should be coded to closed
Excludes1: traumatic amputation of wrist and hand (S68.-)
Excludes2: fracture of distal parts of ulna and radius (S52.-)

> 7th characters for category S62
> A—initial encounter for closed fracture
> B—initial encounter for open fracture
> D—subsequent encounter for fracture with routine healing
> G—subsequent encounter for fracture with delayed healing
> K—subsequent encounter for fracture with nonunion
> P—subsequent encounter for fracture with malunion
> S—sequela

S62.0 `5th` Fracture of navicular [scaphoid] bone of wrist

S62.00 `6th` Unspecified fracture of navicular [scaphoid] bone of wrist

S62.001 `7th` Unspecified fracture of navicular [scaphoid] bone of right wrist

S62.002 `7th` Unspecified fracture of navicular [scaphoid] bone of left wrist

S62.01 `6th` Fracture of distal pole of navicular [scaphoid] bone of wrist
Fracture of volar tuberosity of navicular [scaphoid] bone of wrist

S62.011 `7th` Displaced fracture of distal pole of navicular [scaphoid] bone of right wrist

S62.012 `7th` Displaced fracture of distal pole of navicular [scaphoid] bone of left wrist

S62.014 `7th` Nondisplaced fracture of distal pole of navicular [scaphoid] bone of right wrist

S62.015 `7th` Nondisplaced fracture of distal pole of navicular [scaphoid] bone of left wrist

S62.02 `6th` Fracture of middle third of navicular [scaphoid] bone of wrist

S62.021 `7th` Displaced fracture of middle third of navicular [scaphoid] bone of right wrist

S62.022 `7th` Displaced fracture of middle third of navicular [scaphoid] bone of left wrist

S62.024 `7th` Nondisplaced fracture of middle third of navicular [scaphoid] bone of right wrist

S62.025 `7th` Nondisplaced fracture of middle third of navicular [scaphoid] bone of left wrist

S62.03 `6th` Fracture of proximal third of navicular [scaphoid] bone of wrist

S62.031 `7th` Displaced fracture of proximal third of navicular [scaphoid] bone of right wrist

S62.032 `7th` Displaced fracture of proximal third of navicular [scaphoid] bone of left wrist

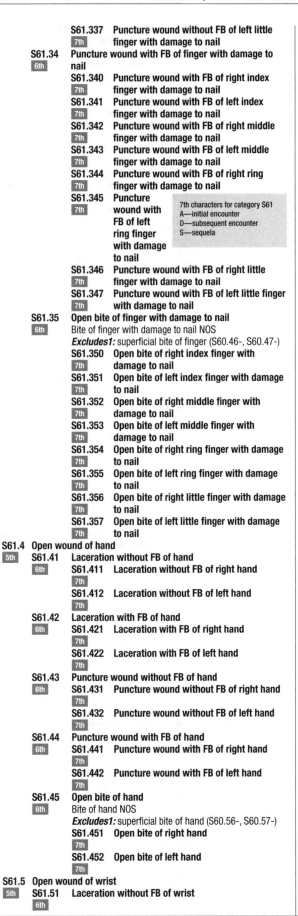

`4th` `5th` `6th` `7th` Additional Character Required   ✓   `3-character code`   Unspecified laterality codes were excluded here.   • =New Code   ▲ =Revised Code   ¤ =Social determinants of health   *Excludes1*—Not coded here, do not use together   *Excludes2*—Not included here

S62.034 `7th` Nondisplaced fracture of proximal third of navicular [scaphoid] bone of right wrist

S62.035 `7th` Nondisplaced fracture of proximal third of navicular [scaphoid] bone of left wrist

S62.1 `5th` **Fracture of other and unspecified carpal bone(s)**

Excludes2: fracture of scaphoid of wrist (S62.0-)

S62.10 `6th` **Fracture of unspecified carpal bone**

Fracture of wrist NOS

S62.101 `7th` **Fracture of unspecified carpal bone, right wrist**

S62.102 `7th` **Fracture of unspecified carpal bone, left wrist**

S62.11 `6th` **Fracture of triquetrum [cuneiform] bone of wrist**

S62.111 `7th` **Displaced fracture of triquetrum [cuneiform] bone, right wrist**

S62.112 `7th` **Displaced fracture of triquetrum [cuneiform] bone, left wrist**

> 7th characters for category S62
> A—initial encounter for closed fracture
> B—initial encounter for open fracture
> D—subsequent encounter for fracture with routine healing
> G—subsequent encounter for fracture with delayed healing
> K—subsequent encounter for fracture with nonunion
> P—subsequent encounter for fracture with malunion
> S—sequela

S62.114 `7th` **Nondisplaced fracture of triquetrum [cuneiform] bone, right wrist**

S62.115 `7th` **Nondisplaced fracture of triquetrum [cuneiform] bone, left wrist**

S62.12 `6th` **Fracture of lunate [semilunar]**

S62.121 `7th` **Displaced fracture of lunate [semilunar], right wrist**

S62.122 `7th` **Displaced fracture of lunate [semilunar], left wrist**

S62.124 `7th` **Nondisplaced fracture of lunate [semilunar], right wrist**

S62.125 `7th` **Nondisplaced fracture of lunate [semilunar], left wrist**

S62.13 `6th` **Fracture of capitate [os magnum] bone**

S62.131 `7th` **Displaced fracture of capitate [os magnum] bone, right wrist**

S62.132 `7th` **Displaced fracture of capitate [os magnum] bone, left wrist**

S62.134 `7th` **Nondisplaced fracture of capitate [os magnum] bone, right wrist**

S62.135 `7th` **Nondisplaced fracture of capitate [os magnum] bone, left wrist**

S62.14 `6th` **Fracture of body of hamate [unciform] bone**

Fracture of hamate [unciform] bone NOS

S62.141 `7th` **Displaced fracture of body of hamate [unciform] bone, right wrist**

S62.142 `7th` **Displaced fracture of body of hamate [unciform] bone, left wrist**

S62.144 `7th` **Nondisplaced fracture of body of hamate [unciform] bone, right wrist**

S62.145 `7th` **Nondisplaced fracture of body of hamate [unciform] bone, left wrist**

S62.15 `6th` **Fracture of hook process of hamate [unciform] bone**

Fracture of unciform process of hamate [unciform] bone

S62.151 `7th` **Displaced fracture of hook process of hamate [unciform] bone, right wrist**

S62.152 `7th` **Displaced fracture of hook process of hamate [unciform] bone, left wrist**

S62.154 `7th` **Nondisplaced fracture of hook process of hamate [unciform] bone, right wrist**

S62.155 `7th` **Nondisplaced fracture of hook process of hamate [unciform] bone, left wrist**

S62.16 `6th` **Fracture of pisiform**

S62.161 `7th` **Displaced fracture of pisiform, right wrist**

S62.162 `7th` **Displaced fracture of pisiform, left wrist**

S62.164 `7th` **Nondisplaced fracture of pisiform, right wrist**

S62.165 `7th` **Nondisplaced fracture of pisiform, left wrist**

S62.17 `6th` **Fracture of trapezium [larger multangular]**

S62.171 `7th` **Displaced fracture of trapezium [larger multangular], right wrist**

S62.172 `7th` **Displaced fracture of trapezium [larger multangular], left wrist**

S62.174 `7th` **Nondisplaced fracture of trapezium [larger multangular], right wrist**

S62.175 `7th` **Nondisplaced fracture of trapezium [larger multangular], left wrist**

S62.18 `6th` **Fracture of trapezoid [smaller multangular]**

S62.181 `7th` **Displaced fracture of trapezoid [smaller multangular], right wrist**

S62.182 `7th` **Displaced fracture of trapezoid [smaller multangular], left wrist**

S62.184 `7th` **Nondisplaced fracture of trapezoid [smaller multangular], right wrist**

S62.185 `7th` **Nondisplaced fracture of trapezoid [smaller multangular], left wrist**

S62.2 `5th` **Fracture of first metacarpal bone**

S62.20 `6th` **Unspecified fracture of first metacarpal bone**

S62.201 `7th` **Unspecified fracture of first metacarpal bone, right hand**

S62.202 `7th` **Unspecified fracture of first metacarpal bone, left hand**

S62.21 `6th` **Bennett's fracture**

S62.211 `7th` **Bennett's fracture, right hand**

S62.212 `7th` **Bennett's fracture, left hand**

S62.22 `6th` **Rolando's fracture**

S62.221 `7th` **Displaced Rolando's fracture, right hand**

S62.222 `7th` **Displaced Rolando's fracture, left hand**

S62.224 `7th` **Nondisplaced Rolando's fracture, right hand**

S62.225 `7th` **Nondisplaced Rolando's fracture, left hand**

S62.23 `6th` **Other fracture of base of first metacarpal bone**

S62.231 `7th` **Other displaced fracture of base of first metacarpal bone, right hand**

S62.232 `7th` **Other displaced fracture of base of first metacarpal bone, left hand**

S62.234 `7th` **Other nondisplaced fracture of base of first metacarpal bone, right hand**

S62.235 `7th` **Other nondisplaced fracture of base of first metacarpal bone, left hand**

S62.24 `6th` **Fracture of shaft of first metacarpal bone**

S62.241 `7th` **Displaced fracture of shaft of first metacarpal bone, right hand**

S62.242 `7th` **Displaced fracture of shaft of first metacarpal bone, left hand**

S62.244 `7th` **Nondisplaced fracture of shaft of first metacarpal bone, right hand**

S62.245 `7th` **Nondisplaced fracture of shaft of first metacarpal bone, left hand**

S62.25 `6th` **Fracture of neck of first metacarpal bone**

S62.251 `7th` **Displaced fracture of neck of first metacarpal bone, right hand**

S62.252 `7th` **Displaced fracture of neck of first metacarpal bone, left hand**

S62.254 `7th` **Nondisplaced fracture of neck of first metacarpal bone, right hand**

S62.255 `7th` **Nondisplaced fracture of neck of first metacarpal bone, left hand**

S62.29 `6th` **Other fracture of first metacarpal bone**

S62.291 `7th` **Other fracture of first metacarpal bone, right hand**

S62.292 `7th` **Other fracture of first metacarpal bone, left hand**

`4th` `5th` `6th` `7th` Additional Character Required   ✔ `3-character code`   Unspecified laterality codes were excluded here.

• =New Code
▲ =Revised Code
▣ =Social determinants of health

Excludes1—Not coded here, do not use together
Excludes2—Not included here

S62.3 **Fracture of other and unspecified metacarpal bone**
`5th`
    Excludes2: fracture of first metacarpal bone (S62.2-)

    S62.30 **Unspecified fracture of other metacarpal bone**
    `6th`
        S62.300 **Unspecified fracture of second metacarpal bone, right hand**
        `7th`
        S62.301 **Unspecified fracture of second metacarpal bone, left hand**
        `7th`
        S62.302 **Unspecified fracture of third metacarpal bone, right hand**
        `7th`
        S62.303 **Unspecified fracture of third metacarpal bone, left hand**
        `7th`
        S62.304 **Unspecified fracture of fourth metacarpal bone, right hand**
        `7th`
        S62.305 **Unspecified fracture of fourth metacarpal bone, left hand**
        `7th`
        S62.306 **Unspecified fracture of fifth metacarpal bone, right hand**
        `7th`
        S62.307 **Unspecified fracture of fifth metacarpal bone, left hand**
        `7th`

> 7th characters for category S62
> A—initial encounter for closed fracture
> B—initial encounter for open fracture
> D—subsequent encounter for fracture with routine healing
> G—subsequent encounter for fracture with delayed healing
> K—subsequent encounter for fracture with nonunion
> P—subsequent encounter for fracture with malunion
> S—sequela

    S62.31 **Displaced fracture of base of other metacarpal bone**
    `6th`
        S62.310 **Displaced fracture of base of second metacarpal bone, right hand**
        `7th`
        S62.311 **Displaced fracture of base of second metacarpal bone, left hand**
        `7th`
        S62.312 **Displaced fracture of base of third metacarpal bone, right hand**
        `7th`
        S62.313 **Displaced fracture of base of third metacarpal bone, left hand**
        `7th`
        S62.314 **Displaced fracture of base of fourth metacarpal bone, right hand**
        `7th`
        S62.315 **Displaced fracture of base of fourth metacarpal bone, left hand**
        `7th`
        S62.316 **Displaced fracture of base of fifth metacarpal bone, right hand**
        `7th`
        S62.317 **Displaced fracture of base of fifth metacarpal bone, left hand**
        `7th`

    S62.32 **Displaced fracture of shaft of other metacarpal bone**
    `6th`
        S62.320 **Displaced fracture of shaft of second metacarpal bone, right hand**
        `7th`
        S62.321 **Displaced fracture of shaft of second metacarpal bone, left hand**
        `7th`
        S62.322 **Displaced fracture of shaft of third metacarpal bone, right hand**
        `7th`
        S62.323 **Displaced fracture of shaft of third metacarpal bone, left hand**
        `7th`
        S62.324 **Displaced fracture of shaft of fourth metacarpal bone, right hand**
        `7th`
        S62.325 **Displaced fracture of shaft of fourth metacarpal bone, left hand**
        `7th`
        S62.326 **Displaced fracture of shaft of fifth metacarpal bone, right hand**
        `7th`
        S62.327 **Displaced fracture of shaft of fifth metacarpal bone, left hand**
        `7th`

    S62.33 **Displaced fracture of neck of other metacarpal bone**
    `6th`
        S62.330 **Displaced fracture of neck of second metacarpal bone, right hand**
        `7th`
        S62.331 **Displaced fracture of neck of second metacarpal bone, left hand**
        `7th`
        S62.332 **Displaced fracture of neck of third metacarpal bone, right hand**
        `7th`
        S62.333 **Displaced fracture of neck of third metacarpal bone, left hand**
        `7th`
        S62.334 **Displaced fracture of neck of fourth metacarpal bone, right hand**
        `7th`
        S62.335 **Displaced fracture of neck of fourth metacarpal bone, left hand**
        `7th`
        S62.336 **Displaced fracture of neck of fifth metacarpal bone, right hand**
        `7th`
        S62.337 **Displaced fracture of neck of fifth metacarpal bone, left hand**
        `7th`

    S62.34 **Nondisplaced fracture of base of other metacarpal bone**
    `6th`
        S62.340 **Nondisplaced fracture of base of second metacarpal bone, right hand**
        `7th`
        S62.341 **Nondisplaced fracture of base of second metacarpal bone left hand**
        `7th`
        S62.342 **Nondisplaced fracture of base of third metacarpal bone, right hand**
        `7th`
        S62.343 **Nondisplaced fracture of base of third metacarpal bone, left hand**
        `7th`
        S62.344 **Nondisplaced fracture of base of fourth metacarpal bone, right hand**
        `7th`
        S62.345 **Nondisplaced fracture of base of fourth metacarpal bone, left hand**
        `7th`
        S62.346 **Nondisplaced fracture of base of fifth metacarpal bone, right hand**
        `7th`
        S62.347 **Nondisplaced fracture of base of fifth metacarpal bone, left hand**
        `7th`

    S62.35 **Nondisplaced fracture of shaft of other metacarpal bone**
    `6th`
        S62.350 **Nondisplaced fracture of shaft of second metacarpal bone, right hand**
        `7th`
        S62.351 **Nondisplaced fracture of shaft of second metacarpal bone, left hand**
        `7th`
        S62.352 **Nondisplaced fracture of shaft of third metacarpal bone, right hand**
        `7th`
        S62.353 **Nondisplaced fracture of shaft of third metacarpal bone, left hand**
        `7th`
        S62.354 **Nondisplaced fracture of shaft of fourth metacarpal bone, right hand**
        `7th`
        S62.355 **Nondisplaced fracture of shaft of fourth metacarpal bone, left hand**
        `7th`
        S62.356 **Nondisplaced fracture of shaft of fifth metacarpal bone, right hand**
        `7th`
        S62.357 **Nondisplaced fracture of shaft of fifth metacarpal bone, left hand**
        `7th`

    S62.36 **Nondisplaced fracture of neck of other metacarpal bone**
    `6th`
        S62.360 **Nondisplaced fracture of neck of second metacarpal bone, right hand**
        `7th`
        S62.361 **Nondisplaced fracture of neck of second metacarpal bone, left hand**
        `7th`
        S62.362 **Nondisplaced fracture of neck of third metacarpal bone, right hand**
        `7th`
        S62.363 **Nondisplaced fracture of neck of third metacarpal bone, left hand**
        `7th`
        S62.364 **Nondisplaced fracture of neck of fourth metacarpal bone, right hand**
        `7th`
        S62.365 **Nondisplaced fracture of neck of fourth metacarpal bone, left hand**
        `7th`
        S62.366 **Nondisplaced fracture of neck of fifth metacarpal bone, right hand**
        `7th`
        S62.367 **Nondisplaced fracture of neck of fifth metacarpal bone, left hand**
        `7th`

    S62.39 **Other fracture of other metacarpal bone**
    `6th`
        S62.390 **Other fracture of second metacarpal bone, right hand**
        `7th`
        S62.391 **Other fracture of second metacarpal bone, left hand**
        `7th`
        S62.392 **Other fracture of third metacarpal bone, right hand**
        `7th`
        S62.393 **Other fracture of third metacarpal bone, left hand**
        `7th`
        S62.394 **Other fracture of fourth metacarpal bone, right hand**
        `7th`

`4th` `5th` `6th` `7th`   Additional Character Required   ✓ 3-character code   Unspecified laterality codes were excluded here.   • =New Code   ▲ =Revised Code   ◘ =Social determinants of health   *Excludes1*—Not coded here, do not use together   *Excludes2*—Not included here

 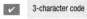

S62.395   Other fracture of fourth metacarpal bone, left hand
`7th`

S62.396   Other fracture of fifth metacarpal bone, right hand
`7th`

S62.397   Other fracture of fifth metacarpal bone, left hand
`7th`

S62.5   **Fracture of thumb**
`5th`

S62.50   Fracture of unspecified phalanx of thumb
`6th`

    S62.501   Fracture of unspecified phalanx of right thumb
`7th`

    S62.502   Fracture of unspecified phalanx of left thumb
`7th`

S62.51   Fracture of proximal phalanx of thumb
`6th`

    S62.511   Displaced fracture of proximal phalanx of right thumb
`7th`

    S62.512   Displaced fracture of proximal phalanx of left thumb
`7th`

    S62.514   Nondisplaced fracture of proximal phalanx of right thumb
`7th`

    S62.515   Nondisplaced fracture of proximal phalanx of left thumb
`7th`

> 7th characters for category S62
> A—initial encounter for closed fracture
> B—initial encounter for open fracture
> D—subsequent encounter for fracture with routine healing
> G—subsequent encounter for fracture with delayed healing
> K—subsequent encounter for fracture with nonunion
> P—subsequent encounter for fracture with malunion
> S—sequela

S62.52   Fracture of distal phalanx of thumb
`6th`

    S62.521   Displaced fracture of distal phalanx of right thumb
`7th`

    S62.522   Displaced fracture of distal phalanx of left thumb
`7th`

    S62.524   Nondisplaced fracture of distal phalanx of right thumb
`7th`

    S62.525   Nondisplaced fracture of distal phalanx of left thumb
`7th`

S62.6   **Fracture of other and unspecified finger(s)**
`5th`

Excludes2: fracture of thumb (S62.5-)

S62.61   Displaced fracture of proximal phalanx of finger
`6th`

    S62.610   Displaced fracture of proximal phalanx of right index finger
`7th`

    S62.611   Displaced fracture of proximal phalanx of left index finger
`7th`

    S62.612   Displaced fracture of proximal phalanx of right middle finger
`7th`

    S62.613   Displaced fracture of proximal phalanx of left middle finger
`7th`

    S62.614   Displaced fracture of proximal phalanx of right ring finger
`7th`

    S62.615   Displaced fracture of proximal phalanx of left ring finger
`7th`

    S62.616   Displaced fracture of proximal phalanx of right little finger
`7th`

    S62.617   Displaced fracture of proximal phalanx of left little finger
`7th`

S62.62   Displaced fracture of middle phalanx of finger
`6th`

    S62.620   Displaced fracture of middle phalanx of right index finger
`7th`

    S62.621   Displaced fracture of middle phalanx of left index finger
`7th`

    S62.622   Displaced fracture of middle phalanx of right middle finger
`7th`

    S62.623   Displaced fracture of middle phalanx of left middle finger
`7th`

    S62.624   Displaced fracture of middle phalanx of right ring finger
`7th`

    S62.625   Displaced fracture of middle phalanx of left ring finger
`7th`

    S62.626   Displaced fracture of middle phalanx of right little finger
`7th`

    S62.627   Displaced fracture of middle phalanx of left little finger
`7th`

S62.63   Displaced fracture of distal phalanx of finger
`6th`

    S62.630   Displaced fracture of distal phalanx of right index finger
`7th`

    S62.631   Displaced fracture of distal phalanx of left index finger
`7th`

    S62.632   Displaced fracture of distal phalanx of right middle finger
`7th`

    S62.633   Displaced fracture of distal phalanx of left middle finger
`7th`

    S62.634   Displaced fracture of distal phalanx of right ring finger
`7th`

    S62.635   Displaced fracture of distal phalanx of left ring finger
`7th`

    S62.636   Displaced fracture of distal phalanx of right little finger
`7th`

    S62.637   Displaced fracture of distal phalanx of left little finger
`7th`

S62.64   Nondisplaced fracture of proximal phalanx of finger
`6th`

    S62.640   Nondisplaced fracture of proximal phalanx of right index finger
`7th`

    S62.641   Nondisplaced fracture of proximal phalanx of left index finger
`7th`

    S62.642   Nondisplaced fracture of proximal phalanx of right middle finger
`7th`

    S62.643   Nondisplaced fracture of proximal phalanx of left middle finger
`7th`

    S62.644   Nondisplaced fracture of proximal phalanx of right ring finger
`7th`

    S62.645   Nondisplaced fracture of proximal phalanx of left ring finger
`7th`

    S62.646   Nondisplaced fracture of proximal phalanx of right little finger
`7th`

    S62.647   Nondisplaced fracture of proximal phalanx of left little finger
`7th`

S62.65   Nondisplaced fracture of medial phalanx of finger
`6th`

    S62.650   Nondisplaced fracture of middle phalanx of right index finger
`7th`

    S62.651   Nondisplaced fracture of middle phalanx of left index finger
`7th`

    S62.652   Nondisplaced fracture of middle phalanx of right middle finger
`7th`

    S62.653   Nondisplaced fracture of middle phalanx of left middle finger
`7th`

    S62.654   Nondisplaced fracture of middle phalanx of right ring finger
`7th`

    S62.655   Nondisplaced fracture of middle phalanx of left ring finger
`7th`

    S62.656   Nondisplaced fracture of middle phalanx of right little finger
`7th`

    S62.657   Nondisplaced fracture of middle phalanx of left little finger
`7th`

S62.66   Nondisplaced fracture of distal phalanx of finger
`6th`

    S62.660   Nondisplaced fracture of distal phalanx of right index finger
`7th`

    S62.661   Nondisplaced fracture of distal phalanx of left index finger
`7th`

    S62.662   Nondisplaced fracture of distal phalanx of right middle finger
`7th`

    S62.663   Nondisplaced fracture of distal phalanx of left middle finger
`7th`

    S62.664   Nondisplaced fracture of distal phalanx of right ring finger
`7th`

    S62.665   Nondisplaced fracture of distal phalanx of left ring finger
`7th`

    S62.666   Nondisplaced fracture of distal phalanx of right little finger
`7th`

    S62.667   Nondisplaced fracture of distal phalanx of left little finger
`7th`

    Additional Character Required   3-character code   Unspecified laterality codes were excluded here.

• =New Code
▲ =Revised Code
¤ =Social determinants of health

Excludes1—Not coded here, do not use together
Excludes2—Not included here

CHAPTER 19. INJURY, POISONING AND CERTAIN OTHER CONSEQUENCES OF EXTERNAL CAUSES   (S63–S63.266)

S63 **DISLOCATION AND SPRAIN OF JOINTS AND LIGAMENTS AT WRIST AND HAND LEVEL**
`4th`

Includes: avulsion of joint or ligament at wrist and hand level
laceration of cartilage, joint or ligament at wrist and hand level
sprain of cartilage, joint or ligament at wrist and hand level
traumatic hemarthrosis of joint or ligament at wrist and hand level
traumatic rupture of joint or ligament at wrist and hand level
traumatic subluxation of joint or ligament at wrist and hand level
traumatic tear of joint or ligament at wrist and hand level

> 7th characters for category S63
> A—initial encounter
> D—subsequent encounter
> S—sequela

Code also any associated open wound
Excludes2: strain of muscle, fascia and tendon of wrist and hand (S66.-)

S63.0 **Subluxation and dislocation of wrist and hand joints**
`5th`

  S63.06 **Subluxation and dislocation of metacarpal (bone), proximal end**
  `6th`

    S63.061 **Subluxation of metacarpal (bone), proximal end of right hand**
    `7th`

    S63.062 **Subluxation of metacarpal (bone), proximal end of left hand**
    `7th`

> 7th characters for category S63
> A—initial encounter
> D—subsequent encounter
> S—sequela

    S63.063 **Subluxation of metacarpal (bone), proximal end of unspecified hand**
    `7th`

    S63.064 **Dislocation of metacarpal (bone), proximal end of right hand**
    `7th`

    S63.065 **Dislocation of metacarpal (bone), proximal end of left hand**
    `7th`

S63.1 **Subluxation and dislocation of thumb**
`5th`

  S63.10 **Unspecified subluxation and dislocation of thumb**
  `6th`

    S63.101 **Unspecified subluxation of right thumb**
    `7th`

    S63.102 **Unspecified subluxation of left thumb**
    `7th`

    S63.104 **Unspecified dislocation of right thumb**
    `7th`

    S63.105 **Unspecified dislocation of left thumb**
    `7th`

  S63.11 **Subluxation and dislocation of metacarpophalangeal joint of thumb**
  `6th`

    S63.111 **Subluxation of metacarpophalangeal joint of right thumb**
    `7th`

    S63.112 **Subluxation of metacarpophalangeal joint of left thumb**
    `7th`

    S63.114 **Dislocation of metacarpophalangeal joint of right thumb**
    `7th`

    S63.115 **Dislocation of metacarpophalangeal joint of left thumb**
    `7th`

  S63.12 **Subluxation and dislocation of interphalangeal joint of thumb**
  `6th`

    S63.121 **Subluxation of interphalangeal joint of right thumb**
    `7th`

    S63.122 **Subluxation of interphalangeal joint of left thumb**
    `7th`

    S63.124 **Dislocation of interphalangeal joint of right thumb**
    `7th`

    S63.125 **Dislocation of interphalangeal joint of left thumb**
    `7th`

S63.2 **Subluxation and dislocation of other finger(s)**
`5th`

Excludes2: subluxation and dislocation of thumb (S63.1-)

  S63.20 **Unspecified subluxation of other finger**
  `6th`

    S63.200 **Unspecified subluxation of right index finger**
    `7th`

    S63.201 **Unspecified subluxation of left index finger**
    `7th`

    S63.202 **Unspecified subluxation of right middle finger**
    `7th`

    S63.203 **Unspecified subluxation of left middle finger**
    `7th`

    S63.204 **Unspecified subluxation of right ring finger**
    `7th`

    S63.205 **Unspecified subluxation of left ring finger**
    `7th`

    S63.206 **Unspecified subluxation of right little finger**
    `7th`

    S63.207 **Unspecified subluxation of left little finge**
    `7th`

  S63.21 **Subluxation of metacarpophalangeal joint of finger**
  `6th`

    S63.210 **Subluxation of metacarpophalangeal joint of right index finger**
    `7th`

    S63.211 **Subluxation of metacar-pophalan-geal joint of left index finger**
    `7th`

    S63.212 **Subluxation of metacarpophalangeal joint of right middle finger**
    `7th`

    S63.213 **Subluxation of metacarpophalangeal joint of left middle finger**
    `7th`

    S63.214 **Subluxation of metacarpophalangeal joint of right ring finger**
    `7th`

    S63.215 **Subluxation of metacarpophalangeal joint of left ring finger**
    `7th`

    S63.216 **Subluxation of metacarpophalangeal joint of right little finger**
    `7th`

    S63.217 **Subluxation of metacarpophalangeal joint of left little finger**
    `7th`

  S63.23 **Subluxation of proximal interphalangeal joint of finger**
  `6th`

    S63.230 **Subluxation of proximal interphalangeal joint of right index finger**
    `7th`

    S63.231 **Subluxation of proximal interphalangeal joint of left index finger**
    `7th`

    S63.232 **Subluxation of proximal interphalangeal joint of right middle finger**
    `7th`

    S63.233 **Subluxation of proximal interphalangeal joint of left middle finger**
    `7th`

    S63.234 **Subluxation of proximal interphalangeal joint of right ring finger**
    `7th`

    S63.235 **Subluxation of proximal interphalangeal joint of left ring finger**
    `7th`

    S63.236 **Subluxation of proximal interphalangeal joint of right little finger**
    `7th`

    S63.237 **Subluxation of proximal interphalangeal joint of left little finger**
    `7th`

  S63.24 **Subluxation of distal interphalangeal joint of finger**
  `6th`

    S63.240 **Subluxation of distal interphalangeal joint of right index finger**
    `7th`

    S63.241 **Subluxation of distal interphalangeal joint of left index finger**
    `7th`

    S63.242 **Subluxation of distal interphalangeal joint of right middle finger**
    `7th`

    S63.243 **Subluxation of distal interphalangeal joint of left middle finger**
    `7th`

    S63.244 **Subluxation of distal interphalangeal joint of right ring finger**
    `7th`

    S63.245 **Subluxation of distal interphalangeal joint of left ring finger**
    `7th`

    S63.246 **Subluxation of distal interphalangeal joint of right little finger**
    `7th`

    S63.247 **Subluxation of distal interphalangeal joint of left little finger**
    `7th`

  S63.26 **Dislocation of metacarpophalangeal joint of finger**
  `6th`

    S63.260 **Dislocation of metacarpophalangeal joint of right index finger**
    `7th`

    S63.261 **Dislocation of metacarpophalangeal joint of left index finger**
    `7th`

    S63.262 **Dislocation of metacarpophalangeal joint of right middle finger**
    `7th`

    S63.263 **Dislocation of metacarpophalangeal joint of left middle finger**
    `7th`

    S63.264 **Dislocation of metacarpophalangeal joint of right ring finger**
    `7th`

    S63.265 **Dislocation of metacarpophalangeal joint of left ring finger**
    `7th`

    S63.266 **Dislocation of metacarpophalangeal joint of right little finger**
    `7th`

`4th` `5th` `6th` `7th` Additional Character Required   ✓ 3-character code   Unspecified laterality codes were excluded here.   • =New Code   ▲ =Revised Code   ◘ =Social determinants of health   **Excludes1**—Not coded here, do not use together   **Excludes2**—Not included here

S63.267 **7th** Dislocation of metacarpophalangeal joint of left little finger

S63.28 **6th** Dislocation of proximal interphalangeal joint of finger

S63.280 **7th** Dislocation of proximal interphalangeal joint of right index finger

S63.281 **7th** Dislocation of proximal interphalangeal joint of left index finger

S63.282 **7th** Dislocation of proximal interphalangeal joint of right middle finger

S63.283 **7th** Dislocation of proximal interphalangeal joint of left middle finger

S63.284 **7th** Dislocation of proximal interphalangeal joint of right ring finger

S63.285 **7th** Dislocation of proximal interphalangeal joint of left ring finger

S63.286 **7th** Dislocation of proximal interphalan-geal joint of right little finger

S63.287 **7th** Dislocation of proximal interphalangeal joint of left little finger

S63.29 **6th** Dislocation of distal interphalangeal joint of finger

> 7th characters for category S63
> A—initial encounter
> D—subsequent encounter
> S—sequela

S63.290 **7th** Dislocation of distal interphalangeal joint of right index finger

S63.291 **7th** Dislocation of distal interphalangeal joint of left index finger

S63.292 **7th** Dislocation of distal interphalangeal joint of right middle finger

S63.293 **7th** Dislocation of distal interphalangeal joint of left middle finger

S63.294 **7th** Dislocation of distal interphalangeal joint of right ring finger

S63.295 **7th** Dislocation of distal interphalangeal joint of left ring finger

S63.296 **7th** Dislocation of distal interphalangeal joint of right little finger

S63.297 **7th** Dislocation of distal inter-phalangeal joint of left little finger

S63.5 **5th** Other and unspecified sprain of wrist

S63.50 **6th** Unspecified sprain of wrist

S63.501 **7th** Unspecified sprain of right wrist

S63.502 **7th** Unspecified sprain of left wrist

S63.51 **6th** Sprain of carpal (joint)

S63.511 **7th** Sprain of carpal joint of right wrist

S63.512 **7th** Sprain of carpal joint of left wrist

S63.52 **6th** Sprain of radiocarpal joint

Excludes1: traumatic rupture of radiocarpal ligament (S63.32-)

S63.521 **7th** Sprain of radiocarpal joint of right wrist

S63.522 **7th** Sprain of radiocarpal joint of left wrist

S63.59 **6th** Other specified sprain of wrist

S63.591 **7th** Other specified sprain of right wrist

S63.592 **7th** Other specified sprain of left wrist

S63.6 **5th** Other and unspecified sprain of finger(s)

Excludes1: traumatic rupture of ligament of finger at metacarpophalangeal and interphalangeal joint(s) (S63.4-)

S63.60 **6th** Unspecified sprain of thumb

S63.601 **7th** Unspecified sprain of right thumb

S63.602 **7th** Unspecified sprain of left thumb

S63.61 **6th** Unspecified sprain of other and unspecified finger(s)

S63.610 **7th** Unspecified sprain of right index finger

S63.611 **7th** Unspecified sprain of left index finger

S63.612 **7th** Unspecified sprain of right middle finger

S63.613 **7th** Unspecified sprain of left middle finger

S63.614 **7th** Unspecified sprain of right ring finger

S63.615 **7th** Unspecified sprain of left ring finger

S63.616 **7th** Unspecified sprain of right little finger

S63.617 **7th** Unspecified sprain of left little finger

S63.62 **6th** Sprain of interphalangeal joint of thumb

S63.621 **7th** Sprain of interphalangeal joint of right thumb

S63.622 **7th** Sprain of interphalangeal joint of left thumb

S63.63 **6th** Sprain of interphalangeal joint of other and unspecified finger(s)

S63.630 **7th** Sprain of interphalangeal joint of right index finger

S63.631 **7th** Sprain of interphalangeal joint of left index finger

S63.632 **7th** Sprain of interphalangeal joint of right middle finger

S63.633 **7th** Sprain of interphalangeal joint of left middle finger

S63.634 **7th** Sprain of interphalangeal joint of right ring finger

S63.635 **7th** Sprain of interphalangeal joint of left ring finger

S63.636 **7th** Sprain of interphalangeal joint of right little finger

S63.637 **7th** Sprain of interphalangeal joint of left little finger

S63.64 **6th** Sprain of metacarpophalangeal joint of thumb

S63.641 **7th** Sprain of metacarpophalangeal joint of right thumb

S63.642 **7th** Sprain of metacarpophalangeal joint of left thumb

S63.65 **6th** Sprain of metacarpophalangeal joint of other and unspecified finger(s)

S63.650 **7th** Sprain of metacarpophalangeal joint of right index finger

S63.651 **7th** Sprain of metacarpophalangeal joint of left index finger

S63.652 **7th** Sprain of metacarpophalangeal joint of right middle finger

S63.653 **7th** Sprain of metacarpophalangeal joint of left middle finger

S63.654 **7th** Sprain of metacarpophalangeal joint of right ring finger

S63.655 **7th** Sprain of metacarpophalangeal joint of left ring finger

S63.656 **7th** Sprain of metacarpophalangeal joint of right little finger

S63.657 **7th** Sprain of metacarpophalangeal joint of left little finger

S63.68 **6th** Other sprain of thumb

S63.681 **7th** Other sprain of right thumb

S63.682 **7th** Other sprain of left thumb

S63.69 **6th** Other sprain of other and unspecified finger(s)

S63.690 **7th** Other sprain of right index finger

S63.691 **7th** Other sprain of left index finger

S63.692 **7th** Other sprain of right middle finger

S63.693 **7th** Other sprain of left middle finger

4th **5th** **6th** **7th** Additional Character Required   ✔   3-character code   Unspecified laterality codes were excluded here.

• =New Code
▲ =Revised Code
▫ =Social determinants of health

Excludes1—Not coded here, do not use together
Excludes2—Not included here

S63.694 Other sprain of right ring finger `7th`

S63.695 Other sprain of left ring finger `7th`

S63.696 Other sprain of right little finger `7th`

S63.697 Other sprain of left little finger `7th`

S63.8 Sprain of other part of wrist and hand `5th`

    S63.8X Sprain of other part of wrist and hand `6th`

        S63.8X1 Sprain of other part of right wrist and hand `7th`

        S63.8X2 Sprain of other part of left wrist and hand `7th`

S63.9 Sprain of unspecified part of wrist and hand `5th`

    S63.91X Sprain of unspecified part of right wrist and hand `7th`

    S63.92X Sprain of unspecified part of left wrist and hand `7th`

S65 `4th` INJURY OF BLOOD VESSELS AT WRIST AND HAND LEVEL

Code also any associated open wound (S61.-)

7th characters for category S63 & S65
A—initial encounter
D—subsequent encounter
S—sequela

S65.2 Injury of superficial palmar arch `5th`

    S65.21 Laceration of superficial palmar arch `6th`

        S65.211 Laceration of superficial palmar arch of right hand `7th`

        S65.212 Laceration of superficial palmar arch of left hand `7th`

    S65.29 Other specified injury of superficial palmar arch `6th`

        S65.291 Other specified injury of superficial palmar arch of right hand `7th`

        S65.292 Other specified injury of superficial palmar arch of left hand `7th`

S65.3 Injury of deep palmar arch `5th`

    S65.30 Unspecified injury of deep palmar arch `6th`

        S65.301 Unspecified injury of deep palmar arch of right hand `7th`

        S65.302 Unspecified injury of deep palmar arch of left hand `7th`

    S65.31 Laceration of deep palmar arch `6th`

        S65.311 Laceration of deep palmar arch of right hand `7th`

        S65.312 Laceration of deep palmar arch of left hand `7th`

    S65.39 Other specified injury of deep palmar arch `6th`

        S65.391 Other specified injury of deep palmar arch of right hand `7th`

        S65.392 Other specified injury of deep palmar arch of left hand `7th`

S65.9 Injury of unspecified blood vessel at wrist and hand level `5th`

    S65.91 Laceration of unspecified blood vessel at wrist and hand level `6th`

        S65.911 Laceration of unspecified blood vessel at wrist and hand level of right arm `7th`

        S65.912 Laceration of unspecified blood vessel at wrist and hand level of left arm `7th`

    S65.99 Other specified injury of unspecified blood vessel at wrist and hand level `6th`

        S65.991 Other specified injury of unspecified blood vessel at wrist and hand of right arm `7th`

        S65.992 Other specified injury of unspecified blood vessel at wrist and hand of left arm `7th`

S66 `4th` INJURY OF MUSCLE, FASCIA AND TENDON AT WRIST AND HAND LEVEL

Code also any associated open wound (S61.-)

Excludes2: sprain of joints and ligaments of wrist and hand (S63.-)

7th characters for categories S65 & S66
A—initial encounter
D—subsequent encounter
S—sequela

S66.0 Injury of long flexor muscle, fascia, and tendon of thumb at wrist and hand level `5th`

S66.01 Strain of long flexor muscle, fascia and tendon of thumb at wrist and hand level `6th`

    S66.011 Strain of long flexor muscle, fascia and tendon of right thumb at wrist and hand level `7th`

    S66.012 Strain of long flexor muscle, fascia and tendon of left thumb at wrist and hand level `7th`

S66.02 Laceration of long flexor muscle, fascia and tendon of thumb at wrist and hand level `6th`

    S66.021 Laceration of long flexor muscle, fascia and tendon of right thumb at wrist and hand level `7th`

    S66.022 Laceration of long flexor muscle, fascia and tendon of left thumb at wrist and hand level `7th`

S66.11 Strain of flexor muscle, fascia and tendon of other and unspecified finger at wrist and hand level `6th`

    S66.110 Strain of flexor muscle, fascia and tendon of right index finger at wrist and hand level `7th`

    S66.111 Strain of flexor muscle, fascia and tendon of left index finger at wrist and hand level `7th`

    S66.112 Strain of flexor muscle, fascia and tendon of right middle finger at wrist and hand level `7th`

    S66.113 Strain of flexor muscle, fascia and tendon of left middle finger at wrist and hand level `7th`

    S66.114 Strain of flexor muscle, fascia and tendon of right ring finger at wrist and hand level `7th`

    S66.115 Strain of flexor muscle, fascia and tendon of left ring finger at wrist and hand level `7th`

    S66.116 Strain of flexor muscle, fascia and tendon of right little finger at wrist and hand level `7th`

    S66.117 Strain of flexor muscle, fascia and tendon of left little finger at wrist and hand level `7th`

S66.21 Strain of extensor muscle, fascia and tendon of thumb at wrist and hand level `6th`

    S66.211 Strain of extensor muscle, fascia and tendon of right thumb at wrist and hand level `7th`

    S66.212 Strain of extensor muscle, fascia and tendon of left thumb at wrist and hand level `7th`

S66.31 Strain of extensor muscle, fascia and tendon of other and unspecified finger at wrist and hand level `6th`

    S66.310 Strain of extensor muscle, fascia and tendon of right index finger at wrist and hand level `7th`

    S66.311 Strain of extensor muscle, fascia and tendon of left index finger at wrist and hand level `7th`

    S66.312 Strain of extensor muscle, fascia and tendon of right middle finger at wrist and hand level `7th`

    S66.313 Strain of extensor muscle, fascia and tendon of left middle finger at wrist and hand level `7th`

    S66.314 Strain of extensor muscle, fascia and tendon of right ring finger at wrist and hand level `7th`

    S66.315 Strain of extensor muscle, fascia and tendon of left ring finger at wrist and hand level `7th`

    S66.316 Strain of extensor muscle, fascia and tendon of right little finger at wrist and hand level `7th`

    S66.317 Strain of extensor muscle, fascia and tendon of left little finger at wrist and hand level `7th`

S66.41 Strain of intrinsic muscle, fascia and tendon of thumb at wrist and hand level `6th`

`4th` `5th` `6th` `7th`   Additional Character Required   ✔   3-character code   Unspecified laterality codes were excluded here.

• =New Code
▲ =Revised Code
▭ =Social determinants of health

Excludes1—Not coded here, do not use together
Excludes2—Not included here

S66.411 **7th** Strain of intrinsic muscle, fascia and tendon of right thumb at wrist and hand level

S66.412 **7th** Strain of intrinsic muscle, fascia and tendon of left thumb at wrist and hand level

S66.51 **6th** Strain of intrinsic muscle, fascia and tendon of other and unspecified finger at wrist and hand level

S66.510 **7th** Strain of intrinsic muscle, fascia and tendon of right index finger at wrist and hand level

S66.511 **7th** Strain of intrinsic muscle, fascia and tendon of left index finger at wrist and hand level

S66.512 **7th** Strain of intrinsic muscle, fascia and tendon of right middle finger at wrist and hand level

S66.513 **7th** Strain of intrinsic muscle, fascia and tendon of left middle finger at wrist and hand level

> 7th characters for category S66
> A—initial encounter
> D—subsequent encounter
> S—sequela

S66.514 **7th** Strain of intrinsic muscle, fascia and tendon of right ring finger at wrist and hand level

S66.515 **7th** Strain of intrinsic muscle, fascia and tendon of left ring finger at wrist and hand level

S66.516 **7th** Strain of intrinsic muscle, fascia and tendon of right little finger at wrist and hand level

S66.517 **7th** Strain of intrinsic muscle, fascia and tendon of left little finger at wrist and hand level

S66.91 **6th** Strain of unspecified muscle, fascia and tendon at wrist and hand level

S66.911 **7th** Strain of unspecified muscle, fascia and tendon at wrist and hand level, right hand

S66.912 **7th** Strain of unspecified muscle, fascia and tendon at wrist and hand level, left hand

S67 **4th** **CRUSHING INJURY OF WRIST, HAND AND FINGERS**
Use additional code for all associated injuries, such as: fracture of wrist and hand (S62.-)
open wound of wrist and hand (S61.-)

> 7th characters for category S67
> A—initial encounter
> D—subsequent encounter
> S—sequela

S67.0 **5th** Crushing injury of thumb

S67.01X **7th** Crushing injury of right thumb

S67.02X **7th** Crushing injury of left thumb

S67.1 **5th** Crushing injury of other and unspecified finger(s)
Excludes2: crushing injury of thumb (S67.0-)

S67.19 **6th** Crushing injury of other finger(s)

S67.190 **7th** Crushing injury of right index finger

S67.191 **7th** Crushing injury of left index finger

S67.192 **7th** Crushing injury of right middle finger

S67.193 **7th** Crushing injury of left middle finger

S67.194 **7th** Crushing injury of right ring finger

S67.195 **7th** Crushing injury of left ring finger

S67.196 **7th** Crushing injury of right little finger

S67.197 **7th** Crushing injury of left little finger, initial encounter

S67.198 **7th** Crushing injury of other finger-
Crushing injury of specified finger with unspecified laterality

S67.2 **5th** Crushing injury of hand
Excludes2: crushing injury of fingers (S67.1-)
crushing injury of thumb (S67.0-)

S67.21X **7th** Crushing injury of right hand

S67.22X **7th** Crushing injury of left hand

S67.3 **5th** Crushing injury of wrist

S67.31X **7th** Crushing injury of right wrist

S67.32X **7th** Crushing injury of left wrist

S67.4 **5th** Crushing injury of wrist and hand
Excludes1: crushing injury of hand alone (S67.2-)
crushing injury of wrist alone (S67.3-)
Excludes2: crushing injury of fingers (S67.1-)
crushing injury of thumb (S67.0-)

S67.41X **7th** Crushing injury of right wrist and hand

S67.42X **7th** Crushing injury of left wrist and hand

(S70–S79) INJURIES TO THE HIP AND THIGH

Excludes2: burns and corrosions (T20–T32)
frostbite (T33–T34)
snake bite (T63.0-)
venomous insect bite or sting (T63.4-)

> 7th characters for category S70
> A—initial encounter
> D—subsequent encounter
> S—sequela

S70 **4th** **SUPERFICIAL INJURY OF HIP AND THIGH**

S70.0 **5th** Contusion of hip

S70.01X **7th** Contusion of right hip

S70.02X **7th** Contusion of left hip

S70.1 **5th** Contusion of thigh

S70.11X **7th** Contusion of right thigh

S70.12X **7th** Contusion of left thigh

S70.2 **5th** Other superficial injuries of hip

S70.21 **6th** Abrasion of hip

S70.211 **7th** Abrasion, right hip

S70.212 **7th** Abrasion, left hip

S70.22 **6th** Blister (nonthermal) of hip

S70.221 **7th** Blister (nonthermal), right hip

S70.222 **7th** Blister (nonthermal), left hip

S70.24 **6th** External constriction of hip

S70.241 **7th** External constriction, right hip

S70.242 **7th** External constriction, left hip

S70.25 **6th** Superficial FB of hip
Splinter in the hip

S70.251 **7th** Superficial FB, right hip

S70.252 **7th** Superficial FB, left hip

S70.26 **6th** Insect bite (nonvenomous) of hip

S70.261 **7th** Insect bite (nonvenomous), right hip

S70.262 **7th** Insect bite (nonvenomous), left hip

S70.27 **6th** Other superficial bite of hip
Excludes1: open bite of hip (S71.05-)

S70.271 **7th** Other superficial bite of hip, right hip

S70.272 **7th** Other superficial bite of hip, left hip

4th **5th** **6th** **7th** Additional Character Required   ✓ 3-character code   Unspecified laterality codes were excluded here.

• =New Code
▲ =Revised Code
▫ =Social determinants of health

Excludes1—Not coded here, do not use together
Excludes2—Not included here

CHAPTER 19. INJURY, POISONING AND CERTAIN OTHER CONSEQUENCES OF EXTERNAL CAUSES   (S66.411–S70.272)

S70.3 Other superficial injuries of thigh

5th S70.31 Abrasion of thigh

6th   **S70.311   Abrasion, right thigh**
7th

         S70.312   Abrasion, left thigh
7th

S70.32 Blister (nonthermal) of thigh
6th   **S70.321   Blister (nonthermal), right thigh**
7th

         S70.322   Blister (nonthermal), left thigh
7th

S70.34 External constriction of thigh
6th   **S70.341   External constriction, right thigh**
7th

         S70.342   External constriction, left thigh
7th

S70.35 Superficial FB of thigh
6th   Splinter in the thigh
         S70.351   Superficial FB, right thigh
7th

         S70.352   Superficial FB, left thigh
7th

S70.36 Insect bite (nonvenomous) of thigh
6th   **S70.361   Insect bite (nonvenomous), right thigh**
7th

         S70.362   Insect bite (nonvenomous), left thigh
7th

S70.37 Other superficial bite of thigh
6th   *Excludes1:* open bite of thigh (S71.15)
         S70.371   Other superficial bite of right thigh
7th

         S70.372   Other superficial bite of left thigh
7th

7th characters for categories S70 & S71
A—initial encounter
D—subsequent encounter
S—sequela

S71 OPEN WOUND OF HIP AND THIGH
4th
Code also any associated wound infection
Excludes1: open fracture of hip and thigh (S72.-)
       traumatic amputation of hip and thigh (S78.-)
Excludes2: bite of venomous animal (T63.-)
       open wound of ankle, foot and toes (S91.-)
       open wound of knee and lower leg (S81.-)

S71.0 Open wound of hip
5th **S71.01 Laceration without FB of hip**
6th   **S71.011   Laceration without FB, right hip**
7th

         S71.012   Laceration without FB, left hip
7th

S71.02 Laceration with FB of hip
6th   **S71.021   Laceration with FB, right hip**
7th

         S71.022   Laceration with FB, left hip
7th

S71.03 Puncture wound without FB of hip
6th   **S71.031   Puncture wound without FB, right hip**
7th

         S71.032   Puncture wound without FB, left hip
7th

S71.04 Puncture wound with FB of hip
6th   **S71.041   Puncture wound with FB, right hip**
7th

         S71.042   Puncture wound with FB, left hip
7th

S71.05 Open bite of hip
6th   Bite of hip NOS
         Excludes1: superficial bite of hip (S70.26, S70.27)
         S71.051   Open bite, right hip
7th

         S71.052   Open bite, left hip
7th

S71.1 Open wound of thigh
5th

S71.11 Laceration without FB of thigh
6th   **S71.111   Laceration without FB, right thigh**
7th

         S71.112   Laceration without FB, left thigh
7th

S71.12 Laceration with FB of thigh
6th   **S71.121   Laceration with FB, right thigh**
7th

         S71.122   Laceration with FB, left thigh
7th

S71.13 Puncture wound without FB of thigh
6th   **S71.131   Puncture wound without FB, right thigh**
7th

         S71.132   Puncture wound without FB, left thigh
7th

S71.14 Puncture wound with FB of thigh
6th   **S71.141   Puncture wound with FB, right thigh**
7th

         S71.142   Puncture wound with FB, left thigh
7th

S71.15 Open bite of thigh
6th   Bite of thigh NOS
         Excludes1: superficial bite of thigh (S70.37-)
         S71.151   Open bite, right thigh
7th

         S71.152   Open bite, left thigh
7th

S72 FRACTURE OF FEMUR
4th
Please see full *ICD-10-CM* manual for seventh characters applicable to open fracture types IIIA, IIIB, or IIIC.
Note: A fracture not indicated as displaced or nondisplaced should be coded to displaced
    A fracture not indicated as open or closed should be coded to closed
    The open fracture designations are based on the Gustilo open fracture classification
Excludes1: traumatic amputation of hip and thigh (S78.-)
Excludes2: fracture of lower leg and ankle (S82.-)
    fracture of foot (S92.-)
    periprosthetic fracture of prosthetic implant of hip (M97.0-)

7th characters for category S72 except S72.47-
A—initial encounter for closed fracture
B—initial encounter for open fracture type I or II initial encounter for open fracture NOS
D—subsequent encounter for closed fracture with routine healing
E—subsequent encounter for open fracture type I or II with routine healing
G—subsequent encounter for closed fracture with delayed healing
H—subsequent encounter for open fracture type I or II with delayed healing
K—subsequent encounter for closed fracture with nonunion
M—subsequent encounter for open fracture type I or II with nonunion
P—subsequent encounter for closed fracture with malunion
Q—subsequent encounter for open fracture type I or II with malunion
S—sequela

S72.0 Fracture of head and neck of femur
5th
    Excludes2: physeal fracture of upper end of femur (S79.0-)
S72.00 Fracture of unspecified part of neck of femur
6th   Fracture of hip NOS
         Fracture of neck of femur NOS
         S72.001   Fracture of unspecified part of neck of right femur
7th   **S72.002   Fracture of unspecified part of neck of left femur**
7th

S72.01 Unspecified intracapsular fracture of femur
6th   Subcapital fracture of femur
         S72.011   Unspecified intracapsular fracture of right femur
7th   **S72.012   Unspecified intracapsular fracture of left femur**
7th

S72.02 Fracture of epiphysis (separation) (upper) of femur
6th   Transepiphyseal fracture of femur
         Excludes1: capital femoral epiphyseal fracture (pediatric) of femur (S79.01-)
         Salter-Harris Type I physeal fracture of upper end of femur (S79.01-)
         S72.021   Displaced fracture of epiphysis (separation) (upper) of right femur
7th

| 4th | 5th | 6th | 7th | Additional Character Required | ✓ 3-character code | Unspecified laterality codes were excluded here. | • =New Code ▲ =Revised Code ▱ =Social determinants of health | *Excludes1*—Not coded here, do not use together *Excludes2*—Not included here |

S72.022 [7th] Displaced fracture of epiphysis (separation) (upper) of left femur

S72.023 [7th] Displaced fracture of epiphysis (separation) (upper) of unspecified femur

S72.024 [7th] Nondisplaced fracture of epiphysis (separation) (upper) of right femur

S72.025 [7th] Nondisplaced fracture of epiphysis (separation) (upper) of left femur

S72.03 [6th] Midcervical fracture of femur
Transcervical fracture of femur NOS

S72.031 [7th] Displaced midcervical fracture of right femur

S72.032 [7th] Displaced midcervical fracture of left femur

S72.034 [7th] Nondisplaced midcervical fracture of right femur

S72.035 [7th] Nondisplaced midcervical fracture of left femur

S72.04 [6th] Fracture of base of neck of femur
Cervicotrochanteric fracture of femur

S72.041 [7th] Displaced fracture of base of neck of right femur

S72.042 [7th] Displaced fracture of base of neck of left femur

S72.044 [7th] Nondisplaced fracture of base of neck of right femur

S72.045 [7th] Nondisplaced fracture of base of neck of left femur

S72.3 [5th] Fracture of shaft of femur

S72.30 [6th] Unspecified fracture of shaft of femur

S72.301 [7th] Unspecified fracture of shaft of right femur

S72.302 [7th] Unspecified fracture of shaft of left femur

S72.32 [6th] Transverse fracture of shaft of femur

S72.321 [7th] Displaced transverse fracture of shaft of right femur

S72.322 [7th] Displaced transverse fracture of shaft of left femur

S72.324 [7th] Nondisplaced transverse fracture of shaft of right femur

S72.325 [7th] Nondisplaced transverse fracture of shaft of left femur

S72.33 [6th] Oblique fracture of shaft of femur

S72.331 [7th] Displaced oblique fracture of shaft of right femur

S72.332 [7th] Displaced oblique fracture of shaft of left femur

S72.334 [7th] Nondisplaced oblique fracture of shaft of right femur

S72.335 [7th] Nondisplaced oblique fracture of shaft of left femur

S72.34 [6th] Spiral fracture of shaft of femur

S72.341 [7th] Displaced spiral fracture of shaft of right femur

S72.342 [7th] Displaced spiral fracture of shaft of left femur

S72.344 [7th] Nondisplaced spiral fracture of shaft of right femur

> 7th characters for category S72 except S72.47-
> A—initial encounter for closed fracture
> B—initial encounter for open fracture type I or II initial encounter for open fracture NOS
> D—subsequent encounter for closed fracture with routine healing
> E—subsequent encounter for open fracture type I or II with routine healing
> G—subsequent encounter for closed fracture with delayed healing
> H—subsequent encounter for open fracture type I or II with delayed healing
> K—subsequent encounter for closed fracture with nonunion
> M—subsequent encounter for open fracture type I or II with nonunion
> P—subsequent encounter for closed fracture with malunion
> Q—subsequent encounter for open fracture type I or II with malunion
> S—sequela

S72.345 [7th] Nondisplaced spiral fracture of shaft of left femur

S72.35 [6th] Comminuted fracture of shaft of femur

S72.351 [7th] Displaced comminuted fracture of shaft of right femur

S72.352 [7th] Displaced comminuted fracture of shaft of left femur

S72.354 [7th] Nondisplaced comminuted fracture of shaft of right femur

S72.355 [7th] Nondisplaced comminuted fracture of shaft of left femur

S72.36 [6th] Segmental fracture of shaft of femur

S72.361 [7th] Displaced segmental fracture of shaft of right femur

S72.362 [7th] Displaced segmental fracture of shaft of left femur

S72.364 [7th] Nondisplaced segmental fracture of shaft of right femur

S72.365 [7th] Nondisplaced segmental fracture of shaft of left femur

S72.39 [6th] Other fracture of shaft of femur

S72.391 [7th] Other fracture of shaft of right femur

S72.392 [7th] Other fracture of shaft of left femur

S72.4 [5th] Fracture of lower end of femur
Fracture of distal end of femur
Excludes2: fracture of shaft of femur (S72.3-)
physeal fracture of lower end of femur (S79.1-)

S72.40 [6th] Unspecified fracture of lower end of femur

S72.401 [7th] Unspecified fracture of lower end of right femur

S72.402 [7th] Unspecified fracture of lower end of left femur

S72.41 [6th] Unspecified condyle fracture of lower end of femur
Condyle fracture of femur NOS

S72.411 [7th] Displaced unspecified condyle fracture of lower end of right femur

S72.412 [7th] Displaced unspecified condyle fracture of lower end of left femur

S72.414 [7th] Nondisplaced unspecified condyle fracture of lower end of right femur

S72.415 [7th] Nondisplaced unspecified condyle fracture of lower end of left femur

S72.42 [6th] Fracture of lateral condyle of femur

S72.421 [7th] Displaced fracture of lateral condyle of right femur

S72.422 [7th] Displaced fracture of lateral condyle of left femur

S72.424 [7th] Nondisplaced fracture of lateral condyle of right femur

S72.425 [7th] Nondisplaced fracture of lateral condyle of left femur

S72.43 [6th] Fracture of medial condyle of femur

S72.431 [7th] Displaced fracture of medial condyle of right femur

S72.432 [7th] Displaced fracture of medial condyle of left femur

S72.434 [7th] Nondisplaced fracture of medial condyle of right femur

S72.435 [7th] Nondisplaced fracture of medial condyle of left femur

S72.44 [6th] Fracture of lower epiphysis (separation) of femur
Excludes1: Salter-Harris Type I physeal fracture of lower end of femur (S79.11-)

S72.441 [7th] Displaced fracture of lower epiphysis (separation) of right femur

S72.442 [7th] Displaced fracture of lower epiphysis (separation) of left femur

S72.444 [7th] Nondisplaced fracture of lower epiphysis (separation) of right femur

S72.445 [7th] Nondisplaced fracture of lower epiphysis (separation) of left femur

---

[4th] [5th] [6th] [7th] Additional Character Required ✓ 3-character code Unspecified laterality codes were excluded here.

• =New Code
▲ =Revised Code
▣ =Social determinants of health

Excludes1—Not coded here, do not use together
Excludes2—Not included here

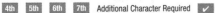

CHAPTER 19. INJURY, POISONING AND CERTAIN OTHER CONSEQUENCES OF EXTERNAL CAUSES   (S72.45–S76.01)

S72.45 [6th] **Supracondylar fracture without intracondylar extension of lower end of femur**
Supracondylar fracture of lower end of femur NOS
Excludes1: supracondylar fracture with intracondylar extension of lower end of femur (S72.46-)

S72.451 [7th] **Displaced supracondylar fracture without intracondylar extension of lower end of right femur**

S72.452 [7th] **Displaced supracondylar fracture without intracondylar extension of lower end of left femur**

S72.454 [7th] **Nondisplaced supracondylar fracture without intracondylar extension of lower end of right femur**

S72.455 [7th] **Nondisplaced supracondylar fracture without intracondylar extension of lower end of left femur**

S72.46 [6th] **Supracondylar fracture with intracondylar extension of lower end of femur**
Excludes1: supracondylar fracture without intracondylar extension of lower end of femur (S72.45-)

S72.461 [7th] **Displaced supracondylar fracture with intracondylar extension of lower end of right femur**

S72.462 [7th] **Displaced supracondylar fracture with intracondylar extension of lower end of left femur**

S72.464 [7th] **Nondisplaced supracondylar fracture with intracondylar extension of lower end of right femur**

S72.465 [7th] **Nondisplaced supracondylar fracture with intracondylar extension of lower end of left femur**

S72.47 [6th] **Torus fracture of lower end of femur**

S72.471 [7th] **Torus fracture of lower end of right femur**

S72.472 [7th] **Torus fracture of lower end of left femur**

> 7th characters for category S72.47-
> A—initial encounter for closed fracture
> D—subsequent encounter for closed fracture with routine healing
> G—subsequent encounter for closed fracture with delayed healing
> K—subsequent encounter for closed fracture with nonunion
> P—subsequent encounter for closed fracture with malunion
> S—sequela

S72.49 [6th] **Other fracture of lower end of femur**

S72.491 [7th] **Other fracture of lower end of right femur**

S72.492 [7th] **Other fracture of lower end of left femur**

S72.8 [5th] **Other fracture of femur**

S72.8X [6th] **Other fracture of femur**

S72.8X1 [7th] **Other fracture of right femur**

S72.8X2 [7th] **Other fracture of left femur**

S72.9 [5th] **Unspecified fracture of femur**
Fracture of thigh NOS
Fracture of upper leg NOS
Excludes1: fracture of hip NOS (S72.00-, S72.01-)

S72.91X [7th] **Unspecified fracture of right femur**

S72.92X [7th] **Unspecified fracture of left femur**

S73 [4th] **DISLOCATION AND SPRAIN OF JOINT AND LIGAMENTS OF HIP**
Includes: avulsion of joint or ligament of hip
laceration of cartilage, joint or ligament of hip
sprain of cartilage, joint or ligament of hip
traumatic hemarthrosis of joint or ligament of hip

> 7th characters for category S73
> A—initial encounter
> D—subsequent encounter
> S—sequela

traumatic rupture of joint or ligament of hip
traumatic subluxation of joint or ligament of hip
traumatic tear of joint or ligament of hip
Code also any associated open wound
Excludes2: strain of muscle, fascia and tendon of hip and thigh (S76.-)

S73.0 [5th] **Subluxation and dislocation of hip**

S73.01 [6th] **Posterior subluxation and dislocation of hip**

S73.011 [7th] **Posterior subluxation of right hip**

S73.012 [7th] **Posterior subluxation of left hip**

S73.014 [7th] **Posterior dislocation of right hip**

S73.015 [7th] **Posterior dislocation of left hip**

S73.02 [6th] **Obturator subluxation and dislocation of hip**

S73.021 [7th] **Obturator subluxation of right hip**

S73.022 [7th] **Obturator subluxation of left hip**

S73.024 [7th] **Obturator dislocation of right hip**

S73.025 [7th] **Obturator dislocation of left hip**

S73.03 [6th] **Other anterior subluxation and dislocation of hip**

S73.031 [7th] **Other anterior subluxation of right hip**

S73.032 [7th] **Other anterior subluxation of left hip**

S73.034 [7th] **Other anterior dislocation of right hip**

S73.035 [7th] **Other anterior dislocation of left hip**

S73.04 [6th] **Central subluxation and dislocation of hip**

S73.041 [7th] **Central subluxation of right hip**

S73.042 [7th] **Central subluxation of left hip**

S73.044 [7th] **Central dislocation of right hip**

S73.045 [7th] **Central dislocation of left hip**

S73.1 [5th] **Sprain of hip**

S73.10 [6th] **Unspecified sprain of hip**

S73.101 [7th] **Unspecified sprain of right hip**

S73.102 [7th] **Unspecified sprain of left hip**

S73.11 [6th] **Iliofemoral ligament sprain of hip**

S73.111 [7th] **Iliofemoral ligament sprain of right hip**

S73.112 [7th] **Iliofemoral ligament sprain of left hip**

S73.12 [6th] **Ischiocapsular (ligament) sprain of hip**

S73.121 [7th] **Ischiocapsular ligament sprain of right hip**

S73.122 [7th] **Ischiocapsular ligament sprain of left hip**

S73.19 [6th] **Other sprain of hip**

S73.191 [7th] **Other sprain of right hip**

S73.192 [7th] **Other sprain of left hip**

S76 [4th] **INJURY OF MUSCLE, FASCIA AND TENDON AT HIP AND THIGH LEVEL**
Code also any associated open wound (S71.-)
Excludes2: injury of muscle, fascia and tendon at lower leg level (S86)
sprain of joint and ligament of hip (S73.1)

> 7th characters for category S76
> A—initial encounter
> D—subsequent encounter
> S—sequela

S76.0 [5th] **Injury of muscle, fascia and tendon of hip**

S76.01 [6th] **Strain of muscle, fascia and tendon of hip**

[4th] [5th] [6th] [7th] Additional Character Required   ✓ 3-character code   Unspecified laterality codes were excluded here.

• =New Code
▲ =Revised Code
✪ =Social determinants of health

Excludes1—Not coded here, do not use together
Excludes2—Not included here

372   PEDIATRIC ICD-10-CM 2022: A MANUAL FOR PROVIDER-BASED CODING

S76.011 `7th` Strain of muscle, fascia and tendon of right hip

S76.012 `7th` Strain of muscle, fascia and tendon of left hip

S76.1 `5th` **Injury of quadriceps muscle, fascia and tendon**
Injury of patellar ligament (tendon)

S76.11 `6th` Strain of quadriceps muscle, fascia and tendon

S76.111 `7th` Strain of right quadriceps muscle, fascia and tendon

S76.112 `7th` Strain of left quadriceps muscle, fascia and tendon

S76.21 `6th` Strain of adductor muscle, fascia and tendon of thigh

S76.211 `7th` Strain of adductor muscle, fascia and tendon of right thigh

S76.212 `7th` Strain of adductor muscle, fascia and tendon of left thigh

S76.31 `6th` Strain of muscle, fascia and tendon of the posterior muscle group at thigh level

S76.311 `7th` Strain of muscle, fascia and tendon of the posterior muscle group at thigh level, right thigh

S76.312 `7th` Strain of muscle, fascia and tendon of the posterior muscle group at thigh level, left thigh

S76.91 `6th` Strain of unspecified muscles, fascia and tendons at thigh level

S76.911 `7th` Strain of unspecified muscles, fascia and tendons at thigh level, right thigh

S76.912 `7th` Strain of unspecified muscles, fascia and tendons at thigh level, left thigh

S79 `4th` **OTHER AND UNSPECIFIED INJURIES OF HIP AND THIGH**
Note: A fracture not indicated as open or closed should be coded to closed

S79.0 `5th` **Physeal fracture of upper end of femur**
Excludes1: apophyseal fracture of upper end of femur (S72.13-) nontraumatic slipped upper femoral epiphysis (M93.0-)

S79.00 `6th` **Unspecified physeal fracture of upper end of femur**

S79.001 `7th` Unspecified physeal fracture of upper end of right femur

S79.002 `7th` Unspecified physeal fracture of upper end of left femur

S79.01 `6th` **Salter-Harris Type I physeal fracture of upper end of femur**
Acute on chronic slipped capital femoral epiphysis (traumatic)
Acute slipped capital femoral epiphysis (traumatic)
Capital femoral epiphyseal fracture
Excludes1: chronic slipped upper femoral epiphysis (nontraumatic) (M93.02-)

S79.011 `7th` Salter-Harris Type I physeal fracture of upper end of right femur,

S79.012 `7th` Salter-Harris Type I physeal fracture of upper end of left femur

S79.09 `6th` **Other physeal fracture of upper end of femur**

S79.091 `7th` Other physeal fracture of upper end of right femur

S79.092 `7th` Other physeal fracture of upper end of left femur

S79.1 `5th` **Physeal fracture of lower end of femur**

S79.10 `6th` **Unspecified physeal fracture of lower end of femur**

S79.101 `7th` Unspecified physeal fracture of lower end of right femur

S79.102 `7th` Unspecified physeal fracture of lower end of left femur

S79.11 `6th` **Salter-Harris Type I physeal fracture of lower end of femur**

> 7th characters for subcategories S79.0–S79.1
> A—initial encounter for closed fracture
> D—subsequent encounter for fracture with routine healing
> G—subsequent encounter for fracture with delayed healing
> K—subsequent encounter for fracture with nonunion
> P—subsequent encounter for fracture with malunion
> S—sequela

S79.111 `7th` Salter-Harris Type I physeal fracture of lower end of right femur

S79.112 `7th` Salter-Harris Type I physeal fracture of lower end of left femur

S79.12 `6th` **Salter-Harris Type II physeal fracture of lower end of femur**

S79.121 `7th` Salter-Harris Type II physeal fracture of lower end of right femur

S79.122 `7th` Salter-Harris Type II physeal fracture of lower end of left femur

S79.13 `6th` **Salter-Harris Type III physeal fracture of lower end of femur**

S79.131 `7th` Salter-Harris Type III physeal fracture of lower end of right femur

S79.132 `7th` Salter-Harris Type III physeal fracture of lower end of left femur

S79.14 `6th` **Salter-Harris Type IV physeal fracture of lower end of femur**

S79.141 `7th` Salter-Harris Type IV physeal fracture of lower end of right femur

S79.142 `7th` Salter-Harris Type IV physeal fracture of lower end of left femur

S79.19 `6th` **Other physeal fracture of lower end of femur**

S79.191 `7th` Other physeal fracture of lower end of right femur

S79.192 `7th` Other physeal fracture of lower end of left femur

S79.8 `5th` **Other specified injuries of hip and thigh**

S79.81 `6th` **Other specified injuries of hip**

S79.811 `7th` Other specified injuries of right hip

> 7th characters for subcategory S79.8
> A—initial encounter
> D—subsequent encounter
> S—sequela

S79.812 `7th` Other specified injuries of left hip

S79.82 `6th` **Other specified injuries of thigh**

S79.821 `7th` Other specified injuries of right thigh

S79.822 `7th` Other specified injuries of left thigh

(S80–S89) INJURIES TO THE KNEE AND LOWER LEG

Excludes2: burns and corrosions (T20–T32)
frostbite (T33–T34)
injuries of ankle and foot, except fracture of ankle and malleolus (S90–S99)
insect bite or sting, venomous (T63.4)

S80 `4th` **SUPERFICIAL INJURY OF KNEE AND LOWER LEG**
Excludes2: superficial injury of ankle and foot (S90.-)

> 7th characters for category S80
> A—initial encounter
> D—subsequent encounter
> S—sequela

S80.0 `5th` **Contusion of knee**

S80.01X `7th` Contusion of right knee

S80.02X `7th` Contusion of left knee

S80.1 `5th` **Contusion of lower leg**

S80.11X `7th` Contusion of right lower leg

S80.12X `7th` Contusion of left lower leg

S80.2 `5th` **Other superficial injuries of knee**

S80.21 `6th` Abrasion of knee

S80.211 `7th` Abrasion, right knee

S80.212 `7th` Abrasion, left knee

S80.22 `6th` Blister (nonthermal) of knee

S80.221 `7th` Blister (nonthermal), right knee

S80.222 `7th` Blister (nonthermal), left knee

`4th` `5th` `6th` `7th` Additional Character Required   ✔ 3-character code   Unspecified laterality codes were excluded here.

• =New Code
▲ =Revised Code
▫ =Social determinants of health

Excludes1—Not coded here, do not use together
Excludes2—Not included here

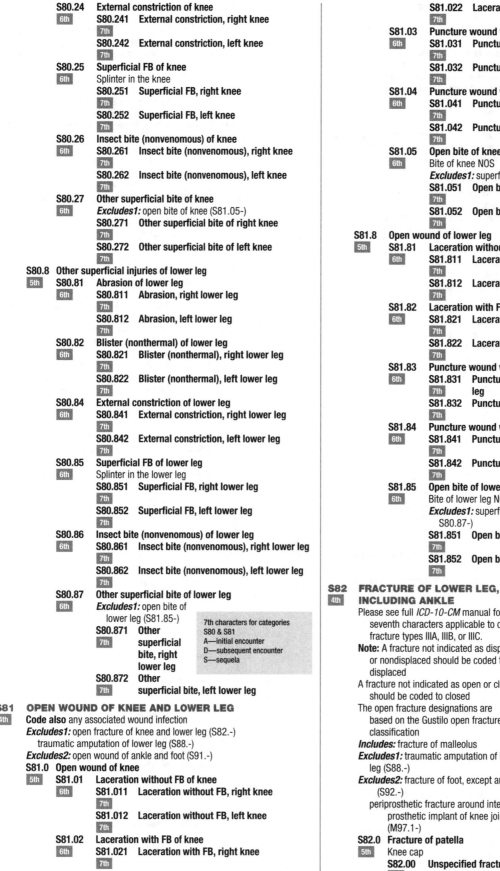

CHAPTER 19. INJURY, POISONING AND CERTAIN OTHER CONSEQUENCES OF EXTERNAL CAUSES   (S80.24–S82.00)

S80.24   **External constriction of knee**
- **6th**   **S80.241**   **External constriction, right knee**   **7th**
- **S80.242**   **External constriction, left knee**   **7th**

S80.25   **Superficial FB of knee**
- **6th**   Splinter in the knee
- **S80.251**   **Superficial FB, right knee**   **7th**
- **S80.252**   **Superficial FB, left knee**   **7th**

S80.26   **Insect bite (nonvenomous) of knee**
- **6th**   **S80.261**   **Insect bite (nonvenomous), right knee**   **7th**
- **S80.262**   **Insect bite (nonvenomous), left knee**   **7th**

S80.27   **Other superficial bite of knee**
- **6th**   *Excludes1:* open bite of knee (S81.05-)
- **S80.271**   **Other superficial bite of right knee**   **7th**
- **S80.272**   **Other superficial bite of left knee**   **7th**

S80.8   **Other superficial injuries of lower leg**
- **5th**

S80.81   **Abrasion of lower leg**
- **6th**   **S80.811**   **Abrasion, right lower leg**   **7th**
- **S80.812**   **Abrasion, left lower leg**   **7th**

S80.82   **Blister (nonthermal) of lower leg**
- **6th**   **S80.821**   **Blister (nonthermal), right lower leg**   **7th**
- **S80.822**   **Blister (nonthermal), left lower leg**   **7th**

S80.84   **External constriction of lower leg**
- **6th**   **S80.841**   **External constriction, right lower leg**   **7th**
- **S80.842**   **External constriction, left lower leg**   **7th**

S80.85   **Superficial FB of lower leg**
- **6th**   Splinter in the lower leg
- **S80.851**   **Superficial FB, right lower leg**   **7th**
- **S80.852**   **Superficial FB, left lower leg**   **7th**

S80.86   **Insect bite (nonvenomous) of lower leg**
- **6th**   **S80.861**   **Insect bite (nonvenomous), right lower leg**   **7th**
- **S80.862**   **Insect bite (nonvenomous), left lower leg**   **7th**

S80.87   **Other superficial bite of lower leg**
- **6th**   *Excludes1:* open bite of lower leg (S81.85-)
- **S80.871**   **Other superficial bite, right lower leg**   **7th**
- **S80.872**   **Other superficial bite, left lower leg**   **7th**

> 7th characters for categories S80 & S81
> A—initial encounter
> D—subsequent encounter
> S—sequela

S81   OPEN WOUND OF KNEE AND LOWER LEG
4th

Code also any associated wound infection
Excludes1: open fracture of knee and lower leg (S82.-)
    traumatic amputation of lower leg (S88.-)
Excludes2: open wound of ankle and foot (S91.-)

S81.0   **Open wound of knee**
- **5th**

S81.01   **Laceration without FB of knee**
- **6th**   **S81.011**   **Laceration without FB, right knee**   **7th**
- **S81.012**   **Laceration without FB, left knee**   **7th**

S81.02   **Laceration with FB of knee**
- **6th**   **S81.021**   **Laceration with FB, right knee**   **7th**
- **S81.022**   **Laceration with FB, left knee**   **7th**

S81.03   **Puncture wound without FB of knee**
- **6th**   **S81.031**   **Puncture wound without FB, right knee**   **7th**
- **S81.032**   **Puncture wound without FB, left knee**   **7th**

S81.04   **Puncture wound with FB of knee**
- **6th**   **S81.041**   **Puncture wound with FB, right knee**   **7th**
- **S81.042**   **Puncture wound with FB, left knee**   **7th**

S81.05   **Open bite of knee**
- **6th**   Bite of knee NOS
- *Excludes1:* superficial bite of knee (S80.27-)
- **S81.051**   **Open bite, right knee**   **7th**
- **S81.052**   **Open bite, left knee**   **7th**

S81.8   **Open wound of lower leg**
- **5th**

S81.81   **Laceration without FB of lower leg**
- **6th**   **S81.811**   **Laceration without FB, right lower leg**   **7th**
- **S81.812**   **Laceration without FB, left lower leg**   **7th**

S81.82   **Laceration with FB of lower leg**
- **6th**   **S81.821**   **Laceration with FB, right lower leg**   **7th**
- **S81.822**   **Laceration with FB, left lower leg**   **7th**

S81.83   **Puncture wound without FB of lower leg**
- **6th**   **S81.831**   **Puncture wound without FB, right lower leg**   **7th**
- **S81.832**   **Puncture wound without FB, left lower leg**   **7th**

S81.84   **Puncture wound with FB of lower leg**
- **6th**   **S81.841**   **Puncture wound with FB, right lower leg**   **7th**
- **S81.842**   **Puncture wound with FB, left lower leg**   **7th**

S81.85   **Open bite of lower leg**
- **6th**   Bite of lower leg NOS
- *Excludes1:* superficial bite of lower leg (S80.86-, S80.87-)
- **S81.851**   **Open bite, right lower leg**   **7th**
- **S81.852**   **Open bite, left lower leg**   **7th**

S82   FRACTURE OF LOWER LEG, INCLUDING ANKLE
4th

Please see full *ICD-10-CM* manual for seventh characters applicable to open fracture types IIIA, IIIB, or IIIC.
Note: A fracture not indicated as displaced or nondisplaced should be coded to displaced
A fracture not indicated as open or closed should be coded to closed
The open fracture designations are based on the Gustilo open fracture classification
Includes: fracture of malleolus
Excludes1: traumatic amputation of lower leg (S88.-)
Excludes2: fracture of foot, except ankle (S92.-)
    periprosthetic fracture around internal prosthetic implant of knee joint (M97.1-)

S82.0   **Fracture of patella**
- **5th**   Knee cap
- **S82.00**   **Unspecified fracture of patella**
- **6th**

> 7th characters for category S82 except S82.16-, S82.31-, S82.81, & S81.82
> A—initial encounter for closed fracture
> B—initial encounter for open fracture type I or II
> C—initial encounter for open fracture NOS
> D—subsequent encounter for closed fracture with routine healing
> E—subsequent encounter for open fracture type I or II with routine healing
> G—subsequent encounter for closed fracture with delayed healing
> H—subsequent encounter for open fracture type I or II with delayed healing
> K—subsequent encounter for closed fracture with nonunion
> M—subsequent encounter for open fracture type I or II with nonunion
> P—subsequent encounter for closed fracture with malunion
> Q—subsequent encounter for open fracture type I or II with malunion
> S—sequela

| 4th | 5th | 6th | 7th | Additional Character Required   ✓   3-character code |

Unspecified laterality codes were excluded here.

● =New Code
▲ =Revised Code
□ =Social determinants of health

Excludes1—Not coded here, do not use together
Excludes2—Not included here

374   **PEDIATRIC ICD-10-CM 2022: A MANUAL FOR PROVIDER-BASED CODING**

S82.001 | Unspecified fracture of right patella
`7th`

S82.002 | Unspecified fracture of left patella
`7th`

S82.1 Fracture of upper end of tibia
`5th` Fracture of proximal end of tibia
Excludes2: fracture of shaft of tibia (S82.2-)
physeal fracture of upper end of tibia (S89.0-)

S82.10 Unspecified fracture of upper end of tibia
`6th`

S82.101 | Unspecified fracture of upper end of right tibia
`7th`

S82.102 | Unspecified fracture of upper end of left tibia
`7th`

S82.16 Torus fracture of upper end of tibia
`6th`

S82.161 | Torus fracture of upper end of right tibia
`7th`

S82.162 | Torus fracture of upper end of left tibia
`7th`

S82.19 Other fracture of upper end of tibia
`6th`

S82.191 | Other fracture of upper end of right tibia
`7th`

S82.192 | Other fracture of upper end of left tibia
`7th`

> 7th characters for category S82 except S82.16-, S82.31-, S82.81, & S81.82
> A—initial encounter for closed fracture
> B—initial encounter for open fracture type I or II
> C—initial encounter for open fracture NOS
> D—subsequent encounter for closed fracture with routine healing
> E—subsequent encounter for open fracture type I or II with routine healing
> G—subsequent encounter for closed fracture with delayed healing
> H—subsequent encounter for open fracture type I or II with delayed healing
> K—subsequent encounter for closed fracture with nonunion
> M—subsequent encounter for open fracture type I or II with nonunion
> P—subsequent encounter for closed fracture with malunion
> Q—subsequent encounter for open fracture type I or II with malunion
> S—sequela

S82.2 Fracture of shaft of tibia
`5th`

S82.20 Unspecified fracture of shaft of tibia
`6th` Fracture of tibia NOS

S82.201 | Unspecified fracture of shaft of right tibia
`7th`

S82.202 | Unspecified fracture of shaft of left tibia
`7th`

S82.24 Spiral fracture of shaft of tibia
`6th` Toddler fracture

S82.241 | Displaced spiral fracture of shaft of right tibia
`7th`

S82.242 | Displaced spiral fracture of shaft of left tibia
`7th`

S82.244 | Nondisplaced spiral fracture of shaft of right tibia
`7th`

S82.245 | Nondisplaced spiral fracture of shaft of left tibia
`7th`

S82.3 Fracture of lower end of tibia
`5th` *Excludes1:* bimalleolar fracture of lower leg (S82.84-)
fracture of medial malleolus alone (S82.5-)
Maisonneuve's fracture (S82.86-)
pilon fracture of distal tibia (S82.87-)
trimalleolar fractures of lower leg (S82.85-)

S82.30 Unspecified fracture of lower end of tibia
`6th`

S82.301 | Unspecified fracture of lower end of right tibia
`7th`

S82.302 | Unspecified fracture of lower end of left tibia
`7th`

S82.31 Torus fracture of lower end of tibia
`6th`

S82.311 | Torus fracture of lower end of right tibia
`7th`

> 7th characters for subcategory S82.31
> A—initial encounter for closed fracture
> D—subsequent encounter for fracture with routine healing
> G—subsequent encounter for fracture with delayed healing
> K—subsequent encounter for fracture with nonunion
> P—subsequent encounter for fracture with malunion
> S—sequela

S82.312 | Torus fracture of lower end of left tibia
`7th`

S82.39 Other fracture of lower end of tibia
`6th`

S82.391 | Other fracture of lower end of right tibia
`7th`

S82.392 | Other fracture of lower end of left tibia
`7th`

S82.4 Fracture of shaft of fibula
`5th` *Excludes2:* fracture of lateral malleolus alone (S82.6-)

S82.40 Unspecified fracture of shaft of fibula
`6th`

S82.401 | Unspecified fracture of shaft of right fibula
`7th`

S82.402 | Unspecified fracture of shaft of left fibula
`7th`

S82.5 Fracture of medial malleolus
`5th` *Excludes1:* pilon fracture of distal tibia (S82.87-)
Salter-Harris type III of lower end of tibia (S89.13-)
Salter-Harris type IV of lower end of tibia (S89.14-)

S82.51X Displaced fracture of medial malleolus of right tibia
`7th`

S82.52X Displaced fracture of medial malleolus of left tibia
`7th`

S82.54X Nondisplaced fracture of medial malleolus of right tibia
`7th`

S82.55X Nondisplaced fracture of medial malleolus of left tibia
`7th`

S82.6 Fracture of lateral malleolus
`5th` *Excludes1:* pilon fracture of distal tibia (S82.87-)

S82.61X Displaced fracture of lateral malleolus of right fibula
`7th`

S82.62X Displaced fracture of lateral malleolus of left fibula
`7th`

S82.64X Nondisplaced fracture of lateral malleolus of right fibula
`7th`

S82.65X Nondisplaced fracture of lateral malleolus of left fibula
`7th`

S82.8 Other fractures of lower leg
`5th`

S82.81 Torus fracture of upper end of fibula
`6th`

S82.811 | Torus fracture of upper end of right fibula
`7th`

S82.812 | Torus fracture of upper end of left fibula
`7th`

> 7th character for subcategories S82.81- & S82.82-
> A—initial encounter for closed fracture
> D—subsequent encounter for fracture with routine healing
> G—subsequent encounter for fracture with delayed healing
> K—subsequent encounter for fracture with nonunion

S82.82 Torus fracture of lower end of fibula
`6th`

S82.821 | Torus fracture of lower end of right fibula
`7th`

S82.822 | Torus fracture of lower end of left fibula
`7th`

> 7th characters for category S82 except S82.16-, S82.31-, S82.81, & S81.82
> A—initial encounter for closed fracture
> B—initial encounter for open fracture type I or II
> C—initial encounter for open fracture NOS
> D—subsequent encounter for closed fracture with routine healing
> E—subsequent encounter for open fracture type I or II with routine healing
> G—subsequent encounter for closed fracture with delayed healing
> H—subsequent encounter for open fracture type I or II with delayed healing
> K—subsequent encounter for closed fracture with nonunion
> M—subsequent encounter for open fracture type I or II with nonunion
> P—subsequent encounter for closed fracture with malunion
> Q—subsequent encounter for open fracture type I or II with malunion
> S—sequela

S82.83 Other fracture of upper and lower end of fibula
`6th`

S82.831 | Other fracture of upper and lower end of right fibula
`7th`

S82.832 | Other fracture of upper and lower end of left fibula
`7th`

S82.84 Bimalleolar fracture of lower leg
`6th`

S82.841 | Displaced bimalleolar fracture of right lower leg
`7th`

`4th` `5th` `6th` `7th` Additional Character Required ✓ 3-character code Unspecified laterality codes were excluded here.

• =New Code
▲ =Revised Code
▢ =Social determinants of health

Excludes1—Not coded here, do not use together
Excludes2—Not included here

S82.842   Displaced bimalleolar fracture of left lower leg
`7th`

S82.844   Nondisplaced bimalleolar fracture of right lower leg
`7th`

S82.845   Nondisplaced bimalleolar fracture of left lower leg
`7th`

S82.85   **Trimalleolar fracture of lower leg**
`6th`

S82.851   Displaced trimalleolar fracture of right lower leg
`7th`

S82.852   Displaced trimalleolar fracture of left lower leg
`7th`

S82.854   Nondisplaced trimalleolar fracture of right lower leg
`7th`

S82.855   Nondisplaced trimalleolar fracture of left lower leg
`7th`

S82.86   **Maisonneuve's fracture**
`6th`

S82.861   Displaced Maisonneuve's fracture of right leg
`7th`

S82.862   Displaced Maisonneuve's fracture of left leg
`7th`

S82.864   Nondisplaced Maisonneuve's fracture of right leg
`7th`

S82.865   Nondisplaced Maisonneuve's fracture of left leg
`7th`

S82.87   **Pilon fracture of tibia**
`6th`

S82.871   Displaced pilon fracture of right tibia
`7th`

S82.872   Displaced pilon fracture of left tibia
`7th`

S82.874   Nondisplaced pilon fracture of right tibia
`7th`

S82.875   Nondisplaced pilon fracture of left tibia
`7th`

S82.89   **Other fractures of lower leg**
`6th`
Fracture of ankle NOS

S82.891   Other fracture of right lower leg
`7th`

S82.892   Other fracture of left lower leg
`7th`

S83   DISLOCATION AND SPRAIN OF JOINTS AND LIGAMENTS OF KNEE
`4th`

Includes: avulsion of joint or ligament of knee
  laceration of cartilage, joint or ligament of knee
  sprain of cartilage, joint or ligament of knee
  traumatic hemarthrosis of joint or ligament of knee
  traumatic rupture of joint or ligament of knee
  traumatic subluxation of joint or ligament of knee
  traumatic tear of joint or ligament of knee

Code also any associated open wound

Excludes1: derangement of patella (M22.0–M22.3)
  injury of patellar ligament (tendon) (S76.1-)
  internal derangement of knee (M23.-)
  old dislocation of knee (M24.36)
  pathological dislocation of knee (M24.36)
  recurrent dislocation of knee (M22.0)

Excludes2: strain of muscle, fascia and tendon of lower leg (S86.-)

> **7th characters for category S83**
> A—initial encounter
> D—subsequent encounter
> S—sequela

S83.0   **Subluxation and dislocation of patella**
`5th`

S83.00   **Unspecified subluxation and dislocation of patella**
`6th`

S83.001   Unspecified subluxation of right patella
`7th`

S83.002   Unspecified subluxation of left patella
`7th`

S83.004   Unspecified dislocation of right patella
`7th`

S83.005   Unspecified dislocation of left patella
`7th`

S83.01   **Lateral subluxation and dislocation of patella**
`6th`

S83.011   Lateral subluxation of right patella
`7th`

S83.012   Lateral subluxation of left patella
`7th`

S83.014   Lateral dislocation of right patella
`7th`

S83.015   Lateral dislocation of left patella
`7th`

S83.09   **Other subluxation and dislocation of patella**
`6th`

S83.091   Other subluxation of right patella
`7th`

S83.092   Other subluxation of left patella
`7th`

S83.094   Other dislocation of right patella
`7th`

S83.095   Other dislocation of left patella
`7th`

S83.1   **Subluxation and dislocation of knee**
`5th`
Excludes2: instability of knee prosthesis (T84.022, T84.023)

S83.10   **Unspecified subluxation and dislocation of knee**
`6th`

S83.101   Unspecified subluxation of right knee
`7th`

S83.102   Unspecified subluxation of left knee
`7th`

S83.104   Unspecified dislocation of right knee
`7th`

S83.105   Unspecified dislocation of left knee
`7th`

S83.11   **Anterior subluxation and dislocation of proximal end of tibia**
`6th`
Posterior subluxation and dislocation of distal end of femur

S83.111   Anterior subluxation of proximal end of tibia, right knee
`7th`

S83.112   Anterior subluxation of proximal end of tibia, left knee
`7th`

S83.114   Anterior dislocation of proximal end of tibia, right knee
`7th`

S83.115   Anterior dislocation of proximal end of tibia, left knee
`7th`

S83.12   **Posterior subluxation and dislocation of proximal end of tibia**
`6th`
Anterior dislocation of distal end of femur

S83.121   Posterior subluxation of proximal end of tibia, right knee
`7th`

S83.122   Posterior subluxation of proximal end of tibia, left knee
`7th`

S83.124   Posterior dislocation of proximal end of tibia, right knee
`7th`

S83.125   Posterior dislocation of proximal end of tibia, left knee
`7th`

S83.13   **Medial subluxation and dislocation of proximal end of tibia**
`6th`

S83.131   Medial subluxation of proximal end of tibia, right knee
`7th`

S83.132   Medial subluxation of proximal end of tibia, left knee
`7th`

S83.134   Medial dislocation of proximal end of tibia, right knee
`7th`

S83.135   Medial dislocation of proximal end of tibia, left knee
`7th`

S83.14   **Lateral subluxation and dislocation of proximal end of tibia**
`6th`

S83.141   Lateral subluxation of proximal end of tibia, right knee
`7th`

S83.142   Lateral subluxation of proximal end of tibia, left knee
`7th`

S83.144   Lateral dislocation of proximal end of tibia, right knee
`7th`

S83.145   Lateral dislocation of proximal end of tibia, left knee
`7th`

S83.19   **Other subluxation and dislocation of knee**
`6th`

S83.191   Other subluxation of right knee
`7th`

S83.192   Other subluxation of left knee
`7th`

`4th` `5th` `6th` `7th`   Additional Character Required   ✔   3-character code   Unspecified laterality codes were excluded here.

● =New Code
▲ =Revised Code
¤ =Social determinants of health

Excludes1—Not coded here, do not use together
Excludes2—Not included here

S83.194 **7th** Other dislocation of right knee

S83.195 **7th** Other dislocation of left knee

S83.4 Sprain of collateral ligament of knee

5th **S83.40** Sprain of unspecified collateral ligament of knee

6th **S83.401** **7th** Sprain of unspecified collateral ligament of right knee

S83.402 **7th** Sprain of unspecified collateral ligament of left knee

6th **S83.41** Sprain of medial collateral ligament of knee
Sprain of tibial collateral ligament

S83.411 **7th** Sprain of medial collateral ligament of right knee

S83.412 **7th** Sprain of medial collateral ligament of left knee

6th **S83.42** Sprain of lateral collateral ligament of knee
Sprain of fibular collateral ligament

> 7th characters for category S83
> A—initial encounter
> D—subsequent encounter
> S—sequela

S83.421 **7th** Sprain of lateral collateral ligament of right knee

S83.422 **7th** Sprain of lateral collateral ligament of left knee

S83.5 Sprain of cruciate ligament of knee

5th **S83.50** Sprain of unspecified cruciate ligament of knee

6th **S83.501** **7th** Sprain of unspecified cruciate ligament of right knee

S83.502 **7th** Sprain of unspecified cruciate ligament of left knee

6th **S83.51** Sprain of anterior cruciate ligament of knee

S83.511 **7th** Sprain of anterior cruciate ligament of right knee

S83.512 **7th** Sprain of anterior cruciate ligament of left knee

6th **S83.52** Sprain of posterior cruciate ligament of knee

S83.521 **7th** Sprain of posterior cruciate ligament of right knee

S83.522 **7th** Sprain of posterior cruciate ligament of left knee

S83.6 Sprain of the superior tibiofibular joint and ligament

5th **S83.60X** **7th** Sprain of the superior tibiofibular joint and ligament, unspecified knee

S83.61X **7th** Sprain of the superior tibiofibular joint and ligament, right knee

S83.62X **7th** Sprain of the superior tibiofibular joint and ligament, left knee

S83.8 Sprain of other specified parts of knee

5th **S83.8X** Sprain of other specified parts of knee

6th **S83.8X1** **7th** Sprain of other specified parts of right knee

S83.8X2 **7th** Sprain of other specified parts of left knee

S83.9 Sprain of unspecified site of knee

5th **S83.91X** **7th** Sprain of unspecified site of right knee

S83.92X **7th** Sprain of unspecified site of left knee

> 7th characters for categories S83 & S86
> A—initial encounter
> D—subsequent encounter
> S—sequela

S86 **4th** **INJURY OF MUSCLE, FASCIA AND TENDON AT LOWER LEG LEVEL**

Code also any associated open wound (S81.-)

Excludes2: injury of muscle, fascia and tendon at ankle (S96.-)
injury of patellar ligament (tendon) (S76.1-)
sprain of joints and ligaments of knee (S83.-)

S86.0 Injury of Achilles tendon

5th **S86.00** Unspecified injury of Achilles tendon

6th **S86.001** **7th** Unspecified injury of right Achilles tendon

S86.002 **7th** Unspecified injury of left Achilles tendon

6th **S86.01** Strain of Achilles tendon

S86.011 **7th** Strain of right Achilles tendon

S86.012 **7th** Strain of left Achilles tendon

6th **S86.02** Laceration of Achilles tendon

S86.021 **7th** Laceration of right Achilles tendon

S86.022 **7th** Laceration of left Achilles tendon

6th **S86.09** Other specified injury of Achilles tendon

S86.091 **7th** Other specified injury of right Achilles tendon

S86.092 **7th** Other specified injury of left Achilles tendon

S86.1 **5th** Injury of other muscle(s) and tendon(s) of posterior muscle group at lower leg level

6th **S86.11** Strain of other muscle(s) and tendon(s) of posterior muscle group at lower leg level

S86.111 **7th** Strain of other muscle(s) and tendon(s) of posterior muscle group at lower leg level, right leg

S86.112 **7th** Strain of other muscle(s) and tendon(s) of posterior muscle group at lower leg level, left leg

S86.2 **5th** Injury of muscle(s) and tendon(s) of anterior muscle group at lower leg level

6th **S86.21** Strain of muscle(s) and tendon(s) of anterior muscle group at lower leg level

S86.211 **7th** Strain of muscle(s) and tendon(s) of anterior muscle group at lower leg level, right leg

S86.212 **7th** Strain of muscle(s) and tendon(s) of anterior muscle group at lower leg level, left leg

S86.3 **5th** Injury of muscle(s) and tendon(s) of peroneal muscle group at lower leg level

6th **S86.31** Strain of muscle(s) and tendon(s) of peroneal muscle group at lower leg level

S86.311 **7th** Strain of muscle(s) and tendon(s) of peroneal muscle group at lower leg level, right leg

S86.312 **7th** Strain of muscle(s) and tendon(s) of peroneal muscle group at lower leg level, left leg

6th **S86.32** Laceration of muscle(s) and tendon(s) of peroneal muscle group at lower leg level

S86.321 **7th** Laceration of mus-cle(s) and tendon(s) of peroneal muscle group at lower leg level, right leg

S86.322 **7th** Laceration of muscle(s) and tendon(s) of peroneal muscle group at lower leg level, left leg

6th **S86.39** Other injury of muscle(s) and tendon(s) of peroneal muscle group at lower leg level

S86.391 **7th** Other injury of muscle(s) and tendon(s) of peroneal muscle group at lower leg level, right leg

S86.392 **7th** Other injury of muscle(s) and tendon(s) of peroneal muscle group at lower leg level, left leg

S86.8 **5th** Injury of other muscles and tendons at lower leg level

6th **S86.81** Strain of other muscles and tendons at lower leg level

S86.811 **7th** Strain of other muscle(s) and tendon(s) at lower leg level, right leg

S86.812 **7th** Strain of other muscle(s) and tendon(s) at lower leg level, left leg

6th **S86.82** Laceration of other muscles and tendons at lower leg level

S86.821 **7th** Laceration of other muscle(s) and tendon(s) at lower leg level, right leg

---

4th **5th** **6th** **7th** Additional Character Required ✔ 3-character code

Unspecified laterality codes were excluded here.

• =New Code
▲ =Revised Code
▫ =Social determinants of health

Excludes1—Not coded here, do not use together
Excludes2—Not included here

S86.822 [7th] Laceration of other muscle(s) and tendon(s) at lower leg level, left leg

S86.89 [6th] Other injury of other muscles and tendons at lower leg level

S86.891 [7th] Other injury of other muscle(s) and tendon(s) at lower leg level, right leg

S86.892 [7th] Other injury of other muscle(s) and tendon(s) at lower leg level, left leg

S86.9 [5th] Injury of unspecified muscle and tendon at lower leg level

S86.91 [6th] Strain of unspecified muscle and tendon at lower leg level

S86.911 [7th] Strain of unspecified muscle(s) and tendon(s) at lower leg level, right leg

S86.912 [7th] Strain of unspecified muscle(s) and tendon(s) at lower leg level, left leg

S89 [4th] **OTHER AND UNSPECIFIED INJURIES OF LOWER LEG**

Note: A fracture not indicated as open or closed should be coded to closed

Excludes2: other and unspecified injuries of ankle and foot (S99.-)

S89.0 [5th] Physeal fracture of upper end of tibia

S89.00 [6th] Unspecified physeal fracture of upper end of tibia

S89.001 [7th] Unspecified physeal fracture of upper end of right tibia

S89.002 [7th] Unspecified physeal fracture of upper end of left tibia

S89.01 [6th] Salter-Harris Type I physeal fracture of upper end of tibia

S89.011 [7th] Salter-Harris Type I physeal fracture of upper end of right tibia

S89.012 [7th] Salter-Harris Type I physeal fracture of upper end of left tibia

> 7th characters for subcategories S89.0, S89.1, S89.2, and S89.3
> A—initial encounter for closed fracture
> D—subsequent encounter for fracture with routine healing
> G—subsequent encounter for fracture with delayed healing
> K—subsequent encounter for fracture with nonunion
> P—subsequent encounter for fracture with malunion
> S—sequela

S89.02 [6th] Salter-Harris Type II physeal fracture of upper end of tibia

S89.021 [7th] Salter-Harris Type II physeal fracture of upper end of right tibia

S89.022 [7th] Salter-Harris Type II physeal fracture of upper end of left tibia

S89.03 [6th] Salter-Harris Type III physeal fracture of upper end of tibia

S89.031 [7th] Salter-Harris Type III physeal fracture of upper end of right tibia

S89.032 [7th] Salter-Harris Type III physeal fracture of upper end of left tibia

S89.04 [6th] Salter-Harris Type IV physeal fracture of upper end of tibia

S89.041 [7th] Salter-Harris Type IV physeal fracture of upper end of right tibia

S89.042 [7th] Salter-Harris Type IV physeal fracture of upper end of left tibia

S89.09 [6th] Other physeal fracture of upper end of tibia

S89.091 [7th] Other physeal fracture of upper end of right tibia

S89.092 [7th] Other physeal fracture of upper end of left tibia

S89.1 [5th] Physeal fracture of lower end of tibia

S89.10 [6th] Unspecified physeal fracture of lower end of tibia

S89.101 [7th] Unspecified physeal fracture of lower end of right tibia

S89.102 [7th] Unspecified physeal fracture of lower end of left tibia

S89.11 [6th] Salter-Harris Type I physeal fracture of lower end of tibia

S89.111 [7th] Salter-Harris Type I physeal fracture of lower end of right tibia

S89.112 [7th] Salter-Harris Type I physeal fracture of lower end of left tibia

S89.12 [6th] Salter-Harris Type II physeal fracture of lower end of tibia

S89.121 [7th] Salter-Harris Type II physeal fracture of lower end of right tibia

S89.122 [7th] Salter-Harris Type II physeal fracture of lower end of left tibia

S89.13 [6th] Salter-Harris Type III physeal fracture of lower end of tibia

Excludes1: fracture of medial malleolus (adult) (S82.5-)

S89.131 [7th] Salter-Harris Type III physeal fracture of lower end of right tibia

S89.132 [7th] Salter-Harris Type III physeal fracture of lower end of left tibia

S89.14 [6th] Salter-Harris Type IV physeal fracture of lower end of tibia

Excludes1: fracture of medial malleolus (adult) (S82.5-)

S89.141 [7th] Salter-Harris Type IV physeal fracture of lower end of right tibia

S89.142 [7th] Salter-Harris Type IV physeal fracture of lower end of left tibia

S89.19 [6th] Other physeal fracture of lower end of tibia

S89.191 [7th] Other physeal fracture of lower end of right tibia

S89.192 [7th] Other physeal fracture of lower end of left tibia

S89.2 [5th] Physeal fracture of upper end of fibula

S89.20 [6th] Unspecified physeal fracture of upper end of fibula

S89.201 [7th] Unspecified physeal fracture of upper end of right fibula

S89.202 [7th] Unspecified physeal fracture of upper end of left fibula

S89.21 [6th] Salter-Harris Type I physeal fracture of upper end of fibula

S89.211 [7th] Salter-Harris Type I physeal fracture of upper end of right fibula

S89.212 [7th] Salter-Harris Type I physeal fracture of upper end of left fibula

S89.22 [6th] Salter-Harris Type II physeal fracture of upper end of fibula

S89.221 [7th] Salter-Harris Type II physeal fracture of upper end of right fibula

S89.222 [7th] Salter-Harris Type II physeal fracture of upper end of left fibula

S89.29 [6th] Other physeal fracture of upper end of fibula

S89.291 [7th] Other physeal fracture of upper end of right fibula

S89.292 [7th] Other physeal fracture of upper end of left fibula

S89.3 [5th] Physeal fracture of lower end of fibula

S89.30 [6th] Unspecified physeal fracture of lower end of fibula

S89.301 [7th] Unspecified physeal fracture of lower end of right fibula

S89.302 [7th] Unspecified physeal fracture of lower end of left fibula

S89.31 [6th] Salter-Harris Type I physeal fracture of lower end of fibula

S89.311 [7th] Salter-Harris Type I physeal fracture of lower end of right fibula

S89.312 [7th] Salter-Harris Type I physeal fracture of lower end of left fibula

S89.32 [6th] Salter-Harris Type II physeal fracture of lower end of fibula

S89.321 [7th] Salter-Harris Type II physeal fracture of lower end of right fibula

S89.322 [7th] Salter-Harris Type II physeal fracture of lower end of left fibula

S89.39 [6th] Other physeal fracture of lower end of fibula

S89.391 [7th] Other physeal fracture of lower end of right fibula

---

[4th] [5th] [6th] [7th] Additional Character Required   [✓]   3-character code   Unspecified laterality codes were excluded here.

• =New Code
▲ =Revised Code
▫ =Social determinants of health

Excludes1—Not coded here, do not use together
Excludes2—Not included here

S89.392 Other physeal fracture of lower end of left fibula
[7th]

S89.8 Other specified injuries of lower leg
[5th]

> 7th characters for subcategory S89.8
> A—initial encounter
> D—subsequent encounter
> S—sequela

S89.81X Other specified injuries of right lower leg
[7th]

S89.82X Other specified injuries of left lower leg
[7th]

(S90–S99) INJURIES TO THE ANKLE AND FOOT

Excludes2: burns and corrosions (T20–T32)
fracture of ankle and malleolus (S82.-)
frostbite (T33–T34)
insect bite or sting, venomous (T63.4)

> 7th characters for category S90
> A—initial encounter
> D—subsequent encounter
> S—sequela

S90 SUPERFICIAL INJURY OF ANKLE, FOOT AND TOES
[4th]

S90.0 Contusion of ankle
[5th]

S90.01X Contusion of right ankle
[7th]

S90.02X Contusion of left ankle
[7th]

S90.1 Contusion of toe without damage to nail
[5th]

S90.11 Contusion of great toe without damage to nail
[6th]

S90.111 Contusion of right great toe without damage to nail
[7th]

S90.112 Contusion of left great toe without damage to nail
[7th]

> 7th characters for category S90
> A—initial encounter
> D—subsequent encounter
> S—sequela

S90.12 Contusion of lesser toe without damage to nail
[6th]

S90.121 Contusion of right lesser toe(s) without damage to nail
[7th]

S90.122 Contusion of left lesser toe(s) without damage to nail
[7th]

S90.2 Contusion of toe with damage to nail
[5th]

S90.21 Contusion of great toe with damage to nail
[6th]

S90.211 Contusion of right great toe with damage to nail
[7th]

S90.212 Contusion of left great toe with damage to nail
[7th]

S90.22 Contusion of lesser toe with damage to nail
[6th]

S90.221 Contusion of right lesser toe(s) with damage to nail
[7th]

S90.222 Contusion of left lesser toe(s) with damage to nail
[7th]

S90.3 Contusion of foot
[5th]
Excludes2: contusion of toes (S90.1-, S90.2-)

S90.31X Contusion of right foot
[7th]

S90.32X Contusion of left foot
[7th]

S90.4 Other superficial injuries of toe
[5th]

S90.41 Abrasion of toe
[6th]

S90.411 Abrasion, right great toe
[7th]

S90.412 Abrasion, left great toe
[7th]

S90.414 Abrasion, right lesser toe(s)
[7th]

S90.415 Abrasion, left lesser toe(s)
[7th]

S90.42 Blister (nonthermal) of toe
[6th]

S90.421 Blister (nonthermal), right great toe
[7th]

S90.422 Blister (nonthermal), left great toe
[7th]

S90.424 Blister (nonthermal), right lesser toe(s)
[7th]

S90.425 Blister (nonthermal), left lesser toe(s)
[7th]

S90.44 External constriction of toe
[6th]
TIP: See category W49 for external cause code (eg, W49.01-, hair causing external constriction).
Hair tourniquet syndrome of toe

S90.441 External constriction, right great toe
[7th]

S90.442 External constriction, left great toe
[7th]

S90.444 External constriction, right lesser toe(s)
[7th]

S90.445 External constriction, left lesser toe(s)
[7th]

S90.45 Superficial FB of toe
[6th]
Splinter in the toe

S90.451 Superficial FB, right great toe
[7th]

S90.452 Superficial FB, left great toe
[7th]

S90.454 Superficial FB, right lesser toe(s)
[7th]

S90.455 Superficial FB, left lesser toe(s)
[7th]

S90.46 Insect bite (nonvenomous) of toe
[6th]

S90.461 Insect bite (nonvenomous), right great toe
[7th]

S90.462 Insect bite (nonvenomous), left great toe
[7th]

S90.464 Insect bite (nonvenomous), right lesser toe(s)
[7th]

S90.465 Insect bite (nonvenomous), left lesser toe(s)
[7th]

S90.47 Other superficial bite of toe
[6th]
Excludes1: open bite of toe (S91.15-, S91.25-)

S90.471 Other superficial bite of right great toe
[7th]

S90.472 Other superficial bite of left great toe
[7th]

S90.474 Other superficial bite of right lesser toe(s)
[7th]

S90.475 Other superficial bite of left lesser toe(s)
[7th]

S90.5 Other superficial injuries of ankle
[5th]

S90.51 Abrasion of ankle
[6th]

S90.511 Abrasion, right ankle
[7th]

S90.512 Abrasion, left ankle
[7th]

S90.52 Blister (nonthermal) of ankle
[6th]

S90.521 Blister (nonthermal), right ankle
[7th]

S90.522 Blister (nonthermal), left ankle
[7th]

S90.54 External constriction of ankle
[6th]

S90.541 External constriction, right ankle
[7th]

S90.542 External constriction, left ankle
[7th]

S90.55 Superficial FB of ankle
[6th]
Splinter in the ankle

S90.551 Superficial FB, right ankle
[7th]

S90.552 Superficial FB, left ankle
[7th]

S90.56 Insect bite (nonvenomous) of ankle
[6th]

S90.561 Insect bite (nonvenomous), right ankle
[7th]

S90.562 Insect bite (nonvenomous), left ankle
[7th]

S90.57 Other superficial bite of ankle
[6th]
Excludes1: open bite of ankle (S91.05-)

S90.571 Other superficial bite of ankle, right ankle
[7th]

S90.572 Other superficial bite of ankle, left ankle
[7th]

[4th] [5th] [6th] [7th] Additional Character Required   ✔ 3-character code   Unspecified laterality codes were excluded here.

• =New Code
▲ =Revised Code
⊡ =Social determinants of health

Excludes1—Not coded here, do not use together
Excludes2—Not included here

S90.8 **Other superficial injuries of foot**

5th **S90.81** **Abrasion of foot**
6th   **S90.811** **Abrasion, right foot**
7th
       S90.812 **Abrasion, left foot**
7th

S90.82 **Blister (nonthermal) of foot**
6th   **S90.821** **Blister (nonthermal), right foot**
7th
       S90.822 **Blister (nonthermal), left foot**
7th

S90.84 **External constriction of foot**
6th   **S90.841** **External constriction, right foot**
7th
       S90.842 **External constriction, left foot**
7th

S90.85 **Superficial FB of foot**
6th   Splinter in the foot
       S90.851 **Superficial FB, right foot**
7th
       S90.852 **Superficial FB, left foot**
7th

S90.86 **Insect bite (nonvenomous) of foot**
6th   **S90.861** **Insect bite (nonvenomous), right foot**
7th
       S90.862 **Insect bite (nonvenomous), left foot**
7th

S90.87 **Other superficial bite of foot**
6th   *Excludes1:* open bite of foot (S91.35-)
       S90.871 **Other superficial bite of right foot**
7th
       S90.872 **Other superficial bite of left foot**
7th

S91 **OPEN WOUND OF ANKLE, FOOT AND TOES**
4th   **Code also** any associated wound infection
       Excludes1: open fracture of ankle, foot
         and toes (S92.-with 7th character B)
         traumatic amputation of ankle and foot
         (S98.-)

| 7th characters for category S91 |
| A—initial encounter |
| D—subsequent encounter |
| S—sequela |

S91.0 **Open wound of ankle**
5th **S91.01** **Laceration without FB of ankle**
6th   **S91.011** **Laceration without FB, right ankle**
7th
       S91.012 **Laceration without FB, left ankle**
7th

S91.02 **Laceration with FB of ankle**
6th   **S91.021** **Laceration with FB, right ankle**
7th
       S91.022 **Laceration with FB, left ankle**
7th

S91.03 **Puncture wound without FB of ankle**
6th   **S91.031** **Puncture wound without FB, right ankle**
7th
       S91.032 **Puncture wound without FB, left ankle**
7th

S91.04 **Puncture wound with FB of ankle**
6th   **S91.041** **Puncture wound with FB, right ankle**
7th
       S91.042 **Puncture wound with FB, left ankle**
7th

S91.05 **Open bite of ankle**
6th   *Excludes1:* superficial bite of ankle (S90.56-, S90.57-)
       S91.051 **Open bite, right ankle**
7th
       S91.052 **Open bite, left ankle**
7th

S91.1 **Open wound of toe without damage to nail**
5th **S91.11** **Laceration without FB of toe without damage to nail**
6th   **S91.111** **Laceration without FB of right great toe**
7th   **without damage to nail**
       S91.112 **Laceration without FB of left great toe**
7th   **without damage to nail**

S91.114 **Laceration without FB of right lesser toe(s)**
7th   **without damage to nail**
S91.115 **Laceration without FB of left lesser toe(s)**
7th   **without damage to nail**

S91.12 **Laceration with FB of toe without damage to nail**
6th   **S91.121** **Laceration with FB of right great toe**
7th   **without damage to nail**
       S91.122 **Laceration with FB of left great toe**
7th   **without damage to nail**
       S91.124 **Laceration with FB of right lesser toe(s)**
7th   **without damage to nail**
       S91.125 **Laceration with FB of left lesser toe(s)**
7th   **without damage to nail**

S91.13 **Puncture wound without FB of toe without damage to nail**
6th   **S91.131** **Puncture wound without FB of right great toe without damage to nail**
7th
       S91.132 **Puncture wound without FB of left great toe without damage to nail**
7th
       S91.134 **Puncture wound without FB of right lesser toe(s) without damage to nail**
7th
       S91.135 **Puncture wound without FB of left lesser toe(s) without damage to nail**
7th

S91.14 **Puncture wound with FB of toe without damage to nail**
6th   **S91.141** **Puncture wound with FB of right great toe without damage to nail**
7th
       S91.142 **Puncture wound with FB of left great toe without damage to nail**
7th
       S91.144 **Puncture wound with FB of right lesser toe(s) without damage to nail**
7th
       S91.145 **Puncture wound with FB of left lesser toe(s) without damage to nail**
7th

S91.15 **Open bite of toe without damage to nail**
6th   Bite of toe NOS
       Excludes1: superficial bite of toe (S90.46-, S90.47-)
       S91.151 **Open bite of right great toe without damage to nail**
7th
       S91.152 **Open bite of left great toe without damage to nail**
7th
       S91.154 **Open bite of right lesser toe(s) without damage to nail**
7th
       S91.155 **Open bite of left lesser toe(s) without damage to nail**
7th

S91.2 **Open wound of toe with damage to nail**
5th **S91.21** **Laceration without FB of toe with damage to nail**
6th   **S91.211** **Laceration without FB of right great toe with damage to nail**
7th
       S91.212 **Laceration without FB of left great toe with damage to nail**
7th
       S91.214 **Laceration without FB of right lesser toe(s) with damage to nail**
7th
       S91.215 **Laceration without FB of left lesser toe(s) with damage to nail**
7th

S91.22 **Laceration with FB of toe with damage to nail**
6th   **S91.221** **Laceration with FB of right great toe with damage to nail**
7th
       S91.222 **Laceration with FB of left great toe with damage to nail**
7th
       S91.224 **Laceration with FB of right lesser toe(s) with damage to nail**
7th
       S91.225 **Laceration with FB of left lesser toe(s) with damage to nail**
7th

S91.23 **Puncture wound without FB of toe with damage to nail**
6th   **S91.231** **Puncture wound without FB of right great toe with damage to nail**
7th
       S91.232 **Puncture wound without FB of left great toe with damage to nail**
7th
       S91.234 **Puncture wound without FB of right lesser toe(s) with damage to nail**
7th
       S91.235 **Puncture wound without FB of left lesser toe(s) with damage to nail**
7th

4th	5th	6th	7th	Additional Character Required	✔	3-character code	Unspecified laterality codes were excluded here.	• =New Code	*Excludes1*—Not coded here, do not use together
								▲ =Revised Code	*Excludes2*—Not included here
								⌑ =Social determinants of health	

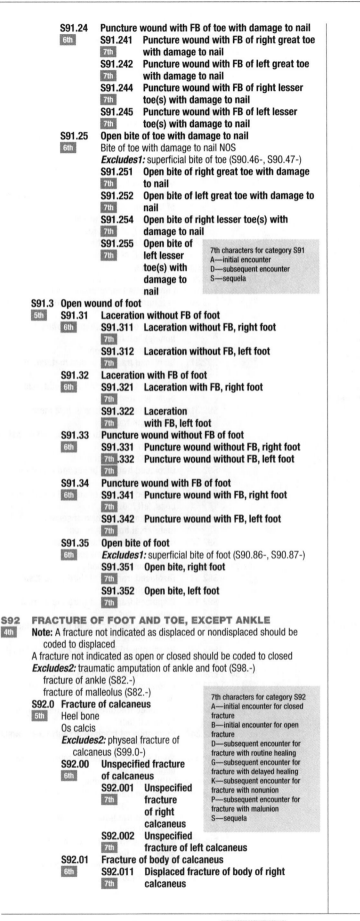

S91.24 Puncture wound with FB of toe with damage to nail
- 6th **S91.241** Puncture wound with FB of right great toe with damage to nail — 7th
- **S91.242** Puncture wound with FB of left great toe with damage to nail — 7th
- **S91.244** Puncture wound with FB of right lesser toe(s) with damage to nail — 7th
- **S91.245** Puncture wound with FB of left lesser toe(s) with damage to nail — 7th

S91.25 Open bite of toe with damage to nail
- 6th Bite of toe with damage to nail NOS
  - *Excludes1:* superficial bite of toe (S90.46-, S90.47-)
  - **S91.251** Open bite of right great toe with damage to nail — 7th
  - **S91.252** Open bite of left great toe with damage to nail — 7th
  - **S91.254** Open bite of right lesser toe(s) with damage to nail — 7th
  - **S91.255** Open bite of left lesser toe(s) with damage to nail — 7th

> 7th characters for category S91
> A—initial encounter
> D—subsequent encounter
> S—sequela

S91.3 Open wound of foot
- 5th **S91.31** Laceration without FB of foot
  - 6th **S91.311** Laceration without FB, right foot — 7th
  - **S91.312** Laceration without FB, left foot — 7th
- **S91.32** Laceration with FB of foot
  - 6th **S91.321** Laceration with FB, right foot — 7th
  - **S91.322** Laceration with FB, left foot — 7th
- **S91.33** Puncture wound without FB of foot
  - 6th **S91.331** Puncture wound without FB, right foot — 7th
  - **S91.332** Puncture wound without FB, left foot — 7th
- **S91.34** Puncture wound with FB of foot
  - 6th **S91.341** Puncture wound with FB, right foot — 7th
  - **S91.342** Puncture wound with FB, left foot — 7th
- **S91.35** Open bite of foot
  - 6th *Excludes1:* superficial bite of foot (S90.86-, S90.87-)
  - **S91.351** Open bite, right foot — 7th
  - **S91.352** Open bite, left foot — 7th

S92   **FRACTURE OF FOOT AND TOE, EXCEPT ANKLE**
- 4th **Note:** A fracture not indicated as displaced or nondisplaced should be coded to displaced
  A fracture not indicated as open or closed should be coded to closed
  - *Excludes2:* traumatic amputation of ankle and foot (S98.-)
    fracture of ankle (S82.-)
    fracture of malleolus (S82.-)

S92.0 Fracture of calcaneus
- 5th Heel bone
  Os calcis
  - *Excludes2:* physeal fracture of calcaneus (S99.0-)
  - **S92.00** Unspecified fracture of calcaneus
    - 6th **S92.001** Unspecified fracture of right calcaneus — 7th
    - **S92.002** Unspecified fracture of left calcaneus — 7th
  - **S92.01** Fracture of body of calcaneus
    - 6th **S92.011** Displaced fracture of body of right calcaneus — 7th

> 7th characters for category S92
> A—initial encounter for closed fracture
> B—initial encounter for open fracture
> D—subsequent encounter for fracture with routine healing
> G—subsequent encounter for fracture with delayed healing
> K—subsequent encounter for fracture with nonunion
> P—subsequent encounter for fracture with malunion
> S—sequela

- **S92.012** Displaced fracture of body of left calcaneus — 7th
- **S92.014** Nondisplaced fracture of body of right calcaneus — 7th
- **S92.015** Nondisplaced fracture of body of left calcaneus — 7th

S92.02 Fracture of anterior process of calcaneus
- 6th **S92.021** Displaced fracture of anterior process of right calcaneus — 7th
- **S92.022** Displaced fracture of anterior process of left calcaneus — 7th
- **S92.024** Nondis-placed fracture of anterior process of right calcaneus — 7th
- **S92.025** Nondisplaced fracture of anterior process of left calcaneus — 7th

S92.03 Avulsion fracture of tuberosity of calcaneus
- 6th **S92.031** Displaced avulsion fracture of tuberosity of right calcaneus — 7th
- **S92.032** Displaced avulsion fracture of tuberosity of left calcaneus — 7th
- **S92.034** Nondisplaced avulsion fracture of tuberosity of right calcaneus — 7th
- **S92.035** Nondisplaced avulsion fracture of tuberosity of left calcaneus — 7th

S92.04 Other fracture of tuberosity of calcaneus
- 6th **S92.041** Displaced other fracture of tuberosity of right calcaneus — 7th
- **S92.042** Displaced other fracture of tuberosity of left calcaneus — 7th
- **S92.044** Nondisplaced other fracture of tuberosity of right calcaneus — 7th
- **S92.045** Nondisplaced other fracture of tuberosity of left calcaneus — 7th

S92.05 Other extraarticular fracture of calcaneus
- 6th **S92.051** Displaced other extraarticular fracture of right calcaneus — 7th
- **S92.052** Displaced other extraarticular fracture of left calcaneus — 7th
- **S92.054** Nondisplaced other extraarticular fracture of right calcaneus — 7th
- **S92.055** Nondisplaced other extraarticular fracture of left calcaneus — 7th

S92.06 Intraarticular fracture of calcaneus
- 6th **S92.061** Displaced intraarticular fracture of right calcaneus — 7th
- **S92.062** Displaced intraarticular fracture of left calcaneus — 7th
- **S92.064** Nondisplaced intraarticular fracture of right calcaneus — 7th
- **S92.065** Nondisplaced intraarticular fracture of left calcaneus — 7th

S92.1 Fracture of talus
- 5th Astragalus
  - **S92.10** Unspecified fracture of talus
    - 6th **S92.101** Unspecified fracture of right talus — 7th
    - **S92.102** Unspecified fracture of left talus — 7th
  - **S92.11** Fracture of neck of talus
    - 6th **S92.111** Displaced fracture of neck of right talus — 7th
    - **S92.112** Displaced fracture of neck of left talus — 7th
    - **S92.114** Nondisplaced fracture of neck of right talus — 7th
    - **S92.115** Nondisplaced fracture of neck of left talus — 7th
  - **S92.12** Fracture of body of talus
    - 6th **S92.121** Displaced fracture of body of right talus — 7th
    - **S92.122** Displaced fracture of body of left talus — 7th
    - **S92.124** Nondisplaced fracture of body of right talus — 7th

---

 4th   5th   6th   7th   Additional Character Required   ✔   3-character code   Unspecified laterality codes were excluded here.   • =New Code   ▲ =Revised Code   ☐ =Social determinants of health   *Excludes1*—Not coded here, do not use together   *Excludes2*—Not included here

S92.125   Nondisplaced fracture of body of left talus
    7th

S92.13   Fracture of posterior process of talus
    6th
     S92.131   Displaced fracture of posterior process of right talus
      7th
     S92.132   Displaced fracture of posterior process of left talus
      7th
     S92.134   Nondisplaced fracture of posterior process of right talus
      7th
     S92.135   Nondisplaced fracture of posterior process of left talus
      7th

S92.14   Dome fracture of talus
    6th
    Excludes1: osteochondritis dissecans (M93.2)
     S92.141   Displaced dome fracture of right talus
      7th
     S92.142   Displaced dome fracture of left talus
      7th
     S92.144   Nondisplaced dome fracture of right talus
      7th
     S92.145   Nondisplaced dome fracture of left talus
      7th

> 7th characters for category S92
> A—initial encounter for closed fracture
> B—initial encounter for open fracture
> D—subsequent encounter for fracture with routine healing
> G—subsequent encounter for fracture with delayed healing
> K—subsequent encounter for fracture with nonunion
> P—subsequent encounter for fracture with malunion
> S—sequela

S92.15   Avulsion fracture (chip fracture) of talus
    6th
     S92.151   Displaced avulsion fracture (chip fracture) of right talus
      7th
     S92.152   Displaced avulsion fracture (chip fracture) of left talus
      7th
     S92.154   Nondisplaced avulsion fracture (chip fracture) of right talus
      7th
     S92.155   Nondisplaced avulsion fracture (chip fracture) of left talus
      7th

S92.19   Other fracture of talus
    6th
     S92.191   Other fracture of right talus
      7th
     S92.192   Other fracture of left talus
      7th

S92.2   Fracture of other and unspecified tarsal bone(s)
    5th
    S92.20   Fracture of unspecified tarsal bone(s)
     6th
      S92.201   Fracture of unspecified tarsal bone(s) of right foot
       7th
      S92.202   Fracture of unspecified tarsal bone(s) of left foot
       7th

    S92.21   Fracture of cuboid bone
     6th
      S92.211   Displaced fracture of cuboid bone of right foot
       7th
      S92.212   Displaced fracture of cuboid bone of left foot
       7th
      S92.214   Nondisplaced fracture of cuboid bone of right foot
       7th
      S92.215   Nondisplaced fracture of cuboid bone of left foot
       7th

    S92.22   Fracture of lateral cuneiform
     6th
      S92.221   Displaced fracture of lateral cuneiform of right foot
       7th
      S92.222   Displaced fracture of lateral cuneiform of left foot
       7th
      S92.224   Nondisplaced fracture of lateral cuneiform of right foot
       7th
      S92.225   Nondisplaced fracture of lateral cuneiform of left foot
       7th

    S92.23   Fracture of intermediate cuneiform
     6th
      S92.231   Displaced fracture of intermediate cuneiform of right foot
       7th
      S92.232   Displaced fracture of intermediate cuneiform of left foot
       7th
      S92.234   Nondisplacedfracture of intermediate cuneiform of right foot
       7th

      S92.235   Nondisplaced fracture of intermediate cuneiform of left foot
       7th

    S92.24   Fracture of medial cuneiform
     6th
      S92.241   Displaced fracture of medial cuneiform of right foot
       7th
      S92.242   Displaced fracture of medial cuneiform of left foot
       7th
      S92.244   Nondisplaced fracture of medial cuneiform of right foot
       7th
      S92.245   Nondisplaced fracture of medial cuneiform of left foot
       7th

    S92.25   Fracture of navicular [scaphoid] of foot
     6th
      S92.251   Displaced fracture of navicular [scaphoid] of right foot
       7th
      S92.252   Displaced fracture of navicular [scaphoid] of left foot
       7th
      S92.254   Nondisplaced fracture of navicular [scaphoid] of right foot
       7th
      S92.255   Nondisplaced fracture of navicular [scaphoid] of left foot
       7th

S92.3   Fracture of metatarsal bone(s)
    5th
    Excludes2: physeal fracture of metatarsal (S99.1-)
    S92.30   Fracture of unspecified metatarsal bone(s)
     6th
      S92.301   Fracture of unspecified metatarsal bone(s), right foot
       7th
      S92.302   Fracture of unspecified metatarsal bone(s), left foot
       7th

    S92.31   Fracture of first metatarsal bone
     6th
      S92.311   Displaced fracture of first metatarsal bone, right foot
       7th
      S92.312   Displaced fracture of first metatarsal bone, left foot
       7th
      S92.314   Nondisplaced fracture of first metatarsal bone, right foot
       7th
      S92.315   Nondisplaced fracture of first metatarsal bone, left foot
       7th

    S92.32   Fracture of second metatarsal bone
     6th
      S92.321   Displaced fracture of second metatarsal bone, right foot
       7th
      S92.322   Displaced fracture of second metatarsal bone, left foot
       7th
      S92.324   Nondisplaced fracture of second metatarsal bone, right foot
       7th
      S92.325   Nondisplaced fracture of second metatarsal bone, left foot
       7th

    S92.33   Fracture of third metatarsal bone
     6th
      S92.331   Displaced fracture of third metatarsal bone, right foot
       7th
      S92.332   Displaced fracture of third metatarsal bone, left foot
       7th
      S92.334   Nondisplaced fracture of third metatarsal bone, right foot
       7th
      S92.335   Nondisplaced fracture of third metatarsal bone, left foot
       7th

    S92.34   Fracture of fourth metatarsal bone
     6th
      S92.341   Displaced fracture of fourth metatarsal bone, right foot
       7th
      S92.342   Displaced fracture of fourth metatarsal bone, left foot
       7th
      S92.344   Nondisplaced fracture of fourth metatarsal bone, right foot
       7th
      S92.345   Nondisplaced fracture of fourth metatarsal bone, left foot
       7th

    S92.35   Fracture of fifth metatarsal bone
     6th
      S92.351   Displaced fracture of fifth metatarsal bone, right foot
       7th
      S92.352   Displaced fracture of fifth metatarsal bone, left foot
       7th
      S92.354   Nondisplaced fracture of fifth metatarsal bone, right foot
       7th
      S92.355   Nondisplaced fracture of fifth metatarsal bone, left foot
       7th

4th   5th   6th   7th   Additional Character Required   ✔   3-character code   Unspecified laterality codes were excluded here.

• =New Code
▲ =Revised Code
▣ =Social determinants of health

Excludes1—Not coded here, do not use together
Excludes2—Not included here

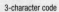

S92.4   **Fracture of great toe**
`5th`   *Excludes2:* physeal fracture of phalanx of toe (S99.2-)

     S92.41   **Fracture of proximal phalanx of great toe**
     `6th`
         S92.411   **Displaced fracture of proximal phalanx of right great toe**
         `7th`
         S92.412   **Displaced fracture of proximal phalanx of left great toe**
         `7th`
         S92.414   **Nondisplaced fracture of proximal phalanx of right great toe**
         `7th`
         S92.415   **Nondisplaced fracture of proximal phalanx of left great toe**
         `7th`

     S92.42   **Fracture of distal phalanx of great toe**
     `6th`
         S92.421   **Displaced fracture of distal phalanx of right great toe**
         `7th`
         S92.422   **Displaced fracture of distal phalanx of left great toe**
         `7th`
         S92.424   **Nondisplaced fracture of distal phalanx of right great toe**
         `7th`
         S92.425   **Nondisplaced fracture of distal phalanx of left great toe**
         `7th`

> **7th characters for category S92**
> A—initial encounter for closed fracture
> B—initial encounter for open fracture
> D—subsequent encounter for fracture with routine healing
> G—subsequent encounter for fracture with delayed healing
> K—subsequent encounter for fracture with nonunion
> P—subsequent encounter for fracture with malunion
> S—sequela

     S92.49   **Other fracture of great toe**
     `6th`
         S92.491   **Other fracture of right great toe**
         `7th`
         S92.492   **Other fracture of left great toe**
         `7th`

S92.5   **Fracture of lesser toe(s)**
`5th`   *Excludes2:* physeal fracture of toe (S99.2-)

     S92.51   **Fracture of proximal phalanx of lesser toe(s)**
     `6th`
         S92.511   **Displaced fracture of proximal phalanx of right lesser toe(s)**
         `7th`
         S92.512   **Displaced fracture of proximal phalanx of left lesser toe(s)**
         `7th`
         S92.514   **Nondisplaced fracture of proximal phalanx of right lesser toe(s)**
         `7th`
         S92.515   **Nondisplaced fracture of proximal phalanx of left lesser toe(s)**
         `7th`

     S92.52   **Fracture of middle phalanx of lesser toe(s)**
     `6th`
         S92.521   **Displaced fracture of middle phalanx of right lesser toe(s)**
         `7th`
         S92.522   **Displaced fracture of middle phalanx of left lesser toe(s)**
         `7th`
         S92.524   **Nondisplaced fracture of middle phalanx of right lesser toe(s)**
         `7th`
         S92.525   **Nondisplaced fracture of middle phalanx of left lesser toe(s)**
         `7th`

     S92.53   **Fracture of distal phalanx of lesser toe(s)**
     `6th`
         S92.531   **Displaced fracture of distal phalanx of right lesser toe(s)**
         `7th`
         S92.532   **Displaced fracture of distal phalanx of left lesser toe(s)**
         `7th`
         S92.534   **Nondisplaced fracture of distal phalanx of right lesser toe(s)**
         `7th`
         S92.535   **Nondisplaced fracture of distal phalanx of left lesser toe(s)**
         `7th`

     S92.59   **Other fracture of lesser toe(s)**
     `6th`
         S92.591   **Other fracture of right lesser toe(s)**
         `7th`
         S92.592   **Other fracture of left lesser toe(s)**
         `7th`

S92.8   **Other fracture of foot**
`5th`
     S92.81   **Other fracture of foot**
     `6th`   Sesamoid fracture of foot
         S92.811   **Other fracture of right foot**
         `7th`

         S92.812   **Other fracture of left foot**
         `7th`

S92.9   **Unspecified fracture of foot and toe**
`5th`
     S92.90   **Unspecified fracture of foot**
     `6th`
         S92.901   **Unspecified fracture of right foot**
         `7th`
         S92.902   **Unspecified fracture of left foot**
         `7th`

     S92.91   **Unspecified fracture of toe**
     `6th`
         S92.911   **Unspecified fracture of right toe(s)**
         `7th`
         S92.912   **Unspecified fracture of left toe(s)**
         `7th`

S93   **DISLOCATION AND SPRAIN OF JOINTS AND LIGAMENTS AT ANKLE, FOOT AND TOE LEVEL**
`4th`
Includes: avulsion of joint or ligament of ankle, foot and toe
     laceration of cartilage, joint or ligament of ankle, foot and toe
     sprain of cartilage, joint or ligament of ankle, foot and toe
     traumatic hemarthrosis of joint or ligament of ankle, foot and toe
     traumatic rupture of joint or ligament of ankle, foot and toe
     traumatic subluxation of joint or ligament of ankle, foot and toe
     traumatic tear of joint or ligament of ankle, foot and toe
Code also any associated open wound
Excludes2: strain of muscle and tendon of ankle and foot (S96.-)

> **7th characters for category S93**
> A—initial encounter
> D—subsequent encounter
> S—sequela

S93.0   **Subluxation and dislocation of ankle joint**
`5th`   Subluxation and dislocation of astragalus
     Subluxation and dislocation of fibula, lower end
     Subluxation and dislocation of talus or of tibia, lower end
     S93.01X   **Subluxation of right ankle joint**
     `7th`
     S93.02X   **Subluxation of left ankle joint**
     `7th`
     S93.04X   **Dislocation of right ankle joint**
     `7th`
     S93.05X   **Dislocation of left ankle joint**
     `7th`

S93.1   **Subluxation and dislocation of toe**
`5th`
     S93.10   **Unspecified subluxation and dislocation of toe**
     `6th`   Dislocation/subluxation of toe NOS
         S93.101   **Unspecified subluxation of right toe(s)**
         `7th`
         S93.102   **Unspecified subluxation of left toe(s)**
         `7th`
         S93.104   **Unspecified dislocation of right toe(s)**
         `7th`
         S93.105   **Unspecified dislocation of left toe(s)**
         `7th`

     S93.11   **Dislocation of interphalangeal joint**
     `6th`
         S93.111   **Dislocation of interphalangeal joint of right great toe**
         `7th`
         S93.112   **Dislocation of interphalangeal joint of left great toe**
         `7th`
         S93.114   **Dislocation of inter-phalangeal joint of right lesser toe(s)**
         `7th`
         S93.115   **Dislocation of interphalangeal joint of left lesser toe(s)**
         `7th`

     S93.12   **Dislocation of metatarsophalangeal joint**
     `6th`
         S93.121   **Dislocation of metatarsophalangeal joint of right great toe**
         `7th`
         S93.122   **Dislocation of metatarsophalangeal joint of left great toe**
         `7th`
         S93.124   **Dislocation of metatarsophalangeal joint of right lesser toe(s)**
         `7th`
         S93.125   **Dislocation of metatarsophalangeal joint of left lesser toe(s)**
         `7th`

     S93.13   **Subluxation of interphalangeal joint**
     `6th`
         S93.131   **Subluxation of interphalangeal joint of right great toe**
         `7th`
         S93.132   **Subluxation of interphalangeal joint of left great toe**
         `7th`

`4th` `5th` `6th` `7th`   Additional Character Required   ✔   3-character code   Unspecified laterality codes were excluded here.

• =New Code
▲ =Revised Code
▣ =Social determinants of health

Excludes1—Not coded here, do not use together
Excludes2—Not included here

CHAPTER 19. INJURY, POISONING AND CERTAIN OTHER CONSEQUENCES OF EXTERNAL CAUSES   (S93.134–S96.01)

S93.134 7th **Subluxation of interphalangeal joint of right lesser toe(s)**

S93.135 7th **Subluxation of interphalangeal joint of left lesser toe(s)**

S93.14 6th **Subluxation of metatarsophalangeal joint**

S93.141 7th **Subluxation of metatarsophalangeal joint of right great toe**

S93.142 7th **Subluxation of metatarsophalangeal joint of left great toe**

S93.144 7th **Subluxation of metatarsophalangeal joint of right lesser toe(s)**

S93.145 7th **Subluxation of metatarsophalangeal joint of left lesser toe(s)**

S93.3 5th **Subluxation and dislocation of foot**
Excludes2: dislocation of toe (S93.1-)

> **7th characters for category S93**
> A—initial encounter
> D—subsequent encounter
> S—sequela

S93.30 6th **Unspecified subluxation and dislocation of foot**
Dislocation of foot NOS
Subluxation of foot NOS

S93.301 7th **Unspecified subluxation of right foot**

S93.302 7th **Unspecified subluxation of left foot**

S93.304 7th **Unspecified dislocation of right foot**

S93.305 7th **Unspecified dislocation of left foot**

S93.31 6th **Subluxation and dislocation of tarsal joint**

S93.311 7th **Subluxation of tarsal joint of right foot**

S93.312 7th **Subluxation of tarsal joint of left foot**

S93.314 7th **Dislocation of tarsal joint of right foot**

S93.315 7th **Dislocation of tarsal joint of left foot**

S93.32 6th **Subluxation and dislocation of tarsometatarsal joint**

S93.321 7th **Subluxation of tarsometa-tarsal joint of right foot**

S93.322 7th **Subluxation of tarsometa-tarsal joint of left foot**

S93.324 7th **Dislocation of tarsometatarsal joint of right foot**

S93.325 7th **Dislocation of tarsometatarsal joint of left foot**

S93.33 6th **Other subluxation and dislocation of foot**

S93.331 7th **Other subluxation of right foot**

S93.332 7th **Other subluxation of left foot**

S93.334 7th **Other dislocation of right foot**

S93.335 7th **Other dislocation of left foot**

S93.4 5th **Sprain of ankle**
Excludes2: injury of Achilles tendon (S86.0-)

S93.40 6th **Sprain of unspecified ligament of ankle**
Sprain of ankle NOS
Sprained ankle NOS

S93.401 7th **Sprain of unspecified ligament of right ankle**

S93.402 7th **Sprain of unspecified ligament of left ankle**

S93.41 6th **Sprain of calcaneofibular ligament**

S93.411 7th **Sprain of calcaneofibular ligament of right ankle**

S93.412 7th **Sprain of calcaneofibular ligament of left ankle**

S93.42 6th **Sprain of deltoid ligament**

S93.421 7th **Sprain of deltoid ligament of right ankle**

S93.422 7th **Sprain of deltoid ligament of left ankle**

S93.43 6th **Sprain of tibiofibular ligament**

S93.431 7th **Sprain of tibiofibular ligament of right ankle**

S93.432 7th **Sprain of tibiofibular ligament of left ankle**

S93.49 6th **Sprain of other ligament of ankle**
Sprain of internal collateral ligament
Sprain of talofibular ligament

S93.491 7th **Sprain of other ligament of right ankle**

S93.492 7th **Sprain of other ligament of left ankle**

S93.5 5th **Sprain of toe**

S93.50 6th **Unspecified sprain of toe**

S93.501 7th **Unspecified sprain of right great toe**

S93.502 7th **Unspecified sprain of left great toe**

S93.504 7th **Unspecified sprain of right lesser toe(s)**

S93.505 7th **Unspecified sprain of left lesser toe(s)**

S93.51 6th **Sprain of interphalangeal joint of toe**

S93.511 7th **Sprain of interphalangeal joint of right great toe**

S93.512 7th **Sprain of interphalangeal joint of left great toe**

S93.514 7th **Sprain of interphalangeal joint of right lesser toe(s)**

S93.515 7th **Sprain of interphalangeal joint of left lesser toe(s)**

S93.52 6th **Sprain of metatarsophalangeal joint of toe**

S93.521 7th **Sprain of metatarsophalangeal joint of right great toe**

S93.522 7th **Sprain of metatarsophalangeal joint of left great toe**

S93.524 7th **Sprain of metatarsophalangeal joint of right lesser toe(s)**

S93.525 7th **Sprain of metatarsophalangeal joint of left lesser toe(s)**

S93.6 5th **Sprain of foot**
Excludes2: sprain of metatarsophalangeal joint of toe (S93.52-)
sprain of toe (S93.5-)

S93.60 6th **Unspecified sprain of foot**

S93.601 7th **Unspecified sprain of right foot**

S93.602 7th **Unspecified sprain of left foot**

S93.61 6th **Sprain of tarsal ligament of foot**

S93.611 7th **Sprain of tarsal ligament of right foot**

S93.612 7th **Sprain of tarsal ligament of left foot**

S93.62 6th **Sprain of tarsometatarsal ligament of foot**

S93.621 7th **Sprain of tarsometatarsal ligament of right foot**

S93.622 7th **Sprain of tarsometatarsal ligament of left foot**

S93.69 6th **Other sprain of foot**

S93.691 7th **Other sprain of right foot**

S93.692 7th **Other sprain of left foot**

S96 4th **INJURY OF MUSCLE AND TENDON AT ANKLE AND FOOT LEVEL**
Code also any associated open wound (S91.-)
Excludes2: injury of Achilles tendon (S86.0-)
sprain of joints and ligaments of ankle and foot (S93.-)

S96.0 5th **Injury of muscle and tendon of long flexor muscle of toe, ankle and foot level**

S96.01 6th **Strain of muscle and tendon of long flexor muscle of toe at ankle and foot level**

| 4th | 5th | 6th | 7th | Additional Character Required | ✔ | 3-character code | Unspecified laterality codes were excluded here. | • =New Code
▲ =Revised Code
⌓ =Social determinants of health | *Excludes1*—Not coded here, do not use together
Excludes2—Not included here |

S96.011 **7th** Strain of muscle and tendon of long flexor muscle of toe at ankle and foot level, right foot

S96.012 **7th** Strain of muscle and tendon of long flexor muscle of toe at ankle and foot level, left foot

S96.02 **6th** Laceration of muscle and tendon of long flexor muscle of toe at ankle and foot level

S96.021 **7th** Laceration of muscle and tendon of long flexor muscle of toe at ankle and foot level, right foot

S96.022 **7th** Laceration of muscle and tendon of long flexor muscle of toe at ankle and foot level, left foot

S96.11 **6th** Strain of muscle and tendon of long extensor muscle of toe at ankle and foot level

S96.111 **7th** Strain of muscle and tendon of long extensor muscle of toe at ankle and foot level, right foot

S96.112 **7th** Strain of muscle and tendon of long extensor muscle of toe at ankle and foot level, left foot

S96.12 **6th** Laceration of muscle and tendon of long extensor muscle of toe at ankle and foot level

S96.121 **7th** Laceration of muscle and tendon of long extensor muscle of toe at ankle and foot level, right foot

S96.122 **7th** Laceration of muscle and tendon of long extensor muscle of toe at ankle and foot level, left foot

S96.21 **6th** Strain of intrinsic muscle and tendon at ankle and foot level

S96.211 **7th** Strain of intrinsic muscle and tendon at ankle and foot level, right foot

S96.212 **7th** Strain of intrinsic muscle and tendon at ankle and foot level, left foot

S96.22 **6th** Laceration of intrinsic muscle and tendon at ankle and foot level

S96.221 **7th** Laceration of intrinsic muscle and tendon at ankle and foot level, right foot

S96.222 **7th** Laceration of intrinsic muscle and tendon at ankle and foot level, left foot

S96.81 **6th** Strain of other specified muscles and tendons at ankle and foot level

S96.811 **7th** Strain of other specified muscles and tendons at ankle and foot level, right foot

S96.812 **7th** Strain of other specified muscles and tendons at ankle and foot level, left foot

S96.91 **6th** Strain of unspecified muscle and tendon at ankle and foot level

S96.911 **7th** Strain of unspecified muscle and tendon at ankle and foot level, right foot

S96.912 **7th** Strain of unspecified muscle and tendon at ankle and foot level, left foot

S96.92 **6th** Laceration of unspecified muscle and tendon at ankle and foot level

S96.921 **7th** Laceration of unspecified muscle and tendon at ankle and foot level, right foot

S96.922 **7th** Laceration of unspecified muscle and tendon at ankle and foot level, left foot

S97 CRUSHING INJURY OF ANKLE AND FOOT
4th **Use additional code(s)** for all associated injuries

7th characters for category S97
A—initial encounter
D—subsequent encounter
S—sequela

S97.0 **Crushing injury of ankle**
5th **S97.01X** Crushing injury of right ankle **7th**
S97.02X Crushing injury of left ankle **7th**

S97.1 **Crushing injury of toe**
5th **S97.10** Crushing injury of unspecified toe(s)
6th **S97.101** Crushing injury of unspecified right toe(s) **7th**

S97.102 Crushing injury of unspecified left toe(s) **7th**

S97.11 **6th** Crushing injury of great toe
S97.111 Crushing injury of right great toe **7th**
S97.112 Crushing injury of left great toe **7th**

S97.12 **6th** Crushing injury of lesser toe(s)
S97.121 Crushing injury of right lesser toe(s) **7th**
S97.122 Crushing injury of left lesser toe(s) **7th**

S97.8 **Crushing injury of foot**
5th **S97.81X** Crushing injury of right foot **7th**
S97.82X Crushing injury of left foot **7th**

S99 OTHER AND UNSPECIFIED
4th **INJURIES OF ANKLE AND FOOT**
S99.0 **Physeal fracture of calcaneus**
5th **S99.00** Unspecified physeal fracture
6th
S99.001 Unspecified physeal fracture of right calcaneus **7th**
S99.002 Unspecified physeal fracture of left calcaneus **7th**

7th characters for subcategories S99.0- and S99.1-
A—initial encounter for closed fracture
B—initial encounter for open fracture
D—subsequent encounter for fracture with routine healing
G—subsequent encounter for fracture with delayed healing
K—subsequent encounter for fracture with nonunion
P—subsequent encounter for fracture with malunion
S—sequela

S99.01 **6th** Salter-Harris Type I physeal fracture
S99.011 Salter-Harris Type I physeal fracture of right calcaneus **7th**
S99.012 Salter-Harris Type I physeal fracture of left calcaneus **7th**

S99.02 **6th** Salter-Harris Type II physeal fracture
S99.021 Salter-Harris Type II physeal fracture of right calcaneus **7th**
S99.022 Salter-Harris Type II physeal fracture of left calcaneus **7th**

S99.03 **6th** Salter-Harris Type III physeal fracture
S99.031 Salter-Harris Type III physeal fracture of right calcaneus **7th**
S99.032 Salter-Harris Type III physeal fracture of left calcaneus **7th**

S99.04 **6th** Salter-Harris Type IV physeal fracture
S99.041 Salter-Harris Type IV physeal fracture of right calcaneus **7th**
S99.042 Salter-Harris Type IV physeal fracture of left calcaneus **7th**

S99.09 **6th** Other physeal fracture
S99.091 Other physeal fracture of right calcaneus **7th**
S99.092 Other physeal fracture of left calcaneus **7th**

S99.1 **Physeal fracture of right metatarsal**
5th **S99.10** Unspecified physeal fracture
6th **S99.101** Unspecified physeal fracture of right metatarsal **7th**
S99.102 Unspecified physeal fracture of left metatarsal **7th**

S99.11 **6th** Salter-Harris Type I physeal fracture of metatarsal
S99.111 Salter-Harris Type I physeal fracture of right metatarsal **7th**
S99.112 Salter-Harris Type I physeal fracture of left metatarsal **7th**

S99.12 **6th** Salter-Harris Type II physeal fracture of metatarsal
S99.121 Salter-Harris Type II physeal fracture of right metatarsal **7th**
S99.122 Salter-Harris Type II physeal fracture of left metatarsal **7th**

S99.13 **6th** Salter-Harris Type III physeal fracture of metatarsal

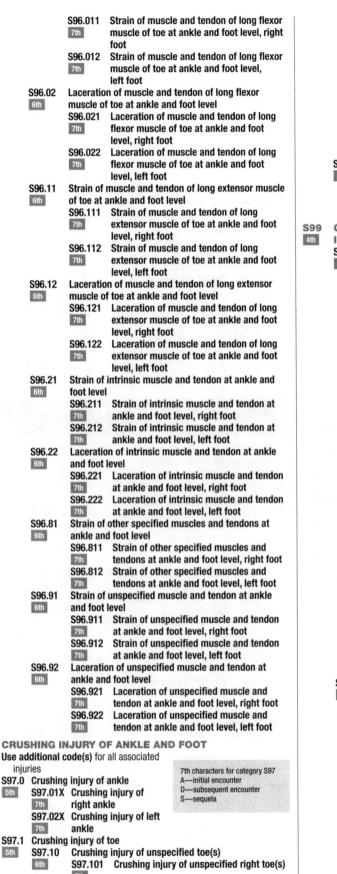

4th **5th** **6th** **7th** Additional Character Required   ✓ 3-character code   Unspecified laterality codes were excluded here.   • =New Code   ▲ =Revised Code   ▫ =Social determinants of health   *Excludes1*—Not coded here, do not use together   *Excludes2*—Not included here

S99.131 **7th** Salter-Harris Type III physeal fracture of right metatarsal

S99.132 **7th** Salter-Harris Type III physeal fracture of left metatarsal

S99.14 **6th** Salter-Harris Type IV physeal fracture of metatarsal

S99.141 **7th** Salter-Harris Type IV physeal fracture of right metatarsal

S99.142 **7th** Salter-Harris Type IV physeal fracture of left metatarsal

S99.19 **6th** Other physeal fracture of metatarsal

S99.191 **7th** Other physeal fracture of right metatarsal

S99.192 **7th** Other physeal fracture of left metatarsal

S99.2 **5th** Physeal fracture of phalanx of toe

S99.20 Unspecified physeal fracture of phalanx of toe

S99.201 **7th** Unspecified physeal fracture of phalanx of right toe

S99.202 **7th** Unspecified physeal fracture of phalanx of left toe

S99.21 **6th** Salter-Harris Type I physeal fracture of phalanx of toe

S99.211 **7th** Salter-Harris Type I physeal fracture of phalanx of right toe

S99.212 **7th** Salter-Harris Type I physeal fracture of phalanx of left toe

S99.22 **6th** Salter-Harris Type II physeal fracture of phalanx of toe

S99.221 **7th** Salter-Harris Type II physeal fracture of phalanx of right toe

S99.222 **7th** Salter-Harris Type II physeal fracture of phalanx of left toe

S99.23 **6th** Salter-Harris Type III physeal fracture of phalanx of toe

S99.231 **7th** Salter-Harris Type III physeal fracture of phalanx of right toe

S99.232 **7th** Salter-Harris Type III physeal fracture of phalanx of left toe

S99.24 **6th** Salter-Harris Type IV physeal fracture of phalanx of toe

S99.241 **7th** Salter-Harris Type IV physeal fracture of phalanx of right toe

S99.242 **7th** Salter-Harris Type IV physeal fracture of phalanx of left toe

S99.29 **6th** Other physeal fracture of phalanx of toe

S99.291 **7th** Other physeal fracture of phalanx of right toe

S99.292 **7th** Other physeal fracture of phalanx of left toe

S99.8 **5th** Other specified injuries of ankle and foot

S99.81 **6th** Other specified injuries of: ankle

S99.811 **7th** right ankle

S99.812 **7th** left ankle

S99.82 **6th** Other specified injuries of foot

S99.821 **7th** Other specified injuries of right foot

S99.822 **7th** Other specified injuries of left foot

> 7th characters for category S99.8- and S99.9-
> A—initial encounter
> D—subsequent encounter
> S—sequela

S99.9 **5th** Unspecified injury of ankle and foot

S99.91 **6th** Unspecified injury of ankle

S99.911 **7th** Unspecified injury of right ankle

S99.912 **7th** Unspecified injury of left ankle

S99.92 **6th** Unspecified injury of foot

S99.921 **7th** Unspecified injury of right foot

S99.922 **7th** Unspecified injury of left foo

(T07–T88) INJURY, POISONING AND CERTAIN OTHER CONSEQUENCES OF EXTERNAL CAUSES

(T07) INJURIES INVOLVING MULTIPLE BODY REGIONS

Excludes1: burns and corrosions (T20–T32)
frostbite (T33–T34)
insect bite or sting, venomous (T63.4)
sunburn (L55.-)

T07 **7th** **UNSPECIFIED MULTIPLE INJURIES**
   Excludes1: injury NOS (T14.90)

> 7th character for T07
> A—initial encounter
> D—subsequent encounter
> S—sequela

(T14) INJURY OF UNSPECIFIED BODY REGION

T14 **4th** **INJURY OF UNSPECIFIED BODY REGION**
   Excludes1: multiple unspecified injuries (T07)

T14.8XX **7th** Other injury of unspecified body region
   Abrasion NOS
   Contusion NOS
   Crush injury NOS
   Fracture NOS
   Skin injury NOS
   Vascular injury NOS
   Wound NOS

> 7th character for T14-
> A—initial encounter
> D—subsequent encounter
> S—sequela

T14.9 **5th** Unspecified injury

T14.90X **7th** Injury, unspecified
   Injury NOS

T14.91X **7th** Suicide attempt
   Attempted suicide NOS

(T15–T19) EFFECTS OF FB ENTERING THROUGH NATURAL ORIFICE

Excludes2: FB accidentally left in operation wound (T81.5-)
FB in penetrating wound—See open wound by body region
residual FB in soft tissue (M79.5)
splinter, without open wound—See superficial injury by body region

T15 **4th** **FB ON EXTERNAL EYE**
   Excludes2: FB in penetrating wound of orbit and eye ball (S05.4-, S05.5-)
   open wound of eyelid and periocular area (S01.1-)
   retained FB in eyelid (H02.8-)
   retained (old) FB in penetrating wound of orbit and eye ball (H05.5-, H44.6-, H44.7-)
   superficial FB of eyelid and periocular area (S00.25-)

T15.0 **5th** FB in cornea

T15.01X **7th** FB in cornea, right eye

T15.02X **7th** FB in cornea, left eye

T15.1 **5th** FB in conjunctival sac

T15.11X **7th** FB in conjunctival sac, right eye

T15.12X **7th** FB in conjunctival sac, left eye

T16 **4th** **FB IN EAR**
   Includes: FB in auditory canal

T16.1XX **7th** FB in right ear

T16.2XX **7th** FB in left ear

T17 **4th** **FB IN RESPIRATORY TRACT**

T17.0XX **7th** FB in nasal sinus

T17.1XX **7th** FB in nostril
   FB in nose NOS

T17.2 **5th** FB in pharynx
   FB in nasopharynx
   FB in throat NOS

> 7th characters for category T17
> A—initial encounter
> D—subsequent encounter
> S—sequela

| **4th** | **5th** | **6th** | **7th** | Additional Character Required | ✓ 3-character code | Unspecified laterality codes were excluded here. | • =New Code
▲ =Revised Code
☐ =Social determinants of health | ***Excludes1***—Not coded here, do not use together
Excludes2—Not included here |

T17.20   **Unspecified FB in pharynx**
6th
   T17.200   **Unspecified FB in pharynx causing asphyxiation**
   7th
   T17.208   **Unspecified FB in pharynx causing other injury**
   7th

T17.21   **Gastric contents in pharynx**
6th
   Aspiration of gastric contents into pharynx
   Vomitus in pharynx
   T17.210   **Gastric contents in pharynx causing asphyxiation**
   7th
   T17.218   **Gastric contents in pharynx causing other injury**
   7th

T17.22   **Food in pharynx**
6th
   Bones in pharynx
   Seeds in pharynx
   T17.220   **Food in pharynx causing asphyxiation**
   7th
   T17.228   **Food in pharynx causing other injury**
   7th

T17.29   **Other foreign object in pharynx**
6th
   T17.290   **Other foreign object in pharynx causing asphyxiation**
   7th
   T17.298   **Other foreign object in pharynx causing other injury**
   7th

T17.3   **FB in larynx**
5th
  T17.30   **Unspecified FB in larynx**
  6th
   T17.300   **Unspecified FB in larynx causing asphyxiation**
   7th
   T17.308   **Unspecified FB in larynx causing other injury**
   7th

  T17.31   **Gastric contents in larynx**
  6th
   Aspiration of gastric contents into larynx
   Vomitus in larynx
   T17.310   **Gastric contents in larynx causing asphyxiation**
   7th

> 7th characters for category T17
> A—initial encounter
> D—subsequent encounter
> S—sequela

   T17.318   **Gastric contents in larynx causing other injury**
   7th

  T17.32   **Food in larynx**
  6th
   Bones in larynx
   Seeds in larynx
   T17.320   **Food in larynx causing asphyxiation**
   7th
   T17.328   **Food in larynx causing other injury**
   7th

  T17.39   **Other foreign object in larynx**
  6th
   T17.390   **Other foreign object in larynx causing asphyxiation**
   7th
   T17.398   **Other foreign object in larynx causing other injury**
   7th

T17.9   **FB in respiratory tract, part unspecified**
5th
  T17.90   **Unspecified FB in respiratory tract, part unspecified**
  6th
   T17.900   **Unspecified FB in respiratory tract, part unspecified causing asphyxiation**
   7th
   T17.908   **Unspecified FB in respiratory tract, part unspecified causing other injury**
   7th

  T17.91   **Gastric contents in respiratory tract, part unspecified**
  6th
   Aspiration of gastric contents into respiratory tract, part unspecified
   Vomitus in trachea respiratory tract, part unspecified
   T17.910   **Gastric contents in respiratory tract, part unspecified causing asphyxiation**
   7th
   T17.918   **Gastric contents in respiratory tract, part unspecified causing other injury**
   7th

  T17.92   **Food in respiratory tract, part unspecified**
  6th
   Bones in respiratory tract, part unspecified
   Seeds in respiratory tract, part unspecified
   T17.920   **Food in respiratory tract, part unspecified causing asphyxiation**
   7th
   T17.928   **Food in respiratory tract, part unspecified causing other injury**
   7th

T17.99   **Other foreign object in respiratory tract, part unspecified**
6th
   T17.990   **Other foreign object in respiratory tract, part unspecified in causing asphyxiation**
   7th
   T17.998   **Other foreign object in respiratory tract, part unspecified causing other injury**
   7th

T18   **FB IN ALIMENTARY TRACT**
4th
Excludes2: FB in pharynx (T17.2-)

T18.0XX   **Foreign body in mouth**
7th

T18.1   **FB in esophagus**
5th
  Excludes2: FB in respiratory tract (T17.-)

  T18.10   **Unspecified FB in esophagus**
  6th
   T18.100   **Unspecified FB in esophagus causing compression of trachea**
   7th
    Unspecified FB in esophagus causing obstruction of respiration
   T18.108   **Unspecified FB in esophagus causing other injury**
   7th

  T18.11   **Gastric contents in esophagus**
  6th
   Vomitus in esophagus
   T18.110   **Gastric contents in esophagus causing compression of trachea**
   7th
    Gastric contents in esophagus causing obstruction of respiration
   T18.118   **Gastric contents in esophagus causing other injury**
   7th

  T18.12   **Food in esophagus**
  6th
   Bones in esophagus
   Seeds in esophagus
   T18.120   **Food in esophagus causing compression of trachea**
   7th
   T18.128   **Food in esophagus causing other injury**
   7th

  T18.19   **Other foreign object in esophagus**
  6th
   T18.190   **Other foreign object in esophagus causing compression of trachea**
   7th
    Other FB in esophagus causing obstruction of respiration
   T18.198   **Other foreign object in esophagus causing other injury**
   7th

T18.2XX   **FB in stomach**
7th

T18.3XX   **FB in small intestine**
7th

T18.4XX   **FB in colon**
7th

T18.5XX   **FB in anus and rectum**
7th
  FB in rectosigmoid (junction)

T18.8XX   **FB in other parts of alimentary tract**
7th

T18.9XX   **FB of alimentary tract, part unspecified**
7th
  FB in digestive system NOS
  Swallowed FB NOS

> 7th characters for category T18
> A—initial encounter
> D—subsequent encounter
> S—sequela

T19   **FB IN GENITOURINARY TRACT**
4th
Excludes2: complications due to implanted mesh (T83.7-)
  mechanical complications of contraceptive device (intrauterine) (vaginal) (T83.3-)
  presence of contraceptive device (intrauterine) (vaginal) (Z97.5)

> 7th characters for category T19
> A—initial encounter
> D—subsequent encounter
> S—sequela

T19.0XX   **FB in urethra**
7th

T19.2XX   **FB in vulva and vagina**
7th

T19.4XX   **FB in penis**
7th

T19.8XX   **FB in other parts of genitourinary tract**
7th

T19.9XX   **FB in genitourinary tract, part unspecified**
7th

4th   **5th**   **6th**   **7th**   Additional Character Required   ✓ 3-character code   Unspecified laterality codes were excluded here.

• =New Code
▲ =Revised Code
▫ =Social determinants of health

Excludes1—Not coded here, do not use together
Excludes2—Not included here

CHAPTER 19. INJURY, POISONING AND CERTAIN OTHER CONSEQUENCES OF EXTERNAL CAUSES   **(T20–T20.15X)**

(T20–T32) BURNS AND CORROSIONS

GUIDELINES

The *ICD-10-CM* makes a distinction between burns and corrosions. The burn codes are for thermal burns, except sunburns, that come from a heat source, such as a fire or hot appliance. The burn codes are also for burns resulting from electricity and radiation. Corrosions are burns due to chemicals. The guidelines are the same for burns and corrosions.

Current burns (T20–T25) are classified by depth, extent and by agent (X code). Burns are classified by depth as first degree (erythema), second degree (blistering), and third degree (full-thickness involvement). Burns of the eye and internal organs (T26–T28) are classified by site, but not by degree.

Sequencing of burn and related condition codes

Sequence first the code that reflects the highest degree of burn when more than one burn is present.

When the reason for the admission or encounter is for treatment of external multiple burns, sequence first the code that reflects the burn of the highest degree.

When a patient has both internal and external burns, the circumstances of admission govern the selection of the principal diagnosis or first-listed diagnosis.

When a patient is admitted for burn injuries and other related conditions such as smoke inhalation and/or respiratory failure, the circumstances of admission govern the selection of the principal or first-listed diagnosis.

Burns of the same anatomical site

Classify burns of the same anatomic site and on the same side but of different degrees to the subcategory identifying the highest degree recorded in the diagnosis (e.g., for second and third degree burns of right thigh, assign only code T24.311-).

Non-healing burns

Non-healing burns are coded as acute burns.
Necrosis of burned skin should be coded as a non-healed burn.

Infected burn

For any documented infected burn site, use an additional code for the infection.

Assign separate codes for each burn site

When coding burns, assign separate codes for each burn site. Category T30, Burn and corrosion, body region unspecified is extremely vague and should rarely be used.

Codes for burns of "multiple sites" should only be assigned when the medical record documentation does not specify the individual sites.

Burns and corrosions classified according to extent of body surface involved

Refer to category T31 for guidelines.

Encounters for treatment of sequela of burns

Encounters for the treatment of the late effects of burns or corrosions (ie, scars or joint contractures) should be coded with a burn or corrosion code with the 7th character S for sequela.

Sequela with a late effect code and current burn

When appropriate, both a code for a current burn or corrosion with 7th character A or D and a burn or corrosion code with 7th character S may be assigned on the same record (when both a current burn and sequela of an old burn exist). Burns and corrosions do not heal at the same rate and a current healing wound may still exist with sequela of a healed burn or corrosion.

Use of an external cause code with burns and corrosions

An external cause code should be used with burns and corrosions to identify the source and intent of the burn, as well as the place where it occurred.

Includes: burns (thermal) from electrical heating appliances
   burns (thermal) from electricity
   burns (thermal) from flame
   burns (thermal) from friction
   burns (thermal) from hot air and hot gases
   burns (thermal) from hot objects
   burns (thermal) from lightning
   burns (thermal) from radiation
   chemical burn [corrosion] (external) (internal)
   scalds
Excludes2: erythema [dermatitis] ab igne (L59.0)
   radiation-related disorders of the skin and subcutaneous tissue (L55–L59)
   sunburn (L55.-)

(T20–T25) BURNS AND CORROSIONS OF EXTERNAL BODY SURFACE, SPECIFIED BY SITE

Includes: burns and corrosions of first degree [erythema]
   burns and corrosions of second degree [blisters] [epidermal loss]
   burns and corrosions of third degree [deep necrosis of underlying tissue] [full-thickness skin loss]

Use additional code from category T31 or T32 to identify extent of body surface involved

> **7th characters for categories T20–T25**
> A—initial encounter
> D—subsequent encounter
> S—sequela

T20   **BURN AND CORROSION OF HEAD, FACE, AND NECK**
`4th`
   Excludes2: burn and corrosion of ear drum (T28.41, T28.91)
      burn and corrosion of eye and adnexa (T26.-)
      burn and corrosion of mouth and pharynx (T28.0)

T20.0   **Burn of unspecified degree of head, face, and neck**
`5th`   **Use additional external cause code** to identify the source, place and intent of the burn (X00–X19, X75–X77, X96–X98, Y92)

T20.00X   **Burn of unspecified degree of head, face, and neck, unspecified site**
`7th`

T20.01   **Burn of unspecified degree of ear [any part, except ear drum]**
`6th`   *Excludes2:* burn of ear drum (T28.41-)

   T20.011   **Burn of unspecified degree of right ear [any part, except ear drum]**
   `7th`

   T20.012   **Burn of unspecified degree of left ear [any part, except ear drum]**
   `7th`

T20.02X   **Burn of unspecified degree of lip(s)**
`7th`

T20.03X   **Burn of unspecified degree of chin**
`7th`

T20.04X   **Burn of unspecified degree of nose (septum)**
`7th`

T20.05X   **Burn of unspecified degree of scalp [any part]**
`7th`

T20.06X   **Burn of unspecified degree of forehead and cheek**
`7th`

T20.07X   **Burn of unspecified degree of neck, initial encounter**
`7th`

T20.09X   **Burn of unspecified degree of multiple sites of head, face, and neck**
`7th`

T20.1   **Burn of first degree of head, face, and neck**
`5th`   **Use additional external cause code** to identify the source, place and intent of the burn (X00–X19, X75–X77, X96–X98, Y92)

T20.10X   **Burn of first degree of head, face, and neck, unspecified site**
`7th`

T20.11   **Burn of first degree of ear [any part, except ear drum]**
`6th`   *Excludes2:* burn of ear drum (T28.41-)

   T20.111   **Burn of first degree of right ear [any part, except ear drum]**
   `7th`

   T20.112   **Burn of first degree of left ear [any part, except ear drum]**
   `7th`

   T20.119   **Burn of first degree of unspecified ear [any part, except ear drum]**
   `7th`

T20.12X   **Burn of first degree of lip(s)**
`7th`

T20.13X   **Burn of first degree of chin**
`7th`

T20.14X   **Burn of first degree of nose (septum)**
`7th`

T20.15X   **Burn of first degree of scalp [any part]**
`7th`

`4th` `5th` `6th` `7th`   Additional Character Required   ✔   3-character code   Unspecified laterality codes were excluded here.

• =New Code
▲ =Revised Code
▣ =Social determinants of health

Excludes1—Not coded here, do not use together
Excludes2—Not included here

T20.16X `7th` Burn of first degree of forehead and cheek

T20.17X `7th` Burn of first degree of neck

T20.19X `7th` Burn of first degree of multiple sites of head, face, and neck

T20.2 `5th` Burn of second degree of head, face, and neck
Use additional external cause code to identify the source, place and intent of the burn (X00–X19, X75–X77, X96–X98, Y92)

T20.20X `7th` Burn of second degree of head, face, and neck, unspecified site

T20.21 `6th` Burn of second degree of ear [any part, except ear drum]
Excludes2: burn of ear drum (T28.41-)

> 7th characters for categories T20–T25
> A—initial encounter
> D—subsequent encounter
> S—sequela

T20.211 `7th` Burn of second degree of right ear [any part, except ear drum]

T20.212 `7th` Burn of second degree of left ear [any part, except ear drum]

T20.219 `7th` Burn of second degree of unspecified ear [any part, except ear drum]

T20.22X `7th` Burn of second degree of lip(s)

T20.23X `7th` Burn of second degree of chin

T20.24X `7th` Burn of second degree of nose (septum)

T20.25X `7th` Burn of second degree of scalp [any part]

T20.26X `7th` Burn of second degree of forehead and cheek

T20.27X `7th` Burn of second degree of neck

T20.29X `7th` Burn of second degree of multiple sites of head, face, and neck

T20.3 `5th` Burn of third degree of head, face, and neck
Use additional external cause code to identify the source, place and intent of the burn (X00–X19, X75–X77, X96–X98, Y92)

T20.30X `7th` Burn of third degree of head, face, and neck, unspecified site

T20.31 `6th` Burn of third degree of ear [any part, except ear drum]
Excludes2: burn of ear drum (T28.41-)

T20.311 `7th` Burn of third degree of right ear [any part, except ear drum]

T20.312 `7th` Burn of third degree of left ear [any part, except ear drum]

T20.319 `7th` Burn of third degree of unspecified ear [any part, except ear drum]

T20.32X `7th` Burn of third degree of lip(s)

T20.33X `7th` Burn of third degree of chin

T20.34X `7th` Burn of third degree of nose (septum)

T20.35X `7th` Burn of third degree of scalp [any part]

T20.36X `7th` Burn of third degree of forehead and cheek

T20.37X `7th` Burn of third degree of neck

T20.39X `7th` Burn of third degree of multiple sites of head, face, and neck

T21 `4th` **BURN AND CORROSION OF TRUNK**
Includes: burns and corrosion of hip region
Excludes2: burns and corrosion of axilla (T22.- with fifth character 4)
burns and corrosion of scapular region (T22.- with fifth character 6)
burns and corrosion of shoulder (T22.- with fifth character 5)

T21.0 Burn of unspecified degree of trunk
`5th` Use additional external cause code to identify the source, place and intent of the burn (X00–X19, X75–X77, X96–X98, Y92)

T21.00X `7th` Burn of unspecified degree of trunk, unspecified site

T21.01X `7th` Burn of unspecified degree of chest wall
Burn of unspecified degree of breast

T21.02X `7th` Burn of unspecified degree of abdominal wall
Burn of unspecified degree of flank or of groin

T21.03X `7th` Burn of unspecified degree of upper back
Burn of unspecified degree of interscapular region

T21.04X `7th` Burn of unspecified degree of lower back

T21.05X `7th` Burn of unspecified degree of buttock
Burn of unspecified degree of anus

T21.06X `7th` Burn of unspecified degree of male genital region
Burn of unspecified degree of penis or of scrotum or of testis

T21.07X `7th` Burn of unspecified degree of female genital region
Burn of unspecified degree of labium (majus) (minus) or of perineum
Burn of unspecified degree of vulva
Excludes2: burn of vagina (T28.3)

T21.09X `7th` Burn of unspecified degree of other site of trunk

T21.1 `5th` Burn of first degree of trunk
Use additional external cause code to identify the source, place and intent of the burn (X00–X19, X75–X77, X96–X98, Y92)

T21.10X `7th` Burn of first degree of trunk, unspecified site

T21.11X `7th` Burn of first degree of chest wall
Burn of first degree of breast

T21.12X `7th` Burn of first degree of abdominal wall
Burn of first degree of flank OR OF GROIN

T21.13X `7th` Burn of first degree of upper back
Burn of first degree of interscapular region

T21.14X `7th` Burn of first degree of lower back

T21.15X `7th` Burn of first degree of buttock
Burn of first degree of anus

T21.16X `7th` Burn of first degree of male genital region
Burn of first degree of penis or of scrotum or of testis

T21.17X `7th` Burn of first degree of female genital region
Burn of first degree of labium (majus) (minus) or of perineum
Burn of first degree of vulva
Excludes2: burn of vagina (T28.3)

T21.19X `7th` Burn of first degree of other site of trunk

T21.2 `5th` Burn of second degree of trunk
Use additional external cause code to identify the source, place and intent of the burn (X00–X19, X75–X77, X96–X98, Y92)

T21.20X `7th` Burn of second degree of trunk, unspecified site

T21.21X `7th` Burn of second degree of chest wall
Burn of second degree of breast

T21.22X `7th` Burn of second degree of abdominal wall
Burn of second degree of flank or of groin

T21.23X `7th` Burn of second degree of upper back
Burn of second degree of interscapular region

T21.24X `7th` Burn of second degree of lower back

T21.25X `7th` Burn of second degree of buttock
Burn of second degree of anus

T21.26X `7th` Burn of second degree of male genital region
Burn of second degree of penis or of scrotum or of testis

T21.27X `7th` Burn of second degree of female genital region
Burn of second degree of labium (majus) (minus) or of perineum
Burn of second degree of vulva
Excludes2: burn of vagina (T28.3)

T21.29X `7th` Burn of second degree of other site of trunk

T21.3 `5th` Burn of third degree of trunk
Use additional external cause code to identify the source, place and intent of the burn (X00–X19, X75–X77, X96–X98, Y92)

CHAPTER 19. INJURY, POISONING AND CERTAIN OTHER CONSEQUENCES OF EXTERNAL CAUSES   (T20.16X–T21.3)

`4th` `5th` `6th` `7th` Additional Character Required   ✔ 3-character code   Unspecified laterality codes were excluded here.   • =New Code   ▲ =Revised Code   ▣ =Social determinants of health   *Excludes1*—Not coded here, do not use together   *Excludes2*—Not included here

T21.30X Burn of third degree of trunk, unspecified site
`7th`

T21.31X Burn of third degree of chest wall
`7th`   Burn of third degree of breast

T21.32X Burn of third degree of abdominal wall
`7th`   Burn of third degree of flank OR GROIN

T21.33X Burn of third degree of upper back
`7th`   Burn of third degree of interscapular region

T21.34X Burn of third degree of lower back
`7th`

T21.35X Burn of third degree of buttock
`7th`   Burn of third degree of anus

T21.36X Burn of third degree of male genital region
`7th`   Burn of third degree of penis or of scrotum or of testis

T21.37X Burn of third degree of female genital region
`7th`   Burn of third degree of labium (majus) (minus)
    Burn of third degree of perineum
    Burn of third degree of vulva
    Excludes2: burn of vagina (T28.3)

T21.39X Burn of third degree of other site of trunk
`7th`

T22 BURN AND CORROSION OF SHOULDER AND UPPER
`4th` LIMB, EXCEPT WRIST AND HAND
    Excludes2: burn and corrosion of interscapular region (T21.-)
    burn and corrosion of wrist and hand (T23.-)

T22.0 Burn of unspecified degree of shoulder and upper limb, except
`5th` wrist and hand
    Use additional external cause code to identify the source, place
    and intent of the burn (X00–X19, X75–X77, X96–X98, Y92)

   T22.00X Burn of unspecified degree of shoulder and upper
   `7th` limb, except wrist and hand, unspecified site

   T22.01 Burn of unspecified
   `6th` degree of forearm
       T22.011 Burn of
       `7th` unspecified
       degree of
       right forearm
       T22.012 Burn of
       `7th` unspecified degree of left forearm

> 7th characters for categories
> T20–T25
> A—initial encounter
> D—subsequent encounter
> S—sequela

   T22.02 Burn of unspecified degree of elbow
   `6th`   **T22.021** Burn of unspecified degree of right elbow
       `7th`
       T22.022 Burn of unspecified degree of left elbow
       `7th`

   T22.03 Burn of unspecified degree of upper arm
   `6th`   **T22.031** Burn of unspecified degree of right upper
       `7th` arm
       T22.032 Burn of unspecified degree of left upper
       `7th` arm

   T22.04 Burn of unspecified degree of axilla
   `6th`   **T22.041** Burn of unspecified degree of right axilla
       `7th`
       T22.042 Burn of unspecified degree of left axilla
       `7th`

   T22.05 Burn of unspecified degree of shoulder
   `6th`   **T22.051** Burn of unspecified degree of right
       `7th` shoulder
       T22.052 Burn of unspecified degree of left shoulder
       `7th`

   T22.06 Burn of unspecified degree of scapular region
   `6th`   **T22.061** Burn of unspecified degree of right
       `7th` scapular region
       T22.062 Burn of unspecified degree of left scapular
       `7th` region

   T22.09 Burn of unspecified degree of multiple sites of
   `6th` shoulder and upper limb, except wrist and hand
       T22.091 Burn of unspecified degree of multiple
       `7th` sites of right shoulder and upper limb,
       except wrist and hand
       T22.092 Burn of unspecified degree of multiple
       `7th` sites of left shoulder and upper limb,
       except wrist and hand

T22.1 Burn of first degree of shoulder and upper limb, except wrist
`5th` and hand
    Use additional external cause code to identify the source, place
    and intent of the burn (X00–X19, X75–X77, X96–X98, Y92)

   T22.10X Burn of first degree of shoulder and upper limb,
   `7th` except wrist and hand, unspecified site

   T22.11 Burn of first degree of forearm
   `6th`   **T22.111** Burn of first degree of right forearm
       `7th`
       T22.112 Burn of first degree of left forearm
       `7th`

   T22.12 Burn of first degree of elbow
   `6th`   **T22.121** Burn of first degree of right elbow
       `7th`
       T22.122 Burn of first degree of left elbow
       `7th`

   T22.13 Burn of first degree of upper arm
   `6th`   **T22.131** Burn of first degree of right upper arm
       `7th`
       T22.132 Burn of first degree of left upper arm
       `7th`

   T22.14 Burn of first degree of axilla
   `6th`   **T22.141** Burn of first degree of right axilla
       `7th`
       T22.142 Burn of first degree of left axilla
       `7th`

   T22.15 Burn of first degree of shoulder
   `6th`   **T22.151** Burn of first degree of right shoulder
       `7th`
       T22.152 Burn of first degree of left shoulder
       `7th`

   T22.16 Burn of first degree of scapular region
   `6th`   **T22.161** Burn of first degree of right scapular
       `7th` region
       T22.162 Burn of first degree of left scapular region
       `7th`

   T22.19 Burn of first degree of multiple sites of shoulder and
   `6th` upper limb, except wrist and hand
       T22.191 Burn of first degree of multiple sites of
       `7th` right shoulder and upper limb, except
       wrist and hand
       T22.192 Burn of first degree of multiple sites of left
       `7th` shoulder and upper limb, except wrist and
       hand
       T22.199 Burn of first degree of multiple sites of
       `7th` unspecified shoulder and upper limb,
       except wrist and hand

T22.2 Burn of second degree of shoulder and upper limb, except
`5th` wrist and hand
    Use additional external cause code to identify the source, place
    and intent of the burn (X00–X19, X75–X77,X96–X98, Y92)

   T22.20X Burn of second degree of shoulder and upper limb,
   `7th` except wrist and hand, unspecified site

   T22.21 Burn of second degree of forearm
   `6th`   **T22.211** Burn of second degree of right forearm
       `7th`
       T22.212 Burn of second degree of left forearm
       `7th`
       T22.219 Burn of second degree of unspecified
       `7th` forearm

   T22.22 Burn of second degree of elbow
   `6th`   **T22.221** Burn of second degree of right elbow
       `7th`
       T22.222 Burn of second degree of left elbow
       `7th`

   T22.23 Burn of second degree of upper arm
   `6th`   **T22.231** Burn of second degree of right upper arm
       `7th`
       T22.232 Burn of second degree of left upper arm
       `7th`

   T22.24 Burn of second degree of axilla
   `6th`   **T22.241** Burn of second degree of right axilla
       `7th`

`4th` `5th` `6th` `7th`   Additional Character Required   ✔   3-character code   Unspecified laterality codes were excluded here.   • =New Code   ▲ =Revised Code   ¤ =Social determinants of health   *Excludes1*—Not coded here, do not use together   *Excludes2*—Not included here

T22.242   Burn of second degree of left axilla
7th

T22.25   Burn of second degree of shoulder
6th

    T22.251   Burn of second degree of right shoulder
    7th

    T22.252   Burn of second degree of left shoulder
    7th

T22.26   Burn of second degree of scapular region
6th

    T22.261   Burn of second degree of right scapular
    7th   region

    T22.262   Burn of second degree of left scapular
    7th   region

T22.29   Burn of second degree of multiple sites of shoulder
6th   and upper limb, except wrist and hand

    T22.291   Burn of second degree of multiple sites
    7th   of right shoulder and upper limb, except
                wrist and hand

    T22.292   Burn of second degree of multiple sites of
    7th   left shoulder and upper limb, except wrist
                and hand

T22.3   Burn of third degree of shoulder and upper limb, except wrist
5th   **and hand**

    Use additional external cause code to identify the source, place
       and intent of the burn (X00–X19, X75–X77, X96–X98, Y92)

T22.31   Burn of third degree of forearm
6th

    T22.311   Burn of third degree of right forearm
    7th

    T22.312   Burn of third degree of left forearm
    7th

    T22.319   Burn of third degree of unspecified
    7th   forearm

T22.32   Burn of third degree of elbow
6th

    T22.321   Burn of third
    7th   degree of right elbow

    T22.322   Burn of third degree of left elbow

T22.33   7th   n of third degree of upper arm
6th

    T22.331   Burn of third degree of right upper arm
    7th

    T22.332   Burn of third
    7th   degree of left upper arm

T22.34   Burn of third degree of axilla
6th

    T22.341   Burn of third degree of right axilla
    7th

    T22.342   Burn of third degree of left axilla
    7th

T22.35   Burn of third degree of shoulder
6th

    T22.351   Burn of third degree of right shoulder
    7th

    T22.352   Burn of third degree of left shoulder
    7th

T22.36   Burn of third degree of scapular region
6th

    T22.361   Burn of third degree of right scapular
    7th   region

    T22.362   Burn of third degree of left scapular region

T22.39   Burn of third degree of multiple sites of shoulder and
6th   upper limb, except wrist and hand

    T22.391   Burn of third degree of multiple sites of
    7th   right shoulder and upper limb, except
                wrist and hand

    T22.392   Burn of third degree of multiple sites of
    7th   left shoulder and upper limb, except wrist
                and hand

T23   BURN AND CORROSION OF WRIST AND HAND
4th

T23.0   Burn of unspecified degree of wrist and hand
5th

    Use additional external cause code to identify the source, place
       and intent of the burn (X00–X19, X75–X77, X96–X98, Y92)

T23.00   Burn of unspecified degree of hand, unspecified site
6th

    T23.001   Burn of unspecified degree of right hand,
    7th   unspecified site

    T23.002   Burn of unspecified degree of left hand,
    7th   unspecified site

    T23.009   Burn of unspecified degree of unspecified
    7th   hand, unspecified site

T23.01   Burn of unspecified degree of thumb (nail)
6th

    T23.011   Burn of unspecified degree of right thumb
    7th   (nail)

    T23.012   Burn of unspecified degree of left thumb
    7th   (nail)

T23.02   Burn of unspecified degree of single finger (nail)
6th   except thumb

    T23.021   Burn of unspecified degree of single right
    7th   finger (nail) except thumb

    T23.022   Burn of unspecified degree of single left
    7th   finger (nail) except thumb

T23.03   Burn of unspecified degree of multiple fingers (nail),
6th   not including thumb

    T23.031   Burn of unspecified degree of multiple
    7th   right fingers (nail), not including thumb

    T23.032   Burn of unspecified degree of multiple left
    7th   fingers (nail), not including thumb

T23.04   Burn of unspecified degree of multiple fingers (nail),
6th   including thumb

    T23.041   Burn of unspecified degree of multiple
    7th   right fingers (nail), including thumb

    T23.042   Burn of unspecified degree of multiple left
    7th   fingers (nail), including thumb

T23.05   Burn of unspecified degree of palm
6th

    T23.051   Burn of unspecified degree of right palm
    7th

    T23.052   Burn of unspecified degree of left palm
    7th

T23.06   Burn of unspecified degree of back of hand
6th

    T23.061   Burn of unspecified degree of back of
    7th   right hand

    T23.062   Burn of unspecified degree of back of left
    7th   hand

T23.07   Burn of unspecified degree of wrist
6th

    T23.071   Burn of unspecified degree of right wrist
    7th

    T23.072   Burn of unspecified degree of left wrist
    7th

T23.09   Burn of unspecified degree of multiple sites of wrist
6th   and hand

    T23.091   Burn of unspecified degree of multiple
    7th   sites of right wrist and hand

    T23.092   Burn of unspecified degree of multiple
    7th   sites of left wrist and hand

T23.1   Burn of first degree of wrist and hand
5th

    Use additional external cause code to identify the source, place
       and intent of the burn (X00–X19, X75–X77, X96–X98, Y92)

T23.10   Burn of first degree of hand, unspecified site
6th

    T23.101   Burn of first degree of right hand,
    7th   unspecified site

    T23.102   Burn of first degree of left hand,
    7th   unspecified site

T23.11   Burn of first degree of thumb (nail)
6th

    T23.111   Burn of first degree of right thumb (nail)
    7th

    T23.112   Burn of first degree of left thumb (nail)
    7th

T23.12   Burn of first degree of single finger (nail) except
6th   thumb

    T23.121   Burn of first degree of single right finger
    7th   (nail) except thumb

    T23.122   Burn of first degree of single left finger
    7th   (nail) except thumb

T23.13   Burn of first degree of multiple fingers (nail), not
6th   including thumb

    T23.131   Burn of first degree of multiple right
    7th   fingers (nail), not including thumb

    T23.132   Burn of first degree of multiple left fingers
    7th   (nail), not including thumb

T23.14   Burn of first degree of multiple fingers (nail),
6th   including thumb

4th   5th   6th   7th   Additional Character Required   ✓   3-character code   Unspecified laterality codes were excluded here.

• =New Code
▲ =Revised Code
◘ =Social determinants of health

Excludes1—Not coded here, do not use together
Excludes2—Not included here

T23.141 `7th` **Burn of first degree of multiple right fingers (nail), including thumb**

T23.142 `7th` **Burn of first degree of multiple left fingers (nail), including thumb**

T23.15 `6th` **Burn of first degree of palm**

    T23.151 `7th` **Burn of first degree of right palm**

    T23.152 `7th` **Burn of first degree of left palm**

T23.16 `6th` **Burn of first degree of back of hand**

    T23.161 `7th` **Burn of first degree of back of right hand**

    T23.162 `7th` **Burn of first degree of back of left hand**

T23.17 `6th` **Burn of first degree of wrist**

    T23.171 `7th` **Burn of first degree of right wrist**

    T23.172 `7th` **Burn of first degree of left wrist**

> 7th characters for categories
> T20–T25
> A—initial encounter
> D—subsequent encounter
> S—sequela

T23.19 `6th` **Burn of first degree of multiple sites of wrist and hand**

    T23.191 `7th` **Burn of first degree of multiple sites of right wrist and hand**

    T23.192 `7th` **Burn of first degree of multiple sites of left wrist and hand**

T23.2 `5th` **Burn of second degree of wrist and hand**

Use additional external cause code to identify the source, place and intent of the burn (X00–X19, X75–X77, X96–X98, Y92)

T23.20 `6th` **Burn of second degree of hand, unspecified site**

    T23.201 `7th` **Burn of second degree of right hand, unspecified site**

    T23.202 `7th` **Burn of second degree of left hand, unspecified site**

T23.21 `6th` **Burn of second degree of thumb (nail)**

    T23.211 `7th` **Burn of second degree of right thumb (nail)**

    T23.212 `7th` **Burn of second degree of left thumb (nail)**

T23.22 `6th` **Burn of second degree of single finger (nail) except thumb**

    T23.221 `7th` **Burn of second degree of single right finger (nail) except thumb**

    T23.222 `7th` **Burn of second degree of single left finger (nail) except thumb**

T23.23 `6th` **Burn of second degree of multiple fingers (nail), not including thumb**

    T23.231 `7th` **Burn of second degree of multiple right fingers (nail), not including thumb**

    T23.232 `7th` **Burn of second degree of multiple left fingers (nail), not including thumb**

T23.24 `6th` **Burn of second degree of multiple fingers (nail), including thumb**

    T23.241 `7th` **Burn of second degree of multiple right fingers (nail), including thumb**

    T23.242 `7th` **Burn of second degree of multiple left fingers (nail), including thumb**

T23.25 `6th` **Burn of second degree of palm**

    T23.251 `7th` **Burn of second degree of right palm**

    T23.252 `7th` **Burn of second degree of left palm**

T23.26 `6th` **Burn of second degree of back of hand**

    T23.261 `7th` **Burn of second degree of back of right hand**

    T23.262 `7th` **Burn of second degree of back of left hand**

T23.27 `6th` **Burn of second degree of wrist**

    T23.271 `7th` **Burn of second degree of right wrist**

    T23.272 `7th` **Burn of second degree of left wrist**

T23.29 `6th` **Burn of second degree of multiple sites of wrist and hand**

    T23.291 `7th` **Burn of second degree of multiple sites of right wrist and hand**

    T23.292 `7th` **Burn of second degree of multiple sites of left wrist and hand**

T23.3 `5th` **Burn of third degree of wrist and hand**

Use additional external cause code to identify the source, place and intent of the burn (X00–X19, X75–X77, X96–X98, Y92)

T23.30 `6th` **Burn of third degree of hand, unspecified site**

    T23.301 `7th` **Burn of third degree of right hand, unspecified site**

    T23.302 `7th` **Burn of third degree of left hand, unspecified site**

T23.31 `6th` **Burn of third degree of thumb (nail)**

    T23.311 `7th` **Burn of third degree of right thumb (nail)**

    T23.312 `7th` **Burn of third degree of left thumb (nail)**

T23.32 `6th` **Burn of third degree of single finger (nail) except thumb**

    T23.321 `7th` **Burn of third degree of single right finger (nail) except thumb**

    T23.322 `7th` **Burn of third degree of single left finger (nail) except thumb**

T23.33 `6th` **Burn of third degree of multiple fingers (nail), not including thumb**

    T23.331 `7th` **Burn of third degree of multiple right fingers (nail), not including thumb**

    T23.332 `7th` **Burn of third degree of multiple left fingers (nail), not including thumb**

T23.34 `6th` **Burn of third degree of multiple fingers (nail), including thumb**

    T23.341 `7th` **Burn of third degree of multiple right fingers (nail), including thumb**

    T23.342 `7th` **Burn of third degree of multiple left fingers (nail), including thumb**

T23.35 `6th` **Burn of third degree of palm**

    T23.351 `7th` **Burn of third degree of right palm**

    T23.352 `7th` **Burn of third degree of left palm**

T23.36 `6th` **Burn of third degree of back of hand**

    T23.361 `7th` **Burn of third degree of back of right hand**

    T23.362 `7th` **Burn of third degree of back of left hand**

T23.37 `6th` **Burn of third degree of wrist**

    T23.371 `7th` **Burn of third degree of right wrist**

    T23.372 `7th` **Burn of third degree of left wrist**

T23.39 `6th` **Burn of third degree of multiple sites of wrist and hand**

    T23.391 `7th` **Burn of third degree of multiple sites of right wrist and hand**

    T23.392 `7th` **Burn of third degree of multiple sites of left wrist and hand**

T24 `4th` **BURN AND CORROSION OF LOWER LIMB, EXCEPT ANKLE AND FOOT**

Excludes2: burn and corrosion of ankle and foot (T25.-)
burn and corrosion of hip region (T21.-)

T24.0 `5th` **Burn of unspecified degree of lower limb, except ankle and foot**

Use additional external cause code to identify the source, place and intent of the burn (X00–X19, X75–X77, X96–X98, Y92)

T24.00 `6th` **Burn of unspecified degree of unspecified site of lower limb, except ankle and foot**

    T24.001 `7th` **Burn of unspecified degree of unspecified site of right lower limb, except ankle and foot**

`4th` `5th` `6th` `7th` Additional Character Required   ✓   3-character code   Unspecified laterality codes were excluded here.

• =New Code
▲ =Revised Code
⌂ =Social determinants of health

Excludes1—Not coded here, do not use together
Excludes2—Not included here

T24.002 Burn of unspecified degree of unspecified site of left lower limb, except ankle and foot
[7th]

> 7th characters for categories T20–T25
> A—initial encounter
> D—subsequent encounter
> S—sequela

T24.01 Burn of unspecified degree of thigh
[6th]
    T24.011 Burn of unspecified degree of right thigh
    [7th]
    T24.012 Burn of unspecified degree of left thigh
    [7th]

T24.02 Burn of unspecified degree of knee
[6th]
    T24.021 Burn of unspecified degree of right knee
    [7th]
    T24.022 Burn of unspecified degree of left knee
    [7th]

T24.03 Burn of unspecified degree of lower leg
[6th]
    T24.031 Burn of unspecified degree of right lower leg
    [7th]
    T24.032 Burn of unspecified degree of left lower leg
    [7th]

T24.09 Burn of unspecified degree of multiple sites of lower limb, except ankle and foot
[6th]
    T24.091 Burn of unspecified degree of multiple sites of right lower limb, except ankle and foot
    [7th]
    T24.092 Burn of unspecified degree of multiple sites of left lower limb, except ankle and foot
    [7th]

T24.1 Burn of first degree of lower limb, except ankle and foot
[5th]
  Use additional external cause code to identify the source, place and intent of the burn (X00–X19, X75–X77, X96–X98, Y92)

T24.10 Burn of first degree of unspecified site of lower limb, except ankle and foot
[6th]
    T24.101 Burn of first degree of unspecified site of right lower limb, except ankle and foot
    [7th]
    T24.102 Burn of first degree of unspecified site of left lower limb, except ankle and foot
    [7th]

T24.11 Burn of first degree of thigh
[6th]
    T24.111 Burn of first degree of right thigh
    [7th]
    T24.112 Burn of first degree of left thigh
    [7th]

T24.12 Burn of first degree of knee
[6th]
    T24.121 Burn of first degree of right knee
    [7th]
    T24.122 Burn of first degree of left knee
    [7th]

T24.13 Burn of first degree of lower leg
[6th]
    T24.131 Burn of first degree of right lower leg
    [7th]
    T24.132 Burn of first degree of left lower leg
    [7th]

T24.19 Burn of first degree of multiple sites of lower limb, except ankle and foot
[6th]
    T24.191 Burn of first degree of multiple sites of right lower limb, except ankle and foot
    [7th]
    T24.192 Burn of first degree of multiple sites of left lower limb, except ankle and foot
    [7th]

T24.2 Burn of second degree of lower limb, except ankle and foot
[5th]
  Use additional external cause code to identify the source, place and intent of the burn (X00–X19, X75–X77, X96–X98, Y92)

T24.20 Burn of second degree of unspecified site of lower limb, except ankle and foot
[6th]
    T24.201 Burn of second degree of unspecified site of right lower limb, except ankle and foot
    [7th]
    T24.202 Burn of second degree of unspecified site of left lower limb, except ankle and foot
    [7th]

T24.21 Burn of second degree of thigh
[6th]
    T24.211 Burn of second degree of right thigh
    [7th]
    T24.212 Burn of second degree of left thigh
    [7th]

T24.22 Burn of second degree of knee
[6th]
    T24.221 Burn of second degree of right knee
    [7th]
    T24.222 Burn of second degree of left knee
    [7th]

T24.23 Burn of second degree of lower leg
[6th]
    T24.231 Burn of second degree of right lower leg
    [7th]
    T24.232 Burn of second degree of left lower leg
    [7th]

T24.29 Burn of second degree of multiple sites of lower limb, except ankle and foot
[6th]
    T24.291 Burn of second degree of multiple sites of right lower limb, except ankle and foot
    [7th]
    T24.292 Burn of second degree of multiple sites of left lower limb, except ankle and foot
    [7th]

T24.3 Burn of third degree of lower limb, except ankle and foot
[5th]
  Use additional external cause code to identify the source, place and intent of the burn (X00–X19, X75–X77, X96–X98, Y92)

T24.30 Burn of third degree of unspecified site of lower limb, except ankle and foot
[6th]
    T24.301 Burn of third degree of unspecified site of right lower limb, except ankle and foot
    [7th]
    T24.302 Burn of third degree of unspecified site of left lower limb, except ankle and foot
    [7th]

T24.31 Burn of third degree of thigh
[6th]
    T24.311 Burn of third degree of right thigh
    [7th]
    T24.312 Burn of third degree of left thigh
    [7th]

T24.32 Burn of third degree of knee
[6th]
    T24.321 Burn of third degree of right knee
    [7th]
    T24.322 Burn of third degree of left knee
    [7th]

T24.33 Burn of third degree of lower leg
[6th]
    T24.331 Burn of third degree of right lower leg
    [7th]
    T24.332 Burn of third degree of left lower leg
    [7th]

T24.39 Burn of third degree of multiple sites of lower limb, except ankle and foot
[6th]
    T24.391 Burn of third degree of multiple sites of right lower limb, except ankle and foot
    [7th]
    T24.392 Burn of third degree of multiple sites of left lower limb, except ankle and foot
    [7th]

T25 BURN AND CORROSION OF ANKLE AND FOOT
[4th]

T25.0 Burn of unspecified degree of ankle and foot
[5th]
  Use additional external cause code to identify the source, place and intent of the burn (X00–X19, X75–X77, X96–X98, Y92)

T25.01 Burn of unspecified degree of ankle
[6th]
    T25.011 Burn of unspecified degree of right ankle
    [7th]
    T25.012 Burn of unspecified degree of left ankle
    [7th]

T25.02 Burn of unspecified degree of foot
[6th]
  Excludes2: burn of unspecified degree of toe(s) (nail) (T25.03-)
    T25.021 Burn of unspecified degree of right foot
    [7th]
    T25.022 Burn of unspecified degree of left foot
    [7th]

T25.03 Burn of unspecified degree of toe(s) (nail)
[6th]
    T25.031 Burn of unspecified degree of right toe(s) (nail)
    [7th]
    T25.032 Burn of unspecified degree of left toe(s) (nail)
    [7th]

T25.09 Burn of unspecified degree of multiple sites of ankle and foot
[6th]
    T25.091 Burn of unspecified degree of multiple sites of right ankle and foot
    [7th]
    T25.092 Burn of unspecified degree of multiple sites of left ankle and foot
    [7th]

[4th] [5th] [6th] [7th] Additional Character Required   ✔ 3-character code   Unspecified laterality codes were excluded here.   • =New Code   ▲ =Revised Code   ⌂ =Social determinants of health   *Excludes1*—Not coded here, do not use together   *Excludes2*—Not included here

T25.1 **Burn of first degree of ankle and foot**
5th **Use additional external cause code** to identify the source, place and intent of the burn (X00–X19, X75–X77, X96–X98, Y92)

    T25.11 **Burn of first degree of ankle**
    6th
        T25.111 **Burn of first degree of right ankle**
        7th
        T25.112 **Burn of first degree of left ankle**
        7th

    T25.12 **Burn of first degree of foot**
    6th
    Excludes2: burn of first degree of toe(s) (nail) (T25.13-)
        T25.121 **Burn of first degree of right foot**
        7th
        T25.122 **Burn of first degree of left foot**
        7th

    T25.13 **Burn of first degree of toe(s) (nail)**
    6th
        T25.131 **Burn of first degree of right toe(s) (nail)**
        7th
        T25.132 **Burn of first degree of left toe(s) (nail)**
        7th

    T25.19 **Burn of first degree of multiple sites of ankle and foot**
    6th
        T25.191 **Burn of first degree of multiple sites of right ankle and foot**
        7th
        T25.192 **Burn of first degree of multiple sites of left ankle and foot**
        7th

T25.2 **Burn of second degree of ankle and foot**
5th **Use additional external cause code** to identify the source, place and intent of the burn (X00–X19, X75–X77, X96–X98, Y92)

    T25.21 **Burn of second degree of ankle**
    6th
        T25.211 **Burn of second degree of right ankle**
        7th
        T25.212 **Burn of second degree of left ankle**
        7th

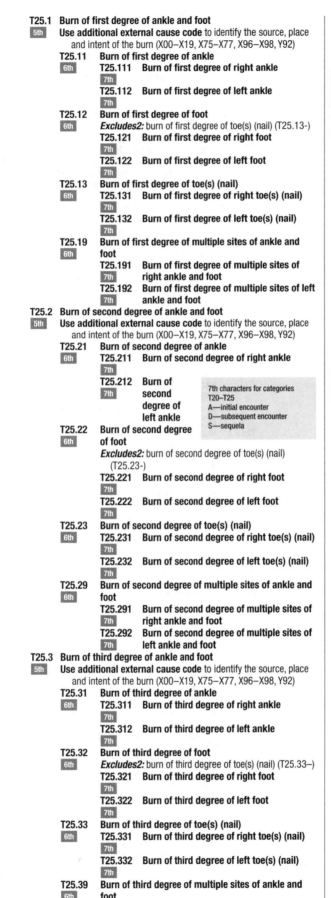

7th characters for categories T20–T25
A—initial encounter
D—subsequent encounter
S—sequela

    T25.22 **Burn of second degree of foot**
    6th
    Excludes2: burn of second degree of toe(s) (nail) (T25.23-)
        T25.221 **Burn of second degree of right foot**
        7th
        T25.222 **Burn of second degree of left foot**
        7th

    T25.23 **Burn of second degree of toe(s) (nail)**
    6th
        T25.231 **Burn of second degree of right toe(s) (nail)**
        7th
        T25.232 **Burn of second degree of left toe(s) (nail)**
        7th

    T25.29 **Burn of second degree of multiple sites of ankle and foot**
    6th
        T25.291 **Burn of second degree of multiple sites of right ankle and foot**
        7th
        T25.292 **Burn of second degree of multiple sites of left ankle and foot**
        7th

T25.3 **Burn of third degree of ankle and foot**
5th **Use additional external cause code** to identify the source, place and intent of the burn (X00–X19, X75–X77, X96–X98, Y92)

    T25.31 **Burn of third degree of ankle**
    6th
        T25.311 **Burn of third degree of right ankle**
        7th
        T25.312 **Burn of third degree of left ankle**
        7th

    T25.32 **Burn of third degree of foot**
    6th
    Excludes2: burn of third degree of toe(s) (nail) (T25.33–)
        T25.321 **Burn of third degree of right foot**
        7th
        T25.322 **Burn of third degree of left foot**
        7th

    T25.33 **Burn of third degree of toe(s) (nail)**
    6th
        T25.331 **Burn of third degree of right toe(s) (nail)**
        7th
        T25.332 **Burn of third degree of left toe(s) (nail)**
        7th

    T25.39 **Burn of third degree of multiple sites of ankle and foot**
    6th

        T25.391 **Burn of third degree of multiple sites of right ankle and foot**
        7th
        T25.392 **Burn of third degree of multiple sites of left ankle and foot**
        7th

(T26–T28) BURNS AND CORROSIONS CONFINED TO EYE AND INTERNAL ORGANS

T26 **BURN AND CORROSION CONFINED TO EYE AND ADNEXA**
4th
    T26.0 **Burn of eyelid and periocular area**
    6th
    Use additional external cause code to identify the source, place and intent of the burn (X00–X19, X75–X77, X96–X98, Y92)

7th characters for categories T26–T28
A—initial encounter
D—subsequent encounter
S—sequela

        T26.01X **Burn of right eyelid and periocular area**
        7th
        T26.02X **Burn of left eyelid and periocular area**
        7th

T28 **BURN AND CORROSION OF OTHER INTERNAL ORGANS**
4th
Use additional external cause code to identify the source and intent of the burn (X00–X19, X75–X77, X96–X98) and external cause code to identify place (Y92)

    T28.0XX **Burn of mouth and pharynx**
    7th
    T28.1XX **Burn of esophagus**
    7th

(T30–T32) BURNS AND CORROSIONS OF MULTIPLE AND UNSPECIFIED BODY REGIONS

T30 **BURN AND CORROSION, BODY REGION UNSPECIFIED**
4th
    T30.0 **Burn of unspecified body region, unspecified degree**
    This code is not for inpatient use. Code to specified site and degree of burns
    Burn NOS
    Multiple burns NOS

Note: No 7th characters are required for categories T30, T31, and T32.

    T30.4 **Corrosion of unspecified body region, unspecified degree**
    This code is not for inpatient use. Code to specified site and degree of corrosion
    Corrosion NOS
    Multiple corrosion NOS

T31 **BURNS CLASSIFIED ACCORDING TO EXTENT OF BODY SURFACE INVOLVED**
4th
Note: This category is to be used as the primary code only when the site of the burn is unspecified. It should be used as a supplementary code with categories T20–T25 when the site is specified.

Please see full *ICD-10-CM* manual if reporting burns classified according to extent of body surface beyond 10% of body surface.

GUIDELINES

Assign codes from category T31, Burns classified according to extent of body surface involved, or T32, Corrosions classified according to extent of body surface involved, **for acute burns or corrosions** when the site of the burn **or corrosion** is not specified or when there is a need for additional data. It is advisable to use category T31 as additional coding when needed to provide data for evaluating burn mortality, such as that needed by burn units. It is also advisable to use category T31 as an additional code for reporting purposes when there is mention of a third-degree burn involving 20 percent or more of the body surface. **Codes from categories T31 and T32 should not be used for sequelae of burns or corrosions.**

Categories T31 and T32 are based on the classic "rule of nines" in estimating body surface involved: head and neck are assigned nine percent, each arm nine percent, each leg 18 percent, the anterior trunk 18 percent, posterior trunk 18 percent, and genitalia one percent. Providers may change these percentage assignments where necessary to accommodate infants and children who have proportionately larger heads than adults, and patients who have large buttocks, thighs, or abdomen that involve burns.

4th 5th 6th 7th Additional Character Required ✔ 3-character code

Unspecified laterality codes were excluded here.

• =New Code
▲ =Revised Code
⌂ =Social determinants of health

Excludes1—Not coded here, do not use together
Excludes2—Not included here

T31.0   **Burns involving less than 10% of body surface**
T31.1   **Burns involving 10–19% of body surface**
  5th   **T31.10**   **Burns involving 10–19% of body surface with 0% to 9% third degree burns**
       Burns involving 10–19% of body surface NOS
       T31.11   **Burns involving 10–19% of body surface with 10–19% third degree burns**

T32   **CORROSIONS CLASSIFIED ACCORDING TO EXTENT OF**
4th   **BODY SURFACE INVOLVED**
     Note: This category is to be used as the primary code only when the site of the corrosion is unspecified. It may be used as a supplementary code with categories T20–T25 when the site is specified.
     T32.0   **Corrosions involving less than 10% of body surface**

(T36–T50) POISONING BY, ADVERSE EFFECTS OF AND UNDERDOSING OF DRUGS, MEDICAMENTS AND BIOLOGICAL SUBSTANCES

GUIDELINES

Codes in categories T36–T65 are combination codes that include the substance that was taken as well as the intent. No additional external cause code is required for poisonings, toxic effects, adverse effects and underdosing codes.

Do not code directly from the Table of Drugs

Do not code directly from the Table of Drugs and Chemicals. Always refer back to the Tabular List. *Refer to the ICD-10-CM manual for the Table of Drugs.*

Use as many codes as necessary to describe

Use as many codes as necessary to describe completely all drugs, medicinal or biological substances.

If the same code would describe the causative agent

If the same code would describe the causative agent for more than one adverse reaction, poisoning, toxic effect or underdosing, assign the code only once.

If two or more drugs, medicinal or biological substances

If two or more drugs, medicinal or biological substances are taken, code each individually unless a combination code is listed in the Table of Drugs and Chemicals. If multiple unspecified drugs, medicinal or biological substances were taken, assign the appropriate code from subcategory T50.91, Poisoning by, adverse effect of and underdosing of multiple unspecified drugs, medicaments and biological substances.

The occurrence of drug toxicity is classified in ICD-10-CM as follows:

ADVERSE EFFECT

When coding an adverse effect of a drug that has been correctly prescribed and properly administered, assign the appropriate code for the nature of the adverse effect followed by the appropriate code for the adverse effect of the drug (T36–T50). The code for the drug should have a 5th or 6th character "5" (for example T36.0X5-). Examples of the nature of an adverse effect are tachycardia, delirium, gastrointestinal hemorrhaging, vomiting, hypokalemia, hepatitis, renal failure, or respiratory failure.

POISONING

When coding a poisoning or reaction to the improper use of a medication (eg, overdose, wrong substance given or taken in error, wrong route of administration), first assign the appropriate code from categories T36–T50. The poisoning codes have an associated intent as their 5th or 6th character (accidental, intentional self-harm, assault and undetermined. **Use additional code(s)** for all manifestations of poisonings.

If there is also a diagnosis of abuse or dependence of the substance, the abuse or dependence is assigned as an additional code.

Examples of poisoning include:

Error was made in drug prescription

Errors made in drug prescription or in the administration of the drug by provider, nurse, patient, or other person.

Overdose of a drug intentionally taken

If an overdose of a drug was intentionally taken or administered and resulted in drug toxicity, it would be coded as a poisoning.

Nonprescribed drug taken with correctly prescribed and properly administered drug

If a nonprescribed drug or medicinal agent was taken in combination with a correctly prescribed and properly administered drug, any drug toxicity or other reaction resulting from the interaction of the two drugs would be classified as a poisoning.

Interaction of drug(s) and alcohol

When a reaction results from the interaction of a drug(s) and alcohol, this would be classified as poisoning.

     See Chapter 4 if poisoning is the result of insulin pump malfunctions.

UNDERDOSING

Underdosing refers to taking less of a medication than is prescribed by a provider or a manufacturer's instruction. Discontinuing the use of a prescribed medication on the patient's own initiative (not directed by the patient's provider) is also classified as an underdosing. For underdosing, assign the code from categories T36–T50 (fifth or sixth character "6").

     Codes for underdosing should never be assigned as principal or first-listed codes. If a patient has a relapse or exacerbation of the medical condition for which the drug is prescribed because of the reduction in dose, then the medical condition itself should be coded.

     Noncompliance (Z91.12-, Z91.13- and Z91.14-) or complication of care (Y63.6–Y63.9) codes are to be used with an underdosing code to indicate intent, if known.

Toxic Effects

When a harmful substance is ingested or comes in contact with a person, this is classified as a toxic effect. The toxic effect codes are in categories T51–T65.

     Toxic effect codes have an associated intent: accidental, intentional self-harm, assault and undetermined.

Includes: adverse effect of correct substance properly administered
     poisoning by overdose of substance
     poisoning by wrong substance given or taken in error
     underdosing by (inadvertently) (deliberately) taking less substance than prescribed or instructed
Code first, for adverse effects, the nature of the adverse effect, such as:
     adverse effect NOS (T88.7)
     aspirin gastritis (K29.-)
     blood disorders (D56–D76)
     contact dermatitis (L23–L25)
     dermatitis due to substances taken internally (L27.-)
     nephropathy (N14.0–N14.2)
Note: The drug giving rise to the adverse effect should be identified by use of codes from categories T36–T50 with fifth or sixth character 5.
Use additional code(s) to specify: manifestations of poisoning
     underdosing or failure in dosage during medical and surgical care (Y63.6, Y63.8–Y63.9)
     underdosing of medication regimen (Z91.12-, Z91.13-)
Excludes1: toxic reaction to local anesthesia in pregnancy (O29.3-)
Excludes2: abuse and dependence of psychoactive substances (F10–F19)
     abuse of non-dependence-producing substances (F55.-)
     drug reaction and poisoning affecting newborn (P00–P96)
     immunodeficiency due to drugs (D84.821)
     pathological drug intoxication (inebriation) (F10–F19)

T36   **POISONING BY, ADVERSE EFFECT OF AND**
4th   **UNDERDOSING OF SYSTEMIC ANTIBIOTICS**
     Excludes1: antineoplastic antibiotics (T45.1-)
         locally applied antibiotic NEC (T49.0)
         topically used antibiotic for ear, nose and throat (T49.6)
         topically used antibiotic for eye (T49.5)
     T36.0   **Poisoning by, adverse effect of**
     5th   **and underdosing of penicillins**
         T36.0X   **Poisoning by,**
         6th **7th**   **adverse effect of and underdosing of penicillins**

> **6th characters for categories T36–T50**
> 1—accidental (unintentional), NOS
> 2—intentional (self-harm)
> 3—assault
> 4—undetermined
> 5—adverse effect
> 6—underdosing
>
> **7th characters for categories T36–T50**
> A—initial encounter
> D—subsequent encounter
> S—sequela

4th **5th** **6th** **7th**   Additional Character Required   ✔   3-character code   Unspecified laterality codes were excluded here.

• =New Code
▲ =Revised Code
▫ =Social determinants of health

Excludes1—Not coded here, do not use together
Excludes2—Not included here

T36.1 Poisoning by, adverse effect of and underdosing of cephalosporins and other beta-lactam antibiotics
- [5th]
  T36.1X [6th] [7th] Poisoning by, adverse effect of and underdosing of cephalosporins and other beta-lactam antibiotics

T36.3 Poisoning by, adverse effect of and underdosing of macrolides
- [5th]
  T36.3X [6th] [7th] Poisoning by, adverse effect of and underdosing of macrolides

T36.6 Poisoning by, adverse effect of and underdosing of rifampicins
- [5th]
  T36.6X [6th] [7th] Poisoning by, adverse effect of and underdosing of rifampicins

T36.8 Poisoning by, adverse effect of and underdosing of other systemic antibiotics
- [5th]
  T36.8X [6th] [7th] Poisoning by, adverse effect of and underdosing of other systemic antibiotics

T37 [4th] POISONING BY, ADVERSE EFFECT OF AND UNDERDOSING OF OTHER SYSTEMIC ANTI-INFECTIVES AND ANTIPARASITICS

Excludes1: anti-infectives topically used for ear, nose and throat (T49.6-)
anti-infectives topically used for eye (T49.5-)
locally applied anti-infectives NEC (T49.0-)

T37.0 [5th] Poisoning by, adverse effect of and underdosing of sulfonamides
  T37.0X [6th] [7th] Poisoning by, adverse effect of and underdosing of sulfonamides

T38 [4th] POISONING BY, ADVERSE EFFECT OF AND UNDERDOSING OF HORMONES AND THEIR SYNTHETIC SUBSTITUTES AND ANTAGONISTS, NEC

Excludes1: mineralocorticoids and their antagonists (T50.0-)
oxytocic hormones (T48.0-)
parathyroid hormones and derivatives (T50.9-)

T38.2 [5th] Poisoning by, adverse effect of and underdosing of antithyroid drugs
  T38.2X [6th] [7th] Poisoning by, adverse effect of and underdosing of antithyroid drugs

T38.3 [5th] Poisoning by, adverse effect of and underdosing of insulin and oral hypoglycemic [antidiabetic] drugs
  T38.3X [6th] [7th] Poisoning by, adverse effect of and underdosing of insulin and oral hypoglycemic [antidiabetic] drugs

T39 [4th] POISONING BY, ADVERSE EFFECT OF AND UNDERDOSING OF NONOPIOID ANALGESICS, ANTIPYRETICS AND ANTIRHEUMATICS

T39.0 [5th] Poisoning by, adverse effect of and underdosing of salicylates
  T39.01 [6th] [7th] Poisoning by, adverse effect of and underdosing of aspirin
  Poisoning by, adverse effect of and underdosing of acetylsalicylic acid
  T39.09 [6th] [7th] Poisoning by, adverse effect of and underdosing of other salicylates

T39.1 [5th] Poisoning by, adverse effect of and underdosing of 4-Aminophenol derivatives
  T39.1X [6th] [7th] Poisoning by, adverse effect of and underdosing of 4-Aminophenol derivatives

T39.3 [5th] Poisoning by, adverse effect of and underdosing of other nonsteroidal anti-inflammatory drugs [NSAID]
  T39.31 [6th] [7th] Poisoning by, adverse effect of and underdosing of propionic acid derivatives
  Poisoning by, adverse effect of and underdosing of fenoprofen/flurbiprofen/ibuprofen/ketoprofen/naproxen/oxaprozin
  T39.39 [6th] [7th] Poisoning by, adverse effect of and under-dosing of other nonsteroidal anti-inflammatory drugs [NSAID]

T40 [4th] POISONING BY, ADVERSE EFFECT OF AND UNDERDOSING OF NARCOTICS AND PSYCHODYSLEPTICS [HALLUCINOGENS]

Excludes2: drug dependence and related mental and behavioral disorders due to psychoactive substance use (F10.–F19.-)

T40.2 [5th] Poisoning by, adverse effect of and underdosing of other opioids
  T40.2X [6th] [7th] Poisoning by, adverse effect of and underdosing of other opioids

T40.4 [5th] Poisoning by, adverse effect of and underdosing of other synthetic narcotics

T40.41 [6th] [7th] Poisoning by fentanyl or fentanyl analogs

T40.42 Poisoning by, adverse effect of and underdosing of tramadol

T40.49 [6th] [7th] Poisoning by, adverse effect of and underdosing of other synthetic narcotics

T40.5 Poisoning by, adverse effect of and underdosing of cocaine
- [5th]
  T40.5X [6th] [7th] Poisoning by, adverse effect of and underdosing of cocaine

T40.7 [5th] Poisoning by, adverse effect of and underdosing of cannabis (derivatives)
  • **T40.71** [6th] [7th] Poisoning by, adverse effect of and underdosing of cannabis (derivatives)
  • **T40.72** [6th] [7th] Poisoning by, adverse effect of and underdosing of synthetic cannabinoids

T42 [4th] POISONING BY, ADVERSE EFFECT OF AND UNDERDOSING OF ANTI-EPILEPTIC, SEDATIVE-HYPNOTIC AND ANTI-PARKINSONISM DRUGS

Excludes2: drug dependence and related mental and behavioral disorders due to psychoactive substance use (F10.- – F19.-)

T42.0 [5th] Poisoning by, adverse effect of and underdosing of hydantoin derivatives
  T42.0X [6th] [7th] Poisoning by, adverse effect of and underdosing of hydantoin derivatives

T42.3 [5th] Poisoning by, adverse effect of and underdosing of barbiturates
  Excludes1: poisoning by, adverse effect of and underdosing of thiobarbiturates (T41.1-)
  T42.3X [6th] [7th] Poisoning by, adverse effect of and underdosing of barbiturates

T42.4 [5th] Poisoning by, adverse effect of and underdosing of benzodiazepines
  T42.4X [6th] [7th] Poisoning by, adverse effect of and underdosing of benzodiazepines

6th characters for categories T36–T50
1—accidental (unintentional), NOS
2—intentional (self-harm)
3—assault
4—undetermined
5—adverse effect
6—underdosing

7th characters for categories T36–T50
A—initial encounter
D—subsequent encounter
S—sequela

T42.6 [5th] Poisoning by, adverse effect of and underdosing of other antiepileptic and sedative-hypnotic drugs
  Poisoning by, adverse effect of and underdosing of methaqualone
  Poisoning by, adverse effect of and underdosing of valproic acid
  Excludes1: poisoning by, adverse effect of and underdosing of carbamazepine (T42.1-)
  T42.6X [6th] [7th] Poisoning by, adverse effect of and underdosing of other antiepileptic and sedative-hypnotic drugs

T43 [4th] POISONING BY, ADVERSE EFFECT OF AND UNDERDOSING OF PSYCHOTROPIC DRUGS, NEC

Excludes1: appetite depressants (T50.5-)
barbiturates (T42.3-)
benzodiazepines (T42.4-)
methaqualone (T42.6-)
psychodysleptics [hallucinogens] (T40.7–T40.9-)

Excludes2: drug dependence and related mental and behavioral disorders due to psychoactive substance use (F10.–-F19.-)

T43.0 [5th] Poisoning by, adverse effect of and underdosing of tricyclic and tetracyclic antidepressants
  T43.01 [6th] [7th] Poisoning by, adverse effect of and underdosing of tricyclic antidepressants
  T43.02 [6th] [7th] Poisoning by, adverse effect of and underdosing of tetracyclic antidepressants

T43.3 [5th] Poisoning by, adverse effect of and underdosing of phenothiazine antipsychotics and neuroleptics
  T43.3X [6th] [7th] Poisoning by, adverse effect of and underdosing of phenothiazine antipsychotics and neuroleptics

T43.6 [5th] Poisoning by, adverse effect of and underdosing of psychostimulants
  Excludes1: poisoning by, adverse effect of and underdosing of cocaine (T40.5-)

[4th] [5th] [6th] [7th] Additional Character Required   ✓   3-character code

Unspecified laterality codes were excluded here.

• =New Code
▲ =Revised Code
▭ =Social determinants of health

Excludes1—Not coded here, do not use together
Excludes2—Not included here

T43.62 `6th` `7th` **Poisoning by, adverse effect of and underdosing of amphetamines**

Poisoning by, adverse effect of and underdosing of methamphetamines

T43.63 `6th` `7th` **Poisoning by, adverse effect of and underdosing of methylphenidate**

T43.64 `6th` `7th` **Poisoning by ecstacy**

Poisoning by MDMA

Poisoning by 3,4-methylenedioxymethamphetamine

T43.9 `5th` **Poisoning by, adverse effect of and underdosing of unspecified psychotropic drug**

T43.91X `7th` **Poisoning by unspecified psychotropic drug, accidental (unintentional)**

Poisoning by psychotropic drug NOS

T43.92X `7th` **Poisoning by unspecified psychotropic drug, intentional self-harm**

T43.95X `7th` **Adverse effect of unspecified psychotropic drug**

T43.96X `7th` **Underdosing of unspecified psychotropic drug**

T44 `4th` **POISONING BY, ADVERSE EFFECT OF AND UNDERDOSING OF DRUGS PRIMARILY AFFECTING THE AUTONOMIC NERVOUS SYSTEM**

T44.5 `5th` **Poisoning by, adverse effect of and underdosing of predominantly beta-adrenoreceptor agonists**

Excludes1: poisoning by, adverse effect of and underdosing of beta-adrenoreceptor agonists used in asthma therapy (T48.6-)

T44.5X `6th` `7th` **Poisoning by, adverse effect of and underdosing of predominantly beta-adrenoreceptor agonists**

T45 `4th` **POISONING BY, ADVERSE EFFECT OF AND UNDERDOSING OF PRIMARILY SYSTEMIC AND HEMATOLOGICAL AGENTS, NEC**

T45.0 `5th` **Poisoning by, adverse effect of and underdosing of antiallergic and antiemetic drugs**

Excludes1: poisoning by, adverse effect of and underdosing of phenothiazine-based neuroleptics (T43.3)

T45.0X `6th` `7th` **Poisoning by, adverse effect of and underdosing of antiallergic and antiemetic drugs**

T45.4 `5th` **Poisoning by, adverse effect of and underdosing of iron and its compounds**

T45.4X `6th` `7th` **Poisoning by, adverse effect of and underdosing of iron and its compounds**

T46 `4th` **POISONING BY, ADVERSE EFFECT OF AND UNDERDOSING OF AGENTS PRIMARILY AFFECTING THE CARDIOVASCULAR SYSTEM**

Excludes1: poisoning by, adverse effect of and underdosing of metaraminol (T44.4)

T46.0 `5th` **Poisoning by, adverse effect of and underdosing of cardiac-stimulant glycosides and drugs of similar action**

T46.0X `6th` `7th` **Poisoning by, adverse effect of and underdosing of cardiac-stimulant glycosides and drugs of similar action**

T47 `4th` **POISONING BY, ADVERSE EFFECT OF AND UNDERDOSING OF AGENTS PRIMARILY AFFECTING THE GASTROINTESTINAL SYSTEM**

T47.8 `5th` **Poisoning by, adverse effect of and underdosing of other agents primarily affecting gastrointestinal system**

T47.8X `6th` `7th` **Poisoning by, adverse effect of and underdosing of other agents primarily affecting gastro-intestinal system**

T48 `4th` **POISONING BY, ADVERSE EFFECT OF AND UNDERDOSING OF AGENTS PRIMARILY ACTING ON SMOOTH AND SKELETAL MUSCLES AND THE RESPIRATORY SYSTEM**

T48.3 `5th` **Poisoning by, adverse effect of and underdosing of antitussives**

T48.3X `6th` `7th` **Poisoning by, adverse effect of and underdosing of antitussives**

T48.5 `5th` **Poisoning by, adverse effect of and underdosing of other anti-common-cold drugs**

Poisoning by, adverse effect of and underdosing of decongestants

Excludes2: poisoning by, adverse effect of and underdosing of antipyretics, NEC (T39.9-)

poisoning by, adverse effect of and underdosing of non-steroidal antiinflammatory drugs (T39.3-)

poisoning by, adverse effect of and underdosing of salicylates (T39.0-)

T48.5X `6th` `7th` **Poisoning by, adverse effect of and underdosing of other anti-common-cold drugs**

T48.6 `5th` **Poisoning by, adverse effect of and underdosing of antiasthmatics, NEC**

Poisoning by, adverse effect of and underdosing of beta-adrenoreceptor agonists used in asthma therapy

Excludes1: poisoning by, adverse effect of and underdosing of beta-adrenoreceptor agonists not used in asthma therapy (T44.5)

poisoning by, adverse effect of and underdosing of anterior pituitary [adenohypophyseal] hormones (T38.8)

T48.6X `6th` `7th` **Poisoning by, adverse effect of and underdosing of antiasthmatics**

T50 `4th` **POISONING BY, ADVERSE EFFECT OF AND UNDERDOSING OF DIURETICS AND OTHER AND UNSPECIFIED DRUGS, MEDICAMENTS AND BIOLOGICAL SUBSTANCES**

T50.0 `5th` **Poisoning by, adverse effect of and underdosing of mineralocorticoids and their antagonists**

T50.0X `6th` `7th` **Poisoning by, adverse effect of and underdosing of mineralocorticoids and their antagonists**

T50.A `5th` **Poisoning by, adverse effect of and underdosing of bacterial vaccines**

T50.A1 `6th` `7th` **Poisoning by, adverse effect of and underdosing of pertussis vaccine, including combinations with a pertussis component**

T50.A2 `6th` `7th` **Poisoning by, adverse effect of and underdosing of mixed bacterial vaccines without a pertussis component**

T50.A9 `6th` `7th` **Poisoning by, adverse effect of and underdosing of other bacterial vaccines**

> 6th characters for categories T36–T50
> 1—accidental (unintentional), NOS
> 2—intentional (self-harm)
> 3—assault
> 4—undetermined
> 5—adverse effect
> 6—underdosing
>
> 7th characters for categories T36–T50
> A—initial encounter
> D—subsequent encounter
> S—sequela

T50.B `5th` **Poisoning by, adverse effect of and underdosing of viral vaccines**

T50.B9 `6th` `7th` **Poisoning by, adverse effect of and underdosing of other viral vaccines**

T50.9 `5th` **Poisoning by, adverse effect of and underdosing of other and unspecified drugs, medicaments and biological substances**

T50.90 `6th` `7th` **Poisoning by, adverse effect of and underdosing of unspecified drugs, medicaments and biological substances**

T50.91 `6th` `7th` **Poisoning by multiple unspecified drugs, medicaments and biological substances**

T50.99 `6th` `7th` **Poisoning by, adverse effect of and underdosing of other drugs, medicaments and biological substances**

(T51–T65) TOXIC EFFECTS OF SUBSTANCES CHIEFLY NONMEDICINAL AS TO SOURCE

Note: When no intent is indicated code to accidental. Undetermined intent is only for use when there is specific documentation in the record that the intent of the toxic effect cannot be determined.

Note: Refer to the Table of Drugs first for a complete listing of chemicals and drugs. If the code is not listed in the tabular, please refer to the complete *ICD-10-CM* Manual.

`4th` `5th` `6th` `7th` Additional Character Required   ✔ 3-character code   Unspecified laterality codes were excluded here.   • =New Code   ▲ =Revised Code   ▢ =Social determinants of health   *Excludes1*—Not coded here, do not use together   *Excludes2*—Not included here

Use additional code(s): for all associated manifestations of toxic effect, such as:
respiratory conditions due to external agents (J60–J70)
personal history of FB fully removed (Z87.821)
to identify any retained FB, if applicable (Z18.-)
Excludes1: contact with and (suspected) exposure to toxic substances (Z77.-)

T52 **TOXIC EFFECT OF ORGANIC SOLVENTS**
`4th`
Excludes1: halogen derivatives of aliphatic
and aromatic hydrocarbons (T53.-)

> 7th characters for categories
> T52–T65
> A—initial encounter
> D—subsequent encounter
> S—sequela

T52.0 **Toxic effects of petroleum products**
`5th`
Toxic effects of gasoline [petrol]
Toxic effects of kerosene [paraffin oil]
Toxic effects of paraffin wax
Toxic effects of ether petroleum
Toxic effects of naphtha petroleum
Toxic effects of spirit petroleum

> **T52.0X** **Toxic effects of petroleum products**
> `6th`
>> **T52.0X1** **Toxic effect of petroleum products, accidental (unintentional)**
>> `7th`
>> Toxic effects of petroleum products NOS
>> **T52.0X2** **Toxic effect of petroleum products, intentional self-harm**
>> `7th`

T52.8 **Toxic effects of other organic solvents**
`5th`
> **T52.8X** **Toxic effects of other organic solvents**
> `6th`
>> **T52.8X1** **Toxic effect of other organic solvents, accidental (unintentional)**
>> `7th`
>> Toxic effects of other organic solvents NOS
>> **T52.8X2** **Toxic effect of other organic solvents, intentional self-harm**
>> `7th`

T54 **TOXIC EFFECT OF CORROSIVE SUBSTANCES**
`4th`
T54.3 **Toxic effects of corrosive alkalis and alkali-like substances**
`5th`
Toxic effects of potassium hydroxide
Toxic effects of sodium hydroxide
> **T54.3X** **Toxic effects of corrosive alkalis and alkali-like substances**
> `6th`
>> **T54.3X1** **Toxic effect of corrosive alkalis and alkali-like substances, accidental (unintentional)**
>> `7th`
>> Toxic effects of corrosive alkalis and alkali-like substances NOS
>> **T54.3X2** **Toxic effect of corrosive alkalis and alkali-like substances, intentional self-harm**
>> `7th`

T56 **TOXIC EFFECT OF METALS**
`4th`
Includes: toxic effects of fumes and vapors of metals
toxic effects of metals from all sources, except medicinal substances
Use additional code to identify any retained metal FB, if applicable (Z18.0-, T18.1-)
Excludes1: arsenic and its compounds (T57.0)
manganese and its compounds (T57.2)
T56.0 **Toxic effects of lead and its compounds**
`5th`
> **T56.0X** **Toxic effects of lead and its compounds**
> `6th`
>> **T56.0X1** **Toxic effect of lead and its compounds, accidental (unintentional)**
>> `7th`
>> Toxic effects of lead and its compounds NOS

T58 **TOXIC EFFECT OF CARBON MONOXIDE**
`4th`
Includes: asphyxiation from carbon monoxide
toxic effect of carbon monoxide from all sources
T58.0 **Toxic effect of carbon monoxide from motor vehicle exhaust**
`5th`
Toxic effect of exhaust gas from gas engine
Toxic effect of exhaust gas from motor pump
> **T58.01X** **Toxic effect of carbon monoxide from motor vehicle exhaust, accidental (unintentional)**
> `7th`
> **T58.02X** **Toxic effect of carbon monoxide from motor vehicle exhaust, intentional self-harm**
> `7th`
> **T58.03X** **Toxic effect of carbon monoxide from motor vehicle exhaust, assault**
> `7th`
> **T58.04X** **Toxic effect of carbon monoxide from motor vehicle exhaust, undetermined**
> `7th`

T58.1 **Toxic effect of carbon monoxide from utility gas**
`5th`
Toxic effect of acetylene
Toxic effect of gas NOS used for lighting, heating, cooking
Toxic effect of water gas
> **T58.11X** **Toxic effect of carbon monoxide from utility gas, accidental (unintentional)**
> `7th`
> **T58.12X** **Toxic effect of carbon monoxide from utility gas, intentional self-harm**
> `7th`
> **T58.13X** **Toxic effect of carbon monoxide from utility gas, assault**
> `7th`
> **T58.14X** **Toxic effect of carbon monoxide from utility gas, undetermined**
> `7th`

T58.9 **Toxic effect of carbon monoxide from unspecified source**
`5th`
> **T58.91X** **Toxic effect of carbon monoxide from unspecified source, accidental (unintentional)**
> `7th`
> **T58.92X** **Toxic effect of carbon monoxide from unspecified source, intentional self-harm**
> `7th`
> **T58.93X** **Toxic effect of carbon monoxide from unspecified source, assault**
> `7th`
> **T58.94X** **Toxic effect of carbon monoxide from unspecified source, undetermined**
> `7th`

T59 **TOXIC EFFECT OF OTHER GASES, FUMES AND VAPORS**
`4th`
Includes: aerosol propellants
Excludes1: chlorofluorocarbons (T53.5)
T59.8 **Toxic effect of other specified gases, fumes and vapors**
`5th`
> **T59.89** **Toxic effect of other specified gases, fumes and vapors**
> `6th`
>> **T59.891** **Toxic effect of other specified gases, fumes and vapors, accidental (unintentional)**
>> `7th`
>> **T59.892** **Toxic effect of other specified gases, fumes and vapors, intentional self-harm**
>> `7th`

> 7th characters for categories
> T52–T65
> A—initial encounter
> D—subsequent encounter
> S—sequela

>> **T59.894** **Toxic effect of other specified gases, fumes and vapors, undetermined**
>> `7th`

T60 **TOXIC EFFECT OF PESTICIDES**
`4th`
Includes: toxic effect of wood preservatives
T60.0 **Toxic effect of organophosphate and carbamate insecticides**
`5th`
> **T60.0X** **Toxic effect of organophosphate and carbamate insecticides**
> `6th`
>> **T60.0X1** **Toxic effect of organophosphate and carbamate insecticides, accidental (unintentional)**
>> `7th`
>> Toxic effect of organophosphate and carbamate insecticides NOS
>> **T60.0X2** **Toxic effect of organophosphate and carbamate insecticides, intentional self-harm**
>> `7th`
>> **T60.0X3** **Toxic effect of organophosphate and carbamate insecticides, assault**
>> `7th`
>> **T60.0X4** **Toxic effect of organophosphate and carbamate insecticides, undetermined**
>> `7th`

T62 **TOXIC EFFECT OF OTHER NOXIOUS SUBSTANCES EATEN AS FOOD**
`4th`
Excludes1: allergic reaction to food, such as:
anaphylactic shock (reaction) due to adverse food reaction (T78.0-)
bacterial food borne intoxications (A05.-)
dermatitis (L23.6, L25.4, L27.2)
food protein-induced enterocolitis syndrome (K52.21)
food protein-induced enteropathy (K52.22)
gastroenteritis (noninfective) (K52.29)
toxic effect of aflatoxin and other mycotoxins (T64)
toxic effect of cyanides (T65.0-)
toxic effect of hydrogen cyanide (T57.3-)
toxic effect of mercury (T56.1-)
T62.0 **Toxic effect of ingested mushrooms**
`5th`
> **T62.0X** **Toxic effect of ingested mushrooms**
> `6th`

| `4th` `5th` `6th` `7th` Additional Character Required | ✓ | 3-character code | Unspecified laterality codes were excluded here. | • =New Code ▲ =Revised Code ▢ =Social determinants of health | *Excludes1*—Not coded here, do not use together *Excludes2*—Not included here |

398   PEDIATRIC ICD-10-CM 2022: A MANUAL FOR PROVIDER-BASED CODING

T62.0X1 `7th` Toxic effect of ingested mushrooms, accidental (unintentional)
Toxic effect of ingested mushrooms NOS

T62.0X2 `7th` Toxic effect of ingested mushrooms, intentional self-harm

T63 `4th` TOXIC EFFECT OF CONTACT WITH VENOMOUS ANIMALS AND PLANTS

Includes: bite or touch of venomous animal
  pricked or stuck by thorn or leaf
Excludes2: ingestion of toxic animal or plant (T61.-, T62.-)

T63.0 `5th` Toxic effect of snake venom

  T63.00 `6th` Toxic effect of unspecified snake venom

    T63.001 `7th` Toxic effect of unspecified snake venom, accidental (unintentional)
     Toxic effect of unspecified snake venom NOS

T63.3 `5th` Toxic effect of venom of spider

  T63.30 `6th` Toxic effect of unspecified spider venom

    T63.301 `7th` Toxic effect of unspecified spider venom, accidental (unintentional)

  T63.33 `6th` Toxic effect of venom of brown recluse spider

    T63.331 `7th` Toxic effect of venom of brown recluse spider, accidental (unintentional)

    T63.332 `7th` Toxic effect of venom of brown recluse spider, intentional self-harm

    T63.333 `7th` Toxic effect of venom of brown recluse spider, assault

    T63.334 `7th` Toxic effect of venom of brown recluse spider, undetermined

T63.4 `5th` Toxic effect of venom of other arthropods

  T63.42 `6th` Toxic effect of venom of ants

    T63.421 `7th` Toxic effect of venom of ants, accidental (unintentional)

  T63.44 `6th` Toxic effect of venom of bees

    T63.441 `7th` Toxic effect of venom of bees, accidental (unintentional)

  T63.45 `6th` Toxic effect of venom of hornets

    T63.451 `7th` Toxic effect of venom of hornets, accidental (unintentional)

  T63.46 `6th` Toxic effect of venom of wasps
    Toxic effect of yellow jacket

    T63.461 `7th` Toxic effect of venom of wasps, accidental (unintentional)

  T63.48 `6th` Toxic effect of venom of other arthropod

    T63.481 `7th` Toxic effect of venom of other arthropod, accidental (unintentional)

T63.6 `5th` Toxic effect of contact with other venomous marine animals

  Excludes1: sea-snake venom (T63.09)
  Excludes2: poisoning by ingestion of shellfish (T61.78-)

  T63.62 `6th` Toxic effect of contact with other jellyfish

    T63.621 `7th` Toxic effect of contact with other jellyfish, accidental (unintentional)

T63.9 `5th` Toxic effect of contact with unspecified venomous animal

  T63.91X `7th` Toxic effect of contact with unspecified venomous animal, accidental (unintentional)

T65 `4th` TOXIC EFFECT OF OTHER AND UNSPECIFIED SUBSTANCES

T65.8 `5th` Toxic effect of other specified substances

  T65.82 `6th` Toxic effect of harmful algae and algae toxins
    Toxic effect of (harmful) algae bloom NOS
    Toxic effect of blue-green algae bloom
    Toxic effect of brown tide
    Toxic effect of cyanobacteria bloom
    Toxic effect of Florida red tide
    Toxic effect of pfiesteria piscicida
    Toxic effect of red tide

    T65.821 `7th` Toxic effect of harmful algae and algae toxins, accidental (unintentional)
     Toxic effect of harmful algae and algae toxins NOS

T65.9 `5th` Toxic effect of unspecified substance

  T65.91X `7th` Toxic effect of unspecified substance, accidental (unintentional)
    Poisoning NOS

T65.92X `7th` Toxic effect of unspecified substance, intentional self-harm

(T66–T78) OTHER AND UNSPECIFIED EFFECTS OF EXTERNAL CAUSES

T67 `4th` EFFECTS OF HEAT AND LIGHT

Excludes1: erythema [dermatitis] ab igne (L59.0)
malignant hyperpyrexia due to anesthesia (T88.3)
radiation-related disorders of the skin and subcutaneous tissue (L55–L59)
Excludes2: burns (T20–T31)
sunburn (L55.-)
sweat disorder due to heat (L74–L75)

7th characters for categories T67–T78
A—initial encounter
D—subsequent encounter
S—sequela

T67.0 `5th` Heatstroke and sunstroke
Use additional code(s) to identify any associated complications of heatstroke, such as:
  coma and stupor (R40.-)
  rhabdomyolysis (M62.82)
  SIRS (R65.1-)

  T67.01X `7th` Heatstroke and sunstroke
    Heat apoplexy
    Heat pyrexia
    Siriasis
    Thermoplegia

  T67.02X `7th` Exertional heatstroke

  T67.09X `7th` Other heatstroke and sunstroke

T67.1XX `7th` Heat syncope
  Heat collapse

T67.2XX `7th` Heat cramp

7th characters for categories T67–T78
A—initial encounter
D—subsequent encounter
S—sequela

T67.3XX `7th` Heat exhaustion, anhydrotic
  Heat prostration due to water depletion
  Excludes1: heat exhaustion due to salt depletion (T67.4)

T67.4XX `7th` Heat exhaustion due to salt depletion
  Heat prostration due to salt (and water) depletion

T67.5XX `7th` Heat exhaustion, unspecified
  Heat prostration NOS

T67.6XX `7th` Heat fatigue, transient

T67.8XX `7th` Other effects of heat and light

T67.9XX `7th` Effect of heat and light, unspecified

T68 `✔` HYPOTHERMIA

Accidental hypothermia
Hypothermia NOS
Use additional code to identify source of exposure:
  Exposure to excessive cold of man-made origin (W93)
  Exposure to excessive cold of natural origin (X31)
Excludes1: hypothermia following anesthesia (T88.51)
  hypothermia not associated with low environmental temperature (R68.0)
  hypothermia of newborn (P80.-)
Excludes2: frostbite (T33–T34)

T70 `4th` EFFECTS OF AIR PRESSURE AND WATER PRESSURE

T70.0XX `7th` Otitic barotrauma
  Aero-otitis media
  Effects of change in ambient atmospheric pressure or water pressure on ears

T70.1XX `7th` Sinus barotrauma
  Aerosinusitis
  Effects of change in ambient atmospheric pressure on sinuses

T70.2 `5th` Other and unspecified effects of high altitude
  Excludes2: polycythemia due to high altitude (D75.1)

  T70.20X `7th` Unspecified effects of high altitude

`4th` `5th` `6th` `7th` Additional Character Required	`✔` 3-character code	Unspecified laterality codes were excluded here.	• =New Code ▲ =Revised Code �़ =Social determinants of health	*Excludes1*—Not coded here, do not use together *Excludes2*—Not included here

T70.29X **Other effects of high altitude**
`7th`
    Alpine sickness
    Anoxia due to high altitude
    Barotrauma NOS
    Hypobaropathy
    Mountain sickness

T71 **ASPHYXIATION**
`4th`
Mechanical suffocation
Traumatic suffocation
Excludes1: acute respiratory distress (syndrome) (J80)
    anoxia due to high altitude (T70.2)
    asphyxia NOS (R09.01)
    asphyxia from carbon monoxide (T58.-)
    asphyxia from inhalation of food or FB (T17.-)
    asphyxia from other gases, fumes and vapors (T59.-)
    respiratory distress (syndrome) in newborn (P22.-)

T71.1 **Asphyxiation due to mechanical threat to breathing**
`5th`
Suffocation due to mechanical threat to breathing

    T71.11 **Asphyxiation due to smothering under pillow**
    `6th`
        T71.111 **Asphyxiation due to smothering under pillow, accidental**
        `7th`
            Asphyxiation due to smothering under pillow NOS
        T71.112 **Asphyxiation due to smothering under pillow, intentional self-harm**
        `7th`
        T71.113 **Asphyxiation due to smothering under pillow, assault**
        `7th`
        T71.114 **Asphyxiation due to smothering under pillow, undetermined, initial encounter**
        `7th`

    T71.12 **Asphyxiation due to plastic bag**
    `6th`
        T71.121 **Asphyxiation due to plastic bag, accidental**
        `7th`
            Asphyxiation due to plastic bag NOS
        T71.122 **Asphyxiation due to plastic bag, intentional self-harm**
        `7th`
        T71.123 **Asphyxiation due to plastic bag, assault**
        `7th`
        T71.124 **Asphyxiation due to plastic bag, undetermined**
        `7th`

    T71.13 **Asphyxiation due to being trapped in bed linens**
    `6th`
        T71.131 **Asphyxiation due to being trapped in bed linens, accidental**
        `7th`
            Asphyxiation due to being trapped in bed linens NOS
        T71.132 **Asphyxiation due to being trapped in bed linens, intentional self-harm**
        `7th`
        T71.133 **Asphyxiation due to being trapped in bed linens, assault**
        `7th`
        T71.134 **Asphyxiation due to being trapped in bed linens, undetermined**
        `7th`

    T71.14 **Asphyxiation due to smothering under another person's body (in bed)**
    `6th`
        T71.141 **Asphyxiation due to smothering under another person's body (in bed), accidental**
        `7th`
            Asphyxiation due to smothering under another person's body (in bed) NOS
        T71.143 **Asphyxiation due to smothering under another person's body (in bed), assault**
        `7th`
        T71.144 **Asphyxiation due to smothering under another person's body (in bed), undetermined**
        `7th`

    T71.15 **Asphyxiation due to smothering in furniture**
    `6th`
        T71.151 **Asphyxiation due to smothering in furniture, accidental**
        `7th`
            Asphyxiation due to smothering in furniture NOS
        T71.152 **Asphyxiation due to smothering in furniture, intentional self-harm**
        `7th`
        T71.153 **Asphyxiation due to smothering in furniture, assault**
        `7th`
        T71.154 **Asphyxiation due to smothering in furniture, undetermined**
        `7th`

    T71.16 **Asphyxiation due to hanging**
    `6th`
    Hanging by window shade cord
    Use additional code for any associated injuries, such as:
        crushing injury of neck (S17.-)
        fracture of cervical vertebrae (S12.0–S12.2-)
        open wound of neck (S11.-)
        T71.161 **Asphyxiation due to hanging, accidental**
        `7th`
            Asphyxiation due to hanging NOS
            Hanging NOS
        T71.162 **Asphyxiation due to hanging, intentional self-harm**
        `7th`
        T71.163 **Asphyxiation due to hanging, assault**
        `7th`
        T71.164 **Asphyxiation due to hanging, undetermined**
        `7th`

    T71.19 **Asphyxiation due to mechanical threat to breathing due to other causes**
    `6th`
        T71.191 **Asphyxiation due to mechanical threat to breathing due to other causes, accidental**
        `7th`
            Asphyxiation due to other causes NOS
        T71.192 **Asphyxiation due to mechanical threat to breathing due to other causes, intentional self-harm**
        `7th`
        T71.193 **Asphyxiation due to mechanical threat to breathing due to other causes, assault**
        `7th`
        T71.194 **Asphyxiation due to mechanical threat to breathing due to other causes, undetermined**
        `7th`

T71.2 **Asphyxiation due to systemic oxygen deficiency due to low oxygen content in ambient air**
`5th`
Suffocation due to systemic oxygen deficiency due to low oxygen content in ambient air

    T71.21X **Asphyxiation due to cave-in or falling earth**
    `7th`
    Use additional code for any associated cataclysm (X34–X38)

    T71.22 **Asphyxiation due to being trapped in a car trunk**
    `6th`
        T71.221 **Asphyxiation due to being trapped in a car trunk, accidental**
        `7th`
        T71.222 **Asphyxiation due to being trapped in a car trunk, intentional self-harm**
        `7th`
        T71.223 **Asphyxiation due to being trapped in a car trunk, assault**
        `7th`
        T71.224 **Asphyxiation due to being trapped in a car trunk, undetermined**
        `7th`

    T71.23 **Asphyxiation due to being trapped in a (discarded) refrigerator**
    `6th`
        T71.231 **Asphyxiation due to being trapped in a (discarded) refrigerator, accidental**
        `7th`
        T71.232 **Asphyxiation due to being trapped in a (discarded) refrigerator, intentional self-harm**
        `7th`
        T71.233 **Asphyxiation due to being trapped in a (discarded) refrigerator, assault**
        `7th`
        T71.234 **Asphyxiation due to being trapped in a (discarded) refrigerator, undetermined**
        `7th`
        T71.29X **Asphyxiation due to being trapped in other low oxygen environment**
        `7th`

    T71.9XX **Asphyxiation due to unspecified cause**
    `7th`
    Suffocation (by strangulation) due to unspecified cause
    Suffocation NOS
    Systemic oxygen deficiency due to low oxygen content in ambient air or due to due to mechanical threat to breathing due to unspecified cause
    Traumatic asphyxia NOS

T73 **EFFECTS OF OTHER DEPRIVATION**
`4th`
    T73.0XX **Starvation**
    `7th`
    Deprivation of food
    T73.1XX **Deprivation of water**
    `7th`

> 7th characters for categories T67–T78
> A—initial encounter
> D—subsequent encounter
> S—sequela

`4th` `5th` `6th` `7th` Additional Character Required   ✔   3-character code   Unspecified laterality codes were excluded here.   • =New Code   ▲ =Revised Code   ⌧ =Social determinants of health   ***Excludes1***—Not coded here, do not use together   ***Excludes2***—Not included here

400   **PEDIATRIC ICD-10-CM 2022: A MANUAL FOR PROVIDER-BASED CODING**

T73.2XX **Exhaustion due to exposure**
`7th`

T73.3XX **Exhaustion due to excessive exertion**
`7th`   Exhaustion due to overexertion

T73.8XX **Other effects of deprivation**
`7th`

T74   ADULT AND CHILD ABUSE, NEGLECT AND OTHER MALTREATMENT, CONFIRMED
`4th`

> **GUIDELINES**
>
> Sequence first the appropriate code from categories T74.- (Adult and child abuse, neglect and other maltreatment, confirmed) or T76.- (Adult and child abuse, neglect and other maltreatment, suspected) for abuse, neglect and other maltreatment, followed by any accompanying mental health or injury code(s).
>
> If the documentation in the medical record states abuse or neglect it is coded as confirmed (T74.-). It is coded as suspected if it is documented as suspected (T76.-).
>
> For cases of confirmed abuse or neglect an external cause code from the assault section (X92–Y08) should be added to identify the cause of any physical injuries. A perpetrator code (Y07) should be added when the perpetrator of the abuse is known. For suspected cases of abuse or neglect, do not report external cause or perpetrator code.
>
> If a suspected case of abuse, neglect or mistreatment is ruled out during an encounter code Z04.71, Encounter for examination and observation following alleged physical adult abuse, ruled out, or code Z04.72, Encounter for examination and observation following alleged child physical abuse, ruled out, should be used, not a code from T76.
>
> If a suspected case of alleged rape or sexual abuse is ruled out during an encounter code Z04.41, Encounter for examination and observation following alleged physical adult abuse, ruled out, or code Z04.42, Encounter for examination and observation following alleged rape or sexual abuse, ruled out, should be used, not a code from T76.
>
> For the victim of a patient suffering from Munchausen syndrome by proxy or Factitious disorder, assign the appropriate code from categories T74, Adult and child abuse, neglect and other maltreatment, confirmed, or T76, Adult and child abuse, neglect and other maltreatment, suspected.
>
> If a suspected case of forced sexual exploitation or forced labor exploitation is ruled out during an encounter, code Z04.81, Encounter for examination and observation of victim following forced sexual exploitation, or code Z04.82, Encounter for examination and observation of victim following forced labor exploitation, should be used, not a code from T76.
>
> **Use additional code,** if applicable, to identify any associated current injury
>   external cause code to identify perpetrator, if known (Y07.-)
>
> ***Excludes1:*** abuse and maltreatment in pregnancy (O9A.3-, O9A.4-, O9A.5-)
>   adult and child maltreatment, suspected (T76.-)

> *7th characters for categories T67–T78*
> A—initial encounter
> D—subsequent encounter
> S—sequela

T74.0 **Neglect or abandonment, confirmed**
`5th` ▫**T74.02X** **Child neglect or abandonment, confirmed**
    `7th`

T74.1 **Physical abuse, confirmed**
`5th`   ***Excludes2:*** sexual abuse (T74.2-)
    ▫**T74.12X** **Child physical abuse, confirmed**
    `7th`   ***Excludes2:*** shaken infant syndrome (T74.4)

T74.2 **Sexual abuse, confirmed**
`5th`   Rape, confirmed
    Sexual assault, confirmed
    ▫**T74.22X** **Child sexual abuse, confirmed**
    `7th`

T74.3 **Psychological abuse, confirmed**
`5th`   ▫**T74.32X** **Child psychological abuse, confirmed**
    `7th`   Bullying and intimidation, confirmed
       Intimidation through social media, confirmed

T74.4XX **Shaken infant syndrome**
`7th`

T74.5 **Forced sexual exploitation, confirmed**
`5th`   ▫**T74.51X** **Adult forced sexual exploitation, confirmed**
    `7th`
    ▫**T74.52X** **Child sexual exploitation, confirmed**
    `7th`

T74.6 **Forced labor exploitation, confirmed**
`5th`   ▫**T74.61X** **Adult forced labor exploitation, confirmed**
    `7th`
    ▫**T74.62X** **Child forced labor exploitation, confirmed**
    `7th`

▫ **T74.9** **Unspecified maltreatment, confirmed**
`5th`   ▫**T74.92X** **Unspecified child maltreatment, confirmed**
    `7th`

T75   OTHER AND UNSPECIFIED EFFECTS OF OTHER EXTERNAL CAUSES
`4th`
Excludes1: adverse effects NEC (T78.-)
Excludes2: burns (electric) (T20–T31)

T75.1XX **Unspecified effects of drowning and nonfatal submersion**
`7th`   Immersion
    Excludes1: specified effects of drowning —*code to* effects

T75.3XX **Motion sickness**
`7th`   Airsickness
    Seasickness
    Travel sickness
    Use additional external cause code to identify vehicle or type of motion (Y92.81-, Y93.5-)

T75.4XX **Electrocution**
`7th`   Shock from electric current
    Shock from electroshock gun (taser)

T75.8 **Other specified effects of external causes**
`5th`   **T75.89X** **Other specified effects of external causes**
    `7th`

T76   ADULT AND CHILD ABUSE, NEGLECT AND OTHER MALTREATMENT, SUSPECTED
`4th`

> **GUIDELINES**
>
> See T74 for full guidelines.
> **Use additional code,** if applicable, to identify any associated current injury
> ***Excludes1:*** adult and child maltreatment, confirmed (T74.-)
>   suspected abuse and maltreatment in pregnancy (O9A.3-, O9A.4-, O9A.5-)
>   suspected adult physical abuse, ruled out (Z04.71)
>   suspected adult sexual abuse, ruled out (Z04.41)
>   suspected child physical abuse, ruled out (Z04.72)
>   suspected child sexual abuse, ruled out (Z04.42)

T76.0 **Neglect or abandonment, suspected**
`5th`   ▫**T76.02X** **Child neglect or abandonment, suspected**
    `7th`

T76.1 **Physical abuse, suspected**
`5th`   ▫**T76.12X** **Child physical abuse, suspected**
    `7th`

T76.2 **Sexual abuse, suspected**
`5th`   Rape, suspected
    Excludes1: alleged abuse, ruled out (Z04.7)
    ▫**T76.22X** **Child sexual abuse, suspected**
    `7th`

T76.3 **Psychological abuse, suspected**
`5th`   ▫**T76.32X** **Child psychological abuse, suspected**
    `7th`   Bullying and intimidation, suspected
       Intimidation through social media, suspected

T76.5 **Forced sexual exploitation, suspected**
`5th`   ▫**T76.52X** **Child sexual exploitation, suspected**
    `7th`

T76.6 **Forced labor exploitation, suspected**
`5th`   ▫**T76.62X** **Child forced labor exploitation, suspected**
    `7th`

T76.9 **Unspecified maltreatment, suspected**
`5th`   ▫**T76.92X** **Unspecified child maltreatment, suspected**
    `7th`

T78   ADVERSE EFFECTS, NEC
`4th`
Excludes2: complications of surgical and medical care NEC (T80–T88)

T78.0 **Anaphylactic reaction due to food**
`5th`   Anaphylactic reaction due to adverse food reaction
    Anaphylactic shock or reaction due to nonpoisonous foods
    Anaphylactoid reaction due to food
    T78.00X **Anaphylactic reaction due to unspecified food**
    `7th`

`4th` `5th` `6th` `7th` Additional Character Required   ✓ 3-character code   Unspecified laterality codes were excluded here.   • =New Code   ▲ =Revised Code   ▫ =Social determinants of health   ***Excludes1***—Not coded here, do not use together   ***Excludes2***—Not included here

  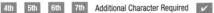

PEDIATRIC ICD-10-CM 2022: A MANUAL FOR PROVIDER-BASED CODING   401

T78.01X `7th` **Anaphylactic reaction due to peanuts**

T78.02X `7th` **Anaphylactic reaction due to shellfish (crustaceans)**

T78.03X `7th` **Anaphylactic reaction due to other fish**

T78.04X `7th` **Anaphylactic reaction due to fruits and vegetables**

T78.05X `7th` **Anaphylactic reaction due to tree nuts and seeds**
Excludes2: anaphylactic reaction due to peanuts (T78.01)

T78.06X `7th` **Anaphylactic reaction due to food additives**

T78.07X `7th` **Anaphylactic reaction due to milk and dairy products**

T78.08X `7th` **Anaphylactic reaction due to eggs**

T78.09X `7th` **Anaphylactic reaction due to other food products**

T78.1XX `7th` **Other adverse food reactions, NEC**
Use additional code to identify the type of reaction, if applicable
Excludes1: anaphylactic reaction or shock due to adverse food reaction (T78.0-)
anaphylactic reaction due to food (T78.0-)
bacterial food borne intoxications (A05.-)
Excludes2: allergic and dietetic gastroenteritis and colitis (K52.29)
allergic rhinitis due to food (J30.5)
dermatitis due to food in contact with skin (L23.6, L24.6, L25.4)
dermatitis due to ingested food (L27.2)
food protein-induced enterocolitis syndrome (K52.21)
food protein-induced enteropathy (K52.22)

T78.2XX `7th` **Anaphylactic shock, unspecified**
Allergic shock
Anaphylactic reaction
Anaphylaxis
Excludes1: anaphylactic reaction or shock due to adverse effect of correct medicinal substance properly administered (T88.6)
anaphylactic reaction or shock due to adverse food reaction (T78.0-)
anaphylactic reaction or shock due to serum (T80.5-)

T78.3XX `7th` **Angioneurotic edema**
Allergic angioedema
Giant urticaria
Quincke's edema
Excludes1: serum urticaria (T80.6-)
urticaria (L50.-)

T78.4 `5th` **Other and unspecified allergy**
Excludes1: specified types of allergic reaction such as:
allergic diarrhea (K52.29)
allergic gastroenteritis and colitis (K52.29)
food protein-induced enterocolitis syndrome (K52.21)
food protein-induced enteropathy (K52.22)
dermatitis (L23–L25, L27.-)
hay fever (J30.1)

T78.40X `7th` **Allergy, unspecified**
Allergic reaction NOS
Hypersensitivity NOS

T78.49X `7th` **Other allergy**

T78.8XX `7th` **Other adverse effects, NEC**

(T79) CERTAIN EARLY COMPLICATIONS OF TRAUMA

T79 `4th` **CERTAIN EARLY COMPLICATIONS OF TRAUMA, NEC**
Excludes2: acute respiratory distress syndrome (J80)
complications occurring during or following medical procedures (T80–T88)
complications of surgical and medical care NEC (T80–T88)

7th characters for category T79
A—initial encounter
D—subsequent encounter
S—sequela

newborn respiratory distress syndrome (P22.0)

T79.4XX `7th` **Traumatic shock**
Shock (immediate) (delayed) following injury
Excludes1: anaphylactic shock due to adverse food reaction (T78.0-)
anaphylactic shock due to correct medicinal substance properlyadministered (T88.6)
anaphylactic shock due to serum (T80.5-)
anaphylactic shock NOS (T78.2)
electric shock (T75.4)
nontraumatic shock NEC (R57.-)
obstetric shock (O75.1)
postprocedural shock (T81.1-)
septic shock (R65.21)
shock complicating abortion or ectopic or molar pregnancy (O00–O07, O08.3)
shock due to anesthetic (T88.2)
shock due to lightning (T75.01)
shock NOS (R57.9)

T79.7XX `7th` **Traumatic subcutaneous emphysema**
Excludes2: emphysema NOS (J43)
emphysema (subcutaneous) resulting from a procedure (T81.82)

(T80–T88) COMPLICATIONS OF SURGICAL AND MEDICAL CARE, NEC

Use additional code for adverse effect, if applicable, to identify drug (T36–T50 with fifth or sixth character 5)
Use additional code(s) to identify the specified condition resulting from the complication
Use additional code to identify devices involved and details of circumstances (Y62–Y82)
Excludes2: any encounters with medical care for postprocedural conditions in which no complications are present, such as:
artificial opening status (Z93.-)
closure of external stoma (Z43.-)
fitting and adjustment of external prosthetic device (Z44.-)
burns and corrosions from local applications and irradiation (T20–T32)
complications of surgical procedures during pregnancy, childbirth and the puerperium (O00–O9A)
mechanical complication of respirator [ventilator] (J95.850)
poisoning and toxic effects of drugs and chemicals (T36–T65 with fifth or sixth character 1–4 or 6)
postprocedural fever (R50.82)
specified complications classified elsewhere, such as:
cerebrospinal fluid leak from spinal puncture (G97.0)
colostomy malfunction (K94.0-)
disorders of fluid and electrolyte imbalance (E86–E87)
functional disturbances following cardiac surgery (I97.0–I97.1)
intraoperative and postprocedural complications of specified body systems (D78.-, E36.-, E89.-, G97.3-, G97.4, H59.3-, H59.-, H95.2-, H95.3, I97.4-, I97.5, J95.6-, J95.7, K91.6-, L76.-, M96.-, N99.-)
ostomy complications (J95.0-, K94.-, N99.5-)
postgastric surgery syndromes (K91.1)
postlaminectomy syndrome NEC (M96.1)
postmastectomy lymphedema syndrome (I97.2)
postsurgical blind-loop syndrome (K91.2)
ventilator associated pneumonia (J95.851)

T80 `4th` **COMPLICATIONS FOLLOWING INFUSION, TRANSFUSION AND THERAPEUTIC INJECTION**
Includes: complications following perfusion
Excludes2: bone marrow transplant rejection (T86.01)
febrile nonhemolytic transfusion reaction (R50.84)
fluid overload due to transfusion (E87.71)
posttransfusion purpura (D69.51)
transfusion associated circulatory overload (TACO) (E87.71)
transfusion (red blood cell) associated hemochromatosis (E83.111)
transfusion related acute lung injury (TRALI) (J95.84)

7th characters for category T80
A—initial encounter
D—subsequent encounter
S—sequela

T80.0XX `7th` **Air embolism following infusion, transfusion and therapeutic injection**

 4th 5th 6th 7th   Additional Character Required   ✔ 3-character code

Unspecified laterality codes were excluded here.

● =New Code
▲ =Revised Code
▣ =Social determinants of health

Excludes1—Not coded here, do not use together
Excludes2—Not included here

T80.2 `5th` **Infections following infusion, transfusion and therapeutic injection**

Use additional code to identify the specific infection, such as:
  sepsis (A41.9)

Use additional code (R65.2-) to identify severe sepsis, if applicable

Excludes2: infections specified as due to prosthetic devices, implants and grafts (T82.6–T82.7, T83.5–T83.6, T84.5–T84.7, T85.7)
  postprocedural infections (T81.4-)

T80.21 `6th` **Infection due to central venous catheter**
  Infection due to pulmonary artery catheter (Swan-Ganz catheter)

  T80.211 `7th` **Bloodstream infection due to central venous catheter**
    Catheter-related bloodstream infection (CRBSI) NOS
    Central line-associated blood-stream infection (CLABSI)
    Bloodstream infection due to Hickman catheter/peripherally inserted central catheter (PICC)/portacath (port-a-cath)/pulmonary artery catheter/triple lumen catheter/umbilical venous catheter

  T80.212 `7th` **Local infection due to central venous catheter**

> 7th characters for category T80
> A—initial encounter
> D—subsequent encounter
> S—sequela

    Exit or insertion site infection
    Local infection due to Hickman catheter/peripherally inserted central catheter (PICC)/portacath (port-a-cath)/pulmonary artery catheter/triple lumen catheter/umbilical venous catheter
    Port or reservoir infection
    Tunnel infection

  T80.218 `7th` **Other infection due to central venous catheter**
    Other central line–associated infection/Hickman catheter/peripherally inserted central catheter (PICC)/portacath (port-a-cath)/pulmonary artery catheter/triple lumen catheter/umbilical venous catheter

  T80.219 `7th` **Unspecified infection due to central venous catheter**
    Central line-associated infection NOS
    Unspecified infection due to Hickman catheter/peripherally inserted central catheter (PICC)/portacath (port-a-cath)/pulmonary artery catheter/triple lumen catheter/umbilical venous catheter

T80.22X `7th` **Acute infection following transfusion, infusion, or injection of blood and blood products**

T80.29X `7th` **Infection following other infusion, transfusion and therapeutic injection**

T80.3 `5th` **ABO incompatibility reaction due to transfusion of blood or blood products**

Excludes1: minor blood group antigens reactions (Duffy) (E) (K(ell)) (Kidd) (Lewis) (M) (N) (P) (S) (T80.A-)

T80.30X `7th` **ABO incompatibility reaction due to transfusion of blood or blood products, unspecified**
  ABO incompatibility blood transfusion NOS
  Reaction to ABO incompatibility from transfusion NOS

T80.5 `5th` **Anaphylactic reaction due to serum**
  Allergic shock due to serum
  Anaphylactic shock due to serum
  Anaphylactoid reaction due to serum
  Anaphylaxis due to serum

Excludes1: ABO incompatibility reaction due to transfusion of blood or blood products (T80.3-)
  allergic reaction or shock NOS (T78.2)

  anaphylactic reaction or shock NOS (T78.2)
  anaphylactic reaction or shock due to adverse effect of correct medicinal substance properly administered (T88.6)
  other serum reaction (T80.6-)

T80.51X `7th` **Anaphylactic reaction due to administration of blood and blood products**

T80.52X `7th` **Anaphylactic reaction due to vaccination**

T80.59X `7th` **Anaphylactic reaction due to other serum**

T80.6 `5th` **Other serum reactions**
  Intoxication by serum
  Protein sickness
  Serum rash
  Serum sickness
  Serum urticaria

Excludes2: serum hepatitis (B16–B19)

T80.61X `7th` **Other serum reaction due to administration of blood and blood products**

T80.62X `7th` **Other serum reaction due to vaccination**

T80.69X `7th` **Other serum reaction due to other serum**
  Code also, if applicable, arthropathy in hypersensitivity reactions classified elsewhere (M36.4)

T80.8 `5th` **Other complications following infusion, transfusion and therapeutic injection**

T80.81 `6th` **Extravasation of vesicant agent**
  Infiltration of vesicant agent

  T80.810 `7th` **Extravasation of vesicant antineoplastic chemotherapy**
    Infiltration of vesicant antineoplastic chemotherapy

  T80.818 `7th` **Extravasation of other vesicant agent**
    Infiltration of other vesicant agent
    Use additional code to identify the specific infection, such as:
    sepsis (A41.9)
    Use additional code (R65.2-) to identify severe sepsis, if applicable
    Excludes2: infections specified as due to prosthetic devices, implants and grafts (T82.6-T82.7, T83.5-T83.6, T84.5-T84.7, T85.7)
    postprocedural infections (T81.4-)

• **T80.82X** `7th` **Complication of immune effector cellular therapy**
  Complication of chimeric antigen receptor (CAR-T) cell therapy
  Complication of IEC therapy
  Excludes2: complication of bone marrow transplant (T86.0)
  Complication of stem cell transplant (T86.5)
  Use additional code to identify the specific complication, such as:
  Cytokine release syndrome (D89.83-)
  Immune effector cell-associated neurotoxicity syndrome (G92.0-)

T80.89X `7th` **Other complications following infusion, transfusion and therapeutic injection**
  Delayed serologic transfusion reaction (DSTR), unspecified incompatibility
  Use additional code to identify graft-versus-host reaction, if applicable, (D89.81-)

T80.9 `5th` **Unspecified complication following infusion, transfusion and therapeutic injection**

T80.90X `7th` **Unspecified complication following infusion and therapeutic injection**

T80.91 `6th` **Hemolytic transfusion reaction, unspecified incompatibility**
  Excludes1: ABO incompatibility with hemolytic transfusion reaction (T80.31-)
  Non-ABO incompatibility with hemolytic transfusion reaction (T80.A1-)
  Rh incompatibility with hemolytic transfusion reaction (T80.41-)

`4th` `5th` `6th` `7th`   Additional Character Required   ✔   3-character code   Unspecified laterality codes were excluded here.   • =New Code   ▲ =Revised Code   ▢ =Social determinants of health   **Excludes1**—Not coded here, do not use together   **Excludes2**—Not included here

CHAPTER 19. INJURY, POISONING AND CERTAIN OTHER CONSEQUENCES OF EXTERNAL CAUSES   (T80.910–T82.898)

T80.910 `7th` **Acute hemolytic transfusion reaction, unspecified incompatibility**

T80.911 `7th` **Delayed hemolytic transfusion reaction, unspecified incompatibility**

T80.919 `7th` **Hemolytic transfusion reaction, unspecified incompatibility, unspecified as acute or delayed**

Hemolytic transfusion reaction NOS

T80.92X `7th` **Unspecified transfusion reaction**

Transfusion reaction NOS

T81 `4th` **COMPLICATIONS OF PROCEDURES, NEC**

Use additional code for adverse effect, if applicable, to identify drug (T36–T50 with fifth or sixth character 5)

Excludes2: complications following immunization (T88.0–T88.1)

complications following infusion, transfusion and therapeutic injection (T80.-)

complications of transplanted organs and tissue (T86.-)

specified complications classified elsewhere, such as:

complication of prosthetic devices, implants and grafts (T82–T85)

dermatitis due to drugs and medicaments (L23.3, L24.4, L25.1, L27.0–L27.1)

endosseous dental implant failure (M27.6-)

floppy iris syndrome (IFIS) (intraoperative) H21.81

intraoperative and postprocedural complications of specific body system (D78.-, E36.-, E89.-, G97.3-, G97.4, H59.3-, H59.-, H95.2-, H95.3, I97.4-, I97.5, J95, K91.-, L76.-, M96.-, N99.-)

ostomy complications (J95.0-, K94.-, N99.5-)

plateau iris syndrome (post-iridectomy) (postprocedural) H21.82

poisoning and toxic effects of drugs and chemicals (T36–T65 with fifth or sixth character 1–4 or 6)

> **7th characters for categories T81–T86**
> A—initial encounter
> D—subsequent encounter
> S—sequela

T81.1 `5th` **Postprocedural shock**

Shock during or resulting from a procedure, NEC

Excludes1: anaphylactic shock NOS (T78.2)

anaphylactic shock due to correct substance properly administered (T88.6)

anaphylactic shock due to serum (T80.5-)

electric shock (T75.4)

obstetric shock (O75.1)

septic shock (R65.21)

shock due to anesthetic (T88.2)

shock following abortion or ectopic or molar pregnancy (O00–O07, O08.3)

traumatic shock (T79.4)

T81.10X `7th` **Postprocedural shock unspecified**

Collapse NOS during or resulting from a procedure, NEC

Postprocedural failure of peripheral circulation

Postprocedural shock NOS

T81.11X `7th` **Postprocedural cardiogenic shock**

T81.12X `7th` **Postprocedural septic shock**

Postprocedural endotoxic shock resulting from a procedure, NEC

Postprocedural gram-negative shock resulting from a procedure, NEC

Code first underlying infection

Use additional code, to identify any associated acute organ dysfunction, if applicable

T81.19X `7th` **Other postprocedural shock**

Postprocedural hypovolemic shock

T81.3 `5th` **Disruption of wound, NEC**

Disruption of any suture materials or other closure methods

Excludes1: breakdown (mechanical) of permanent sutures (T85.612)

displacement of permanent sutures (T85.622)

disruption of cesarean delivery wound (O90.0)

disruption of perineal obstetric wound (O90.1)

mechanical complication of permanent sutures NEC (T85.692)

T81.30X `7th` **Disruption of wound, unspecified**

Disruption of wound NOS

T81.31X `7th` **Disruption of external operation (surgical) wound, NEC**

Dehiscence of operation wound NOS

Disruption of operation wound NOS

Disruption or dehis-cence of closure of cornea

Disruption or dehiscence of closure of mucosa

Disruption or dehiscence of closure of skin and subcutaneous tissue

Full-thickness skin disruption or dehiscence

Superficial disruption or dehiscence of operation wound

Excludes1: dehiscence of amputation stump (T87.81)

T81.33X `7th` **Disruption of traumatic injury wound repair**

Disruption or dehiscence of closure of traumatic laceration (external) (internal)

T81.4 `5th` **Infection following a procedure**

Wound abscess following a procedure

Use additional code to identify infection

Use additional code (R65.2-) to identify severe sepsis, if applicable

Excludes2: bleb associated endophthalmitis (H59.4-)

infection due to infusion, transfusion and therapeutic injection (T80.2-)

infection due to prosthetic devices, implants and grafts (T82.6-T82.7, T83.5-T83.6, T84.5-T84.7,T85.7)

obstetric surgical wound infection (O86.0-)

postprocedural fever NOS (R50.82)

postprocedural retroperitoneal abscess (K68.11)

T81.40X `7th` **Infection following a procedure, unspecified**

T81.41X `7th` **Infection following a procedure, superficial incisional surgical site**

Subcutaneous abscess following a procedure

Stitch abscess following a procedure

T81.42X `7th` **Infection following a procedure, deep incisional surgical site**

Intra-muscular abscess following a procedure

T81.43X `7th` **Infection following a procedure, organ and space surgical site**

Intra-abdominal abscess following a procedure

Subphrenic abscess following a procedure

T81.44X `7th` **Sepsis following a procedure**

Use additional code to identify the sepsis

T81.49X `7th` **Infection following a procedure, other surgical site**

T81.8 `5th` **Other complications of procedures, NEC**

Excludes2: hypothermia following anesthesia (T88.51)

malignant hyperpyrexia due to anesthesia (T88.3)

T81.89X `7th` **Other complications of procedures, NEC**

Use additional code to specify complication, such as: postprocedural delirium (F05)

T81.9XX `7th` **Unspecified complication of procedure**

T82 `4th` **COMPLICATIONS OF CARDIAC AND VASCULAR PROSTHETIC DEVICES, IMPLANTS AND GRAFTS**

Excludes2: failure and rejection of transplanted organs and tissue (T86.-)

T82.7XX `7th` **Infection and inflammatory reaction due to other cardiac and vascular devices, implants and grafts**

Use additional code to identify infection

T82.8 `5th` **Other specified complications of cardiac and vascular prosthetic devices, implants and grafts**

T82.84 `6th` **Pain due to cardiac and vascular prosthetic devices, implants and grafts**

T82.847 `7th` **Pain due to cardiac prosthetic devices, implants and grafts**

T82.848 `7th` **Pain due to vascular prosthetic devices, implants and grafts**

T82.89 `6th` **Other specified complication of cardiac and vascular prosthetic devices, implants and grafts**

T82.897 `7th` **Other specified complication of cardiac prosthetic devices, implants and grafts**

T82.898 `7th` **Other specified complication of vascular prosthetic devices, implants and grafts**

`4th` `5th` `6th` `7th` Additional Character Required   ✔ 3-character code   Unspecified laterality codes were excluded here.

• =New Code
▲ =Revised Code
� =Social determinants of health

Excludes1—Not coded here, do not use together
Excludes2—Not included here

T82.9XX `7th` **Unspecified complication of cardiac and vascular prosthetic device, implant and graft**

T83 `4th` **COMPLICATIONS OF GENITOURINARY PROSTHETIC DEVICES, IMPLANTS AND GRAFTS**

Excludes2: failure and rejection of transplanted organs and tissue (T86.-)

T83.0 **Mechanical complication of urinary catheter**

`5th` **T83.09** `6th` **Other mechanical complication of urinary catheter**

Obstruction (mechanical) of urinary catheter
Perforation of urinary catheter
Protrusion of urinary catheter

T83.090 `7th` **Other mechanical complication of cystostomy catheter**

T83.091 `7th` **Other mechanical complication of indwelling urethral catheter**

> 7th characters for categories
> T81–T86
> A—initial encounter
> D—subsequent encounter
> S—sequela

T83.098 `7th` **Other mechanical complication of other urinary catheter**

Other mechanical complication of Hopkins catheter
Other mechanical complication of ileostomy catheter
Other mechanical complication of urostomy catheter

T83.5 `5th` **Infection and inflammatory reaction due to prosthetic device, implant and graft in urinary system**

Use additional code to identify infection

T83.51 `6th` **Infection and inflammatory reaction due to urinary catheter**

Excludes2: complications of stoma of urinary tract (N99.5-)

T83.510 `7th` **Infection and inflammatory reaction due to cystostomy catheter**

T83.511 `7th` **Infection and inflammatory reaction due to indwelling urethral catheter**

T83.512 `7th` **Infection and inflammatory reaction due to nephrostomy catheter**

T83.518 `7th` **Infection and inflammatory reaction due to other urinary catheter**

Infection and inflammatory reaction due to Hopkins catheter or ileostomy catheter or urostomy catheter

T83.59 `6th` **Infection and inflammatory reaction due to prosthetic device, implant and graft in urinary system**

T83.591 `7th` **Infection and inflammatory reaction due to implanted urinary sphincter**

T83.593 `7th` **Infection and inflammatory reaction due to other urinary stents**

Infection and inflammatory reaction due to ileal conduit stents
Infection and inflammatory reaction due to nephroureteral stent

T83.598 `7th` **Infection and inflammatory reaction due to other prosthetic device, implant and graft in urinary system**

T83.9XX `7th` **Unspecified complication of genitourinary prosthetic device, implant and graft**

T85 `4th` **COMPLICATIONS OF OTHER INTERNAL PROSTHETIC DEVICES, IMPLANTS AND GRAFTS**

Excludes2: failure and rejection of transplanted organs and tissue (T86.-)

T85.0 `5th` **Mechanical complication of ventricular intracranial (communicating) shunt**

T85.01X `7th` **Breakdown (mechanical) of ventricular intracranial (communicating) shunt**

T85.02X `7th` **Displacement of ventricular intracranial (communicating) shunt**

Malposition of ventricular intracranial (communicating) shunt

T85.03X `7th` **Leakage of ventricular intracranial (communicating) shunt**

T85.09X `7th` **Other mechanical complication of ventricular intracranial (communicating) shunt**

Obstruction (mechanical) of ventricular intracranial (communicating) shunt
Perforation of ventricular intracranial (communicating) shunt
Protrusion of ventricular intracranial (communicating) shunt

T85.6 `5th` **Mechanical complication of other specified internal and external prosthetic devices, implants and grafts**

T85.62 `6th` **Displacement of other specified internal prosthetic devices, implants and grafts**

Malposition of other specified internal prosthetic devices, implants and grafts

T85.624 **Displacement of insulin pump**

T85.628 **Displacement of other specified internal prosthetic devices, implants and grafts**

T85.69 `6th` **Other mechanical complication of other specified internal prosthetic devices, implants and grafts**

Obstruction, mechanical of other specified internal prosthetic devices, implants and grafts
Perforation of other specified internal prosthetic devices, implants and grafts
Protrusion of other specified internal prosthetic devices, implants and grafts

T85.694 `7th` **Other mechanical complication of insulin pump**

T85.695 `7th` **Other mechanical complication of other nervous system device, implant or graft**

Other mechanical complication of intrathecal infusion pump

T85.698 `7th` **Other mechanical complication of other specified internal prosthetic devices, implant and grafts**

Mechanical complication of nonabsorbable surgical material NOS

T85.7 `5th` **Infection and inflammatory reaction due to other internal prosthetic devices, implants and grafts**

Use additional code to identify infection

T85.79X `7th` **Infection and inflammatory reaction due to other internal prosthetic devices, implants and grafts**

T86 `4th` **COMPLICATIONS OF TRANSPLANTED ORGANS AND TISSUE**

Codes under category T86, Complications of transplanted organs and tissues, are for use for both complications and rejection of transplanted organs. A transplant complication code is only assigned if the complication affects the function of the transplanted organ. Two codes are required to fully describe a transplant complication: the appropriate code from category T86 and a secondary code that identifies the complication.

Pre-existing conditions or conditions that develop after the transplant are not coded as complications unless they affect the function of the transplanted organs.

See I.C.21 for transplant organ removal status

See I.C.2 for malignant neoplasm associated with transplanted organ.

Use additional code to identify other transplant complications, such as:
graft-versus-host disease (D89.81-)
malignancy associated with organ transplant (C80.2)
post-transplant lymphoproliferative disorders (PTLD) (D47.Z1)

T86.0 **Complications of bone marrow transplant**

`5th` **T86.01X** `7th` **Bone marrow transplant rejection**

T86.02X `7th` **Bone marrow transplant failure**

T86.1 `5th` **Complications of kidney transplant**

Patients who have undergone kidney transplant may still have some form of CKD because the kidney transplant may not fully restore kidney function. Code T86.1- should be assigned for documented complications of a kidney transplant, such as transplant failure or rejection or other transplant complication. Code T86.1- should not be assigned for post kidney transplant patients who have CKD unless a transplant complication such as transplant failure or rejection is documented. If the

---

`4th` `5th` `6th` `7th` Additional Character Required   ✓ 3-character code   Unspecified laterality codes were excluded here.

• =New Code
▲ =Revised Code
▫ =Social determinants of health

Excludes1—Not coded here, do not use together
Excludes2—Not included here

CHAPTER 19. INJURY, POISONING AND CERTAIN OTHER CONSEQUENCES OF EXTERNAL CAUSES (T86.10X–T88.9XX)

documentation is unclear as to whether the patient has a complication of the transplant, query the provider.

Conditions that affect the function of the transplanted kidney, other than CKD, should be assigned a code from subcategory T86.1, Complications of transplanted organ, kidney, and a secondary code that identifies the complication.

For patients with CKD following a kidney transplant, but who do not have a complication such as failure or rejection, see section I.C.14 CKD and kidney transplant status.

T86.10X **Unspecified complication of kidney transplant**
7th

T86.11X **Kidney transplant rejection**
7th

T86.12X **Kidney transplant failure**
7th

T86.13X **Kidney transplant infection**
7th
Use additional code to specify infection

T86.19X **Other complication of kidney transplant**
7th

> 7th characters for categories
> T81–T86
> A—initial encounter
> D—subsequent encounter
> S—sequela

T86.2 **Complications of heart transplant**
5th
Excludes1: complication of:
artificial heart device (T82.5-)
heart-lung transplant (T86.3-)

T86.21X **Heart transplant rejection**
7th

T86.22X **Heart transplant failure**
7th

T86.29 **Other complications of heart transplant**
6th

T86.290 **Cardiac allograft vasculopathy**
7th
Excludes1: atherosclerosis of coronary arteries (I25.75-, I25.76-, I25.81-)

T86.298 **Other complications of heart transplant**
7th

T86.3 **Complications of heart-lung transplant**
5th

T86.30X **Unspecified complication of heart-lung transplant**
7th

T86.31X **Heart-lung transplant rejection**
7th

T86.32X **Heart-lung transplant failure**
7th

T86.33X **Heart-lung transplant infection**
7th
Use additional code to specify infection

T86.39X **Other complications of heart-lung transplant**
7th

T86.4 **Complications of liver transplant**
5th

T86.41X **Liver transplant rejection**
7th

T86.42X **Liver transplant failure**
7th

T86.5XX **Complications of stem cell transplant**
7th
Complications from stem cells from peripheral blood
Complications from stem cells from umbilical cord

T86.8 **Complications of other transplanted organs and tissues**
5th

T86.81 **Complications of lung transplant**
6th
Excludes1: complication of heart-lung transplant (T86.3-)

T86.810 **Lung transplant rejection**
7th

T86.811 **Lung transplant failure**
7th

T86.9 **Complication of unspecified transplanted organ and tissue**
5th

T86.90X **Unspecified complication of unspecified transplanted organ and tissue**
7th

T88 **OTHER COMPLICATIONS OF SURGICAL AND MEDICAL CARE, NEC**
4th
Excludes2: complication following infusion, transfusion and therapeutic injection (T80.-)
complication following procedure NEC (T81.-)
complications of anesthesia in labor and delivery (O74.-)
complications of anesthesia in pregnancy (O29.-)
complications of anesthesia in puerperium (O89.-)
complications of devices, implants and grafts (T82–T85)
complications of obstetric surgery and procedure (O75.4)
dermatitis due to drugs and medicaments (L23.3, L24.4, L25.1, L27.0–L27.1)
poisoning and toxic effects of drugs and chemicals (T36–T65 with fifth or sixth character 1–4 or 6)
specified complications classified elsewhere

T88.0XX **Infection following immunization**
7th
Sepsis following immunization

T88.1XX **Other complications following immunization, NEC**
7th
Generalized vaccinia
Rash following immunization
Excludes1: vaccinia not from vaccine (B08.011)
Excludes2: anaphylactic shock due to serum (T80.5-)
other serum reactions (T80.6-)
postimmunization arthropathy (M02.2)
postimmunization encephalitis (G04.02)
postimmunization fever (R50.83)
Use additional code to identify the complication

T88.6XX **Anaphylactic reaction due to adverse effect of correct drug or medicament properly administered**
7th
Anaphylactic shock due to adverse effect of correct drug or medicament properly administered
Anaphylactoid reaction NOS
Use additional code for adverse effect, if applicable, to identify drug (T36–T50 with fifth or sixth character 5)
Excludes1: anaphylactic reaction due to serum (T80.5-)
anaphylactic shock or reaction due to adverse food reaction (T78.0-)

T88.7XX **Unspecified adverse effect of drug or medicament**
7th
Drug hypersensitivity NOS
Drug reaction NOS
Use additional code for adverse effect, if applicable, to identify drug (T36–T50 with fifth or sixth character 5)
Excludes1: specified adverse effects of drugs and medicaments (A00–R94 and T80–T88.6, T88.8)

T88.8XX **Other specified complications of surgical and medical care, NEC**
7th

T88.9XX **Complication of surgical and medical care, unspecified**
7th

  4th 5th 6th 7th Additional Character Required ✔ 3-character code | Unspecified laterality codes were excluded here. | • =New Code ▲ =Revised Code ▫ =Social determinants of health | *Excludes1*—Not coded here, do not use together *Excludes2*—Not included here

Chapter 20. External causes of morbidity (V00–Y99)

The external causes of morbidity codes should never be sequenced as the first-listed or principal diagnosis.

External cause codes are intended to provide data for injury research and evaluation of injury prevention strategies. These codes capture how the injury or health condition happened (cause), the intent (unintentional or accidental; or intentional, such as suicide or assault), the place where the event occurred, the activity of the patient at the time of the event, and the person's status (eg, civilian, military).

There is no national requirement for mandatory *ICD-10-CM* external cause code reporting. Unless a provider is subject to a state-based external cause code reporting mandate or these codes are required by a particular payer, reporting of *ICD-10-CM* codes in Chapter 20, External Causes of Morbidity, is not required. In the absence of a mandatory reporting requirement, providers are encouraged to voluntarily report external cause codes, as they provide valuable data for injury research and evaluation of injury prevention strategies.

General External Cause Coding Guidelines

USED WITH ANY CODE IN THE RANGE OF A00.0–T88.9, Z00–Z99
An external cause code may be used with any code in the range of A00.0–T88.9, Z00–Z99, classification that **represents** a health condition due to an external cause. Though they are most applicable to injuries, they are also valid for use with such things as infections or diseases due to an external source, and other health conditions, such as a heart attack that occurs during strenuous physical activity.

EXTERNAL CAUSE CODE USED FOR LENGTH OF TREATMENT
Assign the external cause code, with the appropriate 7th character (initial encounter, subsequent encounter or sequela) for each encounter for which the injury or condition is being treated.

Most categories in Chapter 20 have a 7th character requirement for each applicable code. Most categories in this chapter have three 7th character values: A, initial encounter, D, subsequent encounter and S, sequela. While the patient may be seen by a new or different provider over the course of treatment for an injury or condition, assignment of the 7th character for external cause should match the 7th character of the code assigned for the associated injury or condition for the encounter.

USE THE FULL RANGE OF EXTERNAL CAUSE CODES
Use the full range of external cause codes to completely describe the cause, the intent, the place of occurrence, and if applicable, the activity of the patient at the time of the event, and the patient's status, for all injuries, and other health conditions due to an external cause.

ASSIGN AS MANY EXTERNAL CAUSE CODES AS NECESSARY
Assign as many external cause codes as necessary to fully explain each cause. If only one external code can be recorded, assign the code most related to the principal diagnosis.

THE SELECTION OF THE APPROPRIATE EXTERNAL CAUSE CODE
The selection of the appropriate external cause code is guided by the Alphabetic Index of External Causes and by Inclusion and Exclusion notes in the Tabular List.

EXTERNAL CAUSE CODE CAN NEVER BE A PRINCIPAL DIAGNOSIS
An external cause code can never be a principal (first-listed) diagnosis.

COMBINATION EXTERNAL CAUSE CODES
Certain of the external cause codes are combination codes that identify sequential events that result in an injury, such as a fall which results in striking against an object. The injury may be due to either event or both. The combination external cause code used should correspond to the sequence of events regardless of which caused the most serious injury.

NO EXTERNAL CAUSE CODE NEEDED IN CERTAIN CIRCUMSTANCES
No external cause code from Chapter 20 is needed if the external cause and intent are included in a code from another chapter (eg, T36.0X1- Poisoning by penicillins, accidental (unintentional)).

Place of Occurrence Guideline
Refer to category Y92.

Activity Code
Refer to category Y93.

Place of Occurrence, Activity, and Status Codes Used with other External Cause Code
When applicable, place of occurrence, activity, and external cause status codes are sequenced after the main external cause code(s). Regardless of the number of external cause codes assigned, there should be only one place of occurrence code, one activity code, and one external cause status code assigned to an encounter.

If the Reporting Format Limits the Number of External Cause Codes
If the reporting format limits the number of external cause codes that can be used in reporting clinical data, report the code for the cause/intent most related to the principal diagnosis. If the format permits capture of additional external cause codes, the cause/intent, including medical misadventures, of the additional events should be reported rather than the codes for place, activity, or external status.

Multiple External Cause Coding Guidelines
More than one external cause code is required to fully describe the external cause of an illness or injury. The assignment of external cause codes should be sequenced in the following priority:

If two or more events cause separate injuries, an external cause code should be assigned for each cause. The first-listed external cause code will be selected in the following order:

External codes for child and adult abuse take priority over all other external cause codes.

See Chapter 19, Child and Adult abuse guidelines.

External cause codes for terrorism events take priority over all other external cause codes except child and adult abuse.

External cause codes for cataclysmic events take priority over all other external cause codes except child and adult abuse and terrorism.

External cause codes for transport accidents take priority over all other external cause codes except cataclysmic events, child and adult abuse and terrorism.

Activity and external cause status codes are assigned following all causal (intent) external cause codes.

The first-listed external cause code should correspond to the cause of the most serious diagnosis due to an assault, accident, or self-harm, following the order of hierarchy listed above.

Child and Adult Abuse Guideline
Refer to category Y07.

Unknown or Undetermined Intent Guideline
If the intent (accident, self-harm, assault) of the cause of an injury or other condition is unknown or unspecified, code the intent as accidental intent. All transport accident categories assume accidental intent.

USE OF UNDETERMINED INTENT
External cause codes for events of undetermined intent are only for use if the documentation in the record specifies that the intent cannot be determined.

Sequelae (Late Effects) of External Cause Guidelines

SEQUELAE EXTERNAL CAUSE CODES
Sequelae are reported using the external cause code with the 7th character "S" for sequela. These codes should be used with any report of a late effect or sequela resulting from a previous injury.

SEQUELA EXTERNAL CAUSE CODE WITH A RELATED CURRENT INJURY
A sequela external cause code should never be used with a related current nature of injury code.

USE OF SEQUELA EXTERNAL CAUSE CODES FOR SUBSEQUENT VISITS
Use a late effect external cause code for subsequent visits when a late effect of the initial injury is being treated. Do not use a late effect external cause code for subsequent visits for follow-up care (eg, to assess healing, to receive rehabilitative therapy) of the injury when no late effect of the injury has been documented.

4th 5th 6th 7th Additional Character Required   ✓ 3-character code

•=New Code   **Excludes1**—Not coded here, do not use together
▲=Revised Code   **Excludes2**—Not included here

CHAPTER 20. EXTERNAL CAUSES OF MORBIDITY   (V00–V00.188)

Terrorism Guidelines (See *ICD-10-CM* manual for full guidelines.)

Cause of injury identified by the Federal Government (FBI) as terrorism
Cause of an injury is suspected to be the result of terrorism Code Y38.9, Terrorism, secondary effects

External cause status

Refer to category Y99.

Note: This chapter permits the classification of environmental events and circumstances as the cause of injury, and other adverse effects. Where a code from this section is applicable, it is intended that it shall be used secondary to a code from another chapter of the Classification indicating the nature of the condition. Most often, the condition will be classifiable to Chapter 19, Injury, poisoning and certain other consequences of external causes (S00–T88). Other conditions that may be stated to be due to external causes are classified in Chapters 1 to 18. For these conditions, codes from Chapter 20 should be used to provide additional information as to the cause of the condition.

ACCIDENTS (V00–X58)

(V00–V99) TRANSPORT ACCIDENTS

Note: This section is structured in 12 groups. Those relating to land transport accidents (V01–V89) reflect the victim's mode of transport and are subdivided to identify the victim's 'counterpart' or the type of event. The vehicle of which the injured person is an occupant is identified in the first two characters since it is seen as the most important factor to identify for prevention purposes. A transport accident is one in which the vehicle involved must be moving or running or in use for transport purposes at the time of the accident.

Use additional code to identify:
    Airbag injury (W22.1)
    Type of street or road (Y92.4-)
    Use of cellular telephone and other electronic equipment at the time of the transport accident (Y93.C-)

Excludes1: agricultural vehicles in stationary use or maintenance (W31.-)
    assault by crashing of motor vehicle (Y03.-)
    automobile or motor cycle in stationary use or maintenance- code to type of accident
    crashing of motor vehicle, undetermined intent (Y32)
    intentional self-harm by crashing of motor vehicle (X82)

Excludes2: transport accidents due to cataclysm (X34–X38)
    A traffic accident is any vehicle accident occurring on the public highway [ie, originating on, terminating on, or involving a vehicle partially on the highway]. A vehicle accident is assumed to have occurred on the public highway unless another place is specified, except in the case of accidents involving only off-road motor vehicles, which are classified as nontraffic accidents unless the contrary is stated.
    A nontraffic accident is any vehicle accident that occurs entirely in any place other than a public highway. Please see full *ICD-10-CM* manual for definitions of transport vehicles.

(V00–V09) PEDESTRIAN INJURED IN TRANSPORT ACCIDENT

Includes: person changing tire on transport vehicle
    person examining engine of vehicle broken down in (on side of) road
Excludes1: fall due to non-transport collision with other person (W03)
    pedestrian on foot falling (slipping) on ice and snow (W00.-)
    struck or bumped by another person (W51)

V00 **PEDESTRIAN CONVEYANCE ACCIDENT**
[4th]
    Use additional place of occurrence and activity external cause codes, if known (Y92.-, Y93.-)
    Excludes1: collision with another person without fall (W51)
        fall due to person on foot colliding with another person on foot (W03)
        fall from non-moving wheelchair, nonmotorized scooter and motorized mobility scooter without collision (W05.-)
        pedestrian (conveyance) collision with other land transport vehicle (V01–V09)
        pedestrian on foot falling (slipping) on ice and snow (W00.-)

> **7th characters for category V00**
> A—initial encounter
> D—subsequent encounter
> S—sequela

V00.0 **Pedestrian on foot injured in collision with pedestrian conveyance**
[5th]
    V00.01X Pedestrian on foot injured in collision with roller-skater
    [7th]
    V00.02X Pedestrian on foot injured in collision with skateboarder
    [7th]
    V00.031 Pedestrian on foot injured in collision with rider of standing electric scooter
    [7th]
    V00.038 Pedestrian on foot injured in collision with rider of other standing micro-mobility pedestrian conveyance
    [7th]
    V00.09X Pedestrian on foot injured in collision with other pedestrian conveyance
    [7th]

V00.1 **Rolling-type pedestrian conveyance accident**
[5th]
    Excludes1: accident with baby stroller (V00.82-)
        accident with wheelchair (powered) (V00.81-)
        accident with motorized mobility scooter (V00.83-)
    V00.11 **In-line roller-skate accident**
    [6th]   **V00.111** Fall from in-line roller-skates
      [7th]
      V00.112 In-line roller-skater colliding with stationary object
      [7th]
      V00.118 Other in-line roller-skate accident
      [7th]   **Excludes1:** roller-skater collision with other land transport vehicle (V01–V09 with 5th character 1)
    V00.12 **Non–in-line roller-skate accident**
    [6th]   **V00.121** Fall from non–in-line roller-skates
      [7th]
      V00.122 Non–in-line roller-skater colliding with stationary object
      [7th]
      V00.128 Other non–in-line roller-skating accident
      [7th]   **Excludes1:** roller-skater collision with other land transport vehicle (V01–V09 with 5th character 1)
    V00.13 **Skateboard accident**
    [6th]   **V00.131** Fall from skateboard
      [7th]
      V00.132 Skateboarder colliding with stationary object
      [7th]
      V00.138 Other skateboard accident
      [7th]   **Excludes1:** skateboarder collision with other land transport vehicle (V01–V09 with 5th character 2)
    V00.14 **Scooter (nonmotorized) accident**
    [6th]   **Excludes1:** motorscooter accident (V20–V29)
      V00.141 Fall from scooter (nonmotorized)
      [7th]
      V00.142 Scooter (nonmotorized) colliding with stationary object
      [7th]
      V00.148 Other scooter (nonmotorized) accident
      [7th]   **Excludes1:** scooter (nonmotorized) collision with other land transport vehicle (V01–V09 with fifth character 9)
    V00.15 **Heelies accident**
    [6th]   Rolling shoe
      Wheeled shoe
      Wheelies accident
      V00.151 Fall from heelies
      [7th]
      V00.152 Heelies colliding with stationary object
      [7th]
      V00.158 Other heelies accident
      [7th]
    V00.18 **Accident on other rolling-type pedestrian conveyance**
    [6th]   **V00.181** Fall from other rolling-type pedestrian conveyance
      [7th]
      V00.182 Pedestrian on other rolling-type pedestrian conveyance colliding with stationary object
      [7th]
      V00.188 Other accident on other rolling-type pedestrian conveyance
      [7th]

[4th] [5th] [6th] [7th]   Additional Character Required   ✓ 3-character code

•=New Code   **Excludes1**—Not coded here, do not use together
▲=Revised Code   **Excludes2**—Not included here

V00.2 **Gliding-type pedestrian conveyance accident**
`5th`
    V00.21 **Ice-skates accident**
    `6th`

7th characters for categories V00 and V01
A—initial encounter
D—subsequent encounter
S—sequela

        V00.211 **Fall from ice-skates**
        `7th`
        V00.212 **Ice-skater colliding with stationary object**
        `7th`
        V00.218 **Other ice-skates accident**
        `7th`
            Excludes1: ice-skater collision with other land transport vehicle (V01–V09 with 5th character 9)

    V00.22 **Sled accident**
    `6th`
        V00.221 **Fall from sled**
        `7th`
        V00.222 **Sledder colliding with stationary object**
        `7th`
        V00.228 **Other sled accident**
        `7th`
            Excludes1: sled collision with other land transport vehicle (V01–V09 with 5th character 9)

V00.3 **Flat-bottomed pedestrian conveyance accident**
`5th`
    V00.31 **Snowboard accident**
    `6th`
        V00.311 **Fall from snowboard**
        `7th`
        V00.312 **Snowboarder colliding with stationary object**
        `7th`
        V00.318 **Other snowboard accident**
        `7th`
            Excludes1: snowboarder collision with other land transport vehicle (V01–V09 with 5th character 9)

    V00.32 **Snow-ski accident**
    `6th`
        V00.321 **Fall from snow-skis**
        `7th`
        V00.322 **Snow-skier colliding with stationary object**
        `7th`
        V00.328 **Other snow-ski accident**
        `7th`
            Excludes1: snow-skier collision with other land transport vehicle (V01–V09 with 5th character 9)

    V00.38 **Other flat-bottomed pedestrian conveyance accident**
    `6th`
        V00.381 **Fall from other flat-bottomed pedestrian conveyance**
        `7th`
        V00.382 **Pedestrian on other flat-bottomed pedestrian conveyance colliding with stationary object**
        `7th`
        V00.388 **Other accident on other flat-bottomed pedestrian conveyance**
        `7th`

V00.8 **Accident on other pedestrian conveyance**
`5th`
    V00.81 **Accident with wheelchair (powered)**
    `6th`
        V00.811 **Fall from moving wheelchair (powered)**
        `7th`
            Excludes1: fall from non-moving wheelchair (W05.0)
        V00.812 **Wheelchair (powered) colliding with stationary object**
        `7th`
        V00.818 **Other accident with wheelchair (powered)**
        `7th`

    V00.82 **Accident with baby stroller**
    `6th`
        V00.821 **Fall from baby stroller**
        `7th`
        V00.822 **Baby stroller colliding with stationary object**
        `7th`
        V00.828 **Other accident with baby stroller**
        `7th`

    V00.84 **Accident with standing micro-mobility pedestrian conveyance**
    `6th`
        V00.841 **Fall from standing electric scooter**
        `7th`
        V00.842 **Pedestrian on standing electric scooter colliding with stationary object**
        `7th`
        V00.848 **Other accident with standing micro-mobility pedestrian conveyance**
        `7th`
            Accident with hoverboard
            Accident with segway

    V00.89 **Accident on other pedestrian conveyance**
    `6th`
        V00.891 **Fall from other pedestrian conveyance**
        `7th`
        V00.892 **Pedestrian on other pedestrian conveyance colliding with stationary object**
        `7th`
        V00.898 **Other accident on other pedestrian conveyance**
        `7th`
            Excludes1: other pedestrian (conveyance) collision with other land transport vehicle (V01–V09 with 5th character 9)

V01 **PEDESTRIAN INJURED IN COLLISION WITH PEDAL CYCLE**
`4th`
    V01.0 **Pedestrian injured in collision with pedal cycle in nontraffic accident**
    `5th`
        V01.00X **Pedestrian on foot injured in collision with pedal cycle in nontraffic accident**
        `7th`
            Pedestrian NOS injured in collision with pedal cycle in nontraffic accident
        V01.01X **Pedestrian on roller-skates injured in collision with pedal cycle in nontraffic accident**
        `7th`
        V01.02X **Pedestrian on skateboard injured in collision with pedal cycle in nontraffic accident**
        `7th`
        V01.03 **Pedestrian on standing micro-mobility pedestrian conveyance injured in collision with pedal cycle in nontraffic accident**
        `6th`
            V01.031 **Pedestrian on standing electric scooter injured in collision with pedal cycle in nontraffic accident**
            `7th`
            V01.038 **Pedestrian on other standing micro-mobility pedestrian conveyance injured in collision with pedal cycle in nontraffic accident**
            `7th`
                Pedestrian on hoverboard injured in collision with pedal cycle in nontraffic accident
                Pedestrian on segway injured in collision with pedal cycle in nontraffic accident
        V01.09X **Pedestrian with other conveyance injured in collision with pedal cycle in nontraffic accident**
        `7th`
            Pedestrian with baby stroller injured in collision with pedal cycle in nontraffic accident
            Pedestrian on ice-skates or nonmotorized scooter or motorized mobility scooter or sled or snowboard or snow-skis or wheelchair (powered) injured in collision with pedal cycle in nontraffic accident

    V01.1 **Pedestrian injured in collision with pedal cycle in traffic accident**
    `5th`
        V01.10X **Pedestrian on foot injured in collision with pedal cycle in traffic accident**
        `7th`
            Pedestrian NOS injured in collision with pedal cycle in traffic accident
        V01.11X **Pedestrian on roller-skates injured in collision with pedal cycle in traffic accident**
        `7th`
        V01.12X **Pedestrian on skateboard injured in collision with pedal cycle in traffic accident**
        `7th`
        V01.13 **Pedestrian on standing micro-mobility pedestrian conveyance injured in collision with pedal cycle in traffic accident**
        `6th`
            V01.131 **Pedestrian on standing electric scooter injured in collision with pedal cycle in traffic accident**
            `7th`
            V01.138 **Pedestrian on other standing micro-mobility pedestrian conveyance injured in collision with pedal cycle in traffic accident**
            `7th`
        V01.19X **Pedestrian with other conveyance injured in collision with pedal cycle in traffic accident**
        `7th`
            Pedestrian with baby stroller injured in collision with pedal cycle in traffic accident
            Pedestrian on ice-skates or nonmotorized scooter or motorized mobility scooter or sled or snowboard or snow-ski or wheelchair (powered) injured in collision with pedal cycle in traffic accident

---

`4th` `5th` `6th` `7th` Additional Character Required   ✔ 3-character code   •=New Code   ▲=Revised Code   *Excludes1*—Not coded here, do not use together   *Excludes2*—Not included here

CHAPTER 20. EXTERNAL CAUSES OF MORBIDITY   (V01.9–V04.02X)

V01.9 `5th` **Pedestrian injured in collision with pedal cycle, unspecified whether traffic or nontraffic accident**

     V01.90X `7th` **Pedestrian on foot injured in collision with pedal cycle, unspecified whether traffic or nontraffic accident**
       Pedestrian NOS injured in collision with pedal cycle, unspecified whether traffic or nontraffic accident

     V01.91X `7th` **Pedestrian on roller-skates injured in collision with pedal cycle, unspecified whether traffic or nontraffic accident**

     V01.92X `7th` **Pedestrian on skateboard injured in collision with pedal cycle, unspecified whether traffic or nontraffic accident**

     V01.93 `6th` **Pedestrian on standing micro-mobility pedestrian conveyance injured in collision with pedal cycle, unspecified whether traffic or nontraffic accident**

> 7th characters for categories
> V01–V04
> A—initial encounter
> D—subsequent encounter
> S—sequela

       V01.931 `7th` **Pedestrian on standing electric scooter injured in collision with pedal cycle, unspecified whether traffic or nontraffic accident**

       V01.938 `7th` **Pedestrian on other standing micro-mobility pedestrian conveyance injured in collision with pedal cycle, unspecified whether traffic or nontraffic accident**
         Pedestrian on hoverboard or segway injured in collision with pedal cycle, unspecified whether traffic or nontraffic accident

     V01.99X `7th` **Pedestrian with other conveyance injured in collision with pedal cycle, unspecified whether traffic or nontraffic accident**
       Includes: Pedestrian with baby stroller, on ice-skates or nonmotorized scooter or motorized mobility scooter or sled or snowboard or snow-skis or wheelchair (powered) injured in collision with pedal cycle unspecified, whether traffic or nontraffic accident

V02 `4th` **PEDESTRIAN INJURED IN COLLISION WITH TWO- OR THREE-WHEELED MOTOR VEHICLE**
Refer to the External Cause of Injuries Table

V03 `4th` **PEDESTRIAN INJURED IN COLLISION WITH CAR, PICK-UP TRUCK OR VAN**

   V03.0 `5th` **Pedestrian injured in collision with car, pick-up truck or van in nontraffic accident**

     V03.00X `7th` **Pedestrian on foot injured in collision with car, pick-up truck or van in nontraffic accident**
       Pedestrian NOS injured in collision with car, pick-up truck or van in nontraffic accident

     V03.01X `7th` **Pedestrian on roller-skates injured in collision with car, pick-up truck or van in nontraffic accident**

     V03.02X `7th` **Pedestrian on skateboard injured in collision with car, pick-up truck or van in nontraffic accident**

     V03.03 `6th` **Pedestrian on standing micro-mobility pedestrian conveyance injured in collision with car, pick-up or van in nontraffic accident**

       V03.031 `7th` **Pedestrian on standing electric scooter injured in collision with car, pick-up or van in nontraffic accident**

       V03.038 `7th` **Pedestrian on other standing micro-mobility pedestrian conveyance injured in collision with car, pick-up or van in nontraffic accident**

     V03.09X `7th` **Pedestrian with other conveyance injured in collision with car, pick-up truck or van in nontraffic accident**
       Includes: Pedestrian with baby stroller or on ice-skates or nonmotorized scooter or motorized mobility scooter or sled or snowboard or snow-skis or wheelchair (powered) injured

   V03.1 `5th` **Pedestrian injured in collision with car, pick-up truck or van in traffic accident**

     V03.10X `7th` **Pedestrian on foot injured in collision with car, pick-up truck or van in traffic accident**
       Pedestrian NOS injured in collision with car, pick-up truck or van in traffic accident

     V03.11X `7th` **Pedestrian on roller-skates injured in collision with car, pick-up truck or van in traffic accident**

     V03.12X `7th` **Pedestrian on skateboard injured in collision with car, pick-up truck or van in traffic accident**

     V03.13 `6th` **Pedestrian on standing micro-mobility pedestrian conveyance injured in collision with car, pick-up or van in traffic accident**

       V03.131 `7th` **Pedestrian on standing electric scooter injured in collision with car, pick-up or van in traffic accident**

       V03.138 `7th` **Pedestrian on other standing micro-mobility pedestrian conveyance injured in collision with car, pick-up or van in traffic accident**
         Includes: Pedestrian on hoverboard or segway injured

     V03.19X `7th` **Pedestrian with other conveyance injured in collision with car, pick-up truck or van in traffic accident**
       Pedestrian with baby stroller or on ice-skates or nonmotorized scooter or motorized mobility scooter or sled or snowboard or snow-skis or wheelchair (powered) injured in collision with car, pick-up truck or van in traffic accident

   V03.9 `5th` **Pedestrian injured in collision with car, pick-up truck or van, unspecified whether traffic or nontraffic accident**

     V03.90X `7th` **Pedestrian on foot injured in collision with car, pick-up truck or van, unspecified whether traffic or nontraffic accident**
       Pedestrian NOS injured in collision with car, pick-up truck or van, unspecified whether traffic or nontraffic accident

     V03.91X `7th` **Pedestrian on roller-skates injured in collision with car, pick-up truck or van, unspecified whether traffic or nontraffic accident**

     V03.92X `7th` **Pedestrian on skateboard injured in collision with car, pick-up truck or van, unspecified whether traffic or nontraffic accident**

     V03.93 `6th` **Pedestrian on standing micro-mobility pedestrian conveyance injured in collision with car, pick-up or van, unspecified whether traffic or nontraffic accident**

       V03.931 `7th` **Pedestrian on standing electric scooter injured in collision with car, pick-up or van, unspecified whether traffic or nontraffic accident**

       V03.938 `7th` **Pedestrian on other standing micro-mobility pedestrian conveyance injured in collision with car, pick-up or van, unspecified whether traffic or nontraffic accident**
         Includes: Pedestrian on hoverboard or segway injured in collision

     V03.99 **Pedestrian with other conveyance injured in collision with car, pick-up truck or van, unspecified whether traffic or nontraffic accident**

V04 `4th` **PEDESTRIAN INJURED IN COLLISION WITH HEAVY TRANSPORT VEHICLE OR BUS**
Excludes1: pedestrian injured in collision with military vehicle (V09.01, V09.21). Refer to External Cause of Injuries Table

   V04.0 `5th` **Pedestrian injured in collision with heavy transport vehicle or bus in nontraffic accident**

     V04.00X `7th` **Pedestrian on foot injured in collision with heavy transport vehicle or bus in nontraffic accident**
       Pedestrian NOS injured in collision with heavy transport vehicle or bus in nontraffic accident

     V04.01X `7th` **Pedestrian on roller-skates injured in collision with heavy transport vehicle or bus in nontraffic accident**

     V04.02X `7th` **Pedestrian on skateboard injured in collision with heavy transport vehicle or bus in nontraffic accident**

`4th` `5th` `6th` `7th` Additional Character Required   ✓ 3-character code

•=New Code
▲=Revised Code

Excludes1—Not coded here, do not use together
Excludes2—Not included here

V04.03 Pedestrian on standing micro-mobility pedestrian conveyance injured in collision with heavy transport vehicle or bus in nontraffic accident
6th

V04.031 Pedestrian on standing electric scooter injured in collision with heavy transport vehicle or bus in nontraffic accident
7th

V04.038 Pedestrian on other standing micro-mobility pedestrian conveyance injured in collision with heavy transport vehicle or bus in nontraffic accident
7th

Pedestrian on hoverboard or segway injured in collision with heavy transport vehicle or bus in nontraffic accident

V04.09X Pedestrian with other conveyance injured in collision with heavy transport vehicle or bus in nontraffic accident
7th

7th characters for categories V01–V04
A—initial encounter
D—subsequent encounter
S—sequela

Includes: Pedestrian with baby stroller or on ice-skates or nonmotorized scooter or motorized mobility scooter or sled or snowboard or snow-skis or wheelchair (powered) injured

V04.1 Pedestrian injured in collision with heavy transport vehicle or bus in traffic accident
5th

V04.10X Pedestrian on foot injured in collision with heavy transport vehicle or bus in traffic accident
7th

Pedestrian NOS injured in collision with heavy transport vehicle or bus in traffic accident

V04.11X Pedestrian on roller-skates injured in collision with heavy transport vehicle or bus in traffic accident
7th

V04.12X Pedestrian on skateboard injured in collision with heavy transport vehicle or bus in traffic accident
7th

V04.13 Pedestrian on standing micro-mobility pedestrian conveyance injured in collision with heavy transport vehicle or bus in traffic accident
6th

V04.131 Pedestrian on standing electric scooter injured in collision with heavy transport vehicle or bus in traffic accident
7th

V04.138 Pedestrian on other standing micro-mobility pedestrian conveyance injured in collision with heavy transport vehicle or bus in traffic accident
7th

Pedestrian on hoverboard or segway injured in collision with heavy transport vehicle or bus intraffic accident

V04.19X Pedestrian with other conveyance injured in collision with heavy transport vehicle or bus in traffic accident
7th

Includes: Pedestrian with baby stroller or on ice-skates or nonmotorized scooter or motorized mobility scooter or sled or snowboard or snow-skis or wheelchair (powered) injured

V04.9 Pedestrian injured in collision with heavy transport vehicle or bus, unspecified whether traffic or nontraffic accident
7th

Refer to External Cause of Injuries Table

V05 PEDESTRIAN INJURED IN COLLISION WITH RAILWAY TRAIN OR RAILWAY VEHICLE
7th

Refer to the External Cause of Injuries Table

V06 PEDESTRIAN INJURED IN COLLISION WITH OTHER NONMOTOR VEHICLE
7th

Includes: collision with animal-drawn vehicle, animal being ridden, nonpowered streetcar

Excludes1: pedestrian injured in collision with pedestrian conveyance (V00.0-)

Refer to External Cause of Injuries Table

V09 PEDESTRIAN INJURED IN OTHER AND UNSPECIFIED TRANSPORT ACCIDENTS
7th

Refer to External Cause of Injuries Table

(V10–V19) PEDAL CYCLE RIDER INJURED IN TRANSPORT ACCIDENT

Includes: any non-motorized vehicle, excluding an animal-drawn vehicle, or a sidecar or trailer attached to the pedal cycle

Excludes2: rupture of pedal cycle tire (W37.0)

7th characters for categories V10–V18
A—initial encounter
D—subsequent encounter
S—sequela

V10 PEDAL CYCLE RIDER INJURED IN COLLISION WITH PEDESTRIAN OR ANIMAL
4th

Excludes1: pedal cycle rider collision with animal-drawn vehicle or animal being ridden (V16.-)

V10.0XX Pedal cycle driver injured in collision with pedestrian or animal in nontraffic accident
7th

V10.1XX Pedal cycle passenger injured in collision with pedestrian or animal in nontraffic accident
7th

V10.2XX Unspecified pedal cyclist injured in collision with pedestrian or animal in nontraffic accident
7th

V10.3XX Person boarding or alighting a pedal cycle injured in collision with pedestrian or animal
7th

V10.4XX Pedal cycle driver injured in collision with pedestrian or animal in traffic accident
7th

V10.5XX Pedal cycle passenger injured in collision with pedestrian or animal in traffic accident
7th

V10.9XX Unspecified pedal cyclist injured in collision with pedestrian or animal in traffic accident
7th

V11 PEDAL CYCLE RIDER INJURED IN COLLISION WITH OTHER PEDAL CYCLE
4th

V11.0XX Pedal cycle driver injured in collision with other pedal cycle in nontraffic accident
7th

V11.1XX Pedal cycle passenger injured in collision with other pedal cycle in nontraffic accident
7th

V11.2XX Unspecified pedal cyclist injured in collision with other pedal cycle in nontraffic accident
7th

V11.3XX Person boarding or alighting a pedal cycle injured in collision with other pedal cycle
7th

V11.4XX Pedal cycle driver injured in collision with other pedal cycle in traffic accident
7th

V11.5XX Pedal cycle passenger injured in collision with other pedal cycle in traffic accident
7th

V11.9XX Unspecified pedal cyclist injured in collision with other pedal cycle in traffic accident
7th

V12 PEDAL CYCLE RIDER INJURED IN COLLISION WITH TWO- OR THREE-WHEELED MOTOR VEHICLE
7th

Refer to External Cause of Injuries Table

V13 PEDAL CYCLE RIDER INJURED IN COLLISION WITH CAR, PICK-UP TRUCK OR VAN
4th

V13.0XX Pedal cycle driver injured in collision with car, pick-up truck or van in nontraffic accident
7th

V13.1XX Pedal cycle passenger injured in collision with car, pick-up truck or van in nontraffic accident
7th

V13.2XX Unspecified pedal cyclist injured in collision with car, pick-up truck or van in nontraffic accident
7th

V13.3XX Person boarding or alighting a pedal cycle injured in collision with car, pick-up truck or van
7th

V13.4XX Pedal cycle driver injured in collision with car, pick-up truck or van in traffic accident
7th

V13.5XX Pedal cycle passenger injured in collision with car, pick-up truck or van in traffic accident
7th

V13.9XX Unspecified pedal cyclist injured in collision with car, pick-up truck or van in traffic accident
7th

V14 PEDAL CYCLE RIDER INJURED IN COLLISION WITH HEAVY TRANSPORT VEHICLE OR BUS
4th

Excludes1: pedal cycle rider injured in collision with military vehicle (V19.81)

V14.0XX Pedal cycle driver injured in collision with heavy transport vehicle or bus in nontraffic accident
7th

V14.1XX Pedal cycle passenger injured in collision with heavy transport vehicle or bus in nontraffic accident
7th

V14.2XX Unspecified pedal cyclist injured in collision with heavy transport vehicle or bus in nontraffic accident
7th

4th 5th 6th 7th Additional Character Required   ✓ 3-character code

•=New Code
▲=Revised Code

Excludes1—Not coded here, do not use together
Excludes2—Not included here

CHAPTER 20. EXTERNAL CAUSES OF MORBIDITY (V04.03–V14.2XX)

V14.3XX   Person boarding or alighting a pedal cycle injured in
7th   collision with heavy transport vehicle or bus
V14.4XX   Pedal cycle driver injured in collision with heavy transport
7th   vehicle or bus in traffic accident
V14.5XX   Pedal cycle passenger injured in collision with heavy
7th   transport vehicle or bus in traffic accident
V14.9XX   Unspecified pedal cyclist injured in collision with heavy
7th   transport vehicle or bus in traffic accident

V15   **PEDAL CYCLE RIDER INJURED IN COLLISION WITH**
4th   **RAILWAY TRAIN OR RAILWAY VEHICLE**
Refer to External Cause of Injuries Table

V16   **PEDAL CYCLE RIDER INJURED IN COLLISION WITH**
4th   **OTHER NONMOTOR VEHICLE**
Includes: collision with animal-drawn vehicle, animal being ridden,
streetcar
Refer to External Cause of Injuries Table

V17   **PEDAL CYCLE RIDER INJURED IN COLLISION WITH**
4th   **FIXED OR STATIONARY OBJECT**
V17.0XX   Pedal cycle driver injured in
7th   collision with fixed or
stationary object in
nontraffic accident
V17.1XX   Pedal cycle passenger injured
7th   in collision with fixed or
stationary object in nontraffic accident
V17.2XX   Unspecified pedal cyclist injured in collision with fixed or
7th   stationary object in nontraffic accident
V17.3XX   Person boarding or alighting a pedal cycle injured in
7th   collision with fixed or stationary object
V17.4XX   Pedal cycle driver injured in collision with fixed or
7th   stationary object in traffic accident
V17.5XX   Pedal cycle passenger injured in collision with fixed or
7th   stationary object in traffic accident
V17.9XX   Unspecified pedal cyclist injured in collision with fixed or
7th   stationary object in traffic accident

> 7th characters for categories
> V10–V18
> A—initial encounter
> D—subsequent encounter
> S—sequela

V18   **PEDAL CYCLE RIDER INJURED IN NONCOLLISION**
4th   **TRANSPORT ACCIDENT**
Includes: fall or thrown from pedal cycle (without antecedent collision)
overturning pedal cycle NOS
overturning pedal cycle without collision
V18.0XX   Pedal cycle driver injured in noncollision transport accident
7th   in nontraffic accident
V18.1XX   Pedal cycle passenger injured in noncollision transport
7th   accident in nontraffic accident
V18.2XX   Unspecified pedal cyclist injured in noncollision transport
7th   accident in nontraffic accident
V18.3XX   Person boarding or alighting a pedal cycle injured in
7th   noncollision transport accident
V18.4XX   Pedal cycle driver injured in noncollision transport accident
7th   in traffic accident
V18.5XX   Pedal cycle passenger injured in noncollision transport
7th   accident in traffic accident
V18.9XX   Unspecified pedal cyclist injured in noncollision transport
7th   accident in traffic accident

V19   **PEDAL CYCLE RIDER INJURED IN OTHER AND**
4th   **UNSPECIFIED TRANSPORT ACCIDENTS**
Refer to External Cause of Injuries Table

(V20–V29) MOTORCYCLE RIDER INJURED IN TRANSPORT ACCIDENT

Includes: moped
motorcycle with sidecar
motorized bicycle
motor scooter

Excludes1: three-wheeled motor vehicle
(V30–V39)

> 7th characters for categories
> V20–V29
> A—initial encounter
> D—subsequent encounter
> S—sequela

V20   **MOTORCYCLE RIDER INJURED IN COLLISION WITH**
4th   **PEDESTRIAN OR ANIMAL**
Excludes1: motorcycle rider collision with animal-drawn vehicle or animal
being ridden (V26.-)

V20.0XX   Motorcycle driver injured in collision with pedestrian or
7th   animal in nontraffic accident
V20.1XX   Motorcycle passenger injured in collision with pedestrian or
7th   animal in nontraffic accident
V20.2XX   Unspecified motorcycle rider injured in collision with
7th   pedestrian or animal in nontraffic accident
V20.3XX   Person boarding or alighting a motorcycle injured in
7th   collision with pedestrian or animal
V20.4XX   Motorcycle driver injured in
7th   collision with pedestrian or animal in traffic accident
V20.5XX   Motorcycle passenger injured in collision with pedestrian or
7th   animal in traffic accident
V20.9XX   Unspecified motorcycle rider injured in collision with
7th   pedestrian or animal in traffic accident

V21   **MOTORCYCLE RIDER INJURED IN COLLISION WITH**
4th   **PEDAL CYCLE**
Excludes1: motorcycle rider collision with animal-drawn vehicle or animal
being ridden (V26.-)
V21.0XX   Motorcycle driver injured in collision or with pedal cycle in
7th   nontraffic accident
V21.1XX   Motorcycle passenger injured in collision with pedal cycle
7th   in nontraffic accident
V21.2XX   Unspecified motorcycle rider injured in collision with pedal
7th   cycle in nontraffic accident
V21.3XX   Person boarding or alighting a motorcycle injured in
7th   collision with pedal cycle
V21.4XX   Motorcycle driver injured in collision with pedal cycle in
7th   traffic accident
V21.5XX   Motorcycle passenger injured in collision with pedal cycle
7th   in traffic accident
V21.9XX   Unspecified motorcycle rider injured in collision with pedal
7th   cycle in traffic accident

V22   **MOTORCYCLE RIDER INJURED IN COLLISION WITH**
7th   **TWO- OR THREE-WHEELED MOTOR VEHICLE**
Refer to External Cause of Injuries Table

V23   **MOTORCYCLE RIDER INJURED IN COLLISION WITH CAR,**
4th   **PICK-UP TRUCK OR VAN**
V23.0XX   Motorcycle driver injured in collision with car, pick-up truck
7th   or van in nontraffic accident
V23.1XX   Motorcycle passenger injured in collision with car, pick-up
7th   truck or van in nontraffic accident
V23.2XX   Unspecified motorcycle rider injured in collision with car,
7th   pick-up truck or van in nontraffic accident
V23.3XX   Person boarding or alighting a motorcycle injured in
7th   collision with car, pick-up truck or van
V23.4XX   Motorcycle driver injured in collision with car, pick-up truck
7th   or van in traffic accident
V23.5XX   Motorcycle passenger injured in collision with car, pick-up
7th   truck or van in traffic accident
V23.9XX   Unspecified motorcycle rider injured in collision with car,
7th   pick-up truck or van in traffic accident

V24   **MOTORCYCLE RIDER INJURED IN COLLISION WITH**
4th   **HEAVY TRANSPORT VEHICLE OR BUS**
Excludes1: motorcycle rider injured in collision with military vehicle
(V29.81)
V24.0XX   Motorcycle driver injured in collision with heavy transport
7th   vehicle or bus in nontraffic accident
V24.1XX   Motorcycle passenger injured in collision with heavy
7th   transport vehicle or bus in nontraffic accident
V24.2XX   Unspecified motorcycle rider injured in collision with heavy
7th   transport vehicle or bus in nontraffic accident
V24.3XX   Person boarding or alighting a motorcycle injured in
7th   collision with heavy transport vehicle or bus
V24.4XX   Motorcycle driver injured in collision with heavy transport
7th   vehicle or bus in traffic accident
V24.5XX   Motorcycle passenger injured in collision with heavy
7th   transport vehicle or bus in traffic accident
V24.9XX   Unspecified motorcycle rider injured in collision with heavy
7th   transport vehicle or bus in traffic accident

4th   5th   6th   7th   Additional Character Required   ✔   3-character code

•=New Code
▲=Revised Code

Excludes1—Not coded here, do not use together
Excludes2—Not included here

V25 **MOTORCYCLE RIDER INJURED IN COLLISION WITH**
`4th` **RAILWAY TRAIN OR RAILWAY VEHICLE**
Refer to External Cause of Injuries Table

V26 **MOTORCYCLE RIDER INJURED IN COLLISION WITH**
`4th` **OTHER NONMOTOR VEHICLE**
Includes: collision with animal-drawn vehicle, animal being ridden, streetcar
Refer to External Cause of Injuries Table

V27 **MOTORCYCLE RIDER INJURED IN COLLISION WITH**
`4th` **FIXED OR STATIONARY OBJECT**
V27.0XX Motorcycle driver injured in collision with fixed or
`7th` stationary object in nontraffic accident
V27.1XX Motorcycle passenger injured in collision with fixed or
`7th` stationary object in nontraffic accident
V27.2XX Unspecified motorcycle rider injured in collision with fixed
`7th` or stationary object in nontraffic accident
V27.3XX Person boarding or alighting a motorcycle injured in
`7th` collision with fixed or stationary object
V27.4XX Motorcycle driver injured
`7th` in collision with fixed or
stationary object in traffic
accident

> 7th characters for categories
> V20–V29
> A—initial encounter
> D—subsequent encounter
> S—sequela

V27.5XX Motorcycle passenger injured
`7th` in collision with fixed or
stationary object in traffic accident
V27.9XX Unspecified motorcycle rider injured in collision with fixed
`7th` or stationary object in traffic accident

V28 **MOTORCYCLE RIDER INJURED IN NONCOLLISION**
`4th` **TRANSPORT ACCIDENT**
Includes: fall or thrown from motorcycle (without antecedent collision)
overturning motorcycle NOS
overturning motorcycle without collision
V28.0XX Motorcycle driver injured in noncollision transport accident
`7th` in nontraffic accident
V28.1XX Motorcycle passenger injured in noncollision transport
`7th` accident in nontraffic accident
V28.2XX Unspecified motorcycle rider injured in noncollision
`7th` transport accident in nontraffic accident
V28.3XX Person boarding or alighting a motorcycle injured in
`7th` noncollision transport accident
V28.4XX Motorcycle driver injured in noncollision transport accident
`7th` in traffic accident
V28.5XX Motorcycle passenger injured in noncollision transport
`7th` accident in traffic accident
V28.9XX Unspecified motorcycle rider injured in noncollision
`7th` transport accident in traffic accident

V29 **MOTORCYCLE RIDER INJURED IN OTHER AND**
`4th` **UNSPECIFIED TRANSPORT ACCIDENTS**
V29.0 Motorcycle driver injured in collision with other and
`5th` unspecified motor vehicles in nontraffic accident
V29.00X Motorcycle driver injured in collision with
`7th` unspecified motor vehicles in nontraffic accident
V29.09X Motorcycle driver injured in collision with other
`7th` motor vehicles in nontraffic accident
V29.1 Motorcycle passenger injured in collision with other and
`5th` unspecified motor vehicles in nontraffic accident
V29.10X Motorcycle passenger injured in collision with
`7th` unspecified motor vehicles in nontraffic accident
V29.19X Motorcycle passenger injured in collision with other
`7th` motor vehicles in nontraffic accident
V29.2 Unspecified motorcycle rider injured in collision with other and
`5th` unspecified motor vehicles in nontraffic accident
V29.20X Unspecified motorcycle rider injured in collision with
`7th` unspecified motor vehicles in nontraffic accident
Motorcycle collision NOS, nontraffic
V29.29X Unspecified motorcycle rider injured in collision with
`7th` other motor vehicles in nontraffic accident
V29.3XX Motorcycle rider (driver) (passenger) injured in unspecified
`7th` nontraffic accident
Motorcycle accident NOS, nontraffic
Motorcycle rider injured in nontraffic accident NOS

V29.4 Motorcycle driver injured in collision with other and
`5th` unspecified motor vehicles in traffic accident
V29.40X Motorcycle driver injured in collision with
`7th` unspecified motor vehicles in traffic accident
V29.49X Motorcycle driver injured in collision with other
`7th` motor vehicles in traffic accident
V29.5 Motorcycle passenger injured in collision with other and
`5th` unspecified motor vehicles in traffic accident
V29.50X Motorcycle passenger injured in collision with
`7th` unspecified motor vehicles in traffic accident
V29.59X Motorcycle passenger injured in collision with other
`7th` motor vehicles in traffic accident
V29.6 Unspecified motorcycle rider injured in collision with other and
`5th` unspecified motor vehicles in traffic accident
V29.60X Unspecified motorcycle rider injured in collision with
`7th` unspecified motor vehicles in traffic accident
Motorcycle collision NOS (traffic)
V29.69X Unspecified motorcycle rider injured in collision with
`7th` other motor vehicles in traffic accident
V29.8 Motorcycle rider (driver) (passenger) injured in other specified
`5th` transport accidents
V29.81X Motorcycle rider (driver) (passenger) injured in
`7th` transport accident with military vehicle
V29.88X Motorcycle rider (driver) (passenger) injured in other
`7th` specified transport accidents
V29.9XX Motorcycle rider (driver) (passenger) injured in unspecified
`7th` traffic accident
Motorcycle accident NOS

(V30–V39) OCCUPANT OF THREE-WHEELED MOTOR VEHICLE INJURED IN TRANSPORT ACCIDENT

Includes: motorized tricycle
motorized rickshaw
three-wheeled motor car

Excludes1: all-terrain vehicles (V86.-)
motorcycle with sidecar (V20–V29)
vehicle designed primarily for off-road use
(V86.-)

> 7th characters for categories
> V30–V39
> A—initial encounter
> D—subsequent encounter
> S—sequela

V30 **OCCUPANT OF THREE-WHEELED MOTOR VEHICLE**
`4th` **INJURED IN COLLISION WITH PEDESTRIAN OR ANIMAL**
Excludes1: three-wheeled motor vehicle collision with animal-drawn
vehicle or animal being ridden (V36.-)
V30.0XX Driver of three-wheeled motor vehicle injured in collision
`7th` with pedestrian or animal in nontraffic accident
V30.1XX Passenger in three-wheeled motor vehicle injured in
`7th` collision with pedestrian or animal in nontraffic accident
V30.2XX Person on outside of three-wheeled motor vehicle injured in
`7th` collision with pedestrian or animal in nontraffic accident
V30.3XX Unspecified occupant of three-wheeled motor vehicle
`7th` injured in collision with pedestrian or animal in nontraffic
accident
V30.4XX Person boarding or alighting a three-wheeled motor vehicle
`7th` injured in collision with pedestrian or animal
V30.5XX Driver of three-wheeled motor vehicle injured in collision
`7th` with pedestrian or animal in traffic accident
V30.6XX Passenger in three-wheeled motor vehicle injured in
`7th` collision with pedestrian or animal in traffic accident
V30.7XX Person on outside of three-wheeled motor vehicle injured in
`7th` collision with pedestrian or animal in traffic accident
V30.9XX Unspecified occupant of three-wheeled motor vehicle
`7th` injured in collision with pedestrian or animal in traffic
accident

V31 **OCCUPANT OF THREE-WHEELED MOTOR VEHICLE**
`4th` **INJURED IN COLLISION WITH PEDAL CYCLE**
Refer to the External Cause of Injuries Table

V32 **OCCUPANT OF THREE-WHEELED MOTOR VEHICLE**
`4th` **INJURED IN COLLISION WITH TWO- OR THREE-**
WHEELED MOTOR VEHICLE
V32.0XX Driver of three-wheeled motor vehicle injured in collision
`7th` with two- or three-wheeled motor vehicle in nontraffic
accident

`4th` `5th` `6th` `7th`   Additional Character Required   ✔   3-character code

•=New Code
▲=Revised Code

Excludes1—Not coded here, do not use together
Excludes2—Not included here

V32.1XX 7th — Passenger in three-wheeled motor vehicle injured in collision with two- or three-wheeled motor vehicle in nontraffic accident

V32.2XX 7th — Person on outside of three-wheeled motor vehicle injured in collision with two- or three-wheeled motor vehicle in nontraffic accident

V32.3XX 7th — Unspecified occupant of three-wheeled motor vehicle injured in collision with two- or three-wheeled motor vehicle in nontraffic accident

V32.4XX 7th — Person boarding or alighting a three-wheeled motor vehicle injured in collision with two- or three-wheeled motor vehicle

V32.5XX 7th — Driver of three-wheeled motor vehicle injured in collision with two- or three-wheeled motor vehicle in traffic accident

> 7th characters for categories V30–V39
> A—initial encounter
> D—subsequent encounter
> S—sequela

V32.6XX 7th — Passenger in three-wheeled motor vehicle injured in collision with two- or three-wheeled motor vehicle in traffic accident

V32.7XX 7th — Person on outside of three-wheeled motor vehicle injured in collision with two- or three-wheeled motor vehicle in traffic accident

V32.9XX 7th — Unspecified occupant of three-wheeled motor vehicle injured in collision with two- or three-wheeled motor vehicle in traffic accident

V33 4th — **OCCUPANT OF THREE-WHEELED MOTOR VEHICLE INJURED IN COLLISION WITH CAR, PICK-UP TRUCK OR VAN**

V33.0XX 7th — Driver of three-wheeled motor vehicle injured in collision with car, pick-up truck or van in nontraffic accident

V33.1XX 7th — Passenger in three-wheeled motor vehicle injured in collision with car, pick-up truck or van in nontraffic accident

V33.2XX 7th — Person on outside of three-wheeled motor vehicle injured in collision with car, pick-up truck or van in nontraffic accident

V33.3XX 7th — Unspecified occupant of three-wheeled motor vehicle injured in collision with car, pick-up truck or van in nontraffic accident

V33.4XX 7th — Person boarding or alighting a three-wheeled motor vehicle injured in collision with car, pick-up truck or van

V33.5XX 7th — Driver of three-wheeled motor vehicle injured in collision with car, pick-up truck or van in traffic accident

V33.6XX 7th — Passenger in three-wheeled motor vehicle injured in collision with car, pick-up truck or van in traffic accident

V33.7XX 7th — Person on outside of three-wheeled motor vehicle injured in collision with car, pick-up truck or van in traffic accident

V33.9XX 7th — Unspecified occupant of three-wheeled motor vehicle injured in collision with car, pick-up truck or van in traffic accident

V34 4th — **OCCUPANT OF THREE-WHEELED MOTOR VEHICLE INJURED IN COLLISION WITH HEAVY TRANSPORT VEHICLE OR BUS**

Excludes1: occupant of three-wheeled motor vehicle injured in collision with military vehicle (V39.81)

V34.0XX 7th — Driver of three-wheeled motor vehicle injured in collision with heavy transport vehicle or bus in nontraffic accident

V34.1XX 7th — Passenger in three-wheeled motor vehicle injured in collision with heavy transport vehicle or bus in nontraffic accident

V34.2XX 7th — Person on outside of three-wheeled motor vehicle injured in collision with heavy transport vehicle or bus in nontraffic accident

V34.3XX 7th — Unspecified occupant of three-wheeled motor vehicle injured in collision with heavy transport vehicle or bus in nontraffic accident

V34.4XX 7th — Person boarding or alighting a three-wheeled motor vehicle injured in collision with heavy transport vehicle or bus

V34.5XX 7th — Driver of three-wheeled motor vehicle injured in collision with heavy transport vehicle or bus in traffic accident

V34.6XX 7th — Passenger in three-wheeled motor vehicle injured in collision with heavy transport vehicle or bus in traffic accident

V34.7XX 7th — Person on outside of three-wheeled motor vehicle injured in collision with heavy transport vehicle or bus in traffic accident

V34.9XX 7th — Unspecified occupant of three-wheeled motor vehicle injured in collision with heavy transport vehicle or bus in traffic accident

V35 4th — **OCCUPANT OF THREE-WHEELED MOTOR VEHICLE INJURED IN COLLISION WITH RAILWAY TRAIN OR RAILWAY VEHICLE**
Refer to External Cause of Injuries Table

V36 4th — **OCCUPANT OF THREE-WHEELED MOTOR VEHICLE INJURED IN COLLISION WITH OTHER NONMOTOR VEHICLE**
Includes: collision with animal-drawn vehicle, animal being ridden, streetcar
Refer to External Cause of Injuries Table

V37 4th — **OCCUPANT OF THREE-WHEELED MOTOR VEHICLE INJURED IN COLLISION WITH FIXED OR STATIONARY OBJECT**

V37.0XX 7th — Driver of three-wheeled motor vehicle injured in collision with fixed or stationary object in nontraffic accident

V37.1XX 7th — Passenger in three-wheeled motor vehicle injured in collision with fixed or stationary object in nontraffic accident

V37.2XX 7th — Person on outside of three-wheeled motor vehicle injured in collision with fixed or stationary object in nontraffic accident

V37.3XX 7th — Unspecified occupant of three-wheeled motor vehicle injured in collision with fixed or stationary object in nontraffic accident

V37.4XX 7th — Person boarding or alighting a three-wheeled motor vehicle injured in collision with fixed or stationary object

V37.5XX 7th — Driver of three-wheeled motor vehicle injured in collision with fixed or stationary object in traffic accident

V37.6XX 7th — Passenger in three-wheeled motor vehicle injured in collision with fixed or stationary object in traffic accident

V37.7XX 7th — Person on outside of three-wheeled motor vehicle injured in collision with fixed or stationary object in traffic accident

V37.9XX 7th — Unspecified occupant of three-wheeled motor vehicle injured in collision with fixed or stationary object in traffic accident

V38 4th — **OCCUPANT OF THREE-WHEELED MOTOR VEHICLE INJURED IN NONCOLLISION TRANSPORT ACCIDENT**

Includes: fall or thrown from three-wheeled motor vehicle
overturning of three-wheeled motor vehicle NOS
overturning of three-wheeled motor vehicle without collision

V38.0XX 7th — Driver of three-wheeled motor vehicle injured in noncollision transport accident in nontraffic accident

V38.1XX 7th — Passenger in three-wheeled motor vehicle injured in noncollision transport accident in nontraffic accident

V38.2XX 7th — Person on outside of three-wheeled motor vehicle injured in noncollision transport accident in nontraffic accident

V38.3XX 7th — Unspecified occupant of three-wheeled motor vehicle injured in noncollision transport accident in nontraffic accident

V38.4XX 7th — Person boarding or alighting a three-wheeled motor vehicle injured in noncollision transport accident

V38.5XX 7th — Driver of three-wheeled motor vehicle injured in noncollision transport accident in traffic accident

V38.6XX 7th — Passenger in three-wheeled motor vehicle injured in noncollision transport accident in traffic accident

V38.7XX 7th — Person on outside of three-wheeled motor vehicle injured in noncollision transport accident in traffic accident

V38.9XX 7th — Unspecified occupant of three-wheeled motor vehicle injured in noncollision transport accident in traffic accident

V39 4th — **OCCUPANT OF THREE-WHEELED MOTOR VEHICLE INJURED IN OTHER AND UNSPECIFIED TRANSPORT ACCIDENTS**

4th 5th 6th 7th Additional Character Required ✔ 3-character code

•=New Code
▲=Revised Code

Excludes1—Not coded here, do not use together
Excludes2—Not included here

V39.0 Driver of three-wheeled motor vehicle injured in collision with other and unspecified motor vehicles in nontraffic accident
> **V39.00X** Driver of three-wheeled motor vehicle injured in collision with unspecified motor vehicles in nontraffic accident
> **V39.09X** Driver of three-wheeled motor vehicle injured in collision with other motor vehicles in nontraffic accident

V39.1 Passenger in three-wheeled motor vehicle injured in collision with other and unspecified motor vehicles in nontraffic accident
> **V39.10X** Passenger in three-wheeled motor vehicle injured in collision with unspecified motor vehicles in nontraffic accident
> **V39.19X** Passenger in three-wheeled motor vehicle injured in collision with other motor vehicles in nontraffic accident

> **7th characters for categories**
> V30–V39
> A—initial encounter
> D—subsequent encounter
> S—sequela

V39.2 Unspecified occupant of three-wheeled motor vehicle injured in accident
> **V39.20X** Unspecified occupant of three-wheeled motor vehicle injured in collision with unspecified motor vehicles in nontraffic accident
> > Collision NOS involving three-wheeled motor vehicle, nontraffic
> **V39.29X** Unspecified occupant of three-wheeled

V39.3XX Occupant (driver) (passenger) of three-wheeled motor vehicle injured in unspecified nontraffic accident
> Accident NOS involving three-wheeled motor vehicle, nontraffic
> Occupant of three-wheeled motor vehicle injured in nontraffic accident NOS

V39.4 Driver of three-wheeled motor vehicle injured in collision with other and unspecified motor vehicles in traffic accident
> **V39.40X** Driver of three-wheeled motor vehicle injured in collision with unspecified motor vehicles in traffic accident
> **V39.49X** Driver of three-wheeled motor vehicle injured in collision with other motor vehicles in traffic accident

V39.5 Passenger in three-wheeled motor vehicle injured in collision with other and unspecified motor vehicles in traffic accident
> **V39.50X** Passenger in three-wheeled motor vehicle injured in collision with unspecified motor vehicles in traffic accident
> **V39.59X** Passenger in three-wheeled motor vehicle injured in collision with other motor vehicles in traffic accident

V39.6 Unspecified occupant of three-wheeled motor vehicle injured in collision with other and unspecified motor vehicles in traffic accident
> **V39.60X** Unspecified occupant of three-wheeled motor vehicle injured in collision with unspecified motor vehicles in traffic accident
> > Collision NOS involving three-wheeled motor vehicle (traffic)
> **V39.69X** Unspecified occupant of three-wheeled motor vehicle injured in collision with other motor vehicles in traffic accident

V39.8 Occupant (driver) (passenger) of three-wheeled motor vehicle injured in other specified transport accidents
> **V39.81X** Occupant (driver) (passenger) of three-wheeled motor vehicle injured in transport accident with military vehicle
> **V39.89X** Occupant (driver) (passenger) of three-wheeled motor vehicle injured in other specified transport accidents

V39.9XX Occupant (driver) (passenger) of three-wheeled motor vehicle injured in unspecified traffic accident
> Accident NOS involving three-wheeled motor vehicle

(V40–V49) CAR OCCUPANT INJURED IN TRANSPORT ACCIDENT

Includes: a four-wheeled motor vehicle designed primarily for carrying passengers
automobile (pulling a trailer or camper)

Excludes1: bus (V50–V59)
> minibus (V50–V59)
> minivan (V50–V59)
> motorcoach (V70–V79)
> pick-up truck (V50–V59)
> sport utility vehicle (SUV) (V50–V59)

> **7th characters for categories**
> V40–V49
> A—initial encounter
> D—subsequent encounter
> S—sequela

V40 **CAR OCCUPANT INJURED IN COLLISION WITH PEDESTRIAN OR ANIMAL**
> **Excludes1:** car collision with animal-drawn vehicle or animal being ridden (V46.-)
> **V40.0XX** Car driver injured in collision with pedestrian or animal in nontraffic accident
> **V40.1XX** Car passenger injured in collision with pedestrian or animal in nontraffic accident
> **V40.2XX** Person on outside of car injured in collision with pedestrian or animal in nontraffic accident
> **V40.3XX** Unspecified car occupant injured in collision with pedestrian or animal in nontraffic accident
> **V40.4XX** Person boarding or alighting a car injured in collision with pedestrian or animal
> **V40.5XX** Car driver injured in collision with pedestrian or animal in traffic accident
> **V40.6XX** Car passenger injured in collision with pedestrian or animal in traffic accident
> **V40.7XX** Person on outside of car injured in collision with pedestrian or animal in traffic accident
> **V40.9XX** Unspecified car occupant injured in collision with pedestrian or animal in traffic accident

V41 **CAR OCCUPANT INJURED IN COLLISION WITH PEDAL CYCLE**
> Refer to External Cause of Injuries Table

V42 **CAR OCCUPANT INJURED IN COLLISION WITH TWO- OR THREE-WHEELED MOTOR VEHICLE**
> **V42.0XX** Car driver injured in collision with two- or three-wheeled motor vehicle in nontraffic accident
> **V42.1XX** Car passenger injured in collision with two- or three-wheeled motor vehicle in nontraffic accident
> **V42.2XX** Person on outside of car injured in collision with two- or three-wheeled motor vehicle in nontraffic accident
> **V42.3XX** Unspecified car occupant injured in collision with two- or three-wheeled motor vehicle in nontraffic accident
> **V42.4XX** Person boarding or alighting a car injured in collision with two- or three-wheeled motor vehicle
> **V42.5XX** Car driver injured in collision with two- or three-wheeled motor vehicle in traffic accident
> **V42.6XX** Car passenger injured in collision with two- or three-wheeled motor vehicle in traffic accident
> **V42.7XX** Person on outside of car injured in collision with two- or three-wheeled motor vehicle in traffic accident
> **V42.9XX** Unspecified car occupant injured in collision with two- or three-wheeled motor vehicle in traffic accident

V43 **CAR OCCUPANT INJURED IN COLLISION WITH CAR, PICK-UP TRUCK OR VAN**
> **V43.0** Car driver injured in collision with car, pick-up truck or van in nontraffic accident
> > **V43.01X** Car driver injured in collision with sport utility vehicle in nontraffic accident
> > **V43.02X** Car driver injured in collision with other type car in nontraffic accident
> > **V43.03X** Car driver injured in collision with pick-up truck in nontraffic accident
> > **V43.04X** Car driver injured in collision with van in nontraffic accident
> **V43.1** Car passenger injured in collision with car, pick-up truck or van in nontraffic accident

---

4th **5th** **6th** **7th** Additional Character Required   ✓ 3-character code

•=New Code
▲=Revised Code

Excludes1—Not coded here, do not use together
Excludes2—Not included here

V43.11X 7th   Car passenger injured in collision with sport utility vehicle in nontraffic accident

V43.12X 7th   Car passenger injured in collision with other type car in nontraffic accident

V43.13X 7th   Car passenger injured in collision with pick-up in nontraffic accident

V43.14X 7th   Car passenger injured in collision with van in nontraffic accident

V43.2 5th   Person on outside of car injured in collision with car, pick-up truck or van in nontraffic accident

V43.21X 7th   Person on outside of car injured in collision with sport utility vehicle in nontraffic accident

V43.22X 7th   Person on outside of car injured in collision with other type car in nontraffic accident

V43.23X 7th   Person on outside of car injured in collision with pick-up truck in nontraffic accident

V43.24X 7th   Person on outside of car injured in collision with van in nontraffic accident

V43.3 5th   Unspecified car occupant injured in collision with car, pick-up truck or van in nontraffic accident

> 7th characters for categories
> V40–V49
> A—initial encounter
> D—subsequent encounter
> S—sequela

V43.31X 7th   Unspecified car occupant injured in collision with sport utility vehicle in nontraffic accident

V43.32X 7th   Unspecified car occupant injured in collision with other type car in nontraffic accident

V43.33X 7th   Unspecified car occupant injured in collision with pick-up truck in nontraffic accident

V43.34X 7th   Unspecified car occupant injured in collision with van in nontraffic accident

V43.4 5th   Person boarding or alighting a car injured in collision with car, pick-up truck or van

V43.41X 7th   Person boarding or alighting a car injured in collision with sport utility vehicle, initial encounter

V43.42X 7th   Person boarding or alighting a car injured in collision with other type car

V43.43X 7th   Person boarding or alighting a car injured in collision with pick-up truck

V43.44X 7th   Person boarding or alighting a car injured in collision with van

V43.5 5th   Car driver injured in collision with car, pick-up truck or van in traffic accident

V43.51X 7th   Car driver injured in collision with sport utility vehicle in traffic accident

V43.52X 7th   Car driver injured in collision with other type car in traffic accident

V43.53X 7th   Car driver injured in collision with pick-up truck in traffic accident

V43.54X 7th   Car driver injured in collision with van in traffic accident

V43.6 5th   Car passenger injured in collision with car, pick-up truck or van in traffic accident

V43.61X 7th   Car passenger injured in collision with sport utility vehicle in traffic accident

V43.62X 7th   Car passenger injured in collision with other type car in traffic accident

V43.63X 7th   Car passenger injured in collision with pick-up truck in traffic accident

V43.64X 7th   Car passenger injured in collision with van in traffic accident

V43.7 5th   Person on outside of car injured in collision with car, pick-up truck or van in traffic accident

V43.71X 7th   Person on outside of car injured in collision with sport utility vehicle in traffic accident

V43.72X 7th   Person on outside of car injured in collision with other type car in traffic accident

V43.73X 7th   Person on outside of car injured in collision with pick-up truck in traffic accident

V43.74X 7th   Person on outside of car injured in collision with van in traffic accident

V43.9 5th   Unspecified car occupant injured in collision with car, pick-up truck or van in traffic accident

V43.91X 7th   Unspecified car occupant injured in collision with sport utility vehicle in traffic accident

V43.92X 7th   Unspecified car occupant injured in collision with other type car in traffic accident

V43.93X 7th   Unspecified car occupant injured in collision with pick-up truck in traffic accident

V43.94X 7th   Unspecified car occupant injured in collision with van in traffic accident

V44 4th   CAR OCCUPANT INJURED IN COLLISION WITH HEAVY TRANSPORT VEHICLE OR BUS

Excludes1: car occupant injured in collision with military vehicle (V49.81)

V44.0XX 7th   Car driver injured in collision with heavy transport vehicle or bus in nontraffic accident

V44.1XX 7th   Car passenger injured in collision with heavy transport vehicle or bus in nontraffic accident

V44.2XX 7th   Person on outside of car injured in collision with heavy transport vehicle or bus in nontraffic accident

V44.3XX 7th   Unspecified car occupant injured in collision with heavy transport vehicle or bus in nontraffic accident

V44.4XX 7th   Person boarding or alighting a car injured in collision with heavy transport vehicle or bus

V44.5XX 7th   Car driver injured in collision with heavy transport vehicle or bus in traffic accident

V44.6XX 7th   Car passenger injured in collision with heavy transport vehicle or bus in traffic accident

V44.7XX 7th   Person on outside of car injured in collision with heavy transport vehicle or bus in traffic accident

V44.9XX 7th   Unspecified car occupant injured in collision with heavy transport vehicle or bus in traffic accident

V45 4th   CAR OCCUPANT INJURED IN COLLISION WITH RAILWAY TRAIN OR RAILWAY VEHICLE

V45.0XX 7th   Car driver injured in collision with railway train or railway vehicle in nontraffic accident

V45.1XX 7th   Car passenger injured in collision with railway train or railway vehicle in nontraffic accident

V45.2XX 7th   Person on outside of car injured in collision with railway train or railway vehicle in nontraffic accident

V45.3XX 7th   Unspecified car occupant injured in collision with railway train or railway vehicle in nontraffic accident

V45.4XX 7th   Person boarding or alighting a car injured in collision with railway train or railway vehicle

V45.5XX 7th   Car driver injured in collision with railway train or railway vehicle in traffic accident

V45.6XX 7th   Car passenger injured in collision with railway train or railway vehicle in traffic accident

V45.7XX 7th   Person on outside of car injured in collision with railway train or railway vehicle in traffic accident

V45.9XX 7th   Unspecified car occupant injured in collision with railway train or railway vehicle in traffic accident

V46 6th   CAR OCCUPANT INJURED IN COLLISION WITH OTHER NONMOTOR VEHICLE

Includes: collision with animal-drawn vehicle, animal being ridden, streetcar

Refer to External Cause of Injuries Table

V47 4th   CAR OCCUPANT INJURED IN COLLISION WITH FIXED OR STATIONARY OBJECT

V47.0XX 7th   Car driver injured in collision with fixed or stationary object in nontraffic accident

V47.1XX 7th   Car passenger injured in collision with fixed or stationary object in nontraffic accident

V47.2XX 7th   Person on outside of car injured in collision with fixed or stationary object in nontraffic accident

V47.3XX 7th   Unspecified car occupant injured in collision with fixed or stationary object in nontraffic accident

V47.4XX 7th   Person boarding or alighting a car injured in collision with fixed or stationary object

V47.5XX 7th   Car driver injured in collision with fixed or stationary object in traffic accident

V47.6XX 7th   Car passenger injured in collision with fixed or stationary object in traffic accident

---

4th   5th   6th   7th   Additional Character Required   ✔   3-character code

•=New Code   ▲=Revised Code

Excludes1—Not coded here, do not use together
Excludes2—Not included here

V47.7XX Person on outside of car injured in collision with fixed or stationary object in traffic accident
7th

V47.9XX Unspecified car occupant injured in collision with fixed or stationary object in traffic accident
7th

V48 CAR OCCUPANT INJURED IN NONCOLLISION
4th TRANSPORT ACCIDENT
Includes: overturning car NOS
overturning car without collision

V48.0XX Car driver injured in noncollision transport accident in nontraffic accident
7th

V48.1XX Car passenger injured in noncollision transport accident in nontraffic accident
7th

V48.2XX Person on outside of car injured in noncollision transport accident in nontraffic accident
7th

V48.3XX Unspecified car occupant injured in noncollision transport accident in nontraffic accident
7th

V48.4XX Person boarding or alighting a car injured in noncollision transport accident
7th

V48.5XX Car driver injured in noncollision transport accident in traffic accident
7th

V48.6XX Car passenger injured in noncollision transport accident in traffic accident
7th

> 7th characters for categories
> V40–V49
> A—initial encounter
> D—subsequent encounter
> S—sequela

V48.7XX Person on outside of car injured in noncollision transport accident in traffic accident
7th

V48.9XX Unspecified car occupant injured in noncollision transport accident in traffic accident
7th

V49 CAR OCCUPANT INJURED IN OTHER AND UNSPECIFIED
4th TRANSPORT ACCIDENTS

V49.0 Driver injured in collision with other and unspecified motor vehicles in nontraffic accident
5th

  V49.00X Driver injured in collision with unspecified motor vehicles in nontraffic accident
  7th

  V49.09X Driver injured in collision with other motor vehicles in nontraffic accident
  7th

V49.1 Passenger injured in collision with other and unspecified motor vehicles in nontraffic accident
5th

  V49.10X Passenger injured in collision with unspecified motor vehicles in nontraffic accident
  7th

  V49.19X Passenger injured in collision with other motor vehicles in nontraffic accident
  7th

V49.2 Unspecified car occupant injured in collision with other and unspecified motor vehicles in nontraffic accident
5th

  V49.20X Unspecified car occupant injured in collision with unspecified motor vehicles in nontraffic accident
  7th   Car collision NOS, nontraffic

  V49.29X Unspecified car occupant injured in collision with other motor vehicles in nontraffic accident
  7th

V49.3XX Car occupant (driver) (passenger) injured in unspecified nontraffic accident
7th
Car accident NOS, nontraffic
Car occupant injured in nontraffic accident NOS

V49.4 Driver injured in collision with other and unspecified motor vehicles in traffic accident
5th

  V49.40X Driver injured in collision with unspecified motor vehicles in traffic accident
  7th

  V49.49X Driver injured in collision with other motor vehicles in traffic accident
  7th

V49.5 Passenger injured in collision with other and unspecified motor vehicles in traffic accident
5th

  V49.50X Passenger injured in collision with unspecified motor vehicles in traffic accident
  7th

  V49.59X Passenger injured in collision with other motor vehicles in traffic accident
  7th

V49.6 Unspecified car occupant injured in collision with other and unspecified motor vehicles in traffic accident
5th

  V49.60X Unspecified car occupant injured in collision with other and unspecified motor vehicles in traffic accident
  7th   Car collision NOS (traffic)

  V49.69X Unspecified car occupant injured in collision with other motor vehicles in traffic accident
  7th

V49.8 Car occupant (driver) (passenger) injured in other specified transport accidents
5th

  V49.81X Car occupant (driver) (passenger) injured in transport accident with military vehicle
  7th

  V49.88X Car occupant (driver) (passenger) injured in other specified transport accidents
  7th

V49.9XX Car occupant (driver) (passenger) injured in unspecified traffic accident
7th
Car accident NOS

(V50–V59) OCCUPANT OF PICK-UP TRUCK OR VAN OR SUV INJURED IN TRANSPORT ACCIDENT

Includes: a four or six wheel motor vehicle designed primarily for carrying passengers and property but weighing less than the local limit for classification as a heavy goods vehicle
Minibus, minivan, sport utility vehicle (SUV), truck, van

Excludes1: heavy transport vehicle (V60–V69)

> 7th characters for categories
> V50–V59
> A—initial encounter
> D—subsequent encounter
> S—sequela

V50 OCCUPANT OF PICK-UP TRUCK OR VAN OR SUV
4th INJURED IN COLLISION WITH PEDESTRIAN OR ANIMAL
Excludes1: pick-up truck or van collision with animal-drawn vehicle or animal being ridden (V56.-)

V50.0XX Driver of pick-up truck or van injured in collision with pedestrian or animal in nontraffic accident
7th

V50.1XX Passenger in pick-up truck or van injured in collision with pedestrian or animal in nontraffic accident
7th

V50.2XX Person on outside of pick-up truck or van injured in collision with pedestrian or animal in nontraffic accident
7th

V50.3XX Unspecified occupant of pick-up truck or van injured in collision with pedestrian or animal in nontraffic accident
7th

V50.4XX Person boarding or alighting a pick-up truck or van injured in collision with pedestrian or animal
7th

V50.5XX Driver of pick-up truck or van injured in collision with pedestrian or animal in traffic accident
7th

V50.6XX Passenger in pick-up truck or van injured in collision with pedestrian or animal in traffic accident
7th

V50.7XX Person on outside of pick-up truck or van injured in collision with pedestrian or animal in traffic accident
7th

V50.9XX Unspecified occupant of pick-up truck or van injured in collision with pedestrian or animal in traffic accident
7th

V51 OCCUPANT OF PICK-UP TRUCK OR VAN INJURED IN
4th COLLISION WITH PEDAL CYCLE
Refer to External Cause of Injuries Table

V52 OCCUPANT OF PICK-UP TRUCK OR VAN OR SUV
4th INJURED IN COLLISION WITH TWO- OR THREE-
WHEELED MOTOR VEHICLE

V52.0XX Driver of pick-up truck or van injured in collision with two- or three-wheeled motor vehicle in nontraffic accident
7th

V52.1XX Passenger in pick-up truck or van injured in collision with two- or three-wheeled motor vehicle in nontraffic accident
7th

V52.2XX Person on outside of pick-up truck or van injured in collision with two- or three-wheeled motor vehicle in nontraffic accident
7th

V52.3XX Unspecified occupant of pick-up truck or van injured in collision with two- or three-wheeled motor vehicle in nontraffic accident
7th

V52.4XX Person boarding or alighting a pick-up truck or van injured in collision with two- or three-wheeled motor vehicle
7th

V52.5XX Driver of pick-up truck or van injured in collision with two- or three-wheeled motor vehicle in traffic accident
7th

V52.6XX Passenger in pick-up truck or van injured in collision with two- or three-wheeled motor vehicle in traffic accident
7th

V52.7XX Person on outside of pick-up truck or van injured in collision with two- or three-wheeled motor vehicle in traffic accident
7th

V52.9XX Unspecified occupant of pick-up truck or van injured in collision with two- or three-wheeled motor vehicle in traffic accident
7th

4th **5th** **6th** **7th** Additional Character Required   ✔ 3-character code

●=New Code
▲=Revised Code

Excludes1—Not coded here, do not use together
Excludes2—Not included here

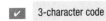

V53 OCCUPANT OF PICK-UP TRUCK OR VAN OR SUV
☐4th☐ INJURED IN COLLISION WITH CAR, PICK-UP TRUCK OR VAN

V53.0XX Driver of pick-up truck or van injured in collision with car,
☐7th☐ pick-up truck or van in nontraffic accident

V53.1XX Passenger in pick-up truck or van injured in collision with
☐7th☐ car, pick-up truck or van in nontraffic accident

V53.2XX Person on outside of pick-up truck or van injured in
☐7th☐ collision with car, pick-up truck or van in nontraffic accident

V53.3XX Unspecified occupant of
☐7th☐ pick-up truck or van injured in collision with car, pick-up truck or van in nontraffic accident

> 7th characters for categories
> V50–V59
> A—initial encounter
> D—subsequent encounter
> S—sequela

V53.4XX Person boarding or alighting
☐7th☐ a pick-up truck or van injured in collision with car, pick-up truck or van

V53.5XX Driver of pick-up truck or van injured in collision with car,
☐7th☐ pick-up truck or van in traffic accident

V53.6XX Passenger in pick-up truck or van injured in collision with
☐7th☐ car, pick-up truck or van in traffic accident

V53.7XX Person on outside of pick-up truck or van injured in
☐7th☐ collision with car, pick-up truck or van in traffic accident

V53.9XX Unspecified occupant of pick-up truck or van injured in
☐7th☐ collision with car, pick-up truck or van in traffic accident

V54 OCCUPANT OF PICK-UP TRUCK OR VAN OR SUV
☐4th☐ INJURED IN COLLISION WITH HEAVY TRANSPORT VEHICLE OR BUS

Excludes1: occupant of pick-up truck or van injured in collision with military vehicle (V59.81)

V54.0XX Driver of pick-up truck or van injured in collision with heavy
☐7th☐ transport vehicle or bus in nontraffic accident

V54.1XX Passenger in pick-up truck or van injured in collision with
☐7th☐ heavy transport vehicle or bus in nontraffic accident

V54.2XX Person on outside of pick-up truck or van injured in
☐7th☐ collision with heavy transport vehicle or bus in nontraffic accident

V54.3XX Unspecified occupant of pick-up truck or van injured in
☐7th☐ collision with heavy transport vehicle or bus in nontraffic accident

V54.4XX Person boarding or alighting a pick-up truck or van injured
☐7th☐ in collision with heavy transport vehicle or bus

V54.5XX Driver of pick-up truck or van injured in collision with heavy
☐7th☐ transport vehicle or bus in traffic accident

V54.6XX Passenger in pick-up truck or van injured in collision with
☐7th☐ heavy transport vehicle or bus in traffic accident

V54.7XX Person on outside of pick-up truck or van injured in
☐7th☐ collision with heavy transport vehicle or bus in traffic accident

V54.9XX Unspecified occupant of pick-up truck or van injured in
☐7th☐ collision with heavy transport vehicle or bus in traffic accident

V55 OCCUPANT OF PICK-UP TRUCK OR VAN OR SUV
☐4th☐ INJURED IN COLLISION WITH RAILWAY TRAIN OR RAILWAY VEHICLE

V55.0XX Driver of pick-up truck or van injured in collision with
☐7th☐ railway train or railway vehicle in nontraffic accident

V55.1XX Passenger in pick-up truck or van injured in collision with
☐7th☐ railway train or railway vehicle in nontraffic accident

V55.2XX Person on outside of pick-up truck or van injured in
☐7th☐ collision with railway train or railway vehicle in nontraffic accident

V55.3XX Unspecified occupant of pick-up truck or van injured in
☐7th☐ collision with railway train or railway vehicle in nontraffic accident

V55.4XX Person boarding or alighting a pick-up truck or van injured
☐7th☐ in collision with railway train or railway vehicle

V55.5XX Driver of pick-up truck or van injured in collision with
☐7th☐ railway train or railway vehicle in traffic accident

V55.6XX Passenger in pick-up truck or van injured in collision with
☐7th☐ railway train or railway vehicle in traffic accident

V55.7XX Person on outside of pick-up truck or van injured in
☐7th☐ collision with railway train or railway vehicle in traffic accident

V55.9XX Unspecified occupant of pick-up truck or van injured in
☐7th☐ collision with railway train or railway vehicle in traffic accident

V56 OCCUPANT OF PICK-UP TRUCK OR VAN INJURED IN
☐4th☐ COLLISION WITH OTHER NONMOTOR VEHICLE

Includes: collision with animal-drawn vehicle, animal being ridden, streetcar

Refer to External Cause of Injuries Table

V57 OCCUPANT OF PICK-UP TRUCK
☐4th☐ OR VAN OR SUV INJURED IN COLLISION WITH FIXED OR STATIONARY OBJECT

V57.0XX Driver of pick-up truck or van injured in collision with fixed
☐7th☐ or stationary object in nontraffic accident

V57.1XX Passenger in pick-up truck or van injured in collision with
☐7th☐ fixed or stationary object in nontraffic accident

V57.2XX Person on outside of pick-up truck or van injured in
☐7th☐ collision with fixed or stationary object in nontraffic accident

V57.3XX Unspecified occupant of pick-up truck or van injured
☐7th☐ in collision with fixed or stationary object in nontraffic accident

V57.4XX Person boarding or alighting a pick-up truck or van injured
☐7th☐ in collision with fixed or stationary object

V57.5XX Driver of pick-up truck or van injured in collision with fixed
☐7th☐ or stationary object in traffic accident

V57.6XX Passenger in pick-up truck or van injured in collision with
☐7th☐ fixed or stationary object in traffic accident

V57.7XX Person on outside of pick-up truck or van injured in
☐7th☐ collision with fixed or stationary object in traffic accident

V57.9XX Unspecified occupant of pick-up truck or van injured in
☐7th☐ collision with fixed or stationary object in traffic accident

V58 OCCUPANT OF PICK-UP TRUCK OR VAN OR SUV
☐4th☐ INJURED IN NONCOLLISION TRANSPORT ACCIDENT

Includes: overturning pick-up truck or van NOS
overturning pick-up truck or van without collision

V58.0XX Driver of pick-up truck or van injured in noncollision
☐7th☐ transport accident in nontraffic accident

V58.1XX Passenger in pick-up truck or van injured in noncollision
☐7th☐ transport accident in nontraffic accident

V58.2XX Person on outside of pick-up truck or van injured in
☐7th☐ noncollision transport accident in nontraffic accident

V58.3XX Unspecified occupant of pick-up truck or van injured in
☐7th☐ noncollision transport accident in nontraffic accident

V58.4XX Person boarding or alighting a pick-up truck or van injured
☐7th☐ in noncollision transport accident

V58.5XX Driver of pick-up truck or van injured in noncollision
☐7th☐ transport accident in traffic accident

V58.6XX Passenger in pick-up truck or van injured in noncollision
☐7th☐ transport accident in traffic accident

V58.7XX Person on outside of pick-up truck or van injured in
☐7th☐ noncollision transport accident in traffic accident

V58.9XX Unspecified occupant of pick-up truck or van injured in
☐7th☐ noncollision transport accident in traffic accident

V59 OCCUPANT OF PICK-UP TRUCK OR VAN OR SUV
☐4th☐ INJURED IN OTHER AND UNSPECIFIED TRANSPORT ACCIDENTS

V59.0 Driver of pick-up truck or van injured in collision with other
☐5th☐ and unspecified motor vehicles in nontraffic accident

V59.00X Driver of pick-up truck or van injured in collision
☐7th☐ with unspecified motor vehicles in nontraffic accident

V59.09X Driver of pick-up truck or van injured in collision
☐7th☐ with other motor vehicles in nontraffic accident

V59.1 Passenger in pick-up truck or van injured in collision with
☐5th☐ other and unspecified motor vehicles in nontraffic accident

V59.10X Passenger in pick-up truck or van injured in collision
☐7th☐ with unspecified motor vehicles in nontraffic accident

☐4th☐ ☐5th☐ ☐6th☐ ☐7th☐ Additional Character Required ✓ 3-character code

•=New Code
▲=Revised Code

Excludes1—Not coded here, do not use together
Excludes2—Not included here

V59.19X **7th** Passenger in pick-up truck or van injured in collision with other motor vehicles in nontraffic accident

V59.2 **5th** Unspecified occupant of pick-up truck or van injured in collision with other and unspecified motor vehicles in nontraffic accident

V59.20X **7th** Unspecified occupant of pick-up truck or van injured in collision with unspecified motor vehicles in nontraffic accident

> 7th characters for categories
> V50–V59
> A—initial encounter
> D—subsequent encounter
> S—sequela

Collision NOS involving pick-up truck or van, nontraffic

V59.29X **7th** Unspecified occupant of pick-up truck or van injured in collision with other motor vehicles in nontraffic accident

V59.3XX **7th** Occupant (driver) (passenger) of pick-up truck or van injured in unspecified nontraffic accident

Accident NOS involving pick-up truck or van, nontraffic
Occupant of pick-up truck or van injured in nontraffic accident NOS

V59.4 **5th** Driver of pick-up truck or van injured in collision with other and unspecified motor vehicles in traffic accident

V59.40X **7th** Driver of pick-up truck or van injured in collision with unspecified motor vehicles in traffic accident

V59.49X **7th** Driver of pick-up truck or van injured in collision with other motor vehicles in traffic accident

V59.5 **5th** Passenger in pick-up truck or van injured in collision with other and unspecified motor vehicles in traffic accident

V59.50X **7th** Passenger in pick-up truck or van injured in collision with unspecified motor vehicles in traffic accident

V59.59X **7th** Passenger in pick-up truck or van injured in collision with other motor vehicles in traffic accident

V59.6 **5th** Unspecified occupant of pick-up truck or van injured in collision with other and unspecified motor vehicles in traffic accident

V59.60X **7th** Unspecified occupant of pick-up truck or van injured in collision with unspecified motor vehicles in traffic accident

Collision NOS involving pick-up truck or van (traffic)

V59.69X **7th** Unspecified occupant of pick-up truck or van injured in collision with other motor vehicles in traffic accident

V59.8 **5th** Occupant (driver) (passenger) of pick-up truck or van injured in other specified transport accidents

V59.81X **7th** Occupant (driver) (passenger) of pick-up truck or van injured in transport accident with military vehicle

V59.88X **7th** Occupant (driver) (passenger) of pick-up truck or van injured in other specified transport accidents

V59.9XX **7th** Occupant (driver) (passenger) of pick-up truck or van injured in unspecified traffic accident

Accident NOS involving pick-up truck or van

(V60–V69) OCCUPANT OF HEAVY TRANSPORT VEHICLE INJURED IN TRANSPORT ACCIDENT

See complete *ICD-10-CM* manual for codes in categories V60–V69.

(V70–V79) BUS OCCUPANT INJURED IN TRANSPORT ACCIDENT

Includes: motorcoach
Excludes1: minibus (V50–V59)

V70 **4th** **BUS OCCUPANT INJURED IN COLLISION WITH PEDESTRIAN OR ANIMAL**

> 7th characters for categories
> V70–V79
> A—initial encounter
> D—subsequent encounter
> S—sequela

Excludes1: bus collision with animal-drawn vehicle or animal being ridden (V76.-)

V70.0XX **7th** Driver of bus injured in collision with pedestrian or animal in nontraffic accident

V70.1XX **7th** Passenger on bus injured in collision with pedestrian or animal in nontraffic accident

V70.2XX **7th** Person on outside of bus injured in collision with pedestrian or animal in nontraffic accident

V70.3XX **7th** Unspecified occupant of bus injured in collision with pedestrian or animal in nontraffic accident

V70.4XX **7th** Person boarding or alighting from bus injured in collision with pedestrian or animal

V70.5XX **7th** Driver of bus injured in collision with pedestrian or animal in traffic accident

V70.6XX **7th** Passenger on bus injured in collision with pedestrian or animal in traffic accident

V70.7XX **7th** Person on outside of bus injured in collision with pedestrian or animal in traffic accident

V70.9XX **7th** Unspecified occupant of bus injured in collision with pedestrian or animal in traffic accident

V71 **BUS OCCUPANT INJURED IN COLLISION WITH PEDAL CYCLE**
Refer to External Cause of Injuries Table

V72 **4th** **BUS OCCUPANT INJURED IN COLLISION WITH TWO- OR THREE-WHEELED MOTOR VEHICLE**

V72.0XX **7th** Driver of bus injured in collision with two- or three-wheeled motor vehicle in nontraffic accident

V72.1XX **7th** Passenger on bus injured in collision with two- or three-wheeled motor vehicle in nontraffic accident

V72.2XX **7th** Person on outside of bus injured in collision with two- or three-wheeled motor vehicle in nontraffic accident

V72.3XX **7th** Unspecified occupant of bus injured in collision with two- or three-wheeled motor vehicle in nontraffic accident

V72.4XX **7th** Person boarding or alighting from bus injured in collision with two- or three-wheeled motor vehicle

V72.5XX **7th** Driver of bus injured in collision with two- or three-wheeled motor vehicle in traffic accident, sequela

V72.6XX **7th** Passenger on bus injured in collision with two- or three-wheeled motor vehicle in traffic accident

V72.7XX **7th** Person on outside of bus injured in collision with two- or three-wheeled motor vehicle in traffic accident

V72.9XX **7th** Unspecified occupant of bus injured in collision with two- or three-wheeled motor vehicle in traffic accident

V73 **4th** **BUS OCCUPANT INJURED IN COLLISION WITH CAR, PICK-UP TRUCK OR VAN**

V73.0XX **7th** Driver of bus injured in collision with car, pick-up truck or van in nontraffic accident

V73.1XX **7th** Passenger on bus injured in collision with car, pick-up truck or van in nontraffic accident

V73.2XX **7th** Person on outside of bus injured in collision with car, pick-up truck or van in nontraffic accident

V73.3XX **7th** Unspecified occupant of bus injured in collision with car, pick-up truck or van in nontraffic accident

V73.4XX **7th** Person boarding or alighting from bus injured in collision with car, pick-up truck or van

V73.5XX **7th** Driver of bus injured in collision with car, pick-up truck or van in traffic accident

V73.6XX **7th** Passenger on bus injured in collision with car, pick-up truck or van in traffic accident

V73.7XX **7th** Person on outside of bus injured in collision with car, pick-up truck or van in traffic accident

V73.9XX **7th** Unspecified occupant of bus injured in collision with car, pick-up truck or van in traffic accident

V74 **4th** **BUS OCCUPANT INJURED IN COLLISION WITH HEAVY TRANSPORT VEHICLE OR BUS**

Excludes1: bus occupant injured in collision with military vehicle (V79.81)

V74.0XX **7th** Driver of bus injured in collision with heavy transport vehicle or bus in nontraffic accident

V74.1XX **7th** Passenger on bus injured in collision with heavy transport vehicle or bus in nontraffic accident

V74.2XX **7th** Person on outside of bus injured in collision with heavy transport vehicle or bus in nontraffic accident

V74.3XX **7th** Unspecified occupant of bus injured in collision with heavy transport vehicle or bus in nontraffic accident

V74.4XX **7th** Person boarding or alighting from bus injured in collision with heavy transport vehicle or bus

V74.5XX **7th** Driver of bus injured in collision with heavy transport vehicle or bus in traffic accident

---

4th **5th** **6th** **7th** Additional Character Required   ✔ 3-character code

•=New Code   **Excludes1**—Not coded here, do not use together
▲=Revised Code   **Excludes2**—Not included here

V74.6XX [7th] Passenger on bus injured in collision with heavy transport vehicle or bus in traffic accident

V74.7XX [7th] Person on outside of bus injured in collision with heavy transport vehicle or bus in traffic accident

V74.9XX [7th] Unspecified occupant of bus injured in collision with heavy transport vehicle or bus in traffic accident

> 7th characters for categories
> V70–V79
> A—initial encounter
> D—subsequent encounter
> S—sequela

V75 [4th] **BUS OCCUPANT INJURED IN COLLISION WITH RAILWAY TRAIN OR RAILWAY VEHICLE**

V75.0XX [7th] Driver of bus injured in collision with railway train or railway vehicle in nontraffic accident

V75.1XX [7th] Passenger on bus injured in collision with railway train or railway vehicle in nontraffic accident

V75.2XX [7th] Person on outside of bus injured in collision with railway train or railway vehicle in nontraffic accident

V75.3XX [7th] Unspecified occupant of bus injured in collision with railway train or railway vehicle in nontraffic accident

V75.4XX [7th] Person boarding or alighting from bus injured in collision with railway train or railway vehicle

V75.5XX [7th] Driver of bus injured in collision with railway train or railway vehicle in traffic accident

V75.6XX [7th] Passenger on bus injured in collision with railway train or railway vehicle in traffic accident

V75.7XX [7th] Person on outside of bus injured in collision with railway train or railway vehicle in traffic accident

V75.9XX [7th] Unspecified occupant of bus injured in collision with railway train or railway vehicle in traffic accident

V76 [7th] **BUS OCCUPANT INJURED IN COLLISION WITH OTHER NONMOTOR VEHICLE**
Refer to External Cause of Injuries Table

V77 [4th] **BUS OCCUPANT INJURED IN COLLISION WITH FIXED OR STATIONARY OBJECT**

V77.0XX [7th] Driver of bus injured in collision with fixed or stationary object in nontraffic accident

V77.1XX [7th] Passenger on bus injured in collision with fixed or stationary object in nontraffic accident

V77.2XX [7th] Person on outside of bus injured in collision with fixed or stationary object in nontraffic accident

V77.3XX [7th] Unspecified occupant of bus injured in collision with fixed or stationary object in nontraffic accident

V77.4XX [7th] Person boarding or alighting from bus injured in collision with fixed or stationary object

V77.5XX [7th] Driver of bus injured in collision with fixed or stationary object in traffic accident

V77.6XX [7th] Passenger on bus injured in collision with fixed or stationary object in traffic accident

V77.7XX [7th] Person on outside of bus injured in collision with fixed or stationary object in traffic accident

V77.9XX [7th] Unspecified occupant of bus injured in collision with fixed or stationary object in traffic accident

V78 [4th] **BUS OCCUPANT INJURED IN NONCOLLISION TRANSPORT ACCIDENT**
Includes: overturning bus NOS
overturning bus without collision

V78.0XX [7th] Driver of bus injured in noncollision transport accident in nontraffic accident

V78.1XX [7th] Passenger on bus injured in noncollision transport accident in nontraffic accident

V78.2XX [7th] Person on outside of bus injured in noncollision transport accident in nontraffic accident

V78.3XX [7th] Unspecified occupant of bus injured in noncollision transport accident in nontraffic accident

V78.4XX [7th] Person boarding or alighting from bus injured in noncollision transport accident

V78.5XX [7th] Driver of bus injured in noncollision transport accident in traffic accident

V78.6XX [7th] Passenger on bus injured in noncollision transport accident in traffic accident

V78.7XX [7th] Person on outside of bus injured in noncollision transport accident in traffic accident

V78.9XX [7th] Unspecified occupant of bus injured in noncollision transport accident in traffic accident

V79 [4th] **BUS OCCUPANT INJURED IN OTHER AND UNSPECIFIED TRANSPORT ACCIDENTS**

V79.0 [5th] Driver of bus injured in collision with other and unspecified motor vehicles in nontraffic accident

V79.00X [7th] Driver of bus injured in collision with unspecified motor vehicles in nontraffic accident

V79.09X [7th] Driver of bus injured in collision with other motor vehicles in nontraffic accident

V79.1 [5th] Passenger on bus injured in collision with other and unspecified motor vehicles in nontraffic accident

V79.10X [7th] Passenger on bus injured in collision with unspecified motor vehicles in nontraffic accident

V79.19X [7th] Passenger on bus injured in collision with other motor vehicles in nontraffic accident

V79.2 [5th] Unspecified bus occupant injured in collision with other and unspecified motor vehicles in nontraffic accident

V79.20X [7th] Unspecified bus occupant injured in collision with unspecified motor vehicles in nontraffic accident
Bus collision NOS, nontraffic

V79.29X [7th] Unspecified bus occupant injured in collision with other motor vehicles in nontraffic accident

V79.3XX [7th] Bus occupant (driver) (passenger) injured in unspecified nontraffic accident
Bus accident NOS, nontraffic
Bus occupant injured in nontraffic accident NOS

V79.4 [5th] Driver of bus injured in collision with other and unspecified motor vehicles in traffic accident

V79.40X [7th] Driver of bus injured in collision with unspecified motor vehicles in traffic accident

V79.49X [7th] Driver of bus injured in collision with other motor vehicles in traffic accident

V79.5 [5th] Passenger on bus injured in collision with other and unspecified motor vehicles in traffic accident

V79.50X [7th] Passenger on bus injured in collision with unspecified motor vehicles in traffic accident

V79.59X [7th] Passenger on bus injured in collision with other motor vehicles in traffic accident

V79.6 [5th] Unspecified bus occupant injured in collision with other and unspecified motor vehicles in traffic accident

V79.60X [7th] Unspecified bus occupant injured in collision with unspecified motor vehicles in traffic accident
Bus collision NOS (traffic)

V79.69X [7th] Unspecified bus occupant injured in collision with other motor vehicles in traffic accident

V79.8 [5th] Bus occupant (driver) (passenger) injured in other specified transport accidents

V79.81X [7th] Bus occupant (driver) (passenger) injured in transport accidents with military vehicle

V79.88X [7th] Bus occupant (driver) (passenger) injured in other specified transport accidents

V79.9XX [7th] Bus occupant (driver) (passenger) injured in unspecified traffic accident
Bus accident NOS

(V80–V89) OTHER LAND TRANSPORT ACCIDENTS

V80 [4th] **ANIMAL-RIDER OR OCCUPANT OF ANIMAL-DRAWN VEHICLE INJURED IN TRANSPORT ACCIDENT**

> 7th characters for categories
> V80–V89
> A—initial encounter
> D—subsequent encounter
> S—sequela

See complete *ICD-10-CM* manual for codes in category V80.

V80.0 [5th] Animal-rider or occupant of animal-drawn vehicle injured by fall from or being thrown from animal or animal-drawn vehicle in noncollision accident

V80.01 [6th] Animal-rider injured by fall from or being thrown from animal in noncollision accident

V80.010 [7th] Animal-rider injured by fall from or being thrown from horse in noncollision accident

---

[4th] [5th] [6th] [7th] Additional Character Required   ✓ 3-character code

•=New Code
▲=Revised Code

Excludes1—Not coded here, do not use together
Excludes2—Not included here

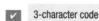

V80.018 Animal-rider injured by fall from or being
7th thrown from other animal in noncollision
accident

V80.02X Occupant of animal-
7th drawn vehicle injured
by fall from or being
thrown from animal-
drawn vehicle in
noncollision accident
Overturning animal-drawn vehicle NOS
Overturning animal-drawn vehicle without collision

7th characters for categories V80–V89
A—initial encounter
D—subsequent encounter
S—sequela

V80.1 Animal-rider or occupant of animal-drawn vehicle injured in
5th collision with pedestrian or animal
Excludes1: animal-rider or occupant of animal-drawn vehicle collision with
animal-drawn vehicle or animal being ridden (V80.7)
V80.11X Animal-rider injured in collision with pedestrian or
7th animal
V80.12X Occupant of animal-drawn vehicle injured in
7th collision with pedestrian or animal
V80.4 Animal-rider or occupant of animal-drawn vehicle injured in
5th collision with car, pick-up truck, van, heavy transport vehicle
or bus
Excludes1: animal-rider injured in collision with military vehicle
(V80.910)
occupant of animal-drawn vehicle injured in collision with
military vehicle (V80.920)
V80.41X Animal-rider injured in collision with car, pick-up
7th truck, van, heavy transport vehicle or bus
V80.42X Occupant of animal-drawn vehicle injured in
7th collision with car, pick-up truck, van, heavy transport
vehicle or bus
V80.7 Animal-rider or occupant of animal-drawn vehicle injured in
5th collision with other nonmotor vehicles
V80.71 Animal-rider or occupant of animal-drawn vehicle
6th injured in collision with animal being ridden
V80.710 Animal-rider injured in collision with other
7th animal being ridden
V80.711 Occupant of animal-drawn vehicle injured
7th in collision with animal being ridden
V80.72 Animal-rider or occupant of animal-drawn vehicle
6th injured in collision with other animal-drawnvehicle
V80.720 Animal-rider injured in collision with
7th animal-drawn vehicle
V80.721 Occupant of animal-drawn vehicle injured
7th in collision with other animal-drawn
vehicle
V80.73 Animal-rider or occupant of animal-drawn vehicle
6th injured in collision with streetcar
V80.730 Animal-rider injured in collision with
7th streetcar
V80.731 Occupant of animal-drawn vehicle injured
7th in collision with streetcar
V80.79 Animal-rider or occupant of animal-drawn vehicle
6th injured in collision with other nonmotorvehicles
V80.790 Animal-rider injured in collision with other
7th nonmotor vehicles
V80.791 Occupant of animal-drawn vehicle injured
7th in collision with other nonmotor vehicles
V80.8 Animal-rider or occupant of animal-drawn vehicle injured in
5th collision with fixed or stationary object
V80.81X Animal-rider injured in collision with fixed or
7th stationary object
V80.82X Occupant of animal-drawn vehicle injured in
7th collision with fixed or stationary object
V80.9 Animal-rider or occupant of animal-drawn vehicle injured in
5th other and unspecified transport accidents
V80.91 Animal-rider injured in other and unspecified
6th transport accidents
V80.918 Animal-rider injured in other transport
7th accident
V80.919 Animal-rider injured in unspecified
7th transport accident
Animal rider accident NOS

V80.92 Occupant of animal-drawn vehicle injured in other
6th and unspecified transport accidents
V80.928 Occupant of animal-drawn vehicle injured
7th in other transport accident
V80.929 Occupant of animal-drawn vehicle injured
7th in unspecified transport accident
Animal-drawn vehicle accident NOS

V81 OCCUPANT OF RAILWAY TRAIN OR RAILWAY VEHICLE
4th INJURED IN TRANSPORT ACCIDENT
Includes: derailment of railway train or railway vehicle
person on outside of train
Excludes1: streetcar (V82.-)
See complete *ICD-10-CM* manual for codes in category V81.

V82 OCCUPANT OF POWERED STREETCAR INJURED IN
4th TRANSPORT ACCIDENT
Includes: interurban electric car
person on outside of streetcar
tram (car)
trolley (car)
Excludes1: bus (V70–V79)
motorcoach (V70–V79)
nonpowered streetcar (V76.-)
train (V81.-)
See complete *ICD-10-CM* manual for codes in category V82.

V83 OCCUPANT OF SPECIAL VEHICLE MAINLY USED ON
4th INDUSTRIAL PREMISES INJURED IN TRANSPORT
ACCIDENT
Includes: battery-powered airport passenger vehicle
battery-powered truck (baggage) (mail)
coal-car in mine
forklift (truck)
logging car
self-propelled industrial truck
station baggage truck (powered)
tram, truck, or tub (powered) in mine or quarry
Excludes1: special construction vehicles (V85.-)
special industrial vehicle in stationary use or maintenance (W31.-)
See complete *ICD-10-CM* manual for codes in category V83.

V84 OCCUPANT OF SPECIAL VEHICLE MAINLY USED IN
4th AGRICULTURE INJURED IN TRANSPORT ACCIDENT
Includes: self-propelled farm machinery
tractor (and trailer)
Excludes1: animal-powered farm machinery accident (W30.8-)
contact with combine harvester (W30.0)
special agricultural vehicle in stationary use or maintenance (W30.-)
V84.0XX Driver of special agricultural vehicle injured in traffic
7th accident
V84.1XX Passenger of special agricultural vehicle injured in traffic
7th accident
V84.2XX Person on outside of special agricultural vehicle injured in
7th traffic accident
V84.3XX Unspecified occupant of special agricultural vehicle injured
7th in traffic accident
V84.4XX Person injured while boarding or alighting from special
7th agricultural vehicle
V84.5XX Driver of special agricultural vehicle injured in nontraffic
7th accident
V84.6XX Passenger of special agricultural vehicle injured in
7th nontraffic accident
V84.7XX Person on outside of special agricultural vehicle injured in
7th nontraffic accident
V84.9XX Unspecified occupant of special agricultural vehicle injured
7th in nontraffic accident

V86 OCCUPANT OF SPECIAL ALL-TERRAIN OR OTHER
4th OFF-ROAD MOTOR VEHICLE, INJURED IN TRANSPORT
ACCIDENT
Excludes1: special all-terrain vehicle in stationary use or maintenance
(W31.-)
sport-utility vehicle (V50–V59)
three-wheeled motor vehicle designed for on-road use (V30–V39)
See complete *ICD-10-CM* manual for codes in category V86.

4th **5th** **6th** **7th** Additional Character Required   ✔ 3-character code

•=New Code   *Excludes1*—Not coded here, do not use together
▲=Revised Code   *Excludes2*—Not included here

V86.0 **Driver of special all-terrain or other off-road motor vehicle injured in traffic accident**
5th

    V86.02X **Driver of snowmobile injured in traffic accident**
    7th

    V86.03X **Driver of dune buggy injured in traffic accident**
    7th

    V86.05X **Driver of 3- or 4- wheeled all-terrain vehicle (ATV) injured in traffic accident**
    7th

    V86.06X **Driver of dirt bike or motor/cross bike injured in traffic accident**
    7th

    V86.09X **Driver of other special all-terrain or other off-road motor vehicle injured in traffic accident**
    7th
        Driver of go cart injured in traffic accident
        Driver of golf cart injured in traffic accident

V86.1 **Passenger of special all-terrain or other off-road motor vehicle injured in traffic accident**
5th

    V86.12X **Passenger of snowmobile injured in traffic accident**
    7th

    V86.13X **Passenger of dune buggy injured in traffic accident**
    7th

    V86.15X **Passenger of 3- or 4- wheeled ATV injured in traffic accident**
    7th

    V86.16X **Passenger of dirt bike or motor/cross bike injured in traffic accident**
    7th

    V86.19X **Passenger of other special all-terrain or other off-road motor vehicle injured in traffic accident**
    7th
        Passenger of go cart injured in traffic accident
        Passenger of golf cart injured in traffic accident

V86.3 **Unspecified occupant of special all-terrain or other off-road motor vehicle injured in traffic accident**
5th

> **7th characters for categories**
> V80–V89
> A—initial encounter
> D—subsequent encounter
> S—sequela

    V86.32X **Unspecific occupant of snowmobile injured in traffic accident**
    7th

    V86.33X **Unspecified occupant of dune buggy injured in traffic accident**
    7th

    V86.35X **Unspecified occupant of 3- or 4- wheeled ATV injured in traffic accident**
    7th

    V86.36X **Unspecified occupant of dirt bike or motor/cross bike injured in traffic accident**
    7th

    V86.39X **Unspecified occupant of other special all-terrain or other off-road motor vehicle injured in traffic accident**
    7th
        Person in go cart or golf cart injured in traffic accident

V86.5 **Driver of special all-terrain or other off-road motor vehicle injured in nontraffic accident**
5th

    V86.52X **Driver of snowmobile injured in nontraffic accident**
    7th

    V86.53X **Driver of dune buggy injured in nontraffic accident**
    7th

    V86.55X **Driver of 3- or 4- wheeled ATV injured in nontraffic accident**
    7th

    V86.56X **Driver of dirt bike or motor/cross bike injured in nontraffic accident**
    7th

    V86.59X **Driver of other special all-terrain or other off-road motor vehicle injured in nontraffic accident**
    7th
        Driver of go cart or golf cart injured in nontraffic accident

V86.6 **Passenger of special all-terrain or other off-road motor vehicle injured in nontraffic accident**
5th

    V86.62X **Passenger of snowmobile injured in nontraffic accident**
    7th

    V86.63X **Passenger of dune buggy injured in nontraffic accident**
    7th

    V86.65X **Passenger of 3- or 4- wheeled ATV injured in nontraffic accident**
    7th

    V86.66X **Passenger of dirt bike or motor/cross bike injured in nontraffic accident**
    7th

    V86.69X **Passenger of other special all-terrain or other off-road motor vehicle injured in nontraffic accident**
    7th
        Passenger of go cart or golf cart injured in nontraffic accident

V86.9 **Unspecified occupant of special all-terrain or other off-road motor vehicle injured in nontraffic accident**
5th

    V86.92X **Unspecific occupant of snowmobile injured in nontraffic accident**
    7th

    V86.93X **Unspecified occupant of dune buggy injured in nontraffic accident**
    7th

    V86.95X **Unspecified occupant of 3- or 4- wheeled ATV injured in nontraffic accident**
    7th

    V86.96X **Unspecified occupant of dirt bike or motor/cross bike injured in nontraffic accident**
    7th

    V86.99X **Unspecified occupant of other special all-terrain or other off-road motor vehicle injured in nontraffic accident**
    7th
        Off-road motor-vehicle accident NOS
        Other motor-vehicle accident NOS
        Unspecified occupant of go cart or golf cart injured in nontraffic accident

V87 **TRAFFIC ACCIDENT OF SPECIFIED TYPE BUT VICTIM'S MODE OF TRANSPORT UNKNOWN**
4th
    Excludes1: collision involving:
        pedal cycle (V10–V19)
        pedestrian (V01–V09)
    See complete *ICD-10-CM* manual for codes in category V87.

V88 **NONTRAFFIC ACCIDENT OF SPECIFIED TYPE BUT VICTIM'S MODE OF TRANSPORT UNKNOWN**
4th
    Excludes1: collision involving:
        pedal cycle (V10–V19)
        pedestrian (V01–V09)
    See complete *ICD-10-CM* manual for codes in category V88.

V89 **MOTOR- OR NONMOTOR-VEHICLE ACCIDENT, TYPE OF VEHICLE UNSPECIFIED**
4th

    V89.0XX **Person injured in unspecified motor-vehicle accident, nontraffic**
    7th
        Motor-vehicle accident NOS, nontraffic

    V89.1XX **Person injured in unspecified nonmotor-vehicle accident, nontraffic**
    7th
        Nonmotor-vehicle accident NOS (nontraffic)

    V89.2XX **Person injured in unspecified motor-vehicle accident, traffic**
    7th
        Motor-vehicle accident [MVA] NOS
        Road (traffic) accident NOS

    V89.3XX **Person injured in unspecified nonmotor-vehicle accident, traffic**
    7th
        Nonmotor-vehicle traffic accident NOS

    V89.9XX **Person injured in unspecified vehicle accident**
    7th
        Collision NOS

(V90–V94) WATER TRANSPORT ACCIDENTS

V90 **DROWNING AND SUBMERSION DUE TO ACCIDENT TO WATERCRAFT**
4th
    Excludes1: fall into water not from watercraft (W16.-)
      water-transport-related drowning or submersion without accident to watercraft (V92.-)

> **7th characters for categories**
> V90–V94
> A—initial encounter
> D—subsequent encounter
> S—sequela

    See complete *ICD-10-CM* manual for subcategory codes V90.1-, V90.2-, V90.3-, and V90.8-.

    V90.0 **Drowning and submersion due to watercraft overturning**
    5th

        V90.01X **Drowning and submersion due to; passenger ship overturning**
        7th
            Drowning and submersion due to Ferry-boat overturning
            Drowning and submersion due to Liner overturning

        V90.02X **fishing boat overturning**
        7th

        V90.03X **other powered watercraft overturning**
        7th
            Drowning and submersion due to Hovercraft (on open water)/Jet ski overturning

        V90.04X **sailboat overturning**
        7th

        V90.05X **canoe or kayak overturning**
        7th

        V90.06X **(nonpowered) inflatable craft overturning**
        7th

4th   5th   6th   7th   Additional Character Required   ✔ 3-character code

•=New Code
▲=Revised Code

Excludes1—Not coded here, do not use together
Excludes2—Not included here

V90.08X **other unpowered watercraft overturning**
7th   Drowning and submersion due to windsurfer overturning
V90.09X **unspecified watercraft overturning**
7th   Drowning and submersion due to boat/ship/watercraft NOS overturning

V91 **OTHER INJURY DUE TO ACCIDENT TO WATERCRAFT**
4th
Includes: any injury except drowning and submersion as a result of an accident to watercraft
Excludes1: civilian water transport accident involving military watercraft (V94.81-)
military watercraft accident in military or war operations (Y36, Y37.-)
Excludes2: drowning and submersion due to accident to watercraft (V90.-)
See complete *ICD-10-CM* manual for codes in category V91.

V92 **DROWNING AND SUBMERSION DUE TO ACCIDENT ON BOARD WATERCRAFT, WITHOUT ACCIDENT TO WATERCRAFT**
4th
Excludes1: civilian water transport accident involving military watercraft (V94.81-)
drowning or submersion due to accident to watercraft (V90-V91)
drowning or submersion of diver who voluntarily jumps from boat not involved in an accident (W16.711, W16.721)
fall into water without watercraft (W16.-)
military watercraft accident in military or war operations (Y36, Y37)
See complete *ICD-10-CM* manual for codes in category V92.

V93 **OTHER INJURY WHILE ON WATERCRAFT, WITHOUT ACCIDENT TO WATERCRAFT**
4th
See complete *ICD-10-CM* manual for subcategory codes V93.0-, V93.1-, V93.2-, V93.4-, V93.5-, V93.6- and V93.8-. codes in category V82.
V93.3 **Fall on board watercraft**
5th
Excludes1: fall due to collision of watercraft (V91.2-)
V93.32X **Fall on board fishing**
7th   **boat**
V93.33X **Fall on board other**
7th   **powered watercraft**
Fall on board Hovercraft/ Jet ski (on open water)

> 7th characters for categories
> V90–V94
> A—initial encounter
> D—subsequent encounter
> S—sequela

V93.34X **Fall on board sailboat**
7th
V93.35X **Fall on board canoe or kayak**
7th
V93.36X **Fall on board (nonpowered) inflatable craft**
7th
V93.38X **Fall on board other unpowered watercraft**
7th
V93.39X **Fall on board unspecified watercraft**
7th   Fall on board boat/ship/watercraft NOS
V93.8 **Other injury due to other accident on board watercraft**
5th
Accidental poisoning by gases or fumes on watercraft
V93.82X **Other injury due to other accident on board fishing**
7th   **boat**
V93.83X **Other injury due to other accident on board other**
7th   **powered watercraft**
Other injury due to other accident on board Hovercraft
Other injury due to other accident on board Jet ski
V93.84X **Other injury due to other accident on board sailboat**
7th
V93.85X **Other injury due to other accident on board canoe or**
7th   **kayak**
V93.86X **Other injury due to other accident on board**
7th   **(nonpowered) inflatable craft**
V93.87X **Other injury due to other accident on board water-**
7th   **skis**
Hit or struck by object while waterskiing
V93.88X **Other injury due to other accident on board other**
7th   **unpowered watercraft**
Hit or struck by object while surfing
Hit or struck by object while on board windsurfer
V93.89X **Other injury due to other accident on board**
7th   **unspecified watercraft**
Other injury due to other accident on board boat/ship/ watercraft NOS

V94 **OTHER AND UNSPECIFIED WATER TRANSPORT**
4th **ACCIDENTS**
Excludes1: military watercraft accidents in military or war operations (Y36, Y37)
V94.0XX **Hitting object or bottom of body of water due to fall from**
7th **watercraft**
Excludes2: drowning and submersion due to fall from watercraft (V92.0-)
V94.1 **Bather struck by watercraft**
5th Swimmer hit by watercraft
V94.11X **Bather struck by powered watercraft**
7th
V94.12X **Bather struck by nonpowered watercraft**
7th
V94.2 **Rider of nonpowered watercraft struck by other watercraft**
5th **V94.21X** **Rider of nonpowered watercraft struck by other**
7th **nonpowered watercraft**
Canoer hit by other nonpowered watercraft
Surfer hit by other nonpowered watercraft
Windsurfer hit by other nonpowered watercraft
V94.22X **Rider of nonpowered watercraft struck by powered**
7th **watercraft**
Canoer hit by motorboat
Surfer hit by motorboat
Windsurfer hit by motorboat
V94.3 **Injury to rider of (inflatable) watercraft being pulled behind**
5th **other watercraft**
V94.31X **Injury to rider of (inflatable) recreational watercraft**
7th **being pulled behind other watercraft**
Injury to rider of inner-tube pulled behind motor boat
V94.32X **Injury to rider of non-recreational watercraft being**
7th **pulled behind other watercraft**
Injury to occupant of dingy being pulled behind boat or ship
Injury to occupant of life-raft being pulled behind boat or ship
V94.4XX **Injury to barefoot water-skier**
7th Injury to person being pulled behind boat or ship
V94.89XX **Other water transport accident**
7th
V94.9XX **Unspecified water transport accident**
7th Water transport accident NOS
initial encounter accident
for definitions of transport

(V95–V97) AIR AND SPACE TRANSPORT ACCIDENTS

Excludes1: military aircraft accidents in military or war operations (Y36, Y37)
See complete *ICD-10-CM* manual for codes in categories V95–V97.

(V98–V99) OTHER AND UNSPECIFIED TRANSPORT ACCIDENTS

See complete *ICD-10-CM* manual for codes in categories V98–V99.

(W00–X58) OTHER EXTERNAL CAUSES OF ACCIDENTAL INJURY

(W00–W19) SLIPPING, TRIPPING, STUMBLING AND FALLS

Excludes1: assault involving a fall (Y01–Y02)
fall from animal (V80.-)
fall (in) (from) machinery (in operation) (W28–W31)
fall (in) (from) transport vehicle (V01–V99)
intentional self-harm involving a fall (X80–X81)

Excludes2: at risk for fall (history of fall) Z91.81 fall (in) (from) burning building (X00.-)
fall into fire (X00–X04, X08)

W00 **FALL DUE TO ICE AND SNOW**
4th
Includes: pedestrian on foot falling (slipping) on ice and snow
Excludes1: fall on (from) ice and snow involving pedestrian conveyance (V00.-)
fall from stairs and steps not due to ice and snow (W10.-)

4th   5th   6th   7th   Additional Character Required   ✔   3-character code

•=New Code   *Excludes1*—Not coded here, do not use together
▲=Revised Code   *Excludes2*—Not included here

CHAPTER 20. EXTERNAL CAUSES OF MORBIDITY   (W00.0XX–W16.02)

W00.0XX [7th] **Fall on same level due to ice and snow**

W00.1XX [7th] **Fall from stairs and steps due to ice and snow**

W00.2XX [7th] **Other fall from one level to another due to ice and snow**

W00.9XX [7th] **Unspecified fall due to ice and snow**

> 7th characters for categories
> W00–W19
> A—initial encounter
> D—subsequent encounter
> S—sequela

W01 [4th] **FALL ON SAME LEVEL FROM SLIPPING, TRIPPING AND STUMBLING**
Includes: fall on moving sidewalk
Excludes1: fall due to bumping (striking) against object (W18.0-)
     fall in shower or bathtub (W18.2-)
     fall on same level NOS (W18.30)
     fall on same level from slipping, tripping and stumbling due to ice or snow (W00.0)
     fall off or from toilet (W18.1-)
     slipping, tripping and stumbling NOS (W18.40)
     slipping, tripping and stumbling without falling (W18.4-)

W01.0XX [7th] **Fall on same level from slipping, tripping and stumbling without subsequent striking against object**
     Falling over animal

W01.1 [5th] **Fall on same level from slipping, tripping and stumbling with subsequent striking against object**
   W01.10X [7th] **Fall on same level from slipping, tripping and stumbling with subsequent striking against unspecified object**
   W01.11 [6th] **Fall on same level from slipping, tripping and stumbling with subsequent striking against sharp object**
     W01.110 [7th] **Fall on same level from slipping, tripping and stumbling with subsequent striking against sharp glass**
     W01.111 [7th] **Fall on same level from slipping, tripping and stumbling with subsequent striking against power tool or machine**
     W01.118 [7th] **Fall on same level from slipping, tripping and stumbling with subsequent striking against other sharp object**
     W01.119 [7th] **Fall on same level from slipping, tripping and stumbling with subsequent striking against unspecified sharp object**
   W01.19 [6th] **Fall on same level from slipping, tripping and stumbling with subsequent striking against other object**
     W01.190 [7th] **Fall on same level from slipping, tripping and stumbling with subsequent striking against furniture**
     W01.198 [7th] **Fall on same level from slipping, tripping and stumbling with subsequent striking against other object**

W03 [7th] **OTHER FALL ON SAME LEVEL DUE TO COLLISION WITH ANOTHER PERSON**
Fall due to non-transport collision with other person
Excludes1: collision with another person without fall (W51)
     crushed or pushed by a crowd or human stampede (W52)
     fall involving pedestrian conveyance (V00-V09)
     fall due to ice or snow (W00)
     fall on same level NOS (W18.30)

W04 [7th] **FALL WHILE BEING CARRIED OR SUPPORTED BY OTHER PERSONS**
Accidentally dropped while being carried

W05 [7th] **FALL FROM NON-MOVING WHEELCHAIR, NONMOTORIZED SCOOTER AND MOTORIZED MOBILITY SCOOTER**
Excludes1: fall from moving wheelchair (powered) (V00.811)
     fall from moving motorized mobility scooter (V00.831)
     fall from nonmotorized scooter (V00.141)

> 7th characters for categories
> W00–W19
> A—initial encounter
> D—subsequent encounter
> S—sequela

W06 [7th] **FALL FROM BED**

W07 [7th] **FALL FROM CHAIR**

W08 [7th] **FALL FROM OTHER FURNITURE**

W09 [4th] **FALL ON AND FROM PLAYGROUND EQUIPMENT**
Excludes1: fall involving recreational machinery (W31)
W09.0XX [7th] **Fall on or from playground slide**
W09.1XX [7th] **Fall from playground swing**
W09.2XX [7th] **Fall on or from jungle gym**
W09.8XX [7th] **Fall on or from other playground equipment**

W10 [4th] **FALL ON AND FROM STAIRS AND STEPS**
Excludes1: Fall from stairs and steps due to ice and snow (W00.1)
W10.0XX [7th] **Fall (on) (from) escalator**
W10.1XX [7th] **Fall (on) (from) sidewalk curb**
W10.2XX [7th] **Fall (on) (from) incline**
     Fall (on) (from) ramp
W10.8XX [7th] **Fall (on) (from) other stairs and steps**
W10.9XX [7th] **Fall (on) (from) unspecified stairs and steps**

W11 [7th] **FALL ON AND FROM LADDER**

W12 [7th] **FALL ON AND FROM SCAFFOLDING**

W13 [4th] **FALL FROM, OUT OF OR THROUGH BUILDING OR STRUCTURE**
W13.0XX [7th] **Fall from, out of or through balcony**
     Fall from, out of or through railing
W13.1XX [7th] **Fall from, out of or through bridge**
W13.2XX [7th] **Fall from, out of or through roof**
W13.3XX [7th] **Fall through floor**
W13.4XX [7th] **Fall from, out of or through window**
     Excludes2: fall with subsequent striking against sharp glass (W01.110-)
W13.8XX [7th] **Fall from, out of or through other building or structure**
     Fall from, out of or through viaduct
     Fall from, out of or through wall
     Fall from, out of or through flag-pole
W13.9XX [7th] **Fall from, out of or through building, not otherwise specified**
     Excludes1: collapse of a building or structure (W20.-)
     fall or jump from burning building or structure (X00.-)

W14 [7th] **FALL FROM TREE**

W15 [7th] **FALL FROM CLIFF**

W16 [4th] **FALL, JUMP OR DIVING INTO WATER**
Excludes1: accidental non-watercraft drowning and submersion not involving fall (W65–W74)
     effects of air pressure from diving (W94.-)
     fall into water from watercraft (V90–V94)
     hitting an object or against bottom when falling from watercraft (V94.0)
Excludes2: striking or hitting diving board (W21.4)
W16.0 [5th] **Fall into swimming pool**
   Excludes1: fall into empty swimming pool (W17.3)
   W16.01 [6th] **Fall into swimming pool striking water surface**
     W16.011 [7th] **Fall into swimming pool striking water surface causing drowning and submersion**
     Excludes1: drowning and submersion while in swimming pool without fall (W67)
     W16.012 [7th] **Fall into swimming pool striking water surface causing other injury**
   W16.02 [6th] **Fall into swimming pool striking bottom**

[4th] [5th] [6th] [7th] Additional Character Required   ✔ 3-character code

•=New Code
▲=Revised Code

Excludes1—Not coded here, do not use together
Excludes2—Not included here

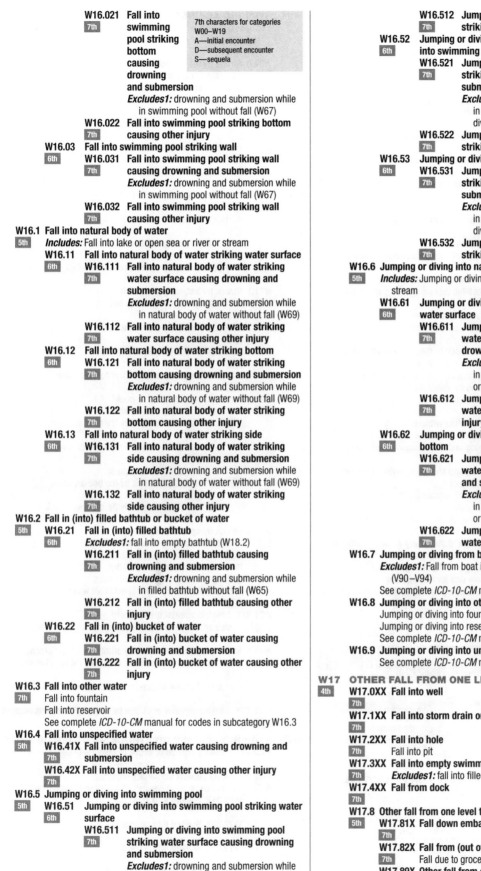

W16.021 `7th` **Fall into swimming pool striking bottom causing drowning and submersion**

> 7th characters for categories W00–W19
> A—initial encounter
> D—subsequent encounter
> S—sequela

> *Excludes1:* drowning and submersion while in swimming pool without fall (W67)

W16.022 `7th` **Fall into swimming pool striking bottom causing other injury**

W16.03 `6th` **Fall into swimming pool striking wall**

  W16.031 `7th` **Fall into swimming pool striking wall causing drowning and submersion**

> *Excludes1:* drowning and submersion while in swimming pool without fall (W67)

  W16.032 `7th` **Fall into swimming pool striking wall causing other injury**

W16.1 `5th` **Fall into natural body of water**

> *Includes:* Fall into lake or open sea or river or stream

  W16.11 `6th` **Fall into natural body of water striking water surface**

    W16.111 `7th` **Fall into natural body of water striking water surface causing drowning and submersion**

> *Excludes1:* drowning and submersion while in natural body of water without fall (W69)

    W16.112 `7th` **Fall into natural body of water striking water surface causing other injury**

  W16.12 `6th` **Fall into natural body of water striking bottom**

    W16.121 `7th` **Fall into natural body of water striking bottom causing drowning and submersion**

> *Excludes1:* drowning and submersion while in natural body of water without fall (W69)

    W16.122 `7th` **Fall into natural body of water striking bottom causing other injury**

  W16.13 `6th` **Fall into natural body of water striking side**

    W16.131 `7th` **Fall into natural body of water striking side causing drowning and submersion**

> *Excludes1:* drowning and submersion while in natural body of water without fall (W69)

    W16.132 `7th` **Fall into natural body of water striking side causing other injury**

W16.2 `5th` **Fall in (into) filled bathtub or bucket of water**

  W16.21 `6th` **Fall in (into) filled bathtub**

> *Excludes1:* fall into empty bathtub (W18.2)

    W16.211 `7th` **Fall in (into) filled bathtub causing drowning and submersion**

> *Excludes1:* drowning and submersion while in filled bathtub without fall (W65)

    W16.212 `7th` **Fall in (into) filled bathtub causing other injury**

  W16.22 `6th` **Fall in (into) bucket of water**

    W16.221 `7th` **Fall in (into) bucket of water causing drowning and submersion**

    W16.222 `7th` **Fall in (into) bucket of water causing other injury**

W16.3 `7th` **Fall into other water**

Fall into fountain

Fall into reservoir

See complete *ICD-10-CM* manual for codes in subcategory W16.3

W16.4 `5th` **Fall into unspecified water**

  W16.41X `7th` **Fall into unspecified water causing drowning and submersion**

  W16.42X `7th` **Fall into unspecified water causing other injury**

W16.5 `5th` **Jumping or diving into swimming pool**

  W16.51 `6th` **Jumping or diving into swimming pool striking water surface**

    W16.511 `7th` **Jumping or diving into swimming pool striking water surface causing drowning and submersion**

> *Excludes1:* drowning and submersion while in swimming pool without jumping or diving (W67)

    W16.512 `7th` **Jumping or diving into swimming pool striking water surface causing other injury**

  W16.52 `6th` **Jumping or diving into swimming pool striking bottom**

    W16.521 `7th` **Jumping or diving into swimming pool striking bottom causing drowning and submersion**

> *Excludes1:* drowning and submersion while in swimming pool without jumping or diving (W67)

    W16.522 `7th` **Jumping or diving into swimming pool striking bottom causing other injury**

  W16.53 `6th` **Jumping or diving into swimming pool striking wall**

    W16.531 `7th` **Jumping or diving into swimming pool striking wall causing drowning and submersion**

> *Excludes1:* drowning and submersion while in swimming pool without jumping or diving (W67)

    W16.532 `7th` **Jumping or diving into swimming pool striking wall causing other injury**

W16.6 `5th` **Jumping or diving into natural body of water**

> *Includes:* Jumping or diving into lake or open sea or river or stream

  W16.61 `6th` **Jumping or diving into natural body of water striking water surface**

    W16.611 `7th` **Jumping or diving into natural body of water striking water surface causing drowning and submersion**

> *Excludes1:* drowning and submersion while in natural body of water without jumping or diving (W69)

    W16.612 `7th` **Jumping or diving into natural body of water striking water surface causing other injury**

  W16.62 `6th` **Jumping or diving into natural body of water striking bottom**

    W16.621 `7th` **Jumping or diving into natural body of water striking bottom causing drowning and submersion**

> *Excludes1:* drowning and submersion while in natural body of water without jumping or diving (W69)

    W16.622 `7th` **Jumping or diving into natural body of water striking bottom causing other injury**

W16.7 **Jumping or diving from boat**

> *Excludes1:* Fall from boat into water -see watercraft accident (V90–V94)

See complete *ICD-10-CM* manual for codes in subcategory W16.7

W16.8 **Jumping or diving into other water**

Jumping or diving into fountain

Jumping or diving into reservoir

See complete *ICD-10-CM* manual for codes in subcategory W16.8

W16.9 **Jumping or diving into unspecified water**

See complete *ICD-10-CM* manual for codes in subcategory W16.9

W17 `4th` **OTHER FALL FROM ONE LEVEL TO ANOTHER**

W17.0XX `7th` **Fall into well**

W17.1XX `7th` **Fall into storm drain or manhole**

W17.2XX `7th` **Fall into hole**

Fall into pit

W17.3XX `7th` **Fall into empty swimming pool**

> *Excludes1:* fall into filled swimming pool (W16.0-)

W17.4XX `7th` **Fall from dock**

W17.8 `5th` **Other fall from one level to another**

  W17.81X `7th` **Fall down embankment (hill)***

  W17.82X `7th` **Fall from (out of) grocery cart**

Fall due to grocery cart tipping over

  W17.89X `7th` **Other fall from one level to another**

Fall from cherry picker/lifting device/sky lift

`4th` `5th` `6th` `7th`   Additional Character Required   ✔   3-character code

• =New Code
▲ =Revised Code

Excludes1—Not coded here, do not use together
Excludes2—Not included here

W18 **OTHER SLIPPING, TRIPPING AND STUMBLING AND FALLS**
`4th`

	7th characters for categories
	W00–W19
	A—initial encounter
	D—subsequent encounter
	S—sequela

W18.0 **Fall due to bumping against object**
`5th`
     Striking against object with subsequent fall
     Excludes1: fall on same level due to slipping, tripping, or stumbling with subsequent striking against object (W01.1-)
     W18.00X **Striking against unspecified object with subsequent fall**
     `7th`
     W18.01X **Striking against sports equipment with subsequent fall**
     `7th`
     W18.02X **Striking against glass with subsequent fall**
     `7th`
     W18.09X **Striking against other object with subsequent fall**
     `7th`

W18.1 **Fall from or off toilet**
`5th`
     W18.11X **Fall from or off toilet without subsequent striking against object**
     `7th`
     Fall from (off) toilet NOS
     W18.12X **Fall from or off toilet with subsequent striking against object**
     `7th`

W18.2XX **Fall in (into) shower or empty bathtub**
`7th`
     Excludes1: fall in full bathtub causing drowning or submersion (W16.21-)

W18.3 **Other and unspecified fall on same level**
`5th`
     W18.30X **Fall on same level, unspecified**
     `7th`
     W18.31X **Fall on same level due to stepping on an object**
     `7th`
     Fall on same level due to stepping on an animal
     Excludes1: slipping, tripping and stumbling without fall due to stepping on animal (W18.41)
     W18.39X **Other fall on same level**
     `7th`

W18.4 **Slipping, tripping and stumbling without falling**
`5th`
     Excludes1: collision with another person without fall (W51)
     W18.40X **Slipping, tripping and stumbling without falling, unspecified**
     `7th`
     W18.41X **Slipping, tripping and stumbling without falling due to stepping on object**
     `7th`
     Slipping, tripping and stumbling without falling due to stepping on animal
     Excludes1: slipping, tripping and stumbling with fall due to stepping on animal (W18.31)
     W18.42X **Slipping, tripping and stumbling without falling due to stepping into hole or opening**
     `7th`
     W18.43X **Slipping, tripping and stumbling without falling due to stepping from one level to another**
     `7th`
     W18.49X **Other slipping, tripping and stumbling without falling**
     `7th`

W19 **UNSPECIFIED FALL**
`7th`
     Accidental fall NOS

(W20–W49) EXPOSURE TO INANIMATE MECHANICAL FORCES

Excludes1: assault (X92–Y08)
     contact or collision with animals or persons (W50–W64)
     exposure to inanimate mechanical forces involving military or war operations (Y36.-, Y37.-)
     intentional self-harm (X71–X83)

	7th characters for categories
	W20–W49
	A—initial encounter
	D—subsequent encounter
	S—sequela

W20 **STRUCK BY THROWN, PROJECTED OR FALLING OBJECT**
`7th`
     Code first any associated:
     cataclysm (X34-X39)
     lightning strike (T75.00)
     Excludes1: falling object in machinery accident (W24, W28-W31)
     falling object in transport accident (V01-V99)
     object set in motion by explosion (W35-W40)
     object set in motion by firearm (W32-W34)
     struck by thrown sports equipment (W21.-)
     See complete *ICD-10-CM* manual for codes in category W20.

W21 **STRIKING AGAINST OR STRUCK BY SPORTS EQUIPMENT**
`4th`
     Excludes1: assault with sports equipment (Y08.0-)
     striking against or struck by sports equipment with subsequent fall (W18.01)

W21.0 **Struck by hit or thrown ball**
`5th`
     W21.00X **Struck by hit or thrown ball, unspecified type**
     `7th`

	7th characters for categories
	W20–W49
	A—initial encounter
	D—subsequent encounter
	S—sequela

     W21.01X **Struck by football**
     `7th`
     W21.02X **Struck by soccer ball**
     `7th`
     W21.03X **Struck by baseball**
     `7th`
     W21.04X **Struck by golf ball**
     `7th`
     W21.05X **Struck by basketball**
     `7th`
     W21.06X **Struck by volleyball**
     `7th`
     W21.07X **Struck by softball**
     `7th`
     W21.09X **Struck by other hit or thrown ball**
     `7th`

W21.1 **Struck by bat, racquet or club**
`5th`
     W21.11X **Struck by baseball bat**
     `7th`
     W21.12X **Struck by tennis racquet**
     `7th`
     W21.13X **Struck by golf club**
     `7th`
     W21.19X **Struck by other bat, racquet or club**
     `7th`

W21.2 **Struck by hockey stick or puck**
`5th`
     W21.21 **Struck by hockey stick**
     `6th`
         W21.210 **Struck by ice hockey stick**
         `7th`
         W21.211 **Struck by field hockey stick**
         `7th`
     W21.22 **Struck by hockey puck**
     `6th`
         W21.220 **Struck by ice hockey puck**
         `7th`
         W21.221 **Struck by field hockey puck**
         `7th`

W21.3 **Struck by sports foot wear**
`5th`
     W21.31X **Struck by shoe cleats**
     `7th`
     Stepped on by shoe cleats
     W21.32X **Struck by skate blades**
     `7th`
     Skated over by skate blades
     W21.39X **Struck by other sports foot wear**
     `7th`

W21.4XX **Striking against diving board**
`7th`
     Use additional code for subsequent falling into water, if applicable (W16.-)

W21.8 **Striking against or struck by other sports equipment**
`5th`
     W21.81X **Striking against or struck by football helmet**
     `7th`
     W21.89X **Striking against or struck by other sports equipment**
     `7th`

W21.9XX **Striking against or struck by unspecified sports equipment**
`7th`

W22 **STRIKING AGAINST OR STRUCK BY OTHER OBJECTS**
`4th`
     Excludes1: striking against or struck by object with subsequent fall (W18.09)

W22.0 **Striking against stationary object**
`5th`
     Excludes1: striking against stationary sports equipment (W21.8)
     W22.01X **Walked into wall**
     `7th`
     W22.02X **Walked into lamppost**
     `7th`
     W22.03X **Walked into furniture**
     `7th`
     W22.04 **Striking against wall of swimming pool**
     `6th`

`4th` `5th` `6th` `7th` Additional Character Required	✓ 3-character code

•=New Code   ***Excludes1***—Not coded here, do not use together
▲=Revised Code   ***Excludes2***—Not included here

W22.041 **Striking against wall of swimming pool causing drowning and submersion**
<small>7th</small>

> 7th characters for categories
> W20–W49
> A—initial encounter
> D—subsequent encounter
> S—sequela

> *Excludes1:* drowning and submersion while swimming without striking against wall (W67)

W22.042 **Striking against wall of swimming pool causing other injury**
<small>7th</small>

W22.09X **Striking against other stationary object**
<small>7th</small>

W22.1 **Striking against or struck by automobile airbag**
<small>5th</small>

W22.10X **Striking against or struck by unspecified automobile airbag**
<small>7th</small>

W22.11X **Striking against or struck by driver side automobile airbag**
<small>7th</small>

W22.12X **Striking against or struck by front passenger side automobile airbag**
<small>7th</small>

W22.19X **Striking against or struck by other automobile airbag**
<small>7th</small>

W22.8XX **Striking against or struck by other objects**
<small>7th</small>
> Striking against or struck by object NOS
> *Excludes1:* struck by thrown, projected or falling object (W20.-)

W23 **CAUGHT, CRUSHED, JAMMED OR PINCHED IN OR BETWEEN OBJECTS**
<small>4th</small>
> *Excludes1:* injury caused by cutting or piercing instruments (W25–W27)
> injury caused by firearms malfunction (W32.1, W33.1-, W34.1-)
> injury caused by lifting and transmission devices (W24.-)
> injury caused by machinery (W28–W31)
> injury caused by nonpowered hand tools (W27.-)
> injury caused by transport vehicle being used as a means of transportation (V01–V99)
> injury caused by struck by thrown, projected or falling object (W20.-)

W23.0XX **Caught, crushed, jammed, or pinched between moving objects**
<small>7th</small>

W23.1XX **Caught, crushed, jammed, or pinched between stationary objects**
<small>7th</small>

W24 **CONTACT WITH LIFTING AND TRANSMISSION DEVICES, NOT ELSEWHERE CLASSIFIED**
<small>4th</small>
> *Excludes1:* transport accidents (V01-V99)

W24.0XX **Contact with lifting devices, not elsewhere classified**
<small>7th</small>
> Contact with chain hoist
> Contact with drive belt
> Contact with pulley (block)

W24.1XX **Contact with transmission devices, not elsewhere classified**
<small>7th</small>
> Contact with transmission belt or cable

W25 **CONTACT WITH SHARP GLASS**
<small>7th</small>
> **Code first** any associated:
> injury due to flying glass from explosion or firearm discharge (W32–W40)
> transport accident (V00-V99)
> *Excludes1:* fall on same level due to slipping, tripping and stumbling with subsequent striking against sharp glass (W01.110-)
> striking against sharp glass with subsequent fall (W18.02-)
> *Excludes 2:* glass embedded in skin (W45)

W26 **CONTACT WITH OTHER SHARP OBJECTS**
<small>4th</small>
> *Excludes 2:* glass embedded in skin (W45.-)

W26.0XX **Contact with knife**
<small>7th</small>

W26.1XX **Contact with sword or dagger**
<small>7th</small>
> *Excludes1:* contact with electric knife (W29.1)

W26.2XX **Contact with edge of stiff paper**
<small>7th</small>
> Paper cut

W26.8XX **Contact with other sharp objects NEC**
<small>7th</small>
> Contact with tin can lid

W26.9XX **Contact with unspecified sharp objects**
<small>7th</small>

W27 **CONTACT WITH NONPOWERED HAND TOOL**
<small>4th</small>

W27.0XX **Contact with workbench tool**
<small>7th</small>
> *Includes:* Contact with auger or axe or chisel or handsaw or screwdriver

W27.1XX **Contact with garden tool**
<small>7th</small>
> *Includes:* Contact with hoe or nonpowered lawn mower or pitchfork or rake

W27.2XX **Contact with scissors**
<small>7th</small>

W27.3XX **Contact with needle (sewing)**
<small>7th</small>
> *Excludes1:* contact with hypodermic needle (W46.-)

W27.4XX **Contact with kitchen utensil**
<small>7th</small>
> *Includes:* Contact with fork or ice-pick or can-opener NOS

W27.5XX **Contact with paper-cutter**
<small>7th</small>

W27.8XX **Contact with other nonpowered hand tool**
<small>7th</small>
> Contact with nonpowered sewing machine or shovel

W28 **CONTACT WITH POWERED LAWN MOWER**
<small>7th</small>
> Powered lawn mower (commercial) (residential)
> *Excludes1:* contact with nonpowered lawn mower (W27.1)
> *Excludes2:* exposure to electric current (W86.-)

(W29–W38)
See complete *ICD-10-CM* manual for codes in categories W29–W38.

W39 **DISCHARGE OF FIREWORK**
<small>7th</small>

(W40, W42)
See complete *ICD-10-CM* manual for codes in categories W40, W42.

W45 **FB OR OBJECT ENTERING THROUGH SKIN**
<small>4th</small>
> *Includes:* foreign body or object embedded in skin
> nail embedded in skin
> *Excludes2:* contact with hand tools (nonpowered) (powered) (W27–W29)
> contact with other sharp object(s) (W26.-)
> contact with sharp glass (W25.-)
> paper cut (W26.2-)
> struck by objects (W20–W22)

W45.0XX **Nail entering through skin**
<small>7th</small>

W45.8XX **Other FB or object entering through skin**
<small>7th</small>
> Splinter in skin NOS

W46 **CONTACT WITH HYPODERMIC NEEDLE**
<small>4th</small>

W46.0XX **Contact with hypodermic needle**
<small>7th</small>
> Hypodermic needle stick NOS

W46.1XX **Contact with contaminated hypodermic needle**
<small>7th</small>

W49 **EXPOSURE TO OTHER INANIMATE MECHANICAL FORCES**
<small>4th</small>
> *Includes:* exposure to abnormal gravitational [G] forces
> exposure to inanimate mechanical forces NEC
> *Excludes1:* exposure to inanimate mechanical forces involving military or war operations (Y36.-, Y37.-)

W49.0 **Item causing external constriction**
<small>5th</small>

W49.01X **Hair causing external constriction**
<small>7th</small>

W49.02X **String or thread causing external constriction**
<small>7th</small>

W49.03X **Rubber band causing external constriction**
<small>7th</small>

W49.04X **Ring or other jewelry causing external constriction**
<small>7th</small>

W49.09X **Other specified item causing external constriction**
<small>7th</small>

W49.9XX **Exposure to other inanimate mechanical forces**
<small>7th</small>

<small>4th</small> <small>5th</small> <small>6th</small> <small>7th</small>   Additional Character Required   ✔   3-character code   •=New Code   ▲=Revised Code   *Excludes1*—Not coded here, do not use together   *Excludes2*—Not included here

CHAPTER 20. EXTERNAL CAUSES OF MORBIDITY   (W22.041–W49.9XX)

CHAPTER 20. EXTERNAL CAUSES OF MORBIDITY　(W50–W61.3)

(W50–W64) EXPOSURE TO ANIMATE MECHANICAL FORCES

Excludes1: Toxic effect of contact with venomous animals and plants (T63.-)

W50 `4th` **ACCIDENTAL HIT, STRIKE, KICK, TWIST, OR SCRATCH BY ANOTHER PERSON**

7th characters for categories
W50–W64
A—initial encounter
D—subsequent encounter
S—sequela

Includes: hit, strike, kick, twist, bite, or scratch by another person NOS
Excludes1: assault by bodily force (Y04)
　　struck by objects (W20–W22)

W50.0XX **Accidental hit or strike by another person**
`7th`　Hit or strike by another person NOS

W50.1XX **Accidental kick by another person**
`7th`　Kick by another person NOS

W50.2XX **Accidental twist by another person**
`7th`　Twist by another person NOS

W50.3XX **Accidental bite by another person**
`7th`　Human bite
　　Bite by another person NOS

W50.4XX **Accidental scratch by another person**
`7th`　Scratch by another person NOS

W51 `7th` **ACCIDENTAL STRIKING AGAINST OR BUMPED INTO BY ANOTHER PERSON**
Excludes1: assault by striking against or bumping into by another person (Y04.2)
　　fall due to collision with another person (W03)

W52 `7th` **CRUSHED, PUSHED OR STEPPED ON BY CROWD OR HUMAN STAMPEDE**
Crushed, pushed or stepped on by crowd or human stampede with or without fall

W53 `4th` **CONTACT WITH RODENT**
Includes: contact with saliva, feces or urine of rodent

W53.0 **Contact with mouse**
`5th`　**W53.01X** **Bitten by mouse**
　　`7th`
　　W53.09X **Other contact with mouse**
　　`7th`

W53.1 **Contact with rat**
`5th`　**W53.11X** **Bitten by rat**
　　`7th`
　　W53.19X **Other contact with rat**
　　`7th`

W53.2 **Contact with squirrel**
`5th`　**W53.21X** **Bitten by squirrel**
　　`7th`
　　W53.29X **Other contact with squirrel**
　　`7th`

W53.8 **Contact with other rodent**
`5th`　**W53.81X** **Bitten by other rodent**
　　`7th`
　　W53.89X **Other contact with other rodent**
　　`7th`

W54 `4th` **CONTACT WITH DOG**
Includes: contact with saliva, feces or urine of dog

W54.0XX **Bitten by dog**
`7th`

Report the injury code as primary

W54.1XX **Struck by dog**
`7th`　Knocked over by dog
W54.8XX **Other contact with dog**
`7th`

W55 `4th` **CONTACT WITH OTHER MAMMALS**
Includes: contact with saliva, feces or urine of mammal
Excludes1: animal being ridden—see transport accidents
　　bitten or struck by dog (W54)
　　bitten or struck by rodent (W53.-)
　　contact with marine mammals (W56.-)
See complete *ICD-10-CM* manual for code subcategories W55.1-, W55.2-, W55.3- W55.4-, W55.5-, and W55.8-.

W55.0 **Contact with cat**
`5th`

W55.01X **Bitten by cat**
`7th`
W55.03X **Scratched by cat**
`7th`
W55.09X **Other contact with cat**
`7th`

W56 `4th` **CONTACT WITH NONVENOMOUS MARINE ANIMAL**
Excludes1: contact with venomous marine animal (T63.-)
See complete *ICD-10-CM* manual for codes in category W56.

W57 `7th` **ACCIDENTAL BITTEN OR STUNG BY NONVENOMOUS INSECT AND OTHER NONVENOMOUS ARTHROPODS**
Excludes1: contact with venomous insects and arthropods (T63.2-, T63.3-, T63.4-)

W58 `4th` **CONTACT WITH CROCODILE OR ALLIGATOR**
See complete *ICD-10-CM* manual for codes in category W58.

W59 `4th` **CONTACT WITH OTHER NONVENOMOUS REPTILES**
Excludes1: contact with venomous reptile (T63.0-, T63.1-)

W59.0 **Contact with nonvenomous lizards**
`5th`　**W59.01X** **Bitten by nonvenomous lizards**
　　`7th`
　　W59.02X **Struck by nonvenomous lizards**
　　`7th`
　　W59.09X **Other contact with nonvenomous lizards**
　　`7th`　Exposure to nonvenomous lizards

W59.1 **Contact with nonvenomous snakes**
`5th`　**W59.11X** **Bitten by nonvenomous snake**
　　`7th`
　　W59.12X **Struck by nonvenomous snake**
　　`7th`
　　W59.13X **Crushed by nonvenomous snake**
　　`7th`
　　W59.19X **Other contact with nonvenomous snake**
　　`7th`

W59.2 **Contact with turtles**
`5th`　Excludes1: contact with tortoises (W59.8-)
　　W59.21X **Bitten by turtle**
　　`7th`
　　W59.22X **Struck by turtle**
　　`7th`
　　W59.29X **Other contact with turtle**
　　`7th`　Exposure to turtles

W59.8 **Contact with other nonvenomous reptiles**
`5th`　**W59.81X** **Bitten by other nonvenomous reptiles**
　　`7th`
　　W59.82X **Struck by other nonvenomous reptiles**
　　`7th`
　　W59.83X **Crushed by other nonvenomous reptiles**
　　`7th`
　　W59.89X **Other contact with other nonvenomous reptiles**
　　`7th`

W60 `7th` **CONTACT WITH NONVENOMOUS PLANT THORNS AND SPINES AND SHARP LEAVES**
Excludes1: Contact with venomous plants (T63.7-)

W61 `4th` **CONTACT WITH BIRDS (DOMESTIC) (WILD)**
Includes: contact with excreta of birds

W61.0 **Contact with parrot**
`5th`　**W61.01X** **Bitten by parrot**
　　`7th`
　　W61.02X **Struck by parrot**
　　`7th`
　　W61.09X **Other contact with parrot**
　　`7th`　Exposure to parrots

W61.1 **Contact with macaw**
`5th`　**W61.11X** **Bitten by macaw**
　　`7th`
　　W61.12X **Struck by macaw**
　　`7th`
　　W61.19X **Other contact with macaw**
　　`7th`　Exposure to macaws

W61.3 **Contact with chicken**
`5th`

 `4th` `5th` `6th` `7th` Additional Character Required　　 3-character code

•=New Code
▲=Revised Code

Excludes1—Not coded here, do not use together
Excludes2—Not included here

W61.32X Struck by chicken
7th

W61.33X Pecked by chicken
7th

W61.39X Other contact with chicken
7th
Exposure to chickens

W61.4 Contact with turkey
5th

W61.42X Struck by turkey
7th

W61.43X Pecked by turkey
7th

W61.49X Other contact with turkey
7th

W61.5 Contact with goose
5th

W61.51X Bitten by goose
7th

W61.52X Struck by goose
7th

W61.59X Other contact with goose
7th

W61.6 Contact with duck
5th

W61.61X Bitten by duck
7th

W61.62X Struck by duck
7th

W61.69X Other contact with duck
7th

W61.9 Contact with other birds
5th

W61.91X Bitten by other birds
7th

W61.92X Struck by other birds
7th

W61.99X Other contact with other birds
7th
Contact with bird NOS

7th characters for categories W50–W64
A—initial encounter
D—subsequent encounter
S—sequela

W62 CONTACT WITH NONVENOMOUS AMPHIBIANS
4th
Excludes1: contact with venomous amphibians (T63.81-R63.83)

W62.0XX Contact with nonvenomous frogs
7th

W62.1XX Contact with nonvenomous toads
7th

W62.9XX Contact with other nonvenomous amphibians
7th

(W65–W74) ACCIDENTAL NON-TRANSPORT DROWNING AND SUBMERSION

Excludes1: accidental drowning and submersion due to fall into water (W16.-)
accidental drowning and submersion due to water transport accident (V90.-, V92.-)
Excludes2: accidental drowning and submersion due to cataclysm (X34–X39)

7th characters for categories W65–W74
A—initial encounter
D—subsequent encounter
S—sequela

W65 ACCIDENTAL DROWNING AND SUBMERSION WHILE IN BATHTUB
7th
Excludes1: accidental drowning and submersion due to fall in (into) bathtub (W16.211)

W67 ACCIDENTAL DROWNING AND SUBMERSION WHILE IN SWIMMING-POOL
7th
Excludes1: accidental drowning and submersion due to fall into swimming pool (W16.011, W16.021, W16.031)
accidental drowning and submersion due to striking into wall of swimming pool (W22.041)

W69 ACCIDENTAL DROWNING AND SUBMERSION WHILE IN NATURAL WATER
7th
Accidental drowning and submersion while in lake/open sea/river/stream
Excludes1: accidental drowning and submersion due to fall into natural body of water (W16.111, W16.121, W16.131)

W74 UNSPECIFIED CAUSE OF ACCIDENTAL DROWNING AND SUBMERSION
7th
Drowning NOS

(W85–W99) EXPOSURE TO ELECTRIC CURRENT, RADIATION AND EXTREME AMBIENT AIR TEMPERATURE AND PRESSURE

Excludes1: exposure to: failure in dosage of radiation or temperature during surgical and medical care (Y63.2–Y63.5)
lightning (T75.0-)
natural cold (X31)
natural heat (X30)
natural radiation NOS (X39)
radiological procedure and radiotherapy (Y84.2)
sunlight (X32)

7th characters for categories W85–W99
A—initial encounter
D—subsequent encounter
S—sequela

W86 EXPOSURE TO OTHER SPECIFIED ELECTRIC CURRENT
4th

W86.0XX Exposure to domestic wiring and appliances
7th

W86.1XX Exposure to industrial wiring, appliances and electrical machinery
7th
Includes: Exposure to conductors or control apparatus or electrical equipment and machinery or transformers

W86.8XX Exposure to other electric current
7th
Includes: Exposure to wiring and appliances in or on farm (not farmhouse) or public building or residential institutions or schools
Exposure to wiring and appliances outdoors

W89 EXPOSURE TO MAN-MADE VISIBLE AND ULTRAVIOLET LIGHT
4th
Includes: exposure to welding light (arc)
Excludes2: exposure to sunlight (X32)

W89.1XX Exposure to tanning bed
7th

W93 EXPOSURE TO EXCESSIVE COLD OF MAN-MADE ORIGIN
4th

W93.0 Contact with or inhalation of dry ice
5th

W93.01X Contact with dry ice
7th

W93.02X Inhalation of dry ice
7th

W93.1 Contact with or inhalation of liquid air
5th

W93.11X Contact with liquid air
7th
Contact with liquid hydrogen
Contact with liquid nitrogen

W93.12X Inhalation of liquid air
7th
Inhalation of liquid hydrogen or nitrogen

W93.2XX Prolonged exposure in deep freeze unit or refrigerator
7th

W93.8XX Exposure to other excessive cold of man-made origin
7th

W94 EXPOSURE TO HIGH AND LOW AIR PRESSURE AND CHANGES IN AIR PRESSURE
4th

W94.0XX Exposure to prolonged high air pressure
7th

W94.1 Exposure to prolonged low air pressure
5th

W94.11X Exposure to residence or prolonged visit at high altitude
7th

W94.12X Exposure to other prolonged low air pressure
7th

W94.2 Exposure to rapid changes in air pressure during ascent
5th

W94.21X Exposure to reduction in atmospheric pressure while surfacing from deep-water diving
7th

W94.22X Exposure to reduction in atmospheric pressure while surfacing from underground
7th

W94.23X Exposure to sudden change in air pressure in aircraft during ascent
7th

W94.29X Exposure to other rapid changes in air pressure during ascent
7th

W94.3 Exposure to rapid changes in air pressure during descent
5th

W94.31X Exposure to sudden change in air pressure in aircraft during descent
7th

W94.32X Exposure to high air pressure from rapid descent in water
7th

W94.39X Exposure to other rapid changes in air pressure during descent
7th

4th 5th 6th 7th   Additional Character Required   ✔   3-character code

•=New Code
▲=Revised Code

Excludes1—Not coded here, do not use together
Excludes2—Not included here

CHAPTER 20. EXTERNAL CAUSES OF MORBIDITY   (X00–X31)

(X00–X08) EXPOSURE TO SMOKE, FIRE AND FLAMES

Excludes1: arson (X97)
Excludes2: explosions (W35–W40)
  lightning (T75.0-)
  transport accident (V01–V99)

> 7th characters for categories
> X00–X08
> A—initial encounter
> D—subsequent encounter
> S—sequela

X00   **EXPOSURE TO UNCONTROLLED FIRE IN BUILDING OR STRUCTURE**
`4th`
  See complete *ICD-10-CM* manual for codes in category X00.
  X00.0XX   Exposure to flames in uncontrolled fire in building or structure
  `7th`
  X00.1XX   Exposure to smoke in uncontrolled fire in building or structure
  `7th`

X01   **EXPOSURE TO UNCONTROLLED FIRE, NOT IN BUILDING OR STRUCTURE**
`4th`
  Includes: exposure to forest fire
  See complete *ICD-10-CM* manual for codes in category X01.

X02   **EXPOSURE TO CONTROLLED FIRE IN BUILDING OR STRUCTURE**
`4th`
  Includes: exposure to fire in fireplace
    exposure to fire in stove
  See complete *ICD-10-CM* manual for codes in category X02.

X03   **EXPOSURE TO CONTROLLED FIRE, NOT IN BUILDING OR STRUCTURE**
`4th`
  Includes: exposure to bon fire or camp-fire or trash fire
  Includes: conflagration in building or structure
  Code first any associated cataclysm
  Excludes2: Exposure to ignition or melting of nightwear (X05)
    Exposure to ignition or melting of other clothing and apparel (X06.-)
    Exposure to other specified smoke, fire and flames (X08.-)
  See complete *ICD-10-CM* manual for codes in category X03.
  X03.0XX   Exposure to flames in controlled fire, not in building or structure
  `7th`
  X03.1XX   Exposure to smoke in controlled fire, not in building or structure
  `7th`

X04   **EXPOSURE TO IGNITION OF HIGHLY FLAMMABLE MATERIAL**
`7th`
  Includes: Exposure to ignition of gasoline or kerosene or petrol
  Excludes2: exposure to ignition or melting of nightwear (X05)
    exposure to ignition or melting of other clothing and apparel (X06)

X05   **EXPOSURE TO IGNITION OR MELTING OF NIGHTWEAR**
`7th`
  Excludes2: exposure to uncontrolled fire in building or structure (X00.-)
    exposure to uncontrolled fire, not in building or structure (X01.-)
    exposure to controlled fire in building or structure (X02.-)
    exposure to controlled fire, not in building or structure (X03.-)
    exposure to ignition of highly flammable materials (X04.-)

X06   **EXPOSURE TO IGNITION OR MELTING OF OTHER CLOTHING AND APPAREL**
`4th`
  X06.0XX   Exposure to ignition of plastic jewelry
  `7th`
  X06.1XX   Exposure to melting of plastic jewelry
  `7th`
  X06.2XX   Exposure to ignition of other clothing and apparel
  `7th`
  X06.3XX   Exposure to melting of other clothing and apparel
  `7th`

X08   **EXPOSURE TO OTHER SPECIFIED SMOKE, FIRE AND FLAMES**
`4th`
  See complete *ICD-10-CM* manual for codes in category X08.

(X10–X19) CONTACT WITH HEAT AND HOT SUBSTANCES

Excludes1: exposure to excessive natural heat (X30)
  exposure to fire and flames (X00–X08)

X10   **CONTACT WITH HOT DRINKS, FOOD, FATS AND COOKING OILS**
`4th`
  X10.0XX   Contact with hot drinks
  `7th`

> 7th characters for categories
> X10–X19
> A—initial encounter
> D—subsequent encounter
> S—sequela

X10.1XX   **Contact with hot food**
`7th`
X10.2XX   **Contact with fats and cooking oils**
`7th`

X11   **CONTACT WITH HOT TAP-WATER**
`4th`
  Includes: contact with boiling tap-water or boiling water NOS
  Excludes1: contact with water heated on stove (X12)
  X11.0XX   Contact with hot water in bath or tub
  `7th`
    Excludes1: contact with running hot water in bath or tub (X11.1)
  X11.1XX   Contact with running hot water
  `7th`
    Contact with hot water running out of hose or tap
  X11.8XX   Contact with other hot tap-water
  `7th`
    Contact with hot water in bucket
    Contact with hot tap-water NOS

X12   **CONTACT WITH OTHER HOT FLUIDS**
`7th`
  Contact with water heated on stove
  Excludes1: hot (liquid) metals (X18)

X13   **CONTACT WITH STEAM AND OTHER HOT VAPORS**
`4th`
  X13.0XX   Inhalation of steam and other hot vapors
  `7th`
  X13.1XX   Other contact with steam and other hot vapors
  `7th`

X15   **CONTACT WITH HOT HOUSEHOLD APPLIANCES**
`4th`
  Excludes1: contact with heating appliances (X16)
    contact with powered household appliances (W29.-)
    exposure to controlled fire in building or structure due to household appliance (X02.8)
    exposure to household appliances electrical current (W86.0)
  X15.0XX   Contact with hot stove (kitchen)
  `7th`
  X15.1XX   Contact with hot toaster
  `7th`
  X15.2XX   Contact with hotplate
  `7th`
  X15.3XX   Contact with hot saucepan or skillet
  `7th`
  X15.8XX   Contact with other hot household appliances
  `7th`
    Contact with cooker/kettle/light bulbs

X16   **CONTACT WITH HOT HEATING APPLIANCES, RADIATORS AND PIPES**
`7th`
  Excludes1: contact with powered appliances (W29.-)
    exposure to controlled fire in building or structure due to appliance (X02.8)
    exposure to industrial appliances electrical current (W86.1)

X17   **CONTACT WITH HOT ENGINES, MACHINERY AND TOOLS**
`7th`
  Excludes1: contact with hot heating appliances, radiators and pipes (X16)
    contact with hot household appliances (X15)

X18   **CONTACT WITH OTHER HOT METALS**
`7th`
  Contact with liquid metal

X19   **CONTACT WITH OTHER HEAT AND HOT SUBSTANCES**
`7th`
  Excludes1: objects that are not normally hot, e.g., an object made hot by a house fire (X00–X08)

(X30–X39) EXPOSURE TO FORCES OF NATURE

X30   **EXPOSURE TO EXCESSIVE NATURAL HEAT**
`7th`
  Exposure to excessive heat as the cause of sunstroke
    Exposure to heat NOS
  Excludes1: excessive heat of man-made origin (W92)
    exposure to man-made radiation (W89)
    exposure to sunlight (X32)
    exposure to tanning bed (W89)

> 7th characters for categories
> X30–X39
> A—initial encounter
> D—subsequent encounter
> S—sequela

X31   **EXPOSURE TO EXCESSIVE NATURAL COLD**
`7th`
  Excessive cold as the cause of chilblains NOS
  Excessive cold as the cause of immersion foot or hand
  Exposure to cold NOS
  Exposure to weather conditions

`4th` `5th` `6th` `7th`   Additional Character Required   ✔   3-character code

•=New Code   **Excludes1**—Not coded here, do not use together
▲=Revised Code   **Excludes2**—Not included here

X32 EXPOSURE TO SUNLIGHT
`7th`   *Excludes1:* man-made radiation (tanning bed) (W89)
   Excludes2: radiation-related disorders of the skin and subcutaneous tissue
    (L55–L59)

X34 EARTHQUAKE
`7th`   *Excludes2:* tidal wave (tsunami) due to earthquake (X37.41)

X35 VOLCANIC ERUPTION
`7th`   *Excludes2:* tidal wave (tsunami) due to volcanic eruption (X37.41)

X36 AVALANCHE, LANDSLIDE AND OTHER EARTH
`7th`   MOVEMENTS
   Includes: victim of mudslide of cataclysmic nature
   Excludes1: earthquake (X34)
   Excludes2: transport accident involving collision with avalanche or
    landslide not in motion (V01–V99)
   See complete *ICD-10-CM* manual for codes in category X36.
   X36.0 Collapse of dam or man-made structure causing earth
    `7th`   movement
   X36.1 Avalanche, landslide, or mudslide
    `7th`

X37 CATACLYSMIC STORM
`4th`   **X37.0XX** Hurricane
    `7th`   Storm surge
   X37.1XX Tornado
    `7th`   Cyclone
    Twister
   X37.2XX Blizzard (snow) (ice)
    `7th`
   X37.3XX Dust storm
    `7th`
   X37.4 Tidal wave
    `5th`   **X37.41X** Tidal wave due to earthquake or volcanic eruption
     `7th`   Tidal wave NOS
     Tsunami
    X37.42X Tidal wave due to storm
     `7th`
    X37.43X Tidal wave due to landslide
     `7th`
   X37.8XX Other cataclysmic storms
    `7th`   Cloudburst
    Torrential rain
    Excludes2: flood (X38)
   X37.9XX Unspecified cataclysmic storm
    `7th`   Storm NOS
    Excludes1: collapse of dam or man-made structure causing
     earth movement (X36.0)

X38 FLOOD
`7th`   Flood arising from remote storm or of nature arising from melting snow
   Flood resulting directly from storm
   Excludes1: collapse of dam or man-made structure causing earth
    movement (X36.0)
    tidal wave NOS (X37.41)
    tidal wave caused by storm (X37.42)

X39 EXPOSURE TO OTHER FORCES OF NATURE
`4th`   **X39.0** Exposure to natural radiation
    `5th`   *Excludes1:* contact with and (suspected) exposure to radon and
     other naturally occurring radiation (Z77.123)
     exposure to man-made radiation (W88–W90)
     exposure to sunlight (X32)
    X39.01X Exposure to radon
     `7th`
    X39.08X Exposure to other natural radiation
     `7th`
   X39.8XX Other exposure to forces of nature
    `7th`

(X50–X58) ACCIDENTAL EXPOSURE TO OTHER SPECIFIED FACTORS

X50 OVEREXERTION FROM MOVEMENT
`4th`   **X50.0XX** Overexertion from strenuous
    `7th`   movement or load
    Lifting heavy objects
    Lifting weights

> 7th characters for category X50
> A—initial encounter
> D—subsequent encounter
> S—sequela

   X50.1XX Overexertion from prolonged
    `7th`   static or awkward postures
    Includes: Prolonged or static bending or kneeling or reaching or
    sitting or standing or twisting
   X50.3XX Overexertion from repetitive movements
    `7th`   Use of hand as hammer
   X50.9XX Other and unspecified overexertion or strenuous
    `7th`   movements or postures
    Contact pressure or contact stress

X58 EXPOSURE TO OTHER
`7th`   SPECIFIED FACTORS
   Accident NOS
   Exposure NOS

> 7th characters for category X58
> A—initial encounter
> D—subsequent encounter
> S—sequela

(X71–X83) INTENTIONAL SELF-HARM

Purposely self-inflicted injury
Suicide (attempted)

X71 INTENTIONAL SELF-HARM BY
`4th`   DROWNING AND SUBMERSION
   See complete *ICD-10-CM* manual for codes
   in category X71.

> 7th characters for category
> X71–X83
> A—initial encounter
> D—subsequent encounter
> S—sequela

X72 INTENTIONAL SELF-HARM BY HANDGUN DISCHARGE
`7th`   Intentional self-harm by gun/pistol/revolver for single hand use
   Excludes1: Very pistol (X74.8)

X73 INTENTIONAL SELF-HARM BY RIFLE, SHOTGUN AND
`4th`   LARGER FIREARM DISCHARGE
   Excludes1: airgun (X74.01)
   See complete *ICD-10-CM* manual for codes in category X73.

X74 INTENTIONAL SELF-HARM BY OTHER AND UNSPECIFIED
`4th`   FIREARM AND GUN DISCHARGE
   See complete *ICD-10-CM* manual for codes in category X74.

X75 INTENTIONAL SELF-HARM BY EXPLOSIVE MATERIAL
`7th`

X76 INTENTIONAL SELF-HARM BY SMOKE, FIRE AND
`7th`   FLAMES

X77 INTENTIONAL SELF-HARM BY STEAM, HOT VAPORS AND
`4th`   HOT OBJECTS
   See complete *ICD-10-CM* manual for codes in category X77.

X78 INTENTIONAL SELF-HARM BY SHARP OBJECT
`4th`   **X78.0XX** Intentional self-harm by sharp glass
    `7th`
   X78.1XX Intentional self-harm by knife
    `7th`
   X78.2XX Intentional self-harm by sword or dagger
    `7th`
   X78.8XX Intentional self-harm by other sharp object
    `7th`
   X78.9XX Intentional self-harm by unspecified sharp object
    `7th`

X79 INTENTIONAL SELF-HARM BY BLUNT OBJECT
`7th`

X80 INTENTIONAL SELF-HARM BY JUMPING FROM A
`7th`   HIGH PLACE
   Intentional fall from one level to another

X81 INTENTIONAL SELF-HARM BY JUMPING OR LYING IN
`4th`   FRONT OF MOVING OBJECT
   See complete *ICD-10-CM* manual for codes in category X81.

`4th` `5th` `6th` `7th`   Additional Character Required   ✓   3-character code

•=New Code
▲=Revised Code

Excludes1—Not coded here, do not use together
Excludes2—Not included here

   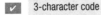

X82 **INTENTIONAL SELF-HARM BY CRASHING OF MOTOR VEHICLE**
4th
See complete *ICD-10-CM* manual for codes in category X82.

X83 **INTENTIONAL SELF-HARM BY OTHER SPECIFIED MEANS**
4th
Excludes1: intentional self-harm by poisoning or contact with toxic substance—See Table of Drugs and Chemicals
See complete *ICD-10-CM* manual for codes in category X83.

(X92–Y09) ASSAULT

Adult and child abuse, neglect and maltreatment are classified as assault. Any of the assault codes may be used to indicate the external cause of any injury resulting from the confirmed abuse.

For confirmed cases of abuse, neglect and maltreatment, when the perpetrator is known, a code from Y07, Perpetrator of maltreatment and neglect, should accompany any other assault codes.

7th characters for categories
X92–Y04
A—initial encounter
D—subsequent encounter
S—sequela

Includes: homicide
injuries inflicted by another person with intent to injure or kill, by any means
Excludes1: injuries due to legal intervention (Y35.-)
injuries due to operations of war (Y36.-)
injuries due to terrorism (Y38.-)

X92 **ASSAULT BY DROWNING AND SUBMERSION**
4th
X92.0XX **Assault by drowning and submersion while in bathtub**
7th
X92.1XX **Assault by drowning and submersion while in swimming pool**
7th
X92.2XX **Assault by drowning and submersion after push into swimming pool**
7th
X92.3XX **Assault by drowning and submersion in natural water**
7th
X92.8XX **Other assault by drowning and submersion**
7th
X92.9XX **Assault by drowning and submersion, unspecified**
7th

X93 **ASSAULT BY HANDGUN DISCHARGE**
7th
Excludes1: Very pistol (X95.8)

X94 **ASSAULT BY RIFLE, SHOTGUN AND LARGER FIREARM DISCHARGE**
4th
Excludes1: airgun (X95.01)
X94.1XX **Assault by hunting rifle**
7th

X95 **ASSAULT BY OTHER AND UNSPECIFIED FIREARM AND GUN DISCHARGE**
4th
X95.0 **Assault by gas, air or spring-operated guns**
5th
X95.01X **Assault by airgun discharge**
7th
Assault by BB or pellet gun discharge
X95.02X **Assault by paintball gun discharge**
7th
X95.09X **Assault by other gas, air or spring-operated gun**
7th
X95.8XX **Assault by other firearm discharge**
7th
Assault by very pistol [flare] discharge
X95.9XX **Assault by unspecified firearm discharge**
7th

X96 **ASSAULT BY EXPLOSIVE MATERIAL**
4th
Excludes1: incendiary device (X97)
terrorism involving explosive material (Y38.2-)
See complete *ICD-10-CM* manual for codes in category X96.

X97 **ASSAULT BY SMOKE, FIRE AND FLAMES**
7th
Assault by arson
Assault by cigarettes

X98 **ASSAULT BY STEAM, HOT VAPORS AND HOT OBJECTS**
4th
X98.0XX **Assault by steam or hot vapors**
7th
X98.1XX **Assault by hot tap water**
7th
X98.2XX **Assault by hot fluids**
7th

7th characters for categories
X92–Y04
A—initial encounter
D—subsequent encounter
S—sequela

X98.3XX **Assault by hot household appliances**
7th
X98.8XX **Assault by other hot objects**
7th
X98.9XX **Assault by unspecified hot objects**
7th

X99 **ASSAULT BY SHARP OBJECT**
4th
Excludes1: assault by strike by sports equipment (Y08.0-)
X99.0XX **Assault by sharp glass**
7th
X99.1XX **Assault by knife**
7th
X99.2XX **Assault by sword or dagger**
7th
X99.8XX **Assault by other sharp object**
7th
X99.9XX **Assault by unspecified sharp object**
7th
Assault by stabbing NOS

Y00 **ASSAULT BY BLUNT OBJECT**
7th
Excludes1: assault by strike by sports equipment (Y08.0-)

Y01 **ASSAULT BY PUSHING FROM HIGH PLACE**
7th

Y02 **ASSAULT BY PUSHING OR PLACING VICTIM IN FRONT OF MOVING OBJECT**
4th
Y02.0XX **Assault by pushing or placing victim in front of motor vehicle**
7th
Y02.1XX **Assault by pushing or placing victim in front of (subway) train**
7th
Y02.8XX **Assault by pushing or placing victim in front of other moving object**
7th

Y03 **ASSAULT BY CRASHING OF MOTOR VEHICLE**
4th
Y03.0XX **Assault by being hit or run over by motor vehicle**
7th
Y03.8XX **Other assault by crashing of motor vehicle**
7th

Y04 **ASSAULT BY BODILY FORCE**
4th
Excludes1: assault by:
submersion (X92.-)
use of weapon (X93–X95, X99, Y00)
Y04.0XX **Assault by unarmed brawl or fight**
7th
Y04.1XX **Assault by human bite**
7th
Y04.2XX **Assault by strike against or bumped into by another person**
7th
Y04.8XX **Assault by other bodily force**
7th
Assault by bodily force NOS

Y07 **PERPETRATOR OF ASSAULT, MALTREATMENT AND NEGLECT**
4th
Adult and child abuse, neglect and maltreatment are classified as assault. Any of the assault codes may be used to indicate the external cause of any injury resulting from the confirmed abuse.

For confirmed cases of abuse, neglect and maltreatment, when the perpetrator is known, a code from Y07, Perpetrator of maltreatment and neglect, should accompany any other assault codes.

See Section I.C.19. Adult and child abuse, neglect and other maltreatment
Note: Codes from this category are for use only in cases of **confirmed abuse** (T74.-)
Selection of the correct perpetrator code is based on the relationship between the perpetrator and the victim
Includes: perpetrator of abandonment
perpetrator of emotional or physical neglect
perpetrator of mental cruelty
perpetrator of physical or sexual abuse
perpetrator of torture
Y07.0 **Spouse or partner, perpetrator of maltreatment and neglect**
5th
Spouse or partner, perpetrator of maltreatment and neglect against spouse or partner
Y07.01 **Husband, perpetrator of maltreatment and neglect**

  Additional Character Required   ✓ 3-character code

•=New Code   *Excludes1*—Not coded here, do not use together
▲=Revised Code   *Excludes2*—Not included here

Y07.02   Wife, perpetrator of maltreatment and neglect
Y07.03   Male partner, perpetrator of maltreatment and neglect
Y07.04   Female partner, perpetrator of maltreatment and neglect

Y07.1 **Parent (adoptive) (biological), perpetrator of maltreatment and neglect** [5th]
    Y07.11   Biological father, perpetrator of maltreatment and neglect
    Y07.12   Biological mother, perpetrator of maltreatment and neglect
    Y07.13   Adoptive father, perpetrator of maltreatment and neglect
    Y07.14   Adoptive mother, perpetrator of maltreatment and neglect

Y07.4 **Other family member, perpetrator of maltreatment and neglect** [5th]
    Y07.41   **Sibling, perpetrator of maltreatment and neglect** [6th]
       Excludes1: stepsibling, perpetrator of maltreatment and neglect (Y07.435, Y07.436)
       Y07.410   Brother, perpetrator of maltreatment and neglect
       Y07.411   Sister, perpetrator of maltreatment and neglect
    Y07.42   **Foster parent, perpetrator of maltreatment and neglect** [6th]
       Y07.420   Foster father, perpetrator of maltreatment and neglect
       Y07.421   Foster mother, perpetrator of maltreatment and neglect
    Y07.43   **Stepparent or stepsibling, perpetrator of maltreatment and neglect** [6th]
       Y07.430   Stepfather, perpetrator of maltreatment and neglect
       Y07.432   Male friend of parent (co-residing in household), perpetrator of maltreatment and neglect
       Y07.433   Stepmother, perpetrator of maltreatment and neglect
       Y07.434   Female friend of parent (co-residing in household), perpetrator of maltreatment and neglect
       Y07.435   Stepbrother, perpetrator or maltreatment and neglect
       Y07.436   Stepsister, perpetrator of maltreatment and neglect
    Y07.49   **Other family member, perpetrator of maltreatment and neglect** [6th]
       Y07.490   Male cousin, perpetrator of maltreatment and neglect
       Y07.491   Female cousin, perpetrator of maltreatment and neglect
       Y07.499   Other family member, perpetrator of maltreatment and neglect

Y07.5 **Non-family member, perpetrator of maltreatment and neglect** [5th]
    Y07.50   Unspecified non-family member, perpetrator of maltreatment and neglect
    Y07.51   **Daycare provider, perpetrator of maltreatment and neglect** [6th]
       Y07.510   At-home childcare provider, perpetrator of maltreatment and neglect
       Y07.511   Daycare center childcare provider, perpetrator of maltreatment and neglect
       Y07.519   Unspecified daycare provider, perpetrator of maltreatment and neglect
    Y07.53   Teacher or instructor, perpetrator of maltreatment and neglect
       Coach, perpetrator of maltreatment and neglect
    Y07.59   Other non-family member, perpetrator of maltreatment and neglect

Y07.6 **Multiple perpetrators of maltreatment and neglect**
Y07.9 **Unspecified perpetrator of maltreatment and neglect**

Y08 **ASSAULT BY OTHER SPECIFIED MEANS** [4th]
    Y08.0 **Assault by strike by sport equipment** [5th]
       Y08.01X   Assault by strike by hockey stick [7th]
       Y08.02X   Assault by strike by baseball bat [7th]
       Y08.09X   Assault by strike by other specified type of sport equipment [7th]
    Y08.8 **Assault by other specified means** [5th]
       Y08.81X   Assault by crashing of aircraft [7th]
       Y08.89X   Assault by other specified means [7th]

Y09 **ASSAULT BY UNSPECIFIED MEANS** [7th]
    Includes: Assassination (attempted) or homicide (attempted), manslaughter (attempted) or murder (attempted) NOS

(Y21–Y33) EVENT OF UNDETERMINED INTENT

Undetermined intent is only for use when there is specific documentation in the record that the intent of the injury cannot be determined. If no such documentation is present, code to accidental (unintentional).
    See complete *ICD-10-CM* manual for codes in categories Y21–Y33.

(Y35–Y38) LEGAL INTERVENTION, OPERATIONS OF WAR, MILITARY OPERATIONS, AND TERRORISM

See complete *ICD-10-CM* manual for codes in categories Y35–Y38.

(Y62–Y69) MISADVENTURES TO PATIENTS DURING SURGICAL AND MEDICAL CARE

Excludes2: breakdown or malfunctioning of medical device (during procedure) (after implantation) (ongoing use) (Y70–Y82)
Excludes 1: surgical and medical procedures as the cause of abnormal reaction of the patient, without mention of misadventure at the time of the procedure (Y83–Y84)
    See complete *ICD-10-CM* manual for codes in categories Y62–Y69.

(Y70–Y82) MEDICAL DEVICES ASSOCIATED WITH ADVERSE INCIDENTS IN DIAGNOSTIC AND THERAPEUTIC USE

Includes: breakdown or malfunction of medical devices (during use) (after implantation) (ongoing use)
Excludes2: misadventure to patients during surgical and medical care, classifiable to (Y62–Y69)
    later complications following use of medical devices without breakdown or malfunctioning of device (Y83–Y84)
    surgical and other medical procedures as the cause of abnormal reaction of the patient, or of later complication, without mention of misadventure at the time of the procedure (Y83–Y84)
    See complete *ICD-10-CM* manual for codes in categories Y70 –Y82.

(Y83–Y84) SURGICAL AND OTHER MEDICAL PROCEDURES AS THE CAUSE OF ABNORMAL REACTION OF THE PATIENT, OR OF LATER COMPLICATION, WITHOUT MENTION OF MISADVENTURE AT THE TIME OF THE PROCEDURE

Excludes1: misadventures to patients during surgical and medical care, classifiable to (Y62–Y69)
Excludes2: breakdown or malfunctioning of medical device (after implantation) (during procedure) (ongoing use) (Y70–Y82)
    See complete *ICD-10-CM* manual for codes in categories Y83–Y84.

(Y90–Y99) SUPPLEMENTARY FACTORS RELATED TO CAUSES OF MORBIDITY CLASSIFIED ELSEWHERE

Note: These categories may be used to provide supplementary information concerning causes of morbidity. They are not to be used for single-condition coding.

Y90 **EVIDENCE OF ALCOHOL INVOLVEMENT DETERMINED BY BLOOD ALCOHOL LEVEL** [4th]
    Code first any associated alcohol related disorders (F10)

[4th] [5th] [6th] [7th] Additional Character Required   [✔] 3-character code   •=New Code   ▲=Revised Code   *Excludes1*—Not coded here, do not use together   *Excludes2*—Not included here

CHAPTER 20. EXTERNAL CAUSES OF MORBIDITY   (Y90.0–Y92.119)

Y90.0   Blood alcohol level of less than 20 mg/100 ml
Y90.1   Blood alcohol level of 20–39 mg/100 ml
Y90.2   Blood alcohol level of 40–59 mg/100 ml
Y90.3   Blood alcohol level of 60–79 mg/100 ml
Y90.4   Blood alcohol level of 80–99 mg/100 ml
Y90.5   Blood alcohol level of 100–119 mg/100 ml
Y90.6   Blood alcohol level of 120–199 mg/100 ml
Y90.7   Blood alcohol level of 200–239 mg/100 ml
Y90.8   Blood alcohol level of 240 mg/100 ml or more
Y90.9   Presence of alcohol in blood, level not specified

Y92   **PLACE OF OCCURRENCE OF THE EXTERNAL CAUSE**
`4th`

> **GUIDELINE**
>
> When applicable, place of occurrence, activity, and external cause status codes are sequenced after the main external cause code(s). Regardless of the number of external cause codes assigned, there should be only one place of occurrence code, one activity code, and one external cause status code assigned to an encounter.
>
> Codes from category Y92, Place of occurrence of the external cause, are secondary codes for use after other external cause codes to identify the location of the patient at the time of injury or other condition.
>
> Generally, a place of occurrence code is assigned only once, at the initial encounter for treatment. However, in the rare instance that a new injury occurs during hospitalization, an additional place of occurrence code may be assigned. No 7th characters are used for Y92.
>
> Do not use place of occurrence code Y92.9 if the place is not stated or is not applicable.

The following category is for use, when relevant, to identify the place of occurrence of the external cause. Use in conjunction with an activity code. Place of occurrence should be recorded only at the **initial encounter** for treatment.

Y92.0   **Non-institutional (private) residence as the place of**
`5th`   **occurrence of the external cause**
     Excludes1: abandoned or derelict house (Y92.89)
     home under construction but not yet occupied (Y92.6-)
     institutional place of residence (Y92.1-)

> Y92 codes are the place of occurrence for the external cause

Y92.00   **Unspecified non-institutional (private) residence**
`6th`
    Y92.000   Kitchen of unspecified non-institutional (private) residence
    Y92.001   Dining room of unspecified non-institutional (private) residence
    Y92.002   Bathroom of unspecified non-institutional (private) residence
    Y92.003   Bedroom of unspecified non-institutional (private) residence
    Y92.007   Garden or yard of unspecified non-institutional (private) residence
    Y92.008   Other place in unspecified non-institutional (private) residence
    Y92.009   Unspecified place in unspecified non-institutional (private) residence
       Home (NOS)

Y92.01   **Single-family non-institutional (private) house**
`6th`
    Farmhouse
    Excludes1: barn (Y92.71)
      chicken coop or hen house (Y92.72) farm field (Y92.73)
      orchard (Y92.74)
      single family mobile home or trailer (Y92.02-)
      slaughter house (Y92.86)
    Y92.010   Kitchen of single-family (private) house
    Y92.011   Dining room of single-family (private) house
    Y92.012   Bathroom of single-family (private) house
    Y92.013   Bedroom of single-family (private) house
    Y92.014   Private driveway to single-family (private) house
    Y92.015   Private garage of single-family (private) house
    Y92.016   Swimming-pool in single-family (private) house or garden
    Y92.017   Garden or yard in single-family (private) house

    Y92.018   Other place in single-family (private) house
    Y92.019   Unspecified place in single-family (private) house

Y92.02   **Mobile home**
`6th`
    Y92.020   Kitchen in mobile home
    Y92.021   Dining room in mobile home
    Y92.022   Bathroom in mobile home
    Y92.023   Bedroom in mobile home
    Y92.024   Driveway of mobile home
    Y92.025   Garage of mobile home
    Y92.026   Swimming-pool of mobile home
    Y92.027   Garden or yard of mobile home
    Y92.028   Other place in mobile home
    Y92.029   Unspecified place in mobile home

Y92.03   **Apartment**
`6th`
    Condominium
    Co-op apartment
    Y92.030   Kitchen in apartment
    Y92.031   Bathroom in apartment
    Y92.032   Bedroom in apartment
    Y92.038   Other place in apartment
    Y92.039   Unspecified place in apartment

Y92.04   **Boarding-house**
`6th`
    Y92.040   Kitchen in boarding-house
    Y92.041   Bathroom in boarding-house
    Y92.042   Bedroom in boarding-house
    Y92.043   Driveway of boarding-house
    Y92.044   Garage of boarding-house
    Y92.045   Swimming-pool of boarding-house
    Y92.046   Garden or yard of boarding-house
    Y92.048   Other place in boarding-house
    Y92.049   Unspecified place in boarding-house

Y92.09   **Other non-institutional residence**
`6th`
    Y92.090   Kitchen in other non-institutional residence
    Y92.091   Bathroom in other non-institutional residence
    Y92.092   Bedroom in other non-institutional residence
    Y92.093   Driveway of other non-institutional residence
    Y92.094   Garage of other non-institutional residence
    Y92.095   Swimming-pool of other non-institutional residence
    Y92.096   Garden or yard of other non-institutional residence
    Y92.098   Other place in other non-institutional residence
    Y92.099   Unspecified place in other non-institutional residence

Y92.1   **Institutional (nonprivate) residence**
`5th`
  Y92.10   **Unspecified residential institution**
  Y92.11   **Children's home and orphanage**
  `6th`
    Y92.110   Kitchen in children's home and orphanage
    Y92.111   Bathroom in children's home and orphanage
    Y92.112   Bedroom in children's home and orphanage
    Y92.113   Driveway of children's home and orphanage
    Y92.114   Garage of children's home and orphanage
    Y92.115   Swimming-pool of children's home and orphanage
    Y92.116   Garden or yard of children's home and orphanage
    Y92.118   Other place in children's home and orphanage
    Y92.119   Unspecified place in children's home and orphanage

---

`4th` `5th` `6th` `7th`   Additional Character Required   ✓ 3-character code

•=New Code
▲=Revised Code

Excludes1—Not coded here, do not use together
Excludes2—Not included here

Y92.12   Nursing home
Home for the sick
Hospice
Refer to the complete *ICD-10-CM* manual for subcategory Y92.12-

Y92.15   Reform school
`6th`
     Y92.150   Kitchen in reform school
     Y92.151   Dining room in reform school
     Y92.152   Bathroom in reform school
     Y92.153   Bedroom in reform school
     Y92.154   Driveway of reform school
     Y92.155   Garage of reform school
     Y92.156   Swimming-pool of reform school
     Y92.157   Garden or yard of reform school
     Y92.158   Other place in reform school
     Y92.159   Unspecified place in reform school

Y92.16   School dormitory
`6th`
     Excludes1: reform school (Y92.15-)
       school buildings and grounds (Y92.2-)
       school sports and athletic areas (Y92.3-)
     Y92.160   Kitchen in school dormitory
     Y92.161   Dining room in school dormitory
     Y92.162   Bathroom in school dormitory
     Y92.163   Bedroom in school dormitory
     Y92.168   Other place in school dormitory
     Y92.169   Unspecified place in school dormitory

Y92.19   Other specified residential institution
Refer to the complete *ICD-10-CM* manual for subcategory Y92.19-

Y92.2   School, other institution and public administrative area
`5th`
Building and adjacent grounds used by the general public or by a particular group of the public
Excludes1: building under construction (Y92.6)
     residential institution (Y92.1)
     school dormitory (Y92.16-)
     sports and athletics area of schools (Y92.3-)

Y92.21   School (private) (public) (state)
`6th`
     Y92.210   Daycare center
     Y92.211   Elementary school
       Kindergarten
     Y92.212   Middle school
     Y92.213   High school
     Y92.214   College
       University
     Y92.215   Trade school
     Y92.218   Other school
     Y92.219   Unspecified school

Y92.22   Religious institution
Church
Mosque
Synagogue

Y92.23   Hospital
`6th`
     Excludes1: ambulatory (outpatient) health services establishments (Y92.53-)
     home for the sick (Y92.12-)
     hospice (Y92.12-)
     nursing home (Y92.12-)
     Y92.230   Patient room in hospital
     Y92.231   Patient bathroom in hospital
     Y92.232   Corridor of hospital
     Y92.233   Cafeteria of hospital
     Y92.234   Operating room of hospital
     Y92.238   Other place in hospital
     Y92.239   Unspecified place in hospital

Y92.24   Public administrative building
`6th`
     Y92.240   Courthouse
     Y92.241   Library
     Y92.242   Post office

Y92.25   Cultural building
`6th`
     Y92.250   Art Gallery
     Y92.251   Museum
     Y92.252   Music hall
     Y92.253   Opera house
     Y92.254   Theater (live)
     Y92.258   Other cultural public building

Y92.26   Movie house or cinema

Y92.29   Other specified public building
Assembly hall
Clubhouse

Y92.3   Sports and athletics area
`5th`

Y92.31   Athletic court
`6th`
     Excludes1: tennis court in private home or garden (Y92.09)
     Y92.310   Basketball court
     Y92.311   Squash court
     Y92.312   Tennis court
     Y92.318   Other athletic court

Y92.32   Athletic field
`6th`
     Y92.320   Baseball field
     Y92.321   Football field
     Y92.322   Soccer field
     Y92.328   Other athletic field
       Cricket field
       Hockey field

Y92.33   Skating rink
`6th`
     Y92.330   Ice skating rink (indoor) (outdoor)
     Y92.331   Roller skating rink

Y92.34   Swimming pool (public)
Excludes1: swimming pool in private home or garden (Y92.016)

Y92.39   Other specified sports and athletic area
Golf-course/gymnasium

Y92.4   Street, highway and other paved roadways
`5th`
Excludes1: private driveway of residence (Y92.014, Y92.024, Y92.043, Y92.093, Y92.113, Y92.123, Y92.154, Y92.194)

Y92.41   Street and highway
`6th`
     Y92.410   Unspecified street and highway
       Road NOS
     Y92.411   Interstate highway
       Freeway/Motorway
     Y92.412   Parkway
     Y92.413   State road
     Y92.414   Local residential or business street
     Y92.415   Exit ramp or entrance ramp of street or highway

Y92.48   Other paved roadways
`6th`
     Y92.480   Sidewalk
     Y92.481   Parking lot
     Y92.482   Bike path
     Y92.488   Other paved roadways

Y92.5   Trade and service area
Excludes1: garage in private home (Y92.015)
     schools and other public administration buildings (Y92.2-)

Y92.51   Private commercial establishments
     Y92.510   Bank
     Y92.511   Restaurant or café
     Y92.512   Supermarket, store or market
     Y92.513   Shop (commercial)

Y92.52   Service areas
     Y92.520   Airport
     Y92.521   Bus station
     Y92.522   Railway station
     Y92.523   Highway rest stop
     Y92.524   Gas station
       Petroleum station
       Service station

Y92.53   Ambulatory health services establishments
     Y92.530   Ambulatory surgery center
       Outpatient surgery center, including that connected with a hospital
       Same day surgery center, including that connected with a hospital
     Y92.531   Health care provider office
       Physician office
     Y92.532   Urgent care center
     Y92.538   Other ambulatory health services establishments

---

`4th` `5th` `6th` `7th`   Additional Character Required   ✓   3-character code

•=New Code
▲=Revised Code

Excludes1—Not coded here, do not use together
Excludes2—Not included here

CHAPTER 20. EXTERNAL CAUSES OF MORBIDITY (Y92.59–Y93.55)

Y92.59 **Other trade areas**
Office building
Casino
Garage (commercial)
Hotel
Radio or television station
Shopping mall
Warehouse

Y92.6 **Industrial and construction area**
Refer to complete *ICD-10-CM* manual for subcategory Y92.6

Y92.7 **Farm**
`5th` Ranch
Excludes1: farmhouse and home premises of farm (Y92.01-)

    Y92.71 **Barn**
    Y92.72 **Chicken coop**
        Hen house
    Y92.73 **Farm field**
    Y92.74 **Orchard**
    Y92.79 **Other farm location**

Y92.8 **Other places**
    Y92.81 **Transport vehicle**
    `6th` ***Excludes1:*** transport accidents (V00-V99)
        Y92.810 **Car**
        Y92.811 **Bus**
        Y92.812 **Truck**
        Y92.813 **Airplane**
        Y92.814 **Boat**
        Y92.815 **Train**
        Y92.816 **Subway car**
        Y92.818 **Other transport vehicle**
    Y92.82 **Wilderness area**
        Y92.820 **Desert**
        Y92.821 **Forest**
        Y92.828 **Other wilderness area**
            Swamp
            Mountain
            Marsh
            Prairie
    Y92.83 **Recreation area**
    `6th` **Y92.830** **Public park**
        Y92.831 **Amusement park**
        Y92.832 **Beach/Seashore**
        Y92.833 **Campsite**
        Y92.834 **Zoological garden (Zoo)**
        Y92.838 **Other recreation area**
    Y92.85 **Railroad track**
    Y92.89 **Other specified places**
        Derelict house

Y92.9 **Unspecified place or not applicable**

Y93 **ACTIVITY CODES**
`4th`

> **GUIDELINE**
>
> Note: Category Y93 is provided for use to indicate the activity of the person seeking healthcare for an injury or health condition, such as a heart attack while shoveling snow, which resulted from, or was contributed to, by the activity. These codes are appropriate for use for both acute injuries, such as those from Chapter 19, and conditions that are due to the long-term, cumulative effects of an activity, such as those from Chapter 13. They are also appropriate for use with external cause codes for cause and intent if identifying the activity provides additional information on the event. These codes should be used in conjunction with codes for external cause status (Y99) and place of occurrence (Y92). See complete *ICD-10-CM* manual for codes in categoriy Y93.
>
> Assign a code from category Y93, Activity code, to describe the activity of the patient at the time the injury or other health condition occurred.
>
> An activity code is used only once, at the initial encounter for treatment. Only one code from Y93 should be recorded on a medical record.
>
> The activity codes are not applicable to poisonings, adverse effects, misadventures or sequela.
>
> Do not assign Y93.9, Unspecified activity, if the activity is not stated.
>
> A code from category Y93 is appropriate for use with external cause and intent codes if identifying the activity provides additional information about the event.
>
> See complete *ICD-10-CM* manual for codes in category Y93.

Y93.0 **Activities involving walking and running**
`5th` ***Excludes1:*** activity, walking an animal (Y93.K1)
    activity, walking or running on a treadmill (Y93.A1)
    Y93.01 **Activity, walking, marching and hiking**
        Activity, walking, marching and hiking on level or elevated terrain
        Excludes1: activity, mountain climbing (Y93.31)
    Y93.02 **Activity, running**

Y93.1 **Activities involving water and water craft**
`5th` ***Excludes1:*** activities involving ice (Y93.2-)
    Y93.11 **Activity, swimming**
    Y93.12 **Activity, springboard and platform diving**
    Y93.13 **Activity, water polo**
    Y93.14 **Activity, water aerobics and water exercise**
    Y93.15 **Activity, underwater diving and snorkeling**
        Activity, SCUBA diving
    Y93.16 **Activity, rowing, canoeing, kayaking, rafting and tubing**
    Y93.17 **Activity, water skiing and wake boarding**
    Y93.18 **Activity, surfing, windsurfing and boogie boarding**
        Activity, water sliding
    Y93.19 **Activity, other involving water and watercraft**
        Activity involving water NOS
        Activity, parasailing
        Activity, water survival training and testing

Y93.2 **Activities involving ice and snow**
`5th` ***Excludes1:*** activity, shoveling ice and snow (Y93.H1)
    Y93.21 **Activity, ice skating**
        Activity, figure skating (singles) (pairs)
        Activity, ice dancing
        Excludes1: activity, ice hockey (Y93.22)
    Y93.22 **Activity, ice hockey**
    Y93.23 **Activity, snow (alpine) (downhill) skiing, snow-boarding, sledding, tobogganing and snow tubing**
        Excludes1: activity, cross country skiing (Y93.24)
    Y93.24 **Activity, cross country skiing**
        Activity, nordic skiing
    Y93.29 **Activity, other involving ice and snow**
        Activity involving ice and snow NOS

Y93.3 **Activities involving climbing, rappelling and jumping off**
`5th` ***Excludes1:*** activity, hiking on level or elevated terrain (Y93.01)
    activity, jumping rope (Y93.56)
    activity, trampoline jumping (Y93.44)
    Y93.31 **Activity, mountain climbing, rock climbing and wall climbing**
    Y93.32 **Activity, rappelling**
    Y93.33 **Activity, BASE jumping**
        Activity, Building, Antenna, Span, Earth jumping
    Y93.34 **Activity, bungee jumping**
    Y93.35 **Activity, hang gliding**
    Y93.39 **Activity, other involving climbing, rappelling and jumping off**

Y93.4 **Activities involving dancing and other rhythmic movement**
`5th` ***Excludes1:*** activity, martial arts (Y93.75)
    Y93.41 **Activity, dancing**
    Y93.42 **Activity, yoga**
    Y93.43 **Activity, gymnastics**
        Activity, rhythmic gymnastics
        Excludes1: activity, trampolining (Y93.44)
    Y93.44 **Activity, trampolining**
    Y93.45 **Activity, cheerleading**
    Y93.49 **Activity, other involving dancing and other rhythmic movements**

Y93.5 **Activities involving other sports and athletics played individually**
`5th` ***Excludes1:*** activity, dancing (Y93.41)
    activity, gymnastic (Y93.43)
    activity, trampoline (Y93.44)
    activity, yoga (Y93.42)
    Y93.51 **Activity, roller skating (inline) and skateboarding**
    Y93.52 **Activity, horseback riding**
    Y93.53 **Activity, golf**
    Y93.54 **Activity, bowling**
    Y93.55 **Activity, bike riding**

`4th` `5th` `6th` `7th` Additional Character Required   ☑ 3-character code

• =New Code
▲ =Revised Code

Excludes1—Not coded here, do not use together
Excludes2—Not included here

Y93.56   **Activity, jumping rope**
Y93.57   **Activity, non-running track and field events**
     Excludes1: activity, running (any form) (Y93.02)
Y93.59   **Activity, other involving other sports and athletics played individually**
     Excludes1: activities involving climbing, rappelling, and jumping (Y93.3-)
       activities involving ice and snow (Y93.2-)
       activities involving walking and running (Y93.0-)
       activities involving water and watercraft (Y93.1-)

Y93.6   **Activities involving other sports and athletics played as a team or group** [5th]
     Excludes1: activity, ice hockey (Y93.22)
       activity, water polo (Y93.13)
Y93.61   **Activity, American tackle football**
     Activity, football NOS
Y93.62   **Activity, American flag or touch football**
Y93.63   **Activity, rugby**
Y93.64   **Activity, baseball**
     Activity, softball
Y93.65   **Activity, lacrosse and field hockey**
Y93.66   **Activity, soccer**
Y93.67   **Activity, basketball**
Y93.68   **Activity, volleyball (beach) (court)**
Y93.6A   **Activity, physical games generally associated with school recess, summer camp and children**
     Including capture the flag/dodge ball/four square/kickball
Y93.69   **Activity, other involving other sports and athletics played as a team or group**
     Activity, cricket

Y93.7   **Activities involving other specified sports and athletics** [5th]
Y93.71   **Activity, boxing**
Y93.72   **Activity, wrestling**
Y93.73   **Activity, racquet and hand sports**
     Activity, handball/racquetball/squash/tennis
Y93.74   **Activity, Frisbee**
Y93.75   **Activity, martial arts**
     Activity, combatives
Y93.79   **Activity, other specified sports and athletics**
     Excludes1: sports and athletics activities specified in categories Y93.0–Y93.6

Y93.B   **Activities involving other muscle strengthening exercises** [5th]
Y93.B1   **Activity, exercise machines primarily for muscle strengthening**
Y93.B2   **Activity, push-ups, pull-ups, sit-ups**
Y93.B3   **Activity, free weights**
     Activity, barbells/dumbbells
Y93.B4   **Activity, pilates**
Y93.B9   **Activity, other involving muscle strengthening exercises**
     Excludes1: activities involving muscle strengthening specified in categories Y93.0–Y93.A

Y93.C   **Activities involving computer technology and electronic devices** [5th]
     Excludes1: activity, electronic musical keyboard or instruments (Y93.J-)
Y93.C1   **Activity, computer keyboarding**
     Activity, electronic game playing using keyboard or other stationary device
Y93.C2   **Activity, hand held interactive electronic device**
     Activity, cellular telephone and communication device
     Activity, electronic game playing using interactive device
     Excludes1: activity, electronic game playing using keyboard or other stationary device (Y93.C1)
Y93.C9   **Activity, other involving computer technology and electronic devices**

Y93.D   **Activities involving arts and handcrafts** [5th]
     Excludes1: activities involving playing musical instrument (Y93.J-)
Y93.D1   **Activity, knitting and crocheting**
Y93.D2   **Activity, sewing**
Y93.D3   **Activity, furniture building and finishing**
     Activity, furniture repair
Y93.D9   **Activity, other involving arts and handcrafts**

Y93.E   **Activities involving personal hygiene and interior property and clothing maintenance** [5th]
     Excludes1: activities involving cooking and grilling (Y93.G-)
       activities involving exterior property and land maintenance, building and construction (Y93.H-)
       activities involving caregiving (Y93.F-)
       activity, dishwashing (Y93.G1)
       activity, food preparation (Y93.G1)
       activity, gardening (Y93.H2)
Y93.E1   **Activity, personal bathing and showering**
Y93.E2   **Activity, laundry**
Y93.E3   **Activity, vacuuming**
Y93.E4   **Activity, ironing**
Y93.E5   **Activity, floor mopping and cleaning**
Y93.E6   **Activity, residential relocation**
     Activity, packing up and unpacking involved in moving to a new residence
Y93.E8   **Activity, other personal hygiene**
Y93.E9   **Activity, other interior property and clothing maintenance**

Y93.G   **Activities involving food preparation, cooking and grilling** [5th]
Y93.G1   **Activity, food preparation and clean up**
     Activity, dishwashing
Y93.G2   **Activity, grilling and smoking food**
Y93.G3   **Activity, cooking and baking**
     Activity, use of stove, oven and microwave oven
Y93.G9   **Activity, other involving cooking and grilling**

Y93.I   **Activities involving roller coasters and other types of external motion** [5th]
Y93.I1   **Activity, roller coaster riding**
Y93.I9   **Activity, other involving external motion**

Y93.J   **Activities involving playing musical instrument** [5th]
     Activity involving playing electric musical instrument
Y93.J1   **Activity, piano playing**
     Activity, musical keyboard (electronic) playing
Y93.J2   **Activity, drum and other percussion instrument playing**
Y93.J3   **Activity, string instrument playing**
Y93.J4   **Activity, winds and brass instrument playing**

Y93.K   **Activities involving animal care** [5th]
     Excludes1: activity, horseback riding (Y93.52)
Y93.K1   **Activity, walking an animal**
Y93.K2   **Activity, milking an animal**
Y93.K3   **Activity, grooming and shearing an animal**
Y93.K9   **Activity, other involving animal care**

Y93.8   **Activities, other specified** [5th]
Y93.81   **Activity, refereeing a sports activity**
Y93.82   **Activity, spectator at an event**
Y93.83   **Activity, rough housing and horseplay**
Y93.84   **Activity, sleeping**
Y93.85   **Activity, choking game**
     Activity, blackout or fainting or pass out game
Y93.89   **Activity, other specified**

Y95   **NOSOCOMIAL CONDITION** [✓]

Y99   **EXTERNAL CAUSE STATUS** [4th]
     GUIDELINE

A code from category Y99, External cause status, should be assigned whenever any other external cause code is assigned for an encounter, including an Activity code, except for the events noted below. Assign a code from category Y99, External cause status, to indicate the work status of the person at the time the event occurred. The status code indicates whether the event occurred during military activity, whether a non-military person was at work, whether an individual including a student or volunteer was involved in a non-work activity at the time of the causal event.

A code from Y99, External cause status, should be assigned, when applicable, with other external cause codes, such as transport accidents and falls. The external cause status codes are not applicable to poisonings, adverse effects, misadventures or late effects.

Do not assign a code from category Y99 if no other external cause codes (cause, activity) are applicable for the encounter.

An external cause status code is used only once, at the initial encounter

---

[4th] [5th] [6th] [7th]   Additional Character Required   [✓]   3-character code

•=New Code   *Excludes1*—Not coded here, do not use together
▲=Revised Code   *Excludes2*—Not included here

for treatment. Only one code from Y99 should be recorded on a medical record.

Do not assign code Y99.9, Unspecified external cause status, if the status is not stated.

Note: A single code from category Y99 should be used in conjunction with the external cause code(s) assigned to a record to indicate the status of the person at the time the event occurred.

Y99.0 Civilian activity done for income or pay

Civilian activity done for financial or other compensation

Excludes1: military activity (Y99.1)

volunteer activity (Y99.2)

Y99.2 Volunteer activity

Excludes1: activity of child or other family member assisting in compensated work of other family member (Y99.8)

Y99.8 Other external cause status

Activity NEC

Activity of child or other family member assisting in compensated work of other family member

Hobby not done for income

Leisure activity

Off-duty activity of military personnel

Recreation or sport not for income or while a student

Student activity

Excludes1: civilian activity done for income or compensation (Y99.0)

military activity (Y99.1)

Y99.9 Unspecified external cause status

Chapter 21. Factors influencing health status and contact with health services (Z00–Z99)

Note: The chapter specific guidelines provide additional information about the use of Z codes for specified encounters.

Use of Z codes in any healthcare setting

Z codes are for use in any healthcare setting. Z codes may be used as either a first-listed (principal diagnosis code in the inpatient setting) or secondary code, depending on the circumstances of the encounter. Certain Z codes may only be used as first-listed or principal diagnosis.

Z codes indicate a reason for an encounter or provide additional information about a patient encounter

Z codes are not procedure codes. A corresponding procedure code must accompany a Z code to describe any procedure performed.

Categories of Z codes

CONTACT/EXPOSURE
Refer to categories Z20 and Z77.

INOCULATIONS AND VACCINATIONS
Refer to category Z23.

STATUS
Status codes indicate that a patient is either a carrier of a disease or has the sequelae or residual of a past disease or condition. This includes such things as the presence of prosthetic or mechanical devices resulting from past treatment. A status code is informative, because the status may affect the course of treatment and its outcome. A status code is distinct from a history code. The history code indicates that the patient no longer has the condition.

A status code should not be used with a diagnosis code from one of the body system chapters, if the diagnosis code includes the information provided by the status code. For example, code Z94.1, Heart transplant status, should not be used with a code from subcategory T86.2, Complications of heart transplant. The status code does not provide additional information. The complication code indicates that the patient is a heart transplant patient.

For encounters for weaning from a mechanical ventilator, assign a code from subcategory J96.1, Chronic respiratory failure, followed by code Z99.11, Dependence on respirator [ventilator] status.

The status Z codes/categories are:
Z14, Z15, Z16, Z17, Z18, Z21, Z22, Z28.3, Z33.1, Z66, Z67, Z68, Z74.01, Z76.82, Z78, Z79, Z88 (Except: Z88.9), Z89, Z90, Z91.0-, Z93, Z94, Z95, Z96, Z97, Z98, Z99

HISTORY (OF)
There are two types of history Z codes, personal and family. *Refer to categories or codes Z80, Z81, Z82, Z83, Z84, Z85, Z86, Z87, Z91.4-, Z91.5, Z91.8- (Except: Z91.83), Z92 (Except: Z92.0 and Z92.82)*

SCREENING
Refer to categories Z11, Z12 and Z13 (except: Z13.9).

OBSERVATION
Refer to categories Z03 and Z04 for further details.

AFTERCARE
Aftercare visit codes cover situations when the initial treatment of a disease has been performed and the patient requires continued care during the healing or recovery phase, or for the long-term consequences of the disease. The aftercare Z code should not be used if treatment is directed at a current, acute disease. The diagnosis code is to be used in these cases. Exceptions to this rule are codes Z51.0, Encounter for antineoplastic radiation therapy, and codes from subcategory Z51.1, Encounter for antineoplastic chemotherapy and immunotherapy. These codes are to be first-listed, followed by the diagnosis code when a patient's encounter is solely to receive radiation therapy, chemotherapy, or immunotherapy for the treatment of a neoplasm. If the reason for the encounter is more than one type of antineoplastic therapy, code Z51.0 and a code from subcategory Z51.1 may be assigned together, in which case one of these codes would be reported as a secondary diagnosis.

The aftercare Z codes should also not be used for aftercare for injuries. For aftercare of an injury, assign the acute injury code with the appropriate 7th character (for subsequent encounter).

The aftercare codes are generally first-listed to explain the specific reason for the encounter. An aftercare code may be used as an additional code when some type of aftercare is provided in addition to the reason for admission and no diagnosis code is applicable. An example of this would be the closure of a colostomy during an encounter for treatment of another condition.

Aftercare codes should be used in conjunction with other aftercare codes or diagnosis codes to provide better detail on the specifics of an aftercare encounter visit, unless otherwise directed by the classification. Should a patient receive multiple types of antineoplastic therapy during the same encounter, code Z51.0, Encounter for antineoplastic radiation therapy, and codes from subcategory Z51.1, Encounter for antineoplastic chemotherapy and immunotherapy, may be used together on a record. The sequencing of multiple aftercare codes depends on the circumstances of the encounter.

Certain aftercare Z code categories need a secondary diagnosis code to describe the resolving condition or sequelae. For others, the condition is included in the code title.

Additional Z code aftercare category terms include fitting and adjustment, and attention to artificial openings.

Status Z codes may be used with aftercare Z codes to indicate the nature of the aftercare. For example code Z95.1, Presence of aortocoronary bypass graft, may be used with code Z48.812, Encounter for surgical aftercare following surgery on the circulatory system, to indicate the surgery for which the aftercare is being performed. A status code should not be used when the aftercare code indicates the type of status, such as using Z43.0, Encounter for attention to tracheostomy, with Z93.0, Tracheostomy status.

The aftercare Z category/codes: Z42, Z43, Z44, Z45, Z46, Z47, Z48, Z49 and Z51

FOLLOW-UP
The follow-up codes are used to explain continuing surveillance following completed treatment of a disease, condition, or injury. *Refer to categories Z08 and Z09.*

DONOR
Refer to the *ICD-10-CM* manual.

COUNSELING
Counseling Z codes are used when a patient or family member receives assistance in the aftermath of an illness or injury, or when support is required in coping with family or social problems. They are not used in conjunction with a diagnosis code when the counseling component of care is considered integral to standard treatment.

The counseling Z codes/categories: Z30.0-, Z31.5, Z31.6-, Z32.2, Z32.3, Z69, Z70, Z71 and Z76.81

NEWBORNS AND INFANTS
Newborn Z codes/categories: Z05, Z76.1, Z00.1- and Z38

ROUTINE AND ADMINISTRATIVE EXAMINATIONS
Pre-operative examination and pre-procedural laboratory examination Z codes are for use only in those situations when a patient is being cleared for a procedure or surgery and no treatment is given.

Refer to the Z codes/categories for routine and administrative examinations: Z00, Z01, Z02 (except: Z02.9) and Z32.0-

MISCELLANEOUS Z CODES
The miscellaneous Z codes capture a number of other health care encounters that do not fall into one of the other categories. Certain of these codes identify the reason for the encounter; others are for use as additional codes that provide useful information on circumstances that may affect a patient's care and treatment.

PROPHYLACTIC ORGAN REMOVAL
For encounters specifically for prophylactic removal of an organ refer to the full *ICD-10-CM* manual guidelines.

MISCELLANEOUS Z CODES/CATEGORIES:
Z28, (except: Z28.3), Z40, Z41 (except: Z41.9), Z53, Z55, Z56, Z57, Z58, Z59, Z60, Z62, Z63, Z64, Z65, Z72, Z73, Z74 (except: Z74.01), Z75, Z76.0, Z76.3, Z76.4, Z76.5, Z91.1-, Z91.84-, Z91.83 and Z91.89

NONSPECIFIC Z CODES
Certain Z codes are so non-specific, or potentially redundant with other codes in the classification, that there can be little justification for their use in the inpatient setting. Their use in the outpatient setting should be limited to those instances

---

| 4th | 5th | 6th | 7th | Additional Character Required | ✔ | 3-character code | Unspecified laterality codes were excluded here. | • =New Code
▲ =Revised Code
◻ =Social determinants of health | *Excludes1*—Not coded here, do not use together
Excludes2—Not included here |

when there is no further documentation to permit more precise coding. Otherwise, any sign or symptom or any other reason for visit that is captured in another code should be used.

NONSPECIFIC Z CODES:

Z02.9, Z04.9, Z13.9, Z41.9, Z52.9, Z86.59, Z88.9 and Z92.0

Z CODES THAT MAY ONLY BE PRINCIPAL/FIRST-LISTED DIAGNOSIS

The following Z codes/categories may only be reported as the principal/first-listed diagnosis, except when there are multiple encounters on the same day and the medical records for the encounters are combined: Z00, Z01, Z02, Z03, Z04, Z33.2, Z31.81, Z31.82, Z31.83, Z31.84, Z34, Z38, Z39, Z40, Z42, Z51.0, Z51.1-, Z52 (except: Z52.9), Z76.1, Z76.2 and Z99.12.

Note: Z codes represent reasons for encounters. A corresponding procedure code must accompany a Z code if a procedure is performed. Categories Z00–Z99 are provided for occasions when circumstances other than a disease, injury or external cause classifiable to categories A00–Y89 are recorded as 'diagnoses' or 'problems.' This can arise in two main ways:

a) When a person who may or may not be sick encounters the health services for some specific purpose, such as to receive limited care or service for a current condition, to donate an organ or tissue, to receive prophylactic vaccination (immunization), or to discuss a problem which is in itself not a disease or injury.

b) When some circumstance or problem is present which influences the person's health status but is not in itself a current illness or injury.

(Z00–Z13) PERSONS ENCOUNTERING HEALTH SERVICES FOR EXAMINATIONS

Note: Nonspecific abnormal findings disclosed at the time of these examinations are classified to categories R70–R94.

Excludes1: examinations related to pregnancy and reproduction (Z30–Z36, Z39.-) Codes in categories Z00–Z04 "may only be reported as the principal/first-listed diagnosis, except when there are multiple encounters on the same day and the medical records for the encounters are combined."

Z00 [4th] ENCOUNTER FOR GENERAL EXAMINATION WITHOUT COMPLAINT, SUSPECTED OR REPORTED DIAGNOSIS

GUIDELINES

The codes are not to be used if the examination is for diagnosis of a suspected condition or for treatment purposes. In such cases the diagnosis code is used. During a routine exam, should a diagnosis or condition be discovered, it should be coded as an additional code. Pre-existing and chronic conditions and history codes may also be included as additional codes as long as the examination is for administrative purposes and not focused on any particular condition.

Some of the codes for routine health examinations distinguish between "with" and "without" abnormal findings. Code assignment depends on the information that is known at the time the encounter is being coded. For example, if no abnormal findings were found during the examination, but the encounter is being coded before test results are back, it is acceptable to assign the code for "without abnormal findings." When assigning a code for "with abnormal findings," additional code(s) should be assigned to identify the specific abnormal finding(s).

Excludes1: encounter for examination for administrative purposes (Z02.-)
Excludes2: encounter for pre-procedural examinations (Z01.81-)
     special screening examinations (Z11–Z13)

Z00.0 **Encounter for general adult medical examination**
[5th] Encounter for adult periodic examination (annual) (physical) and any associated laboratory and radiologic examinations
     Excludes1: encounter for examination of sign or symptom— code to sign or symptom
       general health check-up of infant or child (Z00.12-)
   Z00.00 **Encounter for general adult medical examination without abnormal findings**
     Encounter for adult health check-up NOS
   Z00.01 **Encounter for general adult medical examination with abnormal findings**
     Use additional code to identify abnormal findings

Z00.1 **Encounter for newborn, infant and child health examinations**
[5th]

Z00.11 **Newborn health examination**
[6th] *Refer to Chapter 16 for guidelines.*
   Health check for child under 29 days old
   Use additional code to identify any abnormal findings
   Excludes1: health check for child over 28 days old (Z00.12-)
   Z00.110 **Health examination for newborn; under 8 days old**
     Health check for newborn under 8 days old
   Z00.111 **8 to 28 days old**
     Health check for newborn 8 to 28 days old
     Newborn weight check

Z00.12 **Encounter for routine child health examination;**
[6th] Health check (routine) for child over 28 days old
   Immunizations appropriate for age
   Routine developmental screening of infant or child
   Routine vision and hearing testing

> Tip: An abnormal finding can be defined as an acute illness/injury/finding, unstable chronic illness, or abnormal screen

   Excludes1: health check for child under 29 days old (Z00.11-)
     health supervision of foundling or other healthy infant or child (Z76.1–Z76.2)
     newborn health examination (Z00.11-)
   Z00.121 **with abnormal findings**
     Use additional code to identify abnormal findings
   Z00.129 **without abnormal findings**
     Encounter for routine child health examination NOS

Z00.2 **Encounter for examination for period of rapid growth in childhood**

Z00.3 **Encounter for examination for adolescent development state**
   Encounter for puberty development state

Z00.7 **Encounter for examination for period of delayed growth in**
[5th] **childhood**
   Z00.70 **Encounter for examination for period of delayed growth in childhood without abnormal findings**
   Z00.71 **Encounter for examination for period of delayed growth in childhood with abnormal findings**
     Use additional code to identify abnormal findings

Z01 [4th] ENCOUNTER FOR OTHER SPECIAL EXAMINATION WITHOUT COMPLAINT, SUSPECTED OR REPORTED DIAGNOSIS

GUIDELINES

The codes are not to be used if the examination is for diagnosis of a suspected condition or for treatment purposes. In such cases the diagnosis code is used. During a routine exam, should a diagnosis or condition be discovered, it should be coded as an additional code. Pre-existing and chronic conditions and history codes may also be included as additional codes as long as the examination is for administrative purposes and not focused on any particular condition.

Some of the codes for routine health examinations distinguish between "with" and "without" abnormal findings. Code assignment depends on the information that is known at the time the encounter is being coded. For example, if no abnormal findings were found during the examination, but the encounter is being coded before test results are back, it is acceptable to assign the code for "without abnormal findings." When assigning a code for "with abnormal findings," additional code(s) should be assigned to identify the specific abnormal finding(s).

Includes: routine examination of specific system

Note: Codes from category Z01 represent the reason for the encounter. A separate procedure code is required to identify any examinations or procedures performed

Excludes1: encounter for examination for administrative purposes (Z02.-)
   encounter for examination for suspected conditions, proven not to exist (Z03.-)
   encounter for laboratory and radiologic examinations as a component of general medical examinations (Z00.0-)
   encounter for laboratory, radiologic and imaging examinations for sign(s) and symptom(s)—**code to the sign(s) or symptom(s)**
Excludes2: screening examinations (Z11–Z13)

 4th **5th** **6th** **7th**   Additional Character Required   ✓   3-character code   Unspecified laterality codes were excluded here.

• =New Code
▲ =Revised Code
¤ =Social determinants of health

Excludes1—Not coded here, do not use together
Excludes2—Not included here

Z01.0 **Encounter for examination of eyes and vision;**
`5th`
Excludes1: examination for driving license (Z02.4)

  Z01.00 **without abnormal findings**
    Encounter for examination of eyes and vision NOS

  Z01.01 **with abnormal findings**
    Use additional code to identify abnormal findings

  Z01.02 **Encounter for examination of eyes and vision**
  `6th` **following failed vision screening;**
    Excludes1: encounter for examination of eyes and vision with abnormal findings (Z01.01)
    encounter for examination of eyes and vision without abnormal findings (Z01.00)

    Z01.020 **without abnormal findings**
    Z01.021 **with abnormal findings**

Z01.1 **Encounter for examination of ears and hearing;**
`5th`
  Z01.10 **Encounter for examination of ears and hearing without abnormal findings**
    Encounter for examination of ears and hearing NOS

  Z01.11 **Encounter for examination of ears and hearing with**
  `6th` **abnormal findings**

    Z01.110 **Encounter for hearing examination following failed hearing screening**

    Z01.118 **Encounter for examination of ears and hearing with other abnormal findings**
      Use additional code to identify abnormal findings

  Z01.12 **Encounter for hearing conservation and treatment**

Z01.3 **Encounter for examination of blood pressure**
`5th`
  Z01.30 **Encounter for examination of blood pressure without abnormal findings**
    Encounter for examination of blood pressure NOS

  Z01.31 **Encounter for examination of blood pressure with abnormal findings**
    Use additional code to identify abnormal findings

Z01.4 **Encounter for gynecological examination**
`5th`
Excludes2: pregnancy examination or test (Z32.0-)
  routine examination for contraceptive maintenance (Z30.4-)

  Z01.41 **Encounter for routine gynecological examination**
  `6th` Encounter for general gynecological examination with or without cervical smear
    Encounter for gynecological examination (general) (routine) NOS
    Encounter for pelvic examination (annual) (periodic)
    Use additional code: for screening for human papillomavirus, if applicable, (Z11.51)
    for screening vaginal pap smear, if applicable (Z12.72)
    to identify acquired absence of uterus, if applicable (Z90.71-)
    Excludes1: gynecologic examination status (Z08)
    screening cervical pap smear not a part of a routine gynecological examination (Z12.4)

    Z01.411 **Encounter for gynecological examination (general) (routine); with abnormal findings**
      Use additional code to identify abnormal findings

    Z01.419 **without abnormal findings**

  Z01.42 **Encounter for cervical smear to confirm findings of recent normal smear following initial abnormal smear**

Z01.8 **Encounter for other specified special examinations**
`5th`
  Z01.81 **Encounter for preprocedural examinations**
  `6th` Pre-operative examination and pre-procedural laboratory examination Z codes are for use only in those situations when a patient is being cleared for a procedure or surgery and no treatment is given.
    Encounter for preoperative examinations
    Encounter for radiological and imaging examinations as part of preprocedural examination

    Z01.810 **Encounter for preprocedural; cardiovascular examination**
    Z01.811 **respiratory examination**

    Z01.812 **laboratory examination**
      Blood and urine tests prior to treatment or procedure

    Z01.818 **Encounter for other preprocedural examination**
      Encounter for preprocedural examination NOS
      Encounter for examinations prior to antineoplastic chemotherapy

  Z01.82 **Encounter for allergy testing**
    Excludes1: encounter for antibody response examination (Z01.84)

  Z01.84 **Encounter for antibody response examination**
    Encounter for immunity status testing
    Excludes1: encounter for allergy testing (Z01.82)

  Z01.89 **Encounter for other specified special examinations**

Z02 **ENCOUNTER FOR ADMINISTRATIVE EXAMINATION**
`4th`

GUIDELINES

The codes are not to be used if the examination is for diagnosis of a suspected condition or for treatment purposes. In such cases the diagnosis code is used. During a routine exam, should a diagnosis or condition be discovered, it should be coded as an additional code. Pre-existing and chronic conditions and history codes may also be included as additional codes as long as the examination is for administrative purposes and not focused on any particular condition.

Some of the codes for routine health examinations distinguish between "with" and "without" abnormal findings. Code assignment depends on the information that is known at the time the encounter is being coded. For example, if no abnormal findings were found during the examination, but the encounter is being coded before test results are back, it is acceptable to assign the code for "without abnormal findings." When assigning a code for "with abnormal findings," additional code(s) should be assigned to identify the specific abnormal finding(s).

Z02.0 **Encounter for examination for admission to educational institution**
  Encounter for examination for admission to preschool (education)
  Encounter for examination for re-admission to school following illness or medical treatment

Z02.1 **Encounter for pre-employment examination**

Z02.2 **Encounter for examination for admission to residential institution**
  Excludes1: examination for admission to prison (Z02.89)

Z02.3 **Encounter for examination for recruitment to armed forces**

Z02.4 **Encounter for examination for driving license**

Z02.5 **Encounter for examination for participation in sport**
  Excludes1: blood-alcohol and blood-drug test (Z02.83)

Z02.6 **Encounter for examination for insurance purposes**

Z02.7 **Encounter for issue of medical certificate**
`5th`
Excludes1: encounter for general medical examination (Z00–Z01, Z02.0–Z02.6, Z02.8–Z02.9)

  Z02.71 **Encounter for disability determination**
    Encounter for issue of medical certificate of incapacity or invalidity

  Z02.79 **Encounter for issue of other medical certificate**

Z02.8 **Encounter for other administrative examinations**
`5th`
  Z02.82 **Encounter for adoption services**

  Z02.83 **Encounter for blood-alcohol and blood-drug test**
    Use additional code for findings of alcohol or drugs in blood (R78.-)

  Z02.89 **Encounter for other administrative examinations**
    Encounter for examination for admission to prison
    Encounter for examination for admission to summer camp
    Encounter for immigration or naturalization examination
    Encounter for premarital examination
    Excludes1: health supervision of foundling or other healthy infant or child (Z76.1–Z76.2)

Z02.9 **Encounter for administrative examinations, unspecified**

`4th` `5th` `6th` `7th` Additional Character Required   ✓   3-character code   Unspecified laterality codes were excluded here.   • =New Code   ▲ =Revised Code   ¤ =Social determinants of health   *Excludes1*—Not coded here, do not use together   *Excludes2*—Not included here

Z03 [4th] ENCOUNTER FOR MEDICAL OBSERVATION FOR SUSPECTED DISEASES AND CONDITIONS RULED OUT

GUIDELINES

This observation category is for use in very limited circumstances when a person is being observed for a suspected condition that is ruled out. The observation codes are not for use if an injury or illness or any signs or symptoms related to the suspected condition are present. In such cases the diagnosis/symptom code is used with the corresponding external cause code. The observation codes are primarily to be used as principal/first listed diagnosis. Additional codes may be used in addition to the observation code but only if they are unrelated to the suspected condition being observed.

This category is to be used when a person without a diagnosis is suspected of having an abnormal condition, without signs or symptoms, which requires study, but after examination and observation, is ruled out. This category is also for use for administrative and legal observation status.

An observation code may be assigned as a secondary diagnosis code when the patient is being observed for a condition that is ruled out and is unrelated to the principal/first-listed diagnosis (e.g., patient presents for treatment following injuries sustained in a motor vehicle accident and is also observed for suspected COVID-19 infection that is subsequently ruled out).

Excludes1: contact with and (suspected) exposures hazardous to health (Z77.-)

encounter for observation and evaluation of newborn for suspected diseases and conditions ruled out (Z05.-)

person with feared complaint in whom no diagnosis is made (Z71.1)

signs or symptoms under study—code to signs or symptoms

Z03.6 Encounter for observation for suspected toxic effect from ingested substance ruled out

Encounter for observation for suspected adverse effect from drug

Encounter for observation for suspected poisoning

Z03.7 [5th] Encounter for suspected maternal and fetal conditions ruled out

GUIDELINES

Codes from subcategory Z03.7 may either be used as a first-listed or as an additional code assignment depending on the case. They are for use in very limited circumstances on a maternal record when an encounter is for a suspected maternal or fetal condition that is ruled out during that encounter (for example, a maternal or fetal condition may be suspected due to an abnormal test result). In addition, these codes are not for use if an illness or any signs or symptoms related to the suspected condition or problem are present. In such cases the diagnosis/symptom code is used.

Additional codes may be used in addition to the code from subcategory Z03.7, but only if they are unrelated to the suspected condition being evaluated.

Encounter for suspected maternal and fetal conditions not found

Excludes1: known or suspected fetal anomalies affecting management of mother, not ruled out (O26.-, O35.-, O36.-, O40.-, O41.-)

Z03.73 Encounter for suspected; fetal anomaly ruled out

Z03.74 problem with fetal growth ruled out

Z03.79 maternal and fetal conditions ruled out

Z03.8 [5th] Encounter for observation for other suspected diseases and conditions ruled out

Z03.81 [6th] Encounter for observation for suspected exposure to; biological agents ruled out

Z03.810 anthrax ruled out

Z03.818 other biological agents ruled out

Z03.82 [6th] Encounter for observation for suspected foreign body ruled out

Excludes1: retained foreign body (Z18.-)

retained foreign body in eyelid (H02.81)

residual foreign body in soft tissue (M79.5)

Excludes2: confirmed foreign body ingestion or aspiration including:

foreign body in alimentary tract (T18)

foreign body in ear (T16)

foreign body on external eye (T15)

foreign body in respiratory tract (T17)

• Z03.821 Encounter for observation for suspected ingested foreign body ruled out

Z03.822 Encounter for observation for suspected aspirated (inhaled) foreign body ruled out

Z03.823 Encounter for observation for suspected inserted (injected) foreign body ruled out

Encounter for observation for suspected inserted (injected) foreign body in eye, orifice or skin ruled out

Z03.89 Encounter for observation for other suspected diseases and conditions ruled out

Encounter for observation for suspected inserted (injected) foreign body in eye, orifice or skin ruled out

Z04 [4th] ENCOUNTER FOR EXAMINATION AND OBSERVATION FOR OTHER REASONS

GUIDELINES

This observation category (excludes Z04.9) is for use in very limited circumstances when a person is being observed for a suspected condition that is ruled out. The observation codes are not for use if an injury or illness or any signs or symptoms related to the suspected condition are present. In such cases the diagnosis/symptom code is used with the corresponding external cause code. The observation codes are primarily to be used as principal diagnosis. Additional codes may be used in addition to the observation code but only if they are unrelated to the suspected condition being observed.

An observation code may be assigned as a secondary diagnosis code when the patient is being observed for a condition that is ruled out and is unrelated to the principal/first-listed diagnosis (e.g., patient presents for treatment following injuries sustained in a motor vehicle accident and is also observed for suspected COVID-19 infection that is subsequently ruled out).

Includes: encounter for examination for medicolegal reasons

This category is to be used when a person without a diagnosis is suspected of having an abnormal condition, without signs or symptoms, which requires study, but after examination and observation, is ruled out.

This category is also for use for administrative and legal observation status.

Z04.1 Encounter for examination and observation following; transport accident

Excludes1: encounter for examination and observation following work accident (Z04.2)

Do not report an external cause code with a Z04- code

Z04.2 work accident

Z04.3 other accident

Z04.4 [5th] Encounter for examination and observation following alleged rape

Encounter for examination and observation of victim following alleged rape

Encounter for examination and observation of victim following alleged sexual abuse

Z04.42 Encounter for examination and observation following alleged child rape

Suspected child rape, ruled out

Suspected child sexual abuse, ruled out

Z04.7 [5th] Encounter for examination and observation following alleged; physical abuse

Z04.72 child physical abuse

Suspected child physical abuse, ruled out

Excludes1: confirmed case of child physical abuse (T74.-)

encounter for examination and observation following alleged child sexual abuse (Z04.42)

suspected case of child physical abuse, not ruled out (T76.-)

Z04.8 [5th] Encounter for examination and observation for other specified reasons

Encounter for examination and observation for request for expert evidence

Z04.81 Encounter for examination and observation of victim following forced sexual exploitation

Z04.82 Encounter for examination and observation of victim following forced labor exploitation

Z04.89 Encounter for examination and observation for other specified reasons

| [4th] | [5th] | [6th] | [7th] | Additional Character Required | [✓] | 3-character code | Unspecified laterality codes were excluded here. | • =New Code ▲ =Revised Code ◘ =Social determinants of health | *Excludes1*—Not coded here, do not use together *Excludes2*—Not included here |

442   PEDIATRIC ICD-10-CM 2022: A MANUAL FOR PROVIDER-BASED CODING

Z04.9 Encounter for examination and observation for unspecified reason

Code is a nonspecific Z code, refer to Chapter 21 for guidelines.

Z05 ENCOUNTER FOR OBSERVATION AND EVALUATION OF NEWBORN FOR SUSPECTED DISEASES AND CONDITIONS RULED OUT
4th

GUIDELINES

Use of Z05 codes

Assign a code from category Z05, Observation and evaluation of newborns and infants for suspected conditions ruled out, to identify those instances when a healthy newborn is evaluated for a suspected condition that is determined after study not to be present. Do not use a code from category Z05 when the patient has identified signs or symptoms of a suspected problem; in such cases code the sign or symptom.

Z05 on Other than the Birth Record

A code from category Z05 may also be assigned as a principal or first-listed code for readmissions or encounters when the code from category Z38 code no longer applies. Codes from category Z05 are for use only for healthy newborns and infants for which no condition after study is found to be present.

Z05 on a birth record

A code from category Z05 is to be used as a secondary code after the code from category Z38, Liveborn infants according to place of birth and type of delivery is listed first.

This category is to be used for newborns, within the neonatal period (the first 28 days of life), who are suspected of having an abnormal condition but without signs or symptoms, and which, after examination and observation, is ruled out.

An observation code may be assigned as a secondary diagnosis code when the patient is being observed for a condition that is ruled out and is unrelated to the principal/first-listed diagnosis (e.g., patient presents for treatment following injuries sustained in a motor vehicle accident and is also observed for suspected COVID-19 infection that is subsequently ruled out).

Z05.0 Observation and evaluation of newborn for suspected; cardiac condition ruled out

Z05.1 infectious condition ruled out

Z05.2 neurological condition ruled out

Z05.3 respiratory condition ruled out

Z05.4 genetic, metabolic or immunologic condition ruled out

5th **Z05.41 genetic condition ruled out**

Z05.42 metabolic condition ruled out

Z05.43 immunologic condition ruled out

Z05.5 gastrointestinal condition ruled out

Z05.6 genitourinary condition ruled out

Z05.7 skin and subcutaneous tissue or musculoskeletal condition ruled out

5th

Z05.71 skin and subcutaneous tissue condition ruled out

Z05.72 musculoskeletal condition ruled out

Z05.73 connective tissue condition ruled out

Z05.8 Observation and evaluation of newborn for other specified suspected condition ruled out

Z05.9 Observation and evaluation of newborn for unspecified suspected condition ruled out

Z08 ENCOUNTER FOR FOLLOW-UP EXAMINATION AFTER COMPLETED TREATMENT FOR MALIGNANT NEOPLASM
✓

GUIDELINES

The follow-up codes are used to explain continuing surveillance following completed treatment of a disease, condition, or injury. They imply that the condition has been fully treated and no longer exists. They should not be confused with aftercare codes, or injury codes with a 7th character for subsequent encounter, that explain ongoing care of a healing condition or its sequelae. Follow-up codes may be used in conjunction with history codes to provide the full picture of the healed condition and its treatment. The follow-up code is sequenced first, followed by the history code.

A follow-up code may be used to explain multiple visits. Should a condition be found to have recurred on the follow-up visit, then the diagnosis code for the condition should be assigned in place of the follow-up code.

Medical surveillance following completed treatment

Use additional code to identify any acquired absence of organs (Z90.-)

Use additional code to identify the personal history of malignant neoplasm (Z85.-)

Excludes1: aftercare following medical care (Z43–Z49, Z51)

Z09 ENCOUNTER FOR FOLLOW-UP EXAMINATION AFTER COMPLETED TREATMENT FOR CONDITIONS OTHER THAN MALIGNANT NEOPLASM
✓

GUIDELINES

The follow-up codes are used to explain continuing surveillance following completed treatment of a disease, condition, or injury. They imply that the condition has been fully treated and no longer exists. They should not be confused with aftercare codes, or injury codes with a 7th character for subsequent encounter, that explain ongoing care of a healing condition or its sequelae. Follow-up codes may be used in conjunction with history codes to provide the full picture of the healed condition and its treatment. The follow-up code is sequenced first, followed by the history code.

A follow-up code may be used to explain multiple visits. Should a condition be found to have recurred on the follow-up visit, then the diagnosis code for the condition should be assigned in place of the follow-up code.

Medical surveillance following completed treatment

Use additional code to identify any applicable history of disease code (Z86.-, Z87.-)

Excludes1: aftercare following medical care (Z43–Z49, Z51)
surveillance of contraception (Z30.4-)
surveillance of prosthetic and other medical devices (Z44–Z46)

Z11 ENCOUNTER FOR SCREENING FOR INFECTIOUS AND PARASITIC DISEASES
4th

GUIDELINES

Screening is the testing for disease or disease precursors in seemingly well individuals so that early detection and treatment can be provided for those who test positive for the disease (eg, screening mammogram).

The testing of a person to rule out or confirm a suspected diagnosis because the patient has some sign or symptom is a diagnostic examination, not a screening. In these cases, the sign or symptom is used to explain the reason for the test.

A screening code may be a first-listed code if the reason for the visit is specifically the screening exam. It may also be used as an additional code if the screening is done during an office visit for other health problems. A screening code is not necessary if the screening is inherent to a routine examination, such as a pap smear done during a routine pelvic examination. Should a condition be discovered during the screening then the code for the condition may be assigned as an additional diagnosis.

The Z code indicates that a screening exam is planned. A procedure code is required to confirm that the screening was performed.

Excludes1: encounter for diagnostic examination-code to sign or symptom

Z11.0 Encounter for screening for; intestinal infectious diseases

Z11.1 respiratory tuberculosis

Encounter for screening for active tuberculosis disease

Z11.2 other bacterial diseases

Z11.3 infections with a predominantly sexual mode of transmission

Excludes2: encounter for screening for HIV (Z11.4)
encounter for screening for human papillomavirus (Z11.51)

Z11.4 HIV

Z11.5 Encounter for screening for; other viral diseases

5th ***Excludes2:*** encounter for screening for viral intestinal disease (Z11.0)

Z11.51 human papillomavirus (HPV)

GUIDELINE

During the COVID-19 pandemic, a screening code is generally not appropriate. Do not assign code Z11.52, Encounter for screening for COVID-19. For encounters for COVID-19 testing, including preoperative testing, code as exposure to COVID-19 (guideline I.C.1.g.1.e.).

Coding guidance will be updated as new information concerning any changes in the pandemic status becomes available.

Z11.52 COVID-19

Z11.59 other viral diseases

| 4th | 5th | 6th | 7th | Additional Character Required | ✓ | 3-character code | Unspecified laterality codes were excluded here. | • =New Code ▲ =Revised Code ▣ =Social determinants of health | ***Excludes1***—Not coded here, do not use together ***Excludes2***—Not included here |

PEDIATRIC ICD-10-CM 2022: A MANUAL FOR PROVIDER-BASED CODING   **443**

Z11.6   Encounter for screening for other protozoal diseases and helminthiases

Excludes2: encounter for screening for protozoal intestinal disease (Z11.0)

Z11.7   Encounter for testing for latent tuberculosis infection

Z11.8   Encounter for screening for other infectious and parasitic diseases

Encounter for screening for chlamydia or rickettsial or spirochetal or mycoses

Z11.9   Encounter for screening for infectious and parasitic diseases, unspecified

Z12   ENCOUNTER FOR SCREENING FOR MALIGNANT NEOPLASMS
`4th`

GUIDELINES

Screening is the testing for disease or disease precursors in seemingly well individuals so that early detection and treatment can be provided for those who test positive for the disease (eg, screening mammogram).

The testing of a person to rule out or confirm a suspected diagnosis because the patient has some sign or symptom is a diagnostic examination, not a screening. In these cases, the sign or symptom is used to explain the reason for the test.

A screening code may be a first-listed code if the reason for the visit is specifically the screening exam. It may also be used as an additional code if the screening is done during an office visit for other health problems. A screening code is not necessary if the screening is inherent to a routine examination, such as a pap smear done during a routine pelvic examination. Should a condition be discovered during the screening then the code for the condition may be assigned as an additional diagnosis.

The Z code indicates that a screening exam is planned. A procedure code is required to confirm that the screening was performed.

Use additional code to identify any family history of malignant neoplasm (Z80.-)

Excludes1: encounter for diagnostic examination-code to sign or symptom

Z12.3   Encounter for screening for malignant neoplasm of breast

`5th` **Z12.31   Encounter for screening mammogram for malignant neoplasm of breast**

Excludes1: inconclusive mammogram (R92.2)

Z12.39   Encounter for other screening for malignant neoplasm of breast

Z12.4   Encounter for screening for malignant neoplasm of cervix

Encounter for screening pap smear for malignant neoplasm of cervix

Excludes1: when screening is part of general gynecological examination (Z01.4-)

Excludes2: encounter for screening for human papillomavirus (Z11.51)

Z12.8   Encounter for screening for malignant neoplasm of; other sites

`5th` **Z12.82   nervous system**

Z12.89   other sites

Z12.9   Encounter for screening for malignant neoplasm, site unspecified

Z13   ENCOUNTER FOR SCREENING FOR OTHER DISEASES AND DISORDERS
`4th`

GUIDELINES

Screening is the testing for disease or disease precursors in seemingly well individuals so that early detection and treatment can be provided for those who test positive for the disease (eg, screening mammogram).

The testing of a person to rule out or confirm a suspected diagnosis because the patient has some sign or symptom is a diagnostic examination, not a screening. In these cases, the sign or symptom is used to explain the reason for the test.

A screening code may be a first-listed code if the reason for the visit is specifically the screening exam. It may also be used as an additional code if the screening is done during an office visit for other health problems. A screening code is not necessary if the screening is inherent to a routine examination, such as a pap smear done during a routine pelvic examination. Should a condition be discovered during the screening then the code for the condition may be assigned as an additional diagnosis.

The Z code indicates that a screening exam is planned. A procedure code is required to confirm that the screening was performed. Excludes Z13.9.

Excludes1: encounter for diagnostic examination-code to sign or symptom

Z13.0   Encounter for screening for; diseases of the blood and blood-forming organs and certain disorders involving the immune mechanism

Z13.1   DM

Z13.2   nutritional, metabolic and other endocrine disorders

`5th` **Z13.21   nutritional disorder**

Z13.22   metabolic disorder

`6th` **Z13.220   lipoid disorders**

Encounter for screening for cholesterol level or hypercholesterolemia or hyperlipidemia

Z13.228   other metabolic disorders

Z13.29   other suspected endocrine disorder

Excludes2: encounter for screening for DM (Z13.1)

Z13.3   Encounter for screening for mental health and behavioral disorders
`5th`

Z13.30   Encounter for screening examination for mental health and behavioral disorders, unspecified

Z13.31   Encounter for screening for depression

Encounter for screening for depression, adult

Encounter for screening for depression for child or adolescent

Z13.32   Encounter for screening for maternal depression

Encounter for screening for perinatal depression

> Do not report **Z13.32** on the baby's record

Z13.39   Encounter for screening examination for other mental health and behavioral disorders

Encounter for screening for alcoholism

Encounter for screening for intellectual disabilities

Z13.4   Encounter for screening for certain developmental disorders in childhood
`5th`

Encounter for screening for developmental handicaps in early childhood

Excludes2: encounter for routine child health examination (Z00.12-)

Z13.40   Encounter for screening for unspecified developmental delays

Z13.41   Encounter for autism screening

Z13.42   Encounter for screening for global developmental delays (milestones)

Encounter for screening for developmental handicaps in early childhood

Z13.49   Encounter for screening for other developmental delays

Z13.5   eye and ear disorders

Excludes2: encounter for general hearing examination (Z01.1-) encounter for general vision examination (Z01.0-)

Z13.6   cardiovascular disorders

Z13.7   genetic and chromosomal anomalies

`5th` *Excludes1:* genetic testing for procreative management (Z31.4-)

Z13.71   Encounter for nonprocreative screening for genetic disease carrier status

Z13.79   Encounter for other screening for genetic and chromosomal anomalies

Z13.8   Encounter for screening for; other specified diseases and disorders
`5th`

Excludes2: screening for malignant neoplasms (Z12.-)

Z13.81   digestive system disorders

`6th` **Z13.810   upper gastrointestinal disorder**

Z13.811   lower gastrointestinal disorder

Excludes1: encounter for screening for intestinal infectious disease (Z11.0)

Z13.818   other digestive system disorders

Z13.82   Encounter for screening for musculoskeletal disorder

`6th` **Z13.828   other musculoskeletal disorder**

Z13.83   respiratory disorder NEC

Excludes1: encounter for screening for respiratory tuberculosis (Z11.1)

Z13.84   dental disorders

Z13.85   Encounter for screening for nervous system disorders
`6th`

Z13.850   traumatic brain injury

Z13.858   other nervous system disorders

`4th` `5th` `6th` `7th` Additional Character Required   ✓   3-character code   Unspecified laterality codes were excluded here.

• =New Code
▲ =Revised Code
�Social determinants of health

Excludes1—Not coded here, do not use together
Excludes2—Not included here

444   PEDIATRIC ICD-10-CM 2022: A MANUAL FOR PROVIDER-BASED CODING

Z13.88 **disorder due to exposure to contaminants**
Excludes1: those exposed to contaminants without suspected disorders (Z57.-, Z77.-)

Z13.89 **other disorder**
Encounter for screening for genitourinary disorders

Z13.9 **Encounter for screening, unspecified**
Code is a nonspecific Z code, refer to Chapter 21 for guidelines.

(Z14–Z15) GENETIC CARRIER AND GENETIC SUSCEPTIBILITY TO DISEASE

Z14 `4th` **GENETIC CARRIER**
Genetic carrier status indicates that a person carries a gene, associated with a particular disease, which may be passed to offspring who may develop that disease. The person does not have the disease and is not at risk of developing the disease. Refer to Chapter 21 for status guidelines.

Z14.0 **Hemophilia A carrier**
`5th` **Z14.01** **Asymptomatic hemophilia A carrier**
Z14.02 **Symptomatic hemophilia A carrier**

Z14.1 **Cystic fibrosis carrier**
Z14.8 **Genetic carrier of other disease**

(Z16) RESISTANCE TO ANTIMICROBIAL DRUGS

Z16 `4th` **RESISTANCE TO ANTIMICROBIAL DRUGS**
This code indicates that a patient has a condition that is resistant to antimicrobial drug treatment. Sequence the infection code first. This is a status category, refer to Chapter 21 for status guidelines.
Note: The codes in this category are provided for use as additional codes to identify the resistance and non-responsiveness of a condition to antimicrobial drugs.
Code first the infection
Excludes1: MRSA infection (A49.02)
MRSA infection in diseases classified elsewhere (B95.62)
MRSA pneumonia (J15.212)
Sepsis due to MRSA (A41.02)

Z16.1 **Resistance to beta lactam antibiotics**
`5th` **Z16.10** **Resistance to unspecified beta lactam antibiotics**
Z16.11 **Resistance to penicillins**
Resistance to amoxicillin or ampicillin
Z16.12 **Extended spectrum beta lactamase (ESBL) resistance**
Excludes 2: MRSA infection in diseases classified elsewhere (B95.62)
Z16.19 **other specified beta lactam antibiotics**
Resistance to cephalosporins

Z16.2 **Resistance to; other antibiotics**
`5th` **Z16.20** **unspecified antibiotic**
Resistance to antibiotics NOS
Z16.21 **vancomycin**
Z16.22 **vancomycin related antibiotics**
Z16.23 **quinolones and fluoroquinolones**
Z16.24 **multiple antibiotics**
Z16.29 **other single specified antibiotic**
Resistance to aminoglycosides or macrolides or sulfonamides or tetracyclines

Z16.3 **Resistance to; other antimicrobial drugs**
`5th` *Excludes1:* resistance to antibiotics (Z16.1-, Z16.2-)
Z16.30 **unspecified antimicrobial drugs**
Drug resistance NOS
Z16.32 **antifungal drug(s)**
Z16.33 **antiviral drug(s)**
`6th` **Z16.341** **single antimycobacterial drug**
Resistance to antimycobacterial drug NOS
Z16.342 **multiple antimycobacterial drugs**
Z16.34 **Resistance to antimycobacterial drug(s)**
Resistance to tuberculostatics
Z16.35 **Resistance to multiple antimicrobial drugs**
Excludes1: Resistance to multiple antibiotics only (Z16.24)
Z16.39 **other specified antimicrobial drug**

(Z18) RETAINED FB FRAGMENTS

Z18 `4th` **RETAINED FB FRAGMENTS**
This is a status category, refer to Chapter 21 for status guidelines.
Includes: embedded fragment (status)
embedded splinter (status)
retained FB status
Excludes1: artificial joint prosthesis status (Z96.6-)
FB accidentally left during a procedure (T81.5-)
FB entering through orifice (T15–T19)
in situ cardiac device (Z95.-)
organ or tissue replaced by means other than transplant (Z96.-, Z97.-)
organ or tissue replaced by transplant (Z94.-)
personal history of retained FB fully removed Z87.821
superficial FB (non-embedded splinter)—code to superficial FB, by site

Z18.1 **Retained metal fragments;**
`5th` *Excludes1:* retained radioactive metal fragments (Z18.01–Z18.09)
Z18.10 **Retained metal fragments, unspecified**
Retained metal fragment NOS
Z18.11 **Retained magnetic metal fragments**
Z18.12 **Retained nonmagnetic metal fragments**

Z18.2 **Retained plastic fragments**
Acrylics fragments
Diethylhexyl phthalates fragments
Isocyanate fragments

Z18.3 **Retained organic fragments**
`5th` **Z18.31** **Retained animal quills or spines**
Z18.32 **Retained tooth**
Z18.33 **Retained wood fragments**
Z18.39 **Other retained organic fragments**

Z18.8 **Other specified retained FB**
`5th` **Z18.81** **Retained glass fragments**
Z18.83 **Retained stone or crystalline fragments**
Retained concrete or cement fragments
Z18.89 **Other specified retained FB fragments**

Z18.9 **Retained FB fragments, unspecified material**

(Z20–Z29) PERSONS WITH POTENTIAL HEALTH HAZARDS RELATED TO COMMUNICABLE DISEASES

GUIDELINES

Category Z20 indicates contact with, and suspected exposure to, communicable diseases. These codes are for patients who do not show any sign or symptom of a disease but are suspected to have been exposed to it by close personal contact with an infected individual or are in an area where a disease is epidemic.

Contact/exposure codes may be used as a first-listed code to explain an encounter for testing, or, more commonly, as a secondary code to identify a potential risk.

Z20 `4th` **CONTACT WITH AND (SUSPECTED) EXPOSURE TO COMMUNICABLE DISEASES**
Excludes1: carrier of infectious disease (Z22.-)
diagnosed current infectious or parasitic disease—see Alphabetic Index
Excludes2: personal history of infectious and parasitic diseases (Z86.1-)

Z20.0 **Contact with and (suspected) exposure to intestinal infectious diseases;**
`5th` **Z20.01** **due to E. coli**
Z20.09 **other intestinal infectious diseases**
Z20.1 **Contact with and (suspected) exposure to; tuberculosis**
Z20.2 **infections with a predominantly sexual mode of transmission**
Z20.3 **rabies**
Z20.4 **rubella**
Z20.5 **viral hepatitis**
Z20.6 **HIV**
Excludes1: asymptomatic HIV
HIV infection status (Z21)
Z20.7 **pediculosis, acariasis and other infestations**
Z20.8 **Contact with and (suspected) exposure to; other communicable diseases**
`5th` **Z20.81** **other bacterial communicable diseases**
`6th` **Z20.810** **anthrax**

`4th` `5th` `6th` `7th` Additional Character Required ✓ 3-character code

Unspecified laterality codes were excluded here.

* =New Code
▲ =Revised Code
⬛ =Social determinants of health

Excludes1—Not coded here, do not use together
Excludes2—Not included here

CHAPTER 21. FACTORS INFLUENCING HEALTH STATUS AND CONTACT WITH HEALTH SERVICES   (Z20.811–Z30.015)

> Z20.811   **meningococcus**
> Z20.818   **other bacterial communicable diseases**
> > Use Z20.818 for exposure to strep throat

Z20.82   **Contact with and (suspected) exposure to; other viral communicable diseases** [6th]
> Z20.820   **varicella**
> Z20.821   **Zika virus**

> **GUIDELINE**
> See Code U07.1 for more information.

> Z20.822   **COVID- 19**
> Z20.828   **other viral communicable diseases**

Z20.89   **other communicable diseases**

Z20.9   **unspecified communicable disease**

Z21   **ASYMPTOMATIC HIV INFECTION STATUS** ✔

This code indicates that a patient has tested positive for HIV but has manifested no signs or symptoms of the disease. This is a status code, refer to Chapter 21 for status guidelines.

HIV positive NOS

Code first HIV disease complicating pregnancy, childbirth and the puerperium, if applicable (O98.7-)

Excludes1: acquired immunodeficiency syndrome (B20)
> contact with HIV (Z20.6)
> exposure to HIV (Z20.6)
> HIV disease (B20)
> inconclusive laboratory evidence of HIV (R75)

Z22   **CARRIER OF INFECTIOUS DISEASE** [4th]

Carrier status indicates that a person harbors the specific organisms of a disease without manifest symptoms and is capable of transmitting the infection. This is a status category, refer to Chapter 21 for status guidelines.

Includes: colonization status
> suspected carrier

Excludes2: carrier of viral hepatitis (B18.-)

Z22.1   **Carrier of other intestinal infectious diseases**

Z22.2   **Carrier of diphtheria**

Z22.3   **Carrier of other specified bacterial diseases** [5th]
> Z22.31   **Carrier of bacterial disease due to; meningococci**
> Z22.32   **Carrier of bacterial disease due to staphylococci** [6th]
> > Z22.321   **Carrier or suspected carrier of MSSA**
> > > MSSA colonization
> > Z22.322   **Carrier or suspected carrier of MRSA**
> > > MRSA colonization
> Z22.33   **Carrier of bacterial disease due to streptococci** [6th]
> > Z22.330   **Carrier of Group B streptococcus**
> > > *Excludes1:* carrier of streptococcus group B (GBS) complicating pregnancy, childbirth and the puerperium (O99.82-)
> > Z22.338   **Carrier of other streptococcus**
> Z22.39   **Carrier of other specified bacterial diseases**

Z22.4   **Carrier of infections with a predominantly sexual mode of transmission**

Z22.5   **Carrier of viral hepatitis**

Z22.6   **Carrier of human T-lymphotropic virus type-1 [HTLV-1] infection**

Z22.7   **Latent tuberculosis**
> Latent tuberculosis infection (LTBI)
> *Excludes1:* nonspecific reaction to cell mediated immunity measurement of gamma interferonantigen response without active tuberculosis (R76.12)
> > nonspecific reaction to tuberculin skin test without active tuberculosis (R76.11)

Z22.8   **Carrier of other infectious diseases**

Z22.9   **Carrier of infectious disease, unspecified**

Z23   **ENCOUNTER FOR IMMUNIZATION** ✔

> **GUIDELINES**
> Code Z23 is for encounters for inoculations and vaccinations. It indicates that a patient is being seen to receive a prophylactic inoculation against a disease. Procedure codes are required to identify the actual administration of the injection and the type(s) of immunizations given. Code Z23 may be used as a secondary code if the inoculation is given as a routine part of preventive health care, such as a well-baby visit.

> Tip: Z23 should be reported for every vaccine encounter

Code first any routine childhood examination

Code also, if applicable, encounter for immunization safety counseling (Z71.85)

Note: procedure codes are required to identify the types of immunizations given

Z28   **IMMUNIZATION NOT CARRIED OUT AND UNDERIMMUNIZATION STATUS** [4th]

Includes: vaccination not carried out

Code also, if applicable, encounter for immunization safety counseling (Z71.85)

Z28.0   **Immunization not carried out due to; contraindication** [5th]
> Z28.01   **acute illness of patient**
> Z28.02   **chronic illness or condition of patient**
> Z28.03   **immune compromised state of patient**
> Z28.04   **patient allergy to vaccine or component**
> Z28.09   **other contraindication**

Z28.1   **Immunization not carried out due to patient decision for reasons of belief or group pressure**
> Immunization not carried out because of religious belief

Z28.2   **Immunization not carried out due to; patient decision for other and unspecified reason** [5th]
> Z28.20   **patient decision for unspecified reason**
> Z28.21   **patient refusal**
> Z28.29   **patient decision for other reason**

Z28.3   **Underimmunization status**
> *This is a status code, refer to Chapter 21 for status guidelines.*
> Delinquent immunization status
> Lapsed immunization schedule status

Z28.8   **Immunization not carried out; for other reason** [5th]
> Z28.81   **due to patient having had the disease**
> Z28.82   **because of caregiver refusal**
> > Immunization not carried out because of parental or guardian refusal
> > *Excludes1:* immunization not carried out because of caregiver refusal because of religious belief (Z28.1)
> Z28.83   **due to unavailability of vaccine**
> > Delay in delivery of vaccine
> > Lack of availability of vaccine
> > Manufacturer delay of vaccine
> Z28.89   **for other reason**

Z28.9   **Immunization not carried out for unspecified reason**

Z29   **ENCOUNTER FOR PROPHYLACTIC MEASURES** [4th]

Excludes 1: desensitization to allergens (Z51.6)
> prophylactic surgery (Z40.-)

Z29.1   **Encounter for prophylactic therapy** [5th]
> Encounter for administration of immunoglobulin
> Z29.11   **Encounter for prophylactic immunotherapy for RSV**
> Z29.12   **Encounter for prophylactic antivenin**
> Z29.13   **Encounter for prophylactic Rho(D) immune globulin**
> Z29.14   **Encounter for prophylactic rabies immune globin**

Z29.3   **Encounter for prophylactic fluoride administration**

Z29.8   **Encounter for other specified prophylactic measures**

Z29.9   **Encounter for prophylactic measures, unspecified**

(Z30–Z39) PERSONS ENCOUNTERING HEALTH SERVICES IN CIRCUMSTANCES RELATED TO REPRODUCTION

Z30   **ENCOUNTER FOR CONTRACEPTIVE MANAGEMENT** [4th]

Z30.0   **Encounter for general counseling and advice on contraception** [5th]
> *Refer to Chapter 21 for guidelines on counseling.*
> Z30.01   **Encounter for initial prescription of; contraceptives** [6th]
> > *Excludes1:* encounter for surveillance of contraceptives (Z30.4-)
> > Z30.011   **contraceptive pills**
> > Z30.012   **emergency contraception**
> > > Encounter for postcoital contraception
> > Z30.013   **injectable contraceptive**
> > Z30.014   **intrauterine contraceptive device**
> > > *Excludes1:* encounter for insertion of intrauterine contraceptive device (Z30.430, Z30.432)
> > Z30.015   **vaginal ring hormonal contraceptive**

  [4th] [5th] [6th] [7th] Additional Character Required   3-character code   Unspecified laterality codes were excluded here.   • =New Code   ▲ =Revised Code   ▫ =Social determinants of health   *Excludes1*—Not coded here, do not use together   *Excludes2*—Not included here

Z30.016 transdermal patch hormonal contraceptive device
Z30.017 implantable subdermal contraceptive
Z30.018 other contraceptives
Encounter for initial prescription of barrier contraception or diaphragm
Z30.019 contraceptives, unspecified
Z30.02 Counseling and instruction in natural family planning to avoid pregnancy
Z30.09 Encounter for other general counseling and advice on contraception
Encounter for family planning advice NOS

Z30.4 Encounter for surveillance of contraceptives
[5th] **Z30.40 Encounter for surveillance of unspecified**
Z30.41 Encounter for surveillance of contraceptive pills
Encounter for repeat prescription for contraceptive pill
Z30.42 Encounter for surveillance of injectable contraceptive
Z30.43 Encounter for surveillance of intrauterine contraceptive device
[6th]
  Z30.430 Encounter for insertion of intrauterine contraceptive device
  Z30.431 Encounter for routine checking of intrauterine contraceptive device
  Z30.432 Encounter for removal of intrauterine contraceptive device
  Z30.433 Encounter for removal and reinsertion of intrauterine contraceptive device
  replacement of intrauterine contraceptive device
Z30.44 Encounter for surveillance of vaginal ring hormonal contraceptive device
Z30.45 Encounter for surveillance of transdermal patch hormonal contraceptive device
Z30.46 Encounter for surveillance of implantable subdermal contraceptive
Encounter for checking, reinsertion or removal of implantable subdermal contraceptive
Z30.49 Encounter for surveillance of other contraceptives
Encounter for surveillance of barrier contraception
Encounter for surveillance of diaphragm

Z30.8 Encounter for other contraceptive management
Encounter for postvasectomy sperm count
Encounter for routine examination for contraceptive maintenance
Excludes1: sperm count following sterilization reversal (Z31.42)
sperm count for fertility testing (Z31.41)
Z30.9 Encounter for contraceptive management, unspecified

Z31 ENCOUNTER FOR PROCREATIVE MANAGEMENT
[4th] ***Excludes2:*** complications associated with artificial fertilization (N98.-)
female infertility (N97.-)
male infertility (N46.-)
Z31.5 Encounter for procreative genetic counseling
Refer to Chapter 21 for guidelines on counseling.
Z31.6 Encounter for general counseling and advice on procreation
[5th] *Refer to Chapter 21 for guidelines on counseling.*
  Z31.69 Encounter for other general counseling and advice on procreation

Z32 ENCOUNTER FOR PREGNANCY TEST AND CHILDBIRTH
[4th] **AND CHILDCARE INSTRUCTION**
Z32.0 Encounter for pregnancy test
[5th]
> **GUIDELINES**
>
> The codes are not to be used if the examination is for diagnosis of a suspected condition or for treatment purposes. In such cases the diagnosis code is used. During a routine exam, should a diagnosis or condition be discovered, it should be coded as an additional code. Pre-existing and chronic conditions and history codes may also be included as additional codes as long as the examination is for administrative purposes and not focused on any particular condition.
> Some of the codes for routine health examinations distinguish between "with" and "without" abnormal findings. Code assignment depends on the information that is known at the time the

encounter is being coded. For example, if no abnormal findings were found during the examination, but the encounter is being coded before test results are back, it is acceptable to assign the code for "without abnormal findings." When assigning a code for "with abnormal findings," additional code(s) should be assigned to identify the specific abnormal finding(s).
  Z32.00 Encounter for pregnancy test, result unknown
  Encounter for pregnancy test NOS
  Z32.01 Encounter for pregnancy test, result positive
  Z32.02 Encounter for pregnancy test, result negative
Z32.3 Encounter for childcare instruction
Encounter for prenatal or postpartum childcare instruction

Z33 PREGNANT STATE
[4th] **Z33.1 Pregnant state, incidental**
This is a status code, refer to Chapter 21 for status guidelines.
Pregnancy NOS
Pregnant state NOS
Excludes1: complications of pregnancy (O00–O9A)

Z38 LIVEBORN INFANTS ACCORDING TO PLACE OF BIRTH
[4th] **AND TYPE OF DELIVERY**

> **GUIDELINES**
>
> When coding the birth episode in a newborn record, assign a code from category Z38, Liveborn infants according to place of birth and type of delivery, as the principal diagnosis. A code from category Z38 is assigned only once, to a newborn at the time of birth and throughout the initial stay at the birth hospital. If a newborn is transferred to another institution, a code from category Z38 should not be used at the receiving hospital.
> A code from category Z38 is used only on the newborn record, not on the mother's record. Codes in category Z38 "may only be reported as the principal/first-listed diagnosis, except when there are multiple encounters on the same day and the medical records for the encounters are combined." Refer to Chapter 16 for further guidelines.

Z38.0 Single liveborn infant, born in hospital
[5th] Single liveborn infant, born in birthing center or other health care facility
  Z38.00 Single liveborn infant, delivered vaginally
  Z38.01 Single liveborn infant, delivered by cesarean
Z38.1 Single liveborn infant, born outside hospital
Z38.2 Single liveborn infant, unspecified as to place of birth
Single liveborn infant NOS
Z38.3 Twin liveborn infant, born in hospital
[5th]   **Z38.30 Twin liveborn infant, delivered vaginally**
  Z38.31 Twin liveborn infant, delivered by cesarean
Z38.4 Twin liveborn infant, born outside hospital
Z38.5 Twin liveborn infant, unspecified as to place of birth
Z38.6 Other multiple liveborn infant, born in hospital
[5th]   **Z38.61 Triplet liveborn infant, delivered vaginally**
  Z38.62 Triplet liveborn infant, delivered by cesarean
  Z38.63 Quadruplet liveborn infant, delivered vaginally
  Z38.64 Quadruplet liveborn infant, delivered by cesarean
  Z38.65 Quintuplet liveborn infant, delivered vaginally
  Z38.66 Quintuplet liveborn infant, delivered by cesarean
  Z38.68 Other multiple liveborn infant, delivered vaginally
  Z38.69 Other multiple liveborn infant, delivered by cesarean
Z38.7 Other multiple liveborn infant, born outside hospital
Z38.8 Other multiple liveborn infant, unspecified as to place of birth

Z39 ENCOUNTER FOR MATERNAL POSTPARTUM CARE
[4th] Use only when billing under the mother
Z39.1 Encounter for care and examination of lactating mother
Encounter for supervision of lactation
Excludes1: disorders of lactation (O92.-)

(Z40–Z53) ENCOUNTERS FOR OTHER SPECIFIC HEALTH CARE

Categories Z40–Z53 are intended for use to indicate a reason for care. They may be used for patients who have already been treated for a disease or injury, but who are receiving aftercare or prophylactic care, or care to consolidate the treatment, or to deal with a residual state.

Z41 ENCOUNTER FOR PROCEDURES FOR PURPOSES OTHER
[4th] **THAN REMEDYING HEALTH STATE**
Z41.2 Encounter for routine and ritual male circumcision
Z41.3 Encounter for ear piercing

[4th] [5th] [6th] [7th] Additional Character Required   ✓ 3-character code   Unspecified laterality codes were excluded here.   • =New Code   ▲ =Revised Code   ▣ =Social determinants of health   ***Excludes1***—Not coded here, do not use together   ***Excludes2***—Not included here

CHAPTER 21. FACTORS INFLUENCING HEALTH STATUS AND CONTACT WITH HEALTH SERVICES   (Z41.8–Z48.3)

Z41.8   **Encounter for other procedures for purposes other than remedying health state**

Z41.9   **Encounter for procedure for purposes other than remedying health state, unspecified**

Z43   ENCOUNTER FOR ATTENTION TO ARTIFICIAL OPENINGS
4th

GUIDELINES

Aftercare visit codes cover situations when the initial treatment of a disease has been performed and the patient requires continued care during the healing or recovery phase, or for the long-term consequences of the disease. The aftercare Z code should not be used if treatment is directed at a current, acute disease. The diagnosis code is to be used in these cases. *Refer to Chapter 21 for aftercare guidelines.*

Includes: closure of artificial openings
passage of sounds or bougies through artificial openings
reforming artificial openings
removal of catheter from artificial openings
toilet or cleansing of artificial openings

Excludes1: complications of external stoma (J95.0-, K94.-, N99.5-)

Excludes2: fitting and adjustment of prosthetic and other devices (Z44–Z46)

Z43.0   **Encounter for attention to tracheostomy**

Z43.1   **Encounter for attention to gastrostomy**

     Excludes 2: artificial opening status only, without need for care (Z93.-)

Z43.2   **Encounter for attention to ileostomy**

Z43.3   **Encounter for attention to colostomy**

Z43.4   **Encounter for attention to other artificial openings of digestive tract**

Z43.5   **Encounter for attention to cystostomy**

Z43.6   **Encounter for attention to other artificial openings of urinary tract**

     Encounter for attention to nephrostomy or ureterostomy or urethrostomy

Z43.7   **Encounter for attention to artificial vagina**

Z43.8   **Encounter for attention to other artificial openings**

Z43.9   **Encounter for attention to unspecified artificial opening**

Z45   ENCOUNTER FOR ADJUSTMENT AND MANAGEMENT OF IMPLANTED DEVICE
4th

Includes: removal or replacement of implanted device

Excludes1: malfunction or other complications of device—see Alphabetical Index

Excludes2: encounter for fitting and adjustment of non-implanted device (Z46.-)

Z45.0   **Encounter for adjustment and management of cardiac device**

   5th   **Z45.01**   **Encounter for adjustment and management of cardiac pacemaker**
     6th

     Encounter for adjustment and management of cardiac resynchronization therapy pacemaker (CRT-P)

     Excludes1: encounter for adjustment and management of automatic implantable cardiac defibrillator with synchronous cardiac pacemaker (Z45.02)

     Z45.010   **Encounter for checking and testing of cardiac pacemaker pulse generator [battery]**

       Encounter for replacing cardiac pacemaker pulse generator [battery]

     Z45.018   **Encounter for adjustment and management of other part of cardiac pacemaker**

       Excludes1: presence of other part of cardiac pacemaker (Z95.0)

       Excludes2: presence of prosthetic and other devices (Z95.1–Z95.5, Z95.811–Z97)

   Z45.02   **Encounter for adjustment and management of automatic implantable cardiac defibrillator**

     Encounter for adjustment and management of automatic implantable cardiac defibrillator with synchronous cardiac pacemaker

     Encounter for adjustment and management of cardiac resynchronization therapy defibrillator (CRT-D)

   Z45.09   **Encounter for adjustment and management of other cardiac device**

Z46   ENCOUNTER FOR FITTING AND ADJUSTMENT OF OTHER DEVICES
4th

Includes: removal or replacement of other device

Excludes1: malfunction or other complications of device—see Alphabetical Index

Excludes2: encounter for fitting and management of implanted devices (Z45.-)
issue of repeat prescription only (Z76.0)
presence of prosthetic and other devices (Z95–Z97)

Z46.2   **Encounter for fitting and adjustment of other devices related to nervous system and special senses**

     Excludes2: encounter for adjustment and management of implanted nervous system device (Z45.4-)
encounter for adjustment and management of implanted visual substitution device (Z45.31)

Z46.6   **Encounter for fitting and adjustment of urinary device**

     Excludes2: attention to artificial openings of urinary tract (Z43.5, Z43.6)

Z46.8   **Encounter for fitting and adjustment of other specified devices**

   5th   **Z46.81**   **Encounter for fitting and adjustment of insulin pump**

     Encounter for insulin pump instruction and training
Encounter for insulin pump titration

   Z46.82   **Encounter for fitting and adjustment of non-vascular catheter**

   Z46.89   **Encounter for fitting and adjustment of other specified devices**

     Encounter for fitting and adjustment of wheelchair

Z46.9   **Encounter for fitting and adjustment of unspecified device**

Z48   ENCOUNTER FOR OTHER POSTPROCEDURAL AFTERCARE
4th

GUIDELINES

Aftercare visit codes cover situations when the initial treatment of a disease has been performed and the patient requires continued care during the healing or recovery phase, or for the long-term consequences of the disease. The aftercare Z code should not be used if treatment is directed at a current, acute disease. The diagnosis code is to be used in these cases. *Refer to Chapter 21 for aftercare guidelines.*

Excludes1: encounter for follow-up examination after completed treatment (Z08–Z09)
encounter for aftercare following injury - code to Injury, by site, with appropriate 7th character for subsequent encounter

Excludes2: encounter for attention to artificial openings (Z43.-)
encounter for fitting and adjustment of prosthetic and other devices (Z44–Z46)

Z48.0   **Encounter for; attention to dressings, sutures and drains**

   5th   *Excludes1:* encounter for planned postprocedural wound closure (Z48.1)

     Do not report a Z48 code for an injury. Use the appropriate injury code.

   Z48.00   **change or removal of nonsurgical wound dressing**

     change or removal of wound dressing NOS

   Z48.01   **change or removal of surgical wound dressing**

   Z48.02   **removal of sutures**

     removal of staples

   Z48.03   **change or removal of drains**

Z48.1   **Encounter for planned postprocedural wound closure**

     Excludes1: encounter for attention to dressings and sutures (Z48.0-)

Z48.2   **Encounter for aftercare following; organ transplant**

   5th   **Z48.21**   **heart transplant**

   Z48.22   **kidney transplant**

   Z48.23   **liver transplant**

   Z48.24   **lung transplant**

   Z48.28   **multiple organ transplant**

     6th   **Z48.280**   **heart-lung transplant**

     Z48.288   **multiple organ transplant**

   Z48.29   **other organ transplant**

     6th   **Z48.290**   **bone marrow transplant**

     Z48.298   **other organ transplant**

Z48.3   **Aftercare following surgery for neoplasm**

     Use additional code to identify the neoplasm

 4th *5th* *6th* *7th*   Additional Character Required   ✔   3-character code   Unspecified laterality codes were excluded here.

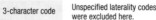 • =New Code   ▲ =Revised Code   ⌑ =Social determinants of health

Excludes1—Not coded here, do not use together
Excludes2—Not included here

Z48.8   Encounter for other specified postprocedural aftercare

Z48.81   Encounter for surgical aftercare following surgery on specified body systems [5th] [6th]

These codes identify the body system requiring aftercare. They are for use in conjunction with other aftercare codes to fully explain the aftercare encounter. The condition treated should also be coded if still present.

Excludes1: aftercare for injury — code the injury with 7th character D
aftercare following surgery for neoplasm (Z48.3)

Excludes2: aftercare following organ transplant (Z48.2-)
orthopedic aftercare (Z47.-)

Z48.810   Encounter for surgical aftercare following surgery on the sense organs

Z48.811   surgery on the nervous system

Excludes2: encounter for surgical aftercare following surgery on the sense organs (Z48.810)

Z48.812   surgery on the circulatory system

Z48.813   surgery on the respiratory system

Z48.814   surgery on the teeth or oral cavity

Z48.815   surgery on the digestive system

Z48.816   surgery on the genitourinary system

Excludes1: encounter for aftercare following sterilization reversal (Z31.42)

Z48.817   surgery on the skin and subcutaneous tissue

Z48.89   Encounter for other specified surgical aftercare

Z51   ENCOUNTER FOR OTHER AFTERCARE AND MEDICAL CARE [4th]

GUIDELINES

Aftercare visit codes cover situations when the initial treatment of a disease has been performed and the patient requires continued care during the healing or recovery phase, or for the long-term consequences of the disease. The aftercare Z code should not be used if treatment is directed at a current, acute disease. The diagnosis code is to be used in these cases. Refer to Chapter 21 for aftercare guidelines.

Code also condition requiring care

Excludes1: follow-up examination after treatment (Z08–Z09)

Excludes2: follow-up examination for medical surveillance after treatment (Z08–Z09)

Z51.0   Encounter for antineoplastic; radiation therapy

May only be reported as the principal/first-listed diagnosis, except when there are multiple encounters on the same day and the medical records for the encounters are combined.

Z51.1   chemotherapy and immunotherapy [5th]

Codes Z51.1- may only be reported as the principal/first-listed diagnosis, except when there are multiple encounters on the same day and the medical records for the encounters are combined.

Excludes2: encounter for chemotherapy and immunotherapy for non-neoplastic condition — code to condition

Z51.11   chemotherapy

Z51.12   immunotherapy

Z51.5   Encounter for palliative care

Z51.6   Encounter for desensitization to allergens

Z51.8   Encounter for other specified aftercare [5th]

Excludes1: holiday relief care (Z75.5)

Z51.81   Encounter for therapeutic drug level monitoring

Code also any long-term (current) drug therapy (Z79.-)

Excludes1: encounter for blood-drug test for administrative or medicolegal reasons (Z02.83)

Z51.89   Encounter for other specified aftercare

Z53   PERSONS ENCOUNTERING HEALTH SERVICES FOR SPECIFIC PROCEDURES AND TREATMENT, NOT CARRIED OUT [4th]

Z53.0   Procedure and treatment not carried out because of contraindication [5th]

Z53.01   Procedure and treatment not carried out due to patient smoking

Z53.09   Procedure and treatment not carried out because of other contraindication

Z53.1   Procedure and treatment not carried out because of patient's decision for reasons of belief and group pressure

Z53.2   Procedure and treatment not carried out because of patient's decision for other and unspecified reasons [5th]

Z53.20   Procedure and treatment not carried out because of patient's decision for unspecified reasons

Z53.21   Procedure and treatment not carried out due to patient leaving prior to being seen by healthcare provider

Z53.29   Procedure and treatment not carried out because of patient's decision for other reasons

Z53.3   Procedure converted to open procedure [5th]

Z53.31   Laparoscopic surgical procedure converted to open procedure

Z53.32   Thoracoscopic surgical procedure converted to open procedure

Z53.33   Arthroscopic surgical procedure converted to open procedure

Z53.39   Other specified procedure converted to open procedure

Z53.8   Procedure and treatment not carried out for other reasons

Z53.9   Procedure and treatment not carried out, unspecified reason

(Z55–Z65) PERSONS WITH POTENTIAL HEALTH HAZARDS RELATED TO SOCIOECONOMIC AND PSYCHOSOCIAL CIRCUMSTANCES

GUIDELINES (HEADER)

Codes describing social determinants of health (SDOH) should be assigned when this information is documented. For social determinants of health, such as information found in categories Z55-Z65, Persons with potential health hazards related to socioeconomic and psychosocial circumstances, code assignment may be based on medical record documentation from clinicians involved in the care of the patient who are not the patient's provider since this information represents social information, rather than medical diagnoses. For example, coding professionals may utilize documentation of social information from social workers, community health workers, case managers, or nurses, if their documentation is included in the official medical record.

Patient self-reported documentation may be used to assign codes for social determinants of health, as long as the patient self-reported information is signed-off by and incorporated into the medical record by either a clinician or provider.

Z55   PROBLEMS RELATED TO EDUCATION AND LITERACY [4th]

Excludes1: disorders of psychological development (F80–F89)

▫**Z55.0   Illiteracy and low-level literacy**

▫**Z55.1   Schooling unavailable and unattainable**

▫**Z55.2   Failed school examinations**

▫**Z55.3   Underachievement in school**

▫**Z55.4   Educational maladjustment and discord with teachers and classmates**

▫●**Z55.5   Less than a high school diploma**

No general equivalence degree (GED)

▫**Z55.8   Other problems related to education and literacy**

Problems related to inadequate teaching

▫**Z55.9   Problems related to education and literacy, unspecified**

Academic problems NOS

Z58   PROBLEMS RELATED TO PHYSICAL ENVIRONMENT

Excludes2: occupational exposure (Z57.-)

▫●**Z58.6   Inadequate drinking-water supply**

Lack of safe drinking water

Excludes2: deprivation of water (T73.1)

Z59   PROBLEMS RELATED TO HOUSING AND ECONOMIC CIRCUMSTANCES [4th]

Excludes2: problems related to upbringing (Z62.-)

▲**Z59.0   Homelessness**

▫●**Z59.00   Homelessness unspecified** [5th]

[4th] [5th] [6th] [7th]   Additional Character Required   ✔   3-character code   Unspecified laterality codes were excluded here.

● =New Code
▲ =Revised Code
▫ =Social determinants of health

Excludes1—Not coded here, do not use together
Excludes2—Not included here

CHAPTER 21. FACTORS INFLUENCING HEALTH STATUS AND CONTACT WITH HEALTH SERVICES (Z59.01–Z63.72)

◻•**Z59.01 Sheltered homelessness**
Doubled up
Living in a shelter such as: motel, scattered site housing, temporary or transitional living situation

◻•**Z59.02 Unsheltered homelessness**
Residing in place not meant for human habitation such as: abandoned buildings, cars, parks, sidewalk
Residing on the street

◻**Z59.1 Inadequate housing**
Lack of heating
Restriction of space
Technical defects in home preventing adequate care
Unsatisfactory surroundings
Excludes1: problems related to the natural and physical environment (Z77.1-)

▲**Z59.4 Lack of adequate food**
Excludes2: deprivation of food/effects of hunger (T73.0)
inappropriate diet or eating habits (Z72.4)
malnutrition (E40-E46)

◻•**Z59.41 Food insecurity**

◻•**Z59.48 Other specified lack of adequate food**
Inadequate food
Lack of food

◻**Z59.5 Extreme poverty**

◻**Z59.6 Low income**

◻**Z59.7 Insufficient social insurance and welfare support**

▲**Z59.8 Other problems related to housing and economic circumstances**
[5th]

Z59.81 Housing instability, housed
[6th]
Foreclosure on home loan
Past due on rent or mortgage
Unwanted multiple moves in the last 12 months

◻•**Z59.811 Housing instability, housed, with risk of homelessness**
Imminent risk of homelessness

◻•**Z59.812 Housing instability, housed, homelessness in past 12 months**

◻•**Z59.819 Housing instability, housed unspecified**

◻•**Z59.89 Other problems related to housing and economic circumstances**
Foreclosure on loan
Isolated dwelling
Problems with creditors

◻**Z59.9 Problem related to housing and economic circumstances, unspecified**

Z60 PROBLEMS RELATED TO SOCIAL ENVIRONMENT
[4th]

Z60.2 Problems related to living alone

◻**Z60.3 Acculturation difficulty**
Problem with migration
Problem with social transplantation

◻**Z60.4 Social exclusion and rejection**
Exclusion and rejection on the basis of personal characteristics, such as unusual physical appearance, illness or behavior
Excludes1: target of adverse discrimination such as for racial or religious reasons (Z60.5)

◻**Z60.5 Target of (perceived) adverse discrimination and persecution**
Excludes1: social exclusion and rejection (Z60.4)

◻**Z60.8 Other problems related to social environment**

◻**Z60.9 Problem related to social environment, unspecified**

Z62 PROBLEMS RELATED TO UPBRINGING
[4th]
Includes: current and past negative life events in childhood
current and past problems of a child related to upbringing
Excludes2: maltreatment syndrome (T74.-)
problems related to housing and economic circumstances (Z59.-)

◻**Z62.0 Inadequate parental supervision and control**

◻**Z62.1 Parental overprotection**

Z62.2 Upbringing away from parents
[5th]
Excludes1: problems with boarding school (Z59.3)

◻**Z62.21 Child in welfare custody**
Child in care of non-parental family member
Child in foster care
Excludes2: problem for parent due to child in welfare custody (Z63.5)

◻**Z62.22 Institutional upbringing**
Child living in orphanage or group home

◻**Z62.29 Other upbringing away from parents**

Z62.8 Other specified problems related to upbringing
[5th] **Z62.81 Personal history of abuse in childhood**
[6th] ◻**Z62.810 Personal history of; physical and sexual abuse in childhood**
Excludes1: current child physical abuse (T74.12, T76.12)
current child sexual abuse (T74.22, T76.22)

◻**Z62.811 psychological abuse in childhood**
Excludes1: current child psychological abuse (T74.32, T76.32)

◻**Z62.812 neglect in childhood**
Excludes1: current child neglect (T74.02, T76.02)

◻**Z62.813 forced labor or sexual exploitation in childhood**
Excludes1: current exploitation or forced labor (T74.52-, T74.62-, T76.52-, T76.62-)

◻**Z62.819 unspecified abuse in childhood**
Excludes1: current child abuse NOS (T74.92, T76.92)

Z62.82 Parent-child conflict
[6th] ◻**Z62.820 Parent-biological child conflict**
Parent-child problem NOS

◻**Z62.821 Parent-adopted child conflict**

◻**Z62.822 Parent-foster child conflict**

Z62.89 Other specified problems related to upbringing
[6th] ◻**Z62.890 Parent-child estrangement NEC**

◻**Z62.891 Sibling rivalry**

◻**Z62.898 Other specified problems related to upbringing**

◻**Z62.9 Problem related to upbringing, unspecified**

Z63 OTHER PROBLEMS RELATED TO PRIMARY SUPPORT GROUP, INCLUDING FAMILY CIRCUMSTANCES
[4th]
Excludes2: maltreatment syndrome (T74.-, T76)
parent-child problems (Z62.-)
problems related to negative life events in childhood (Z62.-)
problems related to upbringing (Z62.-)

Z63.0 Problems in relationship with spouse or partner
Relationship distress with spouse or intimate partner
Excludes1: counseling for spousal or partner abuse problems (Z69.1)
counseling related to sexual attitude, behavior, and orientation (Z70.-)

Z63.3 Absence of family member
[5th] *Excludes1:* absence of family member due to disappearance and death (Z63.4)
absence of family member due to separation and divorce (Z63.5)

◻**Z63.31 Absence of family member due to military deployment**
Individual or family affected by other family member being on military deployment
Excludes1: family disruption due to return of family member from military deployment (Z63.71)

◻**Z63.32 Other absence of family member**

◻**Z63.4 Disappearance and death of family member**
Assumed death of family member
Bereavement

◻**Z63.5 Disruption of family by separation and divorce**

Z63.6 Dependent relative needing care at home

Z63.7 Other stressful life events affecting family and household
[5th] ◻**Z63.71 Stress on family due to return of family member from military deployment**
Individual or family affected by family member having returned from military deployment (current or past conflict)

◻**Z63.72 Alcoholism and drug addiction in family**

[4th] [5th] [6th] [7th] Additional Character Required ✓ 3-character code   Unspecified laterality codes were excluded here.   • =New Code   *Excludes1*—Not coded here, do not use together
▲ =Revised Code   *Excludes2*—Not included here
◻ =Social determinants of health

450   **PEDIATRIC ICD-10-CM 2022: A MANUAL FOR PROVIDER-BASED CODING**

◻**Z63.79** **Other stressful life events affecting family and household**
Anxiety (normal) about sick person in family
Health problems within family
Ill or disturbed family member
Isolated family

◻**Z63.8** **Other specified problems related to primary support group**
Family discord NOS
Family estrangement NOS
High expressed emotional level within family
Inadequate family support NOS
Inadequate or distorted communication within family

◻**Z63.9** **Problem related to primary support group, unspecified**
Relationship disorder NOS

Z64 [4th] **PROBLEMS RELATED TO CERTAIN PSYCHOSOCIAL CIRCUMSTANCES**

Z64.0 **Problems related to unwanted pregnancy**

Z64.4 **Discord with counselors**
Discord with probation officer
Discord with social worker

Z65 [4th] **PROBLEMS RELATED TO OTHER PSYCHOSOCIAL CIRCUMSTANCES**

Z65.3 **Problems related to other legal circumstances**
Arrest
Child custody or support proceedings
Litigation
Prosecution

Z65.4 **Victim of crime and terrorism**
Victim of torture

◻**Z65.8** **Other specified problems related to psychosocial circumstances**
Religious or spiritual problem

◻**Z65.9** **Problem related to unspecified psychosocial circumstances**

(Z66) DO NOT RESUSCITATE STATUS

Z66 **DO NOT RESUSCITATE**
[✓] This code may be used when it is documented by the provider that a patient is on do not resuscitate status at any time during the stay. This is a status code, *refer to Chapter 21 for status guidelines.*
DNR status

(Z67) BLOOD TYPE

Z67 [4th] **BLOOD TYPE**

Z67.1 **Type A blood**
[5th] **Z67.10** **Type A blood, Rh positive**
Z67.11 **Type A blood, Rh negative**

Z67.2 **Type B blood**
[5th] **Z67.20** **Type B blood, Rh positive**
Z67.21 **Type B blood, Rh negative**

Z67.3 **Type AB blood**
[5th] **Z67.30** **Type AB blood, Rh positive**
Z67.31 **Type AB blood, Rh negative**

Z67.4 **Type O blood**
[5th] **Z67.40** **Type O blood, Rh positive**
Z67.41 **Type O blood, Rh negative**

(Z68) BODY MASS INDEX [BMI]

Z68 [4th] **BODY MASS INDEX [BMI]**

GUIDELINES

This is a status category, refer to Chapter 21 for status guidelines. **BMI codes should only be assigned when the associated diagnosis (such as overweight or obesity) meets** the definition of a reportable diagnosis (see Section III, Reporting Additional Diagnoses). **Do not assign BMI codes during pregnancy.** *See Section I.B.14 for BMI documentation by clinicians other than the patient's provider.*
Kilograms per meters squared
Note: BMI adult codes are for use for persons 20 years of age or older.
BMI pediatric codes are for use for persons 2–19 years of age. These percentiles are based on the growth charts published by the Centers for Disease Control and Prevention (CDC)

Z68.1 **BMI 19.9 or less, adult**
Z68.2 **BMI 20-29, adult**
[5th] **Z68.20** **BMI 20.0-20.9, adult**
Z68.21 **BMI 21.0-21.9, adult**
Z68.22 **BMI 22.0-22.9, adult**
Z68.23 **BMI 23.0-23.9, adult**
Z68.24 **BMI 24.0-24.9, adult**
Z68.25 **BMI 25.0-25.9, adult**
Z68.26 **BMI 26.0-26.9, adult**
Z68.27 **BMI 27.0-27.9, adult**
Z68.28 **BMI 28.0-28.9, adult**
Z68.29 **BMI 29.0-29.9, adult**

Z68.3 **BMI 30-39, adult**
[5th] **Z68.30** **BMI 30.0-30.9, adult**
Z68.31 **BMI 31.0-31.9, adult**
Z68.32 **BMI 32.0-32.9, adult**
Z68.33 **BMI 33.0-33.9, adult**
Z68.34 **BMI 34.0-34.9, adult**
Z68.35 **BMI 35.0-35.9, adult**
Z68.36 **BMI 36.0-36.9, adult**
Z68.37 **BMI 37.0-37.9, adult**
Z68.38 **BMI 38.0-38.9, adult**
Z68.39 **BMI 39.0-39.9, adult**

Z68.4 **BMI 40 or greater, adult**
[5th] **Z68.41** **BMI 40.0-44.9, adult**
Z68.42 **BMI 45.0-49.9, adult**
Z68.43 **BMI 50.0-59.9, adult**
Z68.44 **BMI 60.0-69.9, adult**
Z68.45 **BMI 70 or greater, adult**

Z68.5 **BMI pediatric**
[5th] **Z68.51** **BMI pediatric, less than 5th percentile for age**
Z68.52 **BMI pediatric, 5th percentile to less than 85th percentile for age**
Z68.53 **BMI pediatric, 85th percentile to less than 95th percentile for age**
Z68.54 **BMI pediatric, greater than or equal to 95th percentile for age**

(Z69–Z76) PERSONS ENCOUNTERING HEALTH SERVICES IN OTHER CIRCUMSTANCES

Z69 [4th] **ENCOUNTER FOR MENTAL HEALTH SERVICES FOR VICTIM AND PERPETRATOR OF ABUSE**

GUIDELINES

Counseling Z codes are used when a patient or family member receives assistance in the aftermath of an illness or injury, or when support is required in coping with family or social problems.
Includes: counseling for victims and perpetrators of abuse

Z69.0 **Encounter for mental health services for child abuse problems**
[5th] **Z69.01** [6th] **Encounter for mental health services for; parental child abuse**
◻**Z69.010** **victim of parental child abuse**
Encounter for mental health services for victim of child abuse or neglect by parent
Encounter for mental health services for victim of child psychological or sexual abuse by parent
◻**Z69.011** **perpetrator of parental child abuse**
Encounter for mental health services for perpetrator of parental child neglect
Encounter for mental health services for perpetrator of parental child psychological or sexual abuse
Excludes1: encounter for mental health services for non-parental child abuse (Z69.02-)

Z69.02 [6th] **Encounter for mental health services for; non-parental child abuse**

[4th] [5th] [6th] [7th] Additional Character Required | [✓] 3-character code | Unspecified laterality codes were excluded here. | ● =New Code ▲ =Revised Code ◻ =Social determinants of health | *Excludes1*—Not coded here, do not use together *Excludes2*—Not included here

□**Z69.020 victim of non-parental child abuse**
Encounter for mental health services for victim of non-parental child neglect
Encounter for mental health services for victim of non-parental child psychological or sexual abuse

□**Z69.021 perpetrator of non-parental child abuse**
Encounter for mental health services for perpetrator of non-parental child neglect
Encounter for mental health services for perpetrator of non-parental child psychological or sexual abuse

Z69.1 [5th] **Encounter for mental health services for; spousal or partner abuse problems**

Z69.11 victim of spousal or partner abuse
Encounter for mental health services for victim of spouse or partner neglect
Encounter for mental health services for victim of spouse or partner psychological abuse
Encounter for mental health services for victim of spouse or partner violence, physical

Z69.12 perpetrator of spousal or partner abuse
Encounter for mental health services for perpetrator of spouse or partner neglect
Encounter for mental health services for perpetrator of spouse or partner psychological abuse Encounter for mental health services for perpetrator of spouse or partner violence, physical Encounter for mental health services for perpetrator of spouse or partner violence, sexual

Z69.8 [5th] **Encounter for mental health services for victim or perpetrator of other abuse**

□**Z69.81 Encounter for mental health services for victim of other abuse**
Encounter for mental health services for victim of non-spousal adult abuse
Encounter for mental health services for victim of spouse or partner violence, sexual
Encounter for rape victim counseling

Z69.82 Encounter for mental health services for perpetrator of other abuse
Encounter for mental health services for perpetrator of non-spousal adult abuse

Z70 [4th] **COUNSELING RELATED TO SEXUAL ATTITUDE, BEHAVIOR AND ORIENTATION**
Includes: encounter for mental health services for sexual attitude, behavior and orientation
Excludes2: contraceptive or procreative counseling (Z30-Z31)

Z70.0 Counseling related to sexual attitude

Z70.1 Counseling related to patient's sexual behavior and orientation
Patient concerned regarding impotence
Patient concerned regarding non-responsiveness
Patient concerned regarding promiscuity
Patient concerned regarding sexual orientation

Z70.2 Counseling related to sexual behavior and orientation of third party
Advice sought regarding sexual behavior and orientation of child
Advice sought regarding sexual behavior and orientation of partner
Advice sought regarding sexual behavior and orientation of spouse

Z70.3 Counseling related to combined concerns regarding sexual attitude, behavior and orientation

Z70.8 Other sex counseling
Encounter for sex education

Z70.9 Sex counseling, unspecified

Z71 [4th] **PERSONS ENCOUNTERING HEALTH SERVICES FOR OTHER COUNSELING AND MEDICAL ADVICE, NEC**
Refer to category Z69 for guideline.
Excludes2: contraceptive or procreation counseling (Z30–Z31)
sex counseling (Z70.-)

Z71.0 Person encountering health services to consult on behalf of another person
Person encountering health services to seek advice or treatment for non-attending third party
Excludes2: anxiety (normal) about sick person in family (Z63.7)
expectant (adoptive) parent(s) pre-birth pediatrician visit (Z76.81)

Z71.2 Person consulting for explanation of examination or test findings

Z71.3 Dietary counseling and surveillance
Use additional code for any associated underlying medical condition
Use additional code to identify body mass index (BMI), if known (Z68.-)

Z71.4 [5th] **Alcohol abuse counseling and surveillance**
Use additional code for alcohol abuse or dependence (F10.-)

Z71.41 Alcohol abuse counseling and surveillance of alcoholic

□**Z71.42 Counseling for family member of alcoholic**
Counseling for significant other, partner, or friend of alcoholic

Z71.5 [5th] **Drug abuse counseling and surveillance**
Use additional code for drug abuse or dependence (F11–F16, F18–F19)

Z71.51 Drug abuse counseling and surveillance of drug abuser

□**Z71.52 Counseling for family member of drug abuser**
Counseling for significant other, partner, or friend of drug abuser

Z71.6 Tobacco abuse counseling
Use additional code for nicotine dependence (F17.-)

Z71.7 HIV counseling

Z71.8 Other specified counseling
[5th] *Excludes2:* counseling for contraception (Z30.0-)

Z71.81 Spiritual or religious counseling

Z71.82 Exercise counseling

Z71.83 Encounter for nonprocreative genetic counseling
Excludes1: counseling for genetics (Z31.5)
counseling for procreative management (Z31.6)

Z71.84 Encounter for health counseling related to travel
Encounter for health risk and safety counseling for (international) travel
Code also, if applicable, encounter for immunization (Z23)
Excludes2: encounter for administrative examination (Z02.-)
encounter for other special examination without complaint, suspected or reported diagnosis (Z01.-)

GUIDELINE
Code Z71.85, Encounter for immunization safety counseling, is to be used for counseling of the patient or caregiver regarding the safety of a vaccine. This code should not be used for the provision of general information regarding risks and potential side effects during routine encounters for the administration of vaccines.

•**Z71.85 Encounter for immunization safety counseling**
Encounter for vaccine product safety counseling
Code also, if applicable, encounter for vaccine Z23
Code also, if applicable, immunization not carried out (Z28.-)
Excludes1: encounter for health counseling related to travel (Z71.84)

Z71.89 Other specified counseling
Encounter for mental health services for victim of child abuse or neglect by parent
Encounter for mental health services for victim of child psychological or sexual abuse by parent

Z71.9 Counseling, unspecified
Encounter for medical advice NOS

Z72 [4th] **PROBLEMS RELATED TO LIFESTYLE**
Excludes2: problems related to life-management difficulty (Z73.-)
problems related to socioeconomic and psychosocial circumstances (Z55–Z65)

 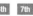 [4th] [5th] [6th] [7th] Additional Character Required 3-character code

Unspecified laterality codes were excluded here.

• =New Code
▲ =Revised Code
□ =Social determinants of health

Excludes1—Not coded here, do not use together
Excludes2—Not included here

Z72.0   **Tobacco use**
Tobacco use NOS
Excludes1: history of tobacco dependence (Z87.891)
    nicotine dependence (F17.2-)
    tobacco dependence (F17.2-)
    tobacco use during pregnancy (O99.33-)

Z72.3   **Lack of physical exercise**

Z72.4   **Inappropriate diet and eating habits**
Excludes1: behavioral eating disorders of infancy or childhood
    (F98.2.–F98.3)
    eating disorders (F50.-)
    lack of adequate food (Z59.48)
    malnutrition and other nutritional deficiencies (E40–E64)

Z72.5   **High risk sexual behavior**
`5th` Promiscuity
Excludes1: paraphilias (F65)
Z72.51   **High risk heterosexual behavior**
Z72.52   **High risk homosexual behavior**
Z72.53   **High risk bisexual behavior**

Z72.6   **Gambling and betting**
Excludes1: compulsive or pathological gambling (F63.0)

Z72.8   **Other problems related to lifestyle**
`5th` **Z72.81**   **Antisocial behavior**
    `6th` *Excludes1:* conduct disorders (F91.-)
      Z72.810   **Child and adolescent antisocial behavior**
       Antisocial behavior (child) (adolescent)
        without manifest psychiatric disorder
       Delinquency NOS
       Group delinquency
       Offenses in the context of gang membership
       Stealing in company with others
       Truancy from school
Z72.82   **Problems related to sleep**
`6th`   **Z72.820**   **Sleep deprivation**
       Lack of adequate sleep
       Excludes1: insomnia (G47.0-)
      Z72.821   **Inadequate sleep hygiene**
       Bad sleep habits
       Irregular sleep habits
       Unhealthy sleep wake schedule
       Excludes1: insomnia (F51.0-, G47.0-)
Z72.89   **Other problems related to lifestyle**
    Self-damaging behavior

Z72.9   **Problem related to lifestyle, unspecified**

Z73   **PROBLEMS RELATED TO LIFE MANAGEMENT**
`4th` **DIFFICULTY**
Excludes2: problems related to socioeconomic and psychosocial
    circumstances (Z55–Z65)
Z73.4   **Inadequate social skills, NEC**
Z73.6   **Limitation of activities due to disability**
Excludes1: care-provider dependency (Z74.-)
Z73.8   **Other problems related to life management difficulty**
`5th` **Z73.81**   **Behavioral insomnia of childhood**
    `6th`   **Z73.810**   **Behavioral insomnia of childhood, sleep-onset association type**
      Z73.811   **Behavioral insomnia of childhood, limit setting type**
      Z73.812   **Behavioral insomnia of childhood, combined type**
      Z73.819   **Behavioral insomnia of childhood, unspecified type**
Z73.82   **Dual sensory impairment**
Z73.89   **Other problems related to life management difficulty**
Z73.9   **Problem related to life management difficulty, unspecified**

Z74   **PROBLEMS RELATED TO CARE PROVIDER DEPENDENCY**
`4th` *Excludes2:* dependence on enabling machines or devices NEC (Z99.-)
Z74.0   **Reduced mobility**
`5th` **Z74.09**   **Other reduced mobility**
    Chair ridden
    Reduced mobility NOS
    Excludes2: wheelchair dependence (Z99.3)
Z74.1   **Need for assistance with personal care**

Z74.2   **Need for assistance at home and no other household member able to render care**
Z74.3   **Need for continuous supervision**
Z74.8   **Other problems related to care provider dependency**
Z74.9   **Problem related to care provider dependency, unspecified**

Z75   **PROBLEMS RELATED TO MEDICAL FACILITIES AND**
`4th` **OTHER HEALTH CARE**
Z75.0   **Medical services not available in home**
Excludes1: no other household member able to render care (Z74.2)
Z75.3   **Unavailability and inaccessibility of health-care facilities**
Excludes1: bed unavailable (Z75.1)

Z76   **PERSONS ENCOUNTERING HEALTH SERVICES IN OTHER**
`4th` **CIRCUMSTANCES**
Z76.0   **Encounter for issue of repeat prescription**
Encounter for issue of repeat prescription for appliance or
    medicaments or spectacles
Excludes2: issue of medical certificate (Z02.7)
    repeat prescription for contraceptive (Z30.4-)
    Codes Z76.1 and Z76.2 may only be reported as the principal/
first-listed diagnosis, except when there are multiple encounters
on the same day and the medical records for the encounters are
combined.
Z76.1   **Encounter for health supervision and care of foundling**
Refer to Chapter 16 for guidelines.
Z76.2   **Encounter for health supervision and care of other healthy infant and child**
Encounter for medical or nursing care or supervision of healthy
infant under circumstances such as adverse socioeconomic
conditions at home or such as awaiting foster or adoptive
placement or such as maternal illness or such as number of
children at home preventing or interfering with normal care
Z76.4   **Other boarder to healthcare facility**
Excludes1: homelessness (Z59.0-)
Z76.5   **Malingerer [conscious simulation]**
Person feigning illness (with obvious motivation)
Excludes1: factitious disorder (F68.1-, F68.A)
    peregrinating patient (F68.1-)
Z76.8   **Persons encountering health services in other specified**
`5th` **circumstances**
Z76.81   **Expectant parent(s) prebirth pediatrician visit**
    Refer to Chapter 21 for guidelines on counseling.
    Pre-adoption pediatrician visit for adoptive parent(s)
Z76.82   **Awaiting organ transplant status**
    This is a status code, refer to Chapter 21 for status guidelines.
    Patient waiting for organ availability
Z76.89   **Persons encountering health services in other specified circumstances**
    Persons encountering health services NOS

(Z77–Z99) PERSONS WITH POTENTIAL HEALTH HAZARDS RELATED TO FAMILY AND PERSONAL HISTORY AND CERTAIN CONDITIONS INFLUENCING HEALTH STATUS

GUIDELINES

Contact/exposure codes may be used as a first-listed code to explain an encounter for testing, or, more commonly, as a secondary code to identify a potential risk. **Code also** any follow-up examination (Z08–Z09)

Z77   **OTHER CONTACT WITH AND (SUSPECTED) EXPOSURES**
`4th` **HAZARDOUS TO HEALTH**
Includes: contact with and (suspected) exposures to potential hazards to
    health
Excludes2: contact with and (suspected) exposure to communicable
    diseases (Z20.-)
    exposure to (parental) (environmental) tobacco smoke in the perinatal
     period (P96.81)
    newborn affected by noxious substances transmitted via placenta or
     breast milk (P04.-)
    occupational exposure to risk factors (Z57.-)
    retained FB (Z18.-)
    retained FB fully removed (Z87.821)
    toxic effects of substances chiefly nonmedicinal as to source (T51–T65)

`4th` `5th` `6th` `7th` Additional Character Required   ✔   3-character code

Unspecified laterality codes were excluded here.

• =New Code
▲ =Revised Code
◰ =Social determinants of health

Excludes1—Not coded here, do not use together
Excludes2—Not included here

Z77.0 **5th** **Contact with and (suspected) exposure to hazardous, chiefly nonmedicinal, chemicals**

    Z77.01 **6th** **Contact with and (suspected) exposure to; hazardous metals**

        Z77.010 **arsenic**

        Z77.011 **lead**

        Z77.012 **uranium**

          Excludes1: retained depleted uranium fragments (Z18.01)

        Z77.018 **other hazardous metals**

          Contact with and (suspected) exposure to chromium compounds or nickel dust

    Z77.02 **6th** **Contact with and (suspected) exposure to; hazardous aromatic compounds**

        Z77.020 **amines**

        Z77.021 **benzene**

        Z77.028 **other hazardous aromatic compounds**

          Aromatic dyes NOS

          Polycyclic aromatic hydrocarbons

    Z77.09 **6th** **Contact with and (suspected) exposure to; other hazardous, chiefly nonmedicinal, chemicals**

        Z77.090 **asbestos**

        Z77.098 **other hazardous, chiefly nonmedicinal, chemicals**

          Dyes NOS

Z77.1 **5th** **Contact with and (suspected) exposure to; environmental pollution and hazards in the physical environment**

    Z77.12 **6th** **hazards in the physical environment**

        Z77.120 **mold (toxic)**

        Z77.128 **other hazards in the physical environment**

Z77.2 **5th** **other hazardous substances**

    Z77.21 **potentially hazardous body fluids**

    Z77.22 **environmental tobacco smoke (acute) (chronic)**

        Exposure to second hand tobacco smoke (acute) (chronic)

        Passive smoking (acute) (chronic)

        Excludes1: nicotine dependence (F17.-)

          tobacco use (Z72.0)

        Excludes2: occupational exposure to environmental tobacco smoke (Z57.31)

    Z77.29 **other hazardous substances**

Z77.9 **Other contact with and (suspected) exposures hazardous to health**

Z78 **4th** **OTHER SPECIFIED HEALTH STATUS**

This is a status category, refer to Chapter 21 for status guidelines.

Excludes2: asymptomatic HIV infection status (Z21)

    postprocedural status (Z93–Z99)

    sex reassignment status (Z87.890)

Z78.1 **Physical restraint status**

    May be used when it is documented by the provider that a patient has been put in restraints during the current encounter. Please note that this code should not be reported when it is documented by the provider that a patient is temporarily restrained during a procedure.

Z78.9 **Other specified health status**

Z79 **4th** **LONG TERM (CURRENT) DRUG THERAPY**

    GUIDELINES

Codes from this category indicate a patient's continuous use of a prescribed drug (including such things as aspirin therapy) for the long-term treatment of a condition or for prophylactic use. It is not for use for patients who have addictions to drugs. This subcategory is not for use of medications for detoxification or maintenance programs to prevent withdrawal symptoms in patients with drug dependence (eg, methadone maintenance for opiate dependence). Assign the appropriate code for the drug dependence instead.

    Assign a code from Z79 if the patient is receiving a medication for an extended period as a prophylactic measure (such as for the prevention of deep vein thrombosis) or as treatment of a chronic condition (such as arthritis) or a disease requiring a lengthy course of treatment (such as cancer). Do not assign a code from category Z79 for medication being administered for a brief period of time to treat an acute illness or injury

(such as a course of antibiotics to treat acute bronchitis). This is a status category, refer to Chapter 21 for status guidelines.

Includes: long term (current) drug use for prophylactic purposes

Code also any therapeutic drug level monitoring (Z51.81)

Excludes2: drug abuse and dependence (F11–F19)

    drug use complicating pregnancy, childbirth, and the puerperium (O99.32-)

Z79.1 **Long term (current) use of; non-steroidal anti-inflammatories (NSAID)**

    Excludes2: long term (current) use of aspirin (Z79.82)

Z79.2 **antibiotics**

Z79.4 **insulin**

    Excludes2: long term (current) use of oral antidiabetic drugs (Z79.84)

        long term (current) use of oral hypoglycemic drugs (Z79.84)

Z79.5 **steroids**

    Z79.51 **inhaled steroids**

    Z79.52 **systemic steroids**

Z79.8 **Other long term (current) drug therapy**

    Z79.82 **Long term (current) use of aspirin**

    Z79.84 **Long term (current) use of oral hypoglycemic drugs**

        Long term use of oral antidiabetic drugs

        Excludes2: long term (current) use of insulin (Z79.4)

    Z79.89 **Other long term (current) drug therapy**

    Z79.899 **6th** **Other long term (current) drug therapy**

Z80 **4th** **FAMILY HISTORY OF PRIMARY MALIGNANT NEOPLASM**

    GUIDELINES

Family history codes are for use when a patient has a family member(s) who has had a particular disease that causes the patient to be at higher risk of also contracting the disease. Family history codes may be used in conjunction with screening codes to explain the need for a test or procedure. History codes are also acceptable on any medical record regardless of the reason for visit. A history of an illness, even if no longer present, is important information that may alter the type of treatment ordered. **The reason for the encounter (for example, screening or counseling) should be sequenced first and the appropriate personal and/or family history code(s) should be assigned as additional diagnos(es).**

Z80.0 **Family history of malignant neoplasm of digestive organs**

    Conditions classifiable to C15-C26

Z80.1 **Family history of malignant neoplasm of trachea, bronchus and lung**

    Conditions classifiable to C33-C34

Z80.2 **Family history of malignant neoplasm of other respiratory and intrathoracic organs**

    Conditions classifiable to C30-C32, C37-C39

Z80.3 **Family history of malignant neoplasm of breast**

    Conditions classifiable to C50.-

Z80.4 **5th** **Family history of malignant neoplasm of genital organs**

    Conditions classifiable to C51-C63

    Z80.41 **Family history of malignant neoplasm of ovary**

    Z80.42 **Family history of malignant neoplasm of prostate**

    Z80.43 **Family history of malignant neoplasm of testis**

    Z80.49 **Family history of malignant neoplasm of other genital organs**

Z80.5 **5th** **Family history of malignant neoplasm of urinary tract**

    Conditions classifiable to C64–C68

    Z80.51 **Family history of malignant neoplasm of kidney**

    Z80.52 **Family history of malignant neoplasm of bladder**

    Z80.59 **Family history of malignant neoplasm of other urinary tract organ**

Z80.6 **Family history of leukemia**

    Conditions classifiable to C91–C95

Z80.7 **Family history of other malignant neoplasms of lymphoid, hematopoietic and related tissues**

    Conditions classifiable to C81–C90, C96.-

Z80.8 **Family history of malignant neoplasm of other organs or systems**

    Conditions classifiable to C00–C14, C40–C49, C69–C79

Z80.9 **Family history of malignant neoplasm, unspecified**

    Conditions classifiable to C80.1

4th **5th** **6th** **7th**   Additional Character Required   ✓   3-character code   Unspecified laterality codes were excluded here.   • =New Code   ▲ =Revised Code   ◘ =Social determinants of health   *Excludes1*—Not coded here, do not use together   *Excludes2*—Not included here

Z81   **FAMILY HISTORY OF MENTAL AND BEHAVIORAL**
`4th`   **DISORDERS**

> **GUIDELINES**
>
> Family history codes are for use when a patient has a family member(s) who has had a particular disease that causes the patient to be at higher risk of also contracting the disease. family history codes may be used in conjunction with screening codes to explain the need for a test or procedure. History codes are also acceptable on any medical record regardless of the reason for visit. A history of an illness, even if no longer present, is important information that may alter the type of treatment ordered.

Z81.0   **Family history of intellectual disabilities**
Conditions classifiable to F70–F79

▫**Z81.1**   **Family history of alcohol abuse and dependence**
Conditions classifiable to F10.

Z81.2   **Family history of tobacco abuse and dependence**
Conditions classifiable to F17.-

Z81.3   **Family history of other psychoactive substance abuse and dependence**
Conditions classifiable to F11-F16, F18-F19

▫**Z81.4**   **Family history of other substance abuse and dependence**
Conditions classifiable to F55

Z81.8   **Family history of other mental and behavioral disorders**
Conditions classifiable elsewhere in F01–F99

Z82   **FAMILY HISTORY OF CERTAIN DISABILITIES AND**
`4th`   **CHRONIC DISEASES (LEADING TO DISABLEMENT)**

> **GUIDELINES**
>
> Family history codes are for use when a patient has a family member(s) who has had a particular disease that causes the patient to be at higher risk of also contracting the disease. Family history codes may be used in conjunction with screening codes to explain the need for a test or procedure. History codes are also acceptable on any medical record regardless of the reason for visit. A history of an illness, even if no longer present, is important information that may alter the type of treatment ordered. **The reason for the encounter (for example, screening or counseling) should be sequenced first and the appropriate personal and/or family history code(s) should be assigned as additional diagnos(es).**

Z82.0   **Family history of; epilepsy and other diseases of the nervous system**
Conditions classifiable to G00–G99

Z82.1   **blindness and visual loss**
Conditions classifiable to H54.-

Z82.2   **deafness and hearing loss**
Conditions classifiable to H90–H91

Z82.3   **Family history of stroke**
Conditions classifiable to I60–I64

Z82.4   **Family history of; ischemic heart disease and other diseases**
`5th`   **of the circulatory system**
Conditions classifiable to I00–I5A, I65–I99

     Z82.41   **sudden cardiac death**
     Z82.49   **ischemic heart disease and other diseases of the circulatory system**

Z82.5   **Family history of asthma and other chronic lower respiratory diseases**
Conditions classifiable to J40–J47
Excludes2: family history of other diseases of the respiratory system (Z83.6)

Z82.6   **Family history of; arthritis and other diseases of the**
`5th`   **musculoskeletal system and connective tissue**
Conditions classifiable to M00–M99

     Z82.61   **arthritis**
     Z82.62   **osteoporosis**
     Z82.69   **other diseases of the musculoskeletal system and connective tissue**

Z82.7   **Family history of; congenital malformations, deformations and**
`5th`   **chromosomal abnormalities**
Conditions classifiable to Q00–Q99

     Z82.71   **polycystic kidney**
     Z82.79   **other congenital malformations, deformations and chromosomal abnormalities**

Z82.8   **Family history of other disabilities and chronic diseases leading to disablement, NEC**

Z83   **FAMILY HISTORY OF OTHER SPECIFIC DISORDERS**
`4th`

> **GUIDELINES**
>
> Family history codes are for use when a patient has a family member(s) who has had a particular disease that causes the patient to be at higher risk of also contracting the disease. family history codes may be used in conjunction with screening codes to explain the need for a test or procedure. History codes are also acceptable on any medical record regardless of the reason for visit. A history of an illness, even if no longer present, is important information that may alter the type of treatment ordered. **The reason for the encounter (for example, screening or counseling) should be sequenced first and the appropriate personal and/or family history code(s) should be assigned as additional diagnos(es).**
> *Excludes2:* contact with and (suspected) exposure to communicable disease in the family (Z20.-)

Z83.0   **Family history of human immunodeficiency virus [HIV] disease**
Conditions classifiable to B20

Z83.1   **Family history of other infectious and parasitic diseases**
Conditions classifiable to A00–B19, B25–B94, B99

Z83.2   **Family history of; diseases of the blood and blood-forming organs and certain disorders involving the immune mechanism**
Conditions classifiable to D50–D89

Z83.3   **DM**
Conditions classifiable to E08–E13

Z83.4   **other endocrine, nutritional and metabolic diseases**
`5th`   Conditions classifiable to E00–E07, E15–E88

     Z83.41   **multiple endocrine neoplasia syndrome**
     Z83.42   **familial hypercholesterolemia**
     Z83.43   **disorders of lipoprotein metabolism and other**
     `6th`   **lipidemia**

         Z83.430   **elevated lipoprotein(a)**
         Family history of elevated Lp(a)
         Z83.438   **other disorder of lipoprotein metabolism and other lipidemia**
         Family history of familial combined hyperlipidemia

     Z83.49   **other endocrine, nutritional and metabolic diseases**

Z83.5   **Family history of eye and ear disorders**
`5th`   **Z83.51**   **Family history of eye disorders**
     `6th`   Conditions classifiable to H00–H53, H55–H59
       Excludes2: family history of blindness and visual loss (Z82.1)

         Z83.511   **Family history of glaucoma**
         Z83.518   **Family history of other specified eye disorder**

     Z83.52   **Family history of ear disorders**
       Conditions classifiable to H60–H83, H92–H95
       Excludes2: family history of deafness and hearing loss (Z82.2)

Z83.6   **Family history of other diseases of the respiratory system**
Conditions classifiable to J00–J39, J60–J99
Excludes2: family history of asthma and other chronic lower respiratory diseases (Z82.5)

Z83.7   **Family history of diseases of the digestive system**
`5th`   Conditions classifiable to K00–K93

     Z83.71   **colonic polyps**
       Excludes2: family history of malignant neoplasm of digestive organs (Z80.0)
     Z83.79   **other diseases of the digestive system**

Z84   **FAMILY HISTORY OF OTHER CONDITIONS**
`4th`

> **GUIDELINES**
>
> Family history codes are for use when a patient has a family member(s) who has had a particular disease that causes the patient to be at higher risk of also contracting the disease. Family history codes may be used in conjunction with screening codes to explain the need for a test or procedure. History codes are also acceptable on any medical record regardless of the reason for visit. A history of an illness, even if no longer present, is important information that may alter the type

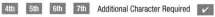

`4th` `5th` `6th` `7th` Additional Character Required   ✔   3-character code   Unspecified laterality codes were excluded here.   • =New Code   ▲ =Revised Code   ▫ =Social determinants of health   *Excludes1*—Not coded here, do not use together   *Excludes2*—Not included here

PEDIATRIC ICD-10-CM 2022: A MANUAL FOR PROVIDER-BASED CODING   **455**

of treatment ordered. **The reason for the encounter (for example, screening or counseling) should be sequenced first and the appropriate personal and/or family history code(s) should be assigned as additional diagnos(es).**

Z84.0   **Family history of diseases of the skin and subcutaneous tissue**
Conditions classifiable to L00–L99

Z84.1   **Family history of disorders of kidney and ureter**
Conditions classifiable to N00–N29

Z84.2   **Family history of other diseases of the genitourinary system**
Conditions classifiable to N30–N99

Z84.3   **Family history of consanguinity**

Z84.8   **Family history of other specified conditions**

    `5th` **Z84.81**   **Family history of carrier of genetic disease**

    Z84.82   **Family history of sudden infant death syndrome**

    Z84.89   **Family history of other specified conditions**

Z85 `4th` PERSONAL HISTORY OF MALIGNANT NEOPLASM

GUIDELINES

Personal history codes explain a patient's past medical condition that no longer exists and is not receiving any treatment, but that has the potential for recurrence, and therefore may require continued monitoring. These codes may be used in conjunction with follow-up codes to explain the need for a test or procedure. History codes are also acceptable on any medical record regardless of the reason for visit. A history of an illness, even if no longer present, is important information that may alter the type of treatment ordered. **The reason for the encounter (for example, screening or counseling) should be sequenced first and the appropriate personal and/or family history code(s) should be assigned as additional diagnos(es).**

Code first any follow-up examination after treatment of malignant neoplasm (Z08)

Use additional code to identify: alcohol use and dependence (F10.-)
    exposure to environmental tobacco smoke (Z77.22)
    history of tobacco dependence (Z87.891)
    occupational exposure to environmental tobacco smoke (Z57.31)
    tobacco dependence (F17.-)
    tobacco use (Z72.0)

Excludes2: personal history of benign neoplasm (Z86.01-)
    personal history of carcinoma-in-situ (Z86.00-)

Z85.5   **Personal history of malignant neoplasm of urinary tract**
  `5th` Conditions classifiable to C64–C68

    Z85.50   **Personal history of malignant neoplasm of; unspecified urinary tract organ**

    Z85.51   **bladder**

    Z85.52   **kidney**

    `6th` *Excludes1:* personal history of malignant neoplasm of renal pelvis (Z85.53)

      Z85.520   **Personal history of; malignant carcinoid tumor of kidney**
Conditions classifiable to C7A.093

      Z85.528   **other malignant neoplasm of kidney**
Conditions classifiable to C64

Z85.6   **Leukemia**
Conditions classifiable to C91–C95
Excludes1: leukemia in remission C91.0–C95.9 with 5th character 1

Z85.7   **Personal history of other malignant neoplasms of lymphoid, hematopoietic and related tissues**
  `5th`

    Z85.71   **Personal history of; Hodgkin lymphoma**
Conditions classifiable to C81

    Z85.72   **non-Hodgkin lymphomas**
Conditions classifiable to C82–C85

    Z85.79   **other malignant neoplasms of lymphoid, hematopoietic and related tissues**
Conditions classifiable to C88–C90, C96
Excludes1: multiple myeloma in remission (C90.01)
    plasma cell leukemia in remission (C90.11)
    plasmacytoma in remission (C90.21)

Z85.8   **Malignant neoplasms of other organs and systems**
  `5th` Conditions classifiable to C00–C14, C40–C49, C69–C79, C7A.098

    Z85.82   **Personal history of malignant neoplasm of skin**

    `6th` **Z85.820**   **Personal history of malignant melanoma of skin**
Conditions classifiable to C43

    Z85.83   **Personal history of malignant neoplasm of; bone and soft tissue**
  `6th` Conditions classifiable to C40–C41; C45–C49

      Z85.830   **bone**

      Z85.831   **soft tissue**
Excludes2: personal history of malignant neoplasm of skin (Z85.82-)

    Z85.84   **Personal history of; malignant neoplasm of eye and nervous tissue**
  `6th` Conditions classifiable to C69–C72

      Z85.840   **eye**

      Z85.841   **brain**

      Z85.848   **other parts of nervous tissue**

    Z85.85   **Personal history of; malignant neoplasm of endocrine glands**
  `6th` Conditions classifiable to C73–C75

      Z85.850   **thyroid**

      Z85.858   **other endocrine glands**

    Z85.89   **other organs and systems**
Conditions classifiable to C7A.098, C76, C77–C79

Z85.9   **Personal history of malignant neoplasm, unspecified**
Conditions classifiable to C7A.00, C80.1

Z86 `4th` PERSONAL HISTORY OF CERTAIN OTHER DISEASES

GUIDELINES

Personal history codes explain a patient's past medical condition that no longer exists and is not receiving any treatment, but that has the potential for recurrence, and therefore may require continued monitoring. These codes may be used in conjunction with follow-up codes to explain the need for a test or procedure. History codes are also acceptable on any medical record regardless of the reason for visit. A history of an illness, even if no longer present, is important information that may alter the type of treatment ordered. **The reason for the encounter (for example, screening or counseling) should be sequenced first and the appropriate personal and/or family history code(s) should be assigned as additional diagnos(es).**

Code first any follow-up examination after treatment (Z09)

Z86.0   **Personal history of in-situ and benign neoplasms and**
  `5th` **neoplasms of uncertain behavior**
Excludes2: personal history of malignant neoplasms (Z85.-)

    Z86.00   **Personal history of in-situ neoplasm**
    `6th` Conditions classifiable to D00–D09

      Z86.000   **Personal history of in-situ neoplasm of breast**
Conditions classifiable to D05

      Z86.001   **Personal history of in-situ neoplasm of cervix uteri**
Conditions classifiable to D06
Personal history of cervical intraepithelial neoplasia III [CIN III]

      Z86.002   **Personal history of in-situ neoplasm of other and unspecified genital organs**
Conditions classifiable to D07
Personal history of high-grade prostatic intraepithelial neoplasia III [HGPIN III]
Personal history of vaginal intraepithelial neoplasia III [VAIN III]
Personal history of vulvar intraepithelial neoplasia III [VIN III]

      Z86.003   **Personal history of in-situ neoplasm of oral cavity, esophagus and stomach**
Conditions classifiable to D00

      Z86.004   **Personal history of in-situ neoplasm of other and unspecified digestive organs**
Conditions classifiable to D01
Personal history of anal intraepithelial neoplasia (AIN III)

      Z86.005   **Personal history of in-situ neoplasm of middle ear and respiratory system**
Conditions classifiable to D02

`4th` `5th` `6th` `7th`   Additional Character Required   ✔   3-character code   Unspecified laterality codes were excluded here.   • =New Code   ▲ =Revised Code   ⌑ =Social determinants of health   *Excludes1*—Not coded here, do not use together   *Excludes2*—Not included here

Z86.006 **Personal history of melanoma in-situ**
Conditions classifiable to D03
Excludes2: sites other than skin—code to personal history of in-situ neoplasm of the site

Z86.007 **Personal history of in-situ neoplasm of skin**
Conditions classifiable to D04
Personal history of carcinoma in situ of skin

Z86.008 **Personal history of in-situ neoplasm of other site**
Conditions classifiable to D09

Z86.03 **Personal history of neoplasm of uncertain behavior**

Z86.1 **Personal history of infectious and parasitic diseases** [5th]
Conditions classifiable to A00–B89, B99
Excludes1: personal history of infectious diseases specific to a body system
sequelae of infectious and parasitic diseases (B90–B94)

Z86.11 **Personal history of; tuberculosis**

Z86.13 **malaria**

Z86.14 **MRSA infection**
Personal history of MRSA infection

Z86.15 **latent tuberculosis infection**

> **GUIDELINE**
> See code U07.1 for more information.

Z86.16 **COVID-19**
Excludes1: post COVID-19 condition (U09.9)

Z86.19 **other infectious and parasitic diseases**

Z86.2 **Personal history of diseases of the blood and blood-forming organs and certain disorders involving the immune mechanism**
Conditions classifiable to D50–D89

Z86.3 **Personal history of endocrine, nutritional and metabolic diseases** [5th]
Conditions classifiable to E00–E88

Z86.39 **other endocrine, nutritional and metabolic disease**

Z86.5 **Personal history of; mental and behavioral disorders** [5th]
Conditions classifiable to F40–F59

Z86.59 **other mental and behavioral disorders**
Code is a nonspecific Z code, refer to Chapter 21 for guidelines.

Z86.6 **Personal history of; diseases of the nervous system and sense organs** [5th]
Conditions classifiable to G00–G99, H00–H95

Z86.61 **infections of the central nervous system**
Personal history of encephalitis
Personal history of meningitis

Z86.69 **other diseases of the nervous system and sense organs**

Z86.7 **Personal history of; diseases of the circulatory system** [5th]
Conditions classifiable to I00–I99

Z86.73 **TIA and cerebral infarction without residual deficits**
Personal history of prolonged reversible ischemic neurological deficit (PRIND)
Personal history of stroke NOS without residual deficits
Excludes1: personal history of traumatic brain injury (Z87.820)
sequelae of cerebrovascular disease (I69.-)

Z86.74 **sudden cardiac arrest**
Personal history of sudden cardiac death successfully resuscitated

Z86.79 **other diseases of the circulatory system**

Z87 **PERSONAL HISTORY OF OTHER DISEASES AND CONDITIONS** [4th]

> **GUIDELINES**
> Personal history codes explain a patient's past medical condition that no longer exists and is not receiving any treatment, but that has the potential for recurrence, and therefore may require continued monitoring. These codes may be used in conjunction with follow-up codes to explain the need for a test or procedure. History codes are also acceptable on any medical record regardless of the reason for visit. A history of an illness, even if no longer present, is important information that may alter the type of treatment ordered. **The reason for the encounter (for example, screening or counseling) should be sequenced first and the appropriate personal and/or family history code(s) should be assigned as additional diagnos(es).**
> **Code first** any follow-up examination after treatment (Z09)

Z87.0 **Personal history of; diseases of the respiratory system** [5th]
Conditions classifiable to J00–J99

Z87.01 **pneumonia (recurrent)**

Z87.09 **other diseases of the respiratory system**

Z87.3 **Personal history of diseases of the musculoskeletal system and connective tissue** [5th]
Conditions classifiable to M00–M99
Excludes2: personal history of (healed) traumatic fracture (Z87.81)

Z87.39 **other diseases of the musculoskeletal system and connective tissue**

Z87.4 **Personal history of; diseases of genitourinary system** [5th]
Conditions classifiable to N00–N99

Z87.44 **diseases of urinary system** [6th]
Excludes1: personal history of malignant neoplasm of cervix uteri (Z85.41)

Z87.440 **urinary (tract) infections**

Z87.441 **nephrotic syndrome**

Z87.442 **urinary calculi**
Personal history of kidney stones

Z87.448 **other diseases of urinary system**

Z87.7 **Personal history of (corrected) congenital malformations** [5th]
Conditions classifiable to Q00–Q89 that have been repaired or corrected
Excludes1: congenital malformations that have been partially corrected or repair but which still require medical treatment—**code to condition**
Excludes2: other postprocedural states (Z98.-)
personal history of medical treatment (Z92.-)
presence of cardiac and vascular implants and grafts (Z95.-)
presence of other devices (Z97.-)
presence of other functional implants (Z96.-)
transplanted organ and tissue status (Z94.-)

Z87.71 **Personal history of; (corrected) congenital malformations of genitourinary system** [6th]

Z87.710 **(corrected) hypospadias**

Z87.718 **other specified (corrected) congenital malformations of genitourinary system**

Z87.72 **Personal history of; (corrected) congenital malformations of nervous system and sense organs** [6th]

Z87.720 **(corrected) congenital malformations of eye**

Z87.721 **(corrected) congenital malformations of ear**

Z87.728 **other specified (corrected) congenital malformations of nervous system and sense organs**

Z87.73 **Personal history of; (corrected) congenital malformations of digestive system** [6th]

Z87.730 **(corrected) cleft lip and palate**

Z87.738 **other specified (corrected) congenital malformations of digestive system**

Z87.74 **Personal history of; (corrected) congenital malformations of heart and circulatory system**

Z87.75 **(corrected) congenital malformations of respiratory system**

Z87.76 **(corrected) congenital malformations of integument, limbs and musculoskeletal system**

Z87.79 **other (corrected) congenital malformations** [6th]

Z87.790 **(corrected) congenital malformations of face and neck**

Z87.798 **other (corrected) congenital malformations**

Z87.8 **Personal history of; other specified conditions** [5th]
Excludes2: personal history of self harm (Z91.5-)

Z87.82 **other (healed) physical injury and trauma** [6th]
Conditions classifiable to S00–T88, except traumatic fractures

---

[4th]	[5th]	[6th]	[7th]	Additional Character Required	✔	3-character code

Unspecified laterality codes were excluded here.

• =New Code
▲ =Revised Code
▢ =Social determinants of health

Excludes1—Not coded here, do not use together
Excludes2—Not included here

 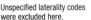

CHAPTER 21. FACTORS INFLUENCING HEALTH STATUS AND CONTACT WITH HEALTH SERVICES (Z87.820–Z91.5)

Z87.820   **traumatic brain injury**
    Excludes1: personal history of TIA, and cerebral infarction without residual deficits (Z86.73)

Z87.821   **retained FB fully removed**

Z87.828   **other (healed) physical injury and trauma**

Z87.89   **Personal history of; other specified conditions**

[6th] Z87.891   **nicotine dependence**
    Excludes1: current nicotine dependence (F17.2-)

Z87.892   **anaphylaxis**
    Code also allergy status such as:
    allergy status to drugs, medicaments and biological substances (Z88.-)
    allergy status, other than to drugs and biological substances (Z91.0-)

Z87.898   **other specified conditions**

Z88 ALLERGY STATUS TO DRUGS, MEDICAMENTS AND [4th] **BIOLOGICAL SUBSTANCES**
This is a status category (excluding Z88.9), refer to Chapter 21 for status guidelines.
Excludes2: Allergy status, other than to drugs and biological substances (Z91.0-)

Z88.0 **Allergy status to; penicillin**
Z88.1 **other antibiotic agents**
Z88.2 **sulfonamides status**
Z88.3 **other anti-infective agents**
Z88.4 **anesthetic agent**
Z88.5 **narcotic agent**
Z88.6 **analgesic agent**
Z88.7 **serum and vaccine**
Z88.8 **other drugs, medicaments and biological substances**
Z88.9 **unspecified drugs, medicaments and biological substances**
    Code is a nonspecific Z code, refer to Chapter 21 for guidelines.

Z90 ACQUIRED ABSENCE OF ORGANS, NEC
[4th] This is a status category, refer to Chapter 21 for status guidelines.
Includes: postprocedural or post-traumatic loss of body part NEC
Excludes1: congenital absence—see Alphabetical Index
Excludes2: postprocedural absence of endocrine glands (E89.-)
Note: Use only if there are no complications or malfunctions of the organ or tissue replaced, the amputation site, or the equipment on which the patient is dependent.

Z90.4 **Acquired absence of; other specified parts of digestive tract**
[5th] Z90.49 **other specified parts of digestive tract**
Z90.5 **Acquired absence of; kidney**
Z90.7 **genital organ(s)**
[5th] *Excludes1:* personal history of sex reassignment (Z87.890)
    Excludes2: female genital mutilation status (N90.81-)
Z90.79 **other genital organ(s)**
Z90.8 **Acquired absence of; other organs**
[5th] Z90.81 **spleen**
Z90.89 **other organs**

Z91 PERSONAL RISK FACTORS, NEC
[4th] *Excludes2:* contact with and (suspected) exposures hazardous to health (Z77.-)
exposure to pollution and other problems related to physical environment (Z77.1-)
personal history of physical injury and trauma (Z87.81, Z87.82-)
occupational exposure to risk factors (Z57.-)

Z91.0 **Allergy status, other than to drugs and biological substances**
[5th] *This is a status sub-category, refer to Chapter 21 for status guidelines.*
Excludes2: Allergy status to drugs, medicaments, and biological substances (Z88.-)

Z91.01 **Food allergy status**
[6th] *Excludes2:* food additives allergy status (Z91.02)
Z91.010 **Allergy to; peanuts**
Z91.011 **milk products**
    Excludes1: lactose intolerance (E73.-)
Z91.012 **eggs**
Z91.013 **seafood**
    Allergy to shellfish or octopus or squid ink

•Z91.014 **mammalian meats**
    Allergy to beef, lamb, pork, red meats
Z91.018 **other foods**
    nuts other than peanuts

Z91.02 **Food additives allergy status**
Z91.03 **Insect allergy status**
[6th] Z91.030 **Bee allergy status**
Z91.038 **Other insect allergy status**
Z91.04 **Nonmedicinal substance allergy status**
[6th] Z91.040 **Latex allergy status**
    Latex sensitivity status
Z91.041 **Radiographic dye allergy status**
    Allergy status to contrast media used for diagnostic X-ray procedure
Z91.048 **Other nonmedicinal substance allergy status**

Z91.1 **Patient's noncompliance with medical treatment and regimen**
[5th] Z91.11 **Patient's noncompliance with dietary regimen**
Z91.12 **Patient's intentional underdosing of medication**
[6th] **regimen**
    Code first underdosing of medication (T36–T50) with fifth or sixth character 6
    Excludes1: adverse effect of prescribed drug taken as directed–code to adverse effect poisoning (overdose)–code to poisoning
Z91.120 **Patient's intentional underdosing of medication regimen due to financial hardship**
Z91.128 **Patient's intentional underdosing of medication regimen for other reason**
Z91.13 **Patient's unintentional underdosing of medication**
[6th] **regimen**
    Code first underdosing of medication (T36–T50) with fifth or sixth character 6
    Excludes1: adverse effect of prescribed drug taken as directed—code to adverse effect poisoning (overdose)—code to poisoning
Z91.138 **Patient's unintentional underdosing of medication regimen for other reason**
Z91.14 **Patient's other noncompliance with medication regimen**
    Patient's underdosing of medication NOS
Z91.15 **Patient's noncompliance with renal dialysis**
Z91.19 **Patient's noncompliance with other medical treatment and regimen**
    Nonadherence to medical treatment

Z91.4 **Personal history of psychological trauma, NEC**
[5th]

GUIDELINES

Personal history codes explain a patient's past medical condition that no longer exists and is not receiving any treatment, but that has the potential for recurrence, and therefore may require continued monitoring. These codes may be used in conjunction with follow-up codes to explain the need for a test or procedure. History codes are also acceptable on any medical record regardless of the reason for visit. A history of an illness, even if no longer present, is important information that may alter the type of treatment ordered. **The reason for the encounter (for example, screening or counseling) should be sequenced first and the appropriate personal and/or family history code(s) should be assigned as additional diagnos(es).**
Z91.49 **Other personal history of psychological trauma, NEC**

▲Z91.5 **Personal history of self-harm**
[5th] **Code also** mental health disorder, if known

GUIDELINES

Personal history codes explain a patient's past medical condition that no longer exists and is not receiving any treatment, but that has the potential for recurrence, and therefore may require continued monitoring. These codes may be used in conjunction with follow-up codes to explain the need for a test or procedure. History codes are also acceptable on any medical record regardless of the reason for visit. A history of an illness, even if no longer present, is important information that may alter the type of treatment ordered. **The reason for the encounter (for**

[4th] [5th] [6th] [7th] Additional Character Required   ✔   3-character code

Unspecified laterality codes were excluded here.

• =New Code
▲ =Revised Code
⌑ =Social determinants of health

Excludes1—Not coded here, do not use together
Excludes2—Not included here

example, screening or counseling) should be sequenced first and the appropriate personal and/or family history code(s) should be assigned as additional diagnos(es).

- **Z91.51** **Personal history of suicidal behavior**
  Personal history of parasuicide
  Personal history of self-poisoning
  Personal history of suicide attempt
- **Z91.52** **Personal history of nonsuicidal self-harm**
  Personal history of nonsuicidal self-injury
  Personal history of self-inflicted injury without suicidal intent
  Personal history of self-mutilation

Z91.8 Other specified personal risk factors, NEC

> **GUIDELINES** `5th`
>
> Personal history codes explain a patient's past medical condition that no longer exists and is not receiving any treatment, but that has the potential for recurrence, and therefore may require continued monitoring. These codes may be used in conjunction with follow-up codes to explain the need for a test or procedure. History codes are also acceptable on any medical record regardless of the reason for visit. A history of an illness, even if no longer present, is important information that may alter the type of treatment ordered. **The reason for the encounter (for example, screening or counseling) should be sequenced first and the appropriate personal and/or family history code(s) should be assigned as additional diagnos(es).** Excludes code Z91.83, Z91.84-.

- **Z91.81** **History of falling**
  At risk for falling
- **Z91.83** **Wandering in diseases classified elsewhere**
  Code first underlying disorder such as:
  Alzheimer's disease (G30.-)
  autism or pervasive developmental disorder (F84.-)
  intellectual disabilities (F70–F79)
  unspecified dementia with behavioral disturbance (F03.9-)
- **Z91.84** **Oral health risk factors**
  - `6th` Z91.841 **Risk for dental caries, low**
  - Z91.842 **Risk for dental caries, moderate**
  - Z91.843 **Risk for dental caries, high**
  - Z91.849 **Unspecified risk for dental caries**
- **Z91.89** **Other specified personal risk factors, NEC**

Z92   PERSONAL HISTORY OF MEDICAL TREATMENT `4th`

> **GUIDELINES**
>
> Personal history codes explain a patient's past medical condition that no longer exists and is not receiving any treatment, but that has the potential for recurrence, and therefore may require continued monitoring. These codes may be used in conjunction with follow-up codes to explain the need for a test or procedure. History codes are also acceptable on any medical record regardless of the reason for visit. A history of an illness, even if no longer present, is important information that may alter the type of treatment ordered. **The reason for the encounter (for example, screening or counseling) should be sequenced first and the appropriate personal and/or family history code(s) should be assigned as additional diagnos(es).** Excludes codes Z92.0 and Z92.82.

Excludes2: postprocedural states (Z98.-)

Z92.2 Personal history of; drug therapy
  `5th` ***Excludes2:*** long term (current) drug therapy (Z79.-)
- Z92.21 **antineoplastic chemotherapy**
- Z92.22 **monoclonal drug therapy**
- Z92.24 **steroid therapy**
  - `6th` Z92.240 **inhaled steroid therapy**
  - Z92.241 **systemic steroid therapy**
    steroid therapy NOS
- Z92.25 **immunosuppression therapy**
  Excludes2: personal history of steroid therapy (Z92.24)
- Z92.29 **other drug therapy**

Z92.8 Personal history of; other medical treatment
- `5th` Z92.81 **extracorporeal membrane oxygenation (ECMO)**
- •Z92.85 **Personal history of cellular therapy**
  `6th`

- •Z92.850 **Personal history of Chimeric Antigen Receptor T-cell therapy**
  Personal history of CAR T-cell therapy
- •Z92.858 **Personal history of other cellular therapy**
- •Z92.859 **Personal history of cellular therapy, unspecified**
- •Z92.86 **Personal history of gene therapy**

Z93   ARTIFICIAL OPENING STATUS `4th`

Note: Use only if there are no complications or malfunctions of the organ or tissue replaced, the amputation site, or the equipment on which the patient is dependent. This is a status category, refer to Chapter 21 for status guidelines.

Excludes1: artificial openings requiring attention or management (Z43.-)
complications of external stoma (J95.0-, K94.-, N99.5-)

Z93.0 Tracheostomy status
Z93.1 Gastrostomy status
Z93.2 Ileostomy status
Z93.3 Colostomy status
Z93.4 Other artificial openings of gastrointestinal tract status
Z93.5 Cystostomy status
  `5th` Z93.50 **Unspecified cystostomy status**
  Z93.51 **Cutaneous-vesicostomy status**
  Z93.52 **Appendico-vesicostomy status**
  Z93.59 **Other cystostomy status**
Z93.8 Other artificial opening status
Z93.9 Artificial opening status, unspecified

Z94   TRANSPLANTED ORGAN AND TISSUE STATUS `4th`

Note: Use only if there are no complications or malfunctions of the organ or tissue replaced, the amputation site, or the equipment on which the patient is dependent. This is a status category, refer to Chapter 21 for status guidelines.

Includes: organ or tissue replaced by heterogenous or homogenous transplant

Excludes1: complications of transplanted organ or tissue—see Alphabetical Index

Excludes2: presence of vascular grafts (Z95.-)

Z94.0 Kidney transplant status
Z94.1 Heart transplant status
  Excludes1: artificial heart status (Z95.812)
  heart-valve replacement status (Z95.2–Z95.4)
Z94.2 Lung transplant status
Z94.3 Heart and lungs transplant status
Z94.4 Liver transplant status
Z94.5 Skin transplant status
  Autogenous skin transplant status
Z94.6 Bone transplant status
Z94.7 Corneal transplant status
Z94.8 Other transplanted organ and tissue status
  `5th` Z94.81 **Bone marrow transplant status**
  Z94.82 **Intestine transplant status**
  Z94.83 **Pancreas transplant status**
  Z94.84 **Stem cells transplant status**
  Z94.89 **Other transplanted organ and tissue status**
Z94.9 Transplanted organ and tissue status, unspecified

Z95   PRESENCE OF CARDIAC AND VASCULAR IMPLANTS AND GRAFTS `4th`

This is a status category, refer to Chapter 21 for status guidelines.

Excludes2: complications of cardiac and vascular devices, implants and grafts (T82.-)

Z95.0 Presence of cardiac pacemaker
  Presence of cardiac resynchronization therapy (CRT-P) pacemaker
  Excludes1: adjustment or management of cardiac pacemaker (Z45.0-)
  presence of automatic (implantable) cardiac defibrillator with synchronous cardiac pacemaker (Z95.810)
Z95.2 Presence of prosthetic heart valve
  Presence of heart valve NOS
Z95.3 Presence of xenogenic heart valve
Z95.4 Presence of other heart-valve replacement
Z95.8 Presence of other cardiac and vascular implants and grafts
  `5th` Z95.81 **Presence of other cardiac implants and grafts**
  `6th`

| `4th` `5th` `6th` `7th` | Additional Character Required | ✔ | 3-character code | Unspecified laterality codes were excluded here. | • =New Code
▲ =Revised Code
▫ =Social determinants of health | ***Excludes1***—Not coded here, do not use together
Excludes2—Not included here |

CHAPTER 21. FACTORS INFLUENCING HEALTH STATUS AND CONTACT WITH HEALTH SERVICES   (Z95.810–Z99.89)

Z95.810   **Presence of automatic (implantable) cardiac defibrillator**

     Presence of automatic (implantable) cardiac defibrillator with synchronous cardiac pacemaker

     Presence of cardiac resynchronization therapy defibrillator (CRT-D)

     Presence of cardioverter-defibrillator (ICD)

Z95.811   **Presence of heart assist device**

Z95.812   **Presence of fully implantable artificial heart**

Z95.818   **Presence of other cardiac implants and grafts**

Z96   PRESENCE OF OTHER FUNCTIONAL IMPLANTS

[4th] **Excludes2:** complications of internal prosthetic devices, implants and grafts (T82-T85)

     fitting and adjustment of prosthetic and other devices (Z44-Z46)

Z96.0   **Presence of urogenital implants**

Z96.1   **Presence of intraocular lens**

     Presence of pseudophakia

Z96.2   **Presence of otological and audiological implants**

[5th]   **Z96.21**   **Cochlear implant status**

     Z96.22   **Myringotomy tube(s) status**

     Z96.29   **Presence of other otological and audiological implants**

       Presence of bone-conduction hearing device

       Presence of eustachian tube stent

       Stapes replacement

Z96.3   **Presence of artificial larynx**

Z96.4   **Presence of endocrine implants**

[5th]   **Z96.41**   **Presence of insulin pump (external) (internal)**

     Z96.49   **Presence of other endocrine implants**

Z96.8   **Presence of other specified functional implants**

[5th]   **Z96.81**   **Presence of artificial skin**

     Z96.82   **Presence of neurostimulator**

       Presence of brain neurostimulator

       Presence of gastric neurostimulator

       Presence of peripheral nerve neurostimulator

       Presence of sacral nerve neurostimulator

       Presence of spinal cord neurostimulator

       Presence of vagus nerve neurostimulator

     Z96.89   **Presence of other specified functional implants**

Z96.9   **Presence of functional implant, unspecified**

Z97   PRESENCE OF OTHER DEVICES

[4th] **Excludes1:** complications of internal prosthetic devices, implants and grafts (T82–T85)

Excludes 2: fitting and adjustment of prosthetic and other devices (Z44–Z46)

Z97.3   **Presence of spectacles and contact lenses**

Z97.4   **Presence of external hearing-aid**

Z97.5   **Presence of (intrauterine) contraceptive device**

     checking, reinsertion or removal of contraceptive device (Z30.43)

     Excludes1: checking, reinsertion or removal of implantable subdermal contraceptive (Z30.46)

     checking, reinsertion or removal of intrauterine contraceptive device (Z30.43-)

Z97.8   **Presence of other specified devices**

Z98   OTHER POSTPROCEDURAL STATES

[4th] This is a status category, refer to Chapter 21 for status guidelines.

Excludes2: aftercare (Z43–Z49, Z51)

     follow-up medical care (Z08–Z09)

     postprocedural complication—see Alphabetical Index

Z98.2   **Presence of cerebrospinal fluid drainage device**

     Presence of CSF shunt

Z98.8   **Other specified postprocedural states**

[5th]   **Z98.85**   **Transplanted organ removal status**

     Assign code Z98.85, Transplanted organ removal status, to indicate that a transplanted organ has been previously removed. This code should not be assigned for the encounter in which the transplanted organ is removed. The complication necessitating removal of the transplant organ should be assigned for that encounter.

     See Chapter 19 for information on the coding of organ transplant complications.

     Transplanted organ previously removed due to complication, failure, rejection or infection

     Excludes1: encounter for removal of transplanted organ—code to complication of transplanted organ (T86.-)

     Z98.87   **Personal history of in utero procedure**

[6th]   **Z98.871**   **Personal history of in utero procedure while a fetus**

     Z98.89   **Other specified postprocedural states**

[6th]   **Z98.890**   **Other specified postprocedural states**

       Personal history of surgery, NEC

Z99   DEPENDENCE ON ENABLING MACHINES AND DEVICES, NEC

[4th] This is a status category, refer to Chapter 21 for status guidelines.

Z99.1   **Dependence on respirator**

[5th]   Dependence on ventilator

     Z99.11   **Dependence on respirator [ventilator] status**

     For encounters for weaning from a mechanical ventilator, assign a code from subcategory J96.1, Chronic respiratory failure, followed by code Z99.11, Dependence on respirator [ventilator] status.

Z99.2   **Dependence on renal dialysis**

     Hemodialysis status

     Peritoneal dialysis status

     Presence of arteriovenous shunt for dialysis

     Renal dialysis status NOS

     Excludes1: encounter for fitting and adjustment of dialysis catheter (Z49.0-)

     Excludes2: noncompliance with renal dialysis (Z91.15)

Z99.3   **Dependence on wheelchair**

     Wheelchair confinement status

     Code first cause of dependence, such as:

       muscular dystrophy (G71.0-)

       obesity (E66.-)

Z99.8   **Dependence on other enabling machines and devices**

[5th]   **Z99.81**   **Dependence on supplemental oxygen**

     Dependence on long-term oxygen

     Z99.89   **Dependence on other enabling machines and devices**

     Dependence on machine or device NOS

[4th] [5th] [6th] [7th]   Additional Character Required   [✓]   3-character code   Unspecified laterality codes were excluded here.   • =New Code   ▲ =Revised Code   ¤ =Social determinants of health   **Excludes1**—Not coded here, do not use together   **Excludes2**—Not included here

460   PEDIATRIC ICD-10-CM 2022: A MANUAL FOR PROVIDER-BASED CODING

Chapter 22. Codes for special purposes (U00–U85)

(U00–U49) PROVISIONAL ASSIGNMENT OF NEW DISEASES OF UNCERTAIN ETIOLOGY OR EMERGENCY USE

U07 EMERGENCY USE OF U07
4th

GUIDELINES

For patients presenting with condition(s) related to vaping, assign code U07.0, Vaping-related disorder, as the principal diagnosis. For lung injury due to vaping, assign only code U07.0. Assign additional codes for other manifestations, such as acute respiratory failure (subcategory J96.0-) or pneumonitis (code J68.0). Associated respiratory signs and symptoms due to vaping, such as cough, shortness of breath, etc., are not coded separately, when a definitive diagnosis has been established. However, it would be appropriate to code separately any gastrointestinal symptoms, such as diarrhea and abdominal pain.

U07.0 Vaping-related disorder
>   Dabbing related lung damage
>   Dabbing related lung injury
>   E-cigarette, or vaping, product use associated lung injury [EVALI]
>   Electronic cigarette related lung damage
>   Electronic cigarette related lung injury
>   **Use additional code** to identify manifestations, such as:
>>   abdominal pain (R10.84)
>>   acute respiratory distress syndrome (J80)
>>   diarrhea (R19.7)
>>   drug-induced interstitial lung disorder (J70.4)
>>   lipoid pneumonia (J69.1)
>>   weight loss (R63.4)

GUIDELINES

COVID-19 infection (infection due to SARS-CoV-2)

Code only confirmed cases

Code only a confirmed diagnosis of the 2019 novel coronavirus disease (COVID-19) as documented by the provider or documentation of a positive COVID-19 test result. For a confirmed diagnosis, assign code U07.1, COVID-19. This is an exception to the hospital inpatient guideline Section II, H. In this context, "confirmation" does not require documentation of a positive test result for COVID-19; the provider's documentation that the individual has COVID-19 is sufficient.

If the provider documents "suspected," "possible," "probable," or "inconclusive" COVID-19, do not assign code U07.1. Instead, code the signs and symptoms reported.

Sequencing of codes

When COVID-19 meets the definition of principal diagnosis, code U07.1, COVID-19, should be sequenced first, followed by the appropriate codes for associated manifestations, except when another guideline requires that certain codes be sequenced first, such as obstetrics, sepsis, or transplant complications.

For a COVID-19 infection that progresses to sepsis, see sepsis guidelines.

See Section I.C.16.h. for COVID-19 infection in newborn.

For a COVID-19 infection in a lung transplant patient, see Section I.C.19.g.3.a. Transplant complications other than kidney.

Acute respiratory manifestations of COVID-19

When the reason for the encounter/admission is a respiratory manifestation of COVID-19, assign code U07.1, COVID-19, as the principal/first-listed diagnosis and assign code(s) for the respiratory manifestation(s) as additional diagnoses.

The following conditions are examples of common respiratory manifestations of COVID-19.

PNEUMONIA

For a patient with pneumonia confirmed as due to COVID-19, assign codes U07.1, COVID-19, and J12.82, Pneumonia due to coronavirus disease 2019.

ACUTE BRONCHITIS

For a patient with acute bronchitis confirmed as due to COVID-19, assign codes U07.1 and J20.8, Acute bronchitis due to other specified organisms. Bronchitis not otherwise specified (NOS) due to COVID-19 should be coded using code U07.1 and J40, Bronchitis, not specified as acute or chronic.

LOWER RESPIRATORY INFECTION

If the COVID-19 is documented as being associated with a lower respiratory infection, not otherwise specified (NOS), or an acute respiratory infection, NOS, codes U07.1 and J22, Unspecified acute lower respiratory infection, should be assigned. If the COVID-19 is documented as being associated with a respiratory infection, NOS, codes U07.1 and J98.8, Other specified respiratory disorders, should be assigned.

ACUTE RESPIRATORY DISTRESS SYNDROME

For acute respiratory distress syndrome (ARDS) due to COVID-19, assign codes U07.1, and J80, Acute respiratory distress syndrome.

ACUTE RESPIRATORY FAILURE

For acute respiratory failure due to COVID-19, assign code U07.1, and code J96.0-, Acute respiratory failure.

NON-RESPIRATORY MANIFESTATIONS OF COVID-19

When the reason for the encounter/admission is a non-respiratory manifestation (e.g., viral enteritis) of COVID-19, assign code U07.1, COVID-19, as the principal/first-listed diagnosis and assign code(s) for the manifestation(s) as additional diagnoses.

Exposure to COVID-19

For asymptomatic individuals with actual or suspected exposure to COVID-19, assign code Z20.828, Contact with and (suspected) exposure to other viral communicable diseases.

For symptomatic individuals with actual or suspected exposure to COVID-19 and the infection has been ruled out, or test results are inconclusive or unknown, assign code Z20.828, Contact with and (suspected) exposure to other viral communicable diseases. See Contact/Exposure guideline, for additional guidance regarding the use of category Z20 codes. If COVID-19 is confirmed see the COVID infection guideline.

Screening for COVID-19

During the COVID-19 pandemic, a screening code is generally not appropriate. Do not assign code Z11.52, Encounter for screening for COVID-19. For encounters for COVID-19 testing, including preoperative testing, code as exposure to COVID-19 (See Exposure guideline).

Coding guidance will be updated as new information concerning any changes in the pandemic status becomes available.

Signs and symptoms without definitive diagnosis of COVID-19

For patients presenting with any signs/symptoms associated with COVID-19 (such as fever, etc.) but a definitive diagnosis has not been established, assign the appropriate code(s) for each of the presenting signs and symptoms such as:
- R05.1 Acute Cough **or R05.9, Cough, unspecified**
- R06.02 Shortness of breath
- R50.9 Fever, unspecified

If a patient with signs/symptoms associated with COVID-19 also has an actual or suspected contact with or exposure to COVID-19, assign Z20.822, Contact with and (suspected) exposure to COVID-19, as an additional code.

Asymptomatic individuals who test positive for COVID-19

For asymptomatic individuals who test positive for COVID-19, see code only confirmed cases guideline. Although the individual is

---

4th **5th** **6th** **7th** Additional Character Required   ✓ 3-character code

•=New Code
▲=Revised Code

Excludes1—Not coded here, do not use together
Excludes2—Not included here

asymptomatic, the individual has tested positive and is considered to have the COVID-19 infection.

Personal history of COVID-19

For patients with a history of COVID-19, assign code Z86.16, Personal history of COVID-19.

Follow-up visits after COVID-19 infection has resolved

For individuals who previously had COVID-19 without residual symptom(s) or condition(s), and are being seen for follow-up evaluation, and COVID-19 test results are negative, assign codes Z09, Encounter for follow-up examination after completed treatment for conditions other than malignant neoplasm, and Z86.16, Personal history of COVID-19.

For follow-up visits for individuals with symptom(s) or condition(s) related to a previous COVID-19 infection, see U07.9

Encounter for antibody testing

For an encounter for antibody testing that is not being performed to confirm a current COVID-19 infection, nor is a follow-up test after resolution of COVID-19, assign Z01.84, Encounter for antibody response examination.

Follow the applicable guidelines above if the individual is being tested to confirm a current COVID-19 infection. For follow-up testing after a COVID-19 infection, see follow-up visits after COVID-19 infection has resolved guideline.

Multisystem Inflammatory Syndrome

For individuals with multisystem inflammatory syndrome (MIS) and COVID-19, assign code U07.1, COVID-19, as the principal/first-listed diagnosis and assign code M35.81, Multisystem inflammatory syndrome, as an additional diagnosis.

If MIS develops as a result of a previous COVID-19 infection, assign codes M35.81, Multisystem inflammatory syndrome, and B94.8, Sequelae of other specified infectious and parasitic diseases.

If an individual with a history of COVID-19 develops MIS and the provider does not indicate the MIS is due to the previous COVID-19 infection, assign codes M35.81, Multisystem inflammatory syndrome, and Z86.16, Personal history of COVID-19.

If an individual with a known or suspected exposure to COVID-19, and no current COVID-19 infection or history of COVID-19, develops MIS, assign codes M35.81, Multisystem inflammatory syndrome, and Z20.822, Contact with and (suspected) exposure to COVID-19.

Additional codes should be assigned for any associated complications of MIS.

U07.1 COVID-19

Use additional code to identify pneumonia or other manifestations

Excludes1: Coronavirus infection, unspecified (B34.2)
Coronavirus as the cause of diseases classified elsewhere (B97.2-)
Pneumonia due to SARS-associated coronavirus (J12.81)

•U09 POST COVID-19 CONDITION

4th **•U09.9 Post COVID-19 condition, unspecified**

Note: This code enables establishment of a link with COVID-19.

This code is not to be used in cases that are still presenting with active COVID-19. However, an exception is made in cases of re-infection with COVID-19, occurring with a condition related to prior COVID-19.

Post-acute sequela of COVID-19

Code first the specific condition related to COVID-19 if known, such as:
chronic respiratory failure (J96.1-)
loss of smell (R43.8)
loss of taste (R43.8)
multisystem inflammatory syndrome (M35.81)
pulmonary embolism (I26.-)
pulmonary fibrosis (J84.10)

 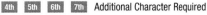 Additional Character Required   ✔ 3-character code   •=New Code   ***Excludes1***—Not coded here, do not use together
▲=Revised Code   ***Excludes2***—Not included here

462   **PEDIATRIC ICD-10-CM 2022: A MANUAL FOR PROVIDER-BASED CODING**

ICD-10-CM EXTERNAL CAUSE OF INJURIES DUE TO COLLISIONS TABLE

These tables are inserted for ease to locate an external cause code from a transport accident.
If not listed here, refer to the index. All codes require additional characters.
4th, 5th, 6th characters are "X" if not listed and all 7th characters (A, D, S) refer to encounter.

ICD-10-CM EXTERNAL CAUSE OF INJURIES DUE TO COLLISIONS TABLE

	Collides with											
	Pedestrian Conveyance	Car/Pick-up Truck/Van	Bike	Bus/HTV	Fixed Object	E-Scooter	Micro-Mobility	Train/Train Car	2 or 3 Motor Wheeler	Non-Motor Vehicle	Other (NOS)	Unspecified
Pedestrian on foot	V00.01 R V00.02 S V00.09 O	V03.00 N V03.10 T V03.90 U	V01.00 N V01.10 T V01.90 U	V04.00 N V04.10 T V04.90 U	Refer to W22	V00.031	V00.038	V05.00 N V05.10 T V05.90 U	V02.00 N V02.10 T V02.90 U	V06.00 N V06.10 T V06.90 U	V09.09 N V09.29 T	V09.00 N V09.20 T

	Collides with									
Activity of the Person Injured	Car/Pick-up Truck/Van	Bike	Bus/HTV	Fixed Object	Pedestrian or Animal	Train/Train Car	2 or 3 Motor Wheeler	Non-Motor Vehicle	Other (NOS)	Unspecified
In-line skater (I)/Roller skater (R)	V03.01 N V03.11 T V03.91 U	V01.01 N V01.11 T V01.91 U	V04.01 N V04.11 T V04.91 U	V00.112 I V00.122 R	V00.118 I V00.128 R	V05.01 N V05.11 T V05.91 U	V02.01 N V02.11 T V02.91 U	V06.01 N V06.11 T V06.91 U	V00.118 I	
Skateboarder	V03.02 N V03.12 T V03.92 U	V01.02 N V01.12 T V01.92 U	V04.02 N V04.12 T V04.92 U	V00.132	V00.138	V05.02 N V05.12 T V05.92 U	V02.02 N V02.12 T V02.92 U	V06.02 N V06.12 T V06.92 U	V00.138	
E-Scooter	V03.031 N V03.131 T V03.931 U	V01.031 N V01.131 T V01.931 U	V04.031 N V04.131 T V04.931 U	V00.842		V05.031 N V05.131 T V05.931 U	V02.031 N V02.131 T V02.931 U	V06.031 N V06.131 T V06.931 U		
Micro-mobility	V03.038 N V03.138 T V03.938 U	V01.038 N V01.138 T V01.938 U	V04.038 N V04.138 T V04.938 U			V05.038 N V05.138 T V05.938 U	V02.038 N V02.138 T V02.938 U	V06.038 N V06.138 T V06.938 U	V00.848	
Other (NOS)	V03.09 N V03.19 T V03.99 U	V01.09 N V01.19 T V01.99 U	V04.09 N V04.19 T V04.99 U			V05.09 N V05.19 T V05.99 U	V02.09 N V02.19 T V02.99 U	V06.09 N V06.19 T V06.99 U		
Scooter (Non-motorized)	V03.09 N V03.19 T V03.99 U	V01.09 N V01.19 T V01.99 U	V04.09 N V04.19 T V04.99 U	V00.142		V05.09 N V05.19 T V05.99 U	V02.09 N V02.19 T V02.99 U	V06.09 N V06.19 T V06.99 U		
Heelies	V03.09 N V03.19 T V03.99 U	V01.09 N V01.19 T V01.99 U	V04.09 N V04.19 T V04.99 U	V00.152		V05.09 N V05.19 T V05.99 U	V02.09 N V02.19 T V02.99 U	V06.09 N V06.19 T V06.99 U		
Ice-skater	V03.09 N V03.19 T V03.99 U	V01.09 N V01.19 T V01.99 U	V04.09 N V04.19 T V04.99 U	V00.212		V05.09 N V05.19 T V05.99 U	V02.09 N V02.19 T V02.99 U	V06.09 N V06.19 T V06.99 U		
Sledder	V03.09 N V03.19 T V03.99 U	V01.09 N V01.19 T V01.99 U	V04.09 N V04.19 T V04.99 U	V00.222		V05.09 N V05.19 T V05.99 U	V02.09 N V02.19 T V02.99 U	V06.09 N V06.19 T V06.99 U		
Snowboarder	V03.09 N V03.19 T V03.99 U	V01.09 N V01.19 T V01.99 U	V04.09 N V04.19 T V04.99 U	V00.312		V05.09 N V05.19 T V05.99 U	V02.09 N V02.19 T V02.99 U	V06.09 N V06.19 T V06.99 U		
Snowskier	V03.09 N V03.19 T V03.99 U	V01.09 N V01.19 T V01.99 U	V04.09 N V04.19 T V04.99 U	V00.322		V05.09 N V05.19 T V05.99 U	V02.09 N V02.19 T V02.99 U	V06.09 N V06.19 T V06.99 U		
Wheelchair	V03.09 N V03.19 T V03.99 U	V01.09 N V01.19 T V01.99 U	V04.09 N V04.19 T V04.99 U	V00.812		V05.09 N V05.19 T V05.99 U	V02.09 N V02.19 T V02.99 U	V06.09 N V06.19 T V06.99 U		

I = In-line skates; R = roller skates; N = nontraffic accident; T = traffic accident; U = unspecified whether traffic or not

Collides with

Activity of the Person Injured	Car/Pick-up Truck/Van	Bike	Bus/HTV	Fixed Object	Pedestrian or Animal	Train/Train Car	2 or 3 Motor Wheeler	Non-Motor Vehicle	Other (NOS)	Unspecified
Bike										
Driver	V13.0 N / V13.4 T	V11.0 N / V11.4 T	V14.0 N / V14.4 T	V17.0 N / V17.4 T	V10.0 N / V10.4 T	V15.0 N / V15.4 T	V12.0 N / V12.4 T	V16.0 N / V16.4 T	V19.09 N / V19.49 T	V19.00 N / V19.40 T
Passenger	V13.1 N / V13.5 T	V11.1 N / V11.5 T	V14.1 N / V14.5 T	V17.1 N / V17.5 T	V10.1 N / V10.5 T	V15.1 N / V15.5 T	V12.1 N / V12.5 T	V16.1 N / V16.5 T	V19.19 N / V19.59 T	V19.10 N / V19.50 T
Boarding	V13.3	V11.3	V14.3	V17.3	V10.3	V15.3	V12.3	V16.3		
Unspecified	V13.2 N / V13.9 T	V11.2 N / V11.9 T	V14.2 N / V14.9 T	V17.2 N / V17.9 T	V10.2 N / V10.9 T	V15.2 N / V15.9 T	V12.2 N / V12.9 T	V16.2 N / V16.9 T	V19.29 N / V19.69 T	V19.20 N / V19.60 T
Motorcycle/Motor Scooter/Moped										
Driver	V23.0 N / V23.4 T	V21.0 N / V21.4 T	V24.0 N / V24.4 T	V27.0 N / V27.4 T	V20.0 N / V20.4 T	V25.0 N / V25.4 T	V22.0 N / V22.4 T	V26.0 N / V26.4 T	V29.09 N / V29.49 T	V29.00 N / V29.40 T
Passenger	V23.1 N / V23.5 T	V21.1 N / V21.5 T	V24.1 N / V24.5 T	V27.1 N / V27.5 T	V20.1 N / V20.5 T	V25.1 N / V25.5 T	V22.1 N / V22.5 T	V26.1 N / V26.5 T	V29.19 N / V29.59 T	V29.10 N / V29.50 T
Boarding	V23.3	V21.3	V24.3	V27.3	V20.3	V25.3	V22.3	V26.3		
Unspecified	V23.2 N / V23.9 T	V21.2 N / V21.9 T	V24.2 N / V24.9 T	V27.2 N / V27.9 T	V20.2 N / V20.9 T	V25.2 N / V25.9 T	V22.2 N / V22.9 T	V26.2 N / V26.9 T	V29.29 N / V29.69 T	V29.20 N / V29.60 T
3-wheel vehicle										
Driver	V33.0 N / V33.5 T	V31.0 N / V31.5 T	V34.0 N / V34.5 T	V37.0 N / V37.5 T	V30.0 N / V30.5 T	V35.0 N / V35.5 T	V32.0 N / V32.5 T	V36.0 N / V36.5 T	V39.09 N / V39.49 T	V39.00 N / V39.40 T
Passenger	V33.1 N / V33.6 T	V31.1 N / V31.6 T	V34.1 N / V34.6 T	V37.1 N / V37.6 T	V30.1 N / V30.6 T	V35.1 N / V35.6 T	V32.1 N / V32.6 T	V36.1 N / V36.6 T	V39.19 N / V39.59 T	V39.10 N / V39.50 T
Rider on outside	V33.2 N / V33.7 T	V31.2 N / V31.7 T	V34.2 N / V34.7 T	V37.2 N / V37.7 T	V30.2 N / V30.7 T	V35.2 N / V35.7 T	V32.2 N / V32.7 T	V36.2 N / V36.7 T		
Boarding	V33.4	V31.4	V34.4	V37.4	V30.4	V35.4	V32.4	V36.4		
Unspecified	V33.3 N / V33.9 T	V31.3 N / V31.9 T	V34.3 N / V34.9 T	V37.3 N / V37.9 T	V30.3 N / V30.9 T	V35.3 N / V35.9 T	V32.3 N / V32.9 T	V36.3 N / V36.9 T	V39.29 N / V39.69 T	V39.20 N / V39.60 T
Car										
Driver	V43.0- N / V43.5- T	V41.0 N / V41.5 T	V44.0 N / V44.5 T	V47.0- N / V47.5- T	V40.0 N / V40.5 T	V45.0 N / V45.5 T	V42.0 N / V42.5 T	V46.0 N / V46.5 T	V49.09 N / V49.49 T	V49.00 N / V49.40 T
Passenger	V43.1- N / V43.6- T	V41.1 N / V41.6 T	V44.1 N / V44.6 T	V47.1- N / V47.6- T	V40.1 N / V40.6 T	V45.1 N / V45.6 T	V42.1 N / V42.6 T	V46.1 N / V46.6 T	V49.19 N / V49.59 T	V49.10 N / V49.50 T
Rider on outside	V43.2- N / V43.7- T	V41.2 N / V41.7 T	V44.2 N / V44.7 T	V47.2- N / V47.7- T	V40.2 N / V40.7 T	V45.2 N / V45.7 T	V42.2 N / V42.7 T	V46.2 N / V46.7 T	V59.3 N / V59.9 T	
Boarding	V43.4-	V41.4	V44.4	V47.4-	V40.4	V45.4	V42.4	V46.4		
Unspecified	V43.3- N / V43.9- T	V41.3 N / V41.9 T	V44.3 N / V44.9 T	V47.3- N / V47.9- T	V40.3 N / V40.9 T	V45.3 N / V45.9 T	V42.3 N / V42.9 T	V46.3 N / V46.9 T	V49.29 N / V49.69 T	V49.20 N / V49.60 T
Pick-up Truck/Van/SUV										
Driver	V53.0 N / V53.5 T	V51.0 N / V51.5 T	V54.0 N / V54.5 T	V57.0 N / V57.5 T	V50.0 N / V50.5 T	V55.0 N / V55.5 T	V52.0 N / V52.5 T	V56.0 N / V56.5 T	V59.09 N / V59.49 T	V59.00 N / V59.40 T
Passenger	V53.1 N / V53.6 T	V51.1 N / V51.6 T	V54.1 N / V54.6 T	V57.1 N / V57.6 T	V50.1 N / V50.6 T	V55.1 N / V55.6 T	V52.1 N / V52.6 T	V56.1 N / V56.6 T	V59.19 N / V59.59 T	V59.10 N / V59.50 T

I = In-line skates; R = roller skates; N = nontraffic accident; T = traffic accident; U = unspecified whether traffic or not

ICD-10-CM EXTERNAL CAUSE OF INJURIES DUE TO COLLISIONS TABLE

Collides with

Activity of the Person Injured	Car/Pick-up Truck/Van	Bike	Bus/HTV	Fixed Object	Pedestrian or Animal	Train/Train Car	2 or 3 Motor Wheeler	Non-Motor Vehicle	Other (NOS)	Unspecified
Rider on outside	V53.2 N V53.7 T	V51.2 N V51.7 T	V54.2 N V54.7 T	V57.2 N V57.7 T	V50.2 N V50.7 T	V55.2 N V55.7 T	V52.2 N V52.7 T	V56.2 N V56.7 T		
Boarding	V53.4	V51.4	V54.4	V57.4	V50.4	V55.4	V52.4	V56.4		
Unspecified	V53.3 N V53.9 T	V51.3 N V51.9 T	V54.3 N V54.9 T	V57.3 N V57.9 T	V50.3 N V50.9 T	V55.3 N V55.9 T	V52.3 N V52.9 T	V56.3 N V56.9 T	V59.29 N V59.69 T	V59.20 N V59.60 T
Bus										
Driver	V73.0 N V73.5 T	V71.0 N V71.5 T	V74.0 N V74.5 T	V77.0 N V77.5 T	V70.0 N V70.5 T	V75.0 N V75.5 T	V72.0 N V72.5 T	V76.0 N V76.5 T	V79.09 N V79.49 T	V79.00 N V79.40 T
Passenger	V73.1 N V73.6 T	V71.1 N V71.6 T	V74.1 N V74.6 T	V77.1 N V77.6 T	V70.1 N V70.6 T	V75.1 N V75.6 T	V72.1 N V72.6 T	V76.1 N V76.6 T	V79.19 N V79.59 T	V79.10 N V79.50 T
Rider on outside	V73.2 N V73.7 T	V71.2 N V71.7 T	V74.2 N V74.7 T	V77.2 N V77.7 T	V70.2 N V70.7 T	V75.2 N V75.7 T	V72.2 N V72.7 T	V76.2 N V76.7 T		V79.3 N V79.9 T
Boarding	V73.4	V71.4	V74.4	V77.4	V70.4	V75.4	V72.4	V76.4		
Unspecified	V73.3 N V73.9 T	V71.3 N V71.9 T	V74.3 N V74.9 T	V77.3 N V77.9 T	V70.3 N V70.9 T	V75.3 N V75.9 T	V72.3 N V72.9 T	V76.3 N V76.9 T	V79.29 N V79.69 T	V79.20 N V79.60 T
Animal Rider	V80.41	V80.21	V80.41	V80.81	V80.710[a] V80.720[a]	V80.61	V80.31	V80.790	V80.51	V80.919
Animal-Drawn Vehicle	V80.42	V80.22	V80.42	V80.82	V80.711[b] V80.721[b]	V80.62	V80.32	V80.791	V80.52	V80.929

Vehicle

Injured Person	Special Agriculture Vehicle	Snowmobile	Dune Buggy	3 or 4 Wheel ATV	Dirt Bike	Other ATV (eg, go-cart, golf cart)
Driver	V84.0 T V84.5 N	V86.02 T V86.52 N	V86.03 T V86.53 N	V86.05 T V86.55 N	V86.06 T V86.56 N	V86.09 T V86.59 N
Passenger	V84.1 T V84.6 N	V86.12 T V86.62 N	V86.13 T V86.63 N	V86.15 T V86.65 N	V86.16 T V86.66 N	V86.19 T V86.69 N
Outside rider	V84.2 T V84.7 N	V86.22 T V86.72 N	V86.23 T V86.73 N	V86.25 T V86.75 N		
Unspecified	V84.3 T V84.9 N	V86.32 T V86.92 N	V86.33 T V86.93 N	V86.35 T V86.95 N	V86.36 T V86.96 N	V86.39 T V86.99 N
Boarding	V84.4	V86.42	V86.43	V86.45	V86.46	V86.49

[a] Collision with other animal being ridden
[b] Collision with animal-drawn vehicle
I = In-line skates; R = roller skates; N = nontraffic accident; T = traffic accident; U = unspecified whether traffic or not

ICD-10-CM EXTERNAL CAUSE
OF INJURIES INDEX

A

Refer to the External Cause of Injury Table **first** for those injuries resulting from a number of collisions (eg, cars, trucks, bikes, e-scooters).

Abandonment (causing exposure to weather conditions) (with intent to injure or kill) NEC X58

Abuse (adult) (child) (mental) (physical) (sexual) X58

Accident (to) X58
- aircraft (in transit) (powered)—*see also* Accident, transport, aircraft
  - due to, caused by cataclysm—*see* Forces of nature, by type
- animal-rider—*see* Accident, transport, animal-rider
- animal-drawn vehicle—*see* Accident, transport, animal-drawn vehicle occupant
- automobile—*see* Accident, transport, car occupant
- bare foot water skier V94.4
- boat, boating—*see also* Accident, watercraft
  - striking swimmer
    - powered V94.11
    - unpowered V94.12
- bus—*see* Accident, transport, bus occupant
- cable car, not on rails V98.0
  - on rails—*see* Accident, transport, streetcar occupant
- car—*see* Accident, transport, car occupant
- caused by, due to
  - chain hoist W24.0
  - cold (excessive)—*see* Exposure, cold
  - corrosive liquid, substance—*see* Table of Drugs and Chemicals
  - cutting or piercing instrument—*see* Contact, with, by type of instrument
  - drive belt W24.0
  - electric
    - current—*see* Exposure, electric current
    - motor (*see also* Contact, with, by type of machine) W31.3
      - current (of) W86.8
  - environmental factor NEC X58
  - explosive material—*see* Explosion
  - fire, flames—*see* Exposure, fire
  - firearm missile—*see* Discharge, firearm by type
  - heat (excessive)—*see* Heat
  - hot—*see* Contact, with, hot
  - ignition—*see* Ignition
  - lifting device W24.0
  - lightning—*see* subcategory T75.0
    - causing fire—*see* Exposure, fire
  - machine, machinery—*see* Contact, with, by type of machine
  - natural factor NEC X58
  - pulley (block) W24.0
  - radiation—*see* Radiation
  - steam X13.1
    - inhalation X13.0
    - pipe X16
  - thunderbolt—*see* subcategory T75.0
    - causing fire—*see* Exposure, fire
  - transmission device W24.1
- diving—*see also* Fall, into, water
  - with
    - drowning or submersion—*see* Drowning
- ice yacht V98.2
- in
  - medical, surgical procedure
    - as, or due to misadventure—*see* Misadventure
    - causing an abnormal reaction or later complication without mention of misadventure (*see also* Complication of or following, by type of procedure) Y84.9
- land yacht V98.1
- late effect of—*see* W00-X58 with 7th character S
- logging car—*see* Accident, transport, industrial vehicle occupant
- machine, machinery—*see also* Contact, with, by type of machine
  - on board watercraft V93.69
    - explosion—*see* Explosion, in, watercraft
    - fire—*see* Burn, on board watercraft
    - powered craft V93.63
      - ferry boat V93.61

Accident (to), *continued*
- ~ fishing boat V93.62
- ~ jet skis V93.63
- ~ liner V93.61
- ~ merchant ship V93.60
- ~ passenger ship V93.61
- ~ sailboat V93.64
- mobility scooter (motorized)—*see* Accident, transport, pedestrian, conveyance, specified type NEC
- motor scooter—*see* Accident, transport, motorcyclist
- motor vehicle NOS (traffic) (*see also* Accident, transport) V89.2
  - nontraffic V89.0
  - three-wheeled NOS—*see* Accident, transport, three-wheeled motor vehicle occupant
- motorcycle NOS—*see* Accident, transport, motorcyclist
- nonmotor vehicle NOS (nontraffic) (*see also* Accident, transport) V89.1
  - traffic NOS V89.3
- nontraffic (victim's mode of transport NOS) V88.9
  - collision (between) V88.7
    - bus and truck V88.5
    - car and:
      - ~ bus V88.3
      - ~ pickup V88.2
      - ~ three-wheeled motor vehicle V88.0
      - ~ train V88.6
      - ~ truck V88.4
      - ~ two-wheeled motor vehicle V88.0
      - ~ van V88.2
    - specified vehicle NEC and:
      - ~ three-wheeled motor vehicle V88.1
      - ~ two-wheeled motor vehicle V88.1
  - known mode of transport—*see* Accident, transport, by type of vehicle
  - noncollision V88.8
- on board watercraft V93.8-
  - inflatable V93.86
    - in tow
      - ~ recreational V94.31
      - ~ specified NEC V94.32
- parachutist V97.29
  - entangled in object V97.21
  - injured on landing V97.22
- pedal cycle—*see* Accident, transport, pedal cyclist
- pedestrian (on foot)
  - with
    - another pedestrian W51
      - ~ with fall W03
        - ◊ due to ice or snow W00.0
    - rider of
      - ~ electric scooter V00.031
      - ~ hoverboard V00.038
      - ~ micro-mobility pedestrian conveyance NEC V00.038
      - ~ Segway V00.038
    - transport vehicle—*see* Accident, transport
  - on pedestrian conveyance—*see* Accident, transport, pedestrian, conveyance
- quarry truck—*see* Accident, transport, industrial vehicle occupant
- railway vehicle (any) (in motion)—*see* Accident, transport, railway vehicle occupant
  - due to cataclysm—*see* Forces of nature, by type
- scooter (non-motorized)—*see* Accident, transport, pedestrian, conveyance, scooter
- skateboard—*see* Accident, transport, pedestrian, conveyance, skateboard
- ski(ing)—*see* Accident, transport, pedestrian, conveyance
  - lift V98.3
- specified cause NEC X58
- streetcar—*see* Accident, transport, streetcar occupant
- traffic (victim's mode of transport NOS) V87.9
  - collision (between) V87.7
    - bus and truck V87.5
    - car and:
      - ~ bus V87.3
      - ~ pickup V87.2
      - ~ three-wheeled motor vehicle V87.0
      - ~ train V87.6
      - ~ truck V87.4

Accident (to), *continued*
- ~ two-wheeled motor vehicle V87.0
- ~ van V87.2
  - specified vehicle NEC V86.39
    - ~ three-wheeled motor vehicle V87.1
    - ~ two-wheeled motor vehicle V87.1
  - known mode of transport—*see* Accident, transport, by type of vehicle
  - noncollision V87.8
- transport (involving injury to) V99
  - agricultural vehicle occupant (nontraffic) V84.-
  - aircraft V97.8-
    - occupant injured (in)
      - ~ nonpowered craft accident V96.9
        - ◊ balloon V96.0-
        - ◊ glider V96.2-
        - ◊ hang glider V96.1-
        - ◊ specified craft NEC V96.8
      - ~ powered craft accident V95.9
        - ◊ fixed wing NEC
          - » commercial V95.3-
          - » private V95.2-
        - ◊ glider (powered) V95.1-
        - ◊ helicopter V95.0-
        - ◊ specified craft NEC V95.8
        - ◊ ultralight V95.1-
      - ~ specified accident NEC V97.0
      - ~ while boarding or alighting V97.1
    - person (injured by)
      - ~ falling from, in or on aircraft V97.0
      - ~ machinery on aircraft V97.89
      - ~ on ground with aircraft involvement V97.39
      - ~ while boarding or alighting aircraft V97.1
  - airport (battery-powered) passenger vehicle—*see* Accident, transport, industrial vehicle occupant
  - all-terrain vehicle occupant (nontraffic) V86.99
    - driver V86.59
    - dune buggy—*see* Accident, transport, dune buggy occupant
    - passenger V86.69
  - animal-drawn vehicle occupant (in) V80.929
    - collision (with)
      - ~ animal V80.12
        - ◊ being ridden V80.711
      - ~ animal-drawn vehicle V80.721
      - ~ fixed or stationary object V80.82
      - ~ nonmotor vehicle V80.791
      - ~ pedestrian V80.12
      - ~ streetcar V80.731
    - noncollision V80.02
    - specified circumstance NEC V80.928
  - animal-rider V80.919
    - collision (with)
      - ~ animal V80.11
        - ◊ being ridden V80.710
      - ~ animal-drawn vehicle V80.720
      - ~ fixed or stationary object V80.81
      - ~ nonmotor vehicle V80.790
      - ~ pedestrian V80.11
      - ~ streetcar V80.730
    - noncollision V80.018
      - ~ specified as horse rider V80.010
    - specified circumstance NEC V80.918
  - bus occupant V79.9
    - collision (with)
    - driver
      - ~ collision (with)
      - ~ noncollision accident (traffic) V78.5
        - ◊ nontraffic V78.0
    - noncollision accident (traffic) V78.9
      - ~ nontraffic V78.3
      - ~ while boarding or alighting V78.4
      - ~ noncollision accident (traffic) V78.7
        - ◊ nontraffic V78.2
    - passenger
      - ~ collision (with)
      - ~ noncollision accident (traffic) V78.6
        - ◊ nontraffic V78.1
    - specified type NEC V79.88
      - ~ military vehicle V79.81
  - cable car, not on rails V98.0
    - on rails—*see* Accident, transport, streetcar occupant

Accident (to), *continued*
- car occupant V49.9
  - ambulance occupant—*see* Accident, transport, ambulance occupant
  - collision (with)
    - ◊ animal being ridden (traffic) V46.9
      - » nontraffic V46.3
      - » while boarding or alighting V46.4
    - ~ animal-drawn vehicle (traffic) V46.9
      - ◊ nontraffic V46.3
      - ◊ while boarding or alighting V46.4
    - ~ car (traffic) V43.92
      - ◊ nontraffic V43.32
      - ◊ while boarding or alighting V43.42
    - ~ motor vehicle NOS (traffic) V49.60
      - ◊ nontraffic V49.20
      - ◊ specified type NEC (traffic) V49.69
        - » nontraffic V49.29
    - ~ pickup truck (traffic) V43.93
      - ◊ nontraffic V43.33
      - ◊ while boarding or alighting V43.43
    - ~ specified vehicle NEC (traffic) V46.9
      - ◊ nontraffic V46.3
      - ◊ while boarding or alighting V46.4
    - ~ sport utility vehicle (traffic) V43.91
      - ◊ nontraffic V43.31
      - ◊ while boarding or alighting V43.41
    - ~ stationary object (traffic) V47.92
      - ◊ while boarding or alighting V47.4
    - ~ streetcar (traffic) V46.9
      - ◊ nontraffic V46.3
      - ◊ while boarding or alighting V46.4
    - ~ van (traffic) V43.94
      - ◊ nontraffic V43.34
      - ◊ while boarding or alighting V43.44
  - driver
    - ~ collision (with)
      - » animal being ridden (traffic) V46.5
        - ❖ nontraffic V46.0
      - ◊ animal-drawn vehicle (traffic) V46.5
        - » nontraffic V46.0
      - ◊ car (traffic) V43.52
        - » nontraffic V43.02
      - ◊ motor vehicle NOS (traffic) V49.40
        - » nontraffic V49.00
        - » specified type NEC (traffic) V49.49
          - ❖ nontraffic V49.09
      - ◊ pickup truck (traffic) V43.53
        - » nontraffic V43.03
      - ◊ specified vehicle NEC (traffic) V46.5
        - » nontraffic V46.0
      - ◊ sport utility vehicle (traffic) V43.51
        - » nontraffic V43.01
      - ◊ streetcar (traffic) V46.5
        - » nontraffic V46.0
      - ◊ van (traffic) V43.54
        - » nontraffic V43.04
    - ~ noncollision accident (traffic) V48.5
      - ◊ nontraffic V48.0
  - noncollision accident (traffic) V48.9
    - ~ nontraffic V48.3
    - ~ while boarding or alighting V48.4
  - nontraffic V49.3
  - hanger-on
    - ~ collision (with)
      - » animal being ridden (traffic) V46.7
        - ❖ nontraffic V46.2
      - ◊ animal-drawn vehicle (traffic) V46.7
        - » nontraffic V46.2
      - ◊ car (traffic) V43.72
        - » nontraffic V43.22
      - ◊ pickup truck (traffic) V43.73
        - » nontraffic V43.23
      - ◊ specified vehicle NEC (traffic) V46.7
        - » nontraffic V46.2
      - ◊ sport utility vehicle (traffic) V43.71
        - » nontraffic V43.21
      - ◊ stationary object (traffic) V47.7
        - » nontraffic V47.2
      - ◊ streetcar (traffic) V46.7
        - » nontraffic V46.2
      - ◊ van (traffic) V43.74
        - » nontraffic V43.24

Accident (to), *continued*
- ~ noncollision accident (traffic) V48.7
  - ◊ nontraffic V48.2
- passenger
  - ~ collision (with)
    - » animal being ridden (traffic) V46.6
      - ❖ nontraffic V46.1
    - ◊ animal-drawn vehicle (traffic) V46.6
      - » nontraffic V46.1
    - ◊ car (traffic) V43.62
      - » nontraffic V43.12
    - ◊ motor vehicle NOS (traffic) V49.50
      - » nontraffic V49.10
      - » specified type NEC (traffic) V49.59
        - ❖ nontraffic V49.19
    - ◊ pickup truck (traffic) V43.63
      - » nontraffic V43.13
    - ◊ specified vehicle NEC (traffic) V46.6
      - » nontraffic V46.1
    - ◊ sport utility vehicle (traffic) V43.61
      - » nontraffic V43.11
    - ◊ streetcar (traffic) V46.6
      - » nontraffic V46.1
    - ◊ van (traffic) V43.64
      - » nontraffic V43.14
  - ~ noncollision accident (traffic) V48.6
    - ◊ nontraffic V48.1
  - specified type NEC V49.88
- due to cataclysm—*see* Forces of nature, by type
- hoverboard V00.848
- ice yacht V98.2
- industrial vehicle occupant (nontraffic) V83.-
- land yacht V98.1
- logging car—*see* Accident, transport, industrial vehicle occupant
- motorcoach—*see* Accident, transport, bus occupant
- motorcyclist V29.9
  - collision (with)
    - ◊ animal being ridden (traffic) V26.9
      - » nontraffic V26.2
      - » while boarding or alighting V26.3
    - ~ animal-drawn vehicle (traffic) V26.9
      - ◊ nontraffic V26.2
      - ◊ while boarding or alighting V26.3
    - ~ motor vehicle NOS (traffic) V29.60
      - ◊ nontraffic V29.20
      - ◊ specified type NEC (traffic) V29.69
        - » nontraffic V29.29
    - ~ specified vehicle NEC (traffic) V26.9
      - ◊ nontraffic V26.2
      - ◊ while boarding or alighting V26.3
    - ~ streetcar (traffic) V26.9
      - ◊ nontraffic V26.2
      - ◊ while boarding or alighting V26.3
  - driver
    - ~ collision (with)
      - » animal being ridden (traffic) V26.4
        - ❖ nontraffic V26.0
      - ◊ animal-drawn vehicle (traffic) V26.4
        - » nontraffic V26.0
      - ◊ specified vehicle NEC (traffic) V26.4
        - » nontraffic V26.0
      - ◊ streetcar (traffic) V26.4
        - » nontraffic V26.0
    - ~ noncollision accident (traffic) V28.4
      - ◊ nontraffic V28.0
  - noncollision accident (traffic) V28.9
    - ~ nontraffic V28.2
    - ~ while boarding or alighting V28.3
  - nontraffic V29.3
  - passenger
    - ~ collision (with)
      - » animal being ridden (traffic) V26.5
        - ❖ nontraffic V26.1
      - ◊ animal-drawn vehicle (traffic) V26.5
        - » nontraffic V26.1
      - ◊ specified vehicle NEC (traffic) V26.5
      - ◊ streetcar (traffic) V26.5
        - » nontraffic V26.1
    - ~ noncollision accident (traffic) V28.5
      - ◊ nontraffic V28.1
  - specified type NEC V29.88
    - ~ military vehicle V29.81

Accident (to), *continued*
- motor vehicle NEC occupant (traffic) V86.39
- occupant (of)
  - aircraft (powered) V95.9
    - ~ nonpowered V96.9
    - ~ specified NEC V95.8
  - airport battery-powered vehicle—*see* Accident, transport, industrial vehicle occupant
  - all-terrain vehicle (ATV)—*see* Accident, transport, all-terrain vehicle occupant
  - animal-drawn vehicle—*see* Accident, transport, animal-drawn vehicle occupant
  - automobile—*see* Accident, transport, car occupant
  - balloon V96.00
  - battery-powered vehicle—*see* Accident, transport, industrial vehicle occupant
  - bicycle—*see* Accident, transport, pedal cyclist
    - ~ motorized—*see* Accident, transport, motorcycle rider
  - boat NEC—*see* Accident, watercraft
  - bus—*see* Accident, transport, bus occupant
  - cable car (on rails)—*see also* Accident, transport, streetcar occupant
    - ~ not on rails V98.0
  - car—*see also* Accident, transport, car occupant
    - ~ cable (on rails)—*see also* Accident, transport, streetcar occupant
      - ◊ not on rails V98.0
  - coach—*see* Accident, transport, bus occupant
  - farm machinery (self-propelled)—*see* Accident, transport, agricultural vehicle occupant
  - forklift—*see* Accident, transport, industrial vehicle occupant
  - glider (unpowered) V96.20
    - ~ hang V96.10
    - ~ powered (microlight) (ultralight)—*see* Accident, transport, aircraft, occupant, powered, glider
  - glider (unpowered) NEC V96.20
  - hang-glider V96.10
  - heavy (transport) vehicle—*see* Accident, transport, truck occupant
  - ice-yacht V98.2
  - kite (carrying person) V96.8
  - land-yacht V98.1
  - microlight—*see* Accident, transport, aircraft, occupant, powered, glider
  - motor scooter—*see* Accident, transport, motorcycle
  - motorcycle (with sidecar)—*see* Accident, transport, motorcycle
  - pedal cycle—*see also* Accident, transport, pedal cyclist
  - pick-up (truck)—*see* Accident, transport, pickup truck occupant
  - railway (train) (vehicle) (subterranean) (elevated)—*see* Accident, transport, railway vehicle occupant
    - ~ motorized—*see* Accident, transport, three-wheeled motor vehicle
    - ~ pedal driven—*see* Accident, transport, pedal cyclist
  - ship NOS V94.9
  - ski-lift (chair) (gondola) V98.3
  - sport utility vehicle—*see* Accident, transport, car occupant
  - streetcar (interurban) (operating on public street or highway)—*see* Accident, transport, streetcar occupant
  - three-wheeled vehicle (motorized)—*see also* Accident, transport, three-wheeled motor vehicle occupant
    - ~ nonmotorized—*see* Accident, transport, pedal cycle
  - tractor (farm) (and trailer)—*see* Accident, transport, agricultural vehicle occupant
  - train—*see* Accident, transport, railway vehicle occupant
  - tram—*see* Accident, transport, streetcar occupant
  - tricycle—*see* Accident, transport, pedal cycle
    - ~ motorized—*see* Accident, transport, three-wheeled motor vehicle

Accident (to), *continued*
◊ two-or three-wheeled motor vehicle (traffic) V87.0
» nontraffic V88.0
~ motor vehicle (traffic) NEC V87.7
◊ nontraffic V88.7
~ two-or three-wheeled vehicle (with) (traffic)
◊ motor vehicle NEC V87.1
» nontraffic V88.1
■ nonmotor vehicle (collision) (noncollision) (traffic) V87.9
~ nontraffic V88.9
– pickup truck occupant V59.9
■ collision (with)
~ animal (traffic) V50.9
◊ animal being ridden (traffic) V56.9
» nontraffic V56.3
» while boarding or alighting V56.4
~ animal-drawn vehicle (traffic) V56.9
◊ nontraffic V56.3
◊ while boarding or alighting V56.4
~ motor vehicle NOS (traffic) V59.60
◊ nontraffic V59.20
◊ specified type NEC (traffic) V59.69
» nontraffic V59.29
~ specified vehicle NEC (traffic) V56.9
◊ nontraffic V56.3
◊ while boarding or alighting V56.4
~ streetcar (traffic) V56.9
◊ nontraffic V56.3
◊ while boarding or alighting V56.4
■ driver
~ collision (with)
» animal being ridden (traffic) V56.5
❖ nontraffic V56.0
◊ animal-drawn vehicle (traffic) V56.5
» nontraffic V56.0
◊ motor vehicle NOS (traffic) V59.40
» nontraffic V59.00
» specified type NEC (traffic) V59.49
❖ nontraffic V59.09
◊ specified vehicle NEC (traffic) V56.5
» nontraffic V56.0
◊ streetcar (traffic) V56.5
» nontraffic V56.0
~ noncollision accident (traffic) V58.5
◊ nontraffic V58.0
■ noncollision accident (traffic) V58.9
~ nontraffic V58.3
~ while boarding or alighting V58.4
■ nontraffic V59.3
■ hanger-on
~ collision (with)
» animal being ridden (traffic) V56.7
❖ nontraffic V56.2
◊ animal-drawn vehicle (traffic) V56.7
» nontraffic V56.2
◊ specified vehicle NEC (traffic) V56.7
» nontraffic V56.2
◊ streetcar (traffic) V56.7
» nontraffic V56.2
~ noncollision accident (traffic) V58.7
◊ nontraffic V58.2
■ passenger
~ collision (with)
» animal being ridden (traffic) V56.6
❖ nontraffic V56.1
◊ animal-drawn vehicle (traffic) V56.6
» nontraffic V56.1
◊ motor vehicle NOS (traffic) V59.50
» nontraffic V59.10
» specified type NEC (traffic) V59.59
❖ nontraffic V59.19
◊ specified vehicle NEC (traffic) V56.6
» nontraffic V56.1
◊ streetcar (traffic) V56.6
» nontraffic V56.1
~ noncollision accident (traffic) V58.6
◊ nontraffic V58.1
■ specified type NEC V59.88
~ military vehicle V59.81

Accident (to), *continued*
– railway vehicle occupant V81.9
■ collision (with) V81.3
~ motor vehicle (non-military) (traffic) V81.1
◊ military V81.83
◊ nontraffic V81.0
~ rolling stock V81.2
~ specified object NEC V81.3
■ during derailment V81.7
■ explosion V81.81
■ fall (in railway vehicle) V81.5
~ during derailment V81.7
~ from railway vehicle V81.6
◊ during derailment V81.7
~ while boarding or alighting V81.4
■ fire V81.81
■ object falling onto train V81.82
■ specified type NEC V81.89
■ while boarding or alighting V81.4
– ski lift V98.3
– specified NEC V98.8
– sport utility vehicle occupant
■ collision (with)
– streetcar occupant V82.9
■ collision (with) V82.3
~ motor vehicle (traffic) V82.1
◊ nontraffic V82.0
~ rolling stock V82.2
■ during derailment V82.7
■ fall (in streetcar) V82.5
~ during derailment V82.7
~ from streetcar V82.6
◊ during derailment V82.7
◊ while boarding or alighting V82.4
~ while boarding or alighting V82.4
■ specified type NEC V82.8
■ while boarding or alighting V82.4
– three-wheeled motor vehicle occupant V39.9
■ collision (with)
~ motor vehicle NOS (traffic) V39.60
◊ nontraffic V39.20
◊ specified type NEC (traffic) V39.69
» nontraffic V39.29
■ driver
~ collision (with)
◊ motor vehicle NOS (traffic) V39.40
» nontraffic V39.00
» specified type NEC (traffic) V39.49
❖ nontraffic V39.09
~ noncollision accident (traffic) V38.5
◊ nontraffic V38.0
■ noncollision accident (traffic) V38.9
~ nontraffic V38.3
~ while boarding or alighting V38.4
■ nontraffic V39.3
■ hanger-on
~ noncollision accident (traffic) V38.7
◊ nontraffic V38.2
■ passenger
~ collision (with)
◊ motor vehicle NOS (traffic) V39.50
» nontraffic V39.10
» specified type NEC (traffic) V39.59
❖ nontraffic V39.19
~ noncollision accident (traffic) V38.6
◊ nontraffic V38.1
■ specified type NEC V39.89
~ military vehicle V39.81
– tractor (farm) (and trailer)—*see* Accident, transport, agricultural vehicle occupant
– tram—*see* Accident, transport, streetcar
– trolley—*see* Accident, transport, streetcar
– truck (heavy) occupant V69.9
■ collision (with)
~ animal (traffic) V60.9
◊ being ridden (traffic) V66.9
» nontraffic V66.3
» while boarding or alighting V66.4
◊ nontraffic V60.3
◊ while boarding or alighting V60.4
~ animal-drawn vehicle (traffic) V66.9
◊ nontraffic V66.3
◊ while boarding or alighting V66.4

Accident (to), *continued*
~ bus (traffic) V64.9
◊ nontraffic V64.3
◊ while boarding or alighting V64.4
~ car (traffic) V63.9
◊ nontraffic V63.3
◊ while boarding or alighting V63.4
~ motor vehicle NOS (traffic) V69.60
◊ nontraffic V69.20
◊ specified type NEC (traffic) V69.69
» nontraffic V69.29
~ pedal cycle (traffic) V61.9
◊ nontraffic V61.3
◊ while boarding or alighting V61.4
~ pickup truck (traffic) V63.9
◊ nontraffic V63.3
◊ while boarding or alighting V63.4
~ railway vehicle (traffic) V65.9
◊ nontraffic V65.3
◊ while boarding or alighting V65.4
~ specified vehicle NEC (traffic) V66.9
◊ nontraffic V66.3
◊ while boarding or alighting V66.4
~ stationary object (traffic) V67.9
◊ nontraffic V67.3
◊ while boarding or alighting V67.4
~ streetcar (traffic) V66.9
◊ nontraffic V66.3
◊ while boarding or alighting V66.4
~ three wheeled motor vehicle (traffic) V62.9
◊ nontraffic V62.3
◊ while boarding or alighting V62.4
~ truck (traffic) V64.9
◊ nontraffic V64.3
◊ while boarding or alighting V64.4
~ two wheeled motor vehicle (traffic) V62.9
◊ nontraffic V62.3
◊ while boarding or alighting V62.4
~ van (traffic) V63.9
◊ nontraffic V63.3
◊ while boarding or alighting V63.4
■ driver
~ collision (with)
◊ animal (traffic) V60.5
» being ridden (traffic) V66.5
❖ nontraffic V66.0
» nontraffic V60.0
◊ animal-drawn vehicle (traffic) V66.5
» nontraffic V66.0
◊ bus (traffic) V64.5
» nontraffic V64.0
◊ car (traffic) V63.5
» nontraffic V63.0
◊ motor vehicle NOS (traffic) V69.40
» nontraffic V69.00
» specified type NEC (traffic) V69.49
❖ nontraffic V69.09
◊ pedal cycle (traffic) V61.5
» nontraffic V61.0
◊ pickup truck (traffic) V63.5
» nontraffic V63.0
◊ railway vehicle (traffic) V65.5
» nontraffic V65.0
◊ specified vehicle NEC (traffic) V66.5
» nontraffic V66.0
◊ stationary object (traffic) V67.5
» nontraffic V67.0
◊ streetcar (traffic) V66.5
» nontraffic V66.0
◊ three wheeled motor vehicle (traffic) V62.5
» nontraffic V62.0
◊ truck (traffic) V64.5
» nontraffic V64.0
◊ two wheeled motor vehicle (traffic) V62.5
» nontraffic V62.0
◊ van (traffic) V63.5
» nontraffic V63.0
~ noncollision accident (traffic) V68.5
◊ nontraffic V68.0
■ hanger-on
~ collision (with)
◊ animal (traffic) V60.7

Accident (to), *continued*
- » being ridden (traffic) V66.7
  - ❖ nontraffic V66.2
  - » nontraffic V60.2
- ◊ animal-drawn vehicle (traffic) V66.7
  - » nontraffic V66.2
- ◊ bus (traffic) V64.7
  - » nontraffic V64.2
- ◊ car (traffic) V63.7
  - » nontraffic V63.2
- ◊ pedal cycle (traffic) V61.7
  - » nontraffic V61.2
- ◊ pickup truck (traffic) V63.7
  - » nontraffic V63.2
- ◊ railway vehicle (traffic) V65.7
  - » nontraffic V65.2
- ◊ specified vehicle NEC (traffic) V66.7
  - » nontraffic V66.2
- ◊ stationary object (traffic) V67.7
  - » nontraffic V67.2
- ◊ streetcar (traffic) V66.7
  - » nontraffic V66.2
- ◊ three wheeled motor vehicle (traffic) V62.7
  - » nontraffic V62.2
- ◊ truck (traffic) V64.7
  - » nontraffic V64.2
- ◊ two wheeled motor vehicle (traffic) V62.7
  - » nontraffic V62.2
- ◊ van (traffic) V63.7
  - » nontraffic V63.2
- ~ noncollision accident (traffic) V68.7
  - ◊ nontraffic V68.2
- ■ noncollision accident (traffic) V68.9
  - ~ nontraffic V68.3
  - ~ while boarding or alighting V68.4
- ■ nontraffic V69.3
- ■ passenger
  - ~ collision (with)
    - ◊ animal (traffic) V60.6
      - » being ridden (traffic) V66.6
        - ❖ nontraffic V66.1
      - » nontraffic V60.1
    - ◊ animal-drawn vehicle (traffic) V66.6
      - » nontraffic V66.1
    - ◊ bus (traffic) V64.6
      - » nontraffic V64.1
    - ◊ car (traffic) V63.6
      - » nontraffic V63.1
    - ◊ motor vehicle NOS (traffic) V69.50
      - » nontraffic V69.10
      - » specified type NEC (traffic) V69.59
        - ❖ nontraffic V69.19
    - ◊ pedal cycle (traffic) V61.6
      - » nontraffic V61.1
    - ◊ pickup truck (traffic) V63.6
      - » nontraffic V63.1
    - ◊ railway vehicle (traffic) V65.6
      - » nontraffic V65.1
    - ◊ specified vehicle NEC (traffic) V66.6
      - » nontraffic V66.1
    - ◊ stationary object (traffic) V67.6
      - » nontraffic V67.1
    - ◊ streetcar (traffic) V66.6
      - » nontraffic V66.1
    - ◊ three wheeled motor vehicle (traffic) V62.6
      - » nontraffic V62.1
    - ◊ truck (traffic) V64.6
      - » nontraffic V64.1
    - ◊ two wheeled motor vehicle (traffic) V62.6
      - » nontraffic V62.1
    - ◊ van (traffic) V63.6
      - » nontraffic V63.1
  - ~ noncollision accident (traffic) V68.6
    - ◊ nontraffic V68.1
- ■ pickup—*see* Accident, transport, pickup truck occupant
- ■ specified type NEC V69.88
  - ~ military vehicle V69.81
- – van occupant V59.9
  - ■ collision (with)
    - ~ animal (traffic) V50.9
      - ◊ being ridden (traffic) V56.9
        - » nontraffic V56.3

Accident (to), *continued*
- » while boarding or alighting V56.4
- ~ animal-drawn vehicle (traffic) V56.9
  - ◊ nontraffic V56.3
  - ◊ while boarding or alighting V56.4
- ~ motor vehicle NOS (traffic) V59.60
  - ◊ nontraffic V59.20
  - ◊ specified type NEC (traffic) V59.69
    - » nontraffic V59.29
- ~ specified vehicle NEC (traffic) V56.9
  - ◊ nontraffic V56.3
  - ◊ while boarding or alighting V56.4
- ~ streetcar (traffic) V56.9
  - ◊ nontraffic V56.3
  - ◊ while boarding or alighting V56.4
- ■ driver
  - ~ collision (with)
    - » animal being ridden (traffic) V56.5
      - ❖ nontraffic V56.0
    - ◊ animal-drawn vehicle (traffic) V56.5
      - » nontraffic V56.0
    - ◊ motor vehicle NOS (traffic) V59.40
      - » nontraffic V59.00
      - » specified type NEC (traffic) V59.49
        - ❖ nontraffic V59.09
    - ◊ specified vehicle NEC (traffic) V56.5
    - ◊ streetcar (traffic) V56.5
      - » nontraffic V56.0
  - ~ noncollision accident (traffic) V58.5
    - ◊ nontraffic V58.0
- ■ noncollision accident (traffic) V58.9
  - ~ nontraffic V58.3
  - ~ while boarding or alighting V58.4
- ■ nontraffic V59.3
- ■ hanger-on
  - ~ collision (with)
    - » animal being ridden (traffic) V56.7
      - ❖ nontraffic V56.2
    - ◊ animal-drawn vehicle (traffic) V56.7
      - » nontraffic V56.2
    - ◊ specified vehicle NEC (traffic) V56.7
      - » nontraffic V56.2
    - ◊ streetcar (traffic) V56.7
      - » nontraffic V56.2
  - ~ noncollision accident (traffic) V58.7
    - ◊ nontraffic V58.2
- ■ passenger
  - ~ collision (with)
    - » animal being ridden (traffic) V56.6
      - ❖ nontraffic V56.1
    - ◊ animal-drawn vehicle (traffic) V56.6
    - ◊ motor vehicle NOS (traffic) V59.50
      - » nontraffic V59.10
      - » specified type NEC (traffic) V59.59
        - ❖ nontraffic V59.19
    - ◊ specified vehicle NEC (traffic) V56.6
      - » nontraffic V56.1
    - ◊ streetcar (traffic) V56.6
      - » nontraffic V56.1
  - ~ noncollision accident (traffic) V58.6
    - ◊ nontraffic V58.1
- ■ specified type NEC V59.88
  - ~ military vehicle V59.81
- – watercraft occupant—*see* Accident, watercraft
- • vehicle NEC V89.9
  - – animal-drawn NEC—*see* Accident, transport, animal-drawn vehicle occupant
  - – special
    - ■ agricultural—*see* Accident, transport, agricultural vehicle occupant
  - – three-wheeled NEC (motorized)—*see* Accident, transport, three-wheeled motor vehicle occupant
- • watercraft V94.9
  - – causing
    - ■ drowning—*see* Drowning, due to, accident to, watercraft
    - ■ injury NEC V91.89
      - ~ crushed between craft and object V91.19
        - ◊ powered craft V91.1-
        - ◊ unpowered craft V91.1-
      - ~ fall on board V91.29
        - ◊ powered craft V91.2-
        - ◊ unpowered craft V91.2-

Accident (to), *continued*
- ~ fire on board causing burn V91.09
  - ◊ powered craft V91.0-
  - ◊ unpowered craft V91.0-
- ~ hit by falling object V91.39
  - ◊ powered craft V91.3-
  - ◊ unpowered craft V91.3-
- ~ specified type NEC V91.89
  - ◊ powered craft V91.8-
  - ◊ unpowered craft V91.8-
- – nonpowered, struck by
  - ■ nonpowered vessel V94.22
  - ■ powered vessel V94.21
- – specified type NEC V94.89
- – striking swimmer
  - ■ powered V94.11
  - ■ unpowered V94.12

Acid throwing (assault) Y08.89

Activity (involving) (of victim at time of event) Y93.9
- • aerobic and step exercise (class) Y93.A3
- • alpine skiing Y93.23
- • animal care NEC Y93.K9
- • arts and handcrafts NEC Y93.D9
- • athletics NEC Y93.79
- • athletics played as a team or group NEC Y93.69
- • athletics played individually NEC Y93.59
- • baking Y93.G3
- • ballet Y93.41
- • barbells Y93.B3
- • BASE (Building, Antenna, Span, Earth) jumping Y93.33
- • baseball Y93.64
- • basketball Y93.67
- • bathing (personal) Y93.E1
- • beach volleyball Y93.68
- • bike riding Y93.55
- • blackout game Y93.85
- • boogie boarding Y93.18
- • bowling Y93.54
- • boxing Y93.71
- • brass instrument playing Y93.J4
- • building construction Y93.H3
- • bungee jumping Y93.34
- • calisthenics Y93.A2
- • canoeing (in calm and turbulent water) Y93.16
- • capture the flag Y93.6A
- • cardiorespiratory exercise NEC Y93.A9
- • caregiving (providing) NEC Y93.F9
  - – bathing Y93.F1
  - – lifting Y93.F2
- • cellular
  - – communication device Y93.C2
  - – telephone Y93.C2
- • challenge course Y93.A5
- • cheerleading Y93.45
- • choking game Y93.85
- • circuit training Y93.A4
- • cleaning
  - – floor Y93.E5
- • climbing NEC Y93.39
  - – mountain Y93.31
  - – rock Y93.31
  - – wall Y93.31
- • clothing care and maintenance NEC Y93.E9
- • combatives Y93.75
- • computer
  - – keyboarding Y93.C1
  - – technology NEC Y93.C9
- • confidence course Y93.A5
- • construction (building) Y93.H3
- • cooking and baking Y93.G3
- • cool down exercises Y93.A2
- • cricket Y93.69
- • crocheting Y93.D1
- • cross country skiing Y93.24
- • dancing (all types) Y93.41
- • digging
  - – dirt Y93.H1
- • dirt digging Y93.H1
- • dishwashing Y93.G1
- • diving (platform) (springboard) Y93.12
  - – underwater Y93.15
- • dodge ball Y93.6A

Activity (involving) (of victim at time of event), *continued*

- downhill skiing Y93.23
- drum playing Y93.J2
- dumbbells Y93.B3
- electronic
  - devices NEC Y93.C9
    - hand held interactive Y93.C2
  - game playing (using) (with)
    - interactive device Y93.C2
    - keyboard or other stationary device Y93.C1
- elliptical machine Y93.A1
- exercise(s)
  - machines ((primarily) for)
    - cardiorespiratory conditioning Y93.A1
    - muscle strengthening Y93.B1
  - muscle strengthening (non-machine) NEC Y93.B9
- external motion NEC Y93.I9
  - rollercoaster Y93.I1
- fainting game Y93.85
- field hockey Y93.65
- figure skating (pairs) (singles) Y93.21
- flag football Y93.62
- floor mopping and cleaning Y93.E5
- food preparation and clean up Y93.G1
- football (American) NOS Y93.61
  - flag Y93.62
  - tackle Y93.61
  - touch Y93.62
- four square Y93.6A
- free weights Y93.B3
- frisbee (ultimate) Y93.74
- furniture
  - building Y93.D3
  - finishing Y93.D3
  - repair Y93.D3
- game playing (electronic)
  - using keyboard or other stationary device Y93.C1
  - using interactive device Y93.C2
- gardening Y93.H2
- golf Y93.53
- grass drills Y93.A6
- grilling and smoking food Y93.G2
- grooming and shearing an animal Y93.K3
- guerilla drills Y93.A6
- gymnastics (rhythmic) Y93.43
- handball Y93.73
- handcrafts NEC Y93.D9
- hand held interactive electronic device Y93.C2
- hang gliding Y93.35
- hiking (on level or elevated terrain) Y93.01
- hockey (ice) Y93.22
  - field Y93.65
- horseback riding Y93.52
- household (interior) maintenance NEC Y93.E9
- ice NEC Y93.29
  - dancing or skating Y93.21
  - hockey Y93.22
- in-line roller skating Y93.51
- ironing Y93.E4
- judo Y93.75
- jumping (off) NEC Y93.39
  - BASE (Building, Antenna, Span, Earth) Y93.33
  - bungee Y93.34
  - jacks Y93.A2
  - rope Y93.56
- jumping jacks Y93.A2
- jumping rope Y93.56
- karate Y93.75
- kayaking (in calm and turbulent water) Y93.16
- keyboarding (computer) Y93.C1
- kickball Y93.6A
- knitting Y93.D1
- lacrosse Y93.65
- land maintenance NEC Y93.H9
- landscaping Y93.H2
- laundry Y93.E2
- machines (exercise)
  - primarily for cardiorespiratory conditioning Y93.A1
  - primarily for muscle strengthening Y93.B1
- maintenance
  - exterior building NEC Y93.H9
  - household (interior) NEC Y93.E9

Activity (involving) (of victim at time of event), *continued*

  - land Y93.H9
  - property Y93.H9
- marching (on level or elevated terrain) Y93.01
- martial arts Y93.75
- microwave oven Y93.G3
- milking an animal Y93.K2
- mopping (floor) Y93.E5
- mountain climbing Y93.31
- muscle strengthening
  - exercises (non-machine) NEC Y93.B9
  - machines Y93.B1
- musical keyboard (electronic) playing Y93.J1
- nordic skiing Y93.24
- obstacle course Y93.A5
- oven (microwave) Y93.G3
- packing up and unpacking in moving to a new residence Y93.E6
- parasailing Y93.19
- percussion instrument playing NEC Y93.J2
- personal
  - bathing and showering Y93.E1
  - hygiene NEC Y93.E8
  - showering Y93.E1
- physical games generally associated with school recess, summer camp and children Y93.6A
- physical training NEC Y93.A9
- piano playing Y93.J1
- pilates Y93.B4
- platform diving Y93.12
- playing musical instrument
  - brass instrument Y93.J4
  - drum Y93.J2
  - musical keyboard (electronic) Y93.J1
  - percussion instrument NEC Y93.J2
  - piano Y93.J1
  - string instrument Y93.J3
  - winds instrument Y93.J4
- property maintenance
  - exterior NEC Y93.H9
  - interior NEC Y93.E9
- pruning (garden and lawn) Y93.H2
- pull-ups Y93.B2
- push-ups Y93.B2
- racquetball Y93.73
- rafting (in calm and turbulent water) Y93.16
- raking (leaves) Y93.H1
- rappelling Y93.32
- refereeing a sports activity Y93.81
- residential relocation Y93.E6
- rhythmic gymnastics Y93.43
- rhythmic movement NEC Y93.49
- riding
  - horseback Y93.52
  - rollercoaster Y93.I1
- rock climbing Y93.31
- rollercoaster riding Y93.I1
- roller skating (in-line) Y93.51
- rough housing and horseplay Y93.83
- rowing (in calm and turbulent water) Y93.16
- rugby Y93.63
- running Y93.02
- SCUBA diving Y93.15
- sewing Y93.D2
- shoveling Y93.H1
  - dirt Y93.H1
  - snow Y93.H1
- showering (personal) Y93.E1
- sit-ups Y93.B2
- skateboarding Y93.51
- skating (ice) Y93.21
  - roller Y93.51
- skiing (alpine) (downhill) Y93.23
  - cross country Y93.24
  - nordic Y93.24
  - water Y93.17
- sledding (snow) Y93.23
- sleeping (sleep) Y93.84
- smoking and grilling food Y93.G2
- snorkeling Y93.15
- snow NEC Y93.29
  - boarding Y93.23
  - shoveling Y93.H1

Activity (involving) (of victim at time of event), *continued*

  - sledding Y93.23
  - tubing Y93.23
- soccer Y93.66
- softball Y93.64
- specified NEC Y93.89
- spectator at an event Y93.82
- sports NEC Y93.79
  - sports played as a team or group NEC Y93.69
  - sports played individually NEC Y93.59
- springboard diving Y93.12
- squash Y93.73
- stationary bike Y93.A1
- step (stepping) exercise (class) Y93.A3
- stepper machine Y93.A1
- stove Y93.G3
- string instrument playing Y93.J3
- surfing Y93.18
  - wind Y93.18
- swimming Y93.11
- tap dancing Y93.41
- tennis Y93.73
- tobogganing Y93.23
- touch football Y93.62
- track and field events (non-running) Y93.57
  - running Y93.02
- trampoline Y93.44
- treadmill Y93.A1
- trimming shrubs Y93.H2
- tubing (in calm and turbulent water) Y93.16
  - snow Y93.23
- ultimate frisbee Y93.74
- underwater diving Y93.15
- unpacking in moving to a new residence Y93.E6
- use of stove, oven and microwave oven Y93.G3
- vacuuming Y93.E3
- volleyball (beach) (court) Y93.68
- wake boarding Y93.17
- walking an animal Y93.K1
- walking (on level or elevated terrain) Y93.01
  - an animal Y93.K1
- wall climbing Y93.31
- warm up and cool down exercises Y93.A2
- water NEC Y93.19
  - aerobics Y93.14
  - craft NEC Y93.19
  - exercise Y93.14
  - polo Y93.13
  - skiing Y93.17
  - sliding Y93.18
  - survival training and testing Y93.19
- weeding (garden and lawn) Y93.H2
- wind instrument playing Y93.J4
- windsurfing Y93.18
- wrestling Y93.72
- yoga Y93.42

Adverse effect of drugs—*see* Table of Drugs and Chemicals

Air
- pressure
  - change, rapid
    - during
      - ascent W94.29
        - while (in) (surfacing from)
          - aircraft W94.23
          - deep water diving W94.21
          - underground W94.22
      - descent W94.39
        - in
          - aircraft W94.31
          - water W94.32
  - high, prolonged W94.0
  - low, prolonged W94.12
    - due to residence or long visit at high altitude W94.11

Alpine sickness W94.11

Altitude sickness W94.11

Anaphylactic shock, anaphylaxis—*see* Table of Drugs and Chemicals

Andes disease W94.11

Arachnidism, arachnoidism X58

Arson (with intent to injure or kill) X97

Asphyxia, asphyxiation
- by
  - food (bone) (seed) (*see* categories T17 and) T18
  - gas—*see also* Table of Drugs and Chemicals
- from
  - fire—*see also* Exposure, fire
  - ignition—*see* Ignition
  - vomitus T17.81

Aspiration
- food (any type) (into respiratory tract) (with asphyxia, obstruction respiratory tract, suffocation) (*see* categories T17 and) T18
- foreign body—*see* Foreign body, aspiration
- vomitus (with asphyxia, obstruction respiratory tract, suffocation) T17.81

Assassination (attempt)—*see* Assault

Assault (homicidal) (by) (in) Y09
- bite (of human being) Y04.1
- bodily force Y04.8
  - bite Y04.1
  - bumping into Y04.2
  - sexual (*see* subcategories T74.0,) T76.0
  - unarmed fight Y04.0
- brawl (hand) (fists) (foot) (unarmed) Y04.0
- burning, burns (by fire) NEC X97
  - acid Y08.89
  - caustic, corrosive substance Y08.89
  - chemical from swallowing caustic, corrosive substance—*see* Table of Drugs and Chemicals
  - cigarette(s) X97
  - hot object X98.9
    - fluid NEC X98.2
    - household appliance X98.3
    - specified NEC X98.8
    - steam X98.0
    - tap water X98.1
    - vapors X98.0
  - scalding X97
  - steam X98.0
  - vitriol Y08.89
- caustic, corrosive substance (gas) Y08.89
- crashing of
  - aircraft Y08.81
  - motor vehicle Y03.8
    - pushed in front of Y02.0
    - run over Y03.0
    - specified NEC Y03.8
- cutting or piercing instrument X99.9
  - dagger X99.2
  - glass X99.0
  - knife X99.1
  - specified NEC X99.8
  - sword X99.2
- dagger X99.2
- drowning (in) X92.9
  - bathtub X92.0
  - natural water X92.3
  - specified NEC X92.8
  - swimming pool X92.1
    - following fall X92.2
- dynamite X96.8
- explosive(s) (material) X96.9
- fight (hand) (fists) (foot) (unarmed) Y04.0
  - with weapon—*see* Assault, by type of weapon
- fire X97
- firearm X95.9
  - airgun X95.01
  - handgun X93
  - hunting rifle X94.1
  - specified NEC X95.8
- gunshot (wound) NEC—*see* Assault, firearm, by type
- incendiary device X97
- injury Y09
  - to child due to criminal abortion attempt NEC Y08.89
- knife X99.1
- late effect of—*see* X92-Y08 with 7th character S
- placing before moving object NEC Y02.8
  - motor vehicle Y02.0
- poisoning—*see* categories T36-T65 with 7th character S
- puncture, any part of body—*see* Assault, cutting or piercing instrument

Assault (homicidal) (by) (in), *continued*
- pushing
  - before moving object NEC Y02.8
    - motor vehicle Y02.0
    - subway train Y02.1
    - train Y02.1
- from high place Y01
- rape T74.2-
- scalding —X97
- sexual (by bodily force) T74.2-
- shooting—*see* Assault, firearm
- specified means NEC Y08.89
- stab, any part of body—*see* Assault, cutting or piercing instrument
- steam X98.0
- striking against
  - other person Y04.2
  - sports equipment Y08.09
    - baseball bat Y08.02
    - hockey stick Y08.01
- struck by
  - sports equipment Y08.09
    - baseball bat Y08.02
    - hockey stick Y08.01
- submersion—*see* Assault, drowning
- violence Y09
- weapon Y09
  - blunt Y00
  - cutting or piercing—*see* Assault, cutting or piercing instrument
  - firearm—*see* Assault, firearm
- wound Y09
  - cutting—*see* Assault, cutting or piercing instrument
  - gunshot—*see* Assault, firearm
  - knife X99.1
  - piercing—*see* Assault, cutting or piercing instrument
  - puncture—*see* Assault, cutting or piercing instrument
  - stab—*see* Assault, cutting or piercing instrument

Attack by mammals NEC W55.89

Avalanche—*see* Landslide

B

Barotitis, barodontalgia, barosinusitis, barotrauma (otitic) (sinus)-—*see* Air, pressure

Battered (baby) (child) (person) (syndrome) X58

Bean in nose (*see* categories T17 and) T18

Bed set on fire NEC—*see* Exposure, fire, uncontrolled, building, bed

Bending, injury in—*see* category Y93

Bends-—*see* Air, pressure, change

Bite, bitten by
- alligator W58.01
- arthropod (nonvenomous) NEC W57
- bull W55.21
- cat W55.01
- cow W55.21
- crocodile W58.11
- dog W54.0
- goat W55.31
- hoof stock NEC W55.31
- horse W55.11
- human being (accidentally) W50.3
  - with intent to injure or kill Y04.1
  - as, or caused by, a crowd or human stampede (with fall) W52
  - assault Y04.1
  - in
    - fight Y04.1
- insect (nonvenomous) W57
- lizard (nonvenomous) W59.01
- mammal NEC W55.81
  - marine W56.31
- marine animal (nonvenomous) W56.81
- millipede W57
- moray eel W56.51
- mouse W53.01
- person(s) (accidentally) W50.3
  - with intent to injure or kill Y04.1

Bite, bitten by, *continued*
  - as, or caused by, a crowd or human stampede (with fall) W52
  - assault Y04.1
  - in
    - fight Y04.1
- pig W55.41
- raccoon W55.51
- rat W53.11
- reptile W59.81
  - lizard W59.01
  - snake W59.11
  - turtle W59.21
    - terrestrial W59.81
- rodent W53.81
  - mouse W53.01
  - rat W53.11
  - specified NEC W53.81
  - squirrel W53.21
- shark W56.41
- sheep W55.31
- snake (nonvenomous) W59.11
- spider (nonvenomous) W57
- squirrel W53.21

Blizzard X37.2

Blood alcohol level Y90.-

Blow X58

Blowing up—*see* Explosion

Brawl (hand) (fists) (foot) Y04.0

Breakage (accidental) (part of)
- ladder (causing fall) W11
- scaffolding (causing fall) W12

Broken
- glass, contact with—*see* Contact, with, glass

Bumping against, into (accidentally)
- object NEC W22.8
  - with fall—*see* Fall, due to, bumping against, object
  - caused by crowd or human stampede (with fall) W52
  - sports equipment W21.9
- person(s) W51
  - with fall W03
    - due to ice or snow W00.0
  - assault Y04.2
  - caused by, a crowd or human stampede (with fall) W52
- sports equipment W21.9

Burn, burned, burning (accidental) (by) (from) (on)
- acid NEC—*see* Table of Drugs and Chemicals
- bed linen—*see* Exposure, fire, uncontrolled, in building, bed
- blowtorch X08.8
  - with ignition of clothing NEC X06.2
    - nightwear X05
- bonfire, campfire (controlled)—*see also* Exposure, fire, controlled, not in building
  - uncontrolled—*see* Exposure, fire, uncontrolled, not in building
- candle X08.8
  - with ignition of clothing NEC X06.2
    - nightwear X05
- caustic liquid, substance (external) (internal) NEC—*see* Table of Drugs and Chemicals
- chemical (external) (internal)—*see also* Table of Drugs and Chemicals
- cigar(s) or cigarette(s) X08.8
  - with ignition of clothing NEC X06.2
    - nightwear X05
- clothes, clothing NEC (from controlled fire) X06.2
  - with conflagration—*see* Exposure, fire, uncontrolled, building
    - not in building or structure—*see* Exposure, fire, uncontrolled, not in building
- cooker (hot) X15.8
  - stated as undetermined whether accidental or intentional Y27.3
- electric blanket X16
- engine (hot) X17
- fire, flames—*see* Exposure, fire
- flare, Very pistol—*see* Discharge, firearm NEC

Burn, burned, burning (accidental) (by) (from) (on), *continued*

- heat
  - from appliance (electrical) (household) (cooking object) X15.-
    - stated as undetermined whether accidental or intentional Y27.3
  - in local application or packing during medical or surgical procedure Y63.5
- heating
  - appliance, radiator or pipe X16
- hot
  - cooker X15.8
  - drink X10.0
  - engine X17
  - fat X10.2
  - fluid NEC X12
  - food X10.1
  - heating appliance X16
  - household appliance NEC X15.8
  - kettle X15.8
  - liquid NEC X12
  - machinery X17
  - metal (molten) (liquid) NEC X18
  - object (not producing fire or flames) NEC X19
  - oil (cooking) X10.2
  - pipe(s) X16
  - radiator X16
  - saucepan (glass) (metal) X15.3
  - stove (kitchen) X15.0
  - substance NEC X19
    - caustic or corrosive NEC—*see* Table of Drugs and Chemicals
  - toaster X15.1
  - tool X17
  - vapor X13.1
  - water (tap)—*see* Contact, with, hot, tap water
- hotplate X15.2
- ignition—*see* Ignition
- inflicted by other person X97
  - by hot objects, hot vapor, and steam—*see* Assault, burning, hot object
- internal, from swallowed caustic, corrosive liquid, substance—*see* Table of Drugs and Chemicals
- iron (hot) X15.8
  - stated as undetermined whether accidental or intentional Y27.3
- kettle (hot) X15.8
  - stated as undetermined whether accidental or intentional Y27.3
- lamp (flame) X08.8
  - with ignition of clothing NEC X06.2
    - nightwear X05
- lighter (cigar) (cigarette) X08.8
  - with ignition of clothing NEC X06.2
    - nightwear X05
- lightning—*see* subcategory T75.0
  - causing fire—*see* Exposure, fire
- liquid (boiling) (hot) NEC X12
  - stated as undetermined whether accidental or intentional Y27.2
- on board watercraft
  - due to
    - accident to watercraft V91.09
      - powered craft V91.0-
      - unpowered craft V91.0-
    - fire on board V93.0-
    - specified heat source NEC on board V93.19
      - ferry boat V93.11
      - fishing boat V93.12
      - jet skis V93.13
      - liner V93.11
      - merchant ship V93.10
      - passenger ship V93.11
      - powered craft NEC V93.13
      - sailboat V93.14
- machinery (hot) X17
- matches X08.8
  - with ignition of clothing NEC X06.2
    - nightwear X05
- mattress—*see* Exposure, fire, uncontrolled, building, bed

Burn, burned, burning (accidental) (by) (from) (on), *continued*

- medicament, externally applied Y63.5
- metal (hot) (liquid) (molten) NEC X18
- nightwear (nightclothes, nightdress, gown, pajamas, robe) X05
- object (hot) NEC X19
- pipe (hot) X16
  - smoking X08.8
    - with ignition of clothing NEC X06.2
      - nightwear X05
- powder—*see* Powder burn
- radiator (hot) X16
- saucepan (hot) (glass) (metal) X15.3
  - stated as undetermined whether accidental or intentional Y27.3
- self-inflicted X76
  - stated as undetermined whether accidental or intentional Y26
- steam X13.1
  - pipe X16
    - stated as undetermined whether accidental or intentional Y27.8
  - stated as undetermined whether accidental or intentional Y27.0
- stove (hot) (kitchen) X15.0
  - stated as undetermined whether accidental or intentional Y27.3
- substance (hot) NEC X19
  - boiling X12
    - stated as undetermined whether accidental or intentional Y27.2
  - molten (metal) X18
  - hot
    - household appliance X77.3
    - object X77.9
- stated as undetermined whether accidental or intentional Y27.0
- therapeutic misadventure
  - heat in local application or packing during medical or surgical procedure Y63.5
  - overdose of radiation Y63.2
- toaster (hot) X15.1
  - stated as undetermined whether accidental or intentional Y27.3
- tool (hot) X17
- torch, welding X08.8
  - with ignition of clothing NEC X06.2
    - nightwear X05
- trash fire (controlled)—*see* Exposure, fire, controlled, not in building
  - uncontrolled—*see* Exposure, fire, uncontrolled, not in building
- vapor (hot) X13.1
  - stated as undetermined whether accidental or intentional Y27.0
- Very pistol—*see* Discharge, firearm NEC

Butted by animal W55-

C

Caisson disease—*see* Air, pressure, change

Campfire (exposure to) (controlled)—*see also* Exposure, fire, controlled, not in building
- uncontrolled—*see* Exposure, fire, uncontrolled, not in building Car sickness T75.3

Cat
- bite W55.01
- scratch W55.03

Cataclysm, cataclysmic (any injury) NEC—*see* Forces of nature

Catching fire—*see* Exposure, fire

Caught
- between
  - folding object W23.0
  - objects (moving) (stationary and moving) W23.0
    - and machinery—*see* Contact, with, by type of machine
    - stationary W23.1
  - sliding door and door frame W23.0

Caught, *continued*
- by, in
  - machinery (moving parts of)—*see* Contact, with, by type of machine
  - washing-machine wringer W23.0
- under packing crate (due to losing grip) W23.1

Cave-in caused by cataclysmic earth surface movement or eruption—*see* Landslide

Change(s) in air pressure—*see* Air, pressure, change

Choked, choking (on) (any object except food or vomitus)
- food (bone) (seed) (*see* categories T17) T18
- vomitus T17.81-

Cloudburst (any injury) X37.8

Cold, exposure to (accidental) (excessive) (extreme) (natural) (place) NEC—*see* Exposure, cold

Collapse
- building W20.1
  - burning (uncontrolled fire) X00.2
- dam or man-made structure (causing earth movement) X36.0
- machinery—*see* Contact, with, by type of machine
- structure W20.1
  - burning (uncontrolled fire) X00.2

Collision (accidental) NEC (*see also* Accident, transport) V89.9
- pedestrian W51
  - with fall W03
    - due to ice or snow W00.0
    - involving pedestrian conveyance—*see* Accident, transport, pedestrian, conveyance
  - and
    - crowd or human stampede (with fall) W52
    - object W22.8
      - with fall—*see* Fall, due to, bumping against, object
- person(s)—*see* Collision, pedestrian
- transport vehicle NEC V89.9
  - and
    - avalanche, fallen or not moving—*see* Accident, transport
      - falling or moving—*see* Landslide
    - landslide, fallen or not moving—*see* Accident, transport
      - falling or moving—*see* Landslide
  - due to cataclysm—*see* Forces of nature, by type

Combustion, spontaneous—*see* Ignition

Complication (delayed) of or following (medical or surgical procedure) Y84.9
- with misadventure—*see* Misadventure
- amputation of limb(s) Y83.5
- anastomosis (arteriovenous) (blood vessel) (gastrojejunal) (tendon) (natural or artificial material) Y83.2
- aspiration (of fluid) Y84.4
  - tissue Y84.8
- biopsy Y84.8
- blood
  - sampling Y84.7
  - transfusion
    - procedure Y84.8
- bypass Y83.2
- catheterization (urinary) Y84.6
  - cardiac Y84.0
- colostomy Y83.3
- cystostomy Y83.3
- dialysis (kidney) Y84.1
- drug—*see* Table of Drugs and Chemicals
- due to misadventure—*see* Misadventure
- duodenostomy Y83.3
- electroshock therapy Y84.3
- external stoma, creation of Y83.3
- formation of external stoma Y83.3
- gastrostomy Y83.3
- graft Y83.2
- hypothermia (medically-induced) Y84.8
- implant, implantation (of)
  - artificial
    - internal device (cardiac pacemaker) (electrodes in brain) (heart valve prosthesis) (orthopedic) Y83.1

Complication (delayed) of or following (medical or surgical procedure), *continued*
- ■ material or tissue (for anastomosis or bypass) Y83.2
  - ~ with creation of external stoma Y83.3
- – natural tissues (for anastomosis or bypass) Y83.2
  - ■ with creation of external stoma Y83.3
- • infusion
  - – procedure Y84.8
- • injection—*see* Table of Drugs and Chemicals
  - – procedure Y84.8
- • insertion of gastric or duodenal sound Y84.5
- • insulin-shock therapy Y84.3
- • paracentesis (abdominal) (thoracic) (aspirative) Y84.4
- • procedures other than surgical operation—*see* Complication of or following, by type of procedure
- • radiological procedure or therapy Y84.2
- • removal of organ (partial) (total) NEC Y83.6
- • sampling
  - – blood Y84.7
  - – fluid NEC Y84.4
  - – tissue Y84.8
- • shock therapy Y84.3
- • surgical operation NEC (*see also* Complication of or following, by type of operation) Y83.9
  - – reconstructive NEC Y83.4
    - ■ with
      - ~ anastomosis, bypass or graft Y83.2
      - ~ formation of external stoma Y83.3
  - – specified NEC Y83.8
- • transfusion—*see also* Table of Drugs and Chemicals
  - – procedure Y84.8
- • transplant, transplantation (heart) (kidney) (liver) (whole organ, any) Y83.0
  - – partial organ Y83.4
- • ureterostomy Y83.3
- • vaccination—*see also* Table of Drugs and Chemicals
  - – procedure Y84.8

Compression
- • divers' squeeze—*see* Air, pressure, change
- • trachea by
  - – food (lodged in esophagus) (*see* categories T17 and T18)
  - – vomitus (lodged in esophagus) T17.81-
    Conflagration—*see* Exposure, fire, uncontrolled
    Constriction (external)
- • hair W49.01
- • jewelry W49.04
- • ring W49.04
- • rubber band W49.03
- • specified item NEC W49.09
- • string W49.02
- • thread W49.02

Contact (accidental)
- • with
  - – abrasive wheel (metalworking) W31.1
  - – alligator W58.0-
  - – amphibian W62.9
    - ■ frog W62.0
    - ■ toad W62.1
  - – animal (nonvenomous) (refer to specific animal by name in alphabetical order under "contact")
    - ■ marine W56.8-
  - – arrow W21.89
    - ■ not thrown, projected or falling W45.8
  - – arthropods (nonvenomous) W57
  - – axe W27.0
  - – band-saw (industrial) W31.2
  - – bayonet—*see* Bayonet wound
  - – bee(s) X58
  - – bench-saw (industrial) W31.2
  - – bird W61.9-
  - – blender W29.0
  - – boiling water X12
    - ■ stated as undetermined whether accidental or intentional Y27.2
  - – bore, earth-drilling or mining (land) (seabed) W31.0
  - – buffalo W55.39
  - – bull W55.2-
  - – bumper cars W31.81
  - – camel W55.39
  - – can

Contact (accidental), *continued*
- ■ lid W26.8
- ■ opener W27.4
  - ~ powered W29.0
- – cat W55.09
  - ■ bite W55.01
  - ■ scratch W55.03
- – caterpillar (venomous) X58
- – centipede (venomous) X58
- – chain
  - ■ hoist W24.0
    - ~ agricultural operations W30.89
  - ■ saw W29.3
- – chicken W61.3-
- – chisel W27.0
- – circular saw W31.2
- – cobra X58
- – combine (harvester) W30.0
- – conveyer belt W24.1
- – cooker (hot) X15.8
  - ■ stated as undetermined whether accidental or intentional Y27.3
- – coral X58
- – cotton gin W31.82
- – cow W55.2-
- – crocodile W58.1-
- – dagger W26.1
  - ■ stated as undetermined whether accidental or intentional Y28.2
- – dairy equipment W31.82
- – dart W21.89
  - ■ not thrown, projected or falling W26.8
- – deer W55.39
- – derrick W24.0
  - ■ agricultural operations W30.89
    - ~ hay W30.2
- – dog W54.-
- – dolphin W56.0-
- – donkey W55.39
- – drill (powered) W29.8
  - ■ earth (land) (seabed) W31.0
  - ■ nonpowered W27.8
- – drive belt W24.0
  - ■ agricultural operations W30.89
- – dry ice—*see* Exposure, cold, man-made
- – dryer (clothes) (powered) (spin) W29.2
- – duck W61.69
- – earth(-)
  - ■ drilling machine (industrial) W31.0
  - ■ scraping machine in stationary use W31.83
- – edge of stiff paper W26.2
- – electric
  - ■ beater W29.0
  - ■ blanket X16
  - ■ fan W29.2
    - ~ commercial W31.82
  - ■ knife W29.1
  - ■ mixer W29.0
- – elevator (building) W24.0
  - ■ agricultural operations W30.89
    - ~ grain W30.3
- – engine(s), hot NEC X17
- – excavating machine W31.0
- – farm machine W30.9
- – feces—*see* Contact, with, by type of animal
- – fer de lance X58
- – fish W56.5-
- – flying horses W31.81
- – forging (metalworking) machine W31.1
- – fork W27.4
- – forklift (truck) W24.0
  - ■ agricultural operations W30.89
- – frog W62.0
- – garden
  - ■ cultivator (powered) W29.3
    - ~ riding W30.89
  - ■ fork W27.1
- – gas turbine W31.3
- – Gila monster X58
- – giraffe W55.39
- – glass (sharp) (broken) W25
  - ■ with subsequent fall W18.02
  - ■ assault X99.0

Contact (accidental), *continued*
- ■ due to fall—*see* Fall, by type
- ■ stated as undetermined whether accidental or intentional Y28.0
- – goat W55.3-
- – goose W61.5-
- – hand
  - ■ saw W27.0
  - ■ tool (not powered) NEC W27.8
    - ~ powered W29.8
- – harvester W30.0
- – hay-derrick W30.2
- – heat NEC X19
  - ■ from appliance (electrical) (household)—*see* Contact, with, hot, household appliance
    - ~ heating appliance X16
- – heating
  - ■ appliance (hot) X16
  - ■ pad (electric) X16
- – hedge-trimmer (powered) W29.3
- – hoe W27.1
- – hoist (chain) (shaft) NEC W24.0
  - ■ agricultural W30.89
- – hoof stock NEC W55.3-
- – hornet(s) X58
- – horse W55.1-
- – hot
  - ■ cooker X15.8
  - ■ drinks X10.0
  - ■ engine X17
  - ■ fats X10.2
  - ■ fluids NEC X12
    - ~ assault X98.2
    - ~ undetermined whether accidental or intentional Y27.2
  - ■ food X10.1
  - ■ heating appliance X16
  - ■ household appliance X15.-
    - ~ assault X98.3
    - ~ object NEC X19
      - ◊ assault X98.8
      - ◊ stated as undetermined whether accidental or intentional Y27.9
    - ~ stated as undetermined whether accidental or intentional Y27.3
  - ■ kettle X15.8
  - ■ light bulb X15.8
  - ■ liquid NEC (*see also* Burn) X12
    - ~ drinks X10.0
    - ~ stated as undetermined whether accidental or intentional Y27.2
    - ~ tap water X11.8
      - ◊ stated as undetermined whether accidental or intentional Y27.1
  - ■ machinery X17
  - ■ metal (molten) (liquid) NEC X18
  - ■ object (not producing fire or flames) NEC X19
  - ■ oil (cooking) X10.2
  - ■ pipe X16
  - ■ plate X15.2
  - ■ radiator X16
  - ■ saucepan (glass) (metal) X15.3
  - ■ skillet X15.3
  - ■ stove (kitchen) X15.0
  - ■ substance NEC X19
  - ■ tap-water X11.8
    - ~ assault X98.1
    - ~ heated on stove X12
      - ◊ stated as undetermined whether accidental or intentional Y27.2
    - ~ in bathtub X11.0
    - ~ running X11.1
    - ~ stated as undetermined whether accidental or intentional Y27.1
  - ■ toaster X15.1
  - ■ tool X17
  - ■ vapors X13.1
    - ~ inhalation X13.0
  - ■ water (tap) X11.8
    - ~ boiling X12
      - ◊ stated as undetermined whether accidental or intentional Y27.2

Contact (accidental), *continued*

- ◊ heated on stove X12
  - ◊ stated as undetermined whether accidental or intentional Y27.2
  - ~ in bathtub X11.0
  - ~ running X11.1
  - ~ stated as undetermined whether accidental or intentional Y27.1
- hotplate X15.2
- ice-pick W27.4
- insect (nonvenomous) NEC W57
- kettle (hot) X15.8
- knife W26.0
  - assault X99.1
  - electric W29.1
  - stated as undetermined whether accidental or intentional Y28.1
  - suicide (attempt) X78.1
- lathe (metalworking) W31.1
  - turnings W45.8
  - woodworking W31.2
- lawnmower (powered) (ridden) W28
  - causing electrocution W86.8
  - unpowered W27.1
- lift, lifting (devices) W24.0
  - agricultural operations W30.89
  - shaft W24.0
- liquefied gas—*see* Exposure, cold, man-made
- liquid air, hydrogen, nitrogen—*see* Exposure, cold, man-made
- lizard (nonvenomous) W59.09
  - bite W59.01
  - strike W59.02
- llama W55.39
- macaw W61.1-
- machine, machinery W31.9
  - abrasive wheel W31.1
  - agricultural including animal-powered W30.-
  - band or bench or circular saw W31.2
  - commercial NEC W31.82
  - drilling, metal (industrial) W31.1
  - earth-drilling W31.0
  - earthmoving or scraping W31.89
  - excavating W31.89
  - forging machine W31.1
  - gas turbine W31.3
  - hot X17
  - internal combustion engine W31.3
  - land drill W31.0
  - lathe W31.1
  - lifting (devices) W24.0
  - metal drill W31.1
  - metalworking (industrial) W31.1
  - milling, metal W31.1
  - mining W31.0
  - molding W31.2
  - overhead plane W31.2
  - power press, metal W31.1
  - prime mover W31.3
  - printing W31.89
  - radial saw W31.2
  - recreational W31.81
  - roller-coaster W31.81
  - rolling mill, metal W31.1
  - sander W31.2
  - seabed drill W31.0
  - shaft
    - ~ hoist W31.0
    - ~ lift W31.0
  - specified NEC W31.89
  - spinning W31.89
  - steam engine W31.3
  - transmission W24.1
  - undercutter W31.0
  - water driven turbine W31.3
  - weaving W31.89
  - woodworking or forming (industrial) W31.2
- mammal (feces) (urine) W55.89
  - marine W56.39 (refer to specific animal by name)
    - ~ specified NEC W56.3-
  - specified NEC W55.8-
- marine
  - animal W56.8- (refer to specific animal by name)

Contact (accidental), *continued*

- meat
  - grinder (domestic) W29.0
    - ~ industrial W31.82
    - ~ nonpowered W27.4
  - slicer (domestic) W29.0
    - ~ industrial W31.82
- merry go round W31.81
- metal, hot (liquid) (molten) NEC X18
- millipede W57
- nail W45.0
  - gun W29.4
- needle (sewing) W27.3
  - hypodermic W46.0
    - ~ contaminated W46.1
- object (blunt) NEC
  - hot NEC X19
  - sharp NEC W26.8
    - ~ inflicted by other person NEC W26.8
    - ~ self-inflicted X78.9
- orca W56.2-
- overhead plane W31.2
- paper (as sharp object) W26.2
- paper-cutter W27.5
- parrot W61.0-
- pig W55.4-
- pipe, hot X16
- pitchfork W27.1
- plane (metal) (wood) W27.0
  - overhead W31.2
- plant thorns, spines, sharp leaves or other mechanisms W60
- powered
  - garden cultivator W29.3
  - household appliance, implement, or machine W29.8
  - saw (industrial) W31.2
    - ~ hand W29.8
- printing machine W31.89
- pulley (block) (transmission) W24.0
  - agricultural operations W30.89
- raccoon W55.5-
- radial-saw (industrial) W31.2
- radiator (hot) X16
- rake W27.1
- rattlesnake X58
- reaper W30.0
- reptile W59.8- (refer to specific reptile by name)
- rivet gun (powered) W29.4
- rodent (feces) (urine) W53.8-
  - mouse W53.0-
  - rat W53.1-
  - specified NEC W53.8-
  - squirrel W53.2-
- roller coaster W31.81
- rope NEC W24.0
  - agricultural operations W30.89
- saliva—*see* Contact, with, by type of animal
- sander W29.8
  - industrial W31.2
- saucepan (hot) (glass) (metal) X15.3
- saw W27.0
  - band (industrial) W31.2
  - bench (industrial) W31.2
  - chain W29.3
  - hand W27.0
- sawing machine, metal W31.1
- scissors W27.2
- scorpion X58
- screwdriver W27.0
  - powered W29.8
- sea
  - anemone, cucumber or urchin (spine) X58
  - lion W56.1-
- sewing-machine (electric) (powered) W29.2
  - not powered W27.8
- shaft (hoist) (lift) (transmission) NEC W24.0
  - agricultural W30.89
- shark W56.4-
- shears (hand) W27.2
  - powered (industrial) W31.1
    - ~ domestic W29.2
- sheep W55.3-

Contact (accidental), *continued*

- shovel W27.8
- snake (nonvenomous) W59.11
- spade W27.1
- spider (venomous) X58
- spin-drier W29.2
- spinning machine W31.89
- splinter W45.8
- sports equipment W21.9
- staple gun (powered) W29.8
- steam X13.1
  - engine W31.3
  - inhalation X13.0
  - pipe X16
  - shovel W31.89
- stove (hot) (kitchen) X15.0
- substance, hot NEC X19
  - molten (metal) X18
- sword W26.1
  - assault X99.2
  - stated as undetermined whether accidental or intentional Y28.2
- tarantula X58
- thresher W30.0
- tin can lid W26.8
- toad W62.1
- toaster (hot) X15.1
- tool W27.8
  - hand (not powered) W27.8
    - ~ auger W27.0
    - ~ axe W27.0
    - ~ can opener W27.4
    - ~ chisel W27.0
    - ~ fork W27.4
    - ~ garden W27.1
    - ~ handsaw W27.0
    - ~ hoe W27.1
    - ~ ice-pick W27.4
    - ~ kitchen utensil W27.4
    - ~ manual
      - ◊ lawn mower W27.1
      - ◊ sewing machine W27.8
    - ~ meat grinder W27.4
    - ~ needle (sewing) W27.3
      - ◊ hypodermic W46.0
        - » contaminated W46.1
    - ~ paper cutter W27.5
    - ~ pitchfork W27.1
    - ~ rake W27.1
    - ~ scissors W27.2
    - ~ screwdriver W27.0
    - ~ specified NEC W27.8
    - ~ workbench W27.0
  - hot X17
  - powered W29.8
    - ~ blender W29.0
      - ◊ commercial W31.82
    - ~ can opener W29.0
      - ◊ commercial W31.82
    - ~ chainsaw W29.3
    - ~ clothes dryer W29.2
      - ◊ commercial W31.82
    - ~ dishwasher W29.2
      - ◊ commercial W31.82
    - ~ edger W29.3
    - ~ electric fan W29.2
      - ◊ commercial W31.82
    - ~ electric knife W29.1
    - ~ food processor W29.0
      - ◊ commercial W31.82
    - ~ garbage disposal W29.0
      - ◊ commercial W31.82
    - ~ garden tool W29.3
    - ~ hedge trimmer W29.3
    - ~ ice maker W29.0
      - ◊ commercial W31.82
    - ~ kitchen appliance W29.0
      - ◊ commercial W31.82
    - ~ lawn mower W28
    - ~ meat grinder W29.0
      - ◊ commercial W31.82
    - ~ mixer W29.0
      - ◊ commercial W31.82

Contact (accidental), *continued*
- ~ rototiller W29.3
- ~ sewing machine W29.2
  - ◊ commercial W31.82
- ~ washing machine W29.2
  - ◊ commercial W31.82
- – transmission device (belt, cable, chain, gear, pinion, shaft) W24.1
  - ■ agricultural operations W30.89
- – turbine (gas) (water-driven) W31.3
- – turkey W61.4-
- – turtle (nonvenomous) W59.2-
  - ■ terrestrial W59.8-
- – under-cutter W31.0
- – vehicle
  - ■ agricultural use (transport)—*see* Accident, transport, agricultural vehicle
    - ~ not on public highway W30.81
  - ■ industrial use (transport)—*see* Accident, transport, industrial vehicle
    - ~ not on public highway W31.83
  - ■ off-road use (transport)—*see* Accident, transport, all-terrain or off-road vehicle
    - ~ not on public highway W31.83
- – venomous animal/plant X58
- – viper X58
- – washing-machine (powered) W29.2
- – wasp X58
- – weaving-machine W31.89
- – winch W24.0
  - ■ agricultural operations W30.89
- – wire NEC W24.0
  - ■ agricultural operations W30.89
- – wood slivers W45.8
- – yellow jacket X58
- – zebra W55.39

Coup de soleil X32

Crash
- • aircraft (in transit) (powered) V95.9
  - – balloon V96.01
  - – fixed wing NEC (private) V95.21
    - ■ commercial V95.31
  - – glider V96.21
    - ■ hang V96.11
    - ■ powered V95.11
  - – helicopter V95.01
  - – microlight V95.11
  - – nonpowered V96.9
    - ■ specified NEC V96.8
  - – powered NEC V95.8
  - – stated as
    - ■ homicide (attempt) Y08.81
    - ■ suicide (attempt) X83.0
  - – ultralight V95.11
- • transport vehicle NEC (*see also* Accident, transport) V89.9

Crushed (accidentally) X58
- • between objects (moving) (stationary and moving) W23.0
  - – stationary W23.1
- • by
  - – alligator W58.03
  - – avalanche NEC—*see* Landslide
  - – cave-in W20.0
    - ■ caused by cataclysmic earth surface movement—*see* Landslide
  - – crocodile W58.13
  - – crowd or human stampede W52
  - – falling
    - ■ aircraft V97.39
    - ■ earth, material W20.0
      - ~ caused by cataclysmic earth surface movement—*see* Landslide
    - ■ object NEC W20.8
  - – landslide NEC—*see* Landslide
  - – lizard (nonvenomous) W59.09
  - – machinery—*see* Contact, with, by type of machine
  - – reptile NEC W59.89
  - – snake (nonvenomous) W59.13
- • in
  - – machinery—*see* Contact, with, by type of machine

Cut, cutting (any part of body) (accidental)—*see also* Contact, with, by object or machine
- • during medical or surgical treatment as misadventure—*see* Index to Diseases and Injuries, Complications
- • inflicted by other person—*see* Assault, cutting or piercing instrument
- • machine NEC (*see also* Contact, with, by type of machine) W31.9
- • self-inflicted—*see* Suicide, cutting or piercing instrument
- • suicide (attempt)—*see* Suicide, cutting or piercing instrument

Cyclone (any injury) X37.1

D

Dehydration from lack of water X58

Deprivation X58

Derailment (accidental)
- • railway (rolling stock) (train) (vehicle) (without antecedent collision) V81.7
  - – with antecedent collision—*see* Accident, transport, railway vehicle occupant
- • streetcar (without antecedent collision) V82.7
  - – with antecedent collision—*see* Accident, transport, streetcar occupant

Descent
- • parachute (voluntary) (without accident to aircraft) V97.29
  - – due to accident to aircraft—*see* Accident, transport, aircraft

Desertion X58

Destitution X58

Disability, late effect or sequela of injury—*see* Sequelae

Discharge (accidental)
- • airgun W34.010
  - – assault X95.01
  - – stated as undetermined whether accidental or intentional Y24.0
- • BB gun—*see* Discharge, airgun
- • firearm (accidental) W34.00
  - – assault X95.9
  - – handgun (pistol) (revolver) W32.0
    - ■ assault X93
    - ■ stated as undetermined whether accidental or intentional Y22
  - – homicide (attempt) X95.9
  - – hunting rifle W33.02
    - ■ assault X94.1
    - ■ stated as undetermined whether accidental or intentional Y23.1
  - – larger W33.00
    - ■ hunting rifle—*see* Discharge, firearm, hunting rifle
    - ■ shotgun—*see* Discharge, firearm, shotgun
    - ■ specified NEC W33.09
      - ~ stated as undetermined whether accidental or intentional Y23.8
    - ■ stated as undetermined whether accidental or intentional Y23.9
    - ■ using rubber bullet
      - ~ injuring
        - ◊ bystander Y35.042
        - ◊ law enforcement personnel Y35.041
        - ◊ suspect Y35.043
  - – machine gun W33.03
    - ■ stated as undetermined whether accidental or intentional Y23.3
  - – pellet gun—*see* Discharge, airgun
  - – shotgun W33.01
    - ■ stated as undetermined whether accidental or intentional Y23.0
  - – specified NEC W34.09
    - ■ assault X95.8
    - ■ stated as undetermined whether accidental or intentional Y24.8
  - – stated as undetermined whether accidental or intentional Y24.9
  - – Very pistol W34.09
    - ■ assault X95.8

Discharge (accidental), *continued*
- ■ stated as undetermined whether accidental or intentional Y24.8
- • firework(s) W39
  - – stated as undetermined whether accidental or intentional Y25
- • gas-operated gun NEC W34.018
  - – airgun—*see* Discharge, airgun
  - – assault X95.09
  - – paintball gun—*see* Discharge, paintball gun
  - – stated as undetermined whether accidental or intentional Y24.8
- • gun NEC—*see also* Discharge, firearm NEC
  - – air—*see* Discharge, airgun
  - – BB—*see* Discharge, airgun
  - – for single hand use—*see* Discharge, firearm, handgun
  - – hand—*see* Discharge, firearm, handgun
  - – machine—*see* Discharge, firearm, machine gun
  - – other specified—*see* Discharge, firearm NEC
  - – paintball—*see* Discharge, paintball gun
  - – pellet—*see* Discharge, airgun
- • handgun—*see* Discharge, firearm, handgun
- • machine gun—*see* Discharge, firearm, machine gun
- • paintball gun W34.011
  - – assault X95.02
  - – stated as undetermined whether accidental or intentional Y24.8
- • rifle (hunting)—*see* Discharge, firearm, hunting rifle
- • shotgun—*see* Discharge, firearm, shotgun
- • spring-operated gun NEC W34.018
  - – assault / homicide (attempt) X95.09
  - – stated as undetermined whether accidental or intentional Y24.8

Diver's disease, palsy, paralysis, squeeze—*see* Air, pressure

Diving (into water)—*see* Accident, diving

Dog bite W54.0

Dragged by transport vehicle NEC (*see also* Accident, transport) V09.9

Drinking poison (accidental)—*see* Table of Drugs and Chemicals

Dropped (accidentally) while being carried or supported by other person W04

Drowning (accidental) W74
- • assault X92.9
- • due to
  - – accident (to)
    - ■ machinery—*see* Contact, with, by type of machine
    - ■ watercraft V90.89
      - ~ burning V90.29
        - ◊ powered V90.2-
        - ◊ unpowered V90.2-
      - ~ crushed V90.39
        - ◊ powered V90.3-
        - ◊ unpowered V90.3-
      - ~ overturning V90.09
        - ◊ powered V90.0-
        - ◊ unpowered V90.0-
      - ~ sinking V90.19
        - ◊ powered V90.1-
        - ◊ unpowered V90.1-
      - ~ specified type NEC V90.89
        - ◊ powered V90.8-
        - ◊ unpowered V90.8-
  - – avalanche—*see* Landslide
  - – cataclysmic
    - ■ earth surface movement NEC—*see* Forces of nature, earth movement
    - ■ storm—*see* Forces of nature, cataclysmic storm
  - – cloudburst X37.8
  - – cyclone X37.1
  - – fall overboard (from) V92.09
    - ■ powered craft V92.0-
    - ■ unpowered craft V92.0-
    - ■ resulting from
      - ~ accident to watercraft—*see* Drowning, due to, accident to, watercraft
      - ~ being washed overboard (from) V92.29
        - ◊ powered craft V92.2-
        - ◊ unpowered craft V92.2-

Explosion (accidental) (of) (with secondary fire), *continued*
- pipe, pressurized W37.8
- pressure, pressurized
  - cooker W38
  - gas tank (in machinery) W36.3
  - hose W37.8
  - pipe W37.8
  - specified device NEC W38
  - tire W37.8
    - bicycle W37.0
  - vessel (in machinery) W38
- propane W40.1
- self-inflicted X75
- steam or water lines (in machinery) W37.8
- stove W40.9
- stated as undetermined whether accidental or intentional Y25
- tire, pressurized W37.8
  - bicycle W37.0
- undetermined whether accidental or intentional Y25
- vehicle tire NEC W37.8
  - bicycle W37.0

Exposure (to) X58
- air pressure change—*see* Air, pressure
- cold (accidental) (excessive) (extreme) (natural) (place) X31
  - assault Y08.89
  - due to
    - man-made conditions W93.8
      - dry ice (contact) W93.01
        - inhalation W93.02
      - liquid air (contact) (hydrogen) (nitrogen) W93.11
        - inhalation W93.12
      - refrigeration unit (deep freeze) W93.2
    - weather (conditions) X31
  - self-inflicted X83.2
- due to abandonment or neglect X58
- electric current W86.8
  - appliance (faulty) W86.8
    - domestic W86.0
  - caused by other person Y08.89
  - conductor (faulty) W86.1
  - control apparatus (faulty) W86.1
  - electric power generating plant, distribution station W86.1
  - electroshock gun—*see* Exposure, electric current, taser
  - lightning—*see* subcategory T75.0
  - live rail W86.8
  - misadventure in medical or surgical procedure in electroshock therapy Y63.4
  - motor (electric) (faulty) W86.8
    - domestic W86.0
  - self-inflicted X83.1
  - specified NEC W86.8
    - domestic W86.0
  - stun gun—*see* Exposure, electric current, taser
  - taser W86.8
    - assault Y08.89
    - self-harm (intentional) X83.8
    - undetermined intent Y33
  - third rail W86.8
  - transformer (faulty) W86.1
- environmental tobacco smoke X58
- excessive
  - cold—*see* Exposure, cold
  - heat (natural) NEC X30
- factor(s) NOS X58
  - environmental NEC X58
    - natural NEC—*see* Forces of nature
  - specified NEC X58
- fire, flames (accidental) X08.8
  - assault X97
  - campfire—*see* Exposure, fire, controlled, not in building
  - controlled (in)
    - with ignition (of) clothing (*see also* Ignition, clothes) X06.2
      - nightwear X05
    - bonfire—*see* Exposure, fire, controlled, not in building

Exposure (to), *continued*
- brazier (in building or structure)—*see also* Exposure, fire, controlled, building
  - not in building or structure—*see* Exposure, fire, controlled, not in building
- building or structure X02.0
  - with
    - fall from building X02.3
    - injury due to building collapse X02.2
    - from building X02.5
    - smoke inhalation X02.1
  - hit by object from building X02.4
  - specified mode of injury NEC X02.8
- fireplace, furnace or stove—*see* Exposure, fire, controlled, building
- not in building or structure X03.0
  - with
    - fall X03.3
    - smoke inhalation X03.1
  - hit by object X03.4
  - specified mode of injury NEC X03.8
- trash—*see* Exposure, fire, controlled, not in building
- fireplace—*see* Exposure, fire, controlled, building
- fittings or furniture (in building or structure) (uncontrolled)—*see* Exposure, fire, uncontrolled, building
- forest (uncontrolled)—*see* Exposure, fire, uncontrolled, not in building
- grass (uncontrolled)—*see* Exposure, fire, uncontrolled, not in building
- hay (uncontrolled)—*see* Exposure, fire, uncontrolled, not in building
- ignition of highly flammable material X04
- in, of, on, starting in
  - machinery—*see* Contact, with, by type of machine
  - motor vehicle (in motion) (*see also* Accident, transport, occupant by type of vehicle) V87.8
    - with collision—*see* Collision
  - railway rolling stock, train, vehicle V81.81
    - with collision—*see* Accident, transport, railway vehicle occupant
  - street car (in motion) V82.8
    - with collision—*see* Accident, transport, streetcar occupant
  - transport vehicle NEC—*see also* Accident, transport
    - with collision—*see* Collision
  - watercraft (in transit) (not in transit) V91.09
    - localized—*see* Burn, on board watercraft, due to, fire on board
    - powered craft V91.03
      - ferry boat V91.01
      - fishing boat V91.02
      - jet skis V91.03
      - liner V91.01
      - merchant ship V91.00
      - passenger ship V91.01
    - unpowered craft V91.08
      - canoe V91.05
      - inflatable V91.06
      - kayak V91.05
      - sailboat V91.04
      - surf-board V91.08
      - waterskis V91.07
      - windsurfer V91.08
- lumber (uncontrolled)—*see* Exposure, fire, uncontrolled, not in building
- prairie (uncontrolled)—*see* Exposure, fire, uncontrolled, not in building
- resulting from
  - explosion—*see* Explosion
  - lightning X08.8
- self-inflicted X76
- specified NEC X08.8
- started by other person X97
- stove—*see* Exposure, fire, controlled, building
- stated as undetermined whether accidental or intentional Y26
- tunnel (uncontrolled)—*see* Exposure, fire, uncontrolled, not in building
- uncontrolled

Exposure (to), *continued*
- in building or structure X00.0
  - with
    - fall from building X00.3
    - injury due to building collapse X00.2
    - jump from building X00.5
    - smoke inhalation X00.1
  - bed X08.00
    - due to
      - cigarette X08.01
      - specified material NEC X08.09
  - furniture NEC X08.20
    - due to
      - cigarette X08.21
      - specified material NEC X08.29
  - hit by object from building X00.4
  - sofa X08.10
    - due to
      - cigarette X08.11
      - specified material NEC X08.19
  - specified mode of injury NEC X00.8
- not in building or structure (any) X01.0
  - with
    - fall X01.3
    - smoke inhalation X01.1
  - hit by object X01.4
  - specified mode of injury NEC X01.8
- undetermined whether accidental or intentional Y26
- forces of nature NEC—*see* Forces of nature
- G-forces (abnormal) W49.9
- gravitational forces (abnormal) W49.9
- heat (natural) NEC—*see* Heat
- high-pressure jet (hydraulic) (pneumatic) W49.9
- hydraulic jet W49.9
- inanimate mechanical force W49.9
- jet, high-pressure (hydraulic) (pneumatic) W49.9
- lightning—*see* subcategory T75.0
  - causing fire—*see* Exposure, fire
- mechanical forces NEC W49.9
  - inanimate NEC W49.9
- noise W42.9
  - supersonic W42.0
- noxious substance—*see* Table of Drugs and Chemicals
- pneumatic jet W49.9
- prolonged in deep-freeze unit or refrigerator W93.2
- radiation—*see* Radiation
- smoke—*see also* Exposure, fire
  - tobacco, second hand Z77.22
- specified factors NEC X58
- sunlight X32
- supersonic waves W42.0
- vibration W49.9
- waves
  - infrasound W49.9
  - sound W42.9
  - supersonic W42.0
- weather NEC—*see* Forces of nature

External cause status Y99.9
- child assisting in compensated work for family Y99.8
- civilian activity done for financial or other compensation Y99.0
- civilian activity done for income or pay Y99.0
- family member assisting in compensated work for other family member Y99.8
- hobby not done for income Y99.8
- leisure activity Y99.8
- off-duty activity of military personnel Y99.8
- recreation or sport not for income or while a student Y99.8
- specified NEC Y99.8
- student activity Y99.8
- volunteer activity Y99.2

F

Factors, supplemental
- alcohol
  - blood level Y90.-
- environmental-pollution-related condition- *see* Z57
- nosocomial condition Y95
- work-related condition Y99.0

Failure
- in suture or ligature during surgical procedure Y65.2
- mechanical, of instrument or apparatus (any) (during any medical or surgical procedure) Y65.8
- sterile precautions (during medical and surgical care)—*see* Misadventure, failure, sterile precautions, by type of procedure
- to
  - introduce tube or instrument Y65.4
    - endotracheal tube during anesthesia Y65.3
  - make curve (transport vehicle) NEC—*see* Accident, transport
  - remove tube or instrument Y65.4

Fall, falling (accidental) W19
- building W20.1
  - burning (uncontrolled fire) X00.3
- down
  - embankment W17.81
  - escalator W10.0
  - hill W17.81
  - ladder W11
  - ramp W10.2
  - stairs, steps W10.9
- due to
  - bumping against
    - object W18.00
      - sharp glass W18.02
      - specified NEC W18.09
      - sports equipment W18.01
    - person W03
      - due to ice or snow W00.0
      - on pedestrian conveyance—*see* Accident, transport, pedestrian, conveyance
  - collision with another person W03
    - due to ice or snow W00.0
    - involving pedestrian conveyance—*see* Accident, transport, pedestrian, conveyance
  - grocery cart tipping over W17.82
  - ice or snow W00.9
    - from one level to another W00.2
      - on stairs or steps W00.1
    - involving pedestrian conveyance—*see* Accident, transport, pedestrian, conveyance
    - on same level W00.0
  - slipping (on moving sidewalk) W01.0
    - with subsequent striking against object W01.10
      - furniture W01.190
      - sharp object W01.119
        - glass W01.110
        - power tool or machine W01.111
        - specified NEC W01.118
      - specified NEC W01.198
  - striking against
    - object W18.00
      - sharp glass W18.02
      - specified NEC W18.09
      - sports equipment W18.01
    - person W03
      - due to ice or snow W00.0
      - on pedestrian conveyance—*see* Accident, transport, pedestrian, conveyance
- earth (with asphyxia or suffocation (by pressure))—*see* Earth, falling
- from, off, out of
  - aircraft NEC (with accident to aircraft NEC) V97.0
    - while boarding or alighting V97.1
  - balcony W13.0
  - bed W06
  - boat, ship, watercraft NEC (with drowning or submersion)—*see* Drowning, due to, fall overboard
    - with hitting bottom or object V94.0
  - bridge W13.1
  - building W13.9
    - burning (uncontrolled fire) X00.3
  - cavity W17.2
  - chair W07
  - cherry picker W17.89
  - cliff W15
  - dock W17.4
  - embankment W17.81
  - escalator W10.0
  - flagpole W13.8

Fall, falling (accidental), *continued*
- furniture NEC W08
- grocery cart W17.82
- haystack W17.89
- high place NEC W17.89
  - stated as undetermined whether accidental or intentional Y30
- hole W17.2
- incline W10.2
- ladder W11
- lifting device W17.89
- machine, machinery—*see also* Contact, with, by type of machine
  - not in operation W17.89
- manhole W17.1
- mobile elevated work platform [MEWP] W17.89
- motorized mobility scooter W05.2
- one level to another NEC W17.89
  - intentional, purposeful, suicide (attempt) X80
  - stated as undetermined whether accidental or intentional Y30
- pit W17.2
- playground equipment W09.8
  - jungle gym W09.2
  - slide W09.0
  - swing W09.1
- quarry W17.89
- railing W13.9
- ramp W10.2
- roof W13.2
- scaffolding W12
- scooter (nonmotorized) W05.1
  - motorized mobility W05.2
- sky lift W17.89
- stairs, steps W10.9
  - curb W10.1
  - due to ice or snow W00.1
  - escalator W10.0
  - incline W10.2
  - ramp W10.2
  - sidewalk curb W10.1
  - specified NEC W10.8
  - standing
    - electric scooter V00.841
    - micro-mobility pedestrian conveyance V00.848
- stepladder W11
- storm drain W17.1
- streetcar NEC V82.6
  - with antecedent collision—*see* Accident, transport, streetcar occupant
  - while boarding or alighting V82.4
- structure NEC W13.8
  - burning (uncontrolled fire) X00.3
- table W08
- toilet W18.11
  - with subsequent striking against object W18.12
- train NEC V81.6
  - during derailment (without antecedent collision) V81.7
    - with antecedent collision—*see* Accident, transport, railway vehicle occupant
  - while boarding or alighting V81.4
- transport vehicle after collision—*see* Accident, transport, by type of vehicle, collision
- tree W14
- vehicle (in motion) NEC (*see also* Accident, transport) V89.9
  - motor NEC (*see also* Accident, transport, occupant, by type of vehicle) V87.8
  - stationary W17.89
    - while boarding or alighting—*see* Accident, transport, by type of vehicle, while boarding or alighting
- viaduct W13.8
- wall W13.8
- watercraft—*see also* Drowning, due to, fall overboard
  - with hitting bottom or object V94.0
- well W17.0
- wheelchair, non-moving W05.0
  - powered—*see* Accident, transport, pedestrian, conveyance occupant, specified type NEC
- window W13.4

Fall, falling (accidental), *continued*
- in, on
  - aircraft NEC V97.0
    - with accident to aircraft V97.0
    - while boarding or alighting V97.1
  - bathtub (empty) W18.2
    - filled W16.212
      - causing drowning W16.211
  - escalator W10.0
  - incline W10.2
  - ladder W11
  - machine, machinery—*see* Contact, with, by type of machine
  - object, edged, pointed or sharp (with cut)—*see* Fall, by type
  - playground equipment W09.8
    - jungle gym W09.2
    - slide W09.0
    - swing W09.1
  - ramp W10.2
  - scaffolding W12
  - shower W18.2
    - causing drowning W16.211
  - staircase, stairs, steps W10.9
    - curb W10.1
    - due to ice or snow W00.1
    - escalator W10.0
    - incline W10.2
    - specified NEC W10.8
  - streetcar (without antecedent collision) V82.5
    - with antecedent collision—*see* Accident, transport, streetcar occupant
    - while boarding or alighting V82.4
  - train (without antecedent collision) V81.5
    - with antecedent collision—*see* Accident, transport, railway vehicle occupant
    - during derailment (without antecedent collision) V81.7
      - with antecedent collision—*see* Accident, transport, railway vehicle occupant
    - while boarding or alighting V81.4
  - transport vehicle after collision—*see* Accident, transport, by type of vehicle, collision
  - watercraft V93.39
    - due to
      - accident to craft V91.29
        - powered craft V91.2-
        - unpowered craft V91.2-
    - powered craft V93.3-
    - unpowered craft V93.3-
- into
  - cavity W17.2
  - dock W17.4
  - fire—*see* Exposure, fire, by type
  - haystack W17.89
  - hole W17.2
  - lake—*see* Fall, into, water
  - manhole W17.1
  - moving part of machinery—*see* Contact, with, by type of machine
  - ocean—*see* Fall, into, water
  - opening in surface NEC W17.89
  - pit W17.2
  - pond—*see* Fall, into, water
  - quarry W17.89
  - river—*see* Fall, into, water
  - shaft W17.89
  - storm drain W17.1
  - stream—*see* Fall, into, water
  - swimming pool—*see also* Fall, into, water, in, swimming pool
    - empty W17.3
  - tank W17.89
  - water W16.42
    - causing drowning W16.41
    - from watercraft—*see* Drowning, due to, fall overboard
    - hitting diving board W21.4
    - in
      - bathtub W16.212
        - causing drowning W16.211
      - bucket W16.222
        - causing drowning W16.221

FAILURE–FALL, FALLING (ACCIDENTAL)

Fall, falling (accidental), *continued*
~ natural body of water W16.112
◊ causing drowning W16.111
◊ striking
» bottom W16.122
❖ causing drowning W16.121
» side W16.132
❖ causing drowning W16.131
~ specified water NEC W16.312
◊ causing drowning W16.311
◊ striking
» bottom W16.322
❖ causing drowning W16.321
» wall W16.332
❖ causing drowning W16.331
~ swimming pool W16.012
◊ causing drowning W16.011
◊ striking
» bottom W16.022
❖ causing drowning W16.021
» wall W16.032
» causing drowning W16.031
~ utility bucket W16.222
◊ causing drowning W16.221
– well W17.0
• involving
– bed W06
– chair W07
– furniture NEC W08
– glass—*see* Fall, by type
– playground equipment W09.8
■ jungle gym W09.2
■ slide W09.0
■ swing W09.1
– roller blades—*see* Accident, transport, pedestrian, conveyance
– skateboard(s)—*see* Accident, transport, pedestrian, conveyance
– skates (ice) (in line) (roller)—*see* Accident, transport, pedestrian, conveyance
– skis—*see* Accident, transport, pedestrian, conveyance
– table W08
– wheelchair, non-moving W05.0
■ powered—*see* Accident, transport, pedestrian, conveyance, specified type NEC
• object—*see* Struck by, object, falling
• off
– toilet W18.11
■ with subsequent striking against object W18.12
• on same level W18.30
– due to
■ specified NEC W18.39
■ stepping on an object W18.31
• out of
– bed W06
– building NEC W13.8
– chair W07
– furniture NEC W08
– wheelchair, non-moving W05.0
■ powered—*see* Accident, transport, pedestrian, conveyance, specified type NEC
– window W13.4
• over
– animal W01.0
– cliff W15
– embankment W17.81
– small object W01.0
• rock W20.8
• same level W18.30
– from
■ being crushed, pushed, or stepped on by a crowd or human stampede W52
■ collision, pushing, shoving, by or with other person W03
■ slipping, stumbling, tripping W01.0
– involving ice or snow W00.0
■ involving skates (ice) (roller), skateboard, skis—*see* Accident, transport, pedestrian, conveyance
• snowslide (avalanche)—*see* Landslide
• stone W20.8

Fall, falling (accidental), *continued*
• structure W20.1
– burning (uncontrolled fire) X00.3
• through
– bridge W13.1
– floor W13.3
– roof W13.2
– wall W13.8
– window W13.4
• timber W20.8
• tree (caused by lightning) W20.8
• while being carried or supported by other person(s) W04
Fallen on by
• animal (not being ridden) NEC W55.89
Felo-de-se—*see* Suicide
Fight (hand) (fists) (foot)—*see* Assault, fight
Fire (accidental)—*see* Exposure, fire
Firearm discharge—*see* Discharge, firearm
Fireworks (explosion) W39
Flash burns from explosion—*see* Explosion
Flood (any injury) (caused by) X38
• collapse of man-made structure causing earth movement X36.0
• tidal wave—*see* Forces of nature, tidal wave
Food (any type) in
• air passages (with asphyxia, obstruction, or suffocation) (*see* categories T17 and) T18
• alimentary tract causing asphyxia (due to compression of trachea) (*see* categories T17 and) T18
Forces of nature X39.8
• avalanche X36.1
– causing transport accident—*see* Accident, transport, by type of vehicle
• blizzard X37.2
• cataclysmic storm X37.9
– with flood X38
– blizzard X37.2
– cloudburst X37.8
– cyclone X37.1
– dust storm X37.3
– hurricane X37.0
– specified storm NEC X37.8
– storm surge X37.0
– tornado X37.1
– twister X37.1
– typhoon X37.0
• cloudburst X37.8
• cold (natural) X31
• cyclone X37.1
• dam collapse causing earth movement X36.0
• dust storm X37.3
• earth movement X36.1
– earthquake X34
– caused by dam or structure collapse X36.0
• earthquake X34
• flood (caused by) X38
– dam collapse X36.0
– tidal wave—*see* Forces of nature, tidal wave
• heat (natural) X30
• hurricane X37.0
• landslide X36.1
– causing transport accident—*see* Accident, transport, by type of vehicle
• lightning—*see* subcategory T75.0
– causing fire—*see* Exposure, fire
• mudslide X36.1
– causing transport accident—*see* Accident, transport, by type of vehicle
• specified force NEC X39.8
• storm surge X37.0
• structure collapse causing earth movement X36.0
• sunlight X32
• tidal wave X37.41
– due to
■ earthquake X37.41
■ landslide X37.43
■ storm X37.42
■ volcanic eruption X37.41
• tornado X37.1
• tsunami X37.41

Forces of nature, *continued*
• twister X37.1
• typhoon X37.0
• volcanic eruption X35
Foreign body
• aspiration—*see* Index to Diseases and Injuries, Foreign body, respiratory tract
• entering through skin W45.8
– can lid W26.8
– nail W45.0
– paper W26.2
– specified NEC W45.8
– splinter W45.8
Forest fire (exposure to)—*see* Exposure, fire, uncontrolled, not in building
Found injured X58
• from exposure (to)—*see* Exposure
• on
– highway, road (way), street V89.9
– railway right of way V81.9
Fracture (circumstances unknown or unspecified) X58
• due to specified cause NEC X58
Frostbite X31
• due to man-made conditions—*see* Exposure, cold, man-made
Frozen—*see* Exposure, cold

G

Gunshot wound W34.00

H

Hailstones, injured by X39.8
Hanged herself or himself—*see* Hanging, self-inflicted
Hanging (accidental) (*see also*** category)** T71
Heat (effects of) (excessive) X30
• due to
– man-made conditions
■ on board watercraft V93.29
~ fishing boat V93.22
~ merchant ship V93.20
~ passenger ship V93.21
~ sailboat V93.24
~ specified powered craft NEC V93.23
– weather (conditions) X30
• from
– electric heating apparatus causing burning X16
• inappropriate in local application or packing in medical or surgical procedure Y63.5
Hemorrhage
• delayed following medical or surgical treatment without mention of misadventure—*see* Index to Diseases and Injuries, Complication(s)
• during medical or surgical treatment as misadventure—*see* Index to Diseases and Injuries, Complication(s)
High
• altitude (effects)—*see* Air, pressure, low
• level of radioactivity, effects—*see* Radiation
• pressure (effects)—*see* Air, pressure, high
• temperature, effects—*see* Heat
• **Hit, hitting (accidental) by**—*see* Struck by
• **Hitting against**—*see* Striking against
• **Hot**
• place, effects—*see also* Heat
• weather, effects X30
House fire (uncontrolled)—*see* Exposure, fire, uncontrolled, building
Humidity, causing problem X39.8
Hunger X58
Hurricane (any injury) X37.0
Hypobarism, hypobaropathy—*see* Air, pressure, low

I

Ictus
• caloris—*see also* Heat
• solaris X30

Ignition (accidental) (*see also* Exposure, fire) X08.8
- anesthetic gas in operating room W40.1
- apparel X06.2
  - from highly flammable material X04
  - nightwear X05
- bed linen (sheets) (spreads) (pillows) (mattress)—*see* Exposure, fire, uncontrolled, building, bed
- benzine X04
- clothes, clothing NEC (from controlled fire) X06.2
  - from
    - highly flammable material X04
- ether X04
  - in operating room W40.1
- explosive material—*see* Explosion
- gasoline X04
- jewelry (plastic) (any) X06.0
- kerosene X04
- material
  - explosive—*see* Explosion
  - highly flammable with secondary explosion X04
- nightwear X05
- paraffin X04
- petrol X04

Immersion (accidental)—*see also* Drowning
- hand or foot due to cold (excessive) X31

Implantation of quills of porcupine W55.89

Inanition (from) (hunger) X58
- thirst X58

Inappropriate operation performed
- correct operation on wrong side or body part (wrong side) (wrong site) Y65.53
- operation intended for another patient done on wrong patient Y65.52
- wrong operation performed on correct patient Y65.51

Incident, adverse
- device
  - anesthesiology Y70.-
  - cardiovascular Y71.-
  - gastroenterology Y73.-
  - general
    - hospital Y74.-
    - surgical Y81.-
  - gynecological Y76.-
  - medical Y82.9
    - specified type NEC Y82.8
  - neurological Y75.-
  - obstetrical Y76.-
  - ophthalmic Y77.-
  - orthopedic Y79.-
  - otorhinolaryngological Y72.-
  - personal use Y74.-
  - physical medicine Y80.-
  - plastic surgical Y81.-
  - radiological Y78.-
  - urology Y73.-

Incineration (accidental)—*see* Exposure, fire

Infanticide—*see* Assault

Infrasound waves (causing injury) W49.9

Ingestion
- foreign body (causing injury) (with obstruction) T17 or T18
- poisonous
  - plant(s) X58
  - substance NEC—*see* Table of Drugs and Chemicals

Inhalation
- excessively cold substance, man-made—*see* Exposure, cold, man-made
- food (any type) (into respiratory tract) (with asphyxia, obstruction respiratory tract, suffocation) (*see* categories T17 and) T18
- foreign body—*see* Foreign body, aspiration
- gastric contents (with asphyxia, obstruction respiratory passage, suffocation) T17.81-
- liquid air, hydrogen, nitrogen W93.12
- steam X13.0
  - assault X98.0
  - stated as undetermined whether accidental or intentional Y27.0

Inhalation, *continued*
- toxic gas—*see* Table of Drugs and Chemicals
- vomitus (with asphyxia, obstruction respiratory passage, suffocation) T17.81-

Injury, injured (accidental(ly)) NOS X58
- by, caused by, from
  - assault—*see* Assault
- homicide (*see also* Assault) Y09
- inflicted (by)
  - other person
    - stated as
      - ~ accidental X58
      - ~ undetermined whether accidental or intentional Y33
- purposely (inflicted) by other person(s)—*see* Assault
- self-inflicted X83.8
  - stated as accidental X58
- specified cause NEC X58
- undetermined whether accidental or intentional Y33

Insolation, effects X30

Insufficient nourishment X58

Interruption of respiration (by)
- food (lodged in esophagus) (*see* categories T17 and) T18
- vomitus (lodged in esophagus) T17.81- Intoxication
- drug—*see* Table of Drugs and Chemicals
- poison—*see* Table of Drugs and Chemicals

J

Jammed (accidentally)
- between objects (moving) (stationary and moving) W23.0
  - stationary W23.1

Jumped, jumping
- before moving object NEC X81.8
  - motor vehicle X81.0
  - subway train X81.1
  - train X81.1
  - undetermined whether accidental or intentional Y31
- from
  - boat (into water) voluntarily, without accident (to or on boat) W16.712
    - with
      - ~ accident to or on boat—*see* Accident, watercraft
      - ~ drowning or submersion W16.711
    - striking bottom W16.722
      - ~ causing drowning W16.721
  - building (*see also* Jumped, from, high place) W13.9
    - burning (uncontrolled fire) X00.5
  - high place NEC W17.89
    - suicide (attempt) X80
    - undetermined whether accidental or intentional Y30
  - structure (*see also* Jumped, from, high place) W13.9
    - burning (uncontrolled fire) X00.5
- into water W16.92
  - causing drowning W16.91
  - from, off watercraft—*see* Jumped, from, boat
  - in
    - natural body W16.612
      - ~ causing drowning W16.611
      - ~ striking bottom W16.622
        - ◊ causing drowning W16.621
    - specified place NEC W16.812
      - ~ causing drowning W16.811
      - ~ striking
        - ◊ bottom W16.822
          - » causing drowning W16.821
        - ◊ wall W16.832
          - » causing drowning W16.831
    - swimming pool W16.512
      - ~ causing drowning W16.511
      - ~ striking
        - ◊ bottom W16.522
          - » causing drowning W16.521
        - ◊ wall W16.532
          - » causing drowning W16.531

K

Kicked by
- animal NEC W55.82
- person(s) (accidentally) W50.1
  - with intent to injure or kill Y04.0
  - as, or caused by, a crowd or human stampede (with fall) W52
  - assault Y04.0
  - in
    - fight Y04.0

Kicking against
- object W22.8
  - sports equipment W21.9
  - stationary W22.09
    - sports equipment W21.89
- person—*see* Striking against, person
- sports equipment W21.9

Knocked down (accidentally) (by) NOS X58
- animal (not being ridden) NEC—*see also* Struck by, by type of animal
- crowd or human stampede W52
- person W51
  - in brawl, fight Y04.0
- transport vehicle NEC (*see also* Accident, transport) V09.9

L

Laceration NEC—*see* Injury

Lack of
- care (helpless person) (infant) (newborn) X58
- food except as result of abandonment or neglect X58
  - due to abandonment or neglect X58
- water except as result of transport accident X58
  - due to transport accident—*see* Accident, transport, by type
  - helpless person, infant, newborn X58

Landslide (falling on transport vehicle) X36.1
- caused by collapse of man-made structure X36.0

Late effect—*see* Sequelae

Lightning (shock) (stroke) (struck by)—*see* subcategory T75.0
- causing fire—*see* Exposure, fire

Loss of control (transport vehicle) NEC—*see* Accident, transport

Lying before train, vehicle or other moving object X81.8
- subway train X81.1
- train X81.1
- undetermined whether accidental or intentional Y31

M

Malfunction (mechanism or component) (of)
- firearm W34.10
  - airgun W34.110
  - BB gun W34.110
  - gas, air or spring-operated gun NEC W34.118
  - handgun W32.1
  - hunting rifle W33.12 larger firearm W33.10
    - specified NEC W33.19
  - machine gun W33.13
  - paintball gun W34.111
  - pellet gun W34.110
  - shotgun W33.11
  - specified NEC W34.19
  - Very pistol [flare] W34.19
- handgun—*see* Malfunction, firearm, handgun

Maltreatment—*see* Perpetrator

Mangled (accidentally) NOS X58

Manhandling (in brawl, fight) Y04.0

Manslaughter (nonaccidental)—*see* Assault

Mauled by animal NEC W55.89

Medical procedure, complication of (delayed or as an abnormal reaction without mention of misadventure)—*see* Complication of or following, by specified type of procedure
- due to or as a result of misadventure—*see* Misadventure

Melting (due to fire)—*see also* Exposure, fire
- apparel NEC X06.3
- clothes, clothing NEC X06.3
  - nightwear X05
- fittings or furniture (burning building) (uncontrolled fire) X00.8
- nightwear X05
- plastic jewelry X06.1

Mental cruelty X58

Military operations (injuries to military and civilians occurring during peacetime on military property and during routine military exercises and operations) (by) (from) (involving)—*Refer to ICD-10-CM Manual*

Misadventure(s) to patient(s) during surgical or medical care Y69
- contaminated medical or biological substance (blood, drug, fluid) Y64.9
  - administered (by) NEC Y64.9
    - immunization Y64.1
    - infusion Y64.0
    - injection Y64.1
    - specified means NEC Y64.8
    - transfusion Y64.0
    - vaccination Y64.1
- excessive amount of blood or other fluid during transfusion or infusion Y63.0
- failure
  - in dosage Y63.9
    - electroshock therapy Y63.4
    - inappropriate temperature (too hot or too cold) in local application and packing Y63.5
    - infusion
      ~ excessive amount of fluid Y63.0
      ~ incorrect dilution of fluid Y63.1
    - insulin-shock therapy Y63.4
    - nonadministration of necessary drug or biological substance Y63.6
    - overdose—*see* Table of Drugs and Chemicals
      ~ radiation, in therapy Y63.2
    - radiation
      ~ overdose Y63.2
    - specified procedure NEC Y63.8
    - transfusion
      ~ excessive amount of blood Y63.0
  - mechanical, of instrument or apparatus (any) (during any procedure) Y65.8
  - sterile precautions (during procedure) Y62.9
    - aspiration of fluid or tissue (by puncture or catheterization, except heart) Y62.6
    - biopsy (except needle aspiration) Y62.8
      ~ needle (aspirating) Y62.6
    - blood sampling Y62.6
    - catheterization Y62.6
      ~ heart Y62.5
    - dialysis (kidney) Y62.2
    - endoscopic examination Y62.4
    - enema Y62.8
    - immunization Y62.3
    - infusion Y62.1
    - injection Y62.3
    - needle biopsy Y62.6
    - paracentesis (abdominal) (thoracic) Y62.6
    - perfusion Y62.2
    - puncture (lumbar) Y62.6
    - removal of catheter or packing Y62.8
    - specified procedure NEC Y62.8
    - surgical operation Y62.0
    - transfusion Y62.1
    - vaccination Y62.3
  - suture or ligature during surgical procedure Y65.2
  - to introduce or to remove tube or instrument—*see* Failure, to
- hemorrhage—*see* Index to Diseases and Injuries, Complication(s)
- inadvertent exposure of patient to radiation Y63.3
- inappropriate
  - operation performed—*see* Inappropriate operation performed
  - temperature (too hot or too cold) in local application or packing Y63.5

Misadventure(s) to patient(s) during surgical or medical care, *continued*
- infusion (*see also* Misadventure, by type, infusion) Y69
  - excessive amount of fluid Y63.0
  - incorrect dilution of fluid Y63.1
  - wrong fluid Y65.1
- nonadministration of necessary drug or biological substance Y63.6
- overdose—*see* Table of Drugs and Chemicals
  - radiation (in therapy) Y63.2
- perforation—*see* Index to Diseases and Injuries, Complication(s)
- performance of inappropriate operation—*see* Inappropriate operation performed
- puncture—*see* Index to Diseases and Injuries, Complication(s)
- specified type NEC Y65.8
  - failure
    - suture or ligature during surgical operation Y65.2
    - to introduce or to remove tube or instrument—*see* Failure, to
  - infusion of wrong fluid Y65.1
  - performance of inappropriate operation—*see* Inappropriate operation performed
  - transfusion of mismatched blood Y65.0
  - wrong
    - fluid in infusion Y65.1
    - placement of endotracheal tube during anesthetic procedure Y65.3
- transfusion—*see* Misadventure, by type, transfusion
  - excessive amount of blood Y63.0
  - mismatched blood Y65.0
- wrong
  - drug given in error—*see* Table of Drugs and Chemicals
  - fluid in infusion Y65.1
  - placement of endotracheal tube during anesthetic procedure Y65.3

Mismatched blood in transfusion Y65.0

Motion sickness T75.3

Mountain sickness W94.11

Mudslide (of cataclysmic nature)—*see* Landslide

N

Nail, contact with W45.0
- gun W29.4

Noise (causing injury) (pollution) W42.9
- supersonic W42.0

Nonadministration (of)
- drug or biological substance (necessary) Y63.6
- surgical and medical care Y66

Nosocomial condition Y95

O

Object
- falling
  - from, in, on, hitting
    - machinery—*see* Contact, with, by type of machine
- set in motion by
  - accidental explosion or rupture of pressure vessel W38
  - firearm—*see* Discharge, firearm, by type
  - machine(ry)—*see* Contact, with, by type of machine

Overdose (drug)—*see* Table of Drugs and Chemicals
- radiation Y63.2

Overexertion
- due to
  - other or unspecified movement X50.9
  - prolonged static or awkward postures X50.1
  - repetitive movements X50.3
  - strenuous movement X50.0

Overexposure (accidental) (to)
- cold (*see also* Exposure, cold) X31
  - due to man-made conditions—*see* Exposure, cold, man-made
- heat (*see also* Heat) X30
- radiation—*see* Radiation
- sun (sunburn) X32

Overexposure (accidental) (to), *continued*
- weather NEC—*see* Forces of nature
- wind NEC—*see* Forces of nature

Overheated—*see* Heat

Overturning (accidental)
- machinery—*see* Contact, with, by type of machine
- transport vehicle NEC (*see also* Accident, transport) V89.9
- watercraft (causing drowning, submersion)—*see also* Drowning, due to, accident to, watercraft, overturning
  - causing injury except drowning or submersion—*see* Accident, watercraft, causing, injury NEC

P

Parachute descent (voluntary) (without accident to aircraft) V97.29
- due to accident to aircraft—*see* Accident, transport, aircraft

Pecked by bird W61.99

Perforation during medical or surgical treatment as misadventure—*see* Index to Diseases and Injuries, Complication(s)

Perpetrator, perpetration, of assault, maltreatment and neglect (by) Y07.-

Piercing—*see* Contact, with, by type of object or machine

Pinched
- between objects (moving) (stationary and moving) W23.0
  - stationary W23.1

Pinned under machine(ry)—*see* Contact, with, by type of machine

Place of occurrence Y92.9
- abandoned house Y92.89
- airplane Y92.813
- airport Y92.520
- ambulatory health services establishment NEC Y92.538
- ambulatory surgery center Y92.530
- amusement park Y92.831
- apartment (co-op) Y92.039
  - bathroom Y92.031
  - bedroom Y92.032
  - kitchen Y92.030
  - specified NEC Y92.038
- assembly hall Y92.29
- bank Y92.510
- barn Y92.71
- baseball field Y92.320
- basketball court Y92.310
- beach Y92.832
- boat Y92.814
- bowling alley Y92.39
- bridge Y92.89
- building under construction Y92.61
- bus Y92.811
  - station Y92.521
- cafe Y92.511
- campsite Y92.833
- campus—*see* Place of occurrence, school
- canal Y92.89
- car Y92.810
- casino Y92.59
- church Y92.22
- cinema Y92.26
- clubhouse Y92.29
- coal pit Y92.64
- college (community) Y92.214
- condominium—*see* apartment
- construction area—Y92.6-
- convalescent home—Y92.129-
- court-house Y92.240
- cricket ground Y92.328
- cultural building Y92.25-
- dancehall Y92.252
- day nursery Y92.210
- dentist office Y92.531
- derelict house Y92.89
- desert Y92.820
- dock NOS Y92.89
- dockyard Y92.62
- doctor's office Y92.531

Poisoning (accidental) (by), *continued*
- fumes or smoke due to
  - explosion (*see also* Explosion) W40.9
  - fire—*see* Exposure, fire
  - ignition—*see* Ignition

Powder burn (by) (from)
- airgun W34.110
- BB gun W34.110
- firearm NEC W34.19
- gas, air or spring-operated gun NEC W34.118
- handgun W32.1
- hunting rifle W33.12
- larger firearm W33.10
  - specified NEC W33.19
- machine gun W33.13
- paintball gun W34.111
- pellet gun W34.110
- shotgun W33.11
- Very pistol [flare] W34.19

Premature cessation (of) surgical and medical care Y66

Privation (food) (water) X58

Procedure (operation)
- correct, on wrong side or body part (wrong side) (wrong site) Y65.53
- intended for another patient done on wrong patient Y65.52
- performed on patient not scheduled for surgery Y65.52
- performed on wrong patient Y65.52
- wrong, performed on correct patient Y65.51

Prolonged
- sitting in transport vehicle—*see* Travel, by type of vehicle
- stay in
  - high altitude as cause of anoxia, barodontalgia, barotitis or hypoxia W94.11

Pulling, excessive—*see* category Y93

Puncture, puncturing—*see also* Contact, with, by type of object or machine
- by
  - plant thorns, spines, sharp leaves or other mechanisms NEC W60
- during medical or surgical treatment as misadventure—*see* Index to Diseases and Injuries, Complication(s)

Pushed, pushing (accidental) (injury in) (overexertion)—*see* category Y93
- by other person(s) (accidental) W51
  - with fall W03
    - due to ice or snow W00.0
  - as, or caused by, a crowd or human stampede (with fall) W52
  - before moving object NEC Y02.8
    - motor vehicle Y02.0
    - subway train Y02.1
    - train Y02.1
  - from
    - high place NEC
      - ~ in accidental circumstances W17.89
      - ~ stated as
        - ◊ intentional, homicide (attempt) Y01
        - ◊ undetermined whether accidental or intentional Y30
    - transport vehicle NEC (*see also* Accident, transport) V89.9

R

Radiation (exposure to) (refer to *ICD-10-CM* manual for more)
- light sources (man-made visible and ultraviolet)
  - natural X32
- misadventure in medical or surgical procedure Y63.2
- natural NEC X39.08
- overdose (in medical or surgical procedure) Y63.2
- sun X32
- ultraviolet (light) (man-made)
  - natural X32

Range disease W94.11

Rape (attempted) T74.2-

Rat bite W53.11

Reaction, abnormal to medical procedure (*see also* Complication of or following, by type of procedure) Y84.9
- with misadventure—*see* Misadventure
- biologicals or drugs or vaccine—*see* Table of Drugs and Chemicals

Recoil
- airgun W34.110
- BB gun W34.110
- firearm NEC W34.19
- gas, air or spring-operated gun NEC W34.118
- handgun W32.1
- hunting rifle W33.12
- larger firearm W33.10
  - specified NEC W33.19
- machine gun W33.13
- paintball gun W34.111
- pellet W34.110
- shotgun W33.11
- Very pistol [flare] W34.19

Reduction in
- atmospheric pressure—*see* Air, pressure, change

Rock falling on or hitting (accidentally) (person) W20.8
- in cave-in W20.0

Run over (accidentally) (by)
- animal (not being ridden) NEC W55.89
- machinery—*see* Contact, with, by specified type of machine
- transport vehicle NEC (*see also* Accident, transport) V09.9
  - motor NEC V09.20

Running
- before moving object X81.8
  - motor vehicle X81.0

Running off, away
- animal (being ridden) (*see also* Accident, transport) V80.918
  - not being ridden W55.89
- animal-drawn vehicle NEC (*see also* Accident, transport) V80.928
- highway, road (way), street
  - transport vehicle NEC (*see also* Accident, transport) V89.9

Rupture pressurized devices—*see* Explosion, by type of device

S

Saturnism—*see* Table of Drugs and Chemicals, lead

Scald, scalding (accidental) (by) (from) (in) X19
- liquid (boiling) (hot) NEC X12
  - stated as undetermined whether accidental or intentional Y27.2
- local application of externally applied substance in medical or surgical care Y63.5
- metal (molten) (liquid) (hot) NEC X18
- self-inflicted X77.9
- stated as undetermined whether accidental or intentional Y27.8
- steam X13.1
  - assault X98.0
  - stated as undetermined whether accidental or intentional Y27.0
- vapor (hot) X13.1
  - assault X98.0
  - stated as undetermined whether accidental or intentional Y27.0

Scratched by
- cat W55.03
- person(s) (accidentally) W50.4
  - with intent to injure or kill Y04.0
  - as, or caused by, a crowd or human stampede (with fall) W52
  - assault Y04.0
  - in
    - fight Y04.0

Seasickness T75.3

Self-harm NEC—*see also* **External cause by type, undetermined whether accidental or intentional**
- intentional—*see* Suicide
- poisoning NEC—*see* Table of Drugs and Chemicals

Self-inflicted (injury) NEC—*see also* External cause by type, undetermined whether accidental or intentional
- intentional—*see* Suicide
- poisoning NEC—*see* Table of Drugs and Chemicals

Sequelae (of)
Use original code to define how the injury occurred with 7th character S

Shock
- electric—*see* Exposure, electric current
- from electric appliance (any) (faulty) W86.8
  - domestic W86.0

Shooting, shot (accidental(ly))—*see also* Discharge, firearm, by type
- herself or himself—*see* Discharge, firearm by type, self-inflicted
- inflicted by other person—*see* Discharge, firearm by type, homicide
  - accidental—*see* Discharge, firearm, by type of firearm
- self-inflicted—*see* Discharge, firearm by type, suicide
  - accidental—*see* Discharge, firearm, by type of firearm
- suicide (attempt)—*see* Discharge, firearm by type, suicide

Shoving (accidentally) by other person—*see* Pushed, by other person

Sickness
- alpine W94.11
- motion—*see* Motion
- mountain W94.11

Sinking (accidental)
- watercraft (causing drowning, submersion)—*see also* Drowning, due to, accident to, watercraft, sinking
  - causing injury except drowning or submersion—*see* Accident, watercraft, causing, injury NEC

Siriasis X32

Slashed wrists—*see* Cut, self-inflicted

Slipping (accidental) (on same level) (with fall) W01.0
- on
  - ice W00.0
    - with skates—*see* Accident, transport, pedestrian, conveyance
  - mud W01.0
  - oil W01.0
  - snow W00.0
    - with skis—*see* Accident, transport, pedestrian, conveyance
  - surface (slippery) (wet) NEC W01.0
- without fall W18.40
  - due to
    - specified NEC W18.49
    - stepping from one level to another W18.43
    - stepping into hole or opening W18.42
    - stepping on object W18.41

Sliver, wood, contact with W45.8

Smoldering (due to fire)—*see* Exposure, fire

Sodomy (attempted) by force T74.2-

Sound waves (causing injury) W42.9
- supersonic W42.0

Splinter, contact with W45.8

Stab, stabbing—*see* Cut

Starvation X58

Status of external cause Y99.-

Stepped on
- by
  - animal (not being ridden) NEC W55.89
  - crowd or human stampede W52
  - person W50.0

Stepping on
- object W22.8
  - with fall W18.31
  - sports equipment W21.9
  - stationary W22.09
    - sports equipment W21.89
- person W51
  - by crowd or human stampede W52
- sports equipment W21.9

Sting
- arthropod, nonvenomous W57
- insect, nonvenomous W57

Storm (cataclysmic)—*see* Forces of nature, cataclysmic storm

Straining, excessive—*see* category Y93

Strangling—*see* Strangulation

Strangulation (accidental)—*see* category T71

Strenuous movements—*see* category Y93

Striking against
- airbag (automobile) W22.10
  - driver side W22.11
  - front passenger side W22.12
  - specified NEC W22.19
- bottom when
  - diving or jumping into water (in) W16.822
    - causing drowning W16.821
    - from boat W16.722
      - causing drowning W16.721
    - natural body W16.622
      - causing drowning W16.821
    - swimming pool W16.522
      - causing drowning W16.521
  - falling into water (in) W16.322
    - causing drowning W16.321
    - fountain—*see* Striking against, bottom when, falling into water, specified NEC
    - natural body W16.122
      - causing drowning W16.121
    - reservoir—*see* Striking against, bottom when, falling into water, specified NEC
    - specified NEC W16.322
      - causing drowning W16.321
    - swimming pool W16.022
      - causing drowning W16.021
- diving board (swimming-pool) W21.4
- object W22.8
  - with
    - drowning or submersion—*see* Drowning
    - fall—*see* Fall, due to, bumping against, object
  - caused by crowd or human stampede (with fall) W52
  - furniture W22.03
  - lamppost W22.02
  - sports equipment W21.9
  - stationary W22.09
    - sports equipment W21.89
  - wall W22.01
- person(s) W51
  - with fall W03
    - due to ice or snow W00.0
  - as, or caused by, a crowd or human stampede (with fall) W52
  - assault Y04.2
- sports equipment W21.9
- wall (when) W22.01
  - diving or jumping into water (in) W16.832
    - causing drowning W16.831
    - swimming pool W16.532
      - causing drowning W16.531
  - falling into water (in) W16.332
    - causing drowning W16.331
    - fountain—*see* Striking against, wall when, falling into water, specified NEC
    - natural body W16.132
      - causing drowning W16.131
    - reservoir—*see* Striking against, wall when, falling into water, specified NEC
    - specified NEC W16.332
      - causing drowning W16.331
    - swimming pool W16.032
      - causing drowning W16.031
  - swimming pool (when) W22.042
    - causing drowning W22.041
    - diving or jumping into water W16.532
      - causing drowning W16.531
    - falling into water W16.032
      - causing drowning W16.031

Struck (accidentally) by
- airbag (automobile) W22.10
  - driver side W22.11

Struck (accidentally) by, *continued*
- front passenger side W22.12
- specified NEC W22.19
- alligator W58.02
- animal (not being ridden) NEC W55.89
- avalanche—*see* Landslide
- ball (hit) (thrown) W21.00
  - assault Y08.09
  - baseball W21.03
  - basketball W21.05
  - golf ball W21.04
  - football W21.01
  - soccer W21.02
  - softball W21.07
  - specified NEC W21.09
  - volleyball W21.06
- bat or racquet
  - baseball bat W21.11
    - assault Y08.02
  - golf club W21.13
    - assault Y08.09
  - specified NEC W21.19
    - assault Y08.09
  - tennis racquet W21.12
    - assault Y08.09
- bullet—*see also* Discharge, firearm by type
- crocodile W58.12
- dog W54.1
- flare, Very pistol—*see* Discharge, firearm NEC
- hailstones X39.8
- hockey (ice)
  - field
    - puck W21.221
    - stick W21.211
  - puck W21.220
  - stick W21.210
    - assault Y08.01
- landslide—*see* Landslide
- lightning—*see* subcategory T75.0
  - causing fire—*see* Exposure, fire
- machine—*see* Contact, with, by type of machine
- mammal NEC W55.89
  - marine W56.32
- marine animal W56.82
- object W22.8
  - blunt W22.8
    - assault Y00
    - undetermined whether accidental or intentional Y29
  - falling W20.8
    - from, in, on
      - building W20.1
        - burning (uncontrolled fire) X00.4
      - cataclysmic
        - earth surface movement NEC—*see* Landslide
        - storm—*see* Forces of nature, cataclysmic storm
      - cave-in W20.0
      - earthquake X34
      - machine (in operation)—*see* Contact, with, by type of machine
      - structure W20.1
        - burning X00.4
      - transport vehicle (in motion)—*see* Accident, transport, by type of vehicle
      - watercraft V93.49
        - due to
          - accident to craft V91.39
            - powered craft V91.3-
            - unpowered craft V91.3-
          - powered craft V93.4-
          - unpowered craft V93.4-
  - moving NEC W20.8
  - projected W20.8
    - assault Y00
    - in sports W21.9
      - assault Y08.09
      - ball W21.00
        - baseball W21.03
        - basketball W21.05
        - football W21.01
        - golf ball W21.04
        - soccer W21.02

Struck (accidentally) by, *continued*
- softball W21.07
- specified NEC W21.09
- volleyball W21.06
- bat or racquet
  - baseball bat W21.11
    - assault Y08.02
  - golf club W21.13
    - assault Y08.09
  - specified NEC W21.19
    - assault Y08.09
  - tennis racquet W21.12
    - assault Y08.09
- hockey (ice)
  - field
    - puck W21.221
    - stick W21.211
  - puck W21.220
  - stick W21.210
    - assault Y08.01
- specified NEC W21.89
  - set in motion by explosion—*see* Explosion
  - thrown W20.8
    - assault Y00
    - in sports W21.9
      - assault Y08.09
      - ball W21.00
        - baseball W21.03
        - basketball W21.05
        - football W21.01
        - golf ball W21.04
        - soccer W21.02
        - soft ball W21.07
        - specified NEC W21.09
        - volleyball W21.06
      - bat or racquet
        - baseball bat W21.11
          - assault Y08.02
        - golf club W21.13
          - assault Y08.09
        - specified NEC W21.19
          - assault Y08.09
        - tennis racquet W21.12
          - assault Y08.09
      - hockey (ice)
        - field
          - puck W21.221
          - stick W21.211
        - puck W21.220
        - stick W21.210
          - assault Y08.01
      - specified NEC W21.89
- other person(s) W50.0
  - with
    - blunt object W22.8
      - intentional, homicide (attempt) Y00
      - sports equipment W21.9
      - undetermined whether accidental or intentional Y29
    - fall W03
      - due to ice or snow W00.0
  - as, or caused by, a crowd or human stampede (with fall) W52
  - assault Y04.2
  - sports equipment W21.9
- sports equipment W21.9
  - assault Y08.09
  - ball W21.00
    - baseball W21.03
    - basketball W21.05
    - football W21.01
    - golf ball W21.04
    - soccer W21.02
    - soft ball W21.07
    - specified NEC W21.09
    - volleyball W21.06
  - bat or racquet
    - baseball bat W21.11
      - assault Y08.02
    - golf club W21.13
      - assault Y08.09
    - specified NEC W21.19

Struck (accidentally) by, *continued*
- ■ tennis racquet W21.12
  - ~ assault Y08.09
- – cleats (shoe) W21.31
- – foot wear NEC W21.39
- – football helmet W21.81
- – hockey (ice)
  - ■ field
    - ~ puck W21.221
    - ~ stick W21.211
  - ■ puck W21.220
  - ■ stick W21.210
    - ~ assault Y08.01
- – skate blades W21.32
- – specified NEC W21.89
  - ■ assault Y08.09
- • thunderbolt—*see* subcategory T75.0
  - – causing fire—*see* Exposure, fire
- • transport vehicle NEC (*see also* Accident, transport) V09.9
  - – intentional, homicide (attempt) Y03.0
  - – motor NEC (*see also* Accident, transport) V09.20
- • vehicle (transport) NEC—*see* Accident, transport, by type of vehicle
  - – stationary (falling from jack, hydraulic lift, ramp) W20.8

Stumbling
- • over
  - – animal NEC W01.0
    - ■ with fall W18.09
  - – carpet, rug or (small) object W22.8
    - ■ with fall W18.09
  - – person W51
    - ■ with fall W03
      - ~ due to ice or snow W00.0
- • without fall W18.40
  - – due to
    - ■ specified NEC W18.49
    - ■ stepping from one level to another W18.43
    - ■ stepping into hole or opening W18.42
    - ■ stepping on object W18.41

Submersion (accidental)—*see* Drowning

Suffocation (accidental) (by external means) (by pressure) (mechanical) (*see also* category) T71
- • due to, by
  - – avalanche—*see* Landslide
  - – explosion—*see* Explosion
  - – fire—*see* Exposure, fire
  - – food, any type (aspiration) (ingestion) (inhalation) (*see* categories T17 and) T18
  - – ignition—*see* Ignition
  - – landslide—*see* Landslide
  - – machine(ry)—*see* Contact, with, by type of machine
  - – vomitus (aspiration) (inhalation) T17.81-
- • in
  - – burning building X00.8

Suicide, suicidal (attempted) (by) X83.8
- • blunt object X79
- • burning, burns X76
  - – hot object X77.9
    - ■ fluid NEC X77.2
    - ■ household appliance X77.3
    - ■ specified NEC X77.8
    - ■ steam X77.0
    - ■ tap water X77.1
    - ■ vapors X77.0
- • caustic substance—*see* Table of Drugs and Chemicals
- • cold, extreme X83.2
- • collision of motor vehicle with
  - – motor vehicle X82.0
  - – specified NEC X82.8
  - – train X82.1
  - – tree X82.2
- • cut (any part of body) X78.9
- • cutting or piercing instrument X78.9
  - – dagger X78.2
  - – glass X78.0
  - – knife X78.1
  - – specified NEC X78.8
  - – sword X78.2

Suicide, suicidal (attempted) (by), *continued*
- • drowning (in) X71.9
  - – bathtub X71.0
  - – natural water X71.3
  - – specified NEC X71.8
  - – swimming pool X71.1
    - ■ following fall X71.2
- • electrocution X83.1
- • explosive(s) (material) X75
- • fire, flames X76
- • firearm X74.9
  - – airgun X74.01
  - – handgun X72
  - – hunting rifle X73.1
  - – larger X73.9
    - ■ specified NEC X73.8
  - – machine gun X73.2
  - -- paintball gun X74.02
  - – shotgun X73.0
  - – specified NEC X74.8
- • hanging X83.8
- • hot object—*see* Suicide, burning, hot object
- • jumping
  - – before moving object X81.8
    - ■ motor vehicle X81.0
    - ■ subway train X81.1
    - ■ train X81.1
  - – from high place X80
- • lying before moving object, train, vehicle X81.8
- • poisoning—*see* Table of Drugs and Chemicals
- • puncture (any part of body)—*see* Suicide, cutting or piercing instrument
- • scald—*see* Suicide, burning, hot object
- • sharp object (any)—*see* Suicide, cutting or piercing instrument
- • shooting—*see* Suicide, firearm
- • specified means NEC X83.8
- • stab (any part of body)—*see* Suicide, cutting or piercing instrument
- • steam, hot vapors X77.0
- • strangulation X83.8
- • submersion—*see* Suicide, drowning
- • suffocation X83.8
- • wound NEC X83.8

Sunstroke X32

Supersonic waves (causing injury) W42.0

Surgical procedure, complication of (delayed or as an abnormal reaction without mention of misadventure)—*see also* Complication of or following, by type of procedure
- • due to or as a result of misadventure—*see* Misadventure

Swallowed, swallowing
- • foreign body T18
- • poison—*see* Table of Drugs and Chemicals
- • substance
  - – caustic or corrosive—*see* Table of Drugs and Chemicals
  - – poisonous—*see* Table of Drugs and Chemicals

T

Tackle in sport W03

Terrorism (involving) Y38.8-

Thirst X58

Thrown (accidentally)
- • against part (any) of or object in transport vehicle (in motion) NEC—*see also* Accident, transport
- • from
  - – high place, homicide (attempt) Y01
  - – machinery—*see* Contact, with, by type of machine
  - – transport vehicle NEC (*see also* Accident, transport) V89.9
- • off—*see* Thrown, from

Thunderbolt—*see* subcategory T75.0
- • causing fire—*see* Exposure, fire

Tidal wave (any injury) NEC—*see* Forces of nature, tidal wave

Took
- • overdose (drug)—*see* Table of Drugs and Chemicals
- • poison—*see* Table of Drugs and Chemicals

Tornado (any injury) X37.1

Torrential rain (any injury) X37.8

Torture X58

Trampled by animal NEC W55.89

Trapped (accidentally)
- • between objects (moving) (stationary and moving)—*see* Caught
- • by part (any) of
  - – motorcycle V29.88
  - – pedal cycle V19.88
  - – transport vehicle NEC (*see also* Accident, transport) V89.9

Travel (effects) (sickness) T75.3

Tree falling on or hitting (accidentally) (person) W20.8

Tripping
- • over
  - – animal W01.0
  - – carpet, rug or (small) object W22.8
    - ■ with fall W18.09
  - – person W51
    - ■ with fall W03
      - ~ due to ice or snow W00.0
- • without fall W18.40
  - – due to
    - ■ specified NEC W18.49
    - ■ stepping from one level to another W18.43
    - ■ stepping into hole or opening W18.42
    - ■ stepping on object W18.41

Twisted by person(s) (accidentally) W50.2
- • with intent to injure or kill Y04.0
- • as, or caused by, a crowd or human stampede (with fall) W52
- • assault Y04.0
- • in fight Y04.0

Twisting, excessive—*see* category Y93

U

Underdosing of necessary drugs, medicaments or biological substances Y63.6

V

Vibration (causing injury) W49.9

Volcanic eruption (any injury) X35

Vomitus, gastric contents in air passages (with asphyxia, obstruction or suffocation) T17.81-

W

Walked into stationary object (any) W22.09
- • furniture W22.03
- • lamppost W22.02
- • wall W22.01

War operations (injuries to military personnel and civilians during war, civil insurrection and peacekeeping missions) (by) (from) (involving)—*Refer to ICD-10-CM Manual*

Washed
- • away by flood—*see* Flood
- • off road by storm (transport vehicle)—*see* Forces of nature, cataclysmic storm

Weather exposure NEC—*see* Forces of nature

Work related condition Y99.0

Wound (accidental) NEC (*see also* Injury) X58
- • battle (*see also* War operations) Y36.90
- • gunshot—*see* Discharge, firearm by type

Wrong
- • device implanted into correct surgical site Y65.51
- • fluid in infusion Y65.1
- • procedure (operation) on correct patient Y65.51
- • patient, procedure performed on Y65.52

Table of Drugs and Chemicals

The following table is a quick reference for all poisonings (accidental/unintentional, intentional/self-harm, assault), adverse effects, and underdosing as a result of a specific drug or chemical. The drugs/chemicals are listed alphabetically with their respective subcategory code. Every code is listed with a dash (-) to indicate that the next character is missing and should be reported with the fifth or sixth character as follows:

1	Poisoning, accidental, unintentional
2	Poisoning, intentional, self-harm
3	Poisoning, assault
4	Poisoning, undetermined
5	Adverse effect
6	Underdosing

DO NOT CODE FROM THE TABLE—ALWAYS REFER TO THE TABULAR. If the code requires an "encounter type," please refer to the tabular for more details.

EXAMPLE

Accidental Poisoning From Lysol—Initial Encounter
Lysol is listed as T54.1X-.
Lysol accidental poisoning would be T54.1X1-.
Lysol accidental poisoning, initial encounter, would be T54.1X1A.

Underdosing of Barbiturate—Follow-up Encounter
Barbiturate is listed as T42.3X-.
Underdosing of barbiturate would be T42.3X6-.
Underdosing of barbiturate, subsequent encounter, would be T42.3X6D.

Drug/Chemical	Code
1-propanol	T51.3X-
2-propanol	T51.2X-
2,4-D (dichlorophen-oxyacetic acid)	T60.3X-
2,4-toluene diisocyanate	T65.0X-
2,4,5-T (trichloro-phenoxyacetic acid)	T60.1X-
14-hydroxydihydro-morphinone	T40.2X-
ABOB	T37.5X-
Abrine	T62.2X-
Abrus (seed)	T62.2X-
Absinthe (beverage)	T51.0X-
Acaricide	T60.8X-
Acebutolol	T44.7X-
Acecarbromal	T42.6X-
Aceclidine	T44.1X-
Acedapsone	T37.0X-
Acefylline piperazine	T48.6X-
Acemorphan	T40.2X-
Acenocoumarin / Acenocoumarol	T45.51-
Acepifylline	T48.6X-
Acepromazine	T43.3X-
Acesulfamethoxypyridazine	T37.0X-
Acetal	T52.8X-
Acetaldehyde (vapor)	T52.8X-
liquid	T65.89-
P-Acetamidophenol	T39.1X-
Acetaminophen	T39.1X-
Acetaminosalol	T39.1X-
Acetanilide	T39.1X-
Acetarsol	T37.3X-
Acetazolamide	T50.2X-
Acetiamine	T45.2X-
Acetic	
acid	T54.2X-
w/sodium acetate (ointment)	T49.3X-
ester (solvent) (vapor)	T52.8X-
irrigating solution	T50.3X-
medicinal (lotion)	T49.2X-
anhydride	T65.89-
ether (vapor)	T52.8X-
Acetohexamide	T38.3X-
Acetohydroxamic acid	T50.99-
Acetomenaphthone	T45.7X-

Drug/Chemical	Code
Acetomorphine	T40.1X-
Acetone (oils)	T52.4X-
Acetonitrile	T52.8X-
Acetophenazine	T43.3X-
Acetophenetedin	T39.1X-
Acetophenone	T52.4X-
Acetorphine	T40.2X-
Acetosulfone (sodium)	T37.1X-
Acetrizoate (sodium)	T50.8X-
Acetrizoic acid	T50.8X-
Acetyl (bromide) (chloride)	T53.6X-
Acetylcarbromal	T42.6X-
Acetylcholine (chloride)	T44.1X-
derivative	T44.1X-
Acetylcysteine	T48.4X-
Acetyldigitoxin	T46.0X-
Acetyldigoxin	T46.0X-
Acetyldihydrocodeine	T40.2X-
Acetyldihydrocodeinone	T40.2X-
Acetylene (gas)	T59.89-
dichloride	T53.6X-
incomplete combustion of	T58.1-
industrial	T59.89-
tetrachloride	T53.6X-
vapor	T53.6X-
Acetylpheneturide	T42.6X-
Acetylphenylhydrazine	T39.8X-
Acetylsalicylic acid (salts)	T39.01-
enteric coated	T39.01-
Acetylsulfamethoxypyridazine	T37.0X-
Achromycin	T36.4X-
ophthalmic preparation	T49.5X-
topical NEC	T49.0X-
Aciclovir	T37.5X-
Acid (corrosive) NEC	T54.2X-
Acidifying agent NEC	T50.90-
Acipimox	T46.6X-
Acitretin	T50.99-
Aclarubicin	T45.1X-
Aclatonium napadisilate	T48.1X-
Aconite (wild)	T46.99-
Aconitine	T46.99-

Drug/Chemical	Code
Aconitum ferox	T46.99-
Acridine	T65.6X-
vapor	T59.89-
Acriflavine	T37.9-
Acriflavinium chloride	T49.0X-
Acrinol	T49.0X-
Acrisorcin	T49.0X-
Acrivastine	T45.0X-
Acrolein (gas)	T59.89-
liquid	T54.1X-
Acrylamide	T65.89-
Acrylic resin	T49.3X-
Acrylonitrile	T65.89-
Actaea spicata	T62.2X-
berry	T62.1X-
Acterol	T37.3X-
ACTH	T38.81-
Actinomycin C	T45.1X-
Actinomycin D	T45.1X-
Activated charcoal—*see also Charcoal, medicinal*	T47.6X-
Acyclovir	T37.5X-
Adenine	T45.2X-
arabinoside	T37.5X-
Adenosine (phosphate)	T46.2X-
ADH	T38.89-
Adhesive NEC	T65.89-
Adicillin	T36.0X-
Adiphenine	T44.3X-
Adipiodone	T50.8X-
Adjunct, pharmaceutical	T50.90-
Adrenal (extract, cortex or medulla) (gluco or mineral corticoids) (hormones)	T38.0X-
ENT agent	T49.6X-
ophthalmic preparation	T49.5X-
topical NEC	T49.0X-
Adrenaline / Adrenalin	T44.5X-
Adrenergic NEC	T44.90-
blocking agent NEC	T44.8X-
beta, heart	T44.7X-
specified NEC	T44.99-
Adrenochrome	
(mono)semicarbazone	T46.99-
derivative	T46.99-
Adrenocorticotrophic hormone	T38.81-
Adrenocorticotrophin	T38.81-
Adriamycin	T45.1X-
Aerosol spray NEC	T65.9-
Aerosporin	T36.8X-
ENT agent	T49.6X-
ophthalmic preparation	T49.5X-
topical NEC	T49.0X-
Aethusa cynapium	T62.2X-
Afghanistan black	T40.71-
Aflatoxin	T64.0-
Afloqualone	T42.8X-

Drug/Chemical	Code
African boxwood	T62.2X-
Agar	T47.4X-
Agonist (predominantly)	
alpha-adrenoreceptor	T44.4X-
beta-adrenoreceptor	T44.5X-
Agricultural agent NEC	T65.9-
Agrypnal	T42.3X-
AHLG	T50.Z1-
Air contaminant(s) type NOS	T65.9-
Ajmaline	T46.2X-
Akee	T62.1X-
Akrinol	T49.0X-
Akritoin	T37.8X-
Alacepril	T46.4X-
Alantolactone	T37.4X-
Albamycin	T36.8X-
Albendazole	T37.4X-
Albumin	T45.8X-
Albuterol	T48.6X-
Albutoin	T42.0X-
Alclometasone	T49.0X-
Alcohol	T51.9-
allyl	T51.8X-
amyl / butyl / propyl	T51.3X-
antifreeze / methyl	T51.1X-
beverage (grain, ethyl)	T51.0X-
dehydrated / denatured	T51.0X-
deterrent NEC	T50.6X-
diagnostic (gastric function)	T50.8X-
industrial	T51.0X-
isopropyl	T51.2X-
preparation for consumption	T51.0X-
radiator	T51.1X-
rubbing	T51.2X-
specified type NEC	T51.8X-
surgical	T51.0X-
vapor (any type of Alcohol)	T59.89-
wood	T51.1X-
Alcuronium (chloride)	T48.1X-
Aldactone	T50.0X-
Aldesulfone sodium	T37.1X-
Aldicarb	T60.0X-
Aldomet	T46.5X-
Aldosterone	T50.0X-
Aldrin (dust)	T60.1X-
Alexitol sodium	T47.1X-
Alfacalcidol	T45.2X-
Alfadolone	T41.1X-
Alfaxalone	T41.1X-
Alfentanil	T40.4X-
Alfuzosin (hydrochloride)	T44.8X-
Algae (harmful) (toxin)	T65.821
Algeldrate	T47.1X-
Algin	T47.8X-
Alglucerase	T45.3X-

Drug/Chemical	Code
Alidase	T45.3X-
Alimemazine	T43.3X-
Aliphatic thiocyanates	T65.0X-
Alizapride	T45.0X-
Alkali (caustic)	T54.3X-
Alkaline antiseptic solution (aromatic)	T49.6X-
Alkalinizing agents (medicinal)	T50.90-
Alkalizing agent NEC	T50.90-
Alka-seltzer	T39.01-
Alkavervir	T46.5X-
Alkonium (bromide)	T49.0X-
Alkylating drug NEC	T45.1X-
antimyeloproliferative or lymphatic	T45.1X-
Alkylisocyanate	T65.0X-
Allantoin	T49.4X-
Allegron	T43.01-
Allethrin	T49.0X-
Allobarbital	T42.3X-
Allopurinol	T50.4X-
Allyl	
Alcohol	T51.8X-
disulfide	T46.6X-
Allylestrenol	T38.5X-
Allylisopropylacetylurea	T42.6X-
Allylisopropylmalonylurea	T42.3X-
Allylthiourea	T49.3X-
Allyltribromide	T42.6X-
Allypropymal	T42.3X-
Almagate	T47.1X-
Almasilate	T47.1X-
Almitrine	T50.7X-
Aloes	T47.2X-
Aloglutamol	T47.1X-
Aloin	T47.2X-
Aloxidone	T42.2X-
Alpha	
acetyldigoxin	T46.0X-
adrenergic blocking drug	T44.6X-
amylase	T45.3X-
tocoferol (acetate) toco	T45.2X-
tocopherol	T45.2X-
Alphadolone	T41.1X-
Alphaprodine	T40.4X-
Alphaxalone	T41.1X-
Alprazolam	T42.4X-
Alprenolol	T44.7X-
Alprostadil	T46.7X-
Alsactide	T38.81-
Alseroxylon	T46.5X-
Alteplase	T45.61-
Altizide	T50.2X-
Altretamine	T45.1X-
Alum (medicinal)	T49.4X-
nonmedicinal (ammonium) (potassium)	T56.89-

Drug/Chemical	Code
Aluminium, aluminum	
acetate / chloride	T49.2X-
solution	T49.0X-
aspirin / bis (acetylsalicylate)	T39.01-
carbonate (gel, basic)	T47.1X-
chlorhydroxide-complex	T47.1X-
clofibrate	T46.6X-
diacetate	T49.2X-
glycinate	T47.1X-
hydroxide (gel)	T47.1X-
hydroxide-magn. carb. gel	T47.1X-
magnesium silicate	T47.1X-
nicotinate	T46.7X-
ointment (surgical) (topical)	T49.3X-
phosphate / silicate (sodium)	T47.1X-
salicylate	T39.09-
subacetate	T49.2X-
sulfate	T49.0X-
tannate	T47.6X-
Alurate	T42.3X-
Alverine	T44.3X-
Alvodine	T40.2X-
Amanita phalloides	T62.0X-
Amanitine	T62.0X-
Amantadine	T42.8X-
Ambazone	T49.6X-
Ambenonium (chloride)	T44.0X-
Ambroxol	T48.4X-
Ambuphylline	T48.6X-
Ambutonium bromide	T44.3X-
Amcinonide	T49.0X-
Amdinocilline	T36.0X-
Ametazole	T50.8X-
Amethocaine (regional, spinal)	T41.3X-
Amethopterin	T45.1X-
Amezinium metilsulfate	T44.99-
Amfebutamone	T43.29-
Amfepramone	T50.5X-
Amfetamine	T43.62-
Amfetaminil	T43.62-
Amfomycin	T36.8X-
Amidefrine mesilate	T48.5X-
Amidone	T40.3X-
Amidopyrine	T39.2X-
Amidotrizoate	T50.8X-
Amiflamine	T43.1X-
Amikacin	T36.5X-
Amikhelline	T46.3X-
Amiloride	T50.2X-
Aminacrine	T49.0X-
Amineptine	T43.01-
Aminitrozole	T37.3X-
Amino acids	T50.3X-
Aminoacetic acid (derivatives)	T50.3X-
Aminoacridine	T49.0X-

Drug/Chemical	Code
Aminobenzoic acid (-p)	T49.3X-
4-Aminobutyric acid	T43.8X-
Aminocaproic acid	T45.62-
Aminoethylisothiourium	T45.8X-
Aminofenazone	T39.2X-
Aminoglutethimide	T45.1X-
Aminohippuric acid	T50.8X-
Aminomethylbenzoic acid	T45.69-
Aminometradine	T50.2X-
Aminopentamide	T44.3X-
Aminophenazone	T39.2X-
Aminophenol	T54.0X-
4-Aminophenol derivatives	T39.1X-
Aminophenylpyridone	T43.59-
Aminophylline	T48.6X-
Aminopterin sodium	T45.1X-
Aminopyrine	T39.2X-
8-Aminoquinoline drugs	T37.2X-
Aminorex	T50.5X-
Aminosalicylic acid	T37.1X-
Aminosalylum	T37.1X-
Amiodarone	T46.2X-
Amiphenazole	T50.7X-
Amiquinsin	T46.5X-
Amisometradine	T50.2X-
Amisulpride	T43.59-
Amitriptyline	T43.01-
Amitriptylinoxide	T43.01-
Amlexanox	T48.6X-
Ammonia (fumes/vapor) (gas)	T59.89-
aromatic spirit	T48.99-
liquid (household)	T54.3X-
Ammoniated mercury	T49.0X-
Ammonium	
acid tartrate	T49.5X-
bromide	T42.6X-
carbonate	T54.3X-
chloride	T50.99-
expectorant	T48.4X-
compounds (household)NEC	T54.3X-
fumes (any usage)	T59.89-
industrial	T54.3X-
ichthyosulronate	T49.4X-
mandelate	T37.9-
sulfamate	T60.3X-
sulfonate resin	T47.8X-
Amobarbital (sodium)	T42.3X-
Amodiaquine	T37.2X-
Amopyroquin (e)	T37.2X-
Amoxapine	T43.01-
Amoxicillin	T36.0X-
Amperozide	T43.59-
Amphenidone	T43.59-
Amphetamine NEC	T43.62-

Drug/Chemical	Code
Amphomycin	T36.8X-
Amphotalide	T37.4X-
Amphotericin B	T36.7X-
topical	T49.0X-
Ampicillin	T36.0X-
Amprotropine	T44.3X-
Amsacrine	T45.1X-
Amygdaline	T62.2X-
Amyl	
acetate	T52.8X-
vapor	T59.89-
alcohol	T51.3X-
chloride	T53.6X-
formate	T52.8X-
nitrite	T46.3X-
propionate	T65.89-
Amylase	T47.5X-
Amyleine, regional	T41.3X-
Amylene	
dichloride	T53.6X-
hydrate	T51.3X-
Amylmetacresol	T49.6X-
Amylobarbitone	T42.3X-
Amylocaine, regional (infiltration) (subcutaneous) (nerve block) (spinal) (topical)	T41.3X-
Amylopectin	T47.6X-
Amytal (sodium)	T42.3X-
Anabolic steroid	T38.7X-
Analeptic NEC	T50.7X-
Analgesic	T39.9-
anti-inflammatory NEC	T39.9-
propionic acid derivative	T39.31-
antirheumatic NEC	T39.4X-
aromatic NEC	T39.1X-
narcotic NEC	T40.60-
non-narcotic NEC	T39.9-
pyrazole	T39.2X-
specified NEC	T39.8X-
Analgin	T39.2X-
Anamirta cocculus	T62.1X-
Ancillin	T36.0X-
Ancrod	T45.69-
Androgen	T38.7X-
Androgen-estrogen mixture	T38.7X-
Androstalone	T38.7X-
Androstanolone	T38.7X-
Androsterone	T38.7X-
Anemone pulsatilla	T62.2X-
Anesthesia	
caudal	T41.3X-
endotracheal	T41.0X-
epidural	T41.3X-
inhalation	T41.0X-
local (nerve or plexus blocking)	T41.3X-
mucosal	T41.3X-

Drug/Chemical	Code
Anesthesia, continued	
muscle relaxation	T48.1X-
potentiated	T41.20-
rectal (general)	T41.20-
local	T41.3X-
regional	T41.3X-
surface	T41.3X-
Anesthetic NEC	T41.41
with muscle relaxant	T41.20-
general	T41.20-
local	T41.3X-
gaseous NEC	T41.0X-
general NEC	T41.20-
halogenated hydrocarbon derivatives NEC	T41.0X-
infiltration NEC	T41.3X-
intravenous NEC	T41.1X-
local NEC	T41.3X-
rectal (general)	T41.20-
local	T41.3X-
regional NEC / spinal NEC	T41.3X-
thiobarbiturate	T41.1X-
topical	T41.3X-
Aneurine	T45.2X-
Angio-Conray	T50.8X-
Angiotensin	T44.5X-
Angiotensinamide	T44.99-
Anhydrohydroxy-progesterone	T38.5X-
Anhydron	T50.2X-
Anileridine	T40.4X-
Aniline (dye) (liquid)	T65.3X-
analgesic	T39.1X-
derivatives, therapeutic NEC	T39.1X-
vapor	T65.3X-
Aniscoropine	T44.3X-
Anise oil	T47.5X-
Anisidine	T65.3X-
Anisindione	T45.51-
Anisotropine methyl-bromide	T44.3X-
Anistreplase	T45.61-
Anorexiant (central)	T50.5X-
Anorexic agents	T50.5X-
Ansamycin	T36.6X-
Ant (bite) (sting)	T63.421
Antabuse	T50.6X-
Antacid NEC	T47.1X-
Antagonist	
Aldosterone	T50.0X-
alpha-adrenoreceptor	T44.6X-
anticoagulant	T45.7X-
beta-adrenoreceptor	T44.7X-
extrapyramidal NEC	T44.3X-
folic acid	T45.1X-
H2 receptor	T47.0X-
heavy metal	T45.8X-
narcotic analgesic	T50.7X-

Drug/Chemical	Code
Antagonist, continued	
opiate	T50.7X-
pyrimidine	T45.1X-
serotonin	T46.5X-
Antazolin (e)	T45.0X-
Anterior pituitary hormone NEC	T38.81-
Anthelmintic NEC	T37.4X-
Anthiolimine	T37.4X-
Anthralin	T49.4X-
Anthramycin	T45.1X-
Antiadrenergic NEC	T44.8X-
Antiallergic NEC	T45.0X-
Anti-anemic (drug) (preparation)	T45.8X-
Antiandrogen NEC	T38.6X-
Antianxiety drug NEC	T43.50-
Antiaris toxicaria	T65.89-
Antiarteriosclerotic drug	T46.6X-
Antiasthmatic drug NEC	T48.6X-
Antibiotic NEC	T36.9-
aminoglycoside	T36.5X-
anticancer	T45.1X-
antifungal	T36.7X-
antimycobacterial	T36.5X-
antineoplastic	T45.1X-
cephalosporin (group)	T36.1X-
chloramphenicol (group)	T36.2X-
ENT	T49.6X-
eye	T49.5X-
fungicidal (local)	T49.0X-
intestinal	T36.8X-
b-lactam NEC	T36.1X-
local	T49.0X-
macrolides	T36.3X-
polypeptide	T36.8X-
specified NEC	T36.8X-
tetracycline (group)	T36.4X-
throat	T49.6X-
Anticancer agents NEC	T45.1X-
Anticholesterolemic drug NEC	T46.6X-
Anticholinergic NEC	T44.3X-
Anticholinesterase	T44.0X-
organophosphorus	T44.0X-
insecticide	T60.0X-
nerve gas	T59.89-
reversible	T44.0X-
ophthalmological	T49.5X-
Anticoagulant NEC	T45.51-
Antagonist	T45.7X-
Anti-common-cold drug NEC	T48.5X-
Anticonvulsant	T42.71
barbiturate	T42.3X-
combination (with barbiturate)	T42.3X-
hydantoin	T42.0X-
hypnotic NEC	T42.6X-
oxazolidinedione	T42.2X-

ANTICONVULSANT–ANTINEOPLASTIC NEC

Drug/Chemical	Code
Anticonvulsant, continued	T42.71
pyrimidinedione	T42.6X-
specified NEC	T42.6X-
succinimide	T42.2X-
Anti-D immunoglobulin (human)	T50.Z1-
Antidepressant	T43.20-
monoamine oxidase inhibitor	T43.1X-
SSNRI	T43.21-
SSRI	T43.22-
specified NEC	T43.29-
tetracyclic	T43.02-
triazolopyridine	T43.21-
tricyclic	T43.01-
Antidiabetic NEC	T38.3X-
biguanide	T38.3X-
and sulfonyl combined	T38.3X-
combined	T38.3X-
sulfonylurea	T38.3X-
Antidiarrheal drug NEC	T47.6X-
absorbent	T47.6X-
Antidiphtheria serum	T50.Z1-
Antidiuretic hormone	T38.89-
Antidote NEC	T50.6X-
heavy metal	T45.8X-
Antidysrhythmic NEC	T46.2X-
Antiemetic drug	T45.0X-
Antiepilepsy agent	T42.71
combination or mixed	T42.5X-
specified, NEC	T42.6X-
Antiestrogen NEC	T38.6X-
Antifertility pill	T38.4X-
Antifibrinolytic drug	T45.62-
Antifilarial drug	T37.4X-
Antiflatulent	T47.5X-
Antifreeze	T65.9-
alcohol	T51.1X-
ethylene glycol	T51.8X-
Antifungal	
antibiotic (systemic)	T36.7X-
anti-infective NEC	T37.9-
disinfectant, local	T49.0X-
nonmedicinal (spray)	T60.3X-
topical	T49.0X-
Anti-gastric-secretion drug NEC	T47.1X-
Antigonadotrophin NEC	T38.6X-
Antihallucinogen	T43.50-
Antihelmintics	T37.4X-
Antihemophilic	
factor	T45.8X-
fraction	T45.8X-
globulin concentrate	T45.7X-
human plasma	T45.8X-
plasma, dried	T45.7X-
Antihemorrhoidal preparation	T49.2X-
Antiheparin drug	T45.7X-

Drug/Chemical	Code
Antihistamine	T45.0X-
Antihookworm drug	T37.4X-
Anti-human lymphocytic globulin	T50.Z1-
Antihyperlipidemic drug	T46.6X-
Antihypertensive drug NEC	T46.5X-
Anti-infective NEC	T37.9-
anthelmintic	T37.4X-
antibiotics	T36.9-
specified NEC	T36.8X-
antimalarial	T37.2X-
antimycobacterial NEC	T37.1X-
antibiotics	T36.5X-
antiprotozoal NEC	T37.3X-
blood	T37.2X-
antiviral	T37.5X-
arsenical	T37.8X-
bismuth, local	T49.0X-
ENT	T49.6X-
eye NEC	T49.5X-
heavy metals NEC	T37.8X-
local NEC	T49.0X-
specified NEC	T49.0X-
mixed	T37.9-
ophthalmic preparation	T49.5X-
topical NEC	T49.0X-
Anti-inflammatory drug NEC	T39.39-
local	T49.0X-
nonsteroidal NEC	T39.39-
propionic acid derivative	T39.31-
specified NEC	T39.39-
Antikaluretic	T50.3X-
Antiknock (tetraethyl lead)	T56.0X-
Antilipemic drug NEC	T46.6X-
Antimalarial	T37.2X-
prophylactic NEC	T37.2X-
pyrimidine derivative	T37.2X-
Antimetabolite	T45.1X-
Antimitotic agent	T45.1X-
Antimony (compounds) (vapor) NEC	T56.89-
anti-infectives	T37.8X-
dimercaptosuccinate	T37.3X-
hydride	T56.89-
pesticide (vapor)	T60.8X-
potassium (sodium)tartrate	T37.8X-
sodium dimercaptosuccinate	T37.3X-
tartrated	T37.8X-
Antimuscarinic NEC	T44.3X-
Antimycobacterial drug NEC	T37.1X-
antibiotics	T36.5X-
combination	T37.1X-
Antinausea drug	T45.0X-
Antinematode drug	T37.4X-
Antineoplastic NEC	T45.1X-
alkaloidal	T45.1X-
antibiotics	T45.1X-

Drug/Chemical	Code
Antineoplastic NEC, continued	T45.1X-
combination	T45.1X-
estrogen	T38.5X-
steroid	T38.7X-
Antiparasitic drug (systemic)	T37.9-
local	T49.0X-
specified NEC	T37.8X-
Antiparkinsonism drug NEC	T42.8X-
Antiperspirant NEC	T49.2X-
Antiphlogistic NEC	T39.4X-
Antiplatyhelmintic drug	T37.4X-
Antiprotozoal drug NEC	T37.3X-
blood	T37.2X-
local	T49.0X-
Antipruritic drug NEC	T49.1X-
Antipsychotic drug	T43.50-
specified NEC	T43.59-
Antipyretic	T39.9-
specified NEC	T39.8X-
Antipyrine	T39.2X-
Antirabies hyperimmune serum	T50.Z1-
Antirheumatic NEC	T39.4X-
Antirigidity drug NEC	T42.8X-
Antischistosomal drug	T37.4X-
Antiscorpion sera	T50.Z1-
Antiseborrheics	T49.4X-
Antiseptics (external) (medicinal)	T49.0X-
Antistine	T45.0X-
Antitapeworm drug	T37.4X-
Antitetanus immunoglobulin	T50.Z1-
Antithrombotic	T45.52-
Antithyroid drug NEC	T38.2X-
Antitoxin	T50.Z1-
Antitrichomonal drug	T37.3X-
Antituberculars	T37.1X-
antibiotics	T36.5X-
Antitussive NEC	T48.3X-
codeine mixture	T40.2X-
opiate	T40.2X-
Antivaricose drug	T46.8X-
Antivenin, antivenom (sera)	T50.Z1-
crotaline	T50.Z1-
spider bite	T50.Z1-
Antivertigo drug	T45.0X-
Antiviral drug NEC	T37.5X-
eye	T49.5X-
Antiwhipworm drug	T37.4X-
Antrol— *see also specific chemical*	T60.9-
fungicide	T60.9-
ANTU (alpha naphthylthiourea)	T60.4X-
Apalcillin	T36.0X-
APC	T48.5X-
Aplonidine	T44.4X-
Apomorphine	T47.7X-

Drug/Chemical	Code
Appetite depressants, central	T50.5X-
Apraclonidine (hydrochloride)	T44.4X-
Apresoline	T46.5X-
Aprindine	T46.2X-
Aprobarbital	T42.3X-
Apronalide	T42.6X-
Aprotinin	T45.62-
Aptocaine	T41.3X-
Aqua fortis	T54.2X-
Ara-A	T37.5X-
Ara-C	T45.1X-
Arachis oil	T49.3X-
cathartic	T47.4X-
Aralen	T37.2X-
Arecoline	T44.1X-
Arginine	T50.99-
glutamate	T50.99-
Argyrol	T49.0X-
ENT agent	T49.6X-
ophthalmic preparation	T49.5X-
Aristocort	T38.0X-
ENT agent	T49.6X-
ophthalmic preparation	T49.5X-
topical NEC	T49.0X-
Aromatics, corrosive	T54.1X-
disinfectants	T54.1X-
Arsenate of lead	T57.0X-
herbicide	T57.0X-
Arsenic, arsenicals (compounds) (dust) (vapor)NEC	T57.0X-
anti-infectives	T37.8X-
pesticide (dust) (fumes)	T57.0X-
Arsine (gas)	T57.0X-
Arsphenamine (silver)	T37.8X-
Arsthinol	T37.3X-
Artane	T44.3X-
Arthropod (venomous) NEC	T63.481
Articaine	T41.3X-
Asbestos	T57.8X-
Ascaridole	T37.4X-
Ascorbic acid	T45.2X-
Asiaticoside	T49.0X-
Asparaginase	T45.1X-
Aspidium (oleoresin)	T37.4X-
Aspirin (aluminum) (soluble)	T39.01-
Aspoxicillin	T36.0X-
Astemizole	T45.0X-
Astringent (local)	T49.2X-
specified NEC	T49.2X-
Astromicin	T36.5X-
Ataractic drug NEC	T43.50-
Atenolol	T44.7X-
Atonia drug, intestinal	T47.4X-
Atophan	T50.4X-
Atracurium besilate	T48.1X-

Drug/Chemical	Code
Atropine	T44.3X-
derivative	T44.3X-
methonitrate	T44.3X-
Attapulgite	T47.6X-
Auramine	T65.89-
dye	T65.6X-
fungicide	T60.3X-
Auranofin	T39.4X-
Aurantiin	T46.99-
Aureomycin	T36.4X-
ophthalmic preparation	T49.5X-
topical NEC	T49.0X-
Aurothioglucose	T39.4X-
Aurothioglycanide	T39.4X-
Aurothiomalate sodium	T39.4X-
Aurotioprol	T39.4X-
Automobile fuel	T52.0X-
Autonomic nervous system agent NEC	T44.90-
Avlosulfon	T37.1X-
Avomine	T42.6X-
Axerophthol	T45.2X-
Azacitidine	T45.1X-
Azacyclonol	T43.59-
Azadirachta	T60.2X-
Azanidazole	T37.3X-
Azapetine	T46.7X-
Azapropazone	T39.2X-
Azaribine	T45.1X-
Azaserine	T45.1X-
Azatadine	T45.0X-
Azatepa	T45.1X-
Azathioprine	T45.1X-
Azelaic acid	T49.0X-
Azelastine	T45.0X-
Azidocillin	T36.0X-
Azidothymidine	T37.5X-
Azinphos (ethyl) (methyl)	T60.0X-
Aziridine (chelating)	T54.1X-
Azithromycin	T36.3X-
Azlocillin	T36.0X-
Azobenzene smoke	T65.3X-
acaricide	T60.8X-
Azosulfamide	T37.0X-
AZT	T37.5X-
Aztreonam	T36.1X-
Azulfidine	T37.0X-
Azuresin	T50.8X-
Bacampicillin	T36.0X-
Bacillus	
lactobacillus	T47.8X-
subtilis	T47.6X-
Bacimycin	T49.0X-
ophthalmic preparation	T49.5X-

Drug/Chemical	Code
Bacitracin zinc	T49.0X-
with neomycin	T49.0X-
ENT agent	T49.6X-
ophthalmic preparation	T49.5X-
topical NEC	T49.0X-
Baclofen	T42.8X-
Baking soda	T50.99-
BAL	T45.8X-
Bambuterol	T48.6X-
Bamethan (sulfate)	T46.7X-
Bamifylline	T48.6X-
Bamipine	T45.0X-
Baneberry— *see Actaea spicata*	
Banewort— *see Belladonna*	
Barbenyl	T42.3X-
Barbexaclone	T42.6X-
Barbital (sodium)	T42.3X-
Barbitone	T42.3X-
Barbiturate NEC	T42.3X-
with tranquilizer	T42.3X-
anesthetic (intravenous)	T41.1X-
Barium (carbonate) (chloride) (sulfite)	T57.8X-
diagnostic agent	T50.8X-
pesticide / rodenticide	T60.4X-
sulfate (medicinal)	T50.8X-
Barrier cream	T49.3X-
Basic fuchsin	T49.0X-
Battery acid or fluid	T54.2X-
Bay rum	T51.8X-
BCG (vaccine)	T50.A9-
BCNU	T45.1X-
Bearsfoot	T62.2X-
Beclamide	T42.6X-
Beclomethasone	T44.5X-
Bee (sting) (venom)	T63.441
Befunolol	T49.5X-
Bekanamycin	T36.5X-
Belladonna— *see Nightshade*	T44.3X-
Bemegride	T50.7X-
Benactyzine	T44.3X-
Benadryl	T45.0X-
Benaprizine	T44.3X-
Benazepril	T46.4X-
Bencyclane	T46.7X-
Bendazol	T46.3X-
Bendrofluazide	T50.2X-
Bendroflumethiazide	T50.2X-
Benemid	T50.4X-
Benethamine penicillin	T36.0X-
Benexate	T47.1X-
Benfluorex	T46.6X-
Benfotiamine	T45.2X-
Benisone	T49.0X-
Benomyl	T60.0X-
Benoquin	T49.8X-

Drug/Chemical	Code
Benoxinate	T41.3X-
Benperidol	T43.4X-
Benproperine	T48.3X-
Benserazide	T42.8X-
Bentazepam	T42.4X-
Bentiromide	T50.8X-
Bentonite	T49.3X-
Benzalbutyramide	T46.6X-
Benzalkonium (chloride)	T49.0X-
ophthalmic preparation	T49.5X-
Benzamidosalicylate (calcium)	T37.1X-
Benzamine	T41.3X-
lactate	T49.1X-
Benzamphetamine	T50.5X-
Benzapril hydrochloride	T46.5X-
Benzathine benzylpenicillin	T36.0X-
Benzathine penicillin	T36.0X-
Benzatropine	T42.8X-
Benzbromarone	T50.4X-
Benzcarbimine	T45.1X-
Benzedrex	T44.99-
Benzedrine (amphetamine)	T43.62-
Benzenamine	T65.3X-
Benzene	T52.1X-
homologues (acetyl) (dimethyl) (methyl) (solvent)	T52.2X-
Benzethonium (chloride)	T49.0X-
Benzfetamine	T50.5X-
Benzhexol	T44.3X-
Benzhydramine (chloride)	T45.0X-
Benzidine	T65.89-
Benzilonium bromide	T44.3X-
Benzimidazole	T60.3X-
Benziodarone	T46.3X-
Benznidazole	T37.3X-
Benzocaine	T41.3X-
Benzodiapin	T42.4X-
Benzodiazepine NEC	T42.4X-
Benzoic acid	T49.0X-
with salicylic acid	T49.0X-
Benzoin (tincture)	T48.5X-
Benzol (benzene)	T52.1X-
vapor	T52.0X-
Benzomorphan	T40.2X-
Benzonatate	T48.3X-
Benzophenones	T49.3X-
Benzopyrone	T46.99-
Benzothiadiazides	T50.2X-
Benzoxonium chloride	T49.0X-
Benzoyl peroxide	T49.0X-
Benzoylpas calcium	T37.1X-
Benzperidin	T43.59-
Benzperidol	T43.59-
Benzphetamine	T50.5X-
Benzpyrinium bromide	T44.1X-
Benzquinamide	T45.0X-

Drug/Chemical	Code
Benzthiazide	T50.2X-
Benztropine	
anticholinergic	T44.3X-
antiparkinson	T42.8X-
Benzydamine	T49.0X-
Benzyl	
acetate	T52.8X-
alcohol	T49.0X-
benzoate	T49.0X-
Benzoic acid	T49.0X-
morphine	T40.2X-
nicotinate	T46.6X-
penicillin	T36.0X-
Benzylhydrochlorthiazide	T50.2X-
Benzylpenicillin	T36.0X-
Benzylthiouracil	T38.2X-
Bephenium hydroxy-naphthoate	T37.4X-
Bepridil	T46.1X-
Bergamot oil	T65.89-
Bergapten	T50.99-
Berries, poisonous	T62.1X-
Beryllium (compounds)	T56.7X-
b-acetyldigoxin	T46.0X-
beta adrenergic blocking agent, heart	T44.7X-
b-benzalbutyramide	T46.6X-
Betacarotene	T45.2X-
b-eucaine	T49.1X-
Beta-Chlor	T42.6X-
b-galactosidase	T47.5X-
Betahistine	T46.7X-
Betaine	T47.5X-
Betamethasone	T49.0X-
topical	T49.0X-
Betamicin	T36.8X-
Betanidine	T46.5X-
b-Sitosterol(s)	T46.6X-
Betaxolol	T44.7X-
Betazole	T50.8X-
Bethanechol	T44.1X-
chloride	T44.1X-
Bethanidine	T46.5X-
Betoxycaine	T41.3X-
Betula oil	T49.3X-
Bevantolol	T44.7X-
Bevonium metilsulfate	T44.3X-
Bezafibrate	T46.6X-
Bezitramide	T40.4X-
BHA	T50.99-
Bhang	T40.71-
BHC (medicinal)	T49.0X-
nonmedicinal (vapor)	T53.6X-
Bialamicol	T37.3X-
Bibenzonium bromide	T48.3X-
Bibrocathol	T49.5X-
Bichloride of mercury— *see Mercury, chloride*	

BICHROMATES (CALCIUM) (POTASSIUM) (SODIUM) (CRYSTALS)–BROMOCHLOROSALICYLANILIDE

Drug/Chemical	Code
Bichromates (calcium) (potassium) (sodium) (crystals)	T57.8X-
fumes	T56.2X-
Biclotymol	T49.6X-
Bicucculine	T50.7X-
Bifemelane	T43.29-
Biguanide derivatives, oral	T38.3X-
Bile salts	T47.5X-
Biligrafin	T50.8X-
Bilopaque	T50.8X-
Binifibrate	T46.6X-
Binitrobenzol	T65.3X-
Bioflavonoid(s)	T46.99-
Biological substance NEC	T50.90-
Biotin	T45.2X-
Biperiden	T44.3X-
Bisacodyl	T47.2X-
Bisbentiamine	T45.2X-
Bisbutiamine	T45.2X-
Bisdequalinium (salts) (diacetate)	T49.6X-
Bishydroxycoumarin	T45.51-
Bismarsen	T37.8X-
Bismuth salts	T47.6X-
aluminate	T47.1X-
anti-infectives	T37.8X-
formic iodide	T49.0X-
glycolylarsenate	T49.0X-
nonmedicinal (compounds)NEC	T65.9-
subcarbonate	T47.6X-
subsalicylate	T37.8X-
sulfarsphenamine	T37.8X-
Bisoprolol	T44.7X-
Bisoxatin	T47.2X-
Bisulepin (hydrochloride)	T45.0X-
Bithionol	T37.8X-
anthelminthic	T37.4X-
Bitolterol	T48.6X-
Bitoscanate	T37.4X-
Bitter almond oil	T62.8X-
Bittersweet	T62.2X-
Black	
flag	T60.9-
henbane	T62.2X-
leaf (40)	T60.9-
widow spider (bite)	T63.31-
antivenin	T50.Z1-
Blast furnace gas (carbon monoxide)	T58.8X-
Bleach	T54.9-
Bleaching agent (medicinal)	T49.4X-
Bleomycin	T45.1X-
Blockain (infiltration) (topical) (subcutaneous) (nerve block)	T41.3X-
Blockers, calcium channel	T46.1X-
Blood (derivatives) (natural) (plasma) (whole) (substitute)	T45.8X-
dried	T45.8X-
drug affecting NEC	T45.9-

Drug/Chemical	Code
Blood (derivatives) (natural) (plasma) (whole) (substitute), continued	T45.8X-
expander NEC	T45.8X-
fraction NEC	T45.8X-
Blue velvet	T40.2X-
Bone meal	T62.8X-
Bonine	T45.0X-
Bopindolol	T44.7X-
Boracic acid	T49.0X-
ENT agent	T49.6X-
ophthalmic preparation	T49.5X-
Borane complex	T57.8X-
Borate(s)	T57.8X-
buffer	T50.99-
cleanser	T54.9-
sodium	T57.8X-
Borax (cleanser)	T54.9-
Bordeaux mixture	T60.3X-
Boric acid	T49.0X-
ENT agent	T49.6X-
ophthalmic preparation	T49.5X-
Bornaprine	T44.3X-
Boron	T57.8X-
hydride NEC	T57.8X-
fumes or gas	T57.8X-
trifluoride	T59.89-
Botox	T48.29-
Botulinus anti-toxin (type A, B)	T50.Z1-
Brake fluid vapor	T59.89-
Brallobarbital	T42.3X-
Bran (wheat)	T47.4X-
Brass (fumes)	T56.89-
Brasso	T52.0X-
Bretylium tosilate	T46.2X-
Brevital (sodium)	T41.1X-
Brinase	T45.3X-
British antilewisite	T45.8X-
Brodifacoum	T60.4X-
Bromal (hydrate)	T42.6X-
Bromazepam	T42.4X-
Bromazine	T45.0X-
Brombenzylcyanide	T59.3X-
Bromelains	T45.3X-
Bromethalin	T60.4X-
Bromhexine	T48.4X-
Bromide salts	T42.6X-
Bromindione	T45.51-
Bromine	
compounds (medicinal)	T42.6X-
sedative	T42.6X-
vapor	T59.89-
Bromisoval	T42.6X-
Bromisovalum	T42.6X-
Bromobenzylcyanide	T59.3X-
Bromochlorosalicylanilide	T49.0X-

Drug/Chemical	Code
Bromocriptine	T42.8X-
Bromodiphenhydramine	T45.0X-
Bromoform	T42.6X-
Bromophenol blue reagent	T50.99-
Bromopride	T47.8X-
Bromosalicylchloranitide	T49.0X-
Bromosalicylhydroxamic acid	T37.1X-
Bromo-seltzer	T39.1X-
Bromoxynil	T60.3X-
Bromperidol	T43.4X-
Brompheniramine	T45.0X-
Bromsulfophthalein	T50.8X-
Bromural	T42.6X-
Bromvaletone	T42.6X-
Bronchodilator NEC	T48.6X-
Brotizolam	T42.4X-
Brovincamine	T46.7X-
Brown recluse spider (bite) (venom)	T63.33-
Brown spider (bite) (venom)	T63.39-
Broxaterol	T48.6X-
Broxuridine	T45.1X-
Broxyquinoline	T37.8X-
Bruceine	T48.29-
Brucia	T62.2X-
Brucine	T65.1X-
Bryonia	T47.2X-
Buclizine	T45.0X-
Buclosamide	T49.0X-
Budesonide	T44.5X-
Budralazine	T46.5X-
Bufferin	T39.01-
Buflomedil	T46.7X-
Buformin	T38.3X-
Bufotenine	T40.99-
Bufrolin	T48.6X-
Bufylline	T48.6X-
Bulk filler	T50.5X-
cathartic	T47.4X-
Bumetanide	T50.1X-
Bunaftine	T46.2X-
Bunamiodyl	T50.8X-
Bunazosin	T44.6X-
Bunitrolol	T44.7X-
Buphenine	T46.7X-
Bupivacaine (infiltration) (Nerve block) (spinal)	T41.3X-
Bupranolol	T44.7X-
Buprenorphine	T40.4X-
Bupropion	T43.29-
Burimamide	T47.1X-
Buserelin	T38.89-
Buspirone	T43.59-
Busulfan, busulphan	T45.1X-
Butabarbital (sodium)	T42.3X-
Butabarbitone	T42.3X-
Butabarpal	T42.3X-

Drug/Chemical	Code
Butacaine	T41.3X-
Butalamine	T46.7X-
Butalbital	T42.3X-
Butallylonal	T42.3X-
Butamben	T41.3X-
Butamirate	T48.3X-
Butane (distributed in mobile container or through pipes)	T59.89-
incomplete combustion	T58.1-
Butanilicaine	T41.3X-
Butanol	T51.3X-
Butanone, 2-butanone	T52.4X-
Butantrone	T49.4X-
Butaperazine	T43.3X-
Butazolidin	T39.2X-
Butetamate	T48.6X-
Butethal	T42.3X-
Butethamate	T44.3X-
Buthalitone (sodium)	T41.1X-
Butisol (sodium)	T42.3X-
Butizide	T50.2X-
Butobarbital (sodium)	T42.3X-
Butobarbitone	T42.3X-
Butoconazole (nitrate)	T49.0X-
Butorphanol	T40.4X-
Butriptyline	T43.01-
Butropium bromide	T44.3X-
Buttercups	T62.2X-
Butyl	
acetate (secondary)	T52.8X-
alcohol	T51.3X-
aminobenzoate	T41.3X-
butyrate	T52.8X-
carbinol or carbitol	T51.3X-
cellosolve	T52.3X-
chloral (hydrate)	T42.6X-
formate or lactate or propionate	T52.8X-
scopolamine bromide	T44.3X-
thiobarbital sodium	T41.1X-
Butylated hydroxy-anisole	T50.99-
Butylchloral hydrate	T42.6X-
Butyltoluene	T52.2X-
Butyn	T41.3X-
Butyrophenone (-based tranquilizers)	T43.4X-
Cabergoline	T42.8X-
Cacodyl, cacodylic acid	T57.0X-
Cactinomycin	T45.1X-
Cade oil	T49.4X-
Cadexomer iodine	T49.0X-
Cadmium (chloride) (fumes) (oxide)	T56.3X-
sulfide (medicinal) NEC	T49.4X-
Cadralazine	T46.5X-
Caffeine	T43.61-
Calabar bean	T62.2X-
Caladium seguinum	T62.2X-

Drug/Chemical	Code
Calamine (lotion)	T49.3X-
Calcifediol	T45.2X-
Calciferol	T45.2X-
Calcitonin	T50.99-
Calcitriol	T45.2X-
Calcium	T50.3X-
actylsalicylate	T39.01-
benzamidosalicylate	T37.1X-
bromide or bromolactobionate	T42.6X-
carbaspirin	T39.01-
carbimide	T50.6X-
carbonate	T47.1X-
chloride (anhydrous)	T50.99-
cyanide	T57.8X-
dioctyl sulfosuccinate	T47.4X-
disodium edathamil	T45.8X-
disodium edetate	T45.8X-
dobesilate	T46.99-
EDTA	T45.8X-
ferrous citrate	T45.4X-
folinate	T45.8X-
glubionate	T50.3X-
gluconate or – gluconogalactogluconate	T50.3X-
hydrate, hydroxide	T54.3X-
hypochlorite	T54.3X-
iodide	T48.4X-
ipodate	T50.8X-
lactate	T50.3X-
leucovorin	T45.8X-
mandelate	T37.9-
oxide	T54.3X-
pantothenate	T45.2X-
phosphate	T50.3X-
salicylate	T39.09-
salts	T50.3X-
Calculus-dissolving drug	T50.99-
Calomel	T49.0X-
Caloric agent	T50.3X-
Calusterone	T38.7X-
Camazepam	T42.4X-
Camomile	T49.0X-
Camoquin	T37.2X-
Camphor	
insecticide	T60.2X-
medicinal	T49.8X-
Camylofin	T44.3X-
Cancer chemo drug regimen	T45.1X-
Candeptin	T49.0X-
Candicidin	T49.0X-
Cannabinoids, synthetic	T40.72-
Cannabinol	T40.71-
Cannabis (derivatives)	T40.71-
Canned heat	T51.1X-
Canrenoic acid	T50.0X-
Canrenone	T50.0X-

Drug/Chemical	Code
Cantharides, cantharidin, cantharis	T49.8X-
Canthaxanthin	T50.99-
Capillary-active drug NEC	T46.90-
Capreomycin	T36.8X-
Capsicum	T49.4X-
Captafol	T60.3X-
Captan	T60.3X-
Captodiame, captodiamine	T43.59-
Captopril	T46.4X-
Caramiphen	T44.3X-
Carazolol	T44.7X-
Carbachol	T44.1X-
Carbacrylamine (resin)	T50.3X-
Carbamate (insecticide)	T60.0X-
Carbamate (sedative)	T42.6X-
herbicide or insecticide	T60.0X-
Carbamazepine	T42.1X-
Carbamide	T47.3X-
peroxide	T49.0X-
topical	T49.8X-
Carbamylcholine chloride	T44.1X-
Carbaril	T60.0X-
Carbarsone	T37.3X-
Carbaryl	T60.0X-
Carbaspirin	T39.01-
Carbazochrome (salicylate) (sodium sulfonate)	T49.4X-
Carbenicillin	T36.0X-
Carbenoxolone	T47.1X-
Carbetapentane	T48.3X-
Carbethyl salicylate	T39.09-
Carbidopa (with levodopa)	T42.8X-
Carbimazole	T38.2X-
Carbinol	T51.1X-
Carbinoxamine	T45.0X-
Carbiphene	T39.8X-
Carbitol	T52.3X-
Carbo medicinalis	T47.6X-
Carbocaine (infiltration) (topical) (subcutaneous) (nerve block)	T41.3X-
Carbocisteine	T48.4X-
Carbocromen	T46.3X-
Carbol fuchsin	T49.0X-
Carbolic acid— *see also Phenol*	T54.0X-
Carbolonium (bromide)	T48.1X-
Carbomycin	T36.8X-
Carbon	
bisulfide (liquid) or vapor	T65.4X-
dioxide (gas)	T59.7X-
medicinal	T41.5X-
nonmedicinal	T59.7X-
snow	T49.4X-
disulfide (liquid) or vapor	T65.4X-
monoxide (from incomplete combustion)	T58.9-
blast furnace gas	T58.8X-
butane (distributed in mobile container or through pipes)	T58.1-

Drug/Chemical	Code
Carbon, continued	
charcoal fumes or coal	T58.2X-
coke (in domestic stoves, fireplaces)	T58.2X-
gas (piped)	T58.1-
solid (in domestic stoves, fireplaces)	T58.2X-
exhaust gas (motor)not in transit	T58.0-
combustion engine, any not in watercraft	T58.0-
farm tractor, not in transit	T58.0-
gas engine / motor pump	T58.01
motor vehicle, not in transit	T58.0-
fuel (in domestic use)	T58.2X-
gas (piped) (natural) or in mobile container	T58.1-
utility	T58.1-
in mobile container	T58.1-
illuminating gas	T58.1-
industrial fuels or gases, any	T58.8X-
kerosene (in domestic stoves, fireplaces)	T58.2X-
kiln gas or vapor	T58.8X-
motor exhaust gas, not in transit	T58.0-
piped gas (manufactured) (natural)	T58.1-
producer gas	T58.8X-
propane (distributed in mobile container)	T58.1-
distributed through pipes	T58.1-
specified source NEC	T58.8X-
stove gas (piped) / utility gas (piped) / water gas	T58.1-
wood (in domestic stoves, fireplaces)	T58.2X-
tetrachloride (vapor) NEC	T53.0X-
Carbonic acid gas	T59.7X-
anhydrase inhibitor NEC	T50.2X-
Carbophenothion	T60.0X-
Carboplatin	T45.1X-
Carboprost	T48.0X-
Carboquone	T45.1X-
Carbowax	T49.3X-
Carboxymethyl-cellulose	T47.4X-
S-Carboxymethyl-cysteine	T48.4X-
Carbrital	T42.3X-
Carbromal	T42.6X-
Carbutamide	T38.3X-
Carbuterol	T48.6X-
Cardiac medications (depressants) (rhythm regulater) NEC	T46.2X-
Cardiografin	T50.8X-
Cardio-green	T50.8X-
Cardiotonic (glycoside)NEC	T46.0X-
Cardiovascular drug NEC	T46.90-
Cardrase	T50.2X-
Carfecillin	T36.0X-
Carfenazine	T43.3X-
Carfusin	T49.0X-
Carindacillin	T36.0X-
Carisoprodol	T42.8X-
Carmellose	T47.4X-
Carminative	T47.5X-
Carmofur	T45.1X-
Carmustine	T45.1X-

Drug/Chemical	Code
Carotene	T45.2X-
Carphenazine	T43.3X-
Carpipramine	T42.4X-
Carprofen	T39.31-
Carpronium chloride	T44.3X-
Carrageenan	T47.8X-
Carteolol	T44.7X-
Carter's Little Pills	T47.2X-
Cascara (sagrada)	T47.2X-
Cassava	T62.2X-
Castellani's paint	T49.0X-
Castor (bean) (oil)	T62.2X-
Catalase	T45.3X-
Caterpillar (sting)	T63.431
Catha (edulis) (tea)	T43.69-
Cathartic NEC	T47.4X-
anthacene derivative	T47.2X-
bulk	T47.4X-
contact	T47.2X-
emollient NEC	T47.4X-
irritant NEC	T47.2X-
mucilage	T47.4X-
saline	T47.3X-
vegetable	T47.2X-
Cathine	T50.5X-
Cathomycin	T36.8X-
Cation exchange resin	T50.3X-
Caustic(s) NEC	T54.9-
alkali	T54.3X-
hydroxide	T54.3X-
potash	T54.3X-
soda	T54.3X-
specified NEC	T54.9-
Ceepryn	T49.0X-
ENT agent	T49.6X-
lozenges	T49.6X-
Cefacetrile	T36.1X-
Cefaclor	T36.1X-
Cefadroxil	T36.1X-
Cefalexin	T36.1X-
Cefaloglycin	T36.1X-
Cefaloridine	T36.1X-
Cefalosporins	T36.1X-
Cefalotin	T36.1X-
Cefamandole	T36.1X-
Cefamycin antibiotic	T36.1X-
Cefapirin	T36.1X-
Cefatrizine	T36.1X-
Cefazedone	T36.1X-
Cefazolin	T36.1X-
Cefbuperazone	T36.1X-
Cefetamet	T36.1X-
Cefixime	T36.1X-
Cefmenoxime	T36.1X-
Cefmetazole	T36.1X-

Drug/Chemical	Code
Cefminox	T36.1X-
Cefonicid	T36.1X-
Cefoperazone	T36.1X-
Ceforanide	T36.1X-
Cefotaxime	T36.1X-
Cefotetan	T36.1X-
Cefotiam	T36.1X-
Cefoxitin	T36.1X-
Cefpimizole	T36.1X-
Cefpiramide	T36.1X-
Cefradine	T36.1X-
Cefroxadine	T36.1X-
Cefsulodin	T36.1X-
Ceftazidime	T36.1X-
Cefteram	T36.1X-
Ceftezole	T36.1X-
Ceftizoxime	T36.1X-
Ceftriaxone	T36.1X-
Cefuroxime	T36.1X-
Cefuzonam	T36.1X-
Celestone	T38.0X-
topical	T49.0X-
Celiprolol	T44.7X-
Cell stimulants and proliferants	T49.8X-
Cellosolve	T52.9-
Cellulose	
cathartic	T47.4X-
hydroxyethyl	T47.4X-
nitrates (topical)	T49.3X-
oxidized	T49.4X-
Centipede (bite)	T63.41-
Central nervous system	
depressants	T42.71
anesthetic (general)NEC	T41.20-
gases NEC	T41.0X-
intravenous	T41.1X-
barbiturates	T42.3X-
benzodiazepines	T42.4X-
bromides	T42.6X-
cannabis sativa	T40.71-
chloral hydrate	T42.6X-
ethanol	T51.0X-
hallucinogenics	T40.90-
hypnotics	T42.71
specified NEC	T42.6X-
muscle relaxants	T42.8X-
paraldehyde	T42.6X-
sedatives; sedative-hypnotics	T42.71
mixed NEC	T42.6X-
specified NEC	T42.6X-
muscle-tone depressants	T42.8X-
stimulants	T43.60-
amphetamines	T43.62-
analeptics	T50.7X-
antidepressants	T43.20-

Drug/Chemical	Code
Central nervous system, continued	
opiate antagonists	T50.7X-
specified NEC	T43.69-
Cephalexin	T36.1X-
Cephaloglycin	T36.1X-
Cephaloridine	T36.1X-
Cephalosporins	T36.1X-
N (adicillin)	T36.0X-
Cephalothin	T36.1X-
Cephalotin	T36.1X-
Cephradine	T36.1X-
Cerbera (odallam)	T62.2X-
Cerberin	T46.0X-
Cerebral stimulants	T43.60-
psychotherapeutic	T43.60-
specified NEC	T43.69-
Cerium oxalate	T45.0X-
Cerous oxalate	T45.0X-
Ceruletide	T50.8X-
Cetalkonium (chloride)	T49.0X-
Cethexonium chloride	T49.0X-
Cetiedil	T46.7X-
Cetirizine	T45.0X-
Cetomacrogol	T50.99-
Cetotiamine	T45.2X-
Cetoxime	T45.0X-
Cetraxate	T47.1X-
Cetrimide	T49.0X-
Cetrimonium (bromide)	T49.0X-
Cetylpyridinium chloride	T49.0X-
ENT agent or lozenges	T49.6X-
Cevitamic acid	T45.2X-
Chalk, precipitated	T47.1X-
Chamomile	T49.0X-
Ch'an su	T46.0X-
Charcoal	T47.6X-
activated— see also Charcoal, medicinal	T47.6X-
fumes (Carbon monoxide)	T58.2X-
industrial	T58.8X-
medicinal (activated)	T47.6X-
antidiarrheal	T47.6X-
poison control	T47.8X-
specified use other than for diarrhea	T47.8X-
topical	T49.8X-
Chaulmosulfone	T37.1X-
Chelating agent NEC	T50.6X-
Chelidonium majus	T62.2X-
Chemical substance NEC	T65.9-
Chenodeoxycholic acid	T47.5X-
Chenodiol	T47.5X-
Chenopodium	T37.4X-
Cherry laurel	T62.2X-
Chinidin (e)	T46.2X-
Chiniofon	T37.8X-
Chlophedianol	T48.3X-

Drug/Chemical	Code
Chloral	T42.6X-
derivative	T42.6X-
hydrate	T42.6X-
Chloralamide	T42.6X-
Chloralodol	T42.6X-
Chloralose	T60.4X-
Chlorambucil	T45.1X-
Chloramine	T57.8X-
topical	T49.0X-
Chloramphenicol	T36.2X-
ENT agent	T49.6X-
ophthalmic preparation	T49.5X-
topical NEC	T49.0X-
Chlorate (potassium) (sodium)NEC	T60.3X-
herbicide	T60.3X-
Chlorazanil	T50.2X-
Chlorbenzene, chlorbenzol	T53.7X-
Chlorbenzoxamine	T44.3X-
Chlorbutol	T42.6X-
Chlorcyclizine	T45.0X-
Chlordan (e) (dust)	T60.1X-
Chlordantoin	T49.0X-
Chlordiazepoxide	T42.4X-
Chlordiethyl benzamide	T49.3X-
Chloresium	T49.8X-
Chlorethiazol	T42.6X-
Chlorethyl— see Ethyl chloride	
Chloretone	T42.6X-
Chlorex	T53.6X-
insecticide	T60.1X-
Chlorfenvinphos	T60.0X-
Chlorhexadol	T42.6X-
Chlorhexamide	T45.1X-
Chlorhexidine	T49.0X-
Chlorhydroxyquinolin	T49.0X-
Chloride of lime (bleach)	T54.3X-
Chlorimipramine	T43.01-
Chlorinated	
camphene	T53.6X-
diphenyl	T53.7X-
hydrocarbons NEC (solvents)	T53.9-
lime (bleach)	T54.3X-
and boric acid solution	T49.0X-
naphthalene (insecticide)	T60.1X-
industrial (non-pesticide)	T53.7X-
pesticide NEC	T60.8X-
solution	T49.0X-
Chlorine (fumes) (gas)	T59.4X-
bleach	T54.3X-
compound gas NEC	T59.4X-
disinfectant	T59.4X-
releasing agents NEC	T59.4X-
Chlorisondamine chloride	T46.99-
Chlormadinone	T38.5X-
Chlormephos	T60.0X-

Drug/Chemical	Code
Chlormerodrin	T50.2X-
Chlormethiazole	T42.6X-
Chlormethine	T45.1X-
Chlormethylenecycline	T36.4X-
Chlormezanone	T42.6X-
Chloroacetic acid	T60.3X-
Chloroacetone	T59.3X-
Chloroacetophenone	T59.3X-
Chloroaniline	T53.7X-
Chlorobenzene, chlorobenzol	T53.7X-
Chlorobromomethane (fire extinguisher)	T53.6X-
Chlorobutanol	T49.0X-
Chlorocresol	T49.0X-
Chlorodehydro-methyltestosterone	T38.7X-
Chlorodinitrobenzene	T53.7X-
Chlorodiphenyl	T53.7X-
Chloroethane— see Ethyl chloride	
Chloroethylene	T53.6X-
Chlorofluorocarbons	T53.5X-
Chloroform (fumes) (vapor)	T53.1X-
anesthetic	T41.0X-
solvent	T53.1X-
water, concentrated	T41.0X-
Chloroguanide	T37.2X-
Chloromycetin	T36.2X-
ENT agent or otic solution	T49.6X-
ophthalmic preparation	T49.5X-
topical NEC	T49.0X-
Chloronitrobenzene	T53.7X-
Chlorophacinone	T60.4X-
Chlorophenol	T53.7X-
Chlorophenothane	T60.1X-
Chlorophyll	T50.99-
Chloropicrin (fumes)	T53.6X-
fumigant / pesticide	T60.8X-
fungicide	T60.3X-
Chloroprocaine (infiltration) (topical) (subcutaneous) (nerve block) (spinal)	T41.3X-
Chloroptic	T49.5X-
Chloropurine	T45.1X-
Chloropyramine	T45.0X-
Chloropyrifos	T60.0X-
Chloropyrilene	T45.0X-
Chloroquine	T37.2X-
Chlorothalonil	T60.3X-
Chlorothen	T45.0X-
Chlorothiazide	T50.2X-
Chlorothymol	T49.4X-
Chlorotrianisene	T38.5X-
Chlorovinyldichloro-arsine	T57.0X-
Chloroxine	T49.4X-
Chloroxylenol	T49.0X-
Chlorphenamine	T45.0X-
Chlorphenesin	T42.8X-
topical (antifungal)	T49.0X-

CHLORPHENIRAMINE–CLIRADON

Drug/Chemical	Code
Chlorpheniramine	T45.0X-
Chlorphenoxamine	T45.0X-
Chlorphentermine	T50.5X-
Chlorproguanil	T37.2X-
Chlorpromazine	T43.3X-
Chlorpropamide	T38.3X-
Chlorprothixene	T43.4X-
Chlorquinaldol	T49.0X-
Chlorquinol	T49.0X-
Chlortalidone	T50.2X-
Chlortetracycline	T36.4X-
Chlorthalidone	T50.2X-
Chlorthion	T60.0X-
Chlorthiophos	T60.0X-
Chlortrianisene	T38.5X-
Chlor-Trimeton	T45.0X-
Chlorzoxazone	T42.8X-
Choke damp	T59.7X-
Cholagogues	T47.5X-
Cholebrine	T50.8X-
Cholecalciferol	T45.2X-
Cholecystokinin	T50.8X-
Cholera vaccine	T50.A9-
Choleretic	T47.5X-
Cholesterol-lowering agents	T46.6X-
Cholestyramine (resin)	T46.6X-
Cholic acid	T47.5X-
Choline	T48.6X-
chloride	T50.99-
dihydrogen citrate	T50.99-
salicylate	T39.09-
theophyllinate	T48.6X-
Cholinergic (drug)NEC	T44.1X-
muscle tone enhancer	T44.1X-
organophosphorus	T44.0X-
insecticide	T60.0X-
nerve gas	T59.89-
trimethyl ammonium propanediol	T44.1X-
Cholinesterase reactivator	T50.6X-
Cholografin	T50.8X-
Chorionic gonadotropin	T38.89-
Chromate	T56.2X-
dust or mist	T56.2X-
lead— see also lead	T56.0X-
paint	T56.0X-
Chromic	
acid	T56.2X-
dust or mist	T56.2X-
phosphate 32P	T45.1X-
Chromium	T56.2X-
compounds— see Chromate	
sesquioxide	T50.8X-
Chromomycin A3	T45.1X-
Chromonar	T46.3X-
Chromyl chloride	T56.2X-

Drug/Chemical	Code
Chrysarobin	T49.4X-
Chrysazin	T47.2X-
Chymar	T45.3X-
ophthalmic preparation	T49.5X-
Chymopapain	T45.3X-
Chymotrypsin	T45.3X-
ophthalmic preparation	T49.5X-
Cianidanol	T50.99-
Cianopramine	T43.01-
Cibenzoline	T46.2X-
Ciclacillin	T36.0X-
Ciclobarbital— see Hexobarbital	
Ciclonicate	T46.7X-
Ciclopirox (olamine)	T49.0X-
Ciclosporin	T45.1X-
Cicuta maculata or virosa	T62.2X-
Cicutoxin	T62.2X-
Cigarette lighter fluid	T52.0X-
Cigarettes (tobacco)	T65.22-
Ciguatoxin	T61.0-
Cilazapril	T46.4X-
Cimetidine	T47.0X-
Cimetropium bromide	T44.3X-
Cinchocaine	T41.3X-
Cinchona	T37.2X-
Cinchonine alkaloids	T37.2X-
Cinchophen	T50.4X-
Cinepazide	T46.7X-
Cinnamedrine	T48.5X-
Cinnarizine	T45.0X-
Cinoxacin	T37.8X-
Ciprofibrate	T46.6X-
Ciprofloxacin	T36.8X-
Cisapride	T47.8X-
Cisplatin	T45.1X-
Citalopram	T43.22-
Citanest (infiltration) (topical) (subcutaneous) (nerve block)	T41.3X-
Citric acid	T47.5X-
Citrovorum (factor)	T45.8X-
Claviceps purpurea	T62.2X-
Clavulanic acid	T36.1X-
Cleaner, cleansing agent, type not specified	T65.89-
of paint or varnish	T52.9-
specified type NEC	T65.89-
Clebopride	T47.8X-
Clefamide	T37.3X-
Clemastine	T45.0X-
Clematis vitalba	T62.2X-
Clemizole (penicillin)	T45.0X-
Clenbuterol	T48.6X-
Clidinium bromide	T44.3X-
Clindamycin	T36.8X-
Clinofibrate	T46.6X-
Clioquinol	T37.8X-
Cliradon	T40.2X-

Drug/Chemical	Code
Clobazam	T42.4X-
Clobenzorex	T50.5X-
Clobetasol	T49.0X-
Clobetasone	T49.0X-
Clobutinol	T48.3X-
Clocortolone	T38.0X-
Clodantoin	T49.0X-
Clodronic acid	T50.99-
Clofazimine	T37.1X-
Clofedanol	T48.3X-
Clofenamide	T50.2X-
Clofenotane	T49.0X-
Clofezone	T39.2X-
Clofibrate	T46.6X-
Clofibride	T46.6X-
Cloforex	T50.5X-
Clomethiazole	T42.6X-
Clometocillin	T36.0X-
Clomifene	T38.5X-
Clomiphene	T38.5X-
Clomipramine	T43.01-
Clomocycline	T36.4X-
Clonazepam	T42.4X-
Clonidine	T46.5X-
Clonixin	T39.8X-
Clopamide	T50.2X-
Clopenthixol	T43.4X-
Cloperastine	T48.3X-
Clophedianol	T48.3X-
Cloponone	T36.2X-
Cloprednol	T38.0X-
Cloral betaine	T42.6X-
Cloramfenicol	T36.2X-
Clorazepate (dipotassium)	T42.4X-
Clorexolone	T50.2X-
Clorfenamine	T45.0X-
Clorgiline	T43.1X-
Clorotepine	T44.3X-
Clorox (bleach)	T54.9-
Clorprenaline	T48.6X-
Clortermine	T50.5X-
Clotiapine	T43.59-
Clotiazepam	T42.4X-
Clotibric acid	T46.6X-
Clotrimazole	T49.0X-
Cloxacillin	T36.0X-
Cloxazolam	T42.4X-
Cloxiquine	T49.0X-
Clozapine	T42.4X-
Coagulant NEC	T45.7X-
Coal (carbon monoxide from)— *see also Carbon, monoxide, coal*	T58.2X-
oil— *see Kerosene*	
tar	T49.1X-
fumes	T59.89-

Drug/Chemical	Code
Coal (carbon monoxide from), continued	T58.2X-
medicinal (ointment)	T49.4X-
analgesics NEC	T39.2X-
naphtha (solvent)	T52.0X-
Cobalamine	T45.2X-
Cobalt (nonmedicinal) (fumes) (industrial)	T56.89-
medicinal (trace) (chloride)	T45.8X-
Cobra (venom)	T63.041
Coca (leaf)	T40.5X-
Cocaine	T40.5X-
topical anesthetic	T41.3X-
Cocarboxylase	T45.3X-
Coccidioidin	T50.8X-
Cocculus indicus	T62.1X-
Cochineal	T65.6X-
medicinal products	T50.99-
Codeine	T40.2X-
Cod-liver oil	T45.2X-
Coenzyme A	T50.99-
Coffee	T62.8X-
Cogalactoiso-merase	T50.99-
Cogentin	T44.3X-
Coke fumes or gas (carbon monoxide)	T58.2X-
industrial use	T58.8X-
Colace	T47.4X-
Colaspase	T45.1X-
Colchicine	T50.4X-
Colchicum	T62.2X-
Cold cream	T49.3X-
Colecalciferol	T45.2X-
Colestipol	T46.6X-
Colestyramine	T46.6X-
Colimycin	T36.8X-
Colistimethate	T36.8X-
Colistin	T36.8X-
sulfate (eye preparation)	T49.5X-
Collagen	T50.99-
Collagenase	T49.4X-
Collodion	T49.3X-
Colocynth	T47.2X-
Colophony adhesive	T49.3X-
Colorant— *see also Dye*	T50.99-
Combustion gas (after combustion) — *see Carbon, monoxide*	
prior to combustion	T59.89-
Compazine	T43.3X-
Compound	
42 (warfarin)	T60.4X-
269 (endrin)	T60.1X-
497 (dieldrin)	T60.1X-
1080 (sodium fluoroacetate)	T60.4X-
3422 (parathion)	T60.0X-
3911 (phorate)	T60.0X-
3956 (toxaphene)	T60.1X-
4049 (malathion)	T60.0X-

Drug/Chemical	Code
Compound, continued	
4069 (malathion)	T60.0X-
4124 (dicapthon)	T60.0X-
E (cortisone)	T38.0X-
F (hydrocortisone)	T38.0X-
Congener, anabolic	T38.7X-
Congo red	T50.8X-
Coniine, conine	T62.2X-
Conium (maculatum)	T62.2X-
Conjugated estrogenic substances	T38.5X-
Contac	T48.5X-
Contact lens solution	T49.5X-
Contraceptive (oral)	T38.4X-
vaginal	T49.8X-
Contrast medium, radiography	T50.8X-
Convallaria glycosides	T46.0X-
Convallaria majalis	T62.2X-
berry	T62.1X-
Copper (dust) (fumes) (nonmedicinal) NEC	T56.4X-
arsenate, arsenite	T57.0X-
insecticide	T60.2X-
emetic	T47.7X-
fungicide	T60.3X-
gluconate	T49.0X-
insecticide	T60.2X-
medicinal (trace)	T45.8X-
oleate	T49.0X-
sulfate	T56.4X-
cupric	T56.4X-
fungicide	T60.3X-
medicinal	
ear	T49.6X-
emetic	T47.7X-
eye	T49.5X-
cuprous	T56.4X-
fungicide	T60.3X-
medicinal	
ear	T49.6X-
emetic	T47.7X-
eye	T49.5X-
Copperhead snake (bite) (venom)	T63.06-
Coral (sting)	T63.69-
snake (bite) (venom)	T63.02-
Corbadrine	T49.6X-
Cordite	T65.89-
vapor	T59.89-
Cordran	T49.0X-
Corn cures	T49.4X-
Corn starch	T49.3X-
Cornhusker's lotion	T49.3X-
Coronary vasodilator NEC	T46.3X-
Corrosive NEC	T54.9-
acid NEC	T54.2X-
aromatics	T54.1X-
disinfectant	T54.1X-

Drug/Chemical	Code
Corrosive NEC, continued	T54.9-
fumes NEC	T54.9-
specified NEC	T54.9-
sublimate	T56.1X-
Cortate	T38.0X-
Cort-Dome	T38.0X-
ENT agent	T49.6X-
ophthalmic preparation	T49.5X-
topical NEC	T49.0X-
Cortef	T38.0X-
ENT agent	T49.6X-
ophthalmic preparation	T49.5X-
topical NEC	T49.0X-
Corticosteroid	T38.0X-
ENT agent	T49.6X-
mineral	T50.0X-
ophthalmic	T49.5X-
topical NEC	T49.0X-
Corticotropin	T38.81-
Cortisol	T49.0X-
ENT agent	T49.6X-
ophthalmic preparation	T49.5X-
topical NEC	T49.0X-
Cortisone (acetate)	T38.0X-
ENT agent	T49.6X-
ophthalmic preparation	T49.5X-
topical NEC	T49.0X-
Cortivazol	T38.0X-
Cortogen	T38.0X-
ENT agent	T49.6X-
ophthalmic preparation	T49.5X-
Cortone	T38.0X-
ENT agent	T49.6X-
ophthalmic preparation	T49.5X-
Cortril	T38.0X-
ENT agent	T49.6X-
ophthalmic preparation	T49.5X-
topical NEC	T49.0X-
Corynebacterium parvum	T45.1X-
Cosmetic preparation	T49.8X-
Cosmetics	T49.8X-
Cosyntropin	T38.81-
Cotarnine	T45.7X-
Co-trimoxazole	T36.8X-
Cottonseed oil	T49.3X-
Cough mixture (syrup)	T48.4X-
containing opiates	T40.2X-
expectorants	T48.4X-
Coumadin	T45.51-
rodenticide	T60.4X-
Coumaphos	T60.0X-
Coumarin	T45.51-
Coumetarol	T45.51-
Cowbane	T62.2X-
Cozyme	T45.2X-

Drug/Chemical	Code
Crack	T40.5X-
Crataegus extract	T46.0X-
Creolin	T54.1X-
disinfectant	T54.1X-
Creosol (compound)	T49.0X-
Creosote (coal tar) (beechwood)	T49.0X-
medicinal (expectorant) (syrup)	T48.4X-
Cresol(s)	T49.0X-
and soap solution	T49.0X-
Cresyl acetate	T49.0X-
Cresylic acid	T49.0X-
Crimidine	T60.4X-
Croconazole	T37.8X-
Cromoglicic acid	T48.6X-
Cromolyn	T48.6X-
Cromonar	T46.3X-
Cropropamide	T39.8X-
with crotethamide	T50.7X-
Crotamiton	T49.0X-
Crotethamide	T39.8X-
with cropropamide	T50.7X-
Croton (oil)	T47.2X-
chloral	T42.6X-
Crude oil	T52.0X-
Cryogenine	T39.8X-
Cryolite (vapor)	T60.1X-
insecticide	T60.1X-
Cryptenamine (tannates)	T46.5X-
Crystal violet	T49.0X-
Cuckoopint	T62.2X-
Cumetharol	T45.51-
Cupric	
acetate	T60.3X-
acetoarsenite	T57.0X-
arsenate	T57.0X-
gluconate	T49.0X-
oleate	T49.0X-
sulfate	T56.4X-
Cuprous sulfate— see also Copper sulfate	T56.4X-
Curare, curarine	T48.1X-
Cyamemazine	T43.3X-
Cyamopsis tetragono-loba	T46.6X-
Cyanacetyl hydrazide	T37.1X-
Cyanic acid (gas)	T59.89-
Cyanide(s) (compounds) (potassium) (sodium)NEC	T65.0X-
dust or gas (inhalation)NEC	T57.3X-
fumigant	T65.0X-
hydrogen	T57.3X-
mercuric— see Mercury	
pesticide (dust) (fumes)	T65.0X-
Cyanoacrylate adhesive	T49.3X-
Cyanocobalamin	T45.8X-
Cyanogen (chloride) (gas)NEC	T59.89-
Cyclacillin	T36.0X-
Cyclaine	T41.3X-

Drug/Chemical	Code
Cyclamate	T50.99-
Cyclamen europaeum	T62.2X-
Cyclandelate	T46.7X-
Cyclazocine	T50.7X-
Cyclizine	T45.0X-
Cyclobarbital	T42.3X-
Cyclobarbitone	T42.3X-
Cyclobenzaprine	T48.1X-
Cyclodrine	T44.3X-
Cycloguanil embonate	T37.2X-
Cyclohexane	T52.8X-
Cyclohexanol	T51.8X-
Cyclohexanone	T52.4X-
Cycloheximide	T60.3X-
Cyclohexyl acetate	T52.8X-
Cycloleucin	T45.1X-
Cyclomethycaine	T41.3X-
Cyclopentamine	T44.4X-
Cyclopenthiazide	T50.2X-
Cyclopentolate	T44.3X-
Cyclophosphamide	T45.1X-
Cycloplegic drug	T49.5X-
Cyclopropane	T41.29-
Cyclopyrabital	T39.8X-
Cycloserine	T37.1X-
Cyclosporin	T45.1X-
Cyclothiazide	T50.2X-
Cycrimine	T44.3X-
Cyhalothrin	T60.1X-
Cymarin	T46.0X-
Cypermethrin	T60.1X-
Cyphenothrin	T60.2X-
Cyproheptadine	T45.0X-
Cyproterone	T38.6X-
Cysteamine	T50.6X-
Cytarabine	T45.1X-
Cytisus	T62.2X-
Cytochrome C	T47.5X-
Cytomel	T38.1X-
Cytosine arabinoside	T45.1X-
Cytoxan	T45.1X-
Cytozyme	T45.7X-
2,4-D	T60.3X-
Dacarbazine	T45.1X-
Dactinomycin	T45.1X-
DADPS	T37.1X-
Dakin's solution	T49.0X-
Dalapon (sodium)	T60.3X-
Dalmane	T42.4X-
Danazol	T38.6X-
Danilone	T45.51-
Danthron	T47.2X-
Dantrolene	T42.8X-
Dantron	T47.2X-

Drug/Chemical	Code
Daphne (gnidium) (mezereum)	T62.2X-
berry	T62.1X-
Dapsone	T37.1X-
Daraprim	T37.2X-
Darnel	T62.2X-
Darvon	T39.8X-
Daunomycin	T45.1X-
Daunorubicin	T45.1X-
DBI	T38.3X-
D-Con	T60.9-
insecticide	T60.2X-
rodenticide	T60.4X-
DDAVP	T38.89-
DDE (bis [chlorophenyl]-dichloroethylene)	T60.2X-
DDS	T37.1X-
DDT (dust)	T60.1X-
Deadly nightshade	T62.2X-
berry	T62.1X-
Deamino-D-arginine vasopressin	T38.89-
Deanol (aceglumate)	T50.99-
Debrisoquine	T46.5X-
Decaborane	T57.8X-
fumes	T59.89-
Decadron	T38.0X-
topical NEC	T49.0X-
Decahydronaphthalene	T52.8X-
Decalin	T52.8X-
Decamethonium (bromide)	T48.1X-
Decholin	T47.5X-
Declomycin	T36.4X-
Decongestant, nasal (mucosa)	T48.5X-
Deet	T60.8X-
Deferoxamine	T45.8X-
Deflazacort	T38.0X-
Deglycyrrhizinized extract of licorice	T48.4X-
Dehydrocholic acid	T47.5X-
Dehydroemetine	T37.3X-
Dekalin	T52.8X-
Delalutin	T38.5X-
Delorazepam	T42.4X-
Delphinium	T62.2X-
Deltamethrin	T60.1X-
Deltasone	T38.0X-
Deltra	T38.0X-
Delvinal	T42.3X-
Demecarium (bromide)	T49.5X-
Demeclocycline	T36.4X-
Demecolcine	T45.1X-
Demegestone	T38.5X-
Demelanizing agents	T49.8X-
Demephion -O and -S	T60.0X-
Demerol	T40.2X-
Demethylchlortetracycline	T36.4X-
Demethyltetracycline	T36.4X-

Drug/Chemical	Code
Demeton -O and -S	T60.0X-
Demulcent (external)	T49.3X-
Demulen	T38.4X-
Denatured alcohol	T51.0X-
Dendrid	T49.5X-
Dental drug, topical application NEC	T49.7X-
Dentifrice	T49.7X-
Deodorant spray (feminine hygiene)	T49.8X-
Deoxycortone	T50.0X-
2-Deoxy-5-fluorouridine	T45.1X-
5-Deoxy-5-fluorouridine	T45.1X-
Deoxyribonuclease (pancreatic)	T45.3X-
Depilatory	T49.4X-
Deprenalin	T42.8X-
Deprenyl	T42.8X-
Depressant, appetite	T50.5X-
Depressant	
appetite (central)	T50.5X-
cardiac	T46.2X-
central nervous system (anesthetic)— *see also Central nervous system, depressants*	T42.7-
general anesthetic	T41.20-
muscle tone	T42.8X-
muscle tone, central	T42.8X-
psychotherapeutic	T43.50-
Deptropine	T45.0X-
Dequalinium (chloride)	T49.0X-
Derris root	T60.2X-
Deserpidine	T46.5X-
Desferrioxamine	T45.8X-
Desipramine	T43.01-
Deslanoside	T46.0X-
Desloughing agent	T49.4X-
Desmethylimipramine	T43.01-
Desmopressin	T38.89-
Desocodeine	T40.2X-
Desogestrel	T38.5X-
Desomorphine	T40.2X-
Desonide	T49.0X-
Desoximetasone	T49.0X-
Desoxycorticosteroid	T50.0X-
Desoxycortone	T50.0X-
Desoxyephedrine	T43.62-
Detaxtran	T46.6X-
Detergent	T49.2X-
external medication	T49.2X-
local	T49.2X-
medicinal	T49.2X-
nonmedicinal	T55.1X-
specified NEC	T55.1X-
Deterrent, alcohol	T50.6X-
Detoxifying agent	T50.6X-
Detrothyronine	T38.1X-
Dettol (external medication)	T49.0X-

Drug/Chemical	Code
Dexamethasone	T38.0X-
ENT agent	T49.6X-
ophthalmic preparation	T49.5X-
topical NEC	T49.0X-
Dexamfetamine	T43.62-
Dexamphetamine	T43.62-
Dexbrompheniramine	T45.0X-
Dexchlorpheniramine	T45.0X-
Dexedrine	T43.62-
Dexetimide	T44.3X-
Dexfenfluramine	T50.5X-
Dexpanthenol	T45.2X-
Dextran (40) (70) (150)	T45.8X-
Dextriferron	T45.4X-
Dextro calcium pantothenate	T45.2X-
Dextro pantothenyl alcohol	T45.2X-
Dextroamphetamine	T43.62-
Dextromethorphan	T48.3X-
Dextromoramide	T40.4X-
topical	T49.8X-
Dextropropoxyphene	T40.4X-
Dextrorphan	T40.2X-
Dextrose	T50.3X-
concentrated solution, intravenous	T46.8X-
Dextrothyroxin	T38.1X-
Dextrothyroxine sodium	T38.1X-
DFP	T44.0X-
DHE	T37.3X-
45	T46.5X-
Diabinese	T38.3X-
Diacetone alcohol	T52.4X-
Diacetyl monoxime	T50.99-
Diacetylmorphine	T40.1X-
Diachylon plaster	T49.4X-
Diaethylstilboestrolum	T38.5X-
Diagnostic agent NEC	T50.8X-
Dial (soap)	T49.2X-
sedative	T42.3X-
Dialkyl carbonate	T52.9-
Diallylbarbituric acid	T42.3X-
Diallymal	T42.3X-
Dialysis solution (intraperitoneal)	T50.3X-
Diaminodiphenylsulfone	T37.1X-
Diamorphine	T40.1X-
Diamox	T50.2X-
Diamthazole	T49.0X-
Dianthone	T47.2X-
Diaphenylsulfone	T37.0X-
Diasone (sodium)	T37.1X-
Diastase	T47.5X-
Diatrizoate	T50.8X-
Diazepam	T42.4X-
Diazinon	T60.0X-
Diazomethane (gas)	T59.89-
Diazoxide	T46.5X-

Drug/Chemical	Code
Dibekacin	T36.5X-
Dibenamine	T44.6X-
Dibenzepin	T43.01-
Dibenzheptropine	T45.0X-
Dibenzyline	T44.6X-
Diborane (gas)	T59.89-
Dibromochloropropane	T60.8X-
Dibromodulcitol	T45.1X-
Dibromoethane	T53.6X-
Dibromomannitol	T45.1X-
Dibromopropamidine isethionate	T49.0X-
Dibrompropamidine	T49.0X-
Dibucaine	T41.3X-
Dibunate sodium	T48.3X-
Dibutoline sulfate	T44.3X-
Dicamba	T60.3X-
Dicapthon	T60.0X-
Dichlobenil	T60.3X-
Dichlone	T60.3X-
Dichloralphenozone	T42.6X-
Dichlorbenzidine	T65.3X-
Dichlorhydrin	T52.8X-
Dichlorhydroxyquinoline	T37.8X-
Dichlorobenzene	T53.7X-
Dichlorobenzyl alcohol	T49.6X-
Dichlorodifluoromethane	T53.5X-
Dichloroethane	T52.8X-
Sym-Dichloroethyl ether	T53.6X-
Dichloroethyl sulfide, not in war	T59.89-
Dichloroethylene	T53.6X-
Dichloroformoxine, not in war	T59.89-
Dichlorohydrin, alpha-dichlorohydrin	T52.8X-
Dichloromethane (solvent) (vapor)	T53.4X-
Dichloronaphthoquinone	T60.3X-
Dichlorophen	T37.4X-
2,4-Dichlorophenoxyacetic acid	T60.3X-
Dichloropropene	T60.3X-
Dichloropropionic acid	T60.3X-
Dichlorphenamide	T50.2X-
Dichlorvos	T60.0X-
Diclofenac	T39.39-
Diclofenamide	T50.2X-
Diclofensine	T43.29-
Diclonixine	T39.8X-
Dicloxacillin	T36.0X-
Dicophane	T49.0X-
Dicoumarol, dicoumarin, dicumarol	T45.51-
Dicrotophos	T60.0X-
Dicyanogen (gas)	T65.0X-
Dicyclomine	T44.3X-
Dicycloverine	T44.3X-
Dideoxycytidine	T37.5X-
Dideoxyinosine	T37.5X-
Dieldrin (vapor)	T60.1X-
Diemal	T42.3X-

Drug/Chemical	Code
Dienestrol	T38.5X-
Dienoestrol	T38.5X-
Dietetic drug NEC	T50.90-
Diethazine	T42.8X-
Diethyl	
barbituric acid / carbinol	T42.3X-
carbamazine	T37.4X-
carbonate / oxide	T52.8X-
ether (vapor)— see also ether	T41.0X-
propion	T50.5X-
stilbestrol	T38.5X-
toluamide (nonmedicinal)	T60.8X-
medicinal	T49.3X-
Diethylcarbamazine	T37.4X-
Diethylene	
dioxide	T52.8X-
glycol (monoacetate) (monobutyl ether) (monoethyl ether)	T52.3X-
Diethylhexylphthalate	T65.89-
Diethylpropion	T50.5X-
Diethylstilbestrol	T38.5X-
Diethylstilboestrol	T38.5X-
Diethylsulfone-diethylmethane	T42.6X-
Diethyltoluamide	T49.0X-
Diethyltryptamine (DET)	T40.99-
Difebarbamate	T42.3X-
Difencloxazine	T40.2X-
Difenidol	T45.0X-
Difenoxin	T47.6X-
Difetarsone	T37.3X-
Diffusin	T45.3X-
Diflorasone	T49.0X-
Diflos	T44.0X-
Diflubenzuron	T60.1X-
Diflucortolone	T49.0X-
Diflunisal	T39.09-
Difluoromethyldopa	T42.8X-
Difluorophate	T44.0X-
Digestant NEC	T47.5X-
Digitalin (e)	T46.0X-
Digitalis (leaf) (glycoside)	T46.0X-
Digitoxin	T46.0X-
Digitoxose	T46.0X-
Digoxin	T46.0X-
Digoxine	T46.0X-
Dihydralazine	T46.5X-
Dihydrazine	T46.5X-
Dihydrocodeine	T40.2X-
Dihydrocodeinone	T40.2X-
Dihydroergocornine	T46.7X-
Dihydroergocristine (mesilate)	T46.7X-
Dihydroergokryptine	T46.7X-
Dihydroergotamine	T46.5X-
Dihydroergotoxine (mesilate)	T46.7X-
Dihydrohydroxycodeinone	T40.2X-
Dihydrohydroxymorphinone	T40.2X-

Drug/Chemical	Code
Dihydroisocodeine	T40.2X-
Dihydromorphine	T40.2X-
Dihydromorphinone	T40.2X-
Dihydrostreptomycin	T36.5X-
Dihydrotachysterol	T45.2X-
Dihydroxyaluminum aminoacetate	T47.1X-
Dihydroxyaluminum sodium carbonate	T47.1X-
Dihydroxyanthraquinone	T47.2X-
Dihydroxycodeinone	T40.2X-
Dihydroxypropyl theophylline	T50.2X-
Diiodohydroxyquin	T37.8X-
topical	T49.0X-
Diiodohydroxyquinoline	T37.8X-
Diiodotyrosine	T38.2X-
Diisopromine	T44.3X-
Diisopropylamine	T46.3X-
Diisopropylfluorophos-phonate	T44.0X-
Dilantin	T42.0X-
Dilaudid	T40.2X-
Dilazep	T46.3X-
Dill	T47.5X-
Diloxanide	T37.3X-
Diltiazem	T46.1X-
Dimazole	T49.0X-
Dimefline	T50.7X-
Dimefox	T60.0X-
Dimemorfan	T48.3X-
Dimenhydrinate	T45.0X-
Dimercaprol (British anti-lewisite)	T45.8X-
Dimercaptopropanol	T45.8X-
Dimestrol	T38.5X-
Dimetane	T45.0X-
Dimethicone	T47.1X-
Dimethindene	T45.0X-
Dimethisoquin	T49.1X-
Dimethisterone	T38.5X-
Dimethoate	T60.0X-
Dimethocaine	T41.3X-
Dimethoxanate	T48.3X-
Dimethyl	
arsine, arsinic acid	T57.0X-
carbinol	T51.2X-
carbonate	T52.8X-
diguanide	T38.3X-
ketone (vapor)	T52.4X-
meperidine	T40.2X-
parathion	T60.0X-
phthlate	T49.3X-
polysiloxane	T47.8X-
sulfate (fumes)	T59.89-
liquid	T65.89-
sulfoxide (nonmedicinal)	T52.8X-
medicinal	T49.4X-
tryptamine	T40.99-
tubocurarine	T48.1X-

Drug/Chemical	Code
Dimethylamine sulfate	T49.4X-
Dimethylformamide	T52.8X-
Dimethyltubocurarinium chloride	T48.1X-
Dimeticone	T47.1X-
Dimetilan	T60.0X-
Dimetindene	T45.0X-
Dimetotiazine	T43.3X-
Dimorpholamine	T50.7X-
Dimoxyline	T46.3X-
Dinitrobenzene	T65.3X-
vapor	T59.89-
Dinitrobenzol	T65.3X-
vapor	T59.89-
Dinitrobutylphenol	T65.3X-
Dinitro (-ortho-) cresol (pesticide) (spray)	T65.3X-
Dinitrocyclohexylphenol	T65.3X-
Dinitrophenol	T65.3X-
Dinoprost	T48.0X-
Dinoprostone	T48.0X-
Dinoseb	T60.3X-
Dioctyl sulfosuccinate (calcium) (sodium)	T47.4X-
Diodone	T50.8X-
Diodoquin	T37.8X-
Dionin	T40.2X-
Diosmin	T46.99-
Dioxane	T52.8X-
Dioxathion	T60.0X-
Dioxin	T53.7X-
Dioxopromethazine	T43.3X-
Dioxyline	T46.3X-
Dipentene	T52.8X-
Diperodon	T41.3X-
Diphacinone	T60.4X-
Diphemanil	T44.3X-
metilsulfate	T44.3X-
Diphenadione	T45.51-
rodenticide	T60.4X-
Diphenhydramine	T45.0X-
Diphenidol	T45.0X-
Diphenoxylate	T47.6X-
Diphenylamine	T65.3X-
Diphenylbutazone	T39.2X-
Diphenylchloroarsine, not in war	T57.0X-
Diphenylhydantoin	T42.0X-
Diphenylmethane dye	T52.1X-
Diphenylpyraline	T45.0X-
Diphtheria	
antitoxin	T50.Z1-
vaccine — See also Vaccines	T50.A9-
Diphylline	T50.2X-
Dipipanone	T40.4X-
Dipivefrine	T49.5X-
Diplovax	T50.B9-
Diprophylline	T50.2X-
Dipropyline	T48.29-

Drug/Chemical	Code
Dipyridamole	T46.3X-
Dipyrone	T39.2X-
Diquat (dibromide)	T60.3X-
Disinfectant	T65.89-
alkaline	T54.3X-
aromatic	T54.1X-
intestinal	T37.8X-
Disipal	T42.8X-
Disodium edetate	T50.6X-
Disoprofol	T41.29-
Disopyramide	T46.2X-
Distigmine (bromide)	T44.0X-
Disulfamide	T50.2X-
Disulfanilamide	T37.0X-
Disulfiram	T50.6X-
Disulfoton	T60.0X-
Dithiazanine iodide	T37.4X-
Dithiocarbamate	T60.0X-
Dithranol	T49.4X-
Diucardin	T50.2X-
Diupres	T50.2X-
Diuretic NEC	T50.2X-
benzothiadiazine	T50.2X-
carbonic acid anhydrase inhibitors	T50.2X-
furfuryl NEC	T50.2X-
loop (high-ceiling)	T50.1X-
mercurial NEC or osmotic	T50.2X-
purine or saluretic NEC	T50.2X-
sulfonamide	T50.2X-
thiazide NEC or xanthine	T50.2X-
Diurgin	T50.2X-
Diuril	T50.2X-
Diuron	T60.3X-
Divalproex	T42.6X-
Divinyl ether	T41.0X-
Dixanthogen	T49.0X-
Dixyrazine	T43.3X-
D-lysergic acid diethylamide	T40.8X-
DMCT	T36.4X-
DMSO— see Dimethyl sulfoxide	
DNBP	T60.3X-
DNOC	T65.3X-
Dobutamine	T44.5X-
DOCA	T38.0X-
Docusate sodium	T47.4X-
Dodicin	T49.0X-
Dofamium chloride	T49.0X-
Dolophine	T40.3X-
Doloxene	T39.8X-
Domestic gas (after combustion)— see Gas, utility	
prior to combustion	T59.89-
Domiodol	T48.4X-
Domiphen (bromide)	T49.0X-
Domperidone	T45.0X-
Dopa	T42.8X-

Drug/Chemical	Code
Dopamine	T44.99-
Doriden	T42.6X-
Dormiral	T42.3X-
Dormison	T42.6X-
Dornase	T48.4X-
Dorsacaine	T41.3X-
Dosulepin	T43.01-
Dothiepin	T43.01-
Doxantrazole	T48.6X-
Doxapram	T50.7X-
Doxazosin	T44.6X-
Doxepin	T43.01-
Doxifluridine	T45.1X-
Doxorubicin	T45.1X-
Doxycycline	T36.4X-
Doxylamine	T45.0X-
Dramamine	T45.0X-
Drano (drain cleaner)	T54.3X-
Dressing, live pulp	T49.7X-
Drocode	T40.2X-
Dromoran	T40.2X-
Dromostanolone	T38.7X-
Dronabinol	T40.71-
Droperidol	T43.59-
Dropropizine	T48.3X-
Drostanolone	T38.7X-
Drotaverine	T44.3X-
Drotrecogin alfa	T45.51-
Drug NEC	T50.90-
specified NEC	T50.99-
DTaP	T50.A1
DTIC	T45.1X-
Duboisine	T44.3X-
Dulcolax	T47.2X-
Duponol (C) (EP)	T49.2X-
Durabolin	T38.7X-
Dyclone	T41.3X-
Dyclonine	T41.3X-
Dydrogesterone	T38.5X-
Dye NEC	T65.6X-
antiseptic	T49.0X-
diagnostic agents	T50.8X-
pharmaceutical NEC	T50.90-
Dyflos	T44.0X-
Dymelor	T38.3X-
Dynamite	T65.3X-
fumes	T59.89-
Dyphylline	T44.3X-
Ear drug NEC	T49.6X-
Ear preparations	T49.6X-
Echothiophate, echothiopate, ecothiopate	T49.5X-
Econazole	T49.0X-
Ecothiopate iodide	T49.5X-
Ecstasy	T43.64-
Ectylurea	T42.6X-

Drug/Chemical	Code
Edathamil disodium	T45.8X-
Edecrin	T50.1X-
Edetate, disodium (calcium)	T45.8X-
Edoxudine	T49.5X-
Edrophonium	T44.0X-
chloride	T44.0X-
EDTA	T50.6X-
Eflornithine	T37.2X-
Efloxate	T46.3X-
Elase	T49.8X-
Elastase	T47.5X-
Elaterium	T47.2X-
Elcatonin	T50.99-
Elder	T62.2X-
berry, (unripe)	T62.1X-
Electrolyte balance drug	T50.3X-
Electrolytes NEC	T50.3X-
Electrolytic agent NEC	T50.3X-
Elemental diet	T50.90-
Elliptinium acetate	T45.1X-
Embramine	T45.0X-
Emepronium (salts) (bromide)	T44.3X-
Emetic NEC	T47.7X-
Emetine	T37.3X-
Emollient NEC	T49.3X-
Emorfazone	T39.8X-
Emylcamate	T43.59-
Enalapril	T46.4X-
Enalaprilat	T46.4X-
Encainide	T46.2X-
Endocaine	T41.3X-
Endosulfan	T60.2X-
Endothall	T60.3X-
Endralazine	T46.5X-
Endrin	T60.1X-
Enflurane	T41.0X-
Enhexymal	T42.3X-
Enocitabine	T45.1X-
Enovid	T38.4X-
Enoxacin	T36.8X-
Enoxaparin (sodium)	T45.51-
Enpiprazole	T43.59-
Enprofylline	T48.6X-
Enprostil	T47.1X-
ENT preparations (anti-infectives)	T49.6X-
Enterogastrone	T38.89-
Enviomycin	T36.8X-
Enzodase	T45.3X-
Enzyme NEC	T45.3X-
depolymerizing	T49.8X-
fibrolytic	T45.3X-
gastric / intestinal	T47.5X-
local action / proteolytic	T49.4X-
thrombolytic	T45.3X-
EPAB	T41.3X-

Drug/Chemical	Code
Epanutin	T42.0X-
Ephedra	T44.99-
Ephedrine	T44.99-
Epichlorhydrin, epichlorohydrin	T52.8X-
Epicillin	T36.0X-
Epiestriol	T38.5X-
Epimestrol	T38.5X-
Epinephrine	T44.5X-
Epirubicin	T45.1X-
Epitiostanol	T38.7X-
Epitizide	T50.2X-
EPN	T60.0X-
EPO	T45.8X-
Epoetin alpha	T45.8X-
Epomediol	T50.99-
Epoprostenol	T45.521
Epoxy resin	T65.89-
Eprazinone	T48.4X-
Epsilon amino-caproic acid	T45.62-
Epsom salt	T47.3X-
Eptazocine	T40.4X-
Equanil	T43.59-
Equisetum	T62.2X-
diuretic	T50.2X-
Ergobasine	T48.0X-
Ergocalciferol	T45.2X-
Ergoloid mesylates	T46.7X-
Ergometrine	T48.0X-
Ergonovine	T48.0X-
Ergot NEC	T64.81
derivative or medicinal (alkaloids) or prepared	T48.0X-
Ergotamine	T46.5X-
Ergotocine	T48.0X-
Ergotrate	T48.0X-
Eritrityl tetranitrate	T46.3X-
Erythrityl tetranitrate	T46.3X-
Erythrol tetranitrate	T46.3X-
Erythromycin (salts)	T36.3X-
ophthalmic preparation	T49.5X-
topical NEC	T49.0X-
Erythropoietin	T45.8X-
human	T45.8X-
Escin	T46.99-
Esculin	T45.2X-
Esculoside	T45.2X-
ESDT (ether-soluble tar distillate)	T49.1X-
Eserine	T49.5X-
Esflurbiprofen	T39.31-
Eskabarb	T42.3X-
Eskalith	T43.8X-
Esmolol	T44.7X-
Estanozolol	T38.7X-
Estazolam	T42.4X-

Drug/Chemical	Code
Estradiol	T38.5X-
with testosterone	T38.7X-
benzoate	T38.5X-
Estramustine	T45.1X-
Estriol	T38.5X-
Estrogen	T38.5X-
Estrone	T38.5X-
Estropipate	T38.5X-
Etacrynate sodium	T50.1X-
Etacrynic acid	T50.1X-
Etafedrine	T48.6X-
Etafenone	T46.3X-
Etambutol	T37.1X-
Etamiphyllin	T48.6X-
Etamivan	T50.7X-
Etamsylate	T45.7X-
Etebenecid	T50.4X-
Ethacridine	T49.0X-
Ethacrynic acid	T50.1X-
Ethadione	T42.2X-
Ethambutol	T37.1X-
Ethamide	T50.2X-
Ethamivan	T50.7X-
Ethamsylate	T45.7X-
Ethanol (beverage)	T51.0X-
Ethanolamine oleate	T46.8X-
Ethaverine	T44.3X-
Ethchlorvynol	T42.6X-
Ethebenecid	T50.4X-
Ether (vapor)	T41.0X-
anesthetic	T41.0X-
divinyl	T41.0X-
ethyl (medicinal)	T41.0X-
nonmedicinal	T52.8X-
solvent	T52.8X-
Ethiazide	T50.2X-
Ethidium chloride (vapor)	T59.89-
Ethinamate	T42.6X-
Ethinylestradiol, ethinyloestradiol	T38.5X-
with	
levonorgestrel or norethisterone	T38.4X-
Ethiodized oil (131 I)	T50.8X-
Ethion	T60.0X-
Ethionamide	T37.1X-
Ethioniamide	T37.1X-
Ethisterone	T38.5X-
Ethobral	T42.3X-
Ethocaine (infiltration) (topical) (nervel block) (spinal)	T41.3X-
Ethoheptazine	T40.4X-
Ethopropazine	T44.3X-
Ethosuximide	T42.2X-
Ethotoin	T42.0X-
Ethoxazene	T37.9-
Ethoxazorutoside	T46.99-
2-Ethoxyethanol	T52.3X-

Drug/Chemical	Code
Ethoxzolamide	T50.2X-
Ethyl	
acetate	T52.8X-
alcohol (beverage)	T51.0X-
aldehyde (vapor)	T59.89-
liquid	T52.8X-
aminobenzoate	T41.3X-
aminophenothiazine	T43.3X-
benzoate	T52.8X-
biscoumacetate	T45.51-
bromide (anesthetic)	T41.0X-
carbamate	T45.1X-
carbinol	T51.3X-
carbonate	T52.8X-
chaulmoograte	T37.1X-
chloride (anesthetic)	T41.0X-
anesthetic (local)	T41.3X-
inhaled	T41.0X-
local	T49.4X-
solvent	T53.6X-
dibunate	T48.3X-
dichloroarsine (vapor)	T57.0X-
estranol	T38.7X-
ether— *see also ether*	T52.8X-
formate NEC (solvent)	T52.0X-
fumarate	T49.4X-
hydroxyisobutyrate NEC (solvent)	T52.8X-
iodoacetate	T59.3X-
lactate NEC (solvent)	T52.8X-
loflazepate	T42.4X-
mercuric chloride	T56.1X-
methylcarbinol	T51.8X-
morphine	T40.2X-
noradrenaline	T48.6X-
oxybutyrate NEC (solvent)	T52.8X-
Ethylene (gas)	T59.89-
anesthetic (general)	T41.0X-
chlorohydrin	T52.8X-
vapor	T53.6X-
dichloride	T52.8X-
vapor	T53.6X-
dinitrate	T52.3X-
glycol(s)	T52.8X-
dinitrate	T52.3X-
monobutyl ether	T52.3X-
imine	T54.1X-
oxide (fumigant) (nonmedicinal)	T59.89-
medicinal	T49.0X-
Ethylenediamine theophylline	T48.6X-
Ethylenediaminetetra-acetic acid	T50.6X-
Ethylenedinitrilotetra-acetate	T50.6X-
Ethylestrenol	T38.7X-
Ethylhydroxycellulose	T47.4X-

Drug/Chemical	Code
Ethylidene	
chloride NEC	T53.6X-
diacetate	T60.3X-
dicoumarin / dicoumarol	T45.51-
diethyl ether	T52.0X-
Ethylmorphine	T40.2X-
Ethylnorepinephrine	T48.6X-
Ethylparachlorophen-oxyisobutyrate	T46.6X-
Ethynodiol	T38.4X-
with mestranol diacetate	T38.4X-
Etidocaine (infiltration) (subcutaneous) (nerve block)	T41.3X-
Etidronate	T50.99-
Etidronic acid (disodium salt)	T50.99-
Etifoxine	T42.6X-
Etilefrine	T44.4X-
Etilfen	T42.3X-
Etinodiol	T38.4X-
Etiroxate	T46.6X-
Etizolam	T42.4X-
Etodolac	T39.39-
Etofamide	T37.3X-
Etofibrate	T46.6X-
Etofylline	T46.7X-
clofibrate	T46.6X-
Etoglucid	T45.1X-
Etomidate	T41.1X-
Etomide	T39.8X-
Etomidoline	T44.3X-
Etoposide	T45.1X-
Etorphine	T40.2X-
Etoval	T42.3X-
Etozolin	T50.1X-
Etretinate	T50.99-
Etryptamine	T43.69-
Etybenzatropine	T44.3X-
Etynodiol	T38.4X-
Eucaine	T41.3X-
Eucalyptus oil	T49.7X-
Eucatropine	T49.5X-
Eucodal	T40.2X-
Euneryl	T42.3X-
Euphthalmine	T44.3X-
Eurax	T49.0X-
Euresol	T49.4X-
Euthroid	T38.1X-
Evans blue	T50.8X-
Evipal	T42.3X-
sodium	T41.1X-
Evipan	T42.3X-
sodium	T41.1X-
Exalamide	T49.0X-
Exalgin	T39.1X-
Excipients, pharmaceutical	T50.90-
Exhaust gas (engine) (motor vehicle)	T58.0-
Ex-Lax (phenolphthalein)	T47.2X-

Drug/Chemical	Code
Expectorant NEC	T48.4X-
Extended insulin zinc suspension	T38.3X-
External medications (skin) (mucous membrane)	T49.9-
dental agent	T49.7X-
ENT agent	T49.6X-
ophthalmic preparation	T49.5X-
specified NEC	T49.8X-
Extrapyramidal antagonist NEC	T44.3X-
Eye agents (anti-infective)	T49.5X-
Eye drug NEC	T49.5X-
FAC (fluorouracil + doxorubicin + cyclophosphamide)	T45.1X-
Factor	
I (fibrinogen)	T45.8X-
III (thromboplastin)	T45.8X-
VIII (antihemophilic Factor) (concentrate)	T45.8X-
IX complex	T45.7X-
human	T45.8X-
Famotidine	T47.0X-
Fat suspension, intravenous	T50.99-
Fazadinium bromide	T48.1X-
Febarbamate	T42.3X-
Fecal softener	T47.4X-
Fedrilate	T48.3X-
Felodipine	T46.1X-
Felypressin	T38.89-
Femoxetine	T43.22-
Fenalcomine	T46.3X-
Fenamisal	T37.1X-
Fenazone	T39.2X-
Fenbendazole	T37.4X-
Fenbutrazate	T50.5X-
Fencamfamine	T43.69-
Fendiline	T46.1X-
Fenetylline	T43.69-
Fenflumizole	T39.39-
Fenfluramine	T50.5X-
Fenobarbital	T42.3X-
Fenofibrate	T46.6X-
Fenoprofen	T39.31-
Fenoterol	T48.6X-
Fenoverine	T44.3X-
Fenoxazoline	T48.5X-
Fenproporex	T50.5X-
Fenquizone	T50.2X-
Fentanyl	T40.4X-
Fentanyl/fentanyl analogs	T40.41-
Fentazin	T43.3X-
Fenthion	T60.0X-
Fenticlor	T49.0X-
Fenylbutazone	T39.2X-
Feprazone	T39.2X-
Fer de lance (bite) (venom)	T63.06-

Drug/Chemical	Code
Ferric— *see also Iron*	
chloride	T45.4X-
citrate	T45.4X-
hydroxide	T45.4X-
pyrophosphate	T45.4X-
Ferritin	T45.4X-
Ferrocholinate	T45.4X-
Ferrodextrane	T45.4X-
Ferropolimaler	T45.4X-
Ferrous— *see also Iron*	T45.4X-
Ferrous fumerate, gluconate, lactate, salt NEC, sulfate (medicinal)	T45.4X-
Ferrovanadium (fumes)	T59.89-
Ferrum— *see Iron*	
Fertilizers NEC	T65.89-
with herbicide mixture	T60.3X-
Fetoxilate	T47.6X-
Fiber, dietary	T47.4X-
Fiberglass	T65.831
Fibrinogen (human)	T45.8X-
Fibrinolysin (human)	T45.69-
Fibrinolysis	
affecting drug	T45.60-
inhibitor NEC	T45.62-
Fibrinolytic drug	T45.61-
Filix mas	T37.4X-
Filtering cream	T49.3X-
Fiorinal	T39.01-
Firedamp	T59.89-
Fish, noxious, nonbacterial	T61.9-
ciguatera	T61.0-
scombroid	T61.1-
shell	T61.781-
specified NEC	T61.771-
Flagyl	T37.3X-
Flavine adenine dinucleotide	T45.2X-
Flavodic acid	T46.99-
Flavoxate	T44.3X-
Flaxedil	T48.1X-
Flaxseed (medicinal)	T49.3X-
Flecainide	T46.2X-
Fleroxacin	T36.8X-
Floctafenine	T39.8X-
Flomax	T44.6X-
Flomoxef	T36.1X-
Flopropione	T44.3X-
Florantyrone	T47.5X-
Floraquin	T37.8X-
Florinef	T38.0X-
ENT agent	T49.6X-
ophthalmic preparation	T49.5X-
topical NEC	T49.0X-
Flowers of sulfur	T49.4X-
Floxuridine	T45.1X-
Fluanisone	T43.4X-

Drug/Chemical	Code
Flubendazole	T37.4X-
Fluclorolone acetonide	T49.0X-
Flucloxacillin	T36.0X-
Fluconazole	T37.8X-
Flucytosine	T37.8X-
Fludeoxyglucose (18F)	T50.8X-
Fludiazepam	T42.4X-
Fludrocortisone	T50.0X-
ENT agent	T49.6X-
ophthalmic preparation	T49.5X-
topical NEC	T49.0X-
Fludroxycortide	T49.0X-
Flufenamic acid	T39.39-
Fluindione	T45.51-
Flumequine	T37.8X-
Flumethasone	T49.0X-
Flumethiazide	T50.2X-
Flumidin	T37.5X-
Flunarizine	T46.7X-
Flunidazole	T37.8X-
Flunisolide	T48.6X-
Flunitrazepam	T42.4X-
Fluocinolone (acetonide)	T49.0X-
Fluocinonide	T49.0X-
Fluocortin (butyl)	T49.0X-
Fluocortolone	T49.0X-
Fluohydrocortisone	T38.0X-
ENT agent	T49.6X-
ophthalmic preparation	T49.5X-
topical NEC	T49.0X-
Fluonid	T49.0X-
Fluopromazine	T43.3X-
Fluoracetate	T60.8X-
Fluorescein	T50.8X-
Fluorhydrocortisone	T50.0X-
Fluoride (nonmedicinal) (pesticide) (sodium) NEC	T60.8X-
medicinal NEC	T50.99-
dental use	T49.7X-
not pesticide NEC	T54.9-
stannous	T49.7X-
Fluorinated corticosteroids	T38.0X-
Fluorine (gas)	T59.5X-
Fluoristan	T49.7X-
Fluormetholone	T49.0X-
Fluoroacetate	T60.8X-
Fluorocarbon monomer	T53.6X-
Fluorocytosine	T37.8X-
Fluorodeoxyuridine	T45.1X-
Fluorometholone	T49.0X-
ophthalmic preparation	T49.5X-
Fluorophosphate insecticide	T60.0X-
Fluorosol	T46.3X-
Fluorouracil	T45.1X-
Fluorphenylalanine	T49.5X-
Fluothane	T41.0X-

Drug/Chemical	Code
Fluoxetine	T43.22-
Fluoxymesterone	T38.7X-
Flupenthixol	T43.4X-
Flupentixol	T43.4X-
Fluphenazine	T43.3X-
Fluprednidene	T49.0X-
Fluprednisolone	T38.0X-
Fluradoline	T39.8X-
Flurandrenolide	T49.0X-
Flurandrenolone	T49.0X-
Flurazepam	T42.4X-
Flurbiprofen	T39.31-
Flurobate	T49.0X-
Fluroxene	T41.0X-
Fluspirilene	T43.59-
Flutamide	T38.6X-
Flutazolam	T42.4X-
Fluticasone propionate	T38.0X-
Flutoprazepam	T42.4X-
Flutropium bromide	T48.6X-
Fluvoxamine	T43.22-
Folacin	T45.8X-
Folic acid	T45.8X-
with ferrous salt	T45.2X-
antagonist	T45.1X-
Folinic acid	T45.8X-
Folium stramoniae	T48.6X-
Follicle-stimulating hormone, human	T38.81-
Folpet	T60.3X-
Fominoben	T48.3X-
Food, foodstuffs, noxious, nonbacterial, NEC	T62.9-
berries	T62.1X-
mushrooms	T62.0X-
plants	T62.2X-
seafood	T61.9-
specified NEC	T61.8X-
seeds	T62.2X-
shellfish	T61.781
specified NEC	T62.8X-
Fool's parsley	T62.2X-
Formaldehyde (solution), gas or vapor	T59.2X-
fungicide	T60.3X-
Formalin	T59.2X-
fungicide	T60.3X-
vapor	T59.2X-
Formic acid	T54.2X-
vapor	T59.89-
Foscarnet sodium	T37.5X-
Fosfestrol	T38.5X-
Fosfomycin	T36.8X-
Fosfonet sodium	T37.5X-
Fosinopril	T46.4X-
sodium	T46.4X-
Fowler's solution	T57.0X-
Foxglove	T62.2X-

Drug/Chemical	Code
Framycetin	T36.5X-
Frangula	T47.2X-
extract	T47.2X-
Frei antigen	T50.8X-
Freon	T53.5X-
Fructose	T50.3X-
Frusemide	T50.1X-
FSH	T38.81-
Ftorafur	T45.1X-
Fuel	
automobile	T52.0X-
exhaust gas, not in transit	T58.0-
vapor NEC	T52.0X-
gas (domestic use) / utility / in mobile container / piped	T59.89-
industrial, incomplete combustion	T58.8X-
Fugillin	T36.8X-
Fulminate of mercury	T56.1X-
Fulvicin	T36.7X-
Fumadil	T36.8X-
Fumagillin	T36.8X-
Fumaric acid	T49.4X-
Fumes (from)	T59.9-
corrosive NEC	T54.9-
freons	T53.5X-
hydrocarbons (all types)	T59.89-
nitrogen dioxide	T59.0X-
petroleum (liquefied) (distributed)	T59.89-
polyester	T59.89-
specified source NEC	T59.89-
sulfur dioxide	T59.1X-
Fumigant NEC	T60.9-
Fungi, noxious, used as food	T62.0X-
Fungicide NEC (nonmedicinal)	T60.3X-
Fungizone	T36.7X-
topical	T49.0X-
Furacin	T49.0X-
Furadantin	T37.9-
Furazolidone	T37.8X-
Furazolium chloride	T49.0X-
Furfural	T52.8X-
Furnace (coal burning) (domestic), gas from	T58.2X-
industrial	T58.8X-
Furniture polish	T65.89-
Furosemide	T50.1X-
Furoxone	T37.9-
Fursultiamine	T45.2X-
Fusafungine	T36.8X-
Fusel oil (any) (amyl) (butyl) (propyl), vapor	T51.3X-
Fusidate (ethanolamine) (sodium)	T36.8X-
Fusidic acid	T36.8X-
Fytic acid, nonasodium	T50.6X-
GABA	T43.8X-
Gadopentetic acid	T50.8X-
Galactose	T50.3X-
b-Galactosidase	T47.5X-

Drug/Chemical	Code
Galantamine	T44.0X-
Gallamine (triethiodide)	T48.1X-
Gallium citrate	T50.99-
Gallopamil	T46.1X-
Gamboge	T47.2X-
Gamimune	T50.Z1-
Gamma globulin	T50.Z1-
Gamma-aminobutyric acid	T43.8X-
Gamma-benzene hexachloride (medicinal)	T49.0X-
nonmedicinal, vapor	T53.6X-
Gamma-BHC (medicinal)	T49.0X-
Gamulin	T50.Z1-
Ganciclovir (sodium)	T37.5X-
Ganglionic blocking drug NEC	T44.2X-
specified NEC	T44.2X-
Ganja	T40.71-
Garamycin	T36.5X-
ophthalmic preparation	T49.5X-
topical NEC	T49.0X-
Gardenal	T42.3X-
Gardepanyl	T42.3X-
Gas NEC	T59.9-
acetylene	T59.89-
incomplete combustion of	T58.1-
air contaminants, source or type not specified	T59.9-
anesthetic	T41.0X-
blast furnace	T58.8X-
chlorine	T59.4X-
coal	T58.2X-
cyanide	T57.3X-
dicyanogen	T65.0X-
exhaust	T58.0-
prior to combustion	T59.89-
from wood- or coal-burning stove or fireplace	T58.2X-
industrial use	T58.8X-
prior to combustion	T59.89-
utility (in mobile container or piped)	T59.89-
garage	T58.0-
hydrocarbon NEC (piped)	T59.89-
hydrocyanic acid	T65.0X-
illuminating (after combustion)	T58.1-
prior to combustion	T59.89-
kiln	T58.8X-
lacrimogenic	T59.3X-
marsh	T59.89-
motor exhaust, not in transit	T58.0-
natural	T59.89-
oil	T52.0X-
petroleum (liquefied) (distributed in mobile containers) (piped)	T59.89-
producer	T58.8X-
refrigerant (chlorofluoro-carbon)	T53.5X-
not chlorofluoro-carbon	T59.89-
sewer	T59.9-
specified source NEC	T59.9-

Drug/Chemical	Code
Gas NEC, continued	T59.9-
stove (after combustion)	T58.1-
prior to combustion	T59.89-
tear	T59.3X-
therapeutic	T41.5X-
utility (for cooking, heating, or lighting) (piped) (mobile container) NEC	T59.89-
water	T58.1-
Gasoline	T52.0X-
vapor	T52.0X-
Gastric enzymes	T47.5X-
Gastrografin	T50.8X-
Gastrointestinal drug	T47.9-
biological	T47.8X-
specified NEC	T47.8X-
Gaultheria procumbens	T62.2X-
Gefarnate	T44.3X-
Gelatin (intravenous)	T45.8X-
absorbable (sponge)	T45.7X-
Gelfilm	T49.8X-
Gelfoam	T45.7X-
Gelsemine	T50.99-
Gelsemium (sempervirens)	T62.2X-
Gemeprost	T48.0X-
Gemfibrozil	T46.6X-
Gemonil	T42.3X-
Gentamicin	T36.5X-
ophthalmic preparation	T49.5X-
topical NEC	T49.0X-
Gentian	T47.5X-
violet	T49.0X-
Gepefrine	T44.4X-
Gestonorone caproate	T38.5X-
Gexane	T49.0X-
Gila monster (venom)	T63.11-
Ginger	T47.5X-
Gitalin	T46.0X-
Gitaloxin	T46.0X-
Gitoxin	T46.0X-
Glafenine	T39.8X-
Glandular extract (medicinal)NEC	T50.Z9-
Glaucarubin	T37.3X-
Glibenclamide	T38.3X-
Glibornuride	T38.3X-
Gliclazide	T38.3X-
Glimidine	T38.3X-
Glipizide	T38.3X-
Gliquidone	T38.3X-
Glisolamide	T38.3X-
Glisoxepide	T38.3X-
Globin zinc insulin	T38.3X-
Globulin (antilymphocytic) (antirhesus) (antivenin) (antiviral)	T50.Z1-
Glucagon	T38.3X-
Glucocorticoids	T38.0X-

Drug/Chemical	Code
Glucocorticosteroid	T38.0X-
Gluconic acid	T50.99-
Glucosamine sulfate	T39.4X-
Glucose	T50.3X-
with sodium chloride	T50.3X-
Glucosulfone sodium	T37.1X-
Glucurolactone	T47.8X-
Glue NEC	T52.8X-
Glutamic acid	T47.5X-
Glutaral (medicinal)	T49.0X-
nonmedicinal	T65.89-
Glutaraldehyde (nonmedicinal)	T65.89-
medicinal	T49.0X-
Glutathione	T50.6X-
Glutethimide	T42.6X-
Glyburide	T38.3X-
Glycerin	T47.4X-
Glycerol	T47.4X-
borax	T49.6X-
intravenous	T50.3X-
iodinated	T48.4X-
Glycerophosphate	T50.99-
Glyceryl	
gualacolate	T48.4X-
nitrate	T46.3X-
triacetate (topical)	T49.0X-
trinitrate	T46.3X-
Glycine	T50.3X-
Glyclopyramide	T38.3X-
Glycobiarsol	T37.3X-
Glycols (ether)	T52.3X-
Glyconiazide	T37.1X-
Glycopyrrolate	T44.3X-
Glycopyrronium (bromide)	T44.3X-
Glycoside, cardiac (stimulant)	T46.0X-
Glycyclamide	T38.3X-
Glycyrrhiza extract	T48.4X-
Glycyrrhizic acid	T48.4X-
Glycyrrhizinate potassium	T48.4X-
Glymidine sodium	T38.3X-
Glyphosate	T60.3X-
Glyphylline	T48.6X-
Gold	
colloidal (I98Au)	T45.1X-
salts	T39.4X-
Golden sulfide of antimony	T56.89-
Goldylocks	T62.2X-
Gonadal tissue extract	T38.90-
female	T38.5X-
male	T38.7X-
Gonadorelin	T38.89-
Gonadotropin	T38.89-
chorionic	T38.89-
pituitary	T38.81-
Goserelin	T45.1X-

Drug/Chemical	Code
Grain alcohol	T51.0X-
Gramicidin	T49.0X-
Granisetron	T45.0X-
Gratiola officinalis	T62.2X-
Grease	T65.89-
Green hellebore	T62.2X-
Green soap	T49.2X-
Grifulvin	T36.7X-
Griseofulvin	T36.7X-
Growth hormone	T38.81-
Guaiac reagent	T50.99-
Guaiacol derivatives	T48.4X-
Guaifenesin	T48.4X-
Guaimesal	T48.4X-
Guaiphenesin	T48.4X-
Guamecycline	T36.4X-
Guanabenz	T46.5X-
Guanacline	T46.5X-
Guanadrel	T46.5X-
Guanatol	T37.2X-
Guanethidine	T46.5X-
Guanfacine	T46.5X-
Guano	T65.89-
Guanochlor	T46.5X-
Guanoclor	T46.5X-
Guanoctine	T46.5X-
Guanoxabenz	T46.5X-
Guanoxan	T46.5X-
Guar gum (medicinal)	T46.6X-
Hachimycin	T36.7X-
Hair	
dye	T49.4X-
preparation NEC	T49.4X-
Halazepam	T42.4X-
Halcinolone	T49.0X-
Halcinonide	T49.0X-
Halethazole	T49.0X-
Hallucinogen NOS	T40.90-
specified NEC	T40.99-
Halofantrine	T37.2X-
Halofenate	T46.6X-
Halometasone	T49.0X-
Haloperidol	T43.4X-
Haloprogin	T49.0X-
Halotex	T49.0X-
Halothane	T41.0X-
Haloxazolam	T42.4X-
Halquinols	T49.0X-
Hamamelis	T49.2X-
Haptendextran	T45.8X-
Harmonyl	T46.5X-
Hartmann's solution	T50.3X-
Hashish	T40.71-
Hawaiian Woodrose seeds	T40.99-
HCB	T60.3X-

Drug/Chemical	Code
HCH	T53.6X-
medicinal	T49.0X-
HCN	T57.3X-
Headache cures, drugs, powders NEC	T50.90-
Heavenly Blue (morning glory)	T40.99-
Heavy metal antidote	T45.8X-
Hedaquinium	T49.0X-
Hedge hyssop	T62.2X-
Heet	T49.8X-
Helenin	T37.4X-
Helium (nonmedicinal)NEC	T59.89-
medicinal	T48.99-
Hellebore (black) (green) (white)	T62.2X-
Hematin	T45.8X-
Hematinic preparation	T45.8X-
Hematological agent	T45.9-
specified NEC	T45.8X-
Hemlock	T62.2X-
Hemostatic	T45.62-
drug, systemic	T45.62-
Hemostyptic	T49.4X-
Henbane	T62.2X-
Heparin (sodium)	T45.51-
action reverser	T45.7X-
Heparin-fraction	T45.51-
Heparinoid (systemic)	T45.51-
Hepatic secretion stimulant	T47.8X-
Hepatitis B	
immune globulin	T50.Z1-
vaccine	T50.B9-
Hepronicate	T46.7X-
Heptabarb	T42.3X-
Heptabarbital	T42.3X-
Heptabarbitone	T42.3X-
Heptachlor	T60.1X-
Heptalgin	T40.2X-
Heptaminol	T46.3X-
Herbicide NEC	T60.3X-
Heroin	T40.1X-
Herplex	T49.5X-
HES	T45.8X-
Hesperidin	T46.99-
Hetacillin	T36.0X-
Hetastarch	T45.8X-
HETP	T60.0X-
Hexachlorobenzene (vapor)	T60.3X-
Hexachlorocyclohexane	T53.6X-
Hexachlorophene	T49.0X-
Hexadiline	T46.3X-
Hexadimethrine (bromide)	T45.7X-
Hexadylamine	T46.3X-
Hexaethyl tetraphos-phate	T60.0X-
Hexafluorenium bromide	T48.1X-
Hexafluronium (bromide)	T48.1X-
Hexa-germ	T49.2X-

HEXAHYDROBENZOL–HYDROCYANIC ACID (LIQUID)

Drug/Chemical	Code
Hexahydrobenzol	T52.8X-
Hexahydrocresol(s)	T51.8X-
arsenide	T57.0X-
arseniurated	T57.0X-
cyanide	T57.3X-
gas	T59.89-
Fluoride (liquid)	T57.8X-
vapor	T59.89-
phophorated	T60.0X-
sulfate	T57.8X-
sulfide (gas)	T59.6X-
arseniurated	T57.0X-
sulfurated	T57.8X-
Hexahydrophenol	T51.8X-
Hexalen	T51.8X-
Hexamethonium bromide	T44.2X-
Hexamethylene	T52.8X-
Hexamethylmelamine	T45.1X-
Hexamidine	T49.0X-
Hexamine (mandelate)	T37.8X-
Hexanone, 2-hexanone	T52.4X-
Hexanuorenium	T48.1X-
Hexapropymate	T42.6X-
Hexasonium iodide	T44.3X-
Hexcarbacholine bromide	T48.1X-
Hexemal	T42.3X-
Hexestrol	T38.5X-
Hexethal (sodium)	T42.3X-
Hexetidine	T37.8X-
Hexobarbital	T42.3X-
rectal	T41.29-
sodium	T41.1X-
Hexobendine	T46.3X-
Hexocyclium (metilsulfate)	T44.3X-
Hexoestrol	T38.5X-
Hexone	T52.4X-
Hexoprenaline	T48.6X-
Hexylcaine	T41.3X-
Hexylresorcinol	T52.2X-
HGH (human growth hormone)	T38.81-
Hinkle's pills	T47.2X-
Histalog	T50.8X-
Histamine (phosphate)	T50.8X-
Histoplasmin	T50.8X-
Holly berries	T62.2X-
Homatropine	T44.3X-
methylbromide	T44.3X-
Homochlorcyclizine	T45.0X-
Homosalate	T49.3X-
Homo-tet	T50.Z1-
Hormone	T38.80-
adrenal cortical steroids	T38.0X-
androgenic	T38.7X-
anterior pituitary NEC	T38.81-
antidiabetic agents	T38.3X-

Drug/Chemical	Code
Hormone, continued	T38.80-
antidiuretic	T38.89-
cancer therapy	T45.1X-
follicle stimulating	T38.81-
gonadotropic	T38.89-
pituitary	T38.81-
growth	T38.81-
luteinizing	T38.81-
ovarian	T38.5X-
oxytocic	T48.0X-
parathyroid (derivatives)	T50.99-
pituitary (posterior)NEC	T38.89-
anterior	T38.81-
specified, NEC	T38.89-
thyroid	T38.1X-
Hornet (sting)	T63.451
Horse anti-human lymphocytic serum	T50.Z1-
Horticulture agent NEC	T65.9-
with pesticide	T60.9-
Human	
albumin	T45.8X-
growth hormone (HGH)	T38.81-
immune serum	T50.Z1-
Hyaluronidase	T45.3X-
Hyazyme	T45.3X-
Hycodan	T40.2X-
Hydantoin derivative NEC	T42.0X-
Hydeltra	T38.0X-
Hydergine	T44.6X-
Hydrabamine penicillin	T36.0X-
Hydralazine	T46.5X-
Hydrargaphen	T49.0X-
Hydrargyri amino-chloridum	T49.0X-
Hydrastine	T48.29-
Hydrazine	T54.1X-
monoamine oxidase inhibitors	T43.1X-
Hydrazoic acid, azides	T54.2X-
Hydriodic acid	T48.4X-
Hydrocarbon gas	T59.89-
Hydrochloric acid (liquid)	T54.2X-
medicinal (digestant)	T47.5X-
vapor	T59.89-
Hydrochlorothiazide	T50.2X-
Hydrocodone	T40.2X-
Hydrocortisone (derivatives)	T49.0X-
aceponate	T49.0X-
ENT agent	T49.6X-
ophthalmic preparation	T49.5X-
topical NEC	T49.0X-
Hydrocortone	T38.0X-
ENT agent	T49.6X-
ophthalmic preparation	T49.5X-
topical NEC	T49.0X-
Hydrocyanic acid (liquid)	T57.3X-
gas	T65.0X-

Drug/Chemical	Code
Hydroflumethiazide	T50.2X-
Hydrofluoric acid (liquid)	T54.2X-
vapor	T59.89-
Hydrogen	T59.89-
arsenide	T57.0X-
arseniureted	T57.0X-
chloride	T57.8X-
cyanide (salts) (gas)	T57.3X-
Fluoride (vapor)	T59.5X-
peroxide	T49.0X-
phosphureted	T57.1X-
sulfide (sulfureted)	T59.6X-
arseniureted	T57.0X-
Hydromethylpyridine	T46.7X-
Hydromorphinol	T40.2X-
Hydromorphinone	T40.2X-
Hydromorphone	T40.2X-
Hydromox	T50.2X-
Hydrophilic lotion	T49.3X-
Hydroquinidine	T46.2X-
Hydroquinone	T52.2X-
vapor	T59.89-
Hydrosulfuric acid (gas)	T59.6X-
Hydrotalcite	T47.1X-
Hydrous wool fat	T49.3X-
Hydroxide, caustic	T54.3X-
Hydroxocobalamin	T45.8X-
Hydroxyamphetamine	T49.5X-
Hydroxycarbamide	T45.1X-
Hydroxychloroquine	T37.8X-
Hydroxydihydrocodeinone	T40.2X-
Hydroxyestrone	T38.5X-
Hydroxyethyl starch	T45.8X-
Hydroxymethylpenta-none	T52.4X-
Hydroxyphenamate	T43.59-
Hydroxyphenylbutazone	T39.2X-
Hydroxyprogesterone	T38.5X-
caproate	T38.5X-
Hydroxyquinoline (derivatives) NEC	T37.8X-
Hydroxystilbamidine	T37.3X-
Hydroxytoluene (nonmedicinal)	T54.0X-
medicinal	T49.0X-
Hydroxyurea	T45.1X-
Hydroxyzine	T43.59-
Hyoscine	T44.3X-
Hyoscyamine	T44.3X-
Hyoscyamus	T44.3X-
dry extract	T44.3X-
Hypaque	T50.8X-
Hypertussis	T50.Z1-
Hypnotic	T42.71
anticonvulsant	T42.71
specified NEC	T42.6X-
Hypochlorite	T49.0X-
Hypophysis, posterior	T38.89-

Drug/Chemical	Code
Hypotensive NEC	T46.5X-
Hypromellose	T49.5X-
Ibacitabine	T37.5X-
Ibopamine	T44.99-
Ibufenac	T39.31-
Ibuprofen	T39.31-
Ibuproxam	T39.31-
Ibuterol	T48.6X-
Ichthammol	T49.0X-
Ichthyol	T49.4X-
Idarubicin	T45.1X-
Idrocilamide	T42.8X-
Ifenprodil	T46.7X-
Ifosfamide	T45.1X-
Iletin	T38.3X-
Ilex	T62.2X-
Illuminating gas (after combustion)	T58.1-
prior to combustion	T59.89-
Ilopan	T45.2X-
Iloprost	T46.7X-
Ilotycin	T36.3X-
ophthalmic preparation	T49.5X-
topical NEC	T49.0X-
Imidazole-4-carboxamide	T45.1X-
Iminostilbene	T42.1X-
Imipenem	T36.0X-
Imipramine	T43.01-
Immu-G	T50.Z1-
Immuglobin	T50.Z1-
Immune (globulin) (serum)	T50.Z1-
Immunoglobin human (intravenous) (normal)	T50.Z1-
Immunosuppressive drug	T45.1X-
Immu-tetanus	T50.Z1-
Indalpine	T43.22-
Indanazoline	T48.5X-
Indandione (derivatives)	T45.51-
Indapamide	T46.5X-
Indendione (derivatives)	T45.51-
Indenolol	T44.7X-
Inderal	T44.7X-
Indian	
hemp	T40.71-
tobacco	T62.2X-
Indigo carmine	T50.8X-
Indobufen	T45.521
Indocin	T39.2X-
Indocyanine green	T50.8X-
Indometacin	T39.39-
Indomethacin	T39.39-
farnesil	T39.4X-
Indoramin	T44.6X-
Industrial	
alcohol	T51.0X-
fumes	T59.89-
solvents (fumes) (vapors)	T52.9-

Drug/Chemical	Code
Influenza vaccine	T50.B9-
Ingested substance NEC	T65.9-
INH	T37.1X-
Inhibitor	
angiotensin-converting enzyme	T46.4X-
carbonic anhydrase	T50.2X-
fibrinolysis	T45.62-
monoamine oxidase NEC	T43.1X-
hydrazine	T43.1X-
postsynaptic	T43.8X-
prothrombin synthesis	T45.51-
Ink	T65.89-
Inorganic substance NEC	T57.9-
Inosine pranobex	T37.5X-
Inositol	T50.99-
nicotinate	T46.7X-
Inproquone	T45.1X-
Insect (sting), venomous	T63.481
ant	T63.421
bee	T63.441
caterpillar	T63.431
hornet	T63.451
wasp	T63.461
Insecticide NEC	T60.9-
carbamate	T60.0X-
chlorinated	T60.1X-
mixed	T60.9-
organochlorine	T60.1X-
organophosphorus	T60.0X-
Insular tissue extract	T38.3X-
Insulin (amorphous) (globin) (isophane) (Lente) (NPH) (Semilente) (Ultralente)	T38.3X-
defalan	T38.3X-
human	T38.3X-
injection, soluble (biphasic)	T38.3X-
intermediate acting	T38.3X-
protamine zinc	T38.3X-
slow acting	T38.3X-
zinc protamine injection/suspension (amorphous) (crystalline)	T38.3X-
Interferon (alpha) (beta) (gamma)	T37.5X-
Intestinal motility control drug	T47.6X-
biological	T47.8X-
Intranarcon	T41.1X-
Intravenous	
amino acids or fat suspensions	T50.99-
Inulin	T50.8X-
Invert sugar	T50.3X-
Iobenzamic acid	T50.8X-
Iocarmic acid	T50.8X-
Iocetamic acid	T50.8X-
Iodamide	T50.8X-

Drug/Chemical	Code
Iodide NEC— *see also Iodine*	T49.0X-
mercury (ointment)	T49.0X-
methylate	T49.0X-
potassium (expectorant)NEC	T48.4X-
Iodinated	
contrast medium	T50.8X-
glycerol	T48.4X-
human serum albumin (131I)	T50.8X-
Iodine (antiseptic, external) (tincture) NEC	T49.0X-
125— *see also Radiation sickness, and Exposure to radioactivce isotopes*	T50.8X-
therapeutic	T50.99-
131— *see also Radiation sickness, and Exposure to radioactivce isotopes*	T50.8X-
therapeutic	T38.2X-
diagnostic	T50.8X-
for thyroid conditions (antithyroid)	T38.2X-
solution	T49.0X-
vapor	T59.89-
Iodipamide	T50.8X-
Iodized (poppy seed) oil	T50.8X-
Iodobismitol	T37.8X-
Iodochlorhydroxyquin	T37.8X-
topical	T49.0X-
Iodochlorhydroxyquinoline	T37.8X-
Iodocholesterol (131I)	T50.8X-
Iodoform	T49.0X-
Iodohippuric acid	T50.8X-
Iodopanoic acid	T50.8X-
Iodophthalein (sodium)	T50.8X-
Iodopyracet	T50.8X-
Iodoquinol	T37.8X-
Iodoxamic acid	T50.8X-
Iofendylate	T50.8X-
Ioglycamic acid	T50.8X-
Iohexol	T50.8X-
Ion exchange resin	
anion	T47.8X-
cation	T50.3X-
cholestyramine	T46.6X-
intestinal	T47.8X-
Iopamidol	T50.8X-
Iopanoic acid	T50.8X-
Iophenoic acid	T50.8X-
Iopodate, sodium	T50.8X-
Iopodic acid	T50.8X-
Iopromide	T50.8X-
Iopydol	T50.8X-
Iotalamic acid	T50.8X-
Iothalamate	T50.8X-
Iothiouracil	T38.2X-
Iotrol	T50.8X-
Iotrolan	T50.8X-
Iotroxate	T50.8X-
Iotroxic acid	T50.8X-

Drug/Chemical	Code
Ioversol	T50.8X-
Ioxaglate	T50.8X-
Ioxaglic acid	T50.8X-
Ioxitalamic acid	T50.8X-
Ipecac	T47.7X-
Ipecacuanha	T48.4X-
Ipodate, calcium	T50.8X-
Ipral	T42.3X-
Ipratropium (bromide)	T48.6X-
Ipriflavone	T46.3X-
Iprindole	T43.01-
Iproclozide	T43.1X-
Iprofenin	T50.8X-
Iproheptine	T49.2X-
Iproniazid	T43.1X-
Iproplatin	T45.1X-
Iproveratril	T46.1X-
Iron (compounds) (medicinal) NEC	T45.4X-
ammonium/dextran injection/salts/sorbitex/sorbitol citric acid complex	T45.4X-
nonmedicinal	T56.89-
Irrigating fluid (vaginal)	T49.8X-
eye	T49.5X-
Isepamicin	T36.5X-
Isoaminile (citrate)	T48.3X-
Isoamyl nitrite	T46.3X-
Isobenzan	T60.1X-
Isobutyl acetate	T52.8X-
Isocarboxazid	T43.1X-
Isoconazole	T49.0X-
Isocyanate	T65.0X-
Isoephedrine	T44.99-
Isoetarine	T48.6X-
Isoethadione	T42.2X-
Isoetharine	T44.5X-
Isoflurane	T41.0X-
Isoflurophate	T44.0X-
Isomaltose, ferric complex	T45.4X-
Isometheptene	T44.3X-
Isoniazid	T37.1X-
with	
rifampicin	T36.6X-
thioacetazone	T37.1X-
Isonicotinic acid hydrazide	T37.1X-
Isonipecaine	T40.4X-
Isopentaquine	T37.2X-
Isophane insulin	T38.3X-
Isophorone	T65.89-
Isophosphamide	T45.1X-
Isopregnenone	T38.5X-
Isoprenaline	T48.6X-
Isopromethazine	T43.3X-
Isopropamide	T44.3X-
iodide	T44.3X-
Isopropanol	T51.2X-

Drug/Chemical	Code
Isopropyl	
acetate	T52.8X-
alcohol	T51.2X-
medicinal	T49.4X-
ether	T52.8X-
Isopropylaminophenazone	T39.2X-
Isoproterenol	T48.6X-
Isosorbide dinitrate	T46.3X-
Isothipendyl	T45.0X-
Isotretinoin	T50.99-
Isoxazolyl penicillin	T36.0X-
Isoxicam	T39.39-
Isoxsuprine	T46.7X-
Ispagula	T47.4X-
husk	T47.4X-
Isradipine	T46.1X-
l-thyroxine sodium	T38.1X-
Itraconazole	T37.8X-
Itramin tosilate	T46.3X-
Ivermectin	T37.4X-
Izoniazid	T37.1X-
with thioacetazone	T37.1X-
Jalap	T47.2X-
Jamaica	
dogwood (bark)	T39.8X-
ginger	T65.89-
root	T62.2X-
Jatropha	T62.2X-
curcas	T62.2X-
Jectofer	T45.4X-
Jellyfish (sting)	T63.62-
Jequirity (bean)	T62.2X-
Jimson weed (stramonium)	T62.2X-
Josamycin	T36.3X-
Juniper tar	T49.1X-
Kallidinogenase	T46.7X-
Kallikrein	T46.7X-
Kanamycin	T36.5X-
Kantrex	T36.5X-
Kaolin	T47.6X-
light	T47.6X-
Karaya (gum)	T47.4X-
Kebuzone	T39.2X-
Kelevan	T60.1X-
Kemithal	T41.1X-
Kenacort	T38.0X-
Keratolytic drug NEC	T49.4X-
anthracene	T49.4X-
Keratoplastic NEC	T49.4X-
Kerosene, kerosine (fuel) (solvent)NEC	T52.0X-
insecticide	T52.0X-
vapor	T52.0X-
Ketamine	T41.29-
Ketazolam	T42.4X-
Ketazon	T39.2X-

KETOBEMIDONE–LEVOPROXYPHYLLINE

Drug/Chemical	Code
Ketobemidone	T40.4X-
Ketoconazole	T49.0X-
Ketols	T52.4X-
Ketone oils	T52.4X-
Ketoprofen	T39.31-
Ketorolac	T39.8X-
Ketotifen	T45.0X-
Khat	T43.69-
Khellin	T46.3X-
Khelloside	T46.3X-
Kiln gas or vapor (carbon monoxide)	T58.8X-
Kitasamycin	T36.3X-
Konsyl	T47.4X-
Kosam seed	T62.2X-
Krait (venom)	T63.09-
Kwell (insecticide)	T60.1X-
anti-infective (topical)	T49.0X-
Labetalol	T44.8X-
Laburnum (seeds)	T62.2X-
leaves	T62.2X-
Lachesine	T49.5X-
Lacidipine	T46.5X-
Lacquer	T65.6X-
Lacrimogenic gas	T59.3X-
Lactated potassic saline	T50.3X-
Lactic acid	T49.8X-
Lactobacillus (all forms or compounds)	T47.6X-
Lactoflavin	T45.2X-
Lactose (as excipient)	T50.90-
Lactuca (virosa) (extract)	T42.6X-
Lactucarium	T42.6X-
Lactulose	T47.3X-
Laevo— see Levo-	
Lanatosides	T46.0X-
Lanolin	T49.3X-
Largactil	T43.3X-
Larkspur	T62.2X-
Laroxyl	T43.01-
Lasix	T50.1X-
Lassar's paste	T49.4X-
Latamoxef	T36.1X-
Latex	T65.81-
Lathyrus (seed)	T62.2X-
Laudanum	T40.0X-
Laudexium	T48.1X-
Laughing gas	T41.0X-
Laurel, black or cherry	T62.2X-
Laurolinium	T49.0X-
Lauryl sulfoacetate	T49.2X-
Laxative NEC	T47.4X-
osmotic	T47.3X-
saline	T47.3X-
stimulant	T47.2X-
L-dopa	T42.8X-

Drug/Chemical	Code
Lead (dust) (fumes) (vapor) NEC	T56.0X-
acetate	T49.2X-
alkyl (fuel additive)	T56.0X-
anti-infectives	T37.8X-
antiknock compound (tetraethyl)	T56.0X-
arsenate, arsenite (dust) (herbicide) (insecticide) (vapor)	T57.0X-
carbonate (paint)	T56.0X-
chromate (paint)	T56.0X-
dioxide	T56.0X-
inorganic	T56.0X-
iodide (pigment) (paint)	T56.0X-
monoxide (dust) (paint)	T56.0X-
organic	T56.0X-
oxide (paint)	T56.0X-
salts	T56.0X-
specified compound NEC	T56.0X-
tetra-ethyl	T56.0X-
Lebanese red	T40.71-
Lefetamine	T39.8X-
Lenperone	T43.4X-
Lente lietin (insulin)	T38.3X-
Leptazol	T50.7X-
Leptophos	T60.0X-
Leritine	T40.2X-
Letosteine	T48.4X-
Letter	T38.1X-
Lettuce opium	T42.6X-
Leucinocaine	T41.3X-
Leucocianidol	T46.99-
Leucovorin (factor)	T45.8X-
Leukeran	T45.1X-
Leuprolide	T38.89-
Levalbuterol	T48.6X-
Levallorphan	T50.7X-
Levamisole	T37.4X-
Levanil	T42.6X-
Levarterenol	T44.4X-
Levdropropizine	T48.3X-
Levobunolol	T49.5X-
Levocabastine (hydrochloride)	T45.0X-
Levocarnitine	T50.99-
Levodopa (w carbidopa)	T42.8X-
Levo-dromoran	T40.2X-
Levoglutamide	T50.99-
Levoid	T38.1X-
Levo-iso-methadone	T40.3X-
Levomepromazine	T43.3X-
Levonordefrin	T49.6X-
Levonorgestrel	T38.4X-
with ethinylestradiol	T38.5X-
Levopromazine	T43.3X-
Levoprome	T42.6X-
Levopropoxyphene	T40.4X-
Levopropylhexedrine	T50.5X-
Levoproxyphylline	T48.6X-

Drug/Chemical	Code
Levorphanol	T40.4X-
Levothyroxine	T38.1X-
sodium	T38.1X-
Levsin	T44.3X-
Levulose	T50.3X-
Lewisite (gas), not in war	T57.0X-
Librium	T42.4X-
Lidex	T49.0X-
Lidocaine	T41.3X-
regional	T41.3X-
spinal	T41.3X-
Lidofenin	T50.8X-
Lidoflazine	T46.1X-
Lighter fluid	T52.0X-
Lignin hemicellulose	T47.6X-
Lignocaine	T41.3X-
regional	T41.3X-
spinal	T41.3X-
Ligroin (e) (solvent)	T52.0X-
vapor	T59.89-
Ligustrum vulgare	T62.2X-
Lily of the valley	T62.2X-
Lime (chloride)	T54.3X-
Limonene	T52.8X-
Lincomycin	T36.8X-
Lindane (insecticide) (nonmedicinal) (vapor)	T53.6X-
medicinal	T49.0X-
Liniments NEC	T49.9-
Linoleic acid	T46.6X-
Linolenic acid	T46.6X-
Linseed	T47.4X-
Liothyronine	T38.1X-
Liotrix	T38.1X-
Lipancreatin	T47.5X-
Lipo-alprostadil	T46.7X-
Lipo-Lutin	T38.5X-
Lipotropic drug NEC	T50.90-
Liquefied petroleum gases	T59.89-
piped (pure or mixed with air)	T59.89-
Liquid	
paraffin	T47.4X-
petrolatum	T47.4X-
topical	T49.3X-
specified NEC	T65.89-
substance	T65.9-
Liquor creosolis compositus	T65.89-
Liquorice	T48.4X-
extract	T47.8X-
Lisinopril	T46.4X-
Lisuride	T42.8X-
Lithane	T43.8X-
Lithium	T56.89-
gluconate	T43.59-
salts (carbonate)	T43.59-
Lithonate	T43.8X-

Drug/Chemical	Code
Liver	
extract	T45.8X-
for parenteral use	T45.8X-
fraction 1	T45.8X-
hydrolysate	T45.8X-
Lizard (bite) (venom)	T63.121
LMD	T45.8X-
Lobelia	T62.2X-
Lobeline	T50.7X-
Local action drug NEC	T49.8X-
Locorten	T49.0X-
Lofepramine	T43.01-
Lolium temulentum	T62.2X-
Lomotil	T47.6X-
Lomustine	T45.1X-
Lonidamine	T45.1X-
Loperamide	T47.6X-
Loprazolam	T42.4X-
Lorajmine	T46.2X-
Loratidine	T45.0X-
Lorazepam	T42.4X-
Lorcainide	T46.2X-
Lormetazepam	T42.4X-
Lotions NEC	T49.9-
Lotusate	T42.3X-
Lovastatin	T46.6X-
Lowila	T49.2X-
Loxapine	T43.59-
Lozenges (throat)	T49.6X-
LSD	T40.8X-
L-Tryptophan— see amino acid	
Lubricant, eye	T49.5X-
Lubricating oil NEC	T52.0X-
Lucanthone	T37.4X-
Luminal	T42.3X-
Lung irritant (gas)NEC	T59.9-
Luteinizing hormone	T38.81-
Lutocylol	T38.5X-
Lutromone	T38.5X-
Lututrin	T48.29-
Lye (concentrated)	T54.3X-
Lygranum (skin test)	T50.8X-
Lymecycline	T36.4X-
Lymphogranuloma venereum antigen	T50.8X-
Lynestrenol	T38.4X-
Lyovac Sodium Edecrin	T50.1X-
Lypressin	T38.89-
Lysergic acid diethylamide	T40.8X-
Lysergide	T40.8X-
Lysine vasopressin	T38.89-
Lysol	T54.1X-
Lysozyme	T49.0X-
Lytta (vitatta)	T49.8X-
Mace	T59.3X-
Macrogol	T50.99-

Drug/Chemical	Code
Macrolide	
anabolic drug	T38.7X-
antibiotic	T36.3X-
Mafenide	T49.0X-
Magaldrate	T47.1X-
Magic mushroom	T40.99-
Magnamycin	T36.8X-
Magnesia magma	T47.1X-
Magnesium NEC	T56.89-
carbonate	T47.1X-
citrate	T47.4X-
hydroxide (oxide)	T47.1X-
peroxide	T49.0X-
salicylate	T39.09-
silicofluoride	T50.3X-
sulfate	T47.4X-
thiosulfate	T45.0X-
trisilicate	T47.1X-
Malathion (medicinal) (insecticide)	T49.0X-
insecticide	T60.0X-
Male fern extract	T37.4X-
M-AMSA	T45.1X-
Mandelic acid	T37.8X-
Manganese (dioxide) (salts)	T57.2X-
medicinal	T50.99-
Mannitol	T47.3X-
hexanitrate	T46.3X-
Mannomustine	T45.1X-
MAO inhibitors	T43.1X-
Mapharsen	T37.8X-
Maphenide	T49.0X-
Maprotiline	T43.02-
Marcaine (infiltration) (subcutaneous) (nerve block)	T41.3X-
Marezine	T45.0X-
Marijuana/Marihuana	T40.71-
Marine (sting)	T63.69-
animals (sting)	T63.69-
plants (sting)	T63.71-
Marplan	T43.1X-
Marsh gas	T59.89-
Marsilid	T43.1X-
Matulane	T45.1X-
Mazindol	T50.5X-
MCPA	T60.3X-
MDMA	T43.64-
Meadow saffron	T62.2X-
Measles virus vaccine (attenuated)	T50.B9-
Meat, noxious	T62.8X-
Meballymal	T42.3X-
Mebanazine	T43.1X-
Mebaral	T42.3X-
Mebendazole	T37.4X-
Mebeverine	T44.3X-
Mebhydrolin	T45.0X-
Mebumal	T42.3X-

Drug/Chemical	Code
Mebutamate	T43.59-
Mecamylamine	T44.2X-
Mechlorethamine	T45.1X-
Mecillinam	T36.0X-
Meclizine (hydrochloride)	T45.0X-
Meclocycline	T36.4X-
Meclofenamate	T39.39-
Meclofenamic acid	T39.39-
Meclofenoxate	T43.69-
Meclozine	T45.0X-
Mecobalamin	T45.8X-
Mecoprop	T60.3X-
Mecrilate	T49.3X-
Mecysteine	T48.4X-
Medazepam	T42.4X-
Medicament NEC	T50.90-
Medinal	T42.3X-
Medomin	T42.3X-
Medrogestone	T38.5X-
Medroxalol	T44.8X-
Medroxyprogesterone acetate (depot)	T38.5X-
Medrysone	T49.0X-
Mefenamic acid	T39.39-
Mefenorex	T50.5X-
Mefloquine	T37.2X-
Mefruside	T50.2X-
Megahallucinogen	T40.90-
Megestrol	T38.5X-
Meglumine	
antimoniate	T37.8X-
diatrizoate	T50.8X-
iodipamide	T50.8X-
iotroxate	T50.8X-
MEK (methyl ethyl ketone)	T52.4X-
Meladinin	T49.3X-
Meladrazine	T44.3X-
Melaleuca alternifolia oil	T49.0X-
Melanizing agents	T49.3X-
Melanocyte-stimulating hormone	T38.89-
Melarsonyl potassium	T37.3X-
Melarsoprol	T37.3X-
Melia azedarach	T62.2X-
Melitracen	T43.01-
Mellaril	T43.3X-
Meloxine	T49.3X-
Melperone	T43.4X-
Melphalan	T45.1X-
Memantine	T43.8X-
Menadiol (sodium sulfate)	T45.7X-
Menadione	T45.7X-
sodium bisulfite	T45.7X-
Menaphthone	T45.7X-
Menaquinone	T45.7X-
Menatetrenone	T45.7X-
Meningococcal vaccine	T50.A9-

Drug/Chemical	Code
Menningovax (-AC) (-C)	T50.A9-
Menotropins	T38.81-
Menthol	T48.5X-
Mepacrine	T37.2X-
Meparfynol	T42.6X-
Mepartricin	T36.7X-
Mepazine	T43.3X-
Mepenzolate	T44.3X-
bromide	T44.3X-
Meperidine	T40.4X-
Mephebarbital	T42.3X-
Mephenamin (e)	T42.8X-
Mephenesin	T42.8X-
Mephenhydramine	T45.0X-
Mephenoxalone	T42.8X-
Mephentermine	T44.99-
Mephenytoin	T42.0X-
with phenobarbital	T42.3X-
Mephobarbital	T42.3X-
Mephosfolan	T60.0X-
Mepindolol	T44.7X-
Mepiperphenidol	T44.3X-
Mepitiostane	T38.7X-
Mepivacaine (epidural)	T41.3X-
Meprednisone	T38.0X-
Meprobam	T43.59-
Meprobamate	T43.59-
Meproscillarin	T46.0X-
Meprylcaine	T41.3X-
Meptazinol	T39.8X-
Mepyramine	T45.0X-
Mequitazine	T43.3X-
Meralluride	T50.2X-
Merbaphen	T50.2X-
Merbromin	T49.0X-
Mercaptobenzothiazole salts	T49.0X-
Mercaptomerin	T50.2X-
Mercaptopurine	T45.1X-
Mercumatilin	T50.2X-
Mercuramide	T50.2X-
Mercurochrome	T49.0X-
Mercurophylline	T50.2X-
Mercury, mercurial, mercuric, mercurous (compounds) (cyanide) (fumes) (nonmedicinal) (vapor) NEC	T56.1X-
ammoniated	T49.0X-
anti-infective	
local	T49.0X-
systemic	T37.8X-
topical	T49.0X-
chloride (ammoniated)	T49.0X-
diuretic NEC	T50.2X-
fungicide (organic)	T56.1X-
oxide, yellow	T49.0X-
Mersalyl	T50.2X-

Drug/Chemical	Code
Merthiolate	T49.0X-
ophthalmic preparation	T49.5X-
Meruvax	T50.B9-
Mesalazine	T47.8X-
Mescal buttons	T40.99-
Mescaline	T40.99-
Mesna	T48.4X-
Mesoglycan	T46.6X-
Mesoridazine	T43.3X-
Mestanolone	T38.7X-
Mesterolone	T38.7X-
Mestranol	T38.5X-
Mesulergine	T42.8X-
Mesulfen	T49.0X-
Mesuximide	T42.2X-
Metabutethamine	T41.3X-
Metactesylacetate	T49.0X-
Metacycline	T36.4X-
Metaldehyde (snail killer) NEC	T60.8X-
Metals (heavy) (nonmedicinal)	T56.9-
dust, fumes, or vapor NEC	T56.9-
light NEC	T56.9-
dust, fumes, or vapor NEC	T56.9-
specified NEC	T56.89-
thallium	T56.81-
Metamfetamine	T43.62-
Metamizole sodium	T39.2X-
Metampicillin	T36.0X-
Metamucil	T47.4X-
Metandienone	T38.7X-
Metandrostenolone	T38.7X-
Metaphen	T49.0X-
Metaphos	T60.0X-
Metapramine	T43.01-
Metaproterenol	T48.29-
Metaraminol	T44.4X-
Metaxalone	T42.8X-
Metenolone	T38.7X-
Metergoline	T42.8X-
Metescufylline	T46.99-
Metetoin	T42.0X-
Metformin	T38.3X-
Methacholine	T44.1X-
Methacycline	T36.4X-
Methadone	T40.3X-
Methallenestril	T38.5X-
Methallenoestril	T38.5X-
Methamphetamine	T43.62-
Methampyrone	T39.2X-
Methandienone	T38.7X-
Methandriol	T38.7X-
Methandrostenolone	T38.7X-
Methane	T59.89-
Methanethiol	T59.89-
Methaniazide	T37.1X-

Drug/Chemical	Code
Methanol (vapor)	T51.1X-
Methantheline	T44.3X-
Methanthelinium bromide	T44.3X-
Methaphenilene	T45.0X-
Methapyrilene	T45.0X-
Methaqualone (compound)	T42.6X-
Metharbital	T42.3X-
Methazolamide	T50.2X-
Methdilazine	T43.3X-
Methedrine	T43.62-
Methenamine (mandelate)	T37.8X-
Methenolone	T38.7X-
Methergine	T48.0X-
Methetoin	T42.0X-
Methiacil	T38.2X-
Methicillin	T36.0X-
Methimazole	T38.2X-
Methiodal sodium	T50.8X-
Methionine	T50.99-
Methisazone	T37.5X-
Methisoprinol	T37.5X-
Methitural	T42.3X-
Methixene	T44.3X-
Methobarbital, methobarbitone	T42.3X-
Methocarbamol	T42.8X-
skeletal muscle relaxant	T48.1X-
Methohexital	T41.1X-
Methohexitone	T41.1X-
Methoin	T42.0X-
Methopholine	T39.8X-
Methopromazine	T43.3X-
Methorate	T48.3X-
Methoserpidine	T46.5X-
Methotrexate	T45.1X-
Methotrimeprazine	T43.3X-
Methoxa-Dome	T49.3X-
Methoxamine	T44.4X-
Methoxsalen	T50.99-
Methoxyaniline	T65.3X-
Methoxybenzyl penicillin	T36.0X-
Methoxychlor	T53.7X-
Methoxy-DDT	T53.7X-
2-Methoxyethanol	T52.3X-
Methoxyflurane	T41.0X-
Methoxyphenamine	T48.6X-
Methoxypromazine	T43.3X-
5-Methoxypsoralen (5-MOP)	T50.99-
8-Methoxypsoralen (8-MOP)	T50.99-
Methscopolamine bromide	T44.3X-
Methsuximide	T42.2X-
Methyclothiazide	T50.2X-
Methyl	
acetate	T52.4X-
acetone	T52.4X-
acrylate	T65.89-

Drug/Chemical	Code
Methyl, continued	
alcohol	T51.1X-
aminophenol	T65.3X-
amphetamine	T43.62-
androstanolone	T38.7X-
atropine	T44.3X-
benzene	T52.2X-
benzoate	T52.8X-
benzol	T52.2X-
bromide (gas)	T59.89-
fumigant	T60.8X-
butanol	T51.3X-
carbinol	T51.1X-
carbonate	T52.8X-
CCNU	T45.1X-
cellosolve	T52.9-
cellulose	T47.4X-
chloride (gas)	T59.89-
chloroformate	T59.3X-
cyclohexane	T52.8X-
cyclohexanol	T51.8X-
cyclohexanone	T52.8X-
cyclohexyl acetate	T52.8X-
demeton	T60.0X-
dihydromorphinone	T40.2X-
ergometrine	T48.0X-
ergonovine	T48.0X-
ethyl ketone	T52.4X-
glucamine antimonate	T37.8X-
hydrazine	T65.89-
iodide	T65.89-
isobutyl ketone	T52.4X-
isothiocyanate	T60.3X-
mercaptan	T59.89-
morphine NEC	T40.2X-
nicotinate	T49.4X-
paraben	T49.0X-
parafynol	T42.6X-
parathion	T60.0X-
peridol	T43.4X-
phenidate	T43.631
ENT agent	T49.6X-
ophthalmic preparation	T49.5X-
topical NEC	T49.0X-
propylcarbinol	T51.3X-
rosaniline NEC	T49.0X-
salicylate	T49.2X-
sulfate (fumes)	T59.89-
liquid	T52.8X-
sulfonal	T42.6X-
testosterone	T38.7X-
thiouracil	T38.2X-
Methylamphetamine	T43.62-
Methylated spirit	T51.1X-
Methylatropine nitrate	T44.3X-

Drug/Chemical	Code
Methylbenactyzium bromide	T44.3X-
Methylbenzethonium chloride	T49.0X-
Methylcellulose	T47.4X-
laxative	T47.4X-
Methylchlorophenoxy-acetic acid	T60.3X-
Methyldopa	T46.5X-
Methyldopate	T46.5X-
Methylene	
blue	T50.6X-
chloride or dichloride (solvent)NEC	T53.4X-
Methylenedioxyamphetamine	T43.62-
Methylenedioxymethamphetamine	T43.64-
Methylergometrine	T48.0X-
Methylergonovine	T48.0X-
Methylestrenolone	T38.5X-
Methylethyl cellulose	T50.99-
Methylhexabital	T42.3X-
Methylmorphine	T40.2X-
Methylparaben (ophthalmic)	T49.5X-
Methylparafynol	T42.6X-
Methylpentynol, methylpenthynol	T42.6X-
Methylphenidate	T43.631
Methylphenobarbital	T42.3X-
Methylpolysiloxane	T47.1X-
Methylprednisolone	T38.0X-
Methylrosaniline	T49.0X-
Methylrosanilinium chloride	T49.0X-
Methyltestosterone	T38.7X-
Methylthionine chloride	T50.6X-
Methylthioninium chloride	T50.6X-
Methylthiouracil	T38.2X-
Methyprylon	T42.6X-
Methysergide	T46.5X-
Metiamide	T47.1X-
Meticillin	T36.0X-
Meticrane	T50.2X-
Metildigoxin	T46.0X-
Metipranolol	T49.5X-
Metirosine	T46.5X-
Metisazone	T37.5X-
Metixene	T44.3X-
Metizoline	T48.5X-
Metoclopramide	T45.0X-
Metofenazate	T43.3X-
Metofoline	T39.8X-
Metolazone	T50.2X-
Metopon	T40.2X-
Metoprine	T45.1X-
Metoprolol	T44.7X-
Metrifonate	T60.0X-
Metrizamide	T50.8X-
Metrizoic acid	T50.8X-
Metronidazole	T37.8X-
Metycaine (infiltration) (topical) (subcutaneous) (nerve block)	T41.3X-

Drug/Chemical	Code
Metyrapone	T50.8X-
Mevinphos	T60.0X-
Mexazolam	T42.4X-
Mexenone	T49.3X-
Mexiletine	T46.2X-
Mezereon	T62.2X-
berries	T62.1X-
Mezlocillin	T36.0X-
Mianserin	T43.02-
Micatin	T49.0X-
Miconazole	T49.0X-
Micronomicin	T36.5X-
Midazolam	T42.4X-
Midecamycin	T36.3X-
Mifepristone	T38.6X-
Milk of magnesia	T47.1X-
Millipede (tropical) (venomous)	T63.41-
Miltown	T43.59-
Milverine	T44.3X-
Minaprine	T43.29-
Minaxolone	T41.29-
Mineral	
acids	T54.2X-
oil (laxative) (medicinal)	T47.4X-
emulsion	T47.2X-
nonmedicinal	T52.0X-
topical	T49.3X-
salt NEC	T50.3X-
spirits	T52.0X-
Mineralocorticosteroid	T50.0X-
Minocycline	T36.4X-
Minoxidil	T46.7X-
Miokamycin	T36.3X-
Miotic drug	T49.5X-
Mipafox	T60.0X-
Mirex	T60.1X-
Mirtazapine	T43.02-
Misonidazole	T37.3X-
Misoprostol	T47.1X-
Mithramycin	T45.1X-
Mitobronitol	T45.1X-
Mitoguazone	T45.1X-
Mitolactol	T45.1X-
Mitomycin	T45.1X-
Mitopodozide	T45.1X-
Mitotane	T45.1X-
Mitoxantrone	T45.1X-
Mivacurium chloride	T48.1X-
Miyari bacteria	T47.6X-
MMR vaccine	T50.B9-
Moclobemide	T43.1X-
Moderil	T46.5X-
Mofebutazone	T39.2X-
Molindone	T43.59-
Molsidomine	T46.3X-

Drug/Chemical	Code
Mometasone	T49.0X-
Monistat	T49.0X-
Monkshood	T62.2X-
Monoamine oxidase inhibitor NEC	T43.1X-
hydrazine	T43.1X-
Monobenzone	T49.4X-
Monochloroacetic acid	T60.3X-
Monochlorobenzene	T53.7X-
Monoethanolamine (oleate)	T46.8X-
Monooctanoin	T50.99-
Monophenylbutazone	T39.2X-
Monosodium glutamate	T65.89-
Monosulfiram	T49.0X-
Monoxidine hydrochloride	T46.1X-
Monuron	T60.3X-
Moperone	T43.4X-
Mopidamol	T45.1X-
MOPP (mechloreth-amine + vincristine + prednisone + procarbazine)	T45.1X-
Morfin	T40.2X-
Morinamide	T37.1X-
Morning glory seeds	T40.99-
Moroxydine	T37.5X-
Morphazinamide	T37.1X-
Morphine	T40.2X-
antagonist	T50.7X-
Morpholinylethylmorphine	T40.2X-
Morsuximide	T42.2X-
Mosapramine	T43.59-
Moth balls (naphthalene)	T60.2X-
paradichlorobenzene	T60.1X-
Motor exhaust gas	T58.0-
Mouthwash (antiseptic)	T49.6X-
Moxastine	T45.0X-
Moxaverine	T44.3X-
Moxisylyte	T46.7X-
Mucilage, plant	T47.4X-
Mucolytic drug	T48.4X-
Mucomyst	T48.4X-
Mucous membrane agents (external)	T49.9-
specified NEC	T49.8X-
Multiple unspec drugs	T50.91-
Mumps	
immune globulin (human)	T50.Z1-
skin test antigen	T50.8X-
Mupirocin	T49.0X-
Muromonab-CD3	T45.1X-
Muscle-action drug NEC	T48.20-
Muscle affecting agents NEC	T48.20-
oxytocic	T48.0X-
relaxants	T48.20-
central nervous system	T42.8X-
skeletal	T48.1X-
smooth	T44.3X-
Mushroom, noxious	T62.0X-

Drug/Chemical	Code
Mussel, noxious	T61.781
Mustard (emetic) (black)	T47.7X-
gas, not in war	T59.9-
nitrogen	T45.1X-
Mustine	T45.1X-
M-vac	T45.1X-
Mycifradin	T36.5X-
topical	T49.0X-
Mycitracin	T36.8X-
ophthalmic preparation	T49.5X-
Mycostatin	T36.7X-
topical	T49.0X-
Mycotoxins (NEC)	T64.81
aflatoxin	T64.0-
Mydriacyl	T44.3X-
Mydriatic drug	T49.5X-
Myelobromal	T45.1X-
Myleran	T45.1X-
Myochrysin (e)	T39.2X-
Myoneural blocking agents	T48.1X-
Myralact	T49.0X-
Myristica fragrans	T62.2X-
Myristicin	T65.89-
Mysoline	T42.3X-
Nabilone	T40.71-
Nabumetone	T39.39-
Nadolol	T44.7X-
Nafcillin	T36.0X-
Nafoxidine	T38.6X-
Naftazone	T46.99-
Naftidrofuryl (oxalate)	T46.7X-
Naftifine	T49.0X-
Nail polish remover	T52.9-
Nalbuphine	T40.4X-
Naled	T60.0X-
Nalidixic acid	T37.8X-
Nalorphine	T50.7X-
Naloxone	T50.7X-
Naltrexone	T50.7X-
Namenda	T43.8X-
Nandrolone	T38.7X-
Naphazoline	T48.5X-
Naphtha (painters') (petroleum)	T52.0X-
solvent	T52.0X-
vapor	T52.0X-
Naphthalene (non-chlorinated)	T60.2X-
chlorinated	T60.1X-
vapor	T60.1X-
insecticide or moth repellent	T60.2X-
chlorinated	T60.1X-
vapor	T60.2X-
chlorinated	T60.1X-
Naphthol	T65.89-
Naphthylamine	T65.89-
Naphthylthiourea (ANTU)	T60.4X-

Drug/Chemical	Code
Naproxen (Naprosyn)	T39.31-
Narcotic (drug)	T40.60-
analgesic NEC	T40.60-
antagonist	T50.7X-
specified NEC	T40.69-
synthetic (other)	T40.49-
Narcotine	T48.3X-
Nardil	T43.1X-
Nasal drug NEC	T49.6X-
Natamycin	T49.0X-
Natural	
blood (product)	T45.8X-
gas (piped)	T59.89-
incomplete combustion	T58.1-
Nealbarbital	T42.3X-
Nectadon	T48.3X-
Nedocromil	T48.6X-
Nefopam	T39.8X-
Nematocyst (sting)	T63.69-
Nembutal	T42.3X-
Nemonapride	T43.59-
Neoarsphenamine	T37.8X-
Neocinchophen	T50.4X-
Neomycin (derivatives)	T36.5X-
with bacitracin	T49.0X-
with neostigmine	T44.0X-
ENT agent	T49.6X-
ophthalmic preparation	T49.5X-
topical NEC	T49.0X-
Neonal	T42.3X-
Neoprontosil	T37.0X-
Neosalvarsan	T37.8X-
Neosilversalvarsan	T37.8X-
Neosporin	T36.8X-
ENT agent	T49.6X-
opthalmic preparation	T49.5X-
topical NEC	T49.0X-
Neostigmine bromide	T44.0X-
Neraval	T42.3X-
Neravan	T42.3X-
Nerium oleander	T62.2X-
Nerve gas, not in war	T59.9-
Nesacaine (infiltration) (subcutaneous) (nerve block)	T41.3X-
Netilmicin	T36.5X-
Neurobarb	T42.3X-
Neuroleptic drug NEC	T43.50-
Neuromuscular blocking drug	T48.1X-
Neutral insulin injection	T38.3X-
Neutral spirits (beverage)	T51.0X-
Niacin	T46.7X-
Niacinamide	T45.2X-
Nialamide	T43.1X-
Niaprazine	T42.6X-
Nicametate	T46.7X-
Nicardipine	T46.1X-

Drug/Chemical	Code
Nicergoline	T46.7X-
Nickel (carbonyl) (tetra-carbonyl) (fumes) (vapor)	T56.89-
Nickelocene	T56.89-
Niclosamide	T37.4X-
Nicofuranose	T46.7X-
Nicomorphine	T40.2X-
Nicorandil	T46.3X-
Nicotiana (plant)	T62.2X-
Nicotinamide	T45.2X-
Nicotine (insecticide) (spray) (sulfate) NEC	T60.2X-
from tobacco	T65.29-
cigarettes	T65.22-
not insecticide	T65.29-
Nicotinic acid	T46.7X-
Nicotinyl alcohol	T46.7X-
Nicoumalone	T45.51-
Nifedipine	T46.1X-
Nifenazone	T39.2X-
Nifuraldezone	T37.9-
Nifuratel	T37.8X-
Nifurtimox	T37.3X-
Nifurtoinol	T37.8X-
Nightshade, deadly (solanum)	T62.2X-
berry	T62.1X-
Nikethamide	T50.7X-
Nilstat	T36.7X-
topical	T49.0X-
Nilutamide	T38.6X-
Nimesulide	T39.39-
Nimetazepam	T42.4X-
Nimodipine	T46.1X-
Nimorazole	T37.3X-
Nimustine	T45.1X-
Niridazole	T37.4X-
Nisentil	T40.2X-
Nisoldipine	T46.1X-
Nitramine	T65.3X-
Nitrate, organic	T46.3X-
Nitrazepam	T42.4X-
Nitrefazole	T50.6X-
Nitrendipine	T46.1X-
Nitric	
acid (liquid)	T54.2X-
vapor	T59.89-
oxide (gas)	T59.0X-
Nitrimidazine	T37.3X-
Nitrite, amyl (medicinal) (vapor)	T46.3X-
Nitroaniline	T65.3X-
vapor	T59.89-
Nitrobenzene, nitrobenzol (vapor)	T65.3X-
Nitrocellulose	T65.89-
lacquer	T65.89-
Nitrodiphenyl	T65.3X-
Nitrofural	T49.0X-
Nitrofurantoin	T37.8X-

NITROFURAZONE–OLEIC ACID

Drug/Chemical	Code
Nitrofurazone	T49.0X-
Nitrogen	T59.0X-
mustard	T45.1X-
Nitroglycerin, nitro-glycerol (medicinal)	T46.3X-
nonmedicinal	T65.5X-
fumes	T65.5X-
Nitroglycol	T52.3X-
Nitrohydrochloric acid	T54.2X-
Nitromersol	T49.0X-
Nitronaphthalene	T65.89-
Nitrophenol	T54.0X-
Nitropropane	T52.8X-
Nitroprusside	T46.5X-
Nitrosodimethylamine	T65.3X-
Nitrothiazol	T37.4X-
Nitrotoluene, nitrotoluol	T65.3X-
vapor	T65.3X-
Nitrous	
acid (liquid)	T54.2X-
fumes	T59.89-
ether spirit	T46.3X-
oxide	T41.0X-
Nitroxoline	T37.8X-
Nitrozone	T49.0X-
Nizatidine	T47.0X-
Nizofenone	T43.8X-
Noctec	T42.6X-
Noludar	T42.6X-
Nomegestrol	T38.5X-
Nomifensine	T43.29-
Nonoxinol	T49.8X-
Nonylphenoxy (polyethoxy-ethanol)	T49.8X-
Noptil	T42.3X-
Noradrenaline	T44.4X-
Noramidopyrine	T39.2X-
methanesulfonate sodium	T39.2X-
Norbormide	T60.4X-
Nordazepam	T42.4X-
Norepinephrine	T44.4X-
Norethandrolone	T38.7X-
Norethindrone	T38.4X-
Norethisterone (acetate) (enantate)	T38.4X-
with ethinylestradiol	T38.5X-
Noretynodrel	T38.5X-
Norfenefrine	T44.4X-
Norfloxacin	T36.8X-
Norgestrel	T38.4X-
Norgestrienone	T38.4X-
Norlestrin	T38.4X-
Norlutin	T38.4X-
Normal serum albumin (human), salt-poor	T45.8X-
Normethandrone	T38.5X-
Normorphine	T40.2X-

Drug/Chemical	Code
Norpseudoephedrine	T50.5X-
Nortestosterone (furanpropionate)	T38.7X-
Nortriptyline	T43.01-
Noscapine	T48.3X-
Nose preparations	T49.6X-
Novobiocin	T36.5X-
Novocain (infiltration) (topical) (spinal)	T41.3X-
Noxious foodstuff	T62.9-
specified NEC	T62.8X-
Noxiptiline	T43.01-
Noxytiolin	T49.0X-
NPH Iletin (insulin)	T38.3X-
Numorphan	T40.2X-
Nunol	T42.3X-
Nupercaine (spinal anesthetic)	T41.3X-
topical (surface)	T41.3X-
Nutmeg oil (liniment)	T49.3X-
Nutritional supplement	T50.90-
Nux vomica	T65.1X-
Nydrazid	T37.1X-
Nylidrin	T46.7X-
Nystatin	T36.7X-
topical	T49.0X-
Nytol	T45.0X-
Obidoxime chloride	T50.6X-
Octafonium (chloride)	T49.3X-
Octamethyl pyrophos-phoramide	T60.0X-
Octanoin	T50.99-
Octatropine methyl-bromide	T44.3X-
Octotiamine	T45.2X-
Octoxinol (9)	T49.8X-
Octreotide	T38.99-
Octyl nitrite	T46.3X-
Oestradiol	T38.5X-
Oestriol	T38.5X-
Oestrogen	T38.5X-
Oestrone	T38.5X-
Ofloxacin	T36.8X-
Oil (of)	T65.89-
bitter almond	T62.8X-
cloves	T49.7X-
colors	T65.6X-
fumes	T59.89-
lubricating	T52.0X-
Niobe	T52.8X-
vitriol (liquid)	T54.2X-
fumes	T54.2X-
wintergreen (bitter) NEC	T49.3X-
Oily preparation (for skin)	T49.3X-
Ointment NEC	T49.3X-
Olanzapine	T43.59-
Oleander	T62.2X-
Oleandomycin	T36.3X-
Oleandrin	T46.0X-
Oleic acid	T46.6X-

Drug/Chemical	Code
Oleovitamin A	T45.2X-
Oleum ricini	T47.2X-
Olive oil (medicinal)NEC	T47.4X-
Olivomycin	T45.1X-
Olsalazine	T47.8X-
Omeprazole	T47.1X-
OMPA	T60.0X-
Oncovin	T45.1X-
Ondansetron	T45.0X-
Ophthaine	T41.3X-
Ophthetic	T41.3X-
Opiate NEC	T40.60-
antagonists	T50.7X-
Opioid NEC	T40.2X-
Opipramol	T43.01-
Opium alkaloids (total)	T40.0X-
Oracon	T38.4X-
Oragrafin	T50.8X-
Oral contraceptives	T38.4X-
Oral rehydration salts	T50.3X-
Orazamide	T50.99-
Orciprenaline	T48.29-
Organidin	T48.4X-
Organonitrate NEC	T46.3X-
Organophosphates	T60.0X-
Orimune	T50.B9-
Orinase	T38.3X-
Ormeloxifene	T38.6X-
Ornidazole	T37.3X-
Ornithine aspartate	T50.99-
Ornoprostil	T47.1X-
Orphenadrine (hydrochloride)	T42.8X-
Ortal (sodium)	T42.3X-
Orthoboric acid	T49.0X-
ENT agent	T49.6X-
ophthalmic preparation	T49.5X-
Orthocaine	T41.3X-
Orthodichlorobenzene	T53.7X-
Ortho-Novum	T38.4X-
Orthotolidine (reagent)	T54.2X-
Osmic acid (liquid) (fumes)	T54.2X-
Osmotic diuretics	T50.2X-
Otilonium bromide	T44.3X-
Otorhinolaryngological drug NEC	T49.6X-
Ouabain (e)	T46.0X-
Ovarian (hormone) (stimulant)	T38.5X-
Ovral	T38.4X-
Ovulen	T38.4X-
Oxacillin	T36.0X-
Oxalic acid	T54.2X-
ammonium salt	T50.99-
Oxamniquine	T37.4X-
Oxanamide	T43.59-
Oxandrolone	T38.7X-
Oxantel	T37.4X-

Drug/Chemical	Code
Oxapium iodide	T44.3X-
Oxaprotiline	T43.02-
Oxaprozin	T39.31-
Oxatomide	T45.0X-
Oxazepam	T42.4X-
Oxazimedrine	T50.5X-
Oxazolam	T42.4X-
Oxazolidine derivatives	T42.2X-
Oxazolidinedione (derivative)	T42.2X-
Oxcarbazepine	T42.1X-
Oxedrine	T44.4X-
Oxeladin (citrate)	T48.3X-
Oxendolone	T38.5X-
Oxetacaine	T41.3X-
Oxethazine	T41.3X-
Oxetorone	T39.8X-
Oxiconazole	T49.0X-
Oxidizing agent NEC	T54.9-
Oxipurinol	T50.4X-
Oxitriptan	T43.29-
Oxitropium bromide	T48.6X-
Oxodipine	T46.1X-
Oxolamine	T48.3X-
Oxolinic acid	T37.8X-
Oxomemazine	T43.3X-
Oxophenarsine	T37.3X-
Oxprenolol	T44.7X-
Oxsoralen	T49.3X-
Oxtriphylline	T48.6X-
Oxybate sodium	T41.29-
Oxybuprocaine	T41.3X-
Oxybutynin	T44.3X-
Oxychlorosene	T49.0X-
Oxycodone	T40.2X-
Oxyfedrine	T46.3X-
Oxygen	T41.5X-
Oxylone	T49.0X-
ophthalmic preparation	T49.5X-
Oxymesterone	T38.7X-
Oxymetazoline	T48.5X-
Oxymetholone	T38.7X-
Oxymorphone	T40.2X-
Oxypertine	T43.59-
Oxyphenbutazone	T39.2X-
Oxyphencyclimine	T44.3X-
Oxyphenisatine	T47.2X-
Oxyphenonium bromide	T44.3X-
Oxypolygelatin	T45.8X-
Oxyquinoline (derivatives)	T37.8X-
Oxytetracycline	T36.4X-
Oxytocic drug NEC	T48.0X-
Oxytocin (synthetic)	T48.0X-
Ozone	T59.89-
PABA	T49.3X-
Packed red cells	T45.8X-

Drug/Chemical	Code
Padimate	T49.3X-
Paint NEC	T65.6X-
cleaner	T52.9-
fumes NEC	T59.89-
lead (fumes)	T56.0X-
solvent NEC	T52.8X-
stripper	T52.8X-
Palfium	T40.2X-
Palm kernel oil	T50.99-
Paludrine	T37.2X-
PAM (pralidoxime)	T50.6X-
Pamaquine (naphthoute)	T37.2X-
Panadol	T39.1X-
Pancreatic	
digestive secretion stimulant	T47.8X-
dornase	T45.3X-
Pancreatin	T47.5X-
Pancrelipase	T47.5X-
Pancuronium (bromide)	T48.1X-
Pangamic acid	T45.2X-
Panthenol	T45.2X-
topical	T49.8X-
Pantopon	T40.0X-
Pantothenic acid	T45.2X-
Panwarfin	T45.51-
Papain (digestant)	T47.5X-
Papaveretum	T40.0X-
Papaverine	T44.3X-
Para-acetamidophenol	T39.1X-
Para-aminobenzoic acid	T49.3X-
Para-aminophenol derivatives	T39.1X-
Para-aminosalicylic acid	T37.1X-
Paracetaldehyde	T42.6X-
Paracetamol	T39.1X-
Parachlorophenol (camphorated)	T49.0X-
Paracodin	T40.2X-
Paradione	T42.2X-
Paraffin(s) (wax)	T52.0X-
liquid (medicinal)	T47.4X-
nonmedicinal	T52.0X-
Paraformaldehyde	T60.3X-
Paraldehyde	T42.6X-
Paramethadione	T42.2X-
Paramethasone	T38.0X-
acetate	T49.0X-
Paraoxon	T60.0X-
Paraquat	T60.3X-
Parasympatholytic NEC	T44.3X-
Parasympathomimetic drug NEC	T44.1X-
Parathion	T60.0X-
Parathormone	T50.99-
Parathyroid extract	T50.99-
Paratyphoid vaccine	T50.A9-
Paredrine	T44.4X-
Paregoric	T40.0X-
Pargyline	T46.5X-
Paris green (insecticide)	T57.0X-
Parnate	T43.1X-
Paromomycin	T36.5X-
Paroxypropione	T45.1X-
Parzone	T40.2X-
PAS	T37.1X-
Pasiniazid	T37.1X-
PBB (polybrominated biphenyls)	T65.89-
PCB	T65.89-
PCP	
meaning pentachlorophenol	T60.1X-
fungicide / herbicide	T60.3X-
insecticide	T60.1X-
meaning phencyclidine	T40.99-
Peach kernel oil (emulsion)	T47.4X-
Peanut oil (emulsion)NEC	T47.4X-
topical	T49.3X-
Pearly Gates (morning glory seeds)	T40.99-
Pecazine	T43.3X-
Pectin	T47.6X-
Pefloxacin	T37.8X-
Pegademase, bovine	T50.Z9-
Pelletierine tannate	T37.4X-
Pemirolast (potassium)	T48.6X-
Pemoline	T50.7X-
Pempidine	T44.2X-
Penamecillin	T36.0X-
Penbutolol	T44.7X-
Penethamate	T36.0X-
Penfluridol	T43.59-
Penflutizide	T50.2X-
Pengitoxin	T46.0X-
Penicillamine	T50.6X-
Penicillin (any)	T36.0X-
Penicillinase	T45.3X-
Penicilloyl polylysine	T50.8X-
Penimepicycline	T36.4X-
Pentachloroethane	T53.6X-
Pentachloronaphthalene	T53.7X-
Pentachlorophenol (pesticide)	T60.1X-
fungicide / herbicide	T60.3X-
insecticide	T60.1X-
Pentaerythritol	T46.3X-
chloral	T42.6X-
tetranitrate NEC	T46.3X-
Pentaerythrityl tetranitrate	T46.3X-
Pentagastrin	T50.8X-
Pentalin	T53.6X-
Pentamethonium bromide	T44.2X-
Pentamidine	T37.3X-
Pentanol	T51.3X-
Pentapyrrolinium (bitartrate)	T44.2X-
Pentaquine	T37.2X-
Pentazocine	T40.4X-

Drug/Chemical	Code
Pentetrazole	T50.7X-
Penthienate bromide	T44.3X-
Pentifylline	T46.7X-
Pentobarbital (sodium)	T42.3X-
Pentobarbitone	T42.3X-
Pentolonium tartrate	T44.2X-
Pentosan polysulfate (sodium)	T39.8X-
Pentostatin	T45.1X-
Pentothal	T41.1X-
Pentoxifylline	T46.7X-
Pentoxyverine	T48.3X-
Pentrinat	T46.3X-
Pentylenetetrazole	T50.7X-
Pentylsalicylamide	T37.1X-
Pentymal	T42.3X-
Peplomycin	T45.1X-
Peppermint (oil)	T47.5X-
Pepsin (digestant)	T47.5X-
Pepstatin	T47.1X-
Peptavlon	T50.8X-
Perazine	T43.3X-
Percaine (spinal)	T41.3X-
topical (surface)	T41.3X-
Perchloroethylene	T53.3X-
medicinal	T37.4X-
vapor	T53.3X-
Percodan	T40.2X-
Percogesic	T45.0X-
Percorten	T38.0X-
Pergolide	T42.8X-
Pergonal	T38.81-
Perhexilene	T46.3X-
Perhexiline (maleate)	T46.3X-
Periactin	T45.0X-
Periciazine	T43.3X-
Periclor	T42.6X-
Perindopril	T46.4X-
Perisoxal	T39.8X-
Peritoneal dialysis solution	T50.3X-
Peritrate	T46.3X-
Perlapine	T42.4X-
Permanganate	T65.89-
Permethrin	T60.1X-
Pernocton	T42.3X-
Pernoston	T42.3X-
Peronine	T40.2X-
Perphenazine	T43.3X-
Pertofrane	T43.01-
Pertussis immune serum (human)	T50.Z1-
Peruvian balsam	T49.0X-
Peruvoside	T46.0X-
Pesticide (dust) (fumes) (vapor) NEC	T60.9-
arsenic	T57.0X-
chlorinated	T60.1X-
cyanide / kerosene	T65.0X-

Drug/Chemical	Code
Pesticide (dust) (fumes) (vapor) NEC, continued	T60.9-
mixture (of compounds)	T60.9-
naphthalene	T60.2X-
organochlorine (compounds)	T60.1X-
petroleum (distillate) (products)NEC	T60.8X-
specified ingredient NEC	T60.8X-
strychnine	T65.1X-
thallium	T60.4X-
Pethidine	T40.4X-
Petrichloral	T42.6X-
Petrol	T52.0X-
vapor	T52.0X-
Petrolatum	T49.3X-
hydrophilic	T49.3X-
liquid	T47.4X-
topical	T49.3X-
nonmedicinal	T52.0X-
red veterinary	T49.3X-
white	T49.3X-
Petroleum (products) NEC	T52.0X-
jelly	T49.3X-
pesticide	T60.8X-
solids	T52.0X-
solvents	T52.0X-
vapor	T52.0X-
Peyote	T40.99-
Phanodorm, phanodorn	T42.3X-
Phanquinone	T37.3X-
Phanquone	T37.3X-
Pharmaceutical (adjunct) (excipient) (sweetner) NEC	T50.90-
Phemitone	T42.3X-
Phenacaine	T41.3X-
Phenacemide	T42.6X-
Phenacetin	T39.1X-
Phenadoxone	T40.2X-
Phenaglycodol	T43.59-
Phenantoin	T42.0X-
Phenaphthazine reagent	T50.99-
Phenazocine	T40.4X-
Phenazone	T39.2X-
Phenazopyridine	T39.8X-
Phenbenicillin	T36.0X-
Phenbutrazate	T50.5X-
Phencyclidine	T40.99-
Phendimetrazine	T50.5X-
Phenelzine	T43.1X-
Phenemal	T42.3X-
Phenergan	T42.6X-
Pheneticillin	T36.0X-
Pheneturide	T42.6X-
Phenformin	T38.3X-
Phenglutarimide	T44.3X-
Phenicarbazide	T39.8X-
Phenindamine	T45.0X-
Phenindione	T45.51-

PHENIPRAZINE–PINKROOT

Drug/Chemical	Code
Pheniprazine	T43.1X-
Pheniramine	T45.0X-
Phenisatin	T47.2X-
Phenmetrazine	T50.5X-
Phenobal	T42.3X-
Phenobarbital	T42.3X-
with mephenytoin	T42.3X-
with phenytoin	T42.3X-
sodium	T42.3X-
Phenobarbitone	T42.3X-
Phenobutiodil	T50.8X-
Phenoctide	T49.0X-
Phenol	T49.0X-
disinfectant	T54.0X-
in oil injection	T46.8X-
medicinal	T49.1X-
nonmedicinal NEC	T54.0X-
pesticide	T60.8X-
red	T50.8X-
Phenolic preparation	T49.1X-
Phenolphthalein	T47.2X-
Phenolsulfonphthalein	T50.8X-
Phenomorphan	T40.2X-
Phenonyl	T42.3X-
Phenoperidine	T40.4X-
Phenopyrazone	T46.99-
Phenoquin	T50.4X-
Phenothiazine (psychotropic)NEC	T43.3X-
insecticide	T60.2X-
Phenothrin	T49.0X-
Phenoxybenzamine	T46.7X-
Phenoxyethanol	T49.0X-
Phenoxymethyl penicillin	T36.0X-
Phenprobamate	T42.8X-
Phenprocoumon	T45.51-
Phensuximide	T42.2X-
Phentermine	T50.5X-
Phenthicillin	T36.0X-
Phentolamine	T46.7X-
Phenyl	
butazone	T39.2X-
enediamine	T65.3X-
hydrazine	T65.3X-
antineoplastic	T45.1X-
salicylate	T49.3X-
Phenylalanine mustard	T45.1X-
Phenylbutazone	T39.2X-
Phenylenediamine	T65.3X-
Phenylephrine	T44.4X-
Phenylethylbiguanide	T38.3X-
Phenylmercuric (acetate) (borate) (nitrate)	T49.0X-
Phenylmethylbarbitone	T42.3X-
Phenylpropanol	T47.5X-
Phenylpropanolamine	T44.99-
Phenylsulfthion	T60.0X-

Drug/Chemical	Code
Phenyltoloxamine	T45.0X-
Phenyramidol, phenyramidon	T39.8X-
Phenytoin	T42.0X-
with Phenobarbital	T42.3X-
pHisoHex	T49.2X-
Pholcodine	T48.3X-
Pholedrine	T46.99-
Phorate	T60.0X-
Phosdrin	T60.0X-
Phosfolan	T60.0X-
Phosgene (gas)	T59.89-
Phosphamidon	T60.0X-
Phosphate	T65.89-
laxative	T47.4X-
organic	T60.0X-
solvent	T52.9-
tricresyl	T65.89-
Phosphine (fumigate)	T57.1X-
Phospholine	T49.5X-
Phosphoric acid	T54.2X-
Phosphorus (compound)NEC	T57.1X-
pesticide	T60.0X-
Phthalates	T65.89-
Phthalic anhydride	T65.89-
Phthalimidoglutarimide	T42.6X-
Phthalylsulfathiazole	T37.0X-
Phylloquinone	T45.7X-
Physeptone	T40.3X-
Physostigma venenosum	T62.2X-
Physostigmine	T49.5X-
Phytolacca decandra	T62.2X-
berries	T62.1X-
Phytomenadione	T45.7X-
Phytonadione	T45.7X-
Picoperine	T48.3X-
Picosulfate (sodium)	T47.2X-
Picric (acid)	T54.2X-
Picrotoxin	T50.7X-
Piketoprofen	T49.0X-
Pilocarpine	T44.1X-
Pilocarpus (jaborandi)extract	T44.1X-
Pilsicainide (hydrochloride)	T46.2X-
Pimaricin	T36.7X-
Pimeclone	T50.7X-
Pimelic ketone	T52.8X-
Pimethixene	T45.0X-
Piminodine	T40.2X-
Pimozide	T43.59-
Pinacidil	T46.5X-
Pinaverium bromide	T44.3X-
Pinazepam	T42.4X-
Pindolol	T44.7X-
Pindone	T60.4X-
Pine oil (disinfectant)	T65.89-
Pinkroot	T37.4X-

Drug/Chemical	Code
Pipadone	T40.2X-
Pipamazine	T45.0X-
Pipamperone	T43.4X-
Pipazetate	T48.3X-
Pipemidic acid	T37.8X-
Pipenzolate bromide	T44.3X-
Piperacetazine	T43.3X-
Piperacillin	T36.0X-
Piperazine	T37.4X-
estrone sulfate	T38.5X-
Piper cubeba	T62.2X-
Piperidione	T48.3X-
Piperidolate	T44.3X-
Piperocaine (all types)	T41.3X-
Piperonyl butoxide	T60.8X-
Pipethanate	T44.3X-
Pipobroman	T45.1X-
Pipotiazine	T43.3X-
Pipoxizine	T45.0X-
Pipradrol	T43.69-
Piprinhydrinate	T45.0X-
Pirarubicin	T45.1X-
Pirazinamide	T37.1X-
Pirbuterol	T48.6X-
Pirenzepine	T47.1X-
Piretanide	T50.1X-
Piribedil	T42.8X-
Piridoxilate	T46.3X-
Piritramide	T40.4X-
Piromidic acid	T37.8X-
Piroxicam	T39.39-
beta-cyclodextrin complex	T39.8X-
Pirozadil	T46.6X-
Piscidia (bark) (erythrina)	T39.8X-
Pitch	T65.89-
Pitkin's solution	T41.3X-
Pitocin	T48.0X-
Pitressin (tannate)	T38.89-
Pituitary extracts (posterior)	T38.89-
anterior	T38.81-
Pituitrin	T38.89-
Pivampicillin	T36.0X-
Pivmecillinam	T36.0X-
Placental hormone	T38.89-
Placidyl	T42.6X-
Plague vaccine	T50.A9-
Plant	
food or fertilizer NEC	T65.89-
containing herbicide	T60.3X-
noxious, used as food	T62.2X-
berries	T62.1X-
seeds	T62.2X-
specified type NEC	T62.2X-
Plasma	T45.8X-
Plasmanate	T45.8X-

Drug/Chemical	Code
Plasminogen (tissue) activator	T45.61-
Plaster dressing	T49.3X-
Plastic dressing	T49.3X-
Plegicil	T43.3X-
Plicamycin	T45.1X-
Podophyllotoxin	T49.8X-
Podophyllum (resin)	T49.4X-
Poison NEC	T65.9-
Poisonous berries	T62.1X-
Pokeweed (any part)	T62.2X-
Poldine metilsulfate	T44.3X-
Polidexide (sulfate)	T46.6X-
Polidocanol	T46.8X-
Poliomyelitis vaccine	T50.B9-
Polish (car) (floor) (furniture) (metal) (porcelain) (silver)	T65.89-
Poloxalkol	T47.4X-
Poloxamer	T47.4X-
Polyaminostyrene resins	T50.3X-
Polycarbophil	T47.4X-
Polychlorinated biphenyl	T65.89-
Polycycline	T36.4X-
Polyester fumes	T59.89-
Polyester resin hardener	T52.9-
fumes	T59.89-
Polyestradiol phosphate	T38.5X-
Polyethanolamine alkyl sulfate	T49.2X-
Polyethylene adhesive	T49.3X-
Polyferose	T45.4X-
Polygeline	T45.8X-
Polymyxin	T36.8X-
B	T36.8X-
ENT agent	T49.6X-
ophthalmic preparation	T49.5X-
topical NEC	T49.0X-
E sulfate (eye preparation)	T49.5X-
Polynoxylin	T49.0X-
Polyoestradiol phosphate	T38.5X-
Polyoxymethyleneurea	T49.0X-
Polysilane	T47.8X-
Polytetrafluoroethylene (inhaled)	T59.89-
Polythiazide	T50.2X-
Polyvidone	T45.8X-
Polyvinylpyrrolidone	T45.8X-
Pontocaine (hydrochloride) (infiltration) (topical)	T41.3X-
Porfiromycin	T45.1X-
Posterior pituitary hormone NEC	T38.89-
Pot	T40.71-
Potash (caustic)	T54.3X-
Potassic saline injection (lactated)	T50.3X-
Potassium (salts) NEC	T50.3X-
aminobenzoate	T45.8X-
aminosalicylate	T37.1X-
antimony ' tartrate'	T37.8X-
arsenite (solution)	T57.0X-
bichromate	T56.2X-

POTASSIUM (SALTS) NEC–PROMAZINE

Drug/Chemical	Code
Potassium (salts) NEC, continued	T50.3X-
bisulfate	T47.3X-
bromide	T42.6X-
canrenoate	T50.0X-
carbonate	T54.3X-
chlorate NEC	T65.89-
chloride	T50.3X-
citrate	T50.99-
cyanide	T65.0X-
ferric hexacyanoferrate (medicinal)	T50.6X-
nonmedicinal	T65.89-
Fluoride	T57.8X-
glucaldrate	T47.1X-
hydroxide	T54.3X-
iodate	T49.0X-
iodide	T48.4X-
nitrate	T57.8X-
oxalate	T65.89-
perchlorate (nonmedicinal)NEC	T65.89-
antithyroid	T38.2X-
medicinal	T38.2X-
Permanganate (nonmedicinal)	T65.89-
medicinal	T49.0X-
sulfate	T47.2X-
Potassium-removing resin	T50.3X-
Potassium-retaining drug	T50.3X-
Povidone	T45.8X-
iodine	T49.0X-
Practolol	T44.7X-
Prajmalium bitartrate	T46.2X-
Pralidoxime (iodide) (chloride)	T50.6X-
Pramiverine	T44.3X-
Pramocaine	T49.1X-
Pramoxine	T49.1X-
Prasterone	T38.7X-
Pravastatin	T46.6X-
Prazepam	T42.4X-
Praziquantel	T37.4X-
Prazitone	T43.29-
Prazosin	T44.6X-
Prednicarbate	T49.0X-
Prednimustine	T45.1X-
Prednisolone	T38.0X-
ENT agent	T49.6X-
ophthalmic preparation	T49.5X-
steaglate	T49.0X-
topical NEC	T49.0X-
Prednisone	T38.0X-
Prednylidene	T38.0X-
Pregnandiol	T38.5X-
Pregneninolone	T38.5X-
Preludin	T43.69-
Premarin	T38.5X-
Premedication anesthetic	T41.20-
Prenalterol	T44.5X-

Drug/Chemical	Code
Prenoxdiazine	T48.3X-
Prenylamine	T46.3X-
Preparation H	T49.8X-
Preparation, local	T49.4X-
Preservative (nonmedicinal)	T65.89-
medicinal	T50.90-
wood	T60.9-
Prethcamide	T50.7X-
Pride of China	T62.2X-
Pridinol	T44.3X-
Prifinium bromide	T44.3X-
Prilocaine	T41.3X-
Primaquine	T37.2X-
Primidone	T42.6X-
Primula (veris)	T62.2X-
Prinadol	T40.2X-
Priscol, Priscoline	T44.6X-
Pristinamycin	T36.3X-
Privet	T62.2X-
berries	T62.1X-
Privine	T44.4X-
Pro-Banthine	T44.3X-
Probarbital	T42.3X-
Probenecid	T50.4X-
Probucol	T46.6X-
Procainamide	T46.2X-
Procaine	T41.3X-
benzylpenicillin	T36.0X-
nerve block (periphreal) (plexus)	T41.3X-
penicillin G	T36.0X-
regional / spinal	T41.3X-
Procalmidol	T43.59-
Procarbazine	T45.1X-
Procaterol	T44.5X-
Prochlorperazine	T43.3X-
Procyclidine	T44.3X-
Producer gas	T58.8X-
Profadol	T40.4X-
Profenamine	T44.3X-
Profenil	T44.3X-
Proflavine	T49.0X-
Progabide	T42.6X-
Progesterone	T38.5X-
Progestin	T38.5X-
oral contraceptive	T38.4X-
Progestogen NEC	T38.5X-
Progestone	T38.5X-
Proglumide	T47.1X-
Proguanil	T37.2X-
Prolactin	T38.81-
Prolintane	T43.69-
Proloid	T38.1X-
Proluton	T38.5X-
Promacetin	T37.1X-
Promazine	T43.3X-

Drug/Chemical	Code
Promedol	T40.2X-
Promegestone	T38.5X-
Promethazine (teoclate)	T43.3X-
Promin	T37.1X-
Pronase	T45.3X-
Pronestyl (hydrochloride)	T46.2X-
Pronetalol	T44.7X-
Prontosil	T37.0X-
Propachlor	T60.3X-
Propafenone	T46.2X-
Propallylonal	T42.3X-
Propamidine	T49.0X-
Propane (in mobile container)	T59.89-
distributed through pipes	T59.89-
incomplete combustion	T58.1-
Propanidid	T41.29-
Propanil	T60.3X-
1-Propanol	T51.3X-
2-Propanol	T51.2X-
Propantheline (bromide)	T44.3X-
Proparacaine	T41.3X-
Propatylnitrate	T46.3X-
Propicillin	T36.0X-
Propiolactone	T49.0X-
Propiomazine	T45.0X-
Propionaidehyde (medicinal)	T42.6X-
Propionate (calcium) (sodium)	T49.0X-
Propion gel	T49.0X-
Propitocaine	T41.3X-
Propofol	T41.29-
Propoxur	T60.0X-
Propoxycaine (infiltration) (spinal) (subcutaneous) (nerve block) (topical)	T41.3X-
Propoxyphene	T40.4X-
Propranolol	T44.7X-
Propyl	
alcohol	T51.3X-
carbinol	T51.3X-
hexadrine	T44.4X-
iodone	T50.8X-
thiouracil	T38.2X-
Propylaminopheno-thiazine	T43.3X-
Propylene	T59.89-
Propylhexedrine	T48.5X-
Propyliodone	T50.8X-
Propylparaben (ophthalmic)	T49.5X-
Propylthiouracil	T38.2X-
Propyphenazone	T39.2X-
Proquazone	T39.39-
Proscillaridin	T46.0X-
Prostacyclin	T45.521
Prostaglandin (I2)	T45.521
E1	T46.7X-
E2	T48.0X-
F2 alpha	T48.0X-

Drug/Chemical	Code
Prostigmin	T44.0X-
Prosultiamine	T45.2X-
Protamine sulfate	T45.7X-
zinc insulin	T38.3X-
Protease	T47.5X-
Protectant, skin NEC	T49.3X-
Protein hydrolysate	T50.99-
Prothiaden— see Dothiepin hydrochloride	
Prothionamide	T37.1X-
Prothipendyl	T43.59-
Prothoate	T60.0X-
Prothrombin	
activator	T45.7X-
synthesis inhibitor	T45.51-
Protionamide	T37.1X-
Protirelin	T38.89-
Protokylol	T48.6X-
Protopam	T50.6X-
Protoveratrine(s) (A) (B)	T46.5X-
Protriptyline	T43.01-
Provera	T38.5X-
Provitamin A	T45.2X-
Proxibarbal	T42.3X-
Proxymetacaine	T41.3X-
Proxyphylline	T48.6X-
Prozac— see Fluoxetine hydrochloride	
Prunus	
laurocerasus	T62.2X-
virginiana	T62.2X-
Prussian blue	
commercial	T65.89-
therapeutic	T50.6X-
Prussic acid	T65.0X-
vapor	T57.3X-
Pseudoephedrine	T44.99-
Psilocin	T40.99-
Psilocybin	T40.99-
Psilocybine	T40.99-
Psoralene (nonmedicinal)	T65.89-
Psoralens (medicinal)	T50.99-
PSP (phenolsulfonphthalein)	T50.8X-
Psychodysleptic drug NOS	T40.90-
specified NEC	T40.99-
Psychostimulant	T43.60-
amphetamine	T43.62-
caffeine	T43.61-
methylphenidate	T43.631
specified NEC	T43.69-
Psychotherapeutic drug NEC	T43.9-
antidepressants	T43.20-
specified NEC	T43.8X-
tranquilizers NEC	T43.50-
Psychotomimetic agents	T40.90-
Psychotropic drug NEC	T43.9-
specified NEC	T43.8X-

PROMEDOL–PSYCHOTROPIC DRUG NEC

Drug/Chemical	Code
Psyllium hydrophilic mucilloid	T47.4X-
Pteroylglutamic acid	T45.8X-
Pteroyltriglutamate	T45.1X-
PTFE— see Polytetrafluoroethylene	
Pulp	
devitalizing paste	T49.7X-
dressing	T49.7X-
Pulsatilla	T62.2X-
Pumpkin seed extract	T37.4X-
Purex (bleach)	T54.9-
Purgative NEC— see also Cathartic	T47.4X-
Purine analogue (antineoplastic)	T45.1X-
Purine diuretics	T50.2X-
Purinethol	T45.1X-
PVP	T45.8X-
Pyrabital	T39.8X-
Pyramidon	T39.2X-
Pyrantel	T37.4X-
Pyrathiazine	T45.0X-
Pyrazinamide	T37.1X-
Pyrazinoic acid (amide)	T37.1X-
Pyrazole (derivatives)	T39.2X-
Pyrazolone analgesic NEC	T39.2X-
Pyrethrin, pyrethrum (nonmedicinal)	T60.2X-
Pyrethrum extract	T49.0X-
Pyribenzamine	T45.0X-
Pyridine	T52.8X-
aldoxime methiodide	T50.6X-
aldoxime methyl chloride	T50.6X-
vapor	T59.89-
Pyridium	T39.8X-
Pyridostigmine bromide	T44.0X-
Pyridoxal phosphate	T45.2X-
Pyridoxine	T45.2X-
Pyrilamine	T45.0X-
Pyrimethamine (w/ sulfadoxine)	T37.2X-
Pyrimidine antagonist	T45.1X-
Pyriminil	T60.4X-
Pyrithione zinc	T49.4X-
Pyrithyldione	T42.6X-
Pyrogallic acid	T49.0X-
Pyrogallol	T49.0X-
Pyroxylin	T49.3X-
Pyrrobutamine	T45.0X-
Pyrrolizidine alkaloids	T62.8X-
Pyrvinium chloride	T37.4X-
PZI	T38.3X-
Quaalude	T42.6X-
Quarternary ammonium	
anti-infective	T49.0X-
ganglion blocking	T44.2X-
parasympatholytic	T44.3X-
Quazepam	T42.4X-
Quicklime	T54.3X-
Quillaja extract	T48.4X-

Drug/Chemical	Code
Quinacrine	T37.2X-
Quinaglute	T46.2X-
Quinalbarbital	T42.3X-
Quinalbarbitone sodium	T42.3X-
Quinalphos	T60.0X-
Quinapril	T46.4X-
Quinestradiol	T38.5X-
Quinestradol	T38.5X-
Quinestrol	T38.5X-
Quinethazone	T50.2X-
Quingestanol	T38.4X-
Quinidine	T46.2X-
Quinine	T37.2X-
Quiniobine	T37.8X-
Quinisocaine	T49.1X-
Quinocide	T37.2X-
Quinoline (derivatives)NEC	T37.8X-
Quinupramine	T43.01-
Quotane	T41.3X-
Rabies	
immune globulin (human)	T50.Z1-
vaccine	T50.B9-
Racemoramide	T40.2X-
Racemorphan	T40.2X-
Racepinefrin	T44.5X-
Raclopride	T43.59-
Radiator alcohol	T51.1X-
Radioactive drug NEC	T50.8X-
Radio-opaque (drugs) (materials)	T50.8X-
Ramifenazone	T39.2X-
Ramipril	T46.4X-
Ranitidine	T47.0X-
Ranunculus	T62.2X-
Rat poison NEC	T60.4X-
Rattlesnake (venom)	T63.01-
Raubasine	T46.7X-
Raudixin	T46.5X-
Rautensin	T46.5X-
Rautina	T46.5X-
Rautotal	T46.5X-
Rauwiloid	T46.5X-
Rauwoldin	T46.5X-
Rauwolfia (alkaloids)	T46.5X-
Razoxane	T45.1X-
Realgar	T57.0X-
Recombinant (R)— see specific protein	
Red blood cells, packed	T45.8X-
Red squill (scilliroside)	T60.4X-
Reducing agent, industrial NEC	T65.89-
Refrigerant gas (CFC)	T53.5X-
not chlorofluoro-carbon	T59.89-
Regroton	T50.2X-
Rehydration salts (oral)	T50.3X-
Rela	T42.8X-

Drug/Chemical	Code
Relaxant, muscle	
anesthetic	T48.1X-
central nervous system	T42.8X-
skeletal NEC	T48.1X-
smooth NEC	T44.3X-
Remoxipride	T43.59-
Renese	T50.2X-
Renografin	T50.8X-
Replacement solution	T50.3X-
Reproterol	T48.6X-
Rescinnamine	T46.5X-
Reserpin (e)	T46.5X-
Resorcin, resorcinol (nonmedicinal)	T65.89-
medicinal	T49.4X-
Respaire	T48.4X-
Respiratory drug NEC	T48.90-
antiasthmatic NEC	T48.6X-
anti-common-cold NEC	T48.5X-
expectorant NEC	T48.4X-
stimulant	T48.90-
Retinoic acid	T49.0X-
Retinol	T45.2X-
Rh (D) immune globulin (human)	T50.Z1-
Rhodine	T39.01-
RhoGAM	T50.Z1-
Rhubarb	
dry extract	T47.2X-
tincture, compound	T47.2X-
Ribavirin	T37.5X-
Riboflavin	T45.2X-
Ribostamycin	T36.5X-
Ricin	T62.2X-
Ricinus communis	T62.2X-
Rickettsial vaccine NEC	T50.A9-
Rifabutin	T36.6X-
Rifamide	T36.6X-
Rifampicin	T36.6X-
with isoniazid	T37.1X-
Rifampin	T36.6X-
Rifamycin	T36.6X-
Rifaximin	T36.6X-
Rimantadine	T37.5X-
Rimazolium metilsulfate	T39.8X-
Rimifon	T37.1X-
Rimiterol	T48.6X-
Ringer (lactate) solution	T50.3X-
Ristocetin	T36.8X-
Ritalin	T43.631
Ritodrine	T44.5X-
Rociverine	T44.3X-
Rocky Mtn spotted fever vaccine	T50.A9-
Rodenticide NEC	T60.4X-
Rohypnol	T42.4X-
Rokitamycin	T36.3X-

Drug/Chemical	Code
Rolaids	T47.1X-
Rolitetracycline	T36.4X-
Romilar	T48.3X-
Ronifibrate	T46.6X-
Rosaprostol	T47.1X-
Rose bengal sodium (131I)	T50.8X-
Rose water ointment	T49.3X-
Rosoxacin	T37.8X-
Rotenone	T60.2X-
Rotoxamine	T45.0X-
Rough-on-rats	T60.4X-
Roxatidine	T47.0X-
Roxithromycin	T36.3X-
Rt-PA	T45.61-
Rubbing alcohol	T51.2X-
Rubefacient	T49.4X-
Rubidium chloride Rb82	T50.8X-
Rubidomycin	T45.1X-
Rue	T62.2X-
Rufocromomycin	T45.1X-
Russel's viper venin	T45.7X-
Ruta (graveolens)	T62.2X-
Rutinum	T46.99-
Rutoside	T46.99-
Sabadilla (plant) (pesticide)	T62.2X-
Saccharated iron oxide	T45.8X-
Saccharin	T50.90-
Saccharomyces boulardii	T47.6X-
Safflower oil	T46.6X-
Safrazine	T43.1X-
Salazosulfapyridine	T37.0X-
Salbutamol	T48.6X-
Salicylamide	T39.09-
Salicylate NEC	T39.09-
methyl	T49.3X-
theobromine calcium	T50.2X-
Salicylazosulfapyridine	T37.0X-
Salicylhydroxamic acid	T49.0X-
Salicylic acid	T49.4X-
with benzoic acid	T49.4X-
congeners/derivatives/salts	T39.09-
Salinazid	T37.1X-
Salmeterol	T48.6X-
Salol	T49.3X-
Salsalate	T39.09-
Salt substitute	T50.90-
Salt-replacing drug	T50.90-
Salt-retaining mineralocorticoid	T50.0X-
Saluretic NEC	T50.2X-
Saluron	T50.2X-
Salvarsan 606 (neosilver) (silver)	T37.8X-
Sambucus canadensis	T62.2X-
berry	T62.1X-
Sandril	T46.5X-
Sanguinaria canadensis	T62.2X-

Drug/Chemical	Code
Saniflush (cleaner)	T54.2X-
Santonin	T37.4X-
Santyl	T49.8X-
Saralasin	T46.5X-
Sarcolysin	T45.1X-
Sarkomycin	T45.1X-
Saroten	T43.01-
Savin (oil)	T49.4X-
Scammony	T47.2X-
Scarlet red	T49.8X-
Scheele's green	T57.0X-
insecticide	T57.0X-
Schizontozide (blood) (tissue)	T37.2X-
Schradan	T60.0X-
Schweinfurth green	T57.0X-
insecticide	T57.0X-
Scilla, rat poison	T60.4X-
Scillaren	T60.4X-
Sclerosing agent	T46.8X-
Scombrotoxin	T61.1-
Scopolamine	T44.3X-
Scopolia extract	T44.3X-
Scouring powder	T65.89-
Sea	
anemone (sting)	T63.631
cucumber (sting)	T63.69-
snake (bite) (venom)	T63.09-
urchin spine (puncture)	T63.69-
Seafood	T61.9-
specified NEC	T61.8X-
Secbutabarbital	T42.3X-
Secbutabarbitone	T42.3X-
Secnidazole	T37.3X-
Secobarbital	T42.3X-
Seconal	T42.3X-
Secretin	T50.8X-
Sedative NEC	T42.71
mixed NEC	T42.6X-
Sedormid	T42.6X-
Seed disinfectant or dressing	T60.8X-
Seeds (poisonous)	T62.2X-
Selegiline	T42.8X-
Selenium NEC (fumes)	T56.89-
disulfide or sulfide	T49.4X-
Selenomethionine (75Se)	T50.8X-
Selsun	T49.4X-
Semustine	T45.1X-
Senega syrup	T48.4X-
Senna	T47.2X-
Sennoside A+B	T47.2X-
Septisol	T49.2X-
Seractide	T38.81-
Serax	T42.4X-
Serenesil	T42.6X-
Serenium (hydrochloride)	T37.9-

Drug/Chemical	Code
Serepax— see Oxazepam	
Sermorelin	T38.89-
Sernyl	T41.1X-
Serotonin	T50.99-
Serpasil	T46.5X-
Serrapeptase	T45.3X-
Serum	
antibotulinus	T50.Z1-
anticytotoxic	T50.Z1-
antidiphtheria	T50.Z1-
antimeningococcus	T50.Z1-
anti-Rh	T50.Z1-
anti-snake-bite	T50.Z1-
antitetanic	T50.Z1-
antitoxic	T50.Z1-
complement (inhibitor)	T45.8X-
convalescent	T50.Z1-
hemolytic complement	T45.8X-
immune (human)	T50.Z1-
protective NEC	T50.Z1-
Setastine	T45.0X-
Setoperone	T43.59-
Sewer gas	T59.9-
Shampoo	T55.0X-
Shellfish, noxious, nonbacterial	T61.781
Sildenafil	T46.7X-
Silibinin	T50.99-
Silicone NEC	T65.89-
medicinal	T49.3X-
Silvadene	T49.0X-
Silver	T49.0X-
anti-infectives	T49.0X-
arsphenamine	T37.8X-
colloidal	T49.0X-
nitrate	T49.0X-
ophthalmic preparation	T49.5X-
toughened (keratolytic)	T49.4X-
nonmedicinal (dust)	T56.89-
protein	T49.5X-
salvarsan	T37.8X-
sulfadiazine	T49.4X-
Silymarin	T50.99-
Simaldrate	T47.1X-
Simazine	T60.3X-
Simethicone	T47.1X-
Simfibrate	T46.6X-
Simvastatin	T46.6X-
Sincalide	T50.8X-
Sinequan	T43.01-
Singoserp	T46.5X-
Sintrom	T45.51-
Sisomicin	T36.5X-
Sitosterols	T46.6X-
Skeletal muscle relaxants	T48.1X-

Drug/Chemical	Code
Skin	
agents (external)	T49.9-
specified NEC	T49.8X-
test antigen	T50.8X-
Sleep-eze	T45.0X-
Sleeping draught, pill	T42.71
Smallpox vaccine	T50.B1-
Smelter fumes NEC	T56.9-
Smog	T59.1X-
Smoke NEC	T59.81-
Smooth muscle relaxant	T44.3X-
Snail killer NEC	T60.8X-
Snake venom or bite	T63.00-
hemocoagulase	T45.7X-
Snuff	T65.21-
Soap (powder) (product)	T55.0X-
enema	T47.4X-
medicinal, soft	T49.2X-
superfatted	T49.2X-
Sobrerol	T48.4X-
Soda (caustic)	T54.3X-
bicarb	T47.1X-
Sodium	
acetosulfone	T37.1X-
acetrizoate	T50.8X-
acid phosphate	T50.3X-
alginate	T47.8X-
amidotrizoate	T50.8X-
aminopterin	T45.1X-
amylosulfate	T47.8X-
amytal	T42.3X-
antimony gluconate	T37.3X-
arsenate	T57.0X-
aurothiomalate	T39.4X-
aurothiosulfate	T39.4X-
barbiturate	T42.3X-
basic phosphate	T47.4X-
bicarbonate	T47.1X-
bichromate	T57.8X-
biphosphate	T50.3X-
bisulfate	T65.89-
borate	
cleanser	T57.8X-
eye	T49.5X-
therapeutic	T49.8X-
bromide	T42.6X-
cacodylate (nonmedicinal)NEC	T50.8X-
anti-infective	T37.8X-
herbicide	T60.3X-
calcium edetate	T45.8X-
carbonate NEC	T54.3X-
chlorate NEC	T65.89-
herbicide	T54.9-

Drug/Chemical	Code
Sodium, continued	
chloride	T50.3X-
with glucose	T50.3X-
chromate	T65.89-
citrate	T50.99-
cromoglicate	T48.6X-
cyanide	T65.0X-
cyclamate	T50.3X-
dehydrocholate	T45.8X-
diatrizoate	T50.8X-
dibunate	T48.4X-
dioctyl sulfosuccinate	T47.4X-
dipantoyl ferrate	T45.8X-
edetate	T45.8X-
ethacrynate	T50.1X-
feredetate	T45.8X-
fluoride— *see Fluoride*	
fluoroacetate (dust) (pesticide)	T60.4X-
free salt	T50.3X-
fusidate	T36.8X-
glucaldrate	T47.1X-
glucosulfone	T37.1X-
glutamate	T45.8X-
hydrogen carbonate	T50.3X-
hydroxide	T54.3X-
hypochlorite (bleach)NEC	T54.3X-
disinfectant	T54.3X-
medicinal (anti-infective) (external)	T49.0X-
vapor	T54.3X-
hyposulfite	T49.0X-
indigotin disulfonate	T50.8X-
iodide	T50.99-
I-131	T50.8X-
therapeutic	T38.2X-
iodohippurate (131I)	T50.8X-
iopodate	T50.8X-
iothalamate	T50.8X-
iron edetate	T45.4X-
lactate (compound solution)	T45.8X-
lauryl (sulfate)	T49.2X-
L-triiodothyronine	T38.1X-
magnesium citrate	T50.99-
mersalate	T50.2X-
metasilicate	T65.89-
metrizoate	T50.8X-
monofluoroacetate (pesticide)	T60.1X-
morrhuate	T46.8X-
nafcillin	T36.0X-
nitrate (oxidizing agent)	T65.89-
nitrite	T50.6X-
nitroferricyanide	T46.5X-
nitroprusside	T46.5X-
oxalate	T65.89-
oxide/peroxide	T65.89-
oxybate	T41.29-

SODIUM–STANOLONE

Drug/Chemical	Code
Sodium, continued	
para-aminohippurate	T50.8X-
perborate (nonmedicinal)NEC	T65.89-
medicinal	T49.0X-
soap	T55.0X-
percarbonate— *see Sodium, perborate*	
pertechnetate Tc99m	T50.8X-
phosphate	
cellulose	T45.8X-
dibasic	T47.2X-
monobasic	T47.2X-
phytate	T50.6X-
picosulfate	T47.2X-
polyhydroxyaluminium monocarbonate	T47.1X-
polystyrene sulfonate	T50.3X-
propionate	T49.0X-
propyl hydroxybenzoate	T50.99-
psylliate	T46.8X-
removing resins	T50.3X-
salicylate	T39.09-
salt NEC	T50.3X-
selenate	T60.2X-
stibogluconate	T37.3X-
sulfate	T47.4X-
sulfoxone	T37.1X-
tetradecyl sulfate	T46.8X-
thiopental	T41.1X-
thiosalicylate	T39.09-
thiosulfate	T50.6X-
tolbutamide	T38.3X-
(L)-triiodothyronine	T38.1X-
tyropanoate	T50.8X-
valproate	T42.6X-
versenate	T50.6X-
Sodium-free salt	T50.90-
Sodium-removing resin	T50.3X-
Soft soap	T55.0X-
Solanine	T62.2X-
berries	T62.1X-
Solanum dulcamara	T62.2X-
berries	T62.1X-
Solapsone	T37.1X-
Solar lotion	T49.3X-
Solasulfone	T37.1X-
Soldering fluid	T65.89-
Solid substance	T65.9-
specified NEC	T65.89-
Solvent, industrial NEC	T52.9-
naphtha	T52.0X-
petroleum	T52.0X-
specified NEC	T52.8X-
Soma	T42.8X-
Somatorelin	T38.89-
Somatostatin	T38.99-
Somatotropin	T38.81-

Drug/Chemical	Code
Somatrem	T38.81-
Somatropin	T38.81-
Sominex	T45.0X-
Somnos	T42.6X-
Somonal	T42.3X-
Soneryl	T42.3X-
Soothing syrup	T50.90-
Sopor	T42.6X-
Soporific	T42.71
Soporific drug	T42.71
specified type NEC	T42.6X-
Sorbide nitrate	T46.3X-
Sorbitol	T47.4X-
Sotalol	T44.7X-
Sotradecol	T46.8X-
Soysterol	T46.6X-
Spacoline	T44.3X-
Spanish fly	T49.8X-
Sparine	T43.3X-
Sparteine	T48.0X-
Spasmolytic	
anticholinergics	T44.3X-
autonomic	T44.3X-
bronchial NEC	T48.6X-
quaternary ammonium	T44.3X-
skeletal muscle NEC	T48.1X-
Spectinomycin	T36.5X-
Speed	T43.62-
Spermicide	T49.8X-
Spider (bite) (venom)	T63.39-
antivenin	T50.Z1-
Spigelia (root)	T37.4X-
Spindle inactivator	T50.4X-
Spiperone	T43.4X-
Spiramycin	T36.3X-
Spirapril	T46.4X-
Spirilene	T43.59-
Spirit(s) (neutral) NEC	T51.0X-
beverage / industrial/ mineral/surgical	T51.0X-
Spironolactone	T50.0X-
Spiroperidol	T43.4X-
Sponge, absorbable (gelatin)	T45.7X-
Sporostacin	T49.0X-
Spray (aerosol)	T65.9-
cosmetic	T65.89-
medicinal NEC	T50.90-
Spurge flax	T62.2X-
Spurges	T62.2X-
Sputum viscosity-lowering drug	T48.4X-
Squill	T46.0X-
rat poison	T60.4X-
Squirting cucumber (cathartic)	T47.2X-
Stains	T65.6X-
Stannous fluoride	T49.7X-
Stanolone	T38.7X-

Drug/Chemical	Code
Stanozolol	T38.7X-
Staphisagria or stavesacre (pediculicide)	T49.0X-
Starch	T50.90-
Stelazine	T43.3X-
Stemetil	T43.3X-
Stepronin	T48.4X-
Sterculia	T47.4X-
Sternutator gas	T59.89-
Steroid	T38.0X-
anabolic	T38.7X-
androgenic	T38.7X-
antineoplastic, hormone	T38.7X-
estrogen	T38.5X-
ENT agent	T49.6X-
ophthalmic preparation	T49.5X-
topical NEC	T49.0X-
Stibine	T56.89-
Stibogluconate	T37.3X-
Stibophen	T37.4X-
Stilbamidine (isetionate)	T37.3X-
Stilbestrol	T38.5X-
Stilboestrol	T38.5X-
Stimulant	
central nervous system	T43.60-
analeptics / opiate antagonist	T50.7X-
psychotherapeutic NEC	T43.60-
specified NEC	T43.69-
respiratory	T48.90-
Stone-dissolving drug	T50.90-
Storage battery (cells) (acid)	T54.2X-
Stovaine (infiltration) (topical) (subcutaneous) (nerve block) (spinal)	T41.3X-
Stovarsal	T37.8X-
Stoxil	T49.5X-
Stramonium	T48.6X-
natural state	T62.2X-
Streptodornase	T45.3X-
Streptoduocin	T36.5X-
Streptokinase	T45.61-
Streptomycin (derivative)	T36.5X-
Streptonivicin	T36.5X-
Streptovarycin	T36.5X-
Streptozocin	T45.1X-
Streptozotocin	T45.1X-
Stripper (paint) (solvent)	T52.8X-
Strobane	T60.1X-
Strofantina	T46.0X-
Strophanthin (g) (k)	T46.0X-
Strophanthus	T46.0X-
Strophantin	T46.0X-
Strophantin-g	T46.0X-
Strychnine (nonmedicinal) (pesticide) (salts)	T65.1X-
medicinal	T48.29-
Styramate	T42.8X-
Styrene	T65.89-

Drug/Chemical	Code
Succinimide, antiepileptic or anticonvulsant	T42.2X-
Succinylcholine	T48.1X-
Succinylsulfathiazole	T37.0X-
Sucralfate	T47.1X-
Sucrose	T50.3X-
Sufentanil	T40.4X-
Sulbactam	T36.0X-
Sulbenicillin	T36.0X-
Sulbentine	T49.0X-
Sulfacetamide	T49.0X-
ophthalmic preparation	T49.5X-
Sulfachlorpyridazine	T37.0X-
Sulfacitine	T37.0X-
Sulfadiasulfone sodium	T37.0X-
Sulfadiazine	T37.0X-
silver (topical)	T49.0X-
Sulfadimethoxine	T37.0X-
Sulfadimidine	T37.0X-
Sulfadoxine	T37.0X-
with pyrimethamine	T37.2X-
Sulfaethidole	T37.0X-
Sulfafurazole	T37.0X-
Sulfaguanidine	T37.0X-
Sulfalene	T37.0X-
Sulfaloxate	T37.0X-
Sulfaloxic acid	T37.0X-
Sulfamazone	T39.2X-
Sulfamerazine	T37.0X-
Sulfameter	T37.0X-
Sulfamethazine	T37.0X-
Sulfamethizole	T37.0X-
Sulfamethoxazole	T37.0X-
with trimethoprim	T36.8X-
Sulfamethoxydiazine	T37.0X-
Sulfamethoxypyridazine	T37.0X-
Sulfamethylthiazole	T37.0X-
Sulfametoxydiazine	T37.0X-
Sulfamidopyrine	T39.2X-
Sulfamonomethoxine	T37.0X-
Sulfamoxole	T37.0X-
Sulfamylon	T49.0X-
Sulfan blue (diagnostic dye)	T50.8X-
Sulfanilamide	T37.0X-
Sulfanilylguanidine	T37.0X-
Sulfaperin	T37.0X-
Sulfaphenazole	T37.0X-
Sulfaphenylthiazole	T37.0X-
Sulfaproxyline	T37.0X-
Sulfapyridine	T37.0X-
Sulfapyrimidine	T37.0X-
Sulfarsphenamine	T37.8X-
Sulfasalazine	T37.0X-
Sulfasuxidine	T37.0X-
Sulfasymazine	T37.0X-
Sulfated amylopectin	T47.8X-

SULFATHIAZOLE–TAR NEC

Drug/Chemical	Code
Sulfathiazole	T37.0X-
Sulfatostearate	T49.2X-
Sulfinpyrazone	T50.4X-
Sulfiram	T49.0X-
Sulfisomidine	T37.0X-
Sulfisoxazole	T37.0X-
ophthalmic preparation	T49.5X-
Sulfobromophthalein (sodium)	T50.8X-
Sulfobromphthalein	T50.8X-
Sulfogaiacol	T48.4X-
Sulfomyxin	T36.8X-
Sulfonal	T42.6X-
Sulfonamide NEC	T37.0X-
eye	T49.5X-
Sulfonazide	T37.1X-
Sulfones	T37.1X-
Sulfonethylmethane	T42.6X-
Sulfonmethane	T42.6X-
Sulfonphthal, sulfonphthol	T50.8X-
Sulfonylurea derivatives, oral	T38.3X-
Sulforidazine	T43.3X-
Sulfoxone	T37.1X-
Sulfur, sulfurated, sulfuric, (compounds NEC) (medicinal)	T49.4X-
acid	T54.2X-
dioxide (gas)	T59.1X-
hydrogen	T59.6X-
ointment	T49.0X-
pesticide (vapor)	T60.9-
vapor NEC	T59.89-
Sulfuric acid	T54.2X-
Sulglicotide	T47.1X-
Sulindac	T39.39-
Sulisatin	T47.2X-
Sulisobenzone	T49.3X-
Sulkowitch's reagent	T50.8X-
Sulmetozine	T44.3X-
Suloctidil	T46.7X-
Sulphadiazine	T37.0X-
Sulphadimethoxine	T37.0X-
Sulphadimidine	T37.0X-
Sulphadione	T37.1X-
Sulphafurazole	T37.0X-
Sulphamethizole	T37.0X-
Sulphamethoxazole	T37.0X-
Sulphan blue	T50.8X-
Sulphaphenazole	T37.0X-
Sulphapyridine	T37.0X-
Sulphasalazine	T37.0X-
Sulphinpyrazone	T50.4X-
Sulpiride	T43.59-
Sulprostone	T48.0X-
Sulpyrine	T39.2X-
Sultamicillin	T36.0X-
Sulthiame	T42.6X-

Drug/Chemical	Code
Sultiame	T42.6X-
Sultopride	T43.59-
Sumatriptan	T39.8X-
Sunflower seed oil	T46.6X-
Superinone	T48.4X-
Suprofen	T39.31-
Suramin (sodium)	T37.4X-
Surfacaine	T41.3X-
Surital	T41.1X-
Sutilains	T45.3X-
Suxamethonium (chloride)	T48.1X-
Suxethonium (chloride)	T48.1X-
Suxibuzone	T39.2X-
Sweet niter spirit	T46.3X-
Sweet oil (birch)	T49.3X-
Sweetener	T50.90-
Sym-dichloroethyl ether	T53.6X-
Sympatholytic NEC	T44.8X-
haloalkylamine	T44.8X-
Sympathomimetic NEC	T44.90-
anti-common-cold	T48.5X-
bronchodilator	T48.6X-
specified NEC	T44.99-
Synagis	T50.B9-
Synalar	T49.0X-
Synthetic cannabinoids	T40.72-
Synthetic narcotics (other)	T40.49-
Synthroid	T38.1X-
Syntocinon	T48.0X-
Syrosingopine	T46.5X-
Systemic drug	T45.9-
specified NEC	T45.8X-
2,4,5-T	T60.3X-
Tablets— *see also specified substance*	T50.90-
Tace	T38.5X-
Tacrine	T44.0X-
Tadalafil	T46.7X-
Talampicillin	T36.0X-
Talbutal	T42.3X-
Talc powder	T49.3X-
Talcum	T49.3X-
Taleranol	T38.6X-
Tamoxifen	T38.6X-
Tamsulosin	T44.6X-
Tandearil, tanderil	T39.2X-
Tannic acid (Tannin)	T49.2X-
medicinal (astringent)	T49.2X-
Tansy	T62.2X-
TAO	T36.3X-
Tapazole	T38.2X-
Tar NEC	T52.0X-
camphor	T60.1X-
distillate	T49.1X-
fumes	T59.89-
medicinal (ointment)	T49.1X-

Drug/Chemical	Code
Taractan	T43.59-
Tarantula (venomous)	T63.321
Tartar emetic	T37.8X-
Tartaric acid	T65.89-
Tartrate, laxative	T47.4X-
Tartrated antimony (anti-infective)	T37.8X-
Tauromustine	T45.1X-
TCA— *see Trichloroacetic acid*	
TCDD	T53.7X-
TDI (vapor)	T65.0X-
Teclothiazide	T50.2X-
Teclozan	T37.3X-
Tegafur	T45.1X-
Tegretol	T42.1X-
Teicoplanin	T36.8X-
Telepaque	T50.8X-
Tellurium	T56.89-
TEM	T45.1X-
Temazepam	T42.4X-
Temocillin	T36.0X-
Tenamfetamine	T43.62-
Teniposide	T45.1X-
Tenitramine	T46.3X-
Tenoglicin	T48.4X-
Tenonitrozole	T37.3X-
Tenoxicam	T39.39-
TEPA	T45.1X-
TEPP	T60.0X-
Teprotide	T46.5X-
Terazosin	T44.6X-
Terbufos	T60.0X-
Terbutaline	T48.6X-
Terconazole	T49.0X-
Terfenadine	T45.0X-
Teriparatide (acetate)	T50.99-
Terizidone	T37.1X-
Terlipressin	T38.89-
Terodiline	T46.3X-
Teroxalene	T37.4X-
Terpin (cis)hydrate	T48.4X-
Terramycin	T36.4X-
Tertatolol	T44.7X-
Tessalon	T48.3X-
Testolactone	T38.7X-
Testosterone	T38.7X-
Tetanus toxoid or vaccine	T50.A9-
antitoxin	T50.Z1-
immune globulin (human)	T50.Z1-
toxoid	T50.A9-
with diphtheria toxoid	T50.A2-
with pertussis	T50.A1-
Tetrabenazine	T43.59-
Tetracaine	T41.3X-
Tetrachlorethylene— *see Tetrachloroethylene*	

Drug/Chemical	Code
Tetrachlormethiazide	T50.2X-
2,3,7,8-Tetrachlorodibenzo-p-dioxin	T53.7X-
Tetrachloroethane	T53.6X-
vapor	T53.6X-
paint or varnish	T53.6X-
Tetrachloroethylene (liquid)	T53.3X-
medicinal	T37.4X-
vapor	T53.3X-
Tetracosactide	T38.81-
Tetracosactrin	T38.81-
Tetracycline	T36.4X-
ophthalmic preparation	T49.5X-
topical NEC	T49.0X-
Tetradifon	T60.8X-
Tetradotoxin	T61.771
Tetraethyl	
lead	T56.0X-
pyrophosphate	T60.0X-
Tetraethylammonium chloride	T44.2X-
Tetraethylthiuram disulfide	T50.6X-
Tetrahydroaminoacridine	T44.0X-
Tetrahydrocannabinol	T40.71-
Tetrahydrofuran	T52.8X-
Tetrahydronaphthalene	T52.8X-
Tetrahydrozoline	T49.5X-
Tetralin	T52.8X-
Tetramethrin	T60.2X-
Tetramethylthiuram (disulfide) NEC	T60.3X-
medicinal	T49.0X-
Tetramisole	T37.4X-
Tetranicotinoyl fructose	T46.7X-
Tetrazepam	T42.4X-
Tetronal	T42.6X-
Tetryl	T65.3X-
Tetrylammonium chloride	T44.2X-
Tetryzoline	T49.5X-
Thalidomide	T45.1X-
Thallium (compounds) (dust) NEC	T56.81-
pesticide	T60.4X-
THC	T40.71-
Thebacon	T48.3X-
Thebaine	T40.2X-
Thenoic acid	T49.6X-
Thenyldiamine	T45.0X-
Theobromine (calcium salicylate)	T48.6X-
sodium salicylate	T48.6X-
Theophyllamine	T48.6X-
Theophylline	T48.6X-
Thiabendazole	T37.4X-
Thialbarbital	T41.1X-
Thiamazole	T38.2X-
Thiambutosine	T37.1X-
Thiamine	T45.2X-
Thiamphenicol	T36.2X-
Thiamylal (sodium)	T41.1X-

Drug/Chemical	Code
Thiazesim	T43.29-
Thiazides (diuretics)	T50.2X-
Thiazinamium metilsulfate	T43.3X-
Thiethylperazine	T43.3X-
Thimerosal	T49.0X-
ophthalmic preparation	T49.5X-
Thioacetazone	T37.1X-
Thiobarbital sodium	T41.1X-
Thiobarbiturate anesthetic	T41.1X-
Thiobismol	T37.8X-
Thiobutabarbital sodium	T41.1X-
Thiocarbamate (insecticide)	T60.0X-
Thiocarbamide	T38.2X-
Thiocarbarsone	T37.8X-
Thiocarlide	T37.1X-
Thioctamide	T50.99-
Thioctic acid	T50.99-
Thiofos	T60.0X-
Thioglycolate	T49.4X-
Thioglycolic acid	T65.89-
Thioguanine	T45.1X-
Thiomercaptomerin	T50.2X-
Thiomerin	T50.2X-
Thiomersal	T49.0X-
Thionazin	T60.0X-
Thiopental (sodium)	T41.1X-
Thiopentone (sodium)	T41.1X-
Thiopropazate	T43.3X-
Thioproperazine	T43.3X-
Thioridazine	T43.3X-
Thiosinamine	T49.3X-
Thiotepa	T45.1X-
Thiothixene	T43.4X-
Thiouracil (benzyl) (methyl) (propyl)	T38.2X-
Thiourea	T38.2X-
Thiphenamil	T44.3X-
Thiram	T60.3X-
medicinal	T49.2X-
Thonzylamine (systemic)	T45.0X-
mucosal decongestant	T48.5X-
Thorazine	T43.3X-
Thorium dioxide suspension	T50.8X-
Thornapple	T62.2X-
Throat drug NEC	T49.6X-
Thrombin	T45.7X-
Thrombolysin	T45.61-
Thromboplastin	T45.7X-
Thurfyl nicotinate	T46.7X-
Thymol	T49.0X-
Thymopentin	T37.5X-
Thymoxamine	T46.7X-
Thymus extract	T38.89-
Thyreotrophic hormone	T38.81-
Thyroglobulin	T38.1X-

Drug/Chemical	Code
Thyroid (hormone)	T38.1X-
Thyrolar	T38.1X-
Thyrotrophin	T38.81-
Thyrotropic hormone	T38.81-
Thyroxine	T38.1X-
Tiabendazole	T37.4X-
Tiamizide	T50.2X-
Tianeptine	T43.29-
Tiapamil	T46.1X-
Tiapride	T43.59-
Tiaprofenic acid	T39.31-
Tiaramide	T39.8X-
Ticarcillin	T36.0X-
Ticlatone	T49.0X-
Ticlopidine	T45.521
Ticrynafen	T50.1X-
Tidiacic	T50.99-
Tiemonium	T44.3X-
iodide	T44.3X-
Tienilic acid	T50.1X-
Tifenamil	T44.3X-
Tigan	T45.0X-
Tigloidine	T44.3X-
Tilactase	T47.5X-
Tiletamine	T41.29-
Tilidine	T40.4X-
Timepidium bromide	T44.3X-
Timiperone	T43.4X-
Timolol	T44.7X-
Tin (chloride) (dust) (oxide) NEC	T56.6X-
anti-infectives	T37.8X-
Tindal	T43.3X-
Tinidazole	T37.3X-
Tinoridine	T39.8X-
Tiocarlide	T37.1X-
Tioclomarol	T45.51-
Tioconazole	T49.0X-
Tioguanine	T45.1X-
Tiopronin	T50.99-
Tiotixene	T43.4X-
Tioxolone	T49.4X-
Tipepidine	T48.3X-
Tiquizium bromide	T44.3X-
Tiratricol	T38.1X-
Tisopurine	T50.4X-
Titanium (compounds) (vapor)	T56.89-
dioxide/ointment/oxide	T49.3X-
tetrachloride	T56.89-
Titanocene	T56.89-
Titroid	T38.1X-
Tizanidine	T42.8X-
TMTD	T60.3X-
TNT (fumes)	T65.3X-
Toadstool	T62.0X-

Drug/Chemical	Code
Tobacco NEC	T65.29-
cigarettes	T65.22-
Indian	T62.2X-
smoke, second-hand	T65.22-
Tobramycin	T36.5X-
Tocainide	T46.2X-
Tocoferol	T45.2X-
Tocopherol (acetate)	T45.2X-
Tocosamine	T48.0X-
Todralazine	T46.5X-
Tofisopam	T42.4X-
Tofranil	T43.01-
Toilet deodorizer	T65.89-
Tolamolol	T44.7X-
Tolazamide	T38.3X-
Tolazoline	T46.7X-
Tolbutamide (sodium)	T38.3X-
Tolciclate	T49.0X-
Tolmetin	T39.39-
Tolnaftate	T49.0X-
Tolonidine	T46.5X-
Toloxatone	T42.6X-
Tolperisone	T44.3X-
Tolserol	T42.8X-
Toluene (liquid)	T52.2X-
diisocyanate	T65.0X-
Toluidine (vapor)	T65.89-
Toluol (liquid)	T52.2X-
vapor	T52.2X-
Toluylenediamine	T65.3X-
Tolylene-2,4-diisocyanate	T65.0X-
Tonic NEC	T50.90-
Topical action drug NEC	T49.9-
ear, nose or throat	T49.6X-
eye	T49.5X-
skin	T49.9-
specified NEC	T49.8X-
Toquizine	T44.3X-
Toremifene	T38.6X-
Tosylchloramide sodium	T49.8X-
Toxaphene (dust) (spray)	T60.1X-
Toxin, diphtheria (Schick Test)	T50.8X-
Tractor fuel NEC	T52.0X-
Tragacanth	T50.99-
Tramadol	T40.42-
Tramazoline	T48.5X-
Tranexamic acid	T45.62-
Tranilast	T45.0X-
Tranquilizer NEC	T43.50-
with hypnotic or sedative	T42.6X-
benzodiazepine NEC	T42.4X-
butyrophenone NEC	T43.4X-
carbamate	T43.59-
dimethylamine / ethylamine	T43.3X-

Drug/Chemical	Code
Tranquilizer NEC, continued	T43.50-
hydroxyzine	T43.59-
major NEC	T43.50-
penothiazine NEC / piperazine NEC	T43.3X-
piperidine / propylamine	T43.3X-
specified NEC	T43.59-
thioxanthene NEC	T43.59-
Tranxene	T42.4X-
Tranylcypromine	T43.1X-
Trapidil	T46.3X-
Trasentine	T44.3X-
Travert	T50.3X-
Trazodone	T43.21-
Trecator	T37.1X-
Treosulfan	T45.1X-
Tretamine	T45.1X-
Tretinoin	T49.0X-
Tretoquinol	T48.6X-
Triacetin	T49.0X-
Triacetoxyanthracene	T49.4X-
Triacetyloleandomycin	T36.3X-
Triamcinolone	T38.0X-
ENT agent	T49.6X-
hexacetonide	T49.0X-
ophthalmic preparation	T49.5X-
topical NEC	T49.0X-
Triampyzine	T44.3X-
Triamterene	T50.2X-
Triazine (herbicide)	T60.3X-
Triaziquone	T45.1X-
Triazolam	T42.4X-
Triazole (herbicide)	T60.3X-
Tribenoside	T46.99-
Tribromacetaldehyde	T42.6X-
Tribromoethanol, rectal	T41.29-
Tribromomethane	T42.6X-
Trichlorethane	T53.2X-
Trichlorethylene	T53.2X-
Trichlorfon	T60.0X-
Trichlormethiazide	T50.2X-
Trichlormethine	T45.1X-
Trichloroacetic acid, Trichloracetic acid	T54.2X-
medicinal	T49.4X-
Trichloroethane	T53.2X-
Trichloroethanol	T42.6X-
Trichloroethyl phosphate	T42.6X-
Trichloroethylene (liquid) (vapor)	T53.2X-
anesthetic (gas)	T41.0X-
Trichlorofluoromethane NEC	T53.5X-
Trichloronate	T60.0X-
2,4,5-Trichlorophen-oxyacetic acid	T60.3X-
Trichloropropane	T53.6X-
Trichlorotriethylamine	T45.1X-
Trichomonacides NEC	T37.3X-
Trichomycin	T36.7X-

Drug/Chemical	Code
Triclobisonium chloride	T49.0X-
Triclocarban	T49.0X-
Triclofos	T42.6X-
Triclosan	T49.0X-
Tricresyl phosphate	T65.89-
solvent	T52.9-
Tricyclamol chloride	T44.3X-
Tridesilon	T49.0X-
Tridihexethyl iodide	T44.3X-
Tridione	T42.2X-
Trientine	T45.8X-
Triethanolamine NEC	T54.3X-
Triethanomelamine	T45.1X-
Triethylenemelamine	T45.1X-
Triethylenephosphoramide	T45.1X-
Triethylenethiophosphoramide	T45.1X-
Trifluoperazine	T43.3X-
Trifluoroethyl vinyl ether	T41.0X-
Trifluperidol	T43.4X-
Triflupromazine	T43.3X-
Trifluridine	T37.5X-
Triflusal	T45.521
Trihexyphenidyl	T44.3X-
Triiodothyronine	T38.1X-
Trilene	T41.0X-
Trilostane	T38.99-
Trimebutine	T44.3X-
Trimecaine	T41.3X-
Trimeprazine (tartrate)	T44.3X-
Trimetaphan camsilate	T44.2X-
Trimetazidine	T46.7X-
Trimethadione	T42.2X-
Trimethaphan	T44.2X-
Trimethidinium	T44.2X-
Trimethobenzamide	T45.0X-
Trimethoprim (w/ sulfamethoxazole)	T37.8X-
Trimethylcarbinol	T51.3X-
Trimethylpsoralen	T49.3X-
Trimeton	T45.0X-
Trimetrexate	T45.1X-
Trimipramine	T43.01-
Trimustine	T45.1X-
Trinitrine	T46.3X-
Trinitrobenzol	T65.3X-
Trinitrophenol	T65.3X-
Trinitrotoluene (fumes)	T65.3X-
Trional	T42.6X-
Triorthocresyl phosphate	T65.89-
Trioxide of arsenic	T57.0X-
Trioxysalen	T49.4X-
Tripamide	T50.2X-
Triparanol	T46.6X-
Tripelennamine	T45.0X-
Triperiden	T44.3X-
Triperidol	T43.4X-

Drug/Chemical	Code
Triphenylphosphate	T65.89-
Triple bromides	T42.6X-
Triple carbonate	T47.1X-
Triprolidine	T45.0X-
Trisodium hydrogen edetate	T50.6X-
Trisoralen	T49.3X-
Trisulfapyrimidines	T37.0X-
Trithiozine	T44.3X-
Tritiozine	T44.3X-
Tritoqualine	T45.0X-
Trofosfamide	T45.1X-
Troleandomycin	T36.3X-
Trolnitrate (phosphate)	T46.3X-
Tromantadine	T37.5X-
Trometamol	T50.2X-
Tromethamine	T50.2X-
Tronothane	T41.3X-
Tropacine	T44.3X-
Tropatepine	T44.3X-
Tropicamide	T44.3X-
Trospium chloride	T44.3X-
Troxerutin	T46.99-
Troxidone	T42.2X-
Tryparsamide	T37.3X-
Trypsin	T45.3X-
Tryptizol	T43.01-
TSH	T38.81-
Tuaminoheptane	T48.5X-
Tuberculin (PPD)	T50.8X-
Tubocurare	T48.1X-
Tubocurarine (chloride)	T48.1X-
Tulobuterol	T48.6X-
Turpentine (spirits of)	T52.8X-
vapor	T52.8X-
Tybamate	T43.59-
Tyloxapol	T48.4X-
Tymazoline	T48.5X-
Tyropanoate	T50.8X-
Tyrothricin	T49.6X-
ENT agent	T49.6X-
ophthalmic preparation	T49.5X-
Ufenamate	T39.39-
Ultraviolet light protectant	T49.3X-
Undecenoic acid	T49.0X-
Undecoylium	T49.0X-
Undecylenic acid (derivatives)	T49.0X-
Unna's boot	T49.3X-
Unsaturated fatty acid	T46.6X-
Unspecified drug or substance	T50.90-
Unspecified drug or substance, multiple	T50.91-
Uracil mustard	T45.1X-
Uramustine	T45.1X-
Urapidil	T46.5X-
Urari	T48.1X-
Urate oxidase	T50.4X-

Drug/Chemical	Code
Urea	T47.3X-
peroxide	T49.0X-
stibamine	T37.4X-
topical	T49.8X-
Urethane	T45.1X-
Uric acid metabolism drug NEC	T50.4X-
Uricosuric agent	T50.4X-
Urinary anti-infective	T37.8X-
Urofollitropin	T38.81-
Urokinase	T45.61-
Urokon	T50.8X-
Ursodeoxycholic acid	T50.99-
Ursodiol	T50.99-
Urtica	T62.2X-
Vaccine NEC	T50.Z9-
antineoplastic	T50.Z9-
bacterial NEC	T50.A9-
with	
other bacterial component	T50.A2-
pertussis component	T50.A1-
viral-rickettsial component	T50.A2-
mixed NEC	T50.A2-
BCG	T50.A9-
cholera	T50.A9-
diphtheria	T50.A9-
with tetanus	T50.A2-
and pertussis	T50.A1-
influenza	T50.B9-
measles, mumps and rubella (MMR)	T50.B9-
meningococcal	T50.A9-
paratyphoid	T50.A9-
plague	T50.A9-
poliomyelitis	T50.B9-
rabies	T50.B9-
respiratory syncytial virus	T50.B9-
rickettsial NEC	T50.A9-
with	
bacterial component	T50.A2-
Rocky Mountain spotted fever	T50.A9-
sabin oral	T50.B9-
smallpox	T50.B1-
TAB	T50.A9-
tetanus	T50.A9-
typhoid	T50.A9-
typhus	T50.A9-
viral NEC	T50.B9-
yellow fever	T50.B9-
Vaccinia immune globulin	T50.Z1-
Vaginal contraceptives	T49.8X-
Valerian (root) (tincture)	T42.6X-
tincture	T42.6X-
Valethamate bromide	T44.3X-
Valisone	T49.0X-
Valium	T42.4X-
Valmid	T42.6X-

Drug/Chemical	Code
Valnoctamide	T42.6X-
Valproate (sodium)	T42.6X-
Valproic acid	T42.6X-
Valpromide	T42.6X-
Vanadium	T56.89-
Vancomycin	T36.8X-
Vapor— see also Gas	T59.9-
kiln (carbon monoxide)	T58.8X-
specified source NEC	T59.89-
Vardenafil	T46.7X-
Varicose reduction drug	T46.8X-
Varnish	T65.4X-
cleaner	T52.9-
Vaseline	T49.3X-
Vasodilan	T46.7X-
Vasodilator	
coronary NEC	T46.3X-
peripheral NEC	T46.7X-
Vasopressin	T38.89-
Vasopressor drugs	T38.89-
Vecuronium bromide	T48.1X-
Vegetable extract, astringent	T49.2X-
Venlafaxine	T43.21-
Venom, venomous (bite) (sting)	T63.9-
amphibian NEC	T63.831
animal NEC	T63.89-
ant	T63.421
arthropod NEC	T63.481
bee	T63.441
centipede	T63.41-
fish	T63.59-
frog	T63.81-
hornet	T63.451
insect NEC	T63.481
lizard	T63.121
marine	
animals	T63.69-
bluebottle	T63.61-
jellyfish NEC	T63.62-
Portugese Man-o-war	T63.61-
sea anemone	T63.631
specified NEC	T63.69-
fish	T63.59-
plants	T63.71-
sting ray	T63.51-
millipede (tropical)	T63.41-
plant NEC	T63.79-
marine	T63.71-
reptile	T63.19-
gila monster	T63.11-
lizard NEC	T63.12-
scorpion	T63.2X-
snake	T63.00-
African NEC	T63.081
American (North) (South)NEC	T63.06-

VENOM, VENOMOUS (BITE) (STING)–WITCH HAZEL

Drug/Chemical	Code
Venom, venomous (bite) (sting), continued	T63.9-
Asian	T63.08-
Australian	T63.07-
cobra	T63.041
coral snake	T63.02-
rattlesnake	T63.01-
specified NEC	T63.09-
taipan	T63.03-
specified NEC	T63.89-
spider	T63.30-
black widow	T63.31-
brown recluse	T63.33-
specified NEC	T63.39-
tarantula	T63.321
sting ray	T63.51-
toad	T63.821
wasp	T63.461
Venous sclerosing drug NEC	T46.8X-
Ventolin— *see Albuterol*	
Veramon	T42.3X-
Verapamil	T46.1X-
Veratrine	T46.5X-
Veratrum	
album	T62.2X-
alkaloids	T46.5X-
viride	T62.2X-
Verdigris	T60.3X-
Veronal	T42.3X-
Veroxil	T37.4X-
Versenate	T50.6X-
Versidyne	T39.8X-
Vetrabutine	T48.0X-
Vidarabine	T37.5X-
Vienna	
green	T57.0X-
insecticide	T60.2X-
red	T57.0X-
pharmaceutical dye	T50.99-
Vigabatrin	T42.6X-
Viloxazine	T43.29-
Viminol	T39.8X-
Vinbarbital, vinbarbitone	T42.3X-
Vinblastine	T45.1X-
Vinburnine	T46.7X-
Vincamine	T45.1X-
Vincristine	T45.1X-
Vindesine	T45.1X-
Vinesthene, vinethene	T41.0X-
Vinorelbine tartrate	T45.1X-
Vinpocetine	T46.7X-
Vinyl	
acetate	T65.89-
bital	T42.3X-
bromide	T65.89-

Drug/Chemical	Code
Vinyl, continued	
chloride	T59.89-
ether	T41.0X-
Vinylbital	T42.3X-
Vinylidene chloride	T65.89-
Vioform	T37.8X-
topical	T49.0X-
Viomycin	T36.8X-
Viosterol	T45.2X-
Viper (venom)	T63.09-
Viprynium	T37.4X-
Viquidil	T46.7X-
Viral vaccine NEC	T50.B9-
Virginiamycin	T36.8X-
Virugon	T37.5X-
Viscous agent	T50.90-
Visine	T49.5X-
Visnadine	T46.3X-
Vitamin NEC	T45.2X-
A, B, B1 or B2 or B6 or B12 or B15, C, D, D2, D3, E (acetate) NEC	T45.2X-
nicotinic acid	T46.7X-
hematopoietic	T45.8X-
K, K1, K2, NEC	T45.7X-
PP	T45.2X-
ulceroprotectant	T47.1X-
Vleminckx's solution	T49.4X-
Voltaren— *see Diclofenac sodium*	
Warfarin	T45.51-
rodenticide	T60.4X-
sodium	T45.51-
Wasp (sting)	T63.461
Water	
balance drug	T50.3X-
distilled	T50.3X-
hemlock	T62.2X-
moccasin (venom)	T63.06-
purified	T50.3X-
Wax (paraffin) (petroleum)	T52.0X-
automobile	T65.89-
Weed killers NEC	T60.3X-
Welldorm	T42.6X-
White	
arsenic	T57.0X-
hellebore	T62.2X-
lotion (keratolytic)	T49.4X-
spirit	T52.0X-
Whitewash	T65.89-
Whole blood (human)	T45.8X-
Wild (black cherry) (poisonous plants NEC)	T62.2X-
Window cleaning fluid	T65.89-
Wintergreen (oil)	T49.3X-
Wisterine	T62.2X-
Witch hazel	T49.2X-

Drug/Chemical	Code
Wood alcohol or spirit	T51.1X-
Wool fat (hydrous)	T49.3X-
Woorali	T48.1X-
Wormseed, American	T37.4X-
Xamoterol	T44.5X-
Xanthine diuretics	T50.2X-
Xanthinol nicotinate	T46.7X-
Xanthotoxin	T49.3X-
Xantinol nicotinate	T46.7X-
Xantocillin	T36.0X-
Xenon (127Xe) (133Xe)	T50.8X-
Xenysalate	T49.4X-
Xibornol	T37.8X-
Xigris	T45.51-
Xipamide	T50.2X-
Xylene (vapor)	T52.2X-
Xylocaine (infiltration) (topical)	T41.3X-
Xylol (vapor)	T52.2X-
Xylometazoline	T48.5X-
Yeast (dried)	T45.2X-
Yellow (jasmine)	T62.2X-
phenolphthalein	T47.2X-
Yew	T62.2X-
Yohimbic acid	T40.99-
Zactane	T39.8X-
Zalcitabine	T37.5X-
Zaroxolyn	T50.2X-
Zephiran (topical)	T49.0X-
ophthalmic preparation	T49.5X-
Zeranol	T38.7X-
Zerone	T51.1X-

Drug/Chemical	Code
Zidovudine	T37.5X-
Zimeldine	T43.22-
Zinc (compounds) (fumes) (vapor)NEC	T56.5X-
anti-infectives (bacitracin)	T49.0X-
antivaricose	T46.8X-
chloride (mouthwash)	T49.6X-
chromate	T56.5X-
gelatin or oxide (plaster)	T49.3X-
peroxide	T49.0X-
pesticides	T56.5X-
phosphide or pyrithionate	T60.4X-
stearate	T49.3X-
sulfate	T49.5X-
ENT agent	T49.6X-
ophthalmic solution	T49.5X-
topical NEC	T49.0X-
undecylenate	T49.0X-
Zineb	T60.0X-
Zinostatin	T45.1X-
Zipeprol	T48.3X-
Zofenopril	T46.4X-
Zolpidem	T42.6X-
Zomepirac	T39.39-
Zopiclone	T42.6X-
Zorubicin	T45.1X-
Zotepine	T43.59-
Zovant	T45.51-
Zoxazolamine	T42.8X-
Zuclopenthixol	T43.4X-
Zygadenus (venenosus)	T62.2X-
Zyprexa	T43.59-

WOOD ALCOHOL OR SPIRIT–ZYPREXA